Foreword I

It is my great pleasure to write the preface to the second new edition of *Classified Dictionary of Traditional Chinese Medicine* (published by Foreign Languages Press). Professor Zhufan Xie, a pioneer in the field of integrated Chinese and western medicine in China, has made many achievements ranging from internal medicine to TCM in both research and clinical treatment.

Graduated from Peking University School of Medicine in 1946, Prof. Xie started his career in internal medicine. It did not take him long to become an expert in the field of renal medicine, including gout nephropathy and renal amyloidosis. With strong theoretical background and rich clinical experiences in western medicine, Prof. Xie started to study traditional Chinese medicine (TCM) systematically in the 1960s, preparing to establish a new branch of medicine at the time – integrated Chinese and western medicine. Since then he has engaged in the teaching, research and clinical practice of integrated traditional Chinese and western medicine. In 1987, Prof. Xie founded the Institute of Integrated Chinese and Western Medicine (now called "Institute of Integrative Medicine") of Peking University and served as its director, leading several research programs on integrated traditional Chinese and western medicine. He has conducted pacesetting modern scientific research on the theory of cold and heat syndromes of TCM eight-class syndrome differentiation, uncovering the relationship between cold-heat syndromes differentiation and the functional activities of the sympathetic-adrenal system – heat syndrome is manifested in hyperactivity of sympathetic-adrenal system, while cold syndrome the opposite. Such a valuable finding has become a general principle that guides TCM doctors to evaluate syndrome differentiation treatment during clinical practice. Prof. Xie also led post-graduate programs on the study of the curative effect mechanism of ancient formulas and achieved outstanding results, earning praises and affirmation from academic circles.

Prof. Xie's proficiency in the English translation of TCM terminology is of great renown both nation- and worldwide. Prof. Xie produced many TCM reference books and clinical literatures and held positions as honorary president of Translation Association of the World Federation of Chinese Medicine Societies and as a WHO consultant. With his tremendous output of works over the years, Prof. Xie has made outstanding contributions in bringing traditional Chinese medicine to the world.

The first edition of *Classified Dictionary of Traditional Chinese Medicine* was published in 2002, which has been receiving a warm welcome in the field of English translation of TCM. This work provides a clearly leveled classification of TCM basic theories, diagnostics, clinical principles, therapeutics, acupuncture, medical history, classic reference works as well as many other aspects of traditional Chinese medicine. It also provides indices by Chinese words, pinyin input, citation and by Chinese character strokes. The entries are carefully selected and the English counterparts are defined in such a way that they are readily acceptable in western mentality and in the meantime full homage is paid to the original thoughts of TCM theories and therapies.

Over the past 16 years, advances have been made in TCM terminology, and Prof. Xie has continued his research in the field, making efforts to refine his previous work. The second edition is not simply a correction of the mistakes in the first one; it has summed up his most recent research achievements.

While remaining the style of "classified dictionary", which offers great convenience for users to look up a term or an expression, the second new edition has collected another 944 entries, making a total of 8330 entries. The addition of the appendix of "Commonly Used Chinese Characters in TCM Terminologies" is of great importance because it convincingly rationalizes the translation of TCM terminologies from etymological origins. In any case, it remains one of the great reference works in the field of traditional Chinese medicine.

Keji Chen, MD
Academician and Master of Chinese Medicine
Chinese Academy of Sciences
November 2018, Beijing

前 言 二

谢竹藩教授学贯中西，业精于勤，不仅以深远的眼界引导了医院中西医结合事业的发展，同时在我国中西医结合事业的起步和发展、中外传统医学的交流和促进，以及中医药文化的传播和语言标准化的进程中做出了卓越的贡献，是推动中医走向世界的先驱。谢竹藩教授自从事中西医结合工作及中医国际交流工作伊始，即对中医名词术语的标准英译工作极为重视，先后主编出版多部中医英语词典，成为中医药名词术语英译领域的领军人物。

《新编汉英中医药分类词典》，简称"《词典》(第一版)"，出版于 2002 年 9 月，出版后深得广大中医界和中西医结合界特别是从事中医对外交流者的好评，并于 2007 年被世界卫生组织选定为制定《西太平洋地区传统医学名词术语国际标准》(以中医学为主)的参考书。此后世界中医学会联合会亦组织各有关国家的专家制定《中医基本名词术语中英对照国际标准》，谢竹藩教授担任审定委员会主任，并根据《词典》(第一版)对各词条逐一进行审核和确定。鉴于谢竹藩教授的优异工作，世界卫生组织和世界中医药学会联合会分别授予其"制定该标准的诸多专家的领军核心"及世界中医学会联合会第一届翻译委员会名誉会长的称号。

在制定上述两本中医名词术语国际标准的过程中，谢竹藩教授得益于《词典》(第一版)的同时，也发现其不足之处。现值该书售罄，准备加印之际，他在我所客座教授谢方的协助下将该书做了修订，使之更加完善，成为《词典》(第二版)。新版增加了收录词条的数量，共收载 8330 条，较第一版增加 944 条；更新了个别词条的译文，使之更加符合上述国际标准和近年来陆续发布的国家标准的译法；逐字逐句审核了各词条的释义并进行了必要的修改；常用引文由原来的 376 句增加到 450 句，并逐句再加斟酌，力求译文既准确反映原意，又通顺易懂，便于读者引用。

《词典》(第二版)的另一项修订工作是编写了中医名词术语中常用字的字义、英译及例证，作为附录刊于书末。中医术语的英译与构成术语的汉字字义密切相关，明确字义是确定英译的关键。例如"三焦"的"焦"字源于"膲"字，后者是体腔及所含内脏的意思，与"火力过猛使东西烧成炭样"无关。明确"焦"的字义，英译不用"burner"或"heater"之类的字样不辩自明。又如古汉语中"能"通"態"，明确"病能"实为"病态"，

“病能”一词的英译问题便迎刃而解。其他如“鼻下口上”称“人中”、“颈动脉”称“人迎”等词条，经解释清楚，其英译即顺理成章。至于同一个字在不同的语词中为何译法可不同，在这里也得到了解释。

在排版上，《词典》（第二版）仍保持了按学科分章节的排列，使之既是一本词典，又可作为一本简要的中医百科全书。

《词典》（第二版）的出版，无疑是中医名词术语标准英译工作与时俱进的直接体现，更是谢竹藩教授笔耕不辍、精勤不倦的治学精神的体现。《词典》（第二版）不仅为广大中医药专业人员、中外医学交流人员提供了一本详尽、准确、实用的参考书，也为新时代的中西医交流、发扬中医药这一中华民族伟大瑰宝的崇高内涵起到了积极的推动作用。

张学智
北京大学中西医结合研究所
北京市中医药薪火传承“3+3”工程“谢竹藩名老中医工作室”

Foreword II

With extraordinary persistence, thorough knowledge of both western and traditional Chinese medicine (TCM), and deep insight into future trend of healthcare, Prof. Zhufan Xie has made tremendous contributions in the field of integration of TCM and western medicine. Not only has he established and directed the Department of Integrative Medicine in Peking University First Hospital, he also founded and promoted this emerging and up-rising medicine nationwide. His exceptional achievements in promoting the communication between the East and West and standardizing the translation of TCM terminologies have made him the pioneer in elucidating TCM to the world. Prof. Xie has been attaching great importance to the standardization of English translation of TCM terminologies since he entered the profession of integrative medicine and international communication. Having authored several TCM English dictionaries, he is well recognized as the core leader in the field of English translation of TCM terminologies.

The first new edition of *Classified Dictionary of Traditional Chinese Medicine*, published in September 2002, has won immense praise from practitioners of TCM and integrative medicine, especially those who were engaged in TCM international communication. It was assigned as the main reference book for the *International Standard Terminologies on Traditional Medicine in the Western Pacific Region* by the World Health Organization (WHO) in 2007. Subsequently, the World Federation of Chinese Medicine Societies invited Prof. Xie along with many other experts worldwide to compile the *International Standard Chinese-English Basic Nomenclature of Chinese Medicine*. As a chairman of the revising-approving committee, Prof. Xie was responsible to proofread every single entry and the Dictionary was referred to most frequently. For his exceptional contributions, Prof. Xie was praised by the WHO as "the leading core among the experts" in making it possible for WHO/WPRO to publish the aforementioned book on terminologies. He was also awarded as the honorary chairman of the first translation committee of the World Federation of Chinese Medicine Societies.

The experiences of preparing these two international standards have also given Prof. Xie the opportunities to re-evaluate the Dictionary. Since then, Prof. Xie has been working on how to correct or modify some individual entries that seem not appropriate, how to make an expression easier to catch, and how to meet the demand of the readers and make it up-to-date. Now that the Dictionary is sold out and ready to be reprinted, he has timely completed the revision of the Dictionary with the assistance of our visiting Prof. Fang Xie. 944 entries have been added, making a total of 8,330; the translations of some entries have been updated to make them more in line with the current national and international standards. The interpretation of each term was reviewed word for word and necessary modifications were made; the entries of common citations were increased from the original 376 to 450, each of which was carefully worded to make sure that it is reflective of the original idea, easy to understand and easy to read, so as to make it as much reader-friendly as possible.

It is noteworthy that a new feature is added by building the appendix of meanings, translations and illustrations of commonly used words in TCM. The translation of a TCM term is closely related to the meaning of the Chinese characters that construct the term. For example, the character "焦" of the term "三焦" is in fact a varied form of the character "膲" which means the body cavity and the internal organs within. Thus it has nothing to do with the meaning of "excessive fire to make things burn into carbon". Obviously, either "burner" or "heater" is an inappropriate term to interpret "焦". For another example, the character "能" is a varied form of "態" in archaic Chinese. So when "病能" is replaced by "病态", the translation of the former is clearer. For other examples, the translation of "人中" into philtrum and the translation of "人迎" into carotid artery become more distinct when the related characters are explained. As for why the same character can be translated differently in different words or phrases, the appendix also provides clear and proper explanations.

Classification of chapters by subjects is maintained in the second new edition, making it both a dictionary and a concise encyclopedia of Chinese medicine.

The publication of the second new edition demonstrates the timely updating of English translation standards of TCM terminology. It is also the embodiment of Prof. Xie's academic spirit of persistence and diligence. The second new edition provides not only a detailed, accurate and practical reference book for domestic and foreign medical practitioners as well as those who are interested in international communication of TCM, but also a great tool for the promotion of communication between Chinese and Western medicine in the new era.

Xuezhi Zhang

Institute of Integrative Medicine, Peking University

Xie Zhufan Studio of "Inheritance Program of TCM Veteran" of

Beijing Traditional Chinese Medicine Administration

凡　例

全书的条目按教材的顺序分类排列共计二十七章，合并为五大门类：基础理论、诊断学、治疗学、临床各科和医学史，不仅便于查找，且可作为微缩的中医全书对待。

各中医学科名词术语的英译和释义是各章节的主体。引文（包括格言、谚语）具有完整句型，不属于名词术语，故另行分出，附于有关章节之后。

每个条目包括汉字原文、注音（汉语拼音加方括号）、对应英译（用黑体字）和释义，但少数名词术语和多数引文因意义不言自明，故无释义。

少数条目有两种以上公认的译法难作取舍者，则予并列，并以分号隔开。

凡一个条目有两种以上含义者，则予并列，用数码分开，并分别释义。

凡一个条目有两种以上含义属不同医学范畴者，则有关章节均可见该条目。

原文和译文中凡用圆括号括起的字属于可加可不加，用方括号括起的字表示可与括号前的字置换。

译文中斜线（即“/”）前后两字可任选一个。

部分名词术语迄今尚无适当英译，只能用汉语拼音。但拼音汉语并非英语，故与其他非英语的文字（如拉丁文）同等对待，用斜体印刷。已被承认为英语者不在此例。

Guide to the Use of the Dictionary

The entries are arranged in 27 sections, which are grouped into five categories: fundamental theories, diagnostics, therapeutics, clinical medicine, and medical history. The arrangement is made basically in accordance with that in the modern series of textbooks of Chinese medicine, so that this book is not only easy to consult, but can also be taken as a mini-encyclopedia of Chinese medicine.

The entries contain technical terms and commonly used citations (including maxims). Since the citations are beyond the scope of terminology, they are separately arranged as attachments to relevant sections.

Each entry consists of the term or citation in Chinese characters, Chinese phonetic transcriptions (pinyin in square brackets), English translation (in boldface) and explanations, but for a few terms and most citations there is no explanation as the translation is self-explanatory.

Some terms may have two or more translations. In this case the translations are placed abreast and separated by semicolons.

If a term has two or more meanings, the different meanings are given separately and marked with numerals to distinguish one from the other(s).

If a term has two or more different meanings belonging to different branches of medicine, the same term will appear in different chapters.

In the original texts and translations, the word put in round brackets can be deleted if necessary and the word put in square brackets can be used to replace the word preceding the brackets.

In the translations, either of the words that precedes and follows a slash, i.e., "/", can be used upon preference.

To date, no equivalents have been found for some terms of Chinese medicine, and only pinyin can be used for the time being. Chinese characters in pinyin are still Chinese language, so they are printed in italics as other foreign languages such as Latin. However, this does not include the words of foreign origin that have already been generally accepted as English.

目 录
Contents

Foreword I

前言二 Foreword II

凡例 Guide to the Use of the Dictionary

基础理论 Fundamental Theories ······ 1

精气学说 Theory of Essential *Qi* ······ 2
阴阳学说 Yin-Yang Theory ······ 5
五行学说 Theory of the Five Elements/Phases ······ 11
天人相应 Correspondence between Nature and Human ······ 17
脏腑 *Zang-Fu* Organs ······ 20
官窍和形体 Sense Organs and Other Body Structures ······ 38
气、血、精、津液 *Qi*, Blood, Essence, and Body Fluids ······ 53
病因 Cause of Disease ······ 62
病机 Mechanism of Disease ······ 78

诊断学 Diagnostics ······ 121

诊法 Diagnostic Methods ······ 123
辨证 Syndrome Differentiation (Pattern Identification) ······ 168
八纲辨证 Eight-principle Syndrome Differentiation (Eight-principle Pattern Identification) ······ 168
六经辨证 Six-meridian/channel Syndrome Differentiation (Six-meridian/channel Pattern Identification) ······ 175
卫气营血辨证 Defense-*qi*-nutrient-blood Syndrome Differentiation (Defense-*qi*-nutrient-blood Pattern Identification) ······ 179
三焦辨证 Triple-energizer Syndrome Differentiation (Triple-energizer Pattern Identification) ······ 181
气血辨证 *Qi*-blood Syndrome Differentiation (*Qi*-blood Pattern Identification) ······ 182
津液辨证 Body Fluid Syndrome Differentiation (Body Fluid Pattern Identification) ······ 187
病因辨证 Disease-cause Syndrome Differentiation (Disease-cause Pattern Identification) ······ 191

脏腑辨证 Visceral Syndrome Differentiation (Visceral Pattern Identification) ······ 200
经络辨证 Meridian/Channel Syndrome Differentiation (Meridian/Channel Pattern Identification) ······ 215

治疗学 Therapeutics ······ 217

治则 Therapeutic Principles ······ 218
治法 Therapeutic Methods ······ 225
中药学 Chinese Pharmaceutics ······ 275
中药的炮制、性能和剂型 Processing, Properties and Dosage Forms of Chinese Medicinals/Drugs ······ 275
中药的分类 Classification of Chinese Medicinals/Drugs ······ 287
常用的中药 Commonly Used Chinese Medicinals/Drugs ······ 295
解表药 Exterior-releasing Medicinals/Drugs ······ 295
止咳化痰平喘药 Antitussives, Expectorants and Antiasthmatics ······ 298
清热药 Heat-clearing Medicinals/Drugs ······ 304
祛风湿药 Wind-dampness-dispelling Medicinals/Drugs (Antirheumatics) ··· 313
温里药 Interior-warming Medicinals/Drugs ······ 317
芳香化湿药 Fragrant Dampness-resolving Medicinals/Drugs ······ 319
利尿逐水药 Diuretics and Hydragogues ······ 320
理气药 *Qi*-regulating Medicinals/Drugs ······ 325
理血药 Blood-regulating Medicinals/Drugs ······ 328
芳香开窍药 Aromatic Stimulants ······ 335
安神药 Tranquilizers ······ 336
平肝熄风药 Liver-pacifying and Wind-extinguishing Medicinals/Drugs ······ 338
补养药 Tonics ······ 340
固涩药 Astringents and Hemostatics ······ 348
消导药 Digestives and Evacuants ······ 351
泻下药 Purgatives ······ 352
驱虫药 Anthelmintics ······ 353
外用药 Medicinals/Drugs for External Use ······ 354
方剂 Formulas ······ 356
成药 Patent Medicines/Drugs ······ 381
针灸学 Acupuncture and Moxibustion ······ 398
经络 Meridians/Channels and Collaterals ······ 398
俞穴 Acupoints ······ 408
针法 Acupuncture ······ 444

灸法及其他由针刺演变之疗法 Moxibustion and Other Techniques Derived from Acupuncture ······ 463
其他疗法与保健 Other Therapies and Health Preservation ······ 480
推拿按摩 *Tuina* and Massage ······ 480
气功 *Qigong* ······ 491
保健 Health Preservation ······ 505

临床各科 Clinical Medicine ······ 513

温病 Warm Diseases ······ 514
内科 Internal Medicine ······ 524
妇产科 Gynecology and Obstetrics ······ 555
儿科 Pediatrics ······ 574
外科 External Medicine ······ 591
眼科 Ophthalmology ······ 607
耳鼻喉科 Otorhinolaryngology ······ 623
口齿科 Stomatology and Dentistry ······ 632
骨伤科 Traumato-orthopedics ······ 635

医学史 Medical History ······ 657

名医 Distinguished Physicians ······ 658
名著 Leading Chinese Medical Works ······ 683

附录 Appendix ······ 707

中医名词术语中常用字的字义、英译及例证
Commonly Used Chinese Characters in TCM Terminologies: Their Meanings, English Translations and Examples ······ 708

索引 Indices ······ 823

中文笔画索引 Chinese Character Stroke Index ······ 824
中文拼音索引 Chinese Character Phonetic Index ······ 885
引文索引 Index of Citations ······ 953
英文索引 Index of Terms in English ······ 959

后记 Afterword

基础理论
Fundamental Theories

精气学说 Theory of Essential *Qi*

精气学说 [jīng qì xué shuō]

theory of essential *qi*: an ancient Chinese philosophical system which explains the formation of the universe by an invisible substance called *qi*. The ceaseless movement of *qi* causes all kinds of changes, and essential *qi* gives rise to life.

精气 [jīng qì]

essential *qi*: the *qi* of the essence, from which life originates and by which it is maintained

精 [jīng]

essence: (1) the essential part or portion of *qi*; (2) all the substances useful for the human body, e.g., food essence from diet; (3) the essential substance stored in the kidney, also called kidney essence (肾精 [shèn jīng])

气 [qì]

***qi*:** the invisible basic substance that forms the universe and produces everything in the world through its movement and changes (cf. 气 [qì] on p. 53)

神 [shén]

vitality; spirit; mind: liveliness derived from essential *qi*, referring to (1) manifestations of vital functioning; (2) domination of all life activities; (3) spiritual and mental activities

三宝 [sān bǎo]

three treasures: collective name for essence, *qi*, and vitality

精气互化 [jīng qì hù huà]

mutual transformation of essence and *qi*: Essence can be transformed into invisible *qi*, and *qi* transformed into visible essence.

气机 [qì jī]

***qi* movement:** constant movement of *qi* in the human body that maintains the vital activities. The basic forms of *qi* movement include ascending, descending, exiting and entering.

气化 [qì huà]

***qi* transformation:** changes produced by the movement of *qi*, viz., metabolism of essence, *qi*, blood, and body fluids as well as their mutual transformation

生化 [shēng huà]

generation and transformation: a term used in traditional Chinese medicine to indicate the production and changes of things, e.g., the process of forming *qi* and blood from food essence

升、降、出、入 [shēng、jiàng、chū、rù]

ascending, descending, exiting and entering: upward, downward, outward and inward directions of *qi* movement, the coordination of which maintains normal life

形 [xíng]

physique: the form or structure of a person's body, opposite to but inseparable from spirit

形气 [xíng qì]

physique and *qi*: Physique refers to the form and/or constitution of a human body, and *qi* refers to the functional activities of the *zang-fu* organs. Normally, physique and *qi* should be kept in coordination.

形气相得 [xíng qì xiāng dé]

equilibrium between physique and *qi*: When a patient's physique and functional activities are in balance, his or her prognosis is usually favorable.

形气相失 [xíng qì xiāng shī]

disequilibrium between physique and *qi*: When a patient's physique and functional activities are not in balance, e.g., an emaciated person with polyphagia and irascibility, and an obese person with shortness of breath and palpitations upon mild exertion, his or her prognosis is usually unfavorable.

形气转化 [xíng qì zhuǎn huà]

conversion between physique and *qi*: a hypothesis that the body makeup may be converted into *qi*, and vice versa

形与神俱 [xíng yǔ shén jù]

harmony between physique and spirit: the healthy state at which one's body and mind are well balanced

常用引文 Commonly Used Citations

万物之生，皆禀元气。

[wàn wù zhī shēng, jiē bǐng yuán qì]

Everything is produced with the endowment of genuine *qi*.

气始而生化，气散而有形，气布而蕃育，气终而象变，其致一也。

[qì shǐ ér shēng huà, qì sàn ér yǒu xíng, qì bù ér fān yù, qì zhōng ér xiàng biàn, qí zhì yī yě]

When *qi* starts, there is generation and transformation; when *qi* moves, the shape of a thing is formed; when *qi* spreads, there is multiplication; when *qi* ends, the shape of a thing is changed: such a correspondence is ubiquitous.

生之来谓之精，两精相搏谓之神。

[shēng zhī lái wèi zhī jīng, liǎng jīng xiāng bó wèi zhī shén]

The original substance of life is called essence, and when yin and yang essence combine, vitality emerges.

积精全神。

[jī jīng quán shén]

Preserve the essence and perfect the spirit.

得神者昌，失神者亡。

[dé shén zhě chāng, shī shén zhě wáng]

Preserving vitality guarantees health while loss of vitality leads to death.

升降出入，无器不有。

[shēng jiàng chū rù, wú qì bù yǒu]

In all visible things, *qi* ascends, descends, goes out and comes in.

根于中者，命曰神机，神去则机息。

根于外者，命曰气立，气止则化绝。

[gēn yú zhōng zhě, mìng yuē shén jī, shén qù zé jī xī。gēn yú wài zhě, mìng yuē qì lì, qì zhǐ zé huà jué]

When the vitality originates inside, it is called the mechanism of the spirit; if the spirit moves away, the mechanism ceases. When the vitality originates outside, it is called the establishment of *qi*; if *qi* stops, transformation ends.

阴阳学说 Yin-Yang Theory

阴阳学说 [yīn yáng xué shuō]

yin-yang theory: an ancient Chinese philosophical concept of naive dialectics, expressing the law of the unity of opposites. Its principle is widely applied to traditional Chinese medicine.

阴阳 [yīn yáng]

yin and yang: the two fundamental principles or properties in the universe, ever opposing and complementing each other, the ceaseless motion of which gives rise to all the changes in the world – an ancient philosophical concept used in traditional Chinese medicine for indicating various antitheses in anatomy, physiology, pathology, diagnosis and treatment, and for explaining the health and disease processes

阴 [yīn]

yin: the female or negative principle, the structural or material aspect of an effective position

阳 [yáng]

yang: the male or positive principle, the active or functional aspect of an effective position

阴中之阳 [yīn zhōng zhī yáng]

yang within yin: Yin may be further divided into yin and yang. The resultant yang is called yang within yin, e.g., night is regarded as yin in relation to day, the period from nightfall to midnight is said to be yang within yin.

阴中之阴 [yīn zhōng zhī yīn]

yin within yin: Yin may be further divided into yin and yang. The resultant yin is called yin within yin, e.g., night is regarded as yin in relation to day, and the period of the small hours is said to be yin within yin.

阳中之阳 [yáng zhōng zhī yáng]

yang within yang: Yang may be further divided into yin and yang. The resultant yang is called yang within yang, e.g., day is regarded as yang in relation to night, and the period from dawn to noon is said to be yang within yang.

阳中之阴 [yáng zhōng zhī yīn]

yin within yang: Yang may be further divided into yin and yang. The resultant yin is called yin within yang, e.g., day is regarded as yang in relation to night, and the period from noon to dusk is said to be yin within yang.

阴阳交感 [yīn yáng jiāo gǎn]

yin-yang interaction: mutual actions of yin and yang, including mutual rooting, opposing, converting, as well as waxing and waning. It is the interaction between yin *qi* and yang *qi* that produces things, living and non-living.

阴阳互根 [yīn yáng hù gēn]

mutual rooting of yin and yang; yin-yang interdependence: the existence of one being the prerequisite for the existence of the other. Without "brightness" (yang), there would be no "darkness" (yin); without "interior" (yin), there would be no "exterior" (yang).

阴阳对立 [yīn yáng duì lì]
yin-yang opposition: the mutually opposing relationship between yin and yang. Yin and yang are always in a state of opposing each other, e.g., feminine, interior, cold, and inhibition being yin while masculine, exterior, heat, and excitement are yang.

阴阳转化 [yīn yáng zhuǎn huà]
yin-yang conversion: The property of the same thing can be converted from yin to yang, or from yang to yin, e.g., the heat syndrome of a disease can be converted into a cold one, and vice versa.

阴阳消长 [yīn yáng xiāo zhǎng]
waxing and waning of yin and yang: Of the two opposites of a single entity, increase of the one is usually associated with decrease of the other, e.g., functional activities (yang) consume nutrient substances (yin) – waning of yin with waxing of yang, and formation and storage of nutrient substances consume functional energy – waxing of yin with waning of yang.

阴阳平衡 [yīn yáng píng héng]
yin-yang balance: the state in which yin and yang are balanced, a harmonious state by which health is guaranteed, also known as yin-yang harmony (阴阳调和 [yīn yáng tiáo hé])

阴阳调和 [yīn yáng tiáo hé]
yin-yang harmony: state of yin and yang by which health is guaranteed, same as yin-yang balance (阴阳平衡 [yīn yáng píng héng])

阴阳失调 [yīn yáng shī tiáo]
yin-yang disharmony: breakdown of the harmonious balance between yin and yang, a state regarded as the general pathogenesis of disease

阴阳不和 [yīn yáng bù hé]
yin-yang disharmony: same as 阴阳失调 [yīn yáng shī tiáo]

阴阳乖戾 [yīn yáng guāi lì]
yin-yang imbalance: state of yin and yang which is regarded as the general pathogenesis of disease, same as yin-yang disharmony (阴阳失调 [yīn yáng shī tiáo] or 阴阳不和[yīn yáng bù hé])

阴阳离决 [yīn yáng lí jué]
separation of yin and yang: state of yin and yang that indicates the end of life

阴阳自和 [yīn yáng zì hé]
spontaneous harmonization of yin and yang: spontaneous recovery from yin-yang imbalance by natural regulatory function, a process indicating recovery of a person from illness

阴阳偏胜 [盛] [yīn yáng piān shèng]
abnormal exuberance of yin or yang: morbid condition marked by yin or yang higher than the normal level – presence of heat when yang is preponderant, and presence of cold when yin is preponderant

阴阳偏衰 [yīn yáng piān shuāi]
abnormal debilitation of yin or yang:

morbid condition marked by yin or yang lower than the normal level – presence of cold when yang is deficient, and presence of heat when yin is deficient

阴阳胜复 [yīn yáng shèng fù]
alternate preponderance of yin and yang: a hypothesis put forward in ancient times to explain natural changes and disease processes such as the periodic changes of seasons and the alternate prevalence of certain diseases

阴阳互损 [yīn yáng hù sǔn]
mutual impairment between yin and yang: collective term for two morbid conditions, namely yang impairment affecting yin and yin impairment affecting yang, resulting in deficiency of both yin and yang

阳损及阴 [yáng sǔn jí yīn]
yang impairment affecting yin: morbid condition in which impairment of yang impedes generation of yin, resulting in deficiency of both yin and yang with a preponderance of yang deficiency, e.g., deficiency of vital function often complicated by deficiency of vital essence in advanced cases

阴损及阳 [yīn sǔn jí yáng]
yin impairment affecting yang: morbid condition in which impairment of yin impedes generation of yang, resulting in deficiency of both yin and yang with a preponderance of yin deficiency, e.g., deficiency of vital essence often complicated by deficiency of vital function in advanced cases

阴极似阳 [yīn jí sì yáng]
extreme yin resembling yang: pathological change in which extremely weakened yang *qi* is expelled by exuberant yin from the interior to float on the body surface, forming a true cold and false heat syndrome/pattern

阳极似阴 [yáng jí sì yīn]
extreme yang resembling yin: pathological change in which exuberant pathogenic heat makes yang *qi* depressed and deeply hidden in the interior, so that yin is restricted to the exterior, forming a true heat and false cold syndrome/pattern

常用引文 Commonly Used Citations

阴阳者，天地之道也，万物之纲纪，变化之父母，生杀之本始。
[yīn yáng zhě, tiān dì zhī dào yě, wàn wù zhī gāng jì, biàn huà zhī fù mǔ, shēng shā zhī běn shǐ]
Yin-yang is the law of nature, the principle of all things, the mother of all changes, and the root of life and death.

天为阳，地为阴；日为阳，月为阴。
[tiān wéi yáng, dì wéi yīn; rì wéi yáng, yuè wéi yīn]
Heaven pertains to yang, while Earth pertains to yin; the sun pertains to yang, while the moon pertains to yin.

水为阴，火为阳。

[shuǐ wéi yīn, huǒ wéi yáng]
Water pertains to yin, while fire pertains to yang.

生之本，本于阴阳。
[shēng zhī běn, běn yú yīn yáng]
The origin of life is yin and yang.

阴阳者，万物之能始也。
[yīn yáng zhě, wàn wù zhī néng shǐ yě]
Yin and yang are the generators of all things.

阳化气，阴成形。
[yáng huà qì, yīn chéng xíng]
Yang produces the vital energy, and yin constructs the physique.

外者为阳，内者为阴。
[wài zhě wéi yáng, nèi zhě wéi yīn]
The external pertains to yang, while the internal pertains to yin.

阴中有阳，阳中有阴。
[yīn zhōng yǒu yáng, yáng zhōng yǒu yīn]
There is yang in yin, and there is yin in yang.

背为阳，阳中之阳，心也。
[bèi wéi yáng, yáng zhōng zhī yáng, xīn yě]
As the back of the body belongs to yang, the yang of yang is the heart.

背为阳，阳中之阴，肺也。
[bèi wéi yáng, yáng zhōng zhī yīn, fèi yě]
As the back of the body belongs to yang, the yin of yang is the lung.

腹为阴，阴中之阴，肾也。
[fù wéi yīn, yīn zhōng zhī yīn, shèn yě]
As the abdomen belongs to yin, the yin of yin is the kidney.

腹为阴，阴中之阳，肝也。
[fù wéi yīn, yīn zhōng zhī yáng, gān yě]
As the abdomen belongs to yin, the yang of yin is the liver.

腹为阴，阴中之至阴，脾也。
[fù wéi yīn, yīn zhōng zhī zhì yīn, pí yě]
As the abdomen belongs to yin, the extreme yin of yin is the spleen.

阴阳之要，阳密乃固。
[yīn yáng zhī yào, yáng mì nǎi gù]
The key to optimize yin and yang is that only when yang is compact can yin be strengthened.

阴在内，阳之守也。阳在外，阴之使也。
[yīn zài nèi, yáng zhī shǒu yě。yáng zài wài, yīn zhī shǐ yě]
Yin resides inside with yang as its defense, while yang stays outside to fulfill the mission of yin.

阳根于阴，阴根于阳。
[yáng gēn yú yīn, yīn gēn yú yáng]
Yang is rooted in yin, and yin is rooted in yang.

阴平阳秘，精神乃治。
[yīn píng yáng mì, jīng shén nǎi zhì]
If one keeps yin even and yang firm, one's spirit will be sound.

阴阳离决，精气乃绝。
[yīn yáng lí jué, jīng qì nǎi jué]

When yin and yang separate, essential *qi* expires.

重阴必阳，重阳必阴。
[chóng yīn bì yáng, chóng yáng bì yīn]
Extreme yin gives rise to yang, and extreme yang gives rise to yin. – a mechanism of yin-yang conversion, e.g., severe loss of fluids (yin) may be manifested by symptoms of yang nature such as feeling hot and restlessness, and intense heat may bring on cold symptoms such as chills and cold limbs

阴胜则阳病，阳胜则阴病。
[yīn shèng zé yáng bìng, yáng shèng zé yīn bìng]
Excess yin makes yang suffer, and excess yang makes yin suffer. – a mechanism of disease explained by yin-yang theory, e.g., excessive cold (yin) impairs yang *qi*, and exuberant heat (yang) consumes body fluids (yin)

阳胜则热，阴胜则寒。
[yáng shèng zé rè, yīn shèng zé hán]
When in predominance, yang makes heat, and yin makes cold.

阴阳者，数之可十，推之可百，数之可千，推之可万，万之大不可胜数，然其要一也。
[yīn yáng zhě, shǔ zhī kě shí, tuī zhī kě bǎi, shǔ zhī kě qiān, tuī zhī kě wàn, wàn zhī dà bù kě shèng shǔ, rán qí yào yī yě]
Yin and yang can be counted from one to ten, and inferred from ten to one hundred, counted from one hundred to one thousand, and inferred from one thousand to ten thousand and even to infinity, but the principle of yin-yang is just one (i.e., the unity of opposites).

谨察阴阳所在而调之，以平为期。
[jǐn chá yīn yáng suǒ zài ér tiáo zhī, yǐ píng wéi qī]
One must carefully observe the positions of yin and yang, and apply appropriate treatment until they are balanced.

阳常有余，阴常不足。
[yáng cháng yǒu yú, yīn cháng bù zú]
Yang is usually redundant while yin is ever deficient. – a theory advocated by Zhu Danxi (1281–1358), according to which the method of replenishing yin is recommended as a basic principle for treating disease

阴静阳躁，阳生阴长。
[yīn jìng yáng zào, yáng shēng yīn zhǎng]
Yin is quiescent, while yang is vigorous. Yang produces birth, while yin nurtures growth.

阳生于阴。
[yáng shēng yú yīn]
Yang originates from yin.

阴生于阳。
[yīn shēng yú yáng]
Yin originates from yang.

孤阳不生，独阴不长。
[gū yáng bù shēng, dú yīn bù zhǎng]
Solitary yang can never be born, and solitary yin never grows.

阳为气，阴为味。

[yáng wéi qì, yīn wéi wèi]

Yang refers to property, and yin to flavor (in the case of a medicinal).

辛甘发散为阳，酸苦涌泄为阴。

[xīn gān fā sàn wéi yáng, suān kǔ yǒng xiè wéi yīn]

The pungent and sweet with dispersing effect pertain to yang, while the sour and bitter with emetic and purgative effects pertain to yin.

五行学说 Theory of the Five Elements/Phases

五行学说 [wǔ xíng xué shuō]

five-element/phase theory: one of the basic theories in traditional Chinese medicine, introduced from ancient natural philosophy concerning the composition and evolution of the physical universe

五行 [wǔ xíng]

five elements/phases: wood, fire, earth, metal and water with their characteristic properties and their generating and restricting relationships – an ancient natural philosophical concept to explain the composition and phenomena of the physical universe, used in traditional Chinese medicine to expound the correspondence between man and the universe, and the physiological and pathological relationships among the internal organs

五行归类 [wǔ xíng guī lèi]

categorization according to the five elements/phases: classification or grouping of things and phenomena into five categories by comparing their structures, properties and actions with those of the five elements/phases, e.g., the liver, heart, spleen, lung, and kidney are classified into the categories of wood, fire, earth, metal, and water, respectively. The relevant methods usually include analogy and deduction.

五行相生 [wǔ xíng xiāng shēng]

generation among the five elements/phases: the relationship among the five elements in which each element/phase or its associated phenomena give rise to or promote another element/phase in the following sequence – wood generating fire, fire generating earth, earth generating metal, metal generating water and water generating wood

木生火 [mù shēng huǒ]

wood generating fire: The category of wood generates or promotes the category of fire. In medicine, this saying usually refers to the physiological process in which normal liver (wood) function supports healthy activities of the heart (fire).

火生土 [huǒ shēng tǔ]

fire generating earth: The category of fire generates or promotes the category of earth. In medicine, this saying usually refers to the physiological process in which normal functioning of the spleen (earth) relies upon sound activities of the vital fire (fire of the life gate).

土生金 [tǔ shēng jīn]

earth generating metal: The category of earth generates or promotes the category of metal. In medicine, this saying refers to the physiological process in which the spleen (earth) sends food essence to nourish the lung (metal).

金生水 [jīn shēng shuǐ]

metal generating water: The category of metal generates or promotes the category of water. In medicine, this saying refers to the physiological process in which the lung (metal) distributes fluids to nourish the kidney (water).

水生木 [shuǐ shēng mù]
water generating wood: The category of water generates or promotes the category of wood. In medicine, this saying refers to the physiological process in which sufficient kidney yin (water) guarantees normal functioning of the liver (wood).

五行相克 [wǔ xíng xiāng kè]
restriction among the five elements/phases: the relationship in which each element/phase or its associated phenomena restrict or suppress another element/phase in the following sequence – water restricting fire, fire restricting metal, metal restricting wood, wood restricting earth, and earth restricting water

木克土 [mù kè tǔ]
wood restricting earth: The category of wood restricts or suppresses the category of earth. In medicine, this saying refers to: (1) the physiological relationship between the liver (wood) and the spleen and stomach (earth); (2) a pathological condition, also called wood overrestricting earth (木乘土 [mù chèng tǔ]).

土克水 [tǔ kè shuǐ]
earth restricting water: The category of earth restricts or suppresses the category of water. In medicine, this saying usually refers to the physiological process in which the function of the spleen (earth) controls water metabolism.

水克火 [shuǐ kè huǒ]
water restricting fire: The category of water restricts or suppresses the category of fire. In medicine, this saying refers to: (1) the physiological process in which the function of the kidney yin (water) restricts the heart fire to prevent the latter's over-exuberance; (2) the pathological process in which excess water in the body impairs the function of the heart (fire).

火克金 [huǒ kè jīn]
fire restricting metal: The category of fire restricts or suppresses the category of metal. In medicine, this saying refers to: (1) the physiological process in which the function of the heart (fire) regulates the activities of the lung (metal); (2) the pathological process in which excessive liver fire aggravates a disease of the lung (metal).

金克木 [jīn kè mù]
metal restricting wood: The category of metal restricts or suppresses the category of wood. In medicine, this saying refers to the physiological process in which the function of the lung (metal) prevents hyperactivity of the liver.

五行制化 [wǔ xíng zhì huà]
inhibition and generation among the five elements/phases: the generating and restricting relationships among the five elements/phases which form a self-limiting balanced process, e.g., wood restricting earth which generates metal that will restrict wood in turn, and so forth

五行相乘 [wǔ xíng xiāng chèng]
over-restriction among the five elements/

phases: abnormally severe restriction of the five elements/phases in the same sequence as ordinary restriction

五行相侮 [wǔ xíng xiāng wǔ]
counter-restriction among the five elements/phases: restriction opposed to that of the ordinary restricting sequence of the five elements/phases

五行母子相及 [wǔ xíng mǔ zǐ xiāng jí]
"mother-child" relationship in the five elements/phases: Disease of the "mother" may involve the "child", and vice versa.

母 [mǔ]
mother (element/phase): the element/phase that generates in the sequence of the five elements/phases, e.g., wood being the "mother" of fire

母气 [mǔ qì]
mother (element/phase) *qi*: *qi* of a *zang* organ that generates in the sequence of the five elements/phases, e.g., the liver (wood) *qi* being the mother *qi* of the heart (fire), and the kidney (water) *qi* being the mother *qi* of the liver (wood), and so forth

子 [zǐ]
child (element/phase): the element that is generated in the sequence of the five elements/phases, e.g., fire being the "child" of wood, and so forth

子气 [zǐ qì]
child (element/phase) *qi*: *qi* of a *zang* organ that is generated in the sequence of the five elements/phases, e.g., the spleen (earth) *qi* being the child *qi* of the heart (fire), and the lung (metal) *qi* being the child *qi* of the spleen (earth), and so forth

木乘土 [mù chèng tǔ]
wood overrestricting earth: pathological condition in which a hyperactive liver impairs the functions of the spleen and stomach

木旺乘土 [mù wàng chèng tǔ]
exuberant wood overrestricting earth: pathological change bringing about disharmony between the liver and the spleen and stomach, in which hyperactivity of the former is primary while insufficiency of the latter is secondary (cf. 土虚木乘 [tǔ xū mù chèng])

土虚木乘 [tǔ xū mù chèng]
wood overrestricting asthenic earth: pathological change of disharmony between the liver and the spleen and stomach, in which hyperactivity of the former is secondary, while insufficiency of the latter is primary (cf. 木旺乘土 [mù wàng chèng tǔ])

木火刑金 [mù huǒ xíng jīn]
wood fire tormenting metal: pathological change expressed in the light of the five-element/phase theory that excessive liver fire consumes lung yin, causing dry cough and chest pain or even hemoptysis accompanied by irritability, bitterness in the mouth and blood-shot eyes

火不生土 [huǒ bù shēng tǔ]
fire failing to generate earth: pathological change expressed in the light of the five-element/phase theory that fire of the life gate (i.e., kidney yang) is insufficient to warm the spleen and stomach, bringing on

such symptoms as diarrhea, indigestion, intolerance of cold and edema

土不制水 [tǔ bù zhì shuǐ]
earth failing to control water: pathological change expressed in the light of the five-element/phase theory that a weak spleen unable to control the water flow may lead to edema or retained fluid

土虚水侮 [tǔ xū shuǐ wǔ]
reversed restriction of water on asthenic earth: expression for insufficiency of the spleen with anasarca according to the five-element/phase theory

金寒水冷 [jīn hán shuǐ lěng]
coldness of metal and water: figurative expression for deficiency-cold of both the lung and kidney

水不涵木 [shuǐ bù hán mù]
water failing to nourish wood: pathological change expressed in the light of the five-element/phase theory that kidney yin deficiency deprives the liver of its nourishment, resulting in insufficiency of liver yin with stirring of liver wind

五时 [wǔ shí]
five seasons: collective term referring to spring, summer, late summer, autumn and winter

五气 [wǔ qì]
five *qi*: (1) collective term referring to five climatic factors, i.e., wind, summerheat, dampness, dryness, and cold; (2) collective term for the *qi* of the five circuits, i.e., *qi* of wood, fire, earth, metal and water

五化 [wǔ huà]
five evolutive phases: collective term referring to the generating, growing, changing, collecting, and storing phases of evolution

五声 [wǔ shēng]
five voices: collective term referring to shouting, laughing, singing, crying and moaning

五官 [wǔ guān]
five (sense) organs: collective term referring to the eyes, tongue, mouth, nose and ears

五方 [wǔ fāng]
five directions: collective term referring to east, south, middle, west and north

常用引文 Commonly Used Citations

木曰曲直。
[mù yuē qū zhí]
Wood is that which can be bent and straightened.

火曰炎上。
[huǒ yuē yán shàng]
Fire is that which flames upward.

土爰稼啬。
[tǔ yuán jià sè]
Earth is the ground of sowing and reaping.

金曰从革。
[jīn yuē cóng gé]
Metal is that which changes itself and others.

水曰润下。
[shuǐ yuē rùn xià]
Water is that which moistens and descends. – a metaphor to explain the downward tendency of pathological changes due to dampness, such as diarrhea and edema of the lower extremities, also known as 水性流下 [shuǐ xìng liú xià]

水性流下。
[shuǐ xìng liú xià]
Water tends to flow downwards.

木喜条达。
[mù xǐ tiáo dá]
Wood (or tree) tends to spread out freely. – a figure of speech to explain the physiological function of the liver in smoothing the flow of *qi* and blood

土喜温燥。
[tǔ xǐ wēn zào]
Earth prefers warmth and dryness. – a figure of speech to explain the physiological property of the spleen, which functions well in warm and dry conditions and is liable to be impaired by cold and dampness

土生万物。
[tǔ shēng wàn wù]
Earth engenders the myriad things. – a metaphor to explain that the spleen and stomach provide the material foundation for the whole body by digesting food and supplying nutrients

金气肃降。
[jīn qì sù jiàng]
Metal *qi* is depurative and descending. – a figure of speech to explain the functional property of the lung, disorder of which often leads to cough, dyspnea and expectoration

金破不鸣。
[jīn pò bù míng]
"A broken gong does not sound." – an expression figuratively referring to hoarseness due to deficiency of the lung

金实不鸣。
[jīn shí bù míng]
"A muffled gong does not sound." – an expression figuratively referring to sudden onset of hoarseness due to attack of the lung by exogenous pathogens such as wind-cold or wind-heat

亢则害，承乃制。
[kàng zé hài, chéng nǎi zhì]
Hyperactivity harms, but harmonization will restrict it.

所不胜，克我者也。
[suǒ bù shèng, kè wǒ zhě yě]
The unrestrained is what restricts me.

所胜，我所克也。
[suǒ shèng, wǒ suǒ kè yě]
The restrained is what I restrict.

木为金之所胜。
[mù wéi jīn zhī suǒ shèng]
Wood is restricted by metal.

金为火之所胜。
[jīn wéi huǒ zhī suǒ shèng]

Metal is restricted by fire.

火为水之所胜。
[huǒ wéi shuǐ zhī suǒ shèng]
Fire is restricted by water.

水为土之所胜。
[shuǐ wéi tǔ zhī suǒ shèng]
Water is restricted by earth.

土为木之所胜。
[tǔ wéi mù zhī suǒ shèng]
Earth is restricted by wood.

木为土之所不胜。
[mù wéi tǔ zhī suǒ bù shèng]
Wood is what earth cannot restrict.

土为水之所不胜。
[tǔ wéi shuǐ zhī suǒ bù shèng]
Earth is what water cannot restrict.

水为火之所不胜。
[shuǐ wéi huǒ zhī suǒ bù shèng]
Water is what fire cannot restrict.

火为金之所不胜。
[huǒ wéi jīn zhī suǒ bù shèng]
Fire is what metal cannot restrict.

金为木之所不胜。
[jīn wéi mù zhī suǒ bù shèng]
Metal is what wood cannot restrict.

母病及子。
[mǔ bìng jí zǐ]
Disorder of a mother organ afflicts its child organ. – an explanation of such pathological conditions, using the five-element/phase theory, as hyperactivity of liver yang developing into exuberant heart fire and weakness of spleen *qi*, as well as the consequent deficiency of lung *qi*

子病及母。
[zǐ bìng jí mǔ]
Disorder of a child organ afflicts its mother organ. – an explanation of such pathological conditions, using the five-element/phase theory, as lung *qi* deficiency developing into spleen *qi* deficiency with failure of the transporting function

子盗母气。
[zǐ dào mǔ qì]
A child organ robs its mother organ of *qi*. – another expression for "disorder of a child organ afflicts its mother organ" (子病及母 [zǐ bìng jí mǔ])

天人相应
Correspondence between Nature and Human

天人相应 [tiān rén xiāng yìng]
correspondence between nature and human: one of the basic theories in traditional Chinese medicine, according to which the physical structure and physiological phenomena of the human body as well as its pathological changes are in adaptive conformity with the variations of the natural environment, and hence in diagnosis and treatment the influences of environmental factors such as climatic conditions and geographical localities should be taken into account

顺应四时 [shùn yìng sì shí]
adaptation to seasonal changes: one of the major points in the theory of correspondence between nature and human that the human body should keep in adaptation to the climatic changes of the four seasons

因时制宜 [yīn shí zhì yí]
taking measures that are suited to the time: a principle of treatment developed on the basis of the correspondence between nature and human that the patient should be treated in accordance with the climatic variations of the four seasons

因地制宜 [yīn dì zhì yí]
taking measures that are suited to the place: a principle of treatment developed on the basis of the correspondence between nature and human that the patient should be treated in accordance with the geographical and climatic features of the relevalent area

运气学说 [yùn qì xué shuō]
theory of the circuits and *qi*: the study of climatic changes and their relation to the occurrence of disease in terms of the five circuits and six *qi*

五运 [wǔ yùn]
five circuits: collective term for the wood, fire, earth, metal and water circuits

六气 [liù qì]
six *qi*: collective term for the six climatic phenomena, i.e., wind, cold, summerheat, dampness, dryness, and fire (heat)

五运六气 [wǔ yùn liù qì]
five circuits and six *qi*: a traditional Chinese doctrine, based upon which meteorological features and changes as well as their effects on the human body can be predicted and calculated in terms of the Heavenly Stems and Earthly Branches

运气 [yùn qì]
(I) circuit-*qi*: abbreviation for the five circuits and six *qi* (五运六气 [wǔ yùn liù qì]); **(II) moving *qi*** (see p. 503)

岁运 [suì yùn]
circuit of year: the circuit *qi* that controls the meteorological features and changes of a given year as well as the corresponding prevalence of disease

主运 [zhǔ yùn]
dominant circuit: the circuit of the regular seasonal changes of the climate

客运 [kè yùn]
guest circuit: the circuit of the seasonal changes of the climate in a particular year

主气 [zhǔ qì]
dominant *qi*: the *qi* that controls the regular seasonal changes of the climate

客气 [kè qì]
guest *qi*: the *qi* that controls the seasonal changes of the climate in a particular year

间气 [jiān qì]
intermediate *qi*: that part of guest *qi*, other than the *qi* responsible for celestial control and the *qi* with terrestrial effect, existing between Heaven and Earth

司天 [sī tiān]
celestial control; controlling Heaven: the guest *qi*'s control of the climatic changes in the first half of the year

在泉 [zài quán]
terrestrial effect; affecting Earth: the guest *qi*'s control of the climatic changes in the latter half of the year

岁会 [suì huì]
annual congruence: periodic meeting of the circuit *qi* of the year with an earthly branch in terms of the five phases, happening in eight years of a sixty-year cycle

天符 [tiān fú]
coincidence of heavenly *qi*: meeting of the circuit *qi* of the year with the *qi* controlling Heaven in terms of the five phases

平气 [píng qì]
normal circuit *qi*: circuit *qi* that is neither excessive nor insufficient, rarely causing disease

天年 [tiān nián]
natural life span: the length of time that a person is expected to live

天干 [tiān gān]
heavenly stems: a sequence of ten symbols used as serial numbers and also in combination with the twelve earthly branches to designate years, months, days and hours

地支 [dì zhī]
earthly branches: a sequence of twelve symbols used in combination with the ten heavenly stems to designate years, months, days and hours

✦ 常用引文 Commonly Used Citations ✦

人与天地相参。
[rén yǔ tiān dì xiāng cān]
Human corresponds to Heaven and Earth.

人以天地之气生，四时之法成。
[rén yǐ tiān dì zhī qì shēng, sì shí zhī fǎ chéng]
Human is born by the *qi* of Heaven and

Earth, and develops along with the law of the four seasons.

天食人以五气，地食人以五味。

[tiān sì rén yǐ wǔ qì, dì sì rén yǐ wǔ wèi]

Heaven provides human with five kinds of *qi* (i.e., wind, heat, dampness, dryness and cold), **and Earth provides human with five kinds of flavors** (i.e., sour, sweet, bitter, salty and pungent flavors).

五脏应四时。

[wǔ zàng yìng sì shí]

The five *zang* organs correspond to the four seasons.

春夏养阳，秋冬养阴。

[chūn xià yǎng yáng, qiū dōng yǎng yīn]

One should cultivate yang in spring and summer, and nourish yin in autumn and winter.

四变之动，脉与之上下，以春应中规，夏应中矩，秋应中衡，冬应中权。

[sì biàn zhī dòng, mài yǔ zhī shàng xià, yǐ chūn yīng zhòng guī, xià yīng zhòng jù, qiū yīng zhòng héng, dōng yīng zhòng quán]

A normal pulse varies with the seasonal changes: It should be round and smooth in spring, square and full in summer, float to the surface in autumn, and sink to the interior in winter.

冬伤于寒，春必温病。

[dōng shāng yú hán, chūn bì wēn bìng]

Attack by cold in winter will inevitably lead to seasonal febrile disease in spring.

必先岁气，无伐天和。

[bì xiān suì qì, wú fá tiān hé]

One must know in advance the condition of the *qi* of the year to avoid punishment for violation of the natural harmony.

夫百病者，多以旦慧昼安，夕加夜甚。

[fū bǎi bìng zhě, duō yǐ dàn huì zhòu ān, xī jiā yè shèn]

Most diseases are light in the morning, calm in the daytime, aggravated in the evening, and worse at night.

脏腑 *Zang-Fu* Organs

脏象学说 [zàng xiàng xué shuō]
visceral manifestation theory: theory that deals with the physiological functions and pathological changes of the internal organs, as well as the relationship with their external manifestations. It is a unique TCM theory that correlates internal mechanisms with external phenomena.

脏象 [zàng xiàng]
visceral manifestation: external manifestation of an internal organ through which a physiological function or a pathological change can be detected

脏腑 [zàng fǔ]
***zang-fu* organs; viscera and bowels:** collective term for all internal organs, including *zang* organs, *fu* organs and extra *fu* organs

脏 [zàng]
***zang* organ; viscus:** any of the internal organs that produce, transform and store essential *qi*

腑 [fǔ]
***fu* organ; bowel:** any of the internal organs that receive, contain and transmit food and drink

五脏 [wǔ zàng]
five *zang* organs; five viscera: collective term for the heart, liver, spleen, lung and kidney

六腑 [liù fǔ]
six *fu* organs; six bowels: collective term for the gallbladder, stomach, large intestine, small intestine, urinary bladder and triple energizer – all related to food digestion and fluid transmission

阳脏 [yáng zàng]
yang *zang* organs; yang viscera: the *zang* organs (or viscera) of yang nature, referring to the heart and the liver, distinguished for their preponderant yang quality, also known as male *zang* organs (牡脏 [mǔ zàng])

牡脏 [mǔ zàng]
male *zang* organs; male viscera: another name for yang *zang* organs (阳脏 [yáng zàng])

阴脏 [yīn zàng]
yin *zang* organs; yin viscera: the *zang* organs (or viscera) of yin nature, referring to the spleen, the lung and the kidney, distinguished for their preponderant yin quality, also known as female *zang* organs (牝脏 [pìn zàng])

牝脏 [pìn zàng]
female *zang* organs; yin viscera: another name for yin *zang* organs (阴脏 [yīn zàng])

心 [xīn]
heart: the organ located in the thoracic cavity above the diaphragm, which controls blood circulation and mental

activities, and serves as the "supreme ruler" of all the *zang-fu* organs

心气 [xīn qì]
heart *qi*: essential *qi* of the heart, which propels the blood through the vessels and also serves as the motive force of mental activities

心血 [xīn xuè]
heart blood: the blood governed by the heart, which circulates all over the body, particularly the portion of the blood that nourishes the heart, and serves as the material basis of its physiological activities, including mental activities

心阴 [xīn yīn]
heart yin: the yin-fluid of the heart, closely related to heart blood both physiologically and pathologically

心阳 [xīn yáng]
heart yang: the yang-*qi* of the heart, which stimulates the activities of the heart and mind, promotes blood circulation and provides heat to the body

心火 [xīn huǒ]
heart fire: (1) a byword for the heart (心 [xīn]) because the heart pertains to fire according to the five-element/phase theory; (2) a synonym for heart yang (心阳 [xīn yáng])

君火 [jūn huǒ]
sovereign fire: a synonym for heart fire (心火[xīn huǒ])

肝 [gān]
liver: the organ located in the right hypochondrium below the diaphragm, which stores blood, facilitates the flow of *qi*, and is closely related to the functions of the tendons and eyes

肝气 [gān qì]
liver *qi*: (1) the visceral *qi* that serves as the motive force of the functional activities of the liver; (2) abbreviation for liver *qi* stagnation (肝气郁滞 [gān qì yù zhì])

肝血 [gān xuè]
liver blood: the blood stored in the liver that nourishes the liver system, including the liver itself, liver meridian, eyes, tendons and nails

肝阴 [gān yīn]
liver yin: the blood and fluid of the liver that coordinate with liver yang

肝阳 [gān yáng]
liver yang: yang-*qi* of the liver, referring chiefly to the flourishing and *qi*-smoothing function of the liver

脾 [pí]
spleen: the *zang* organ in the middle energizer, which shares with the stomach the function of digesting food, transports and distributes nutrients and water, reinforces *qi*, keeps blood flowing within the vessels, and is closely related to the limbs and muscles

脾气 [pí qì]
spleen *qi*: essential *qi* of the spleen that serves as the dynamic force for the transportation, distribution and ascension of nutrients and water, and keeps blood flowing within the blood vessels

脾阳 [pí yáng]

spleen yang: the yang aspect of the spleen, referring to the promotion of the spleen functions including transportation, transformation, ascension and warming

脾阴 [pí yīn]

spleen yin: (1) yin-fluid of the spleen; (2) the yin aspect of the spleen, opposite to spleen yang, referring to the moistening and nourishing effect of the spleen; (3) a term referring to the spleen itself as the stomach pertaining to yang and the spleen to yin

肺 [fèi]

lung: a pair of organs located in the thoracic cavity, that control respiration, dominate *qi*, regulate water passage, and are closely related to the functions of the nose and skin surface

肺气 [fèi qì]

lung *qi*: dynamic force of the various functions of the lung

肺阴 [fèi yīn]

lung yin: essence and fluid that nourish the lung, coordinating with lung *qi*

肺津 [fèi jīn]

lung fluid: fluid that moistens the lung, pertaining to lung yin

肺阳 [fèi yáng]

lung yang: the yang aspect of the lung, referring to the warming, moving, ascending and diffusing functions of the lung

肾 [shèn]

kidney: a *zang* organ that stores vital essence, controls the growth, development, reproduction and urinary functions, and also has a direct effect on the conditions of the bones and marrow, the activities of the brain, the hearing, and the inspiratory function of the respiratory system

肾阴 [shèn yīn]

kidney yin: the yin aspect of the kidney including the yin-fluid as well as the essence stored in the kidney, the material basis of the functional activities of kidney yang, which has a moistening and nourishing effect on all the organs; also called kidney water (肾水 [shèn shuǐ]), genuine water (真水 [zhēn shuǐ]), original yin (元阴 [yuán yīn]) or genuine yin (真阴 [zhēn yīn]). Since yin and yang counterbalance each other, when kidney yin is insufficient, kidney yang is bound to be hyperactive, even to the extent of frenetic stirring of the ministerial fire. On the other hand, frenetic stirring of the ministerial fire may further consume kidney yin.

肾水 [shèn shuǐ]

(I) kidney water: another name for kidney yin (肾阴 [shèn yīn]); **(II) kidney edema:** edema due to kidney yang deficiency

真水 [zhēn shuǐ]

genuine water: another name for kidney yin (肾阴 [shèn yīn])

元阴 [yuán yīn]

original yin: another name for kidney yin (肾阴 [shèn yīn]), stressing the latter's importance

真阴 [zhēn yīn]

genuine yin: another name for kidney yin

(肾阴 [shèn yīn]), stressing the latter's importance

肾阳 [shèn yáng]
kidney yang: the yang aspect of the kidney, which warms and activates all the organs including the kidney, serving as the dynamic force of the functional activities of the kidney as well as the source of human life; also called original yang (元阳 [yuán yáng]), genuine yang (真阳 [zhēn yáng]) or genuine fire (真火 [zhēn huǒ])

元阳 [yuán yáng]
original yang: another name for kidney yang (肾阳 [shèn yáng]), stressing the latter's importance

真阳 [zhēn yáng]
genuine yang: another name for kidney yang (肾阳 [shèn yáng]), stressing the latter's importance

真火 [zhēn huǒ]
genuine fire: another name for kidney yang (肾阳 [shèn yáng])

心包络 [xīn bāo luò]
pericardium: the sac that surrounds the heart and protects the latter against attack by exogenous pathogenic factors, usually abbreviated as 心包 [xīn bāo]

心包 [xīn bāo]
pericardium: same as 心包络 [xīn bāo luò]

命门 [mìng mén]
(I) life gate: the home of water and fire as the root of life, closely related to the kidney both physiologically and pathologically. The genuine fire in the life gate, i.e., life gate fire, refers to kidney fire, and the genuine water in the life gate refers to kidney yin. **(II) *Mingmen* (GV4):** an acupoint on the lower back and on the posterior midline, in the depression below the spinous process of the 2nd lumbar vertebra

胆 [dǎn]
gallbladder: a *fu* organ connected with the liver, which stores and discharges bile

胃 [wèi]
stomach: a *fu* organ that receives and preliminarily digests food, and expels the chyme into the small intestine

胃脘 [wèi wǎn]
stomach cavity: the space or potential space within the stomach extending from the cardia to the pylorus

脘 [wǎn]
stomach cavity: abbreviation for 胃脘 [wèi wǎn]

上脘 [shàng wǎn]
(I) upper stomach cavity: the upper part of the stomach cavity, including the cardia; **(II) *Shangwan* (CV13):** an acupoint on the upper abdomen and on the anterior midline, 5 *cun* above the center of the umbilicus

中脘 [zhōng wǎn]
(I) middle stomach cavity: the middle part of the stomach cavity; **(II) *Zhongwan* (CV12):** an acupoint on the upper abdomen and on the anterior midline, 4 *cun* above the center of the umbilicus

下脘 [xià wǎn]
(I) lower stomach cavity: the lower part of the stomach cavity, including the pylorus; **(II) *Xiawan* (CV10):** an acupoint on the upper abdomen and on the anterior midline, 2 *cun* above the center of the umbilicus

胃气 [wèi qì]
stomach *qi*: (1) referring to the function of food intake and preliminary digestion; (2) referring to the material basis of the normal pulse

胃阳 [wèi yáng]
stomach yang: the yang aspect of the stomach, referring to the warming and digestive functions of the stomach

胃阴 [wèi yīn]
stomach yin: the yin aspect the stomach, referring to (1) the fluid produced by the stomach necessary for performing normal food intake and preliminary digestion in coordination with stomach yang; (2) the fluid of the whole alimentary canal

胃津 [wèi jīn]
stomach fluid: fluid produced by the stomach, a part of stomach yin

大肠 [dà cháng]
large intestine: a *fu* organ that has the function of passing the waste through the alimentary canal

小肠 [xiǎo cháng]
small intestine: a *fu* organ that receives food content from the stomach, further digests it, absorbs the nourishing and excretes the waste

膀胱 [páng guāng]
bladder: a *fu* organ that stores and discharges urine

三焦 [sān jiāo]
triple energizer: collective term for the three portions of the body cavity, through which the visceral *qi* is transformed and fluids are transmitted

上焦 [shàng jiāo]
upper energizer: the upper portion of the body cavity, i.e., the portion above the diaphragm housing the heart and lung

中焦 [zhōng jiāo]
middle energizer: the middle portion of the body cavity, i.e., the portion between the diaphragm and the umbilicus housing the spleen and stomach

下焦 [xià jiāo]
lower energizer: the lower portion of the body cavity, i.e., the portion below the umbilicus housing the bladder and intestines, also including the liver and kidney in the case of syndrome differentiation or pattern identification of warm diseases

形脏 [xíng zàng]
organs containing visible substances: a group of visceral organs including the stomach, small and large intestines, and bladder

奇恒之腑 [qí héng zhī fǔ]
extraordinary organs: collective term for the brain, marrow, bones, blood vessels,

gallbladder and uterus. They are so called because their physiological properties are different from those of both ordinary *zang* and *fu* organs.

脑 [nǎo]
brain: one of the extraordinary organs contained within the cranium where the marrow converges and where spiritual and mental activities take place, also known as sea of marrow (髓海 [suǐ hǎi])

髓海 [suǐ hǎi]
sea of marrow: another name for the brain (脑 [nǎo])

元神之府 [yuán shén zhī fǔ]
house of the original spirit: euphemistic name for the brain

髓 [suǐ]
marrow: an extraordinary organ including bone marrow and spinal marrow, both of which are nourished by kidney essence

骨 [gǔ]
bone: one of the extraordinary organs forming the framework of the body, which protects the internal organs and facilitates movement, closely related to the kidney function and nourished by the marrow

髓之府 [suǐ zhī fǔ]
house of marrow: euphemistic name for bones

脉 [mài]
(I) vessel: the conduit through which *qi* and blood pass; **(II) pulse:** beating of the artery as felt at the wrist

血之府 [xuè zhī fǔ]
house of blood: euphemistic name for blood vessels

女子胞 [nǚ zǐ bāo]
uterus; womb: an organ in the female for carrying and nourishing offspring during fetal development, also called 胞宫 [bāo gōng],子脏 [zǐ zàng] and 胞脏 [bāo zàng]

胞宫 [bāo gōng]
womb: another name for the uterus (女子胞 [nǚ zǐ bāo])

子脏 [zǐ zàng]
viscus for offspring: another name for the uterus (女子胞 [nǚ zǐ bāo])

胞脏 [bāo zàng]
viscus for fetus: another name for the uterus (女子胞 [nǚ zǐ bāo])

四海 [sì hǎi]
four seas; four reservoirs: collective term for the sea or reservoir of marrow (the brain), the sea or reservoir of blood (the conception vessel), the sea or reservoir of *qi* (the pectoral region) and the sea or reservoir of food and drink (the stomach)

气海 [qì hǎi]
(I) sea of *qi*; reservoir of *qi*: the central part of the chest or the pectoral region as the upper one and the region just below the umbilicus as the lower one; **(II) *Qihai* (CV6):** an acupoint on the conception vessel, 1.5 *cun* below the umbilicus

血海 [xuè hǎi]
(I) sea of blood; reservoir of blood: (1) the conception vessel; (2) the liver;

(II) ***Xuehai*** **(SP10):** an acupoint on the medial side of the thigh, 2 *cun* above the superior medial corner of the patella, on the prominence of the medial head of the quadriceps muscle of the thigh

水谷之海 [shuǐ gǔ zhī hǎi]
reservoir of food and drink: euphemistic term for the stomach

血室 [xuè shì]
blood chamber: term referring to (1) the uterus; (2) the liver; (3) the thoroughfare vessel

脏象 [zàng xiàng]
visceral manifestation: the outward manifestation of internal organs through which physiological functions as well as pathological changes can be detected and the state of health judged

传化之腑 [chuán huà zhī fǔ]
fu **organs of conveyance and transformation:** *fu* organs that have the function of conveying and transforming food and drink, i.e., the stomach, small intestine, large intestine, triple energizer, and bladder

五脏所恶 [wǔ zàng suǒ wù]
aversions of the five *zang* organs: collective term referring to heat, cold, wind, dampness and dryness in relation to the five *zang* organs, the elements that the heart, lung, liver, spleen and kidney are averse to, respectively

五脏所主 [wǔ zàng suǒ zhǔ]
charges of the five *zang* organs: collective term referring to the vessels, skin, sinews/tendons, muscles and bones in relation to the five *zang* organs, the body parts that the heart, lung, liver, spleen and kidney are in charge of, respectively

五脏所藏 [wǔ zàng suǒ cáng]
storage of the five *zang* organs: collective term referring to the mind, corporeal soul, ethereal soul, thought and will in relation to the five *zang* organs, the spiritual and mental activities that the heart, lung, liver, spleen and kidney store, respectively

五味所入 [wǔ wèi suǒ rù]
accessibility of the five flavors: collective term referring to the liver, heart, spleen, lung and kidney, the *zang* organs which the sour, bitter, sweet, pungent and salty flavors can reach and enter, respectively

五志 [wǔ zhì]
five emotions; five minds: collective term for joy, anger, thought, anxiety, and fear assigned to the heart, liver, spleen, lung and kidney, respectively

脏腑相合 [zàng fǔ xiāng hé]
pairing of *zang* and *fu* organs; pairing of visceral organs: the interrelation and mutual influence between the *zang* and *fu* organs, which are connected by the corresponding meridians/channels. The heart is paired with the small intestine, the lung with the large intestine, the spleen with the stomach, the liver with the gallbladder, and the kidney with the bladder.

脏气 [zàng qì]
qi **of *zang* organs; visceral *qi*:** (1) the *qi* that enables the visceral organs to perform their activities; (2) the functional activities

of the visceral organs

心肾相交 [xīn shèn xiāng jiāo]
heart-kidney interaction: mutual assisting and suppressing relationship between the heart and the kidney, also known as 水火相济 [shuǐ huǒ xiāng jì]

水火相济 [shuǐ huǒ xiāng jì]
water-fire coordination: an expression synonymous with heart-kidney interaction (心肾相交 [xīn shèn xiāng jiāo]) for the heart corresponds to fire and the kidney to water

中精之腑 [zhōng jīng zhī fǔ]
***fu* organ with refined juice:** the gallbladder that contains bile, a clear and pure juice. All other *fu* organs contain and convey turbid substances.

中清之腑 [zhōng qīng zhī fǔ]
***fu* organ with clear juice:** the gallbladder that contains bile, a clear and pure juice, same as 中精之腑 [zhōng jīng zhī fǔ]

传导之腑 [chuán dǎo zhī fǔ]
***fu* organ of conveyance:** the large intestine that conveys the waste, also called organ of conveyance (传导之官 [chuán dǎo zhī guān])

传导之官 [chuán dǎo zhī guān]
organ of conveyance: same as *fu* organ of conveyance (传导之腑 [chuán dǎo zhī fǔ])

命门之火 [mìng mén zhī huǒ]
life gate fire: synonym for kidney yang (肾阳 [shèn yáng]), the basic fire of life, staying within kidney yin. It is the basis of the sexual and reproductive functions and is intimately involved in growth, development and aging. It warms and nourishes all the visceral organs. In particular, the spleen and stomach rely upon its warming effect to carry out their normal transportation and transformation functions.

命火 [mìng huǒ]
life fire: abbreviation for life gate fire (命门之火 [mìng mén zhī huǒ])

先天之火 [xiān tiān zhī huǒ]
inborn fire: another name for kidney yang (肾阳 [shèn yáng])

肾之府 [shèn zhī fǔ]
house of the kidney: the lumbar region where the kidneys are situated

相火 [xiàng huǒ]
ministerial fire: (1) a kind of physiological fire originating in the kidney and attached to the liver, gallbladder and triple energizer, which, in cooperation with the sovereign fire from the heart warms the viscera and promotes their activities; (2) the part of the fire controlled by the kidney that promotes sexual potency

三焦气化 [sān jiāo qì huà]
activity of the triple energizer: distribution, dissemination and excretion of fluid and movement of *qi* that depend on the normal functioning of the triple energizer

中渎之腑 [zhōng dú zhī fǔ]
***fu* organ for water communication:** a euphemism for the triple energizer

常用引文 Commonly Used Citations

五脏为实，藏而不泄。
[wǔ zàng wéi shí, cáng ér bù xiè]
The five *zang* organs are solid. They have the function of storing but not discharging.

六腑为空，泄而不藏。
[liù fǔ wéi kōng, xiè ér bù cáng]
The six *fu* organs are hollow. They have the function of discharging but not storing.

脏行气于腑。
[zàng xíng qì yú fǔ]
The *zang* organs provide *qi* to the *fu* organs.

腑输精于脏。
[fǔ shū jīng yú zàng]
The *fu* organs supply nutrients to the *zang* organs.

五脏藏精气而不泄。
[wǔ zàng cáng jīng qì ér bù xiè]
The five *zang* organs store up the essential *qi*, but hardly discharge any.

六腑传化物而不藏。
[liù fǔ chuán huà wù ér bù cáng]
The six *fu* organs transport the digested food, but hardly store any.

心属火。
[xīn shǔ huǒ]
The heart pertains to fire.

心者，君主之官，神明出焉。
[xīn zhě, jūn zhǔ zhī guān, shén míng chū yān]
The heart plays the role of the supreme commander of the human body, out of whom mental and spiritual activities come.

心主血脉。
[xīn zhǔ xuè mài]
The heart controls blood circulation.

心主神明。
[xīn zhǔ shén míng]
The heart controls spiritual and mental activities.

心者，其华在面。
[xīn zhě, qí huá zài miàn]
The heart manifests its splendor in the complexion: The condition of the heart is often reflected in the complexion.

心开窍于舌。
[xīn kāi qiào yú shé]
The heart opens into the tongue: The condition of the heart is often reflected in the tongue.

舌为心之苗。
[shé wéi xīn zhī miáo]
The tongue behaves as the sign of the heart: another expression for 心开窍于舌 [xīn kāi qiào yú shé]

心藏神。
[xīn cáng shén]
The heart houses the mind.

心在志为喜。
[xīn zài zhì wéi xǐ]
The emotion apt to affect the heart is joy.

心恶热。
[xīn wù rè]
The heart is intolerant of heat.

心合小肠。
[xīn hé xiǎo cháng]
The heart is paired with the small intestine. (cf. 心与小肠相表里 [xīn yǔ xiǎo cháng xiāng biǎo lǐ])

心与小肠相表里。
[xīn yǔ xiǎo cháng xiāng biǎo lǐ]
The heart and small intestine are interior-exteriorly related: The heart and the small intestine are connected with each other via the heart and the small intestine meridians/channels. This relationship is manifested in heart fire spreading to the small intestine, which leads to bloody urine.

小肠者，受盛之官，化物出焉。
[xiǎo cháng zhě, shòu chéng zhī guān, huà wù chū yān]
The small intestine acts like an officer in charge of reception and is responsible for further digestion of food.

小肠主受盛。
[xiǎo cháng zhǔ shòu chéng]
The small intestine is responsible for receiving food contents (from the stomach).

小肠主化物。
[xiǎo cháng zhǔ huà wù]
The small intestine is responsible for digesting food.

小肠化食，泌别清浊。
[xiǎo cháng huà shí, mì bié qīng zhuó]
The small intestine digests food, and separates the clear/useful from the turbid/waste.

肝者，将军之官，谋虑出焉。
[gān zhě, jiāng jūn zhī guān, móu lǜ chū yān]
The liver acts like a general who is valiant and resourceful.

肝属木。
[gān shǔ mù]
The liver pertains to wood.

肝藏血。
[gān cáng xuè]
The liver stores blood.

肝主疏泄。
[gān zhǔ shū xiè]
The liver governs free flow of *qi*.

肝主升发。
[gān zhǔ shēng fā]
The liver governs flourishing growth.

肝主筋。
[gān zhǔ jīn]
The liver governs the sinews/tendons: Only when liver blood is abundant can its nourishing action influence the sinews/tendons and enable them to move normally.

肝者，其华在爪。
[gān zhě, qí huá zài zhǎo]

The liver manifests its splendor in the nails: Lustrous nails signify a sound liver.

爪为筋之余。

[zhǎo wéi jīn zhī yú]

The nails are the odds and ends of the sinews/tendons: The nails reflect the condition of the liver which supplies the sinews/tendons with blood and nutrients.

肝开窍于目。

[gān kāi qiào yú mù]

The liver opens into the eyes: Normal eyesight depends upon proper functioning of the liver.

肝主目。

[gān zhǔ mù]

The liver governs the eyes.

肝藏魂。

[gān cáng hún]

The liver houses the ethereal soul: Patients with liver disease often complain of nightmares and restlessness.

肝主怒。

[gān zhǔ nù]

Irritability is a chief symptom of liver disease.

肝在志为怒。

[gān zài zhì wéi nù]

The emotion apt to affect the liver is anger.

肝恶风。

[gān wù fēng]

The liver is intolerant of wind.

肝为风木之脏。

[gān wéi fēng mù zhī zàng]

The liver is a viscus of wind and wood. It is so said because the liver smooths the flow of *qi* and blood，like a tree branching out freely and, if diseased, the symptoms of wind such as vertigo, tremors, or even convulsions arise.

肝为血海。

[gān wéi xuè hǎi]

The liver is a sea of blood: The liver has the function of storing blood and regulating the volume of circulating blood.

发为血之余。

[fà wéi xuè zhī yú]

Hair is the odds and ends of blood. It is so said because the hair is nourished by blood, and it grows thick and shiny in youth when blood supply is abundant, but turns grey or falls out in the aged when the supply is insufficient.

肝为刚脏。

[gān wéi gāng zàng]

The liver is a viscus of the temperament. It is so said because a patient with liver disease is apt to become excited, fiery, and hard to control or restrain.

肝为牡脏。

[gān wéi mǔ zàng]

The liver is a male viscus/*zang* organ. It is so said because the liver is preponderantly of an active and effective disposition, in contrast to the spleen and the lung (e.g., the liver suppresses the function of the spleen, and its fire can make the lung suffer).

肝体阴而用阳。

[gān tǐ yīn ér yòng yáng]
The liver is substantially yin but functionally yang. It is so said because the liver stores blood (yin factor) and, on the other hand, its physiological functions and pathological manifestations (e.g., normal and abnormal motility) pertain to yang nature.

肝肾同源。
[gān shèn tóng yuán]
The liver and kidney share a source. It is so said because: (1) the liver and kidney store, respectively, the blood and the vital essence, which have a common source; (2) the essence of the liver and kidney can back up each other, and deficiency of one will result in deficiency of the other.

肝合胆。
[gān hé dǎn]
The liver is paired with the gallbladder.

肝与胆相表里。
[gān yǔ dǎn xiāng biǎo lǐ]
The liver and gallbladder are interior-exteriorly related.

胆主决断。
[dǎn zhǔ jué duàn]
The gallbladder dominates decision making: The gallbladder is in charge of making proper judgment in the face of adversity, ensuring invulnerability to such stimuli as fear or fright.

胆者，中正之官。
[dǎn zhě, zhōng zhèng zhī guān]
The gallbladder is analogous to a mediator. (cf. 胆主决断 [dǎn zhǔ jué duàn])

脾属土。
[pí shǔ tǔ]
The spleen pertains to earth.

脾胃者，仓廪之官，五味出焉。
[pí wèi zhě, cāng lǐn zhī guān, wǔ wèi chū yān]
The spleen and stomach act like granary officers who are responsible for storing and supplying (food of) **the five flavors.**

脾主运化。
[pí zhǔ yùn huà]
The spleen governs transportation and transformation: The spleen has the function of digestion, assimilation and distribution of nutrients.

脾藏营。
[pí cáng yíng]
The spleen stores nutrients.

脾气主升。
[pí qì zhǔ shēng]
Spleen *qi* ascends: Spleen *qi* sends nutrients upward to the heart and lung, and provides lifting power to prevent visceroptosis.

脾主升清。
[pí zhǔ shēng qīng]
The spleen sends clarity upward: The functions of the spleen include sending nutrients, i.e., clarity upward to the heart and lung to produce *qi* and blood.

脾统血。
[pí tǒng xuè]
The spleen controls the blood: The spleen keeps blood within the vessels.

脾主肌肉。

[pí zhǔ jī ròu]

The spleen governs the flesh: A healthy spleen usually makes a person display a full figure, while a diseased spleen makes one lose flesh.

脾主四肢。

[pí zhǔ sì zhī]

The spleen governs the limbs: The strength of the limbs depends upon the nourishment guaranteed by the normal functioning of the spleen. A diseased spleen usually causes weakness of the limbs.

脾者，其华在唇。

[pí zhě, qí huá zài chún]

The spleen manifests its splendor in the lips: Red and lustrous lips signify normal functioning of the spleen.

脾开窍于口。

[pí kāi qiào yú kǒu]

The spleen opens into the mouth: A person whose spleen functions well always has a good appetite and normal taste in the mouth.

脾藏意。

[pí cáng yì]

The spleen stores thoughts: Excessive scrupulosities may impair the spleen, bringing on such symptoms as anorexia.

脾在志为思。

[pí zài zhì wéi sī]

The emotion apt to affect the spleen is pensiveness.

脾恶湿。

[pí wù shī]

The spleen is intolerant of dampness: Dampness is apt to impair the transporting and transforming functions of the spleen, leading to diarrhea, lassitude, edema, etc.

脾为气血生化之源。

[pí wéi qì xuè shēng huà zhī yuán]

The spleen is the source of *qi*-blood formation: This is because the spleen has the functions of digestion, assimilation, transportation and distribution of nutrients.

脾为生痰之源。

[pí wéi shēng tán zhī yuán]

The spleen is the source of phlegm formation: Phlegm is formed when dysfunction of the spleen leads to accumulation of dampness.

脾主后天。

[pí zhǔ hòu tiān]

The spleen determines the acquired constitution.

脾胃为后天之本。

[pí wèi wéi hòu tiān zhī běn]

The spleen and stomach provide the material basis of the acquired constitution.

脾合胃。

[pí hé wèi]

The spleen is paired with the stomach: The spleen and stomach are connected by a meridian/channel and are complementary in their functions.

脾与胃相表里。

[pí yǔ wèi xiāng biǎo lǐ]

The spleen and stomach are interior-exteriorly related.

胃主受纳。
[wèi zhǔ shòu nà]
The stomach governs the food intake.

胃为水谷之海。
[wèi wéi shuǐ gǔ zhī hǎi]
The stomach serves as the reservoir of food and drink.

胃主腐熟。
[wèi zhǔ fǔ shú]
The stomach digests food into chyme.

胃主降浊。
[wèi zhǔ jiàng zhuó]
The stomach sends the chyme downward.

胃气主降。
[wèi qì zhǔ jiàng]
Stomach *qi* descends: The stomach sends its contents downward to the intestines.

肺属金。
[fèi shǔ jīn]
The lung pertains to metal.

肺主气，司呼吸。
[fèi zhǔ qì, sī hū xī]
The lung governs *qi* and performs respiration.

肺为气之主。
[fèi wéi qì zhī zhǔ]
The lung is the governor of *qi*.

肺主宣发。
[fèi zhǔ xuān fā]
The lung governs diffusion and dissemination: The lung has the function of exhaling turbid air, diffusing defense *qi*, and disseminating body fluid, *qi* and blood.

肺主肃降。
[fèi zhǔ sù jiàng]
The lung governs purification and descending: The lung has the function of inhaling the clean air, sending the fluid downward, purifying the airway and moving the *qi* downward.

肺朝百脉。
[fèi cháo bǎi mài]
The lung faces all blood vessels. It is so said because the blood of the whole body must pass through the lung.

肺主行水。
[fèi zhǔ xíng shuǐ]
The lung controls the water flow: Water metabolism in the human body is associated with the descending and purifying functions of the lung.

肺主通调水道。
[fèi zhǔ tōng tiáo shuǐ dào]
The lung regulates the water passage: The lung constantly sends fluid downward to the kidney for the excretion of urine. Impairment of lung *qi* may lead to obstruction of the water passage, manifested by oliguria and edema.

肺为水之上源。
[fèi wéi shuǐ zhī shàng yuán]
The lung is the upper source of water. It is so said because the lung which regulates the water passage is situated in the upper energizer.

肺合皮毛。
[fèi hé pí máo]
The lung is paired with the skin and body hair: The skin and hair refer to the

body's surface as well as body resistance to external pathogenic factors.

肺主皮毛。
[fèi zhǔ pí máo]
The lung controls the skin and body hair.

肺主一身之表。
[fèi zhǔ yī shēn zhī biǎo]
The lung is in charge of the body surface: Sound lung *qi* strengthens superficial defense *qi*. If lung *qi* is insufficient, the body's resistance is weakened, followed by vulnerability to colds.

肺主声。
[fèi zhǔ shēng]
The lung controls the voice.

肺者，其华在毛。
[fèi zhě, qí huá zài máo]
The lung manifests its splendor in the hair of the body.

肺开窍于鼻。
[fèi kāi qiào yú bí]
The lung opens into the nose.

肺为华盖。
[fèi wéi huá gài]
The lung is the canopy of the viscera: The lung with its lobes stretches like a cover, being situated above all the other visceral organs.

肺为娇脏。
[fèi wéi jiāo zàng]
The lung is a delicate organ: The lung is vulnerable to attack by exogenous pathogens.

肺为贮痰之器。
[fèi wéi zhù tán zhī qì]
The lung is a container of phlegm: The lung is the main organ where phlegm is retained.

肺藏魄。
[fèi cáng pò]
The lung houses the corporeal soul.

肺在志为悲。
[fèi zài zhì wéi bēi]
The emotion apt to affect the lung is sorrow.

肺在志为忧。
[fèi zài zhì wéi yōu]
The emotion apt to affect the lung is anxiety.

肺恶寒。
[fèi wù hán]
The lung is intolerant of cold.

肺与大肠相表里。
[fèi yǔ dà cháng xiāng biǎo lǐ]
The lung and large intestine are interior-exteriorly related. (cf. 肺合大肠 [fèi hé dà cháng])

肺合大肠。
[fèi hé dà cháng]
The lung is paired with the large intestine: The lung and large intestine are connected with each other via the lung and the large intestine meridians/channels, enabling close functional interactions between the two internal organs. In clinical practice, purging the bowels clears lung heat, and some types of constipation are best treated by reinforcing lung *qi*.

大肠者，传导之官，变化出焉。
[dà cháng zhě, chuán dǎo zhī guān, biàn huà chū yān]
The large intestine is an organ in charge of transportation. It transforms food drosses into feces and excretes the latter out of the body.

大肠主传导。
[dà cháng zhǔ chuán dǎo]
The large intestine governs conveyance of waste.

肾属水。
[shèn shǔ shuǐ]
The kidney pertains to water.

肾者，作强之官，伎巧出焉。
[shèn zhě, zuò qiáng zhī guān, jì qiǎo chū yān]
The kidney is an organ of strength and energy, from which skillfulness and cleverness stem.

肾为气之根。
[shèn wéi qì zhī gēn]
The kidney is the root of *qi*. (cf. 肾主纳气 [shèn zhǔ nà qì])

肾主纳气。
[shèn zhǔ nà qì]
The kidney controls the reception of *qi*/air: The kidney promotes inspiration.

肾主生殖。
[shèn zhǔ shēng zhí]
The kidney is in charge of reproduction.

肾为先天之本。
[shèn wéi xiān tiān zhī běn]
The kidney is the foundation of the inborn constitution. It is so said because the kidney plays a key role in growth, development and reproduction.

腰为肾之府。
[yāo wéi shèn zhī fǔ]
The lumbus is the house of the kidney.

肾藏志。
[shèn cáng zhì]
The kidney houses the will (memory).

肾在志为恐。
[shèn zài zhì wéi kǒng]
The emotion apt to affect the kidney is fear.

肾藏精。
[shèn cáng jīng]
The kidney stores essence.

肾主水。
[shèn zhǔ shuǐ]
The kidney governs water.

肾司开阖。
[shèn sī kāi hé]
The kidney regulates excretion and retention (of water).

肾为水脏。
[shèn wéi shuǐ zàng]
The kidney is an organ of water. It is so said because the kidney pertains to water according to the five element/phase theory, and regulates water metabolism in the body.

肾其充在骨，骨充则髓实。
[shèn qí chōng zài gǔ, gǔ chōng zé suǐ shí]

The kidney supplies the bones with marrow, and healthy bones indicate the fullness of marrow.

肾主骨。
[shèn zhǔ gǔ]
The kidney governs the bones.

齿为骨之余。
[chǐ wéi gǔ zhī yú]
The teeth are the odds and ends of the bones.

肾主命门之火。
[shèn zhǔ mìng mén zhī huǒ]
The kidney controls the fire of the life gate.

肾司二阴。
[shèn sī èr yīn]
The kidney controls the two private parts (i.e., the urethra or uro-genital orifice and anus).

肾恶燥。
[shèn wù zào]
The kidney is intolerant of dryness: As the kidney stores essence and controls fluid metabolism, dryness which is incompatible with essence and fluid is apt to disturb the function of the kidney.

肾开窍于二阴。
[shèn kāi qiào yú èr yīn]
The kidney opens into the two private parts (i.e., the uro-genital orifice and the anus**).**

肾与膀胱相表里。
[shèn yǔ páng guāng xiāng biǎo lǐ]
The kidney and bladder are interior-exteriorly related.

肾合膀胱。
[shèn hé páng guāng]
The kidney is paired with the bladder.

肾者，其华在发。
[shèn zhě, qí huá zài fà]
The kidney manifests its splendor in the hair of the head: The function of the kidney is reflected in the thickness and glossiness of the hair of the head.

肾开窍于耳。
[shèn kāi qiào yú ěr]
The kidney opens into the ears: Healthy kidney ensures acute hearing, while kidney dysfunction is often accompanied by impaired hearing and tinnitus.

肾气通于耳。
[shèn qì tōng yú ěr]
Kidney *qi* reaches the ears.

六腑以通为用。
[liù fǔ yǐ tōng wéi yòng]
The six *fu* organs function well when they are unobstructed.

六腑以降为顺。
[liù fǔ yǐ jiàng wéi shùn]
The normal function of the six *fu* organs is to send the contents downwards.

膀胱者，州都之官。
[páng guāng zhě, zhōu dū zhī guān]
The bladder is an organ that controls a reservoir.

膀胱主藏津液。
[páng guāng zhǔ cáng jīn yè]

The bladder is in charge of storing fluid (i.e., urine).

心包络与三焦相表里。

[xīn bāo luò yǔ sān jiāo xiāng biǎo lǐ]

The pericardium and triple energizer are interior-exteriorly related.

三焦者，决渎之官，水道出焉。

[sān jiāo zhě, jué dú zhī guān, shǔi dào chū yān]

The triple energizer is the organ in charge of dredging the water passage.

三焦有名无形。

[sān jiāo yǒu míng wú xíng]

The triple energizer is an insubstantial organ.

上焦如雾。

[shàng jiāo rú wù]

The upper energizer works like a sprayer (to spread nutrients and *qi* throughout the body).

中焦如沤。

[zhōng jiāo rú òu]

The middle energizer works like a fermentor (to digest food).

下焦如渎。

[xià jiāo rú dú]

The lower energizer works like a drainer (to drain off waste and surplus water.)

三焦为营卫之源。

[sān jiāo wéi yíng wèi zhī yuán]

The triple energizer is the source of both nutrient and defensive *qi*.

上焦主纳。

[shàng jiāo zhǔ nà]

The upper energizer is in charge of reception (namely, intake of air and food).

中焦主化。

[zhōng jiāo zhǔ huà]

The middle energizer is in charge of transformation (namely, transforming food and drink into nutrients).

下焦主出。

[xià jiāo zhǔ chū]

The lower energizer is in charge of excretion.

髓海有余，则轻劲多力，自过其度。

[suǐ hǎi yǒu yú, zé qīng jìn duō lì, zì guò qí dù]

If one's sea of marrow is superabundant, one will be nimble and vigorous, and able to endure unusually hard work.

髓海不足，则脑转耳鸣。

[suǐ hǎi bù zú, zé nǎo zhuàn ěr míng]

If the sea of marrow is insufficient, vertigo and tinnitus will arise.

官窍和形体 Sense Organs and Other Body Structures

五官 [wǔ guān]
five (sense) organs: collective term for the nose, eyes, ears, mouth and throat

孔窍 [kǒng qiào]
orifice: an outer opening in the body, e.g., the nasal orifices

七窍 [qī qiào]
seven orifices: collective term for the eyes, ears, nostrils and mouth

九窍 [jiǔ qiào]
nine orifices: (1) collective term for the eyes, ears, nostrils and mouth, plus the urethral orifice and anus; (2) collective term for the eyes, ears, nostrils and mouth, plus the tongue and throat

上窍 [shàng qiào]
upper orifices: the orifices on the head

下窍 [xià qiào]
lower orifices: the urethral opening and anus

苗窍 [miáo qiào]
signal orifices: the body openings serving as windows, through which pathological changes of the internal organs can be detected. The nose, eyes, mouth (lips), tongue and ears are the specific body openings (or windows) of the lung, liver, spleen, heart and kidney, respectively.

鼻 [bí]
nose: the part of the face above the mouth, used for breathing, smelling, and assisting in vocalization, and taken as the specific opening of the lung

鼻窍 [bí qiào]
nasal orifice: the outer opening of the nasal cavity, taken as a specific opening related to the lung

鼻孔 [bí kǒng]
nostril: either of the two openings at the end of the nose through which the breath passes, also known as the opening of the nasal cavity (鼻洞 [bí dòng])

鼻洞 [bí dòng]
opening of the nasal cavity: same as nostril (鼻孔 [bí kǒng])

鼻翼 [bí yì]
ala nasi: the expanded outer wall on each side of the nose

方上 [fāng shàng]
ala nasi area: the area of the outer wall of each nostril, the inspection of which may provide information about the condition of the stomach

鼻准 [bí zhǔn]
apex nasi: the tip of the nose, also called 鼻尖 [bí jiān]

鼻尖 [bí jiān]
tip of the nose: same as apex nasi (鼻准 [bí zhǔn])

鼻根 [bí gēn]
radix nasi: the root of the nose

鼻隧 [bí suì]
nasal passage: the part of the nose including the nasal vestibule and the posterior naris

鼻梁 [bí liáng]
dorsum nasi: the part of the nose formed by the junction of the lateral surfaces, also known as the bridge of the nose (鼻茎 [bí jīng])

鼻茎 [bí jīng]
bridge of the nose: same as dorsum nasi (鼻梁 [bí liáng])

鼻柱 [bí zhù]
(I) dorsum of the nose: same as dorsum nasi (鼻梁 [bí liáng]); **(II) nasal septum:** the dividing wall between the nasal cavities

鼻柱骨 [bí zhù gǔ]
bony nasal septum: the bony part of the nasal septum

鼻毛 [bí máo]
vibrissa: the hair growing in the nasal cavity

口 [kǒu]
mouth: the opening through which one takes in food, regarded as the specific orifice for the spleen

唇 [chún]
lip: the fleshy margin of the mouth, also called "flying door" (飞门 [fēi mén]), the color and luster of which reflect the condition of the spleen

飞门 [fēi mén]
"flying door": another name for lip (唇 [chún])

齿 [chǐ]
tooth: hard bony structure rooted in the gum, used for biting, chewing and assisting in vocalization

真牙 [zhēn yá]
wisdom tooth: the third molar tooth

龈 [yín]
gum: the flesh at the base of the teeth, pertaining to the stomach meridian/channel

舌 [shé]
tongue: the movable organ in the mouth, used in tasting and assisting in swallowing, mastication and vocalization

舌旁 [shé páng]
side of the tongue: also known as the edge of the tongue (舌边 [she biān])

舌边 [shé biān]
edge of the tongue; border of the tongue: the outside boundary of the tongue, the color and luster of which may reflect the condition of the liver and gallbladder

舌端 [shé duān]
tip of the tongue: also known as 舌尖 [shé jiān]

舌尖 [shé jiān]
tip of the tongue: the point or thin end of the tongue, the color and luster of which may reflect the condition of the heart and lung

咽 [yān]
pharynx: the passage between the mouth and the larynx and esophagus, also called 嗌 [yì]

嗌 [yì]
pharynx: same as 咽 [yān]

咽门 [yān mén]
opening of the pharynx: the part of the throat through which food passes from the mouth into the esophagus

咽底 [yān dǐ]
retropharynx: the posterior pharyngeal wall

咽喉 [yān hóu]
laryngopharynx; throat: the potential cavity at the back of the root of the tongue, connected with the mouth, nose, and the respiratory and digestive tracts, and through which many meridians/channels run

悬雍垂 [xuán yōng chuí]
palatine uvula: the small fleshy mass hanging from the soft palate above the root of the tongue, also called "small tongue" (小舌 [xiǎo shé]), or uvula (蒂丁 [dì dīng]; 蒂中 [dì zhōng])

小舌 [xiǎo shé]
"small tongue": a popular name for the palatine uvula (悬雍垂 [xuán yōng chuí])

蒂丁 [dì dīng]
uvula: a pendent fleshy lobe, usually referring to the palatine uvula (悬雍垂 [xuán yōng chuí]), also called 蒂中 [dì zhōng]

蒂中 [dì zhōng]
uvula: same as 蒂丁[dì dīng]

颃颡 [háng sǎng]
nasopharynx: the upper part of the pharynx continuous with the nasal passages

喉核 [hóu hé]
tonsils: a pair of prominent masses that lie one on each side of the throat

喉关 [hóu guān]
faucial isthmus: the part of the throat formed by the tonsils, uvula and back of the tongue

肺系 [fèi xì]
(I) lung system: collective term for the lung and its appendages, including nose, larynx, trachea and bronchi; **(II) lung tract:** (1) the tract connecting the lung with the larynx; (2) the larynx and trachea

会厌 [huì yàn]
epiglottis: a thin lamella of cartilage that serves to cover the glottis during an act of swallowing

七冲门 [qī chōng mén]
seven portals; seven gates: seven important doorways or openings along the alimentary tract – the lips (飞门 [fēi mén]), teeth (户门 [hù mén]), epiglottis (吸门 [xī mén]), cardia (贲门 [bēn mén]), pylorus (幽门 [yōu mén]), ileocecal conjunction (阑门 [lán mén]), and anus (魄门 [pò mén])

户门 [hù mén]
"entrance doors"; teeth: the bodily

appendage on the jaws designed for mastication, one of the seven portals (七冲门 [qī chōng mén])

吸门 [xī mén]

"breath gate"; epiglottis: the thin piece of tissue at the back of the throat that prevents food and drink entering the trachea, one of the seven portals (七冲门 [qī chōng mén])

贲门 [bēn mén]

"rushing gate"; cardia: the orifice between the esophagus and the stomach, one of the seven portals (七冲门 [qī chōng mén])

幽门 [yōu mén]

"serene gate"; pylorus: the distal (duodenal) aperture of the stomach, one of the seven portals (七冲门 [qī chōng mén])

阑门 [lán mén]

"screen gate"; ileocecal conjunction: the part of the intestines where the small and large intestines join, one of the seven portals (七冲门 [qī chōng mén])

魄门 [pò mén]

"corporeal-soul gate"; anus: one of the seven portals (七冲门 [qī chōng mén]). It is so called because the anus is the lower opening of the large intestine, which is exterior-interiorly related to the lung – the *zang* organ that stores the corporeal soul.

皮毛 [pí máo]

skin and body hair: the body surface which is associated with the lung in function

毫毛 [háo máo]

down: fine hair of the skin

腠［凑］理 [còu lǐ]

(I) interstitial striae: collective term referring to the striae of the skin, muscles and visceral organs; **(II) subcutaneous interstice:** term referring to the superficial layer of the body, including the sweat pore

肌腠［凑］[jī còu]

muscular striae: a general term for the superficial layer of the human body under the skin

肌 [jī]

muscle: tissue that produces movement and strength

肉 [ròu]

flesh: soft tissue between the skin and bones, consisting of muscle and fat

分肉 [fēn ròu]

muscle boundary: the boundary between muscles and subcutaneous fat

玄府 [xuán fǔ]

sweat pore: the opening of the duct of the sweat gland on the surface of the skin, literally meaning "mysterious residence", so named because the opening is too minute to be visible, also called 元府 [yuán fǔ] and known as 气门 [qì mén] or 鬼门[guǐ mén]

元府 [yuán fǔ]

sweat pore: same as 玄府 [xuán fǔ]

气门 [qì mén]

"*qi* portal": another name for sweat pore (玄府 [xuán fǔ])

鬼门 [guǐ mén]
"ghost gate": another name for sweat pore (玄府 [xuán fǔ])

膈 [鬲] [gé]
diaphragm: the musculo-membranous partition separating the chest and abdomen

筋 [jīn]
sinew; tendon: the tough band or cord of tissue that joins muscle to bone

膜原 [mó yuán]
(I) pleurodiaphragmatic interspace: the space between the pleura and diaphragm; **(II) interior-exterior interspace:** the space between the interior and exterior of the body, a concept used in the diagnosis of febrile diseases

募原 [mù yuán]
same as 膜原 [mó yuán]

膏肓 [gāo huāng]
(I) infracardio-supradiaphragmatic space: the space below the heart and above the diaphragm, the innermost part of the body. A disease involving this part is believed to be life-threatening and beyond cure. **(II) *Gaohuang* (BL43):** an acupoint on the bladder meridian/channel

丹田 [dān tián]
elixir fields; *dantian*: three regions of the body to which one's mind is focused while practicing *qigong*: the lower elixir field – the region located on the upper 2/3 of the line joining the umbilicus and symphysis pubis; the middle elixir field – the xiphoid area; and the upper elixir field – the region between the eyebrows

精明之府 [jīng míng zhī fǔ]
house of intelligence: euphemistic term for the head

诸阳之会 [zhū yáng zhī huì]
confluence of all the yang meridians/channels: the site where all the yang meridians/channels meet, i.e., the head

头颅骨 [tóu lú gǔ]
cranium; skull: the bone structure that forms the head and encloses and protects the brain

巅顶 [diān dǐng]
vertex cranii: the top of the head, the highest point of the skull, often abbreviated as 巅 [diān]

巅 [diān]
vertex: abbreviation for vertex cranii (top of the head) (巅顶 [diān dǐng])

囟门 [xìn mén]
fontanel: membrane-covered space remaining in incompletely ossified skull of an infant

囟 [xìn]
fontanel: abbreviation for囟门 [xìn mén]

发际 [fà jì]
hairline: edge of the scalp round the face and over the neck

前发际 [qián fà jì]
anterior hairline: edge of the scalp on the forehead

后发际 [hòu fà jì]
posterior hairline: edge of the scalp above the neck

天庭 [tiān tíng]
mid-frons: central region of the forehead

阙中 [què zhōng]; 阙 [què]
ophryon: the mid-point between the eyebrows, inspection of which provides guidance for diagnosing lung diseases

印堂 [yìn táng]
(I) ophryon: same as 阙中 [què zhōng]; **(II)** ***Yintang*** **(EX-HN 3):** an acupoint located in between the eyebrows

阙上 [què shàng]
supra-ophryon area: the area above the mid-point in between the eyebrows and below the mid-frons, inspection of which provides guidance for diagnosing diseases of the throat

额 [é]
forehead: the part of the face above the eyebrows and below the hairline, also known as frons (额颅 [é lú])

额颅 [é lú]
frons: same as forehead (额 [é])

额角 [é jiǎo]
forehead corner: the area where the corner of the forehead meets the hairline

颞颥 [niè rú]
anterior temple: the region lateral and posterior to the orbit, corresponding to the temporal side of the sphenoid bone

太阳 [tài yáng]
(I) temporal region: the flattened region on each side of the forehead; **(II)** ***Taiyang*** **(EX-HN 5):** an acupoint on the temporal region of the head; **(III) greater yang:** abbreviation for the greater yang meridian/channel of the hand and the greater yang meridian/channel of the foot, referring to the small intestinal meridian/channel and the bladder meridian/channel, respectively

锐发 [ruì fà]
sideburns: patches of hair growing on the face in front of the ears

眉棱骨 [méi léng gǔ]
supra-orbital ridge: the prominence of the frontal bone over the supra-orbital arch

眉心 [méi xīn]
center of the eyebrows; glabella: midpoint between the eyebrows

目 [mù]
eye: the organ of sight, functionally associated with all *zang-fu* organs and meridians/channels, particularly the liver

目眶 [mù kuàng]
eye socket; orbit: the bony cavity beneath the frontal bone on each side, which encloses and protects the eye

泪窍 [lèi qiào]
lacrimal punctum: the opening of the lacrimal duct at the inner canthus of the eye

五轮 [wǔ lún]
five orbiculi: collective term for the eyelid, canthus, white of the eye, black of the eye and pupil. A TCM theory of ophthalmology holds that each of the

zang organs has a specific physio-pathological association with one of the orbiculi. (cf. 肉轮 [ròu lún], 血轮 [xuè lún], 气轮 [qì lún], 风轮 [fēng lún], 水轮 [shuǐ lún])

肉轮 [ròu lún]
flesh orbiculus: the eyelid, one of the five orbiculi, believed to be associated with the spleen

血轮 [xuè lún]
blood orbiculus: the canthus, one of the five orbiculi, believed to be associated with the heart

气轮 [qì lún]
***qi* orbiculus:** the white of the eye, one of the five orbiculi, believed to be associated with the lung

风轮 [fēng lún]
wind orbiculus: the black of the eye, one of the five orbiculi, believed to be associated with the liver

水轮 [shuǐ lún]
water orbiculus: the pupil, one of the five orbiculi, believed to be associated with the kidney

八廓 [bā kuò]
eight regions of the eye: an ancient hypothesis of dividing the eye into eight regions, each of which is thought to be associated with a particular internal organ pathologically. This hypothesis is obsolete because of controversies over the location of the regions and their relationship to the internal organs.

胞睑 [bāo jiǎn]
palpebra: the eyelid

目眦 [mù zì]
canthus (of the eye): the corner of the eye formed by the meeting of the upper and lower eyelids

目内眦 [mù nèi zì]
inner canthus (of the eye): the medial corner of the eye, also called medial canthus

目锐眦 [mù ruì zì]
lateral canthus (of the eye): the lateral corner of the eye, also called outer canthus (外眦 [wài zì])

内眦 [nèi zì]
inner canthus: abbreviation for 目内眦 [mù nèi zì]

外眦 [wài zì]
outer canthus: same as lateral canthus (目锐眦 [mù ruì zì])

目纲 [mù gāng]
tarsal plate: the plate that forms the framework of the eyelid

睑弦 [jiǎn xián]
palpebral margin: the edge of the free margin of the eyelid, from which the eyelashes grow

目弦 [mù xián]
margin of the eyelid: same as palpebral margin (睑弦 [jiǎn xián])

目上胞 [mù shàng bāo]
upper eyelid: the superior of the paired

movable folds that protect the anterior surface of the eyeball

目上弦 [mù shàng xián]
margin of the upper eyelid: the edge of the free margin of the upper eyelid

目下胞 [mù xià bāo]
lower eyelid: the inferior of the paired movable folds that protect the anterior surface of the eyeball

目下弦 [mù xià xián]
margin of the lower eyelid: the edge of the free margin of the lower eyelid

睑内 [jiǎn nèi]
palpebral conjunctiva: the membrane that lines the inner side of the eyelid

白睛 [bái jīng]
white of the eye: the white part of the eyeball, also called 白仁 [bái rén]

白仁 [bái rén]
white kernel: another name for the white of the eye (白睛 [bái jīng])

目系 [mù xì]
eye connector: the cord connecting the eye with the brain, including the ocular nerve and blood vessels associated with the eye

耳 [ěr]
ear: the organ of hearing, to which kidney *qi* flows, also known as the orifice of the kidney

耳廓 [ěr kuò]
auricle: the portion of the external ear not contained within the head, including the helix, anthelix and earlobe, also known as 耳壳 [ěr qiào]

耳壳 [ěr qiào]
auricle: same as 耳廓 [ěr kuò]

耳轮 [ěr lún]
helix: the incurved rim of the external ear

耳垂 [ěr chuí]
earlobe: the pendent part of the external ear

耳孔 [ěr kǒng]
ear-hole: opening of the external ear

耳道 [ěr dào]
external acoustic meatus: the auditory canal leading from the opening of the external ear to the eardrum, also called 耳窍 [ěr qiào]

耳窍 [ěr qià]
external acoustic meatus: same as 耳道 [ěr dào]

耳膜 [ěr mó]
eardrum: the tympanic membrane

耳门 [ěr mén]
(I) tragus: the small projection in front of the external meatus of the ear; **(II)** ***Ermen*** **(TE 21):** an acupoint on the face, anterior to the supratragic notch, in the depression behind the posterior border of the condyloid process of the mandible

颧 [quán]
malar eminence: the prominence of the cheekbone

颊 [jiá]
cheek: the area of the face inferior and

lateral to the malar eminence and anterior to the ear lobe

颊车 [jiá chē]
(I) mandibular angle: the angle formed by the junction of the posterior and lower borders of the lower jaw; **(II) *Jiache* (ST 6):** an acupoint on the face, in the depression where the masseter muscle is prominent

曲颊 [qū jiá]
(I) mandibular arch: the curved structure of the lower jaw; **(II) mandibular angle**

颐 [yí]
lower cheek: the portion of the face between the corner of the mouth and the mandibular angle

人中 [rén zhōng]
(I) philtrum: the middle vertical groove below the nose and above the upper lip; **(II) *Renzhong* (GV 26):** an acupoint on the face, at the junction of the upper third and middle third of the philtrum, also called *Shuigou* (GV 26) (水沟 [shuǐ gōu])

承浆 [chéng jiāng]
(I) middle of the mentolabial groove: the middle portion of the groove or sulcus lying between the chin and lower lip; **(II) *Chengjiang* (CV 24):** an acupoint located at the middle of mentolabial groove

吻 [wěn]
corner of the mouth: the part of the mouth where the upper and lower lips meet

颌 [hé]
jaw: the lower part of the face formed by the bones containing the teeth and the surrounding soft tissues

颔 [hàn]
chin: the lower portion of the face below the lower lip, including the front part of the lower jaw

颈 [jǐng]
neck: the part of the body that connects the head to the shoulders

结喉 [jié hóu]
laryngeal prominence: "Adam's apple"

枕骨 [zhěn gǔ]
occipital bone: the bone that forms the posterior part of the cranium, also called 玉枕骨[yù zhěn gǔ]

玉枕骨 [yù zhěn gǔ]
occipital bone: same as 枕骨[zhěn gǔ]

完骨 [wán gǔ]
mastoid process: the process of the temporary bone behind the ear

曲牙 [qū yá]
mandibular angle: the angle formed by the junction of the posterior and lower borders of the lower jaw, also called 曲颊 [qū jiá]

曲颊 [qū jiá]
mandibular angle: same as 曲牙 [qū yá]

项 [xiàng]
nape: the back part of the neck

肩 [jiān]
shoulder: the part of the body by which the arm is connected to the trunk

肩胛 [jiān jiǎ]

scapula; shoulder blade: the flat bone on either side of the upper back

胂 [shèn]

prominent muscle: (1) the paravertebral muscle; (2) the muscle below the iliac crest

手骨 [shǒu gǔ]

hand bones: collective term for the metacarpal and digital bones of the hand

臂 [bì]

(I) arm: the upper limb from the shoulder to the hand; **(II) forearm:** the part of the arm from the elbow to the wrist

臂内廉 [bì nèi lián]

inner aspect of the arm: (1) the medial aspect of the forearm; (2) the medial aspect of the entire upper limb

臂外廉 [bì wài lián]

outer aspect of the arm: (1) the lateral aspect of the forearm; (2) the lateral aspect of the entire upper limb

臑 [nào]

(I) humeral region: the region of the arm below the shoulder and above the elbow; **(II) anterior brachial muscle:** the biceps muscle of the arm

臑骨 [nào gǔ]

humerus: the bone extending from the shoulder to the elbow

肱 [gōng]

upper arm: the part of the arm from the shoulder to the elbow

缺盆 [quē pén]

(I) supraclavicular fossa: depression on either side of the neck behind the clavicle; **(II) *Quepen* (ST 12):** an acupoint at the center of the supraclavicular fossa

上横骨 [shàng héng gǔ]

manubrium of the sternum: the cephalic segment of the sternum

虚里 [xū lǐ]

***Xuli*:** (1) the area of the apex beat; (2) the great collateral of the spleen

膻中 [dàn zhōng]

(I) thoracic center: the central part of the chest, between the nipples; **(II) *Danzhong* (GV 17):** an acupoint on the chest, where the anterior midline and the line connecting the nipples cross each other

鸠尾 [jiū wěi]

(I) xiphoid process: the pointed process of cartilage, connected with the lower part of the sternum; **(II) *Jiuwei* (CV 15):** an acupoint on the anterior midline, 1 *cun* below the xiphisternal synchondrosis

膺 [yīng]

chest: frontal area of the thorax

臆 [yì]

pectoral muscle: muscle on the ventral side of the thorax

胁 [xié]

lateral pectoral region: the upper lateral region of the human body from the armpit to the 12th rib

季肋 [jì lèi]
hypochondrium; hypochondriac region: either of the superolateral regions of the abdomen, lateral to the epigastric region, overlying the costal cartilages of the 11th and 12th ribs, also called 季胁 [jì xié]

季胁 [jì xié]
hypochondrium: same as 季肋 [jì lèi]

腹 [fù]
abdomen: the portion of the body which lies between the thorax and the pelvis

大腹 [dà fù]
(I) whole abdomen: all of the abdomen; **(II) upper abdomen:** the part of the abdomen above the umbilicus

小腹 [xiǎo fù]
lower abdomen: the part of the abdomen below the umbilicus

少腹 [shào fù]
(I) lateral lower abdomen: either of the lateral regions of the lower abdomen; **(II) lower abdomen:** same as 小腹 [xiǎo fù]

脐腹 [qí fù]
peri-umbilical abdomen: the part of the abdomen around the umbilicus

神阙 [shén què]
(I) umbilicus: the navel; **(II) *Shenque* (CV8):** an acupoint at the center of the umbilicus

横骨 [héng gǔ]
(I) pubic bone: the anterior inferior part of the hip bone on either side, articulating with its fellow in the anterior midline at the pubic symphysis; **(II) *Henggu* (KI 11):** a pair of acupoints on the lower abdomen, 5 *cun* below the center of the umbilicus and 0.5 *cun* lateral to the anterior midline

曲骨 [qū gǔ]
(I) pubic symphysis: the joint formed by the union of the pubic bones; **(II) *Qugu* (CV2):** an acupoint on the anterior midline at the midpoint of the upper border of the pubic symphysis

会阴 [huì yīn]
(I) perineum: the area between the anus and the posterior part of the external genitalia; **(II) *Huiyin* (CV1):** an acupoint in the center of perineum

毛际 [máo jì]
suprapubic margin: the upper border of the region where the pubic hair grows

气街 [qì jiē]
***qi* pathway:** (1) the pathway along which *qi* flows; (2) the area of the pulsating vessel (i.e., femoral artery) in the groin

前阴 [qián yīn]
anterior yin: the external genitalia including external orifice of the urethra

后阴 [hòu yīn]
posterior yin: the anus

二阴 [èr yīn]
two yin; two private parts: the external genitalia and anus

产门 [chǎn mén]
vaginal orifice (of a paturient): the external opening of the vagina during childbirth

阴户 [yīn hù]
(I) vaginal orifice: the external opening of the vagina; **(II) vulva:** see p. 555

阴门 [yīn mén]
vaginal orifice: same as 阴户 [yīn hù]

子门 [zǐ mén]
cervical orifice: orifice of the uterine cervix, the opening through which the fetus passes out of the uterus during delivery

廷孔 [tíng kǒng]
(I) external urethral orifice (of the female)**:** the opening of the urethra on the female body surface through which urine is discharged; **(II) vaginal orifice**

阴器 [yīn qì]
external genitals: external male genital organs, comprising the penis and scrotum

阴囊 [yīn náng]
scrotum: the external pouch that contains the testes, also called 肾囊 [shèn náng]

肾囊 [shèn náng]
scrotum: same as 阴囊 [yīn náng]

睾 [gāo]
testis; testicle: the male reproductive organ where the sperms are produced

阴茎 [yīn jīng]
penis: the cylindrical organ with which a male copulates and urinates

茎 [jīng]
penis: abbreviation for 阴茎 [yīn jīng]

茎垂 [jīng chuí]
penis and testes

宗筋 [zōng jīn]
ancestral sinew: (1) collective term for the sinews that control the articular movement; (2) euphemistic expression for penis

宗筋之会 [zōng jīn zhī huì]
confluence of ancestral sinews: a term referring to the male genitals

精窍 [jīng qiào]
male urinary meatus: the external orifice of the male urethra

肛门 [gāng mén]
anus: the lower opening of the large intestine through which the stool is discharged, also called the corporeal-soul gate (魄门 [pò mén])

腰 [yāo]
lumbus; lower back: the part of the back between the thorax and the pelvis

精室 [jīng shì]
essence chamber: the part of a male body where semen is stored

交骨 [jiāo gǔ]
union bone: (1) the sacrococcygeal joint; (2) the pubic bone

股 [gǔ]
thigh: the part of the leg between the knee and the hip

膝 [xī]
knee: the joint between the thigh and the lower part of the leg

筋之府 [jīn zhī fǔ]
house of sinews/tendons: a euphemistic name for the knee where *Yanglingquan* (GB 34), the most influential acupoint of sinews/tendons is located

膝髌 [xī bìn]
kneecap; patella: a thick flat movable bone situated at the front of the knee

膝腘 [xī guó]
post-patellar fossa: the popliteal fossa, same as 腘 [guó]

腘 [guó]
popliteal fossa: the depression in the posterior region of the knee

胫 [jìng]
shin: (1) the part of the lower limb between the knee and the ankle; (2) the anterior aspect of the leg; (3) abbreviation for shinbone (胫骨 [jìng gǔ])

胫骨 [jìng gǔ]
shinbone; tibia: the bone in the front of the leg

腓腨 [féi shuàn]
calf: the fleshy back part of the leg below the knee, also known as 腨 [shuàn]

腨 [shuàn]
calf: abbreviation for 腓腨 [féi shuàn]

内踝 [nèi huái]
internal malleolus; medial malleolus: the process of the tibia that projects on the medial side of its lower extremity at the ankle, also known as 合骨[hé gǔ]

合骨 [hé gǔ]
internal malleolus: another name for 内踝 [nèi huái]

外踝 [wài huái]
external malleolus; lateral malleolus: the expanded projection of the fibula on the lateral side of the leg at the ankle, also known as 核骨 [hé gǔ]

核骨 [hé gǔ]
external malleolus: another name for 外踝 [wài huái]

踵 [zhǒng]
heel: the back part of the human foot below the ankle and behind the arch

跖 [zhí]
metatarsus: the part of the human foot between the tarsus and phalanges

百骸 [bǎi hái]
skeleton: the bones collectively forming the framework supporting the human body

脊 [jǐ]
spine: the spinal column

颈骨 [jǐng gǔ]
neck bone: the cervical vertebra

柱骨 [zhù gǔ]
columnar bone: (1) the clavicle; (2) the cervical vertebra

腰骨 [yāo gǔ]
lumbar bone: collective term for the 3rd, 4th and 5th lumbar vertebrae

髋骨 [kuān gǔ]
(I) hipbone: the pelvic bone which is composed of the ilium, ischium, and pubis, also called 髁骨 [kē gǔ] or 胯骨 [kuà gǔ]; **(II) *Kuangu* (EX-LE 1):** the pair of acupoints located at 1.5 *cun* lateral and medial to *Liangqiu* (ST 34), symmetrically and on each thigh

髁骨 [kē gǔ]
hipbone: same as 髋骨 [kuān gǔ]

胯骨 [kuà gǔ]
hipbone: same as 髋骨 [kuān gǔ]

高骨 [gāo gǔ]
protruding bone: (1) the styloid process of the radius; (2) the lumbar vertebra

辅骨 [fǔ gǔ]
assisting bone: (1) the radius and fibula; (2) the condyle at the knee

髀 [bì]
thigh: the part of the leg from the hip to the knee

髀骨 [bì gǔ]
thighbone; femur: the proximal bone of the lower limb extending from the hip to the knee, also called 楗 [jiàn]

楗 [jiàn]
thighbone: another name for 髀骨 [bì gǔ]

髀枢 [bì shū]
trochanter: a rough prominence at the upper part of the femur

尾骶 [wěi dǐ]
sacrococcygeal region: the region of the back overlying the sacrum and coccyx

尾骶骨 [wěi dǐ gǔ]
sacrococcyx: the caudal extremity of the vertebral column formed by the union of the five fused vertebrae and the coccygeal bone

尾闾骨 [wěi lǘ gǔ]
coccyx: the small bone caudad to the sacrum

尻 [kāo]
sacral region: the region of the back overlying the sacrum

尻骨 [kāo gǔ]
sacrum: the part of the spinal column that forms the dorsal wall of the pelvis and consists of five fused vertebrae

骺骨 [héng gǔ]
shank bone: collective term for fibula and tibia

胫骨 [jìng gǔ]
shinbone; tibia: the inner and larger of the two bones of the leg between the knee and the ankle, also called 骭骨 [gàn gǔ]

骭骨 [gàn gǔ]
shinbone: same as 胫骨 [jìng gǔ]

外辅骨 [wài fǔ gǔ]
fibula: the outer of the two bones of the leg below the knee

足跗 [zú fū]
instep: the top part of the foot, abbreviated as 跗 [fū]

跗 [fū]
instep: abbreviation for 足跗 [zú fū]

跗骨 [fū gǔ]
metatarsal bones: the five bones extending from the tarsus to the phalanges of the toes

骨空 [gǔ kōng]
"bony space": anatomical term referring to (1) interosseous space; (2) bone marrow cavity; (3) articular cavity

骨解 [gǔ jiě]
joint: any part of the body where two bones meet

百节 [bǎi jié]
all joints: the joints of the body as a whole

十二节 [shí èr jié]
twelve joints: the joints of the shoulder, elbow and wrist on the upper limbs and those of the thigh, knee and ankle on the lower limbs, altogether twelve in number

大节 [dà jié]
large joints: (1) the large joints of the human skeleton; (2) the proximal joints of the fingers and toes

八溪 [bā xī]
eight transverse markings: the transverse markings across the skin surface formed at the elbow, wrist, knee and ankle joints

本节 [běn jié]
basic (digital) joints: the eminences of the metacarpophalangeal and metatarsophalangeal joints

虎口 [hǔ kǒu]
"tiger's mouth"; thumb web: the region between the thumb and the index finger, so called because it looks like the opening mouth of a tiger when the hand opens

赤白肉际 [chì bái ròu jì]
"border of the red and white flesh"; dorsoventral boundary (of the hand or foot): the boundary between the palm or sole (red in color) and the back of the hand or foot (white in color), respectively

丛毛 [cóng máo]
clustered hair: the hairs growing on the back of the proximal phalange of the big toe

气、血、精、津液
Qi, Blood, Essence, and Body Fluids

气 [qì]

***qi*:** the basic element that constitutes the cosmos and which through its movements, changes and transformations, produces everything in the world, including the human body and life activities. In the field of medicine, *qi* in its physiological sense is referred to as the basic element or energy which makes up the human body and supports its vital activities, such as 水谷之气 [shuǐ gǔ zhī qì], *qi* of food and drink, i.e., the nutrient or the nutritive action, and 呼吸之气 [hū xī zhī qì], *qi* of respiration, i.e., the breathed air. Since *qi* is invisible and its existence in the human body can only be perceived through its resultant activities as expressed through organs and tissues, it is more frequently used in the sense of functional activities, such as 脏腑之气 [zàng fǔ zhī qì], *qi* of the *zang-fu* organs, i.e., the physical substrata and dynamic force of the functional activities of the *zang-fu* organs, or simply the functional activities of the *zang-fu* organs. The term *qi* can also be used in a pathological sense, e.g., 邪气 [xié qì], pathogenic *qi* which means pathogenic factor or pathogen.

水谷之气 [shuǐ gǔ zhī qì]

***qi* of water and grain; *qi* of food and drink:** the essential substance and energy derived from food and drink

谷气 [gǔ qì]

food *qi*: abbreviation for *qi* of food and drink (水谷之气 [shuǐ gǔ zhī qì])

水谷 [shuǐ gǔ]

water and grain; food and drink: the diet

大气 [dà qì]

air: the earth's atmosphere, especially that which is breathed

呼吸之气 [hū xī zhī qì]

breathed air: air inhaled and exhaled through respiration

先天之气 [xiān tiān zhī qì]

innate *qi*; prenatal *qi*: the *qi* that exists in a person from birth and is stored in the kidney

后天之气 [hòu tiān zhī qì]

acquired *qi*; postnatal *qi*: the *qi* that is acquired after birth and formed from food *qi* obtained in the spleen and stomach in combination with the fresh air (oxygen) inhaled into the lung

元气 [yuán qì]

original *qi*: the *qi* derived from the innate essence and supplemented by acquired *qi*, acting as the primary dynamic force for life activities, also called 原气 [yuán qì]

原气 [yuán qì]

original *qi*: same as 元气 [yuán qì]

真气 [zhēn qì]

genuine *qi*: combination of innate *qi* and

acquired *qi*, serving as the dynamic force of all vital functions

正气 [zhèng qì]
(I) healthy *qi*: collective term for the physical substrata and dynamic forces of all normal functions of the human body, including such health-sustaining abilities as adaptation to the environments, resistance against pathogens, and self-recovery from illnesses; **(II) normal weather**

宗气 [zōng qì]
pectoral *qi*; ancestral *qi*: combination of essential *qi* derived from food with the inhaled air, stored in the chest, serving as the dynamic force for blood circulation, respiration, voice, and body movements

营气 [yíng qì]
nutrient *qi*: the *qi* that moves within the vessels and nourishes all the organs and tissues

营阴 [yíng yīn]
nutrient yin: another name for nutrient *qi*, as the *qi* that moves inside the vessels pertains to yin while that which moves outside the vessels pertains to yang

卫气 [wèi qì]
defense *qi*: the *qi* that moves outside the vessels, protecting the body surface and warding off exogenous pathogens

卫阳 [wèi yáng]
defense yang: another name for defense *qi*, as the *qi* that moves outside the vessels pertains to yang while that which moves inside the vessels pertains to yin

津气 [jīn qì]
(I) fluid *qi*: synonym for 津 [jīn], i.e., fluid; **(II) fluid-*qi*:** collective term for body fluid and yang *qi*

精气 [jīng qì]
essential *qi*: the *qi* of the essence, from which life originates and by which life is maintained, including the *qi* derived from reproductive essence, food essence, and essence of the *zang-fu* organs

肾间动气 [shèn jiān dòng qì]
motive *qi* between the kidneys: the part of the genuine *qi* stored between the kidneys as the motive force necessary for the activities of the *zang-fu* organs and meridian/channel system

脏气 [zàng qì]
***zang*-organ *qi*:** the physical substrata and dynamic forces of the functional activities of a *zang* organ

腑气 [fǔ qì]
***fu*-organ *qi*:** the physical substrata and dynamic forces of the functional activities of a *fu* organ

心气 [xīn qì]
heart *qi*: the physical substrata and dynamic forces of the functional activities of the heart

肝气 [gān qì]
liver *qi*: (1) the physical substrata and dynamic forces of the functional activities of the liver; (2) abbreviation for liver *qi* depression (肝气郁结 [gān qì yù jié])

脾气 [pí qì]
spleen *qi*: the physical substrata and

dynamic forces of the functional activities of the spleen

肺气 [fèi qì]
lung *qi*: (1) the physical substrata and dynamic forces of the functional activities of the lung; (2) the breathed air

肾气 [shèn qì]
kidney *qi*: the physical substrata and dynamic forces of the functional activities of the kidney

胆气 [dǎn qì]
gallbladder *qi*: the physical substrata and dynamic forces of the functional activities of the gallbladder

胃气 [wèi qì]
stomach *qi*: (1) the physical substrata and dynamic forces of the functional activities of the stomach; (2) the reflection of basic vitality detected by examination of the radial pulse

清气 [qīng qì]
clear *qi*: (1) fresh air, usually referring to the air inspired into the lung, especially oxygen; (2) the clarified thin part of food essence, i.e., the nutrient; (3) to clear up the *qi* aspect, a method of treating febrile disease with heat in the *qi* aspect

浊气 [zhuó qì]
turbid *qi*: (1) the dense part of food essence; (2) waste gas, e.g., air expired or flatus discharged

阳气 [yáng qì]
yang *qi*: the yang aspect of *qi*, often referring to functional activities in opposition to yin *qi* as physical substrata

阴气 [yīn qì]
yin *qi*: the yin aspect of *qi*, often referring to physical substrata in opposition to yang *qi* as functional activities

清阳 [qīng yáng]
clear yang: light and clear yang *qi* that usually exists in the upper or exterior part of the body, including the fresh air inhaled and the superficial resistance

经络之气 [jīng luò zhī qì]
meridian/channel *qi*: the *qi* that flows through the meridians/channels

经气 [jīng qì]
meridian/channel *qi*: abbreviation for 经络之气 [jīng luò zhī qì]

卫气营血 [wèi qì yíng xuè]
defense, *qi*, nutrient and blood: four aspects denoting the four portions or strata of the body from the superficial to the deep, to show the location, seriousness, stage or phase of an acute febrile disease as a guide to diagnosis

卫分 [wèi fèn]
defense aspect: the most superficial stratum of the body apt to be invaded at the initial stage of an acute febrile disease, often abbreviated as 卫 [wèi]

卫 [wèi]
defense: (1) abbreviation for defense aspect (卫分 [wèi fèn]); (2) abbreviation for defense *qi* (卫气 [wèi qì])

气分 [qì fèn]
***qi* aspect:** the second stratum of the body deeper than the superficial defense aspect, often referring to the lung, gallbladder, spleen, stomach and large intestine

营分 [yíng fèn]
nutrient aspect: the stratum of the body between the *qi* and blood aspects, often abbreviated as 营 [yíng]

营 [yíng]
nutrient: (1) abbreviation for the nutrient aspect (营分 [yíng fèn]); (2) abbreviation for nutrient *qi* (营气 [yíng qì]) or nutritive yin (营阴 [yíng yīn])

血分 [xuè fèn]
blood aspect: the deepest stratum of the body involved in the severest stage of an acute febrile disease, often abbreviated as 血 [xuè]

气机 [qì jī]
***qi* movement; *qi* activity:** the constant movement of *qi* (ascending, descending, exiting and entering as its basic forms) that promotes and facilitates various physiological activities, maintaining life

气化 [qì huà]
***qi* transformation:** a general term referring to various transforming changes through the activity of *qi*, namely the metabolism of essence, *qi*, blood and fluids, as well as their mutual transformations. In other words, *qi* transformation corresponds to metabolism, substance transformation and energy transformation.

中气 [zhōng qì]
middle *qi*: abbreviation for *qi* of the middle energizer, i.e., *qi* of the spleen and stomach

血 [xuè]
blood: the red fluid circulating through the blood vessels and nourishing the body tissues

精血 [jīng xuè]
essence-blood: combined term indicating both the essence and blood owing to their kinship, and often representing all the nourishing substances necessary for maintaining human life

营血 [yíng xuè]
(I) nutrient-blood: (1) collective term for nutrient and blood; (2) the later stage of an acute febrile disease involving both the nutrient and blood aspects; **(II) nutrient blood:** synonym for blood as blood furnishes nourishment

血脉 [xuè mài]
blood vessel: the vessel in which blood circulates

血气 [xuè qì]
blood *qi*: the *qi* of blood, referring to the functions of blood

精 [jīng]
(I) essence: the fundamental substance that builds up the physical structure and maintains the body functions; **(II) semen:** the whitish liquid containing sperm, also known as reproductive essence 生殖之精 [shēng zhí zhī jīng]

水谷之精 [shuǐ gǔ zhī jīng]

food essence: the essential substance derived from food, which is required for the maintenance of life activities and the metabolism of the human body, also known as 水谷精微 [shuǐ gǔ jīng wēi]

水谷精微 [shuǐ gǔ jīng wēi]

food essence: same as 水谷之精 [shuǐ gǔ zhī jīng]

精微 [jīng wēi]

refined essence: a figurative term usually referring to the refined nutritious substances derived from foodstuffs through digestion

先天之精 [xiān tiān zhī jīng]

innate essence: the original substance which is responsible for construction of the body and generation of offspring, often referring to the reproductive essence (生殖之精 [shēng zhí zhī jīng])

后天之精 [hòu tiān zhī jīng]

acquired essence: the essential substance derived from food after digestion and absorption, to maintain the body functions and replenish the physical construction

生殖之精 [shēng zhí zhī jīng]

reproductive essence: the fundamental substance for reproduction, referring to semen and ovum

肾精 [shèn jīng]

kidney essence: the original essence stored in the kidney, including the reproductive essence

浊阴 [zhuó yīn]

turbid yin: heavy and turbid matter in the body, chiefly referring to the urine and feces, also to the concentrated and turbid part of food essence

精汁 [jīng zhī]

refined juice: the juice contained in the gallbladder, referring to bile

神 [shén]

(I) mind: condition of one's mental faculties, including consciousness, attention, and thinking; **(II) spirit:** condition of one's spiritual activities, including mind, feelings and character; **(III) vitality:** liveliness or vigor, the manifestation of vital functioning

形体 [xíng tǐ]

configuration and constitution; physique: the general appearance and condition of a person's body

形 [xíng]

physique: abbreviation for 形体 [xíng tǐ]

精神 [jīng shén]

spirit: the state of mind, mood or feelings

魂 [hún]

ethereal soul: the moral and spiritual part of a human being

魄 [pò]

corporeal soul: the animating part of the mind

意 [yì]

thought: act or power of thinking and forming ideas

志 [zhì]

(I) will: mental power by which a person can direct thoughts and actions; **(II) emotion:** a strong feeling such as fear or anger; **(III) mind:** thinking process including remembering

津 [jīn]

(I) (thin) fluid: the fluid that circulates with *qi* and blood. It is mainly distributed over the exterior part of the body, and can be secreted as tears, saliva, sweat, etc.; **(II) saliva:** the fluid that is secreted into the mouth

液 [yè]

(thick) liquid: the fluid that does not circulate together with *qi* and blood, but is stored in body cavities such as the articular and cranial cavities

津液 [jīn yè]

body fluids: a general term for all kinds of fluids required by the normal functioning of the body, including secretions such as saliva, tears, and sweat

阴液 [yīn yè]

yin liquid: nutrient fluid in the body, especially that of or for the internal organs

清浊 [qīng zhuó]

clarity and turbidity: a term that often refers to the essence and the waste of digested food

五液 [wǔ yè]

five kinds of liquid: collective term for sweat, tears, snivel, slobber and spittle

五脏化液 [wǔ zàng huà yè]

secretion from the five *zang* organs: sweat derived from the heart, tears from the liver, saliva from the spleen, snivel from the lung, and spittle from the kidney

汗 [hàn]

sweat: the liquid on the skin discharged from the pores

泪 [lèi]

tears: one of the five kinds of liquid, which cleanses and moistens the eyeballs, and excessive discharge of which, if not during weeping, is often related to the function of the liver

涎 [xián]

drool; (thin) saliva: a part of liquid produced in the mouth that helps one chew and digest, one of the five kinds of fluid associated with the function of the spleen

涕 [tì]

snivel: the liquid that exudates from the nose

唾 [tuò]

spittle; (thick) saliva: a part of liquid produced in the mouth, one of the five kinds of fluid associated with the function of the kidney

常用引文 Commonly Used Citations

泪为肝液。

[lèi wéi gān yè]

Tears are the fluid of the liver. It is so said because tears come from the eyes, which reflect the condition of the liver as its specific opening. Lack of tears with dry eyes is a common symptom indicating deficiency of essence and blood in the liver.

汗为心液。

[hàn wéi xīn yè]

Sweat is the fluid of the heart. It is so said because sweat comes from the blood, and the heart controls the blood. Clinically, spontaneous sweating is commonly seen when heart yang is insufficient, while night sweating usually suggests heart yin deficiency.

涎为脾液。

[xián wéi pí yè]

Drool is the fluid of the spleen. It is so said because the spleen has its specific body opening in the mouth. Clinically, a dry mouth is frequently seen in cases of inadequacy of fluid in the spleen and stomach, and dysfunction of the spleen in sending up fluid.

涕为肺液。

[tì wéi fèi yè]

Snivel is the fluid of the lung. It is so said because the nose is the specific body opening of the lung. Clinically, a dry nose is usually due to heat or dryness in the lung, while patients with impeded function of the lung often have a runny nose.

唾为肾液。

[tuò wéi shèn yè]

Spittle is the fluid of the kidney. It is so said because the kidney meridian/channel runs through the sublingual area. Clinically, excessive spittle can be cured by using kidney tonics.

血汗同源。

[xuè hàn tóng yuán]

Blood and sweat share a common source. It is so said because sweat comes from the blood.

精血同源。

[jīng xuè tóng yuán]

Essence and blood share a common source: Both essence and blood constitute the material basis of the human body; blood comes from innate essence and is nourished by acquired food essence.

津血同源。

[jīn xuè tóng yuán]

Body fluids and blood share a common source: Both body fluids and blood are derived from drink and food, and they are associated with each other physiologically and pathologically.

气为血帅。

[qì wéi xuè shuài]

***Qi* is the commander of blood.** It is so

said because *qi* provides the dynamic force of blood flow, maintains blood circulation within the vessels, and promotes blood regeneration; on the other hand, *qi* stagnation is apt to cause blood stasis, and *qi* deficiency may lead to chronic bleeding or blood deficiency.

血为气母。

[xuè wéi qì mǔ]

Blood is the mother of *qi*. It is so said because blood is the material basis of *qi*; deficiency of blood usually leads to deficiency of *qi*, and massive loss of blood may cause prostration of *qi* as manifested by collapse.

气行血行。

[qì xíng xuè xíng]

When *qi* moves, blood circulates.

卫气者，所以温分肉，充皮肤，肥腠理，司开合者也。

[wèi qì zhě, suǒ yǐ wēn fēn ròu, chōng pí fū, féi còu lǐ, sī kāi hé zhě yě]

Defense *qi* warms the flesh, flushes the skin, replenishes the interstices and controls the opening and closing of the pores.

宗气积于胸中，出于喉咙，以贯心脉，而行呼吸。

[zōng qì jī yú xiōng zhōng, chū yú hóu lóng, yǐ guàn xīn mài, ér xíng hū xī]

Accumulating in the chest and issuing from the throat, pectoral *qi* runs through the heart and vessels and conducts respiration.

营气者，泌其津液，注之于脉，化以为血，以荣四末，内注五脏六腑。

[yíng qì zhě, mì qí jīn yè, zhù zhī yú mài, huà yǐ wéi xuè, yǐ róng sì mò, nèi zhù wǔ zàng liù fǔ]

Nutrient *qi* secretes fluid, pours it into the vessels and transforms it into blood so that the limbs and the *zang-fu* organs are nourished.

夫精者，身之本也。

[fū jīng zhě, shēn zhī běn yě]

Essence is the foundation of the body.

生之来谓之精，两精相搏谓之神。

[shēng zhī lái wèi zhī jīng, liǎng jīng xiāng bó wèi zhī shén]

What enables the generation of a human being is called essence; what the combination of yin and yang essence brings about is called spirit (life activity).

随神往来谓之魂。

[suí shén wǎng lái wèi zhī hún]

The function of consciousness that comes and goes with the spiritual activities is called soul.

并精出入者谓之魄。

[bìng jīng chū rù zhě wèi zhī pò]

The instinctive faculty attached to the configurations is called corporeal soul.

心有所忆谓之意。

[xīn yǒu suǒ yì wèi zhī yì]

The reflection in the heart (mind) is called idea.

意之所存谓之志。

[yì zhī suǒ cún wèi zhī zhì]

Persistent idea is called will.

因志而存变谓之思。

[yīn zhì ér cún biàn wèi zhī sī]

Study of change according to will is called thinking.

因思而远慕谓之虑。

[yīn sī ér yuǎn mù wèi zhī lǜ]

Careful thinking for long-term planning is called consideration.

因虑而处物谓之智。

[yīn lǜ ér chǔ wù wèi zhī zhì]

Proper management of different things after consideration is called wisdom.

恬淡虚无，真气从之，精神内守，病安从来。

[tián dàn xū wú, zhēn qì cóng zhī, jīng shén nèi shǒu, bìng ān cóng lái]

If one has a tranquil mind content in nothingness, in the wake of which genuine *qi* will come and keep the spirit strong internally, how can any illness occur?

病因 Cause of Disease

病因 [bìng yīn]
cause of disease: that which produces disease

三因 [sān yīn]
three categories of disease cause: external cause, internal cause, and cause neither internal nor external – an ancient classification of causes of disease

外因 [wài yīn]
exogenous cause; external cause: cause of disease that originates outside the body, referring chiefly to the six excessive and untimely climatic influences and pestilential pathogens

内因 [nèi yīn]
endogenous cause; internal cause: cause of disease that arises within the body, referring chiefly to excessive emotional changes

不内外因 [bù nèi wài yīn]
non-exo-endogenous cause; cause neither internal nor external: etiological factors other than the exogenous and endogenous, referring chiefly to such factors as improper diet, overwork, trauma, sexual overindulgence, animal bite, etc.

邪气 [xié qì]
pathogenic *qi*; pathogen: an agent that is harmful to the body and capable of causing disease

邪 [xié]
pathogen: abbreviation for pathogenic *qi* (邪气 [xié qì])

外邪 [wài xié]
external pathogen: any pathogenic factor that originates outside the body, including the six excesses and various infectious factors

客邪 [kè xié]
intruding pathogen: pathogenic factor from without, same as external pathogen (外邪 [wài xié])

时邪 [shí xié]
seasonal pathogen: general term for the pathogenic factors that cause seasonal diseases

外感 [wài gǎn]
external contraction: catching or developing a disease caused by any of the external pathogens

六气 [liù qì]
six *qi*: (1) the six vital substances for human life: essence, *qi*, nutrient, fluid, blood and vessel; (2) the six normal climatic phenomena: wind, cold, summerheat, dampness, dryness, and fire (heat)

六淫 [liù yín]
six excesses: (1) the six excessive or untimely climatic influences as external pathogenic factors: wind, cold, summerheat, dampness, dryness, and fire; (2) the six pathogenic factors: wind, cold, heat, dampness,

dryness, and fire either exogenous or endogenous

淫气 [yín qì]
excessive *qi*: excessive climatic influence or overabundance of yin or yang of the body which causes disease

四时不正之气 [sì shí bù zhèng zhī qì]
abnormal weather in the four seasons: that which disturbs the normal biorhythm of human beings, enhances the virulence of pathogens and often causes disease

疠气；戾气 [lì qì]
pestilential *qi*; epidemic pathogen: the pathogen that causes a virulent contagious or infectious disease affecting a large number of individuals at the same time, also called 疫疠之气 [yì lì zhī qì], 疫毒 [yì dú], 异气 [yì qì] , or 杂气 [zá qì]

疫疠之气 [yì lì zhī qì]
the full name of 疠气 [lì qì]

疫毒 [yì dú]
pestilential toxin; epidemic toxin: another name for epidemic pathogen (疠气[lì qì])

异气 [yì qì]
abnormal *qi*: another name for epidemic pathogen (疠气 [lì qì])

杂气 [zá qì]
impure *qi*: another name for epidemic pathogen (疠气 [lì qì])

时行戾气 [shí xíng lì qì]
seasonal epidemic pathogen: a pathogen that causes the epidemic of an infectious disease prevalent only in some particular season

恶气 [è qì]
malign *qi*: (1) a general term for pathogenic *qi*, including the six excesses and pestilential pathogens; (2) a pathological product derived from the stagnation of *qi* and blood

虚邪 [xū xié]
deficiency-exploiting pathogen: any pathogen that invades the human body when the latter's healthy *qi* is insufficient

贼风 [zéi fēng]
stealthy wind: wind as a pathogenic factor that invades an unprotected body

阴邪 [yīn xié]
yin pathogen: (1) pathogen of yin nature, i.e., cold and dampness, which tends to impede and injure yang; (2) pathogen that attacks the yin meridians/channels

阳邪 [yáng xié]
yang pathogen: (1) pathogen of yang nature, i.e., wind, summerheat, dryness or fire, which tends to take the form of heat and injures yin (body fluid and/or essence); (2) pathogen that attacks the yang meridians/channels

合邪 [hé xié]
combined pathogen: a combination of two or more pathogens invading the human body simultaneously

伏气 [fú qì]
latent *qi*: (1) latent pathogen, another name for 伏邪 [fú xié]; (2) abbreviation

for 伏气温病 [fú qì wēn bìng], i.e., a warm disease caused by a latent pathogen

伏邪 [fú xié]

latent pathogen: pathogen concealed in the body, which causes disease after an incubation period, also called latent *qi* (伏气 [fú qì])

风 [fēng]

wind: (1) one of the six excesses as a pathogenic factor characterized by rapid movements, swift changes, and ascending and opening actions, also called pathogenic wind (风邪 [fēng xié]); (2) abbreviation for wind syndrome/pattern (风证 [fēng zhèng])

风邪 [fēng xié]

pathogenic wind: full name of wind (风 [fēng]) as a pathogenic factor

风燥 [fēng zào]

wind-dryness: a combined pathogen of external wind and dryness, which usually prevails in autumn

风痰 [fēng tán]

wind-phlegm: (1) a combined pathogen of wind and phlegm; (2) a syndrome/pattern due to wind-phlegm, marked by vertigo, numbness, hemiplegia, and phlegmatic sounds in the throat

内风 [nèi fēng]

internal wind: (1) a morbid condition caused by excessive heat or deficiency of blood or essence in the liver and marked by dizziness, fainting, convulsions, tremor, numbness, hemiplegia, etc., also known as liver wind; (2) the pathogenetic factor that produces such a condition

外风 [wài fēng]

external wind: wind as one of the six excesses that causes external wind syndrome/pattern

寒 [hán]

cold: (1) one of the six excesses as a pathogenic factor characterized by damage to yang *qi*, deceleration of activities, and congealing and contracting actions, also called 寒邪 [hán xié]; (2) abbreviation for cold syndrome/pattern (寒证 [hán zhèng]), usually marked by intolerance of cold, cold limbs, preference for warmth, loose stools, and pale tongue with whitish coating

寒邪 [hán xié]

pathogenic cold: full name of cold (寒 [hán]) as a pathogenic factor

外寒 [wài hán]

external cold: (1) cold pathogen from outside in an external contraction; (2) outer manifestation of yang *qi* insufficiency, such as cold limbs and intolerance of cold

内寒 [nèi hán]

internal cold: (1) a morbid condition caused by yang *qi* insufficiency of the *zang-fu* organs, especially of the kidney and spleen, marked by watery diarrhea, abdominal pain, cold limbs, intolerance of cold, and slow and sunken pulse; (2) the pathogenetic factor that produces such a condition

中寒 [zhòng hán]

cold stroke: attack of cold directly to

the stomach and intestines, marked by abdominal pain, borborygmi, and diarrhea, accompanied by chills or cold limbs

暑 [shǔ]

summerheat: one of the six excesses as a pathogenic factor, which exists only in summer and brings on symptoms such as fever, headache, thirst, fidgetiness, sweating, and rapid gigantic pulse, also called summerheat *qi* (暑气 [shǔ qì]) or pathogenic summerheat (暑邪 [shǔ xié])

暑气 [shǔ qì]

summerheat *qi*: summerheat as a pathogenic factor or pathogenic summerheat, often abbreviated as summerheat (暑 [shǔ])

暑邪 [shǔ xié]

pathogenic summerheat: summerheat as a pathogenic factor, often abbreviated as summerheat (暑 [shǔ])

暑热 [shǔ rè]

summerheat: (1) same as 暑邪 [shǔ xié]; (2) heat syndrome/pattern due to the invasion of pathogenic summerheat

暑湿 [shǔ shī]

summerheat-dampness: (1) a combined pathogenic factor in summer causing fever with stuffiness sensation in the chest and epigastrium, and yellow greasy tongue coating; (2) disease caused by summerheat and dampness

湿 [shī]

dampness: (1) one of the six excesses as a pathogenic factor, which is apt to disturb the flow of *qi* and the normal functioning of the spleen and stomach, also called dampness *qi* (湿气 [shī qì]); (2) pathological product due to disordered water metabolism, which may in turn become a pathogenic factor, also called internal dampness (内湿 [nèi shī])

湿气 [shī qì]

dampness (*qi*): (1) dampness as a pathogenic factor; (2) disease caused by dampness

湿浊 [shī zhuó]

dampness turbidity: synonym for dampness *qi* (湿气 [shī qì]), so named because of the turbid and sticky property of pathogenic dampness

湿邪 [shī xié]

pathogenic dampness: dampness as a pathogenic factor, often abbreviated as dampness (湿 [shī])

外湿 [wài shī]

external dampness: a pathogenic factor that attacks a person living and working in damp places, bringing on symptoms such as headache as if the head were tightly bound, lassitude, heaviness in the limbs, fullness in the chest, joint pains and swelling with a heavy sensation

内湿 [nèi shī]

internal dampness: (1) retention of water within the body caused by deficiency of spleen and kidney yang with disturbance in the water metabolism and distribution, manifested by loss of appetite, diarrhea, abdominal distension, oliguria and edema; (2) the pathological product due to disordered water metabolism, which turns to be a pathogenic factor affecting the functions of the *zang-fu* organs, particularly the spleen and stomach

中湿 [zhòng shī]
dampness stroke: (1) a pathological change attributed to dampness attack, either from without or from within; (2) a type of apoplexy due to contraction of dampness, marked by sudden attack of vertigo or loss of consciousness along with phlegmatic sounds in the throat, also called phlegm stroke (痰中 [tán zhòng])

水气 [shuǐ qì]
water *qi*; pathogenic water: (1) pathogenetic factor derived from water retention in a case of kidney insufficiency, causing edema; (2) edema

燥 [zào]
dryness: (1) one of the six pathogenic factors, which prevails in autumn and impairs body fluids, bringing on dryness of the nasal cavity, parched lips, dry cough, and constipation, also called dryness *qi* (燥气 [zào qì]); (2) abbreviation for dryness syndrome/pattern (燥证 [zào zhèng])

燥气 [zào qì]
dryness *qi*: dryness as a pathogenic factor or pathogenic dryness

燥邪 [zào xié]
pathogenic dryness: dryness as a pathogenic factor

凉燥 [liáng zào]
cool dryness: (1) disease marked by a syndrome/pattern of wind-cold together with dryness; (2) pathogenic factor that causes such a disease

温燥 [wēn zào]
warm dryness: (1) disease marked by a syndrome/pattern of wind-heat together with dryness; (2) pathogenic factor that causes such a disease

燥热 [zào rè]
dryness-heat: pathogenic heat transformed from dryness

燥火 [zào huǒ]
dryness-fire: pathogenic fire transformed from dryness

外燥 [wài zào]
external dryness: climatic influence as a pathogenic factor that causes external dryness syndrome/pattern

内燥 [nèi zào]
internal dryness: dryness in the interior due to consumption of body fluids

火 [huǒ]
fire: (1) one of the five elements; (2) physiological energy of life; (3) one of the six excesses as a pathogenic factor characterized by intense heat that is apt to damage fluid, consume *qi*, engender wind, induce bleeding, and disturb mental activities, also called pathogenic fire (火邪 [huǒ xié]); (4) pathological manifestation of intense heat such as flushed face, bloodshot eyes, acute local inflammation

火邪 [huǒ xié]
pathogenic fire: fire as a pathogenic factor

热 [rè]
heat: (1) one of the six excesses as a pathogenic factor of the same property as

fire, also called pathogenic heat (热邪 [rè xié]); (2) abbreviation for heat syndrome/pattern (热证 [rè zhèng]), usually marked by fever, aversion to heat, thirst with desire for cold drinks, scanty concentrated urine, constipation, reddened tongue with yellow coating, and rapid pulse

热邪 [rè xié]
pathogenic heat; heat pathogen: heat as a pathogenic factor

温热 [wēn rè]
(I) warmth-heat: pathogenic factor causing febrile diseases, same as pathogenic warmth (温邪 [wēn xié]) and pathogenic heat (热邪 [rè xié]). In the strict sense, pathogenic warmth attacks insidiously, causes milder diseases, and prevails in winter and spring, while pathogenic heat causes severe diseases with sudden onset and prevails in summer. **(II) warmth-heat disease:** any externally contracted febrile disease, same as warm disease (温病 [wēn bìng])

温邪 [wēn xié]
pathogenic warmth; warmth pathogen: collective term for various pathogens causing externally contracted acute febrile diseases

风温 [fēng wēn]
wind-warmth: (1) combined pathogenic factor of external wind and warmth, also called 风温邪气 [fēng wēn xié qì]; (2) disease caused by wind-warmth pathogen

风温邪气 [fēng wēn xié qì]
pathogenic wind-warmth; wind-warmth pathogen: full name of wind-warmth (风温 [fēng wēn]) as a pathogenic factor

风寒 [fēng hán]
wind-cold: (1) combined pathogenic factor of external wind and cold, also called pathogenic wind-cold (风寒邪气 [fēng hán xié qì]), which causes marked chilliness with mild fever, headache, general aching, nasal congestion and discharge, and floating, tense pulse when invading the exterior of the body; (2) abbreviation for wind-cold syndrome/pattern (风寒证 [fēng hán zhèng]), i.e., syndrome/pattern caused by attack of wind and cold in combination

风寒邪气 [fēng hán xié qì]
pathogenic wind-cold; wind-cold pathogen: full name of wind-cold (风寒 [fēng hán]) as a pathogenic factor

风热 [fēng rè]
wind-heat: (1) combined pathogenic factor of external wind and heat, also called pathogenic wind-heat (风热邪气 [fēng rè xié qì]), which causes high fever with slight aversion to wind, mild thirst, and floating, rapid pulse when invading the exterior of the body; (2) abbreviation of wind-heat syndrome/pattern (风热证 [fēng rè zhèng]), i.e., syndrome/pattern caused by attack of external wind and heat in combination

风热邪气 [fēng rè xié qì]
pathogenic wind-heat; wind-heat pathogen: full name of wind-heat (风热 [fēng rè]) as a pathogenic factor

风火 [fēng huǒ]
wind-fire: combined pathogenic factor of wind and fire

风湿 [fēng shī]

wind-dampness: (1) combined pathogenic factor of wind and dampness, also called pathogenic wind-dampness (风湿邪气 [fēng shī xié qì]), which often blocks the collateral meridians/channels, causing general aching, arthralgia and impaired movements; (2) abbreviation for wind-dampness syndrome/pattern (风湿证 [fēng shī zhèng]), i.e., syndrome/pattern caused by attack of wind and dampness in combination

风湿邪气 [fēng shī xié qì]

pathogenic wind-dampness; wind-dampness pathogen, see wind-dampness (风湿 [fēng shī])

风寒湿 [fēng hán shī]

wind-cold-dampness: combined pathogenic factor of wind, cold and dampness, which often causes rheumatic and rheumatoid arthritis, also called pathogenic wind-cold-dampness (风寒湿邪 [fēng hán shī xié])

风寒湿邪 [fēng hán shī xié]

pathogenic wind-cold-dampness: full name of wind-cold-dampness (风寒湿 [fēng hán shī]) as a pathogenic factor

寒湿 [hán shī]

cold-dampness: (1) combined pathogenic factor of cold and dampness; (2) abbreviation of cold-dampness syndrome/pattern (寒湿证 [hán shī zhèng])

湿热 [shī rè]

dampness-heat: (1) combined pathogenic factor of dampness and heat; (2) abbreviation of dampness-heat disease (湿热病 [shī rè bìng]) or dampnessheat syndrome/pattern (湿热证 [shī rè zhèng])

湿火 [shī huǒ]

dampness-fire: fire that comes from stagnant dampness and impairs spleen and stomach yin

风燥 [fēng zào]

wind-dryness: (1) combined pathogenic factor of external wind and dryness, generally prevailing in autumn; (2) abbreviation for wind-dryness syndrome/pattern 风燥证 [fēng zào zhèng]

燥热 [zào rè]

dryness-heat: (1) combined pathogenic factor of dryness and heat, also called dryness-fire (燥火 [zào huǒ]); (2) abbreviation of dryness-heat syndrome/pattern (燥热证 [zào rè zhèng])

燥火 [zào huǒ]

dryness-fire: (1) combined pathogenic factor of dryness and fire; (2) abbreviation for dryness-fire syndrome/pattern (燥火证 [zào huǒ zhèng])

毒 [dú]

(I) toxin: any virulent pathogen that causes a fulminating disease; **(II) poison:** substance that kills or harms an organism

热毒 [rè dú]

heat toxin: a virulent pathogen derived from retained pathogenic heat

火毒 [huǒ dú]

fire toxin: (1) toxin that originates from stagnation of pathogenic fire or heat, mostly occurring in inflammations of external diseases; (2) toxin that causes infection of burns

湿毒 [shī dú]
dampness toxin: toxin that comes from retained dampness and causes an intractable lesion with abundant exudation

寒毒 [hán dú]
cold toxin: pathogen of cold-induced diseases

麻毒 [má dú]
measles toxin: the pathogen that causes measles

内毒 [nèi dú]
endogenous toxin: toxin arising inside the body, which may cause abscess, eruption, bleeding, and even impairment of consciousness

胎毒 [tāi dú]
fetal toxin: toxin that affects the fetus and causes a variety of inflammatory or eruptive diseases of the infant after birth

蛊毒 [gǔ dú]
parasitic toxin: the pathogenic factor derived from parasitic infestation, which causes diseases marked by abdominal lumps, tympanites and ascites

内伤 [nèi shāng]
(I) endogenous damage: a general term for pathogenic factors such as emotions, overstrain, and dietary irregularities that impair the internal organs; **(II) internal injury:** a term designating injury to the deep tissue or internal organs

七情 [qī qíng]
seven emotions: joy, anger, anxiety, thought (or pensiveness), sorrow, fear and fright taken as endogenous factors causing disease if in excess

五志 [wǔ zhì]
five emotions; five minds: collective term for joy, anger, thought (or pensiveness), sorrow and fear, which may turn into fire if in excess

喜 [xǐ]
joy: one of the seven emotions that in excess may make the heart *qi* sluggish, resulting in absent-mindedness, palpitations, insomnia and even mental disturbance

怒 [nù]
anger: one of the seven emotions that in excess may cause liver *qi* to ascend, resulting in headache, flushed face, bloodshot eyes, or hematemesis, and even sudden fainting

忧 [yōu]
anxiety: one of the seven emotions that in excess may cause injury to the lung, and in combination with pensivenss may injure the spleen

思 [sī]
thought; pensiveness: one of the seven emotions that in excess may cause stagnation of spleen *qi*, resulting in anorexia, abdominal distension, and loose stools

悲 [bēi]
sorrow: one of the seven emotions that in excess may consume lung *qi*, resulting in shortness of breath, listlessness and fatigue

恐 [kǒng]
fear: one of the seven emotions that in excess may cause kidney *qi* to sink, resulting in incontinence of urine and stool, or even syncope

惊 [jīng]
fright: one of the seven emotions that in excess may disturb heart *qi*, resulting in palpitations or mental confusion

五志过极 [wǔ zhì guò jí]
five emotions/minds in excess: excessive joy, anger, thought, sorrow and fear, which may disturb the normal flow of *qi* and blood of the internal organs

五志化火 [wǔ zhì huà huǒ]
transformation of the five emotions/minds into fire: Uncontrolled overflow of the five emotions (joy, anger, thought, sorrow and fear) may disturb the natural flow of *qi* and injure genuine yin, giving rise to fire symptoms, such as irritability, insomnia, bitterness in the mouth, chest pain, and hemoptysis.

邪火 [xié huǒ]
morbid fire: pathogenic or pathological fire, as opposed to physiological fire

郁火 [yù huǒ]
stagnant fire: fire derived from stagnancy of yang *qi*

六郁 [liù yù]
six stagnations: collective term for stagnation of *qi* , blood, dampness, fire, phlegm and food

饮食劳倦 [yǐn shí láo juàn]
improper diet and overstrain: a group of pathogenic factors that cause internal injuries, including dietary irregularities, abnormal degree of fatigue, etc.

饮食不节 [yǐn shí bù jié]
dietary irregularities: diet harmful to health, including ingestion of raw, cold or unclean food, voracious eating or excessive hunger, predilection for a special food, alcohol addiction, etc.

饮食不洁 [yǐn shí bù jié]
contaminated food: food contaminated by disease-carrying substances

贪食生冷 [tān shí shēng lěng]
overindulgence in raw and cold food: eating too much cold and uncooked food, which is apt to impair the function of the spleen and stomach

膏粱厚味 [gāo liáng hòu wèi]
rich and flavored food: food containing a large amount of fat and spices, which may produce phlegm and heat

五味偏嗜 [wǔ wèi piān shì]
flavor predilection: habitual preference for a particular flavor or taste that may give rise to disease, e.g., partiality for pungent food that induces oral ulceration, constipation and hemorrhoids

癖嗜 [pǐ shì]
addiction: habitual preference

酒癖 [jiǔ pǐ]
alcohol addiction: the state of heavy dependence on alcohol

劳倦 [láo juàn]
overstrain: abnormal degree of fatigue brought about by excessive exertion, one of the common causes of deficiency syndromes/patterns, also called 劳伤 [láo shāng]

劳伤 [láo shāng]
overstrain: same as 劳倦 [láo juàn]

房事过度 [fáng shì guò dù]
excess of sexual activity: excessive sexual intercourse that consumes the kidney essence

房事不节 [fáng shì bù jié]
intemperance in sexual life: synonymous with excess of sexual activity (房事过度 [fáng shì guò dù])

房劳 [fáng láo]
sexual consumption: exhaustion due to sexual overindulgence

劳复 [láo fù]
relapse due to overexertion: relapse of disease due to overexertion and fatigue

女劳复 [nǚ láo fù]
relapse due to sex: relapse of disease due to intemperance in sexual life

食复 [shí fù]
relapse due to diet: relapse of disease due to improper diet

跌打损伤 [diē dǎ sǔn shāng]
(injury from) knocks and falls: a wound or damage to some part of the body caused by a knock or fall

烫火伤 [tàng huǒ shāng]
scald and burn: an injury caused by fire or heat

虫兽伤 [chóng shòu shāng]
insect or animal bite: a wound made by an animal or insect

癫狗咬伤 [diān gǒu yǎo shāng]
rabid dog bite: a wound made by the bite of a rabid dog

瘀血 [yū xuè]
static blood: a pathological product of blood stasis, including extravasated blood, sluggish circulation or congested blood in a viscus, all of which may turn into pathogenic factors

痰 [tán]
phlegm: (1) pathologic secretions of the diseased respiratory organs, also called "visible phlegm" (有形之痰 [yǒu xíng zhī tán]) since it is visible when expectorated; (2) the turbid pathological product of a diseased visceral organ, especially the spleen, which, in turn, may cause various troubles, e.g., nausea and vomiting when the stomach is affected; palpitations, impairment of consciousness or even mania when the heart is invaded, and scrofula when accumulating subcutaneously, also known as "invisible phlegm" (无形之痰 [wú xíng zhī tán]) in these cases

有形之痰 [yǒu xíng zhī tán]
visible phlegm: phlegm in the respiratory tract, especially expectorated sputum

无形之痰 [wú xíng zhī tán]
invisible phlegm: phlegm that exists in

the body except for the respiratory tract

湿痰 [shī tán]

dampness-phlegm: phlegm as a pathogenic factor produced by long-standing retention of dampness due to deficiency of spleen *qi*, which brings on such symptoms as profuse frothy sputum, nausea, fullness in the chest, cough and dyspnea, and plump tongue with slippery or greasy coating, also called phlegm-dampness (痰湿 [tán shī])

痰湿 [tán shī]

phlegm-dampness: same as 湿痰 [shī tán]

痰浊 [tán zhuó]

phlegm turbidity: a term referring chiefly to stagnant phlegm, particularly phlegm that causes apoplexy, epilepsy or mania

顽痰 [wán tán]

obstinate phlegm: phlegm existing persistently and difficult to get rid of, serving as the cause of a stubborn illness

饮 [yǐn]

(I) retained fluid: the clear and watery product due to disordered fluid metabolism, which, in turn, serves as a pathogenic factor; **(II) fluid retention:** abbreviation for fluid retention syndrome (饮证 [yǐn zhèng]), a general term for various syndromes/patterns caused by retained fluid; **(III) cold decoction:** decoction to be taken cold

浊邪 [zhuó xié]

turbid pathogen: pathogenic dampness-turbidity or phlegm-turbidity, usually impeding the movement of yang *qi*

秽浊 [huì zhuó]

filthy turbidity: a common term for various turbid pathogens and filthy *qi* that cause diseases, including miasma

中毒 [zhòng dú]

poisoning: illness caused by poison

中恶 [zhòng è]

attack of noxious factor: a condition occurring in children, characterized by sudden onset of syncope or mental disorder

水土不服 [shuǐ tǔ bù fú]

non-acclimatization: illness due to failure to acclimatize to a new environment bringing on such symptoms as loss of appetite, abdominal distension, diarrhea, menstrual complaints (in women), etc.

诸虫 [zhū chóng]

parasitic worms: worms living in the human body, especially in the intestines

瘴气 [zhàng qì]

miasma: noxious vapor present in mountainous regions, alleged to be the cause of certain kinds of malaria, also known as miasmic toxin (瘴毒 [zhàng dú]) or mountain miasma (山岚瘴气 [shān lán zhàng qì])

瘴毒 [zhàng dú]

miasmic toxin: same as miasma (瘴气 [zhàng qì])

山岚瘴气 [shān lán zhàng qì]

mountain miasma: same as miasma (瘴气 [zhàng qì])

先天不足 [xiān tiān bù zú]
congenital defect: imperfection existing before birth

后天失调 [hòu tiān shī tiáo]
lack of proper postnatal care: lack of proper care after birth

体质学说 [tǐ zhì xué shuō]
constitution theory; theory of physical constitution: a theory that studies the formation, characteristics and categorization of human constitutions and their relationship with pathogenesis, diagnosis, prevention and treatment of diseases

体质 [tǐ zhì]
constitution: the physical makeup and functional features of the body, determined by inborn endowment and modified by acquired nurture

阴阳平和质 [yīn yáng píng hé zhì]
balanced yin-yang constitution: constitution with harmonious and balanced yin and yang, marked by robust physique full of vigor, easy-going personality, and sleek complexion with implicit expression

偏阴质 [piān yīn zhì]
yin-preponderant constitution: constitution with inhibited, weak, quiescent, gloomy and cold features, marked by plump physique inclined to tiredness, introversion, quiescence, immovability, and lusterless complexion

偏阳质 [piān yáng zhì]
yang-preponderant constitution: constitution with excited, strong, active and fervent features, marked by robust but slender physique full of vigor, extroversion, restlessness, irascibility and reddish complexion

木形之人 [mù xíng zhī rén]
wood-featured person: person characterized by bluish complexion, small head, long face, broad shoulders and back, straight body, small hands and feet, and intelligence, usually a mental worker with weak physical strength, tolerant of warmth but intolerant of cold, and hence subject to pathogenic attacks in autumn and winter

火形之人 [huǒ xíng zhī rén]
fire-featured person: person characterized by ruddy complexion, broad and revealing teeth, narrow forehead and small head, well developed shoulders, back, thighs and abdomen, small hands and feet, stable steps and swaying shoulders when walking, plump muscles over the shoulders and back, boldness of vision and generosity, inconsistency and suspiciousness, quick comprehension, dandyism, hastiness, short lifespan and susceptibility to sudden death, tolerant of the weather in spring and summer, but intolerant of the weather in autumn and winter, and hence subject to pathogenic attacks in the latter two seasons

土形之人 [tǔ xíng zhī rén]
earth-featured person: person characterized by sallow complexion, round face, large head, well developed shoulders and back, strong figure, stable steps, small hands and feet, mental calmness, tendency to help others, averse to power and influence, tolerant of the weather in autumn and winter, but intolerant of the weather in spring and summer, and hence

subject to pathogenic attacks in spring and autumn

金形之人 [jīn xíng zhī rén]

metal-featured person: person characterized by whitish complexion, square face, small head, small shoulders and back, strong heels, nimble limbs, short-temperedness, calmness when quiet and intrepid when active, tolerant of the weather in autumn and winter, and vulnerable to pathogenic attacks in spring and summer

水形之人 [shǔi xíng zhī rén]

water-featured person: person characterized by dark complexion, wrinkled face, large head, broad cheeks, small shoulders, big abdomen, swaying body when walking, long back with longer length from the waist to the sacral region, tolerant of the weather in autumn and winter, and vulnerable to pathogenic attacks in spring and summer

阴阳五态人 [yīn yáng wǔ tài rén]

five yin-yang dispositions: collective term for five categories of dispositions according to relative preponderance of yin or yang – *taiyin* (greater yin), *shaoyin* (lesser yin), *taiyang* (greater yang), *shaoyang* (lesser yang) and balanced yin-yang dispositions

太阴之人 [tài yīn zhī rén]

***taiyin* person; person of greater yin:** person who is greedy and unkind, fond of taking and averse to giving, poker-faced and slow in action in order to take advantage of others

少阴之人 [shào yīn zhī rén]

***shaoyin* person; person of lesser yin:** person who likes to covet small advantages and harbors vicious intentions, takes pleasure in another's misfortune, and jealous of another's success

太阳之人 [tài yáng zhī rén]

***taiyang* person; person of greater yang:** person who is usually self-satisfied and likes to boast, often aims too high, acts carelessly, and does not feel regret even when he has failed.

少阳之人 [shào yáng zhī rén]

***shaoyang* person; person of lesser yang:** person who is sociable, likes to exaggerate his reputation and ability, and tends to face upward when standing and shake the body when walking.

阴阳和平之人 [yīn yáng hé píng zhī rén]

balanced yin-yang person: person who lives in quietness with a peaceful and fearless mind in accordance with the law of Nature, doesn't care about fame and wealth, and remains modest even though exalted

病理体质 [bìng lǐ tǐ zhì]

pathological diathesis: constitutional disposition toward a particular abnormal state or condition of yin-yang disharmony or deficient *qi*-blood coordination

阳热质 [yáng rè zhì]

yang-heat diathesis: pathological diathesis with preponderance of yang heat, manifested by strong physique, flushed face and eyes, thirst with a desire for cold drinks, aversion to heat and liking for cold, short voiding of deep-colored urine, dry stools, reddened tongue with yellow coating, and rapid pulse

阴寒质 [yīn hán zhì]
yin-cold diathesis: pathological diathesis with preponderance of yin cold, manifested by plump physique, white complexion, aversion to cold and liking for warmth, lusterless complexion, lack of energy, constipated or loose stools, long voiding of clear urine, pale tongue, and slow sunken pulse

血瘀质 [xuè yū zhì]
blood stasis diathesis: pathological diathesis with the characteristics of blood stasis, manifested by cyanotic lips, blackish eye sockets, rough and scaly skin, purple tongue or purple spots on the tongue, and choppy pulse

痰湿质 [tán shī zhì]
phlegm-dampness diathesis: pathological diathesis with the characteristics of phlegm-dampness, manifested by obesity, heaviness of the body and feeling as if tightly bound, dry mouth with no desire for drink, greasy tongue coating, and slippery pulse

阴虚质 [yīn xū zhì]
yin deficiency diathesis: pathological diathesis with the characteristics of yin deficiency, manifested by slender physique, flushed cheeks, dry mouth and throat, vexing heat in the palms of the hands and soles of the feet, reddened tongue with scanty moisture, and rapid thready pulse

阳虚质 [yáng xū zhì]
yang deficiency diathesis: pathological diathesis with the characteristics of yang deficiency manifested by cold body and limbs, bright-pale complexion, listlessness, loose stools, long voiding of clear urine, pale tongue, and slow sunken pulse

气血两虚质 [qì xuè liǎng xū zhì]
***qi*-blood deficiency diathesis:** pathological diathesis with the characteristics of deficiency of both *qi* and blood, manifested by pale complexion, shortness of breath, lack of energy, palpitations, forgetfulness, pale lips, tongue and nails, and weak, thready and sunken pulse

肥膏肉人 [féi gāo ròu rén]
plump, fat and stout persons: Overweight persons can be classified into three groups, i.e., plump, fat and stout persons.

肥人 [féi rén]
plump person: an overweight person of small figure with thick skeletal muscles and rich subcutaneous fat, also called 脂人 [zhī rén]

脂人 [zhī rén]
plump person: same as 肥人 [féi rén]

膏人 [gāo rén]
fat person: an overweight person with loose skin and sagging bulging abdomen

肉人 [ròu rén]
stout person: an overweight and muscular person with a large physique

✦ 常用引文 Commonly Used Citations ✦

风善行而数变。
[fēng shàn xíng ér shuò biàn]
Wind moves swiftly and capriciously.

风胜则动。
[fēng shèng zé dòng]
When wind prevails, involuntary movements occur.

风为百病之长。
[fēng wéi bǎi bìng zhī zhǎng]
Wind is the primary cause of various diseases.

寒为阴邪，易伤阳气。
[hán wéi yīn xié, yì shāng yáng qì]
Cold, as a yin pathogen, is likely to damage yang *qi*.

寒性凝滞。
[hán xìng níng zhì]
Cold is characterized by congealing and stagnation.

寒性收引。
[hán xìng shōu yǐn]
Cold is characterized by contraction.

湿性重浊。
[shī xìng zhòng zhuó]
Dampness is characterized by heaviness and turbidity.

湿性黏滞。
[shī xìng nián zhì]
Dampness is characterized by stickiness and stagnation.

湿易伤阳。
[shī yì shāng yáng]
Dampness tends to damage yang.

湿胜则阳微。
[shī shèng zé yáng wēi]
When dampness prevails, yang is debilitated.

湿胜则濡泻。
[shī shèng zé rú xiè]
When dampness prevails, soggy diarrhea occurs.

燥胜则干。
[zào shèng zé gān]
When dryness prevails, desiccation occurs.

上燥则咳。
[shàng zào zé ké]
Dryness in the upper (part of the body) **leads to cough.**

中燥则渴。
[zhōng zào zé kě]
Dryness in the middle (part of the body) **leads to thirst.**

下燥则结。
[xià zào zé jié]
Dryness in the lower (part of the body) **leads to constipation.**

火性炎上。
[huǒ xìng yán shàng]
Fire is characterized by flaring up.

热胜则肿。
[rè shèng zé zhǒng]
When heat predominates, swelling occurs.

喜伤心。
[xǐ shāng xīn]
(Excessive) joy damages the heart.

喜则气缓。
[xǐ zé qì huǎn]
Joy makes (heart) *qi* relax. (or **Joy relaxes *qi*.**)

怒伤肝。
[nù shāng gān]
Anger damages the liver.

怒则气上。
[nù zé qì shàng]
Anger makes (liver) *qi* rise. (or **Anger raises *qi*.**)

忧伤肺。
[yōu shāng fèi]
Anxiety damages the lung.

忧则气郁。
[yōu zé qì yù]
Anxiety makes *qi* depressed. (or **Anxiety depresses *qi*.**)

悲则气消。
[bēi zé qì xiāo]
Sorrow makes (lung) *qi* disperse. (or **Sorrow disperses *qi*.**)

思伤脾。
[sī shāng pí]
Pensiveness damages the spleen.

思则气结。
[sī zé qì jié]
Pensiveness makes (spleen) *qi* stagnate. (or **Pensiveness stalls *qi*.**)

恐伤肾。
[kǒng shāng shèn]
Fear damages the kidney.

恐则气下。
[kǒng zé qì xià]
Fear makes *qi* descend. (or **Fear sinks *qi*.**)

惊则气乱。
[jīng zé qì luàn]
Fright makes *qi* disturbed. (or **Fright disturbs *qi*.**)

寒则气收。
[hán zé qì shōu]
Cold makes *qi* contract. (or **Cold contracts *qi*.**)

炅则气泄。
[jiǒng zé qì xiè]
Overheatedness makes *qi* dissipate. (or **Overheatedness dissipates *qi*.**)

劳则气耗。
[láo zé qì hào]
Strain makes *qi* decrease. (or **Strain consumes *qi*.**)

病机 Mechanism of Disease

病机 [bìng jī]
mechanism of disease; pathomechanism: the mechanism of the origination, development and outcome of a disease

病机十九条 [bìng jī shí jiǔ tiáo]
nineteen guiding rules of pathomechanism: the general rules of the origination and development of diseases as summarized in *The Yellow Emperor's Internal Classic*

病能 [态] [bìng tài]
pathological state of a disease: an ancient term referring comprehensively to clinical manifestations, cause and mechanism of a disease

正邪相争 [zhèng xié xiāng zhēng]
struggle between healthy and pathogenic *qi*: fundamental view of mechanism of disease that any disease is a process of struggle between healthy *qi* and pathogenic *qi*, also known as 正邪分争 [zhèng xié fēn zhēng]

正邪分争 [zhèng xié fēn zhēng]
struggle between healthy and pathogenic *qi*: same as 正邪相争 [zhèng xié xiāng zhēng]

邪正盛衰 [xié zhèng shèng shuāi]
exuberance and debilitation between pathogenic and healthy *qi*: the law that determines a disease process and its prognosis, namely, rise of healthy *qi* with decline of pathogenic *qi* leading to improvement and recovery, while exuberance of pathogenic *qi* with debilitation of healthy *qi* resulting in deterioration and even death

邪正消长 [xié zhèng xiāo zhǎng]
rise and decline between pathogenic and healthy *qi*: same as exuberance and debilitation between pathogenic and healthy *qi* (邪正盛衰 [xié zhèng shèng shuāi])

正虚邪实 [zhèng xū xié shí]
insufficiency of healthy *qi* and excessiveness of pathogenic *qi*: pathological change in which healthy *qi* is undermined while pathogenic *qi* prevails, denoting that the patient is in an unfavorable state with lowered body resistance

阳虚阴盛 [yáng xū yīn shèng]
yang deficiency with yin exuberance: a pathological change in which yin cold becomes excessive due to insufficient yang of the spleen and kidney which fails to warm up all the *zang-fu* organs, usually manifested as intolerance of cold, cold limbs, diarrhea and edema

阴盛阳衰 [yīn shèng yáng shuāi]
yin exuberance with yang debilitation: pathological change in which yang declines due to endogenous excessive yin cold, usually manifested as aversion to cold, cold limbs, and diarrhea

阳盛 [yáng shèng]
yang exuberance: pathological change

characterized by preponderance of yang, such as excessive functional activity, increased metabolism, enhanced body reactivity, and surplus of heat, occurring typically in excess heat syndromes/patterns

阴盛 [yīn shèng]

yin exuberance: pathological change characterized by preponderance of yin, such as decreased function, insufficient heat production, and accumulation of disease products, occurring typically in excess cold syndromes/patterns

阳虚 [yáng xū]

yang deficiency: (1) pathological change characterized by insufficiency of yang *qi*, usually associated with decline of warming, driving, and moving actions; (2) abbreviation for yang deficiency syndrome/pattern (阳虚证 [yáng xū zhèng])

阳衰 [yáng shuāi]

decline of yang: synonymous with yang deficiency (阳虚 [yáng xū])

阴虚 [yīn xū]

yin deficiency: (1) pathological change characterized by consumption of yin fluid, usually associated with internal heat and dryness; (2) abbreviation for yin deficiency syndrome/pattern (阴虚证 [yīn xū zhèng])

阴衰 [yīn shuāi]

decline of yin: synonymous with yin deficiency (阴虚 [yīn xū])

阴虚阳亢 [yīn xū yáng kàng]

yin deficiency with yang hyperactivity: pathologcial change in which yang becomes hyperactive due to yin deficiency. Deficiency of vital essence, blood or body fluids may lead to breakdown of the equilibrium between yin and yang, resulting in increased activity of the latter, bringing on such symptoms as headache, dizziness, malar flush, heat sensation in the chest, palms of the hands and soles of the feet, afternoon fever, night sweats, hemoptysis, irritability, insomnia, increased libido, or nocturnal emission.

阴虚火旺 [yīn xū huǒ wàng]

yin deficiency with effulgent fire: pathologcial change in which fire becomes exuberant due to deficiency of yin, often bringing on such symptoms as flushed cheeks, irritability, sore throat or increased libido

阴阳格拒 [yīn yáng gé jù]

yin-yang repulsion: a serious pathological change in which extremely excessive yin in the interior forces asthenic yang to spread outward or extremely exuberant yang in the interior keeps insufficient yin on the outside, bringing about pseudo-heat or pseudo-cold manifestations

阳盛格阴 [yáng shèng gé yīn]

exuberant yang repelling yin: pathological change in which extremely exuberant yang trapped in the interior keeps insufficient yin in the exterior, usually referring to high fever with pseudo-cold symptoms

格阴 [gé yīn]

repulsion of yin: abbreviation for exuberant yang repelling yin (阳盛格阴 [yáng shèng gé yīn])

阴盛格阳 [yīn shèng gé yáng]
exuberant yin repelling yang: a pathological change in which extremely excessive yin entrenched in the interior forces asthenic yang to stay at the surface of the body, usually referring to intense endogenous cold with pseudo-heat symptoms

格阳 [gé yáng]
repulsion of yang: abbreviation for exuberant yin repelling yang (阴盛格阳 [yīn shèng gé yáng])

阴阳两虚 [yīn yáng liǎng xū]
dual deficiency of yin-yang: pathological change characterized by deficiency of both yin and yang

亡阴 [wáng yīn]
yin exhaustion: pathological change characterized by excessive loss of essence and fluid due to high fever, profuse sweating, vomiting, diarrhea, bleeding, or other consumptive conditions, usually manifested by sudden deterioration of eyesight, impaired consciousness or delirium, also known as yin collapse (脱阴 [tuō yīn] or 阴脱 [yīn tuō])

脱阴 [tuō yīn]
yin collapse: same as yin exhaustion (亡阴 [wáng yīn])

阴脱 [yīn tuō]
yin collapse: same as yin exhaustion (亡阴 [wáng yīn])

亡阳 [wáng yáng]
yang exhaustion: (1) pathological change characterized by excessive loss of yang *qi*, due to high fever, profuse perspiration, drastic vomiting and diarrhea, massive bleeding, and other consumptive conditions; (2) abbreviation for yang exhaustion syndrome/pattern (亡阳证 [wáng yáng zhèng])

脱阳 [tuō yáng]
yang collapse: (1) same as yang exhaustion (亡阳 [wáng yáng]); (2) prostration of the male during or after sexual intercourse

阳脱 [yáng tuō]
yang collapse: same as 脱阳 [tuō yáng]

阴竭阳脱 [yīn jié yáng tuō]
yin exhaustion and yang collapse: pathological change in which both yin and yang are exhausted

虚阳上浮 [xū yáng shàng fú]
asthenic yang floating upward: pathological change in which consumption of essence and blood deprives yang of its base, causing it to float at the upper part of the body, leading to tidal fever with malar flush and thirst

孤阳上越 [gū yáng shàng yuè]
solitary yang floating upward: same as 虚阳上浮 [xū yáng shàng fú]

伤阴 [shāng yīn]
damage to yin: pathological change characterized by impairment of yin, especially that of the liver and kidney in advanced cases of febrile disease, usually manifested by low fever, heat sensation in the palms of the hands and soles of the feet, emaciation, thirst, malar flush, dry and scarlet red tongue, and fine, feeble and rapid pulse

伤津 [shāng jīn]
damage to fluid: pathological change characterized by impairment of body fluids, especially that of the lung and stomach, usually manifested by thirst, dry cough, irritability, scanty urine, and constipation

津脱 [jīn tuō]
fluid collapse: a severe form of damage to body fluids, usually due to profuse sweating, excessive vomiting or diarrhea, also called fluid exhaustion (亡津液 [wáng jīn yè])

亡津液 [wáng jīn yè]
fluid exhaustion: synonymous with fluid collapse (津脱 [jīn tuō])

脏腑津亏 [zàng fǔ jīn kuī]
fluid insufficiency of visceral organs: general term for fluid insufficiency involving visceral organs

肺津亏损 [fèi jīn kuī sǔn]
lung fluid depletion: pathological change characterized by insufficiency of fluid in the lung

胃津亏损 [wèi jīn kuī sǔn]
stomach fluid depletion: pathological change characterized by insufficiency of fluid in the stomach

大肠津亏 [dà cháng jīn kuī]
large intestinal fluid depletion: pathological change characterized by severe insufficiency of fluid in the large intestine, often seen in the aged, postpartum or at late stage of a febrile disease

津亏血燥 [jīn kuī xuè zào]
fluid depletion with blood dryness: pathological change marked by withered skin, dry throat, thirst, oliguria, reddened tongue without saliva, and thready and rapid pulse

津亏热结 [jīn kuī rè jié]
fluid depletion with retained heat: (1) pathological change characterized by insufficiency of fluid with retention of heat in the interior; (2) abbreviation for syndrome/pattern of fluid depletion with retained heat (津亏热结证 [jīn kuī rè jié zhèng])

津亏火炽 [jīn kuī huǒ chì]
fluid depletion with exuberant fire: pathological change marked by fever, fidgeting, insomnia, dry and sore throat, constipation, reddened tongue, and thready, rapid pulse

伤阳 [shāng yáng]
damage to yang: pathological change characterized by impairment of yang, resulting from various causes such as excessive use of cold-nature medicinals and attack of cold on meridians/channels, usually manifested by aversion to cold, cold extremities and other symptoms of yang deficiency

阴脱 [yīn tuō]
yin collapse: synonym for yin exhaustion (亡阴 [wáng yīn])

表里病机 [biǎo lǐ bìng jī]
pathogenesis of the exterior and interior: pathogenesis of a disease in terms of the depth of its location, including

cold or heat of the exterior or interior, deficiency or excess of the exterior or interior, and disease of both the exterior and interior

表里寒热 [biǎo lǐ hán rè]

cold or heat of the exterior and interior: pathogenesis involving cold or heat changes of the outer and inner parts of the body

表寒 [biǎo hán]

exterior cold: (1) attack of the outer part of the body by wind-cold; (2) abbreviation for exterior cold syndrome/pattern (表寒证 [biǎo hán zhèng])

表热 [biǎo rè]

exterior heat: (1) attack on the outer part of the body by wind-heat; (2) abbreviation for exterior heat syndrome/pattern (表热证 [biǎo rè zhèng])

里寒 [lǐ hán]

interior cold: (1) pathological change characterized by preponderance of yin cold or decline of yang *qi* in the interior; (2) abbreviation for interior cold syndrome/pattern (里寒证 [lǐ hán zhèng])

里热 [lǐ rè]

interior heat: (1) pathological change characterized by heat in the interior due to either exuberance of pathogenic heat or yin deficiency; (2) abbreviation for interior heat syndrome/pattern (里热证 [lǐ rè zhèng])

表里虚实 [biǎo lǐ xū shí]

deficiency or excess of the exterior and interior: pathogenesis involving deficiency or excess changes of the outer and inner parts of the body

表虚 [biǎo xū]

exterior deficiency: (1) deficiency of defense *qi* in the superficial part of the body, marked by spontaneous sweating or sweating accompanied by aversion to wind, and floating, feeble pulse; (2) abbreviation for exterior deficiency syndrome/pattern (表虚证 [biǎo xū zhèng])

表实 [biǎo shí]

exterior excess: (1) invasion of exogenous pathogens that causes gathering of defense *qi* in the skin and muscles and blockage of the interstices and pores; (2) abbreviation for exterior excess syndrome/pattern (表实证 [biǎo shí zhèng])

里虚 [lǐ xū]

interior deficiency: a general term for deficiency of *qi*, blood, yin, and yang of the internal organs

里实 [lǐ shí]

interior excess: (1) a general term denoting accumulation of pathological products in the body, such as phlegm, retained fluid, stagnant *qi* and blood, intestinal parasites, and undigested food; (2) abbreviation for interior excess syndrome/pattern (里实证 [lǐ shí zhèng])

表里出入 [biǎo lǐ chū rù]

entering the interior and exiting to the exterior: transmission of pathogen in the course of a disease from the exterior to the interior part of the body and vice versa

由表入里 [yóu biǎo rù lǐ]

entering the interior from the exterior:

development of a disease with the pathogen penetrating from the exterior to the interior of the body

由里出表 [yóu lǐ chū biǎo]
exiting to the exterior from the interior: process of a disease where the pathogen goes from the interior out to the body's surface, e.g., appearance of skin eruption followed by abatement of fever in the course of measles, indicating improvement of the case

表热传里 [biǎo rè chuán lǐ]
inward transmission of exterior heat: process of a disease where interior heat syndrome/pattern develops along with disappearance of exterior heat symptoms, also known as transmission of pathogenic heat into the interior (热邪传里 [rè xié chuán lǐ])

热邪传里 [rè xié chuán lǐ]
transmission of pathogenic heat into the interior: another way of expressing inward transmission of exterior heat (表热传里 [biǎo rè chuán lǐ])

寒热转化 [hán rè zhuǎn huà]
conversion of cold and heat: conversion of a cold syndrome/pattern into a heat syndrome/pattern, and vice versa

入里化热 [rù lǐ huà rè]
conversion into heat after entering the interior: transformation of exogenous pathogenic factors into heat after having penetrated into the interior of the body

半表半里 [bàn biǎo bàn lǐ]
half-exterior half-interior: (1) location of a disease between the exterior and the interior; (2) abbreviation for half-exterior half-interior syndrome/pattern (半表半里证 [bàn biǎo bàn lǐ zhèng])

表里同病 [biǎo lǐ tóng bìng]
disease involving both the exterior and interior: disease developed in both the exterior and interior parts of the body

表寒里热 [biǎo hán lǐ rè]
exterior cold and interior heat: (1) pathological change characterized by cold in the exterior part and heat in the interior part of the body; (2) abbreviation for syndrome/pattern of exterior cold and interior heat (表寒里热证 [biǎo hán lǐ rè zhèng])

表热里寒 [biǎo rè lǐ hán]
exterior heat and interior cold: (1) pathological change characterized by heat in the exterior and cold in the interior of the body; (2) abbreviation for syndrome/pattern of exterior heat and interior cold (表热里寒证 [biǎo rè lǐ hán zhèng])

表里俱寒 [biǎo lǐ jù hán]
cold in both the exterior and interior: pathological change characterized by presence of cold in both the exterior and interior parts of the body

表里俱热 [biǎo lǐ jù rè]
heat in both the exterior and interior: pathological change characterized by presence of heat in both the exterior and interior parts of the body

表虚里实 [biǎo xū lǐ shí]
exterior deficiency and interior excess:

(1) pathological change characterized by simultaneous presence of deficiency in the exterior and excess in the interior; (2) abbreviation for syndrome/pattern of exterior deficiency and interior excess (表虚里实证 [biǎo xū lǐ shí zhèng])

表实里虚 [biǎo shí lǐ xū]
exterior excess and interior deficiency: (1) pathological change characterized by simultaneous presence of excess in the exterior and deficiency in the interior; (2) abbreviation for syndrome/pattern of exterior excess and interior deficiency (表实里虚证 [biǎo shí lǐ xū zhèng])

上虚下实 [shàng xū xià shí]
upper deficiency and lower excess: (1) pathological change characterized by deficiency of healthy *qi* in the upper part of the body and excess of pathogenic *qi* in the lower; (2) abbreviation for upper-deficiency and lower-excess syndrome/pattern (上虚下实证 [shàng xū xià shí zhèng])

上实下虚 [shàng shí xià xū]
upper excess and lower deficiency: (1) pathological change characterized by excess of pathogenic *qi* in the upper part of the body and deficiency of healthy *qi* in the lower, also called upper preponderance and lower deficiency (上盛下虚 [shàng shèng xià xū]); (2) abbreviation for upper-excess and lower-deficiency syndrome/pattern (上实下虚证 [shàng shí xià xū zhèng])

上盛下虚 [shàng shèng xià xū]
upper preponderance and lower deficiency: synonymous with upper excess and lower deficiency (上实下虚 [shàng shí xià xū])

虚实夹杂 [xū shí jiá zá]
deficiency-excess in complexity: pathological state in which both excess of pathogenic *qi* and deficiency of healthy *qi* occur in a disease process

虚中夹实 [xū zhōng jiá shí]
deficiency complicated by excess: deficiency condition complicated by excess symptoms while the former is dominant, e.g., a case of consumptive disease with emaciation and other deficiency symptoms complicated by blood stasis with amenorrhea

实中夹虚 [shí zhōng jiá xū]
excess complicated by deficiency: excess syndrome/pattern complicated by deficiency symptoms while the former is dominant, e.g., a case of ascites with abdominal distension complicated by emaciation, lassitude, loss of appetite and other deficiency symptoms

由实转虚 [yóu shí zhuǎn xū]
conversion of excess into deficiency: (syndrome/pattern) turning from excess of pathogenic *qi* into deficiency of healthy *qi* during the process of a disease

由虚转实 [yóu xū zhuǎn shí]
conversion of deficiency into excess: (syndrome/pattern) turning from deficiency of healthy *qi* into excess of pathogenic *qi* during the process of a disease

虚实真假 [xū shí zhēn jiǎ]
true or false deficiency and excess:

appearance of deficiency or excess manifestations opposite to the true nature of the disease

真实假虚 [zhēn shí jiǎ xū]
true excess with false deficiency: (1) pathological change, excess in nature with pseudo-deficiency symptoms, e.g., accumulation of dampness-heat with such signs as lack of strength and weak limbs, also known as "great excessiveness looking like debilitation" (大实如羸状 [dà shí rú léi zhuàng]); (2) abbreviation for syndrome/pattern of true excess with false deficiency (真实假虚证 [zhēn shí jiǎ xū zhèng])

真虚假实 [zhēn xū jiǎ shí]
true deficiency with false excess: (1) pathological change, deficient in nature with pseudo-excess symptoms, e.g., severe decline of *zang-fu* functions with such manifestations as abdominal distension, panting and constipation, also known as "extreme insufficiency presenting signs of exuberance" (至虚有盛候 [zhì xū yǒu shèng hòu]); (2) abbreviation for syndrome/pattern of true deficiency with false excess (真虚假实证 [zhēn xū jiǎ shí zhèng])

表里俱虚 [biǎo lǐ jù xū]
deficiency in both the exterior and interior: pathological change characterized by deficiency in both the exterior and interior parts of the body

表里俱实 [biǎo lǐ jù shí]
excess in both the exterior and interior: pathological change characterized by presence of excess in both the exterior and interior parts of the body

表气不固 [biǎo qì bù gù]
insecurity of exterior *qi*: failure to protect the superficies of the body by insufficient defense *qi*, which makes one susceptible to exogenous pathogenic factors, especially cold, and liable to perspire spontaneously, also called insecurity of defense *qi* (卫气不固 [wèi qì bù gù])

卫气不固 [wèi qì bù gù]
insecurity of defense *qi*: same as insecurity of exterior *qi* (表气不固 [biǎo qì bù gù])

卫阳被遏 [wèi yáng bèi è]
defense yang being depressed: pathological change in which depressed yang *qi* fails to warm and protect the body surface

温邪上受 [wēn xié shàng shòu]
attack of warm pathogen on the upper: mechanism of the onset of most acute febrile diseases starting from the upper respiratory tract

温邪犯肺 [wēn xié fàn fèi]
warm pathogen invading the lung: mechanism of the initial stage of an acute febrile disease when a warm pathogen invades the lung and the superficial defensive system, causing fever, cough, sore throat, thirst, and rapid floating pulse

逆传心包 [nì chuán xīn bāo]
adverse transmission to the pericardium: mechanism of impairment of consciousness or coma occurring soon after onset of an acute febrile disease when a warm pathogen

is transmitted directly to the pericardium instead of the *qi* aspect

阳虚水泛 [yáng xū shuǐ fàn]
yang deficiency with water flood; edema due to yang deficiency: mechanism of generalized edema when yang deficiency of the spleen and kidney leads to retention of water in the body

营卫不和 [yíng wèi bù hé]
disharmony between nutrient and defense *qi*: mechanism that explains certain forms of abnormal sweating, particularly spontaneous sweating in an exterior syndrome, as the defense aspect regulates the excretion of sweat while the nutrient aspect provides fluid for the formation of sweat

卫弱营强 [wèi ruò yíng qiáng]
weak defense *qi* with strong nutrient: mechanism of spontaneous sweating without fever in an exterior syndrome/pattern

卫强营弱 [wèi qiáng yíng ruò]
strong defense *qi* with weak nutrient: mechanism of sweating that occurs only during fever in an exterior syndrome/pattern

卫气同病 [wèi qì tóng bìng]
disease of both defense and *qi* (aspects): pathological change that causes high fever, thirst, and irritability together with chills and general aching in the case of an acute febrile disease

卫营同病 [wèi yíng tóng bìng]
disease of both defense and nutrient (aspects): pathological change that causes high fever and delirium together with chills, headache, and general aching in the case of an acute febrile disease

气营两燔 [qì yíng liǎng fán]
blazing in both *qi* and nutrient: intense heat in both *qi* and nutrient aspects, causing high fever, thirst, mental irritability, delirium, and barely visible skin eruption in the case of an acute febrile disease

气血两燔 [qì xuè liǎng fán]
blazing in both *qi* and blood: intense heat in both *qi* and blood aspects, causing high fever, delirium, hemoptysis, epistaxis, skin eruptions, and even convulsions in the case of an acute febrile disease

热邪阻肺 [rè xié zǔ fèi]
heat pathogen obstructing the lung: pathological change that causes fever, cough, thick, yellowish or blood-stained sputum, dyspnea, chest pain, reddened tip of the tongue with dry yellow coating, and full and rapid pulse

热迫大肠 [rè pò dà cháng]
heat distressing the large intestine: pathological change in which pathogenic heat impairs the function of the large intestine, causing acute diarrhea with abdominal pain, burning sensation of the anus, scanty dark urine, and dry yellow coating of the tongue

热入心包 [rè rù xīn bāo]
heat entering the pericardium: pathological change that causes high fever with delirium or even coma in the case of an acute febrile disease

热入营血 [rè rù yíng xuè]
heat entering nutrient-blood: (1) pathological change in which pathogenic heat enters the nutrient-blood and disturbs the heart (mind); (2) abbreviation for syndrome/pattern of heat entering nutrientblood (热入营血证 [rè rù yíng xuè zhèng])

血热动血 [xuè rè dòng xuè]
blood heat stirring blood: (1) pathological change characterized by blood heat causing frenetic movement of blood; (2) abbreviation for syndrome/pattern of blood heat stirring blood (血热动血证 [xuè rè dòng xuè zhèng])

血热风盛 [xuè rè fēng shèng]
blood heat with raging wind: (1) pathological change characterized by extremely exuberant pathogenic heat which enters the blood aspect and stirs up violent wind; (2) abbreviation for syndrome/pattern of blood heat with raging wind (血热风盛证[xuè rè fēng shèng zhèng])

血热化燥 [xuè rè huà zào]
blood heat transforming into dryness: (1) pathological change in which the pathogenic heat entering the blood, impairs yin and induces dryness transformation; (2) abbreviation for syndrome/pattern of blood heat with dryness transformation (血热化燥证 [xuè rè huà zào zhèng])

热入血分 [rè rù xuè fèn]
heat entering the blood aspect: pathological change that causes fever, restlessness, delirium, skin eruption, and bleeding (hematemesis, epistaxis or hematochezia) in late and severest stage of an acute febrile disease

血分热毒 [xuè fèn rè dú]
heat toxin in the blood aspect: (1) penetration of heat into the blood aspect in the case of an epidemic febrile disease, causing high fever, delirium, skin eruption, or hematuria; (2) common mechanism of acute pyogenic infections marked by recurrent local inflammation or boil formation

热入血室 [rè rù xuè shì]
heat entering the blood chamber: pathological change in which pathogenic heat enters the blood chamber during menstruation or after childbirth and contends with the blood, usually causing abdominal pain, menstrual disturbances, alternate fever and chills, and delirium at night

热伏冲任 [rè fú chōng rèn]
heat hiding in the thoroughfare and conception vessels: pathological change in which heat stays in the thoroughfare and conception vessels

热邪内结 [rè xié nèi jié]
heat accumulation in the interior: a general term referring to accumulation of pathogenic heat in *zang-fu* organs

热结 [rè jié]
heat accumulation: abbreviation for heat accumulation in the interior (热邪内结 [rè xié nèi jié])

热结下焦 [rè jié xià jiāo]
heat accumulation in the lower energizer: accumulation of heat in the intestines

and bladder that causes lower abdominal distension and pain, constipation, short voiding of dark urine or even hematuria, and sometimes tenderness of the lower abdomen accompanied by restlessness

热盛伤津 [rè shèng shāng jīn]
exuberant heat damaging fluid: process by which excess heat dissipates body fluids, causing fluid consumption syndrome/pattern

热灼肾阴 [rè zhuó shèn yīn]
heat scorching kidney yin: pathological change with consumption of kidney yin by pathogenic heat, which causes low fever, heat sensation in the palms of the hands and soles of the feet, dry mouth, impairment of hearing, dry and deep reddened tongue without coating, and thready and rapid pulse, occurring at the advanced stage of an acute febrile disease

热伤筋脉 [rè shāng jīn mài]
heat damaging muscles and sinews/ tendons: pathological change that leads to cramps, flaccidity or paralysis of limbs in the case of high or prolonged fever

瘀热 [yū rè]
stagnant heat: (1) heat combined with phlegm-dampness retained in the body and causing jaundice; (2) heat produced by static blood

伏热 [fú rè]
latent heat: pathological change occurring in the case of a febrile disease with the heat pathogen hidden deeply in the interior

伏热在里 [fú rè zài lǐ]
latent heat in the interior: pathological change that usually causes dry throat, foul breath, reddened tongue, constipation and scanty dark urine

血分瘀热 [xuè fèn yū rè]
stagnant heat in the blood aspect: (1) pathological change characterized by stagnation of heat in the blood aspect with deep penetration into the *zang-fu* organs including the heart, liver and kidney; (2) heat produced by static blood

热极生风 [rè jí shēng fēng]
extreme heat engendering wind: pathological change referring to the occurrence of convulsions and opisthotonus in a case of high fever

热盛风动 [rè shèng fēng dòng]
exuberant heat stirring up wind: same as 热极生风 [rè jí shēng fēng]

血虚生风 [xuè xū shēng fēng]
blood deficiency engendering wind: pathological change referring to dizziness, twitching or tremor resulting from persisting anemia or profuse bleeding

血燥生风 [xuè zào shēng fēng]
blood dryness engendering wind: pathological change in which the skin becomes rough and dry, with cracks and fissures because of dryness in the blood

风寒束表 [fēng hán shù biǎo]
wind-cold fettering the exterior: pathological change in which external wind-cold attacks the superficial aspect of the body, causing chills with mild fever, headache or general aching, stuffy and runny nose, and lack of sweating

风湿相搏 [fēng shī xiāng bó]
mutual contention of wind and dampness: pathological change resulting in muscle ache and joint pain, usually occurring in cases of wind-dampness contraction

风火相煽 [fēng huǒ xiāng shān]
mutual incitement of wind and fire: pathological change that causes hyperexia and convulsions in the most advanced stage of an acute febrile disease

风火内旋 [fēng huǒ nèi xuán]
wind-fire whirling internally: pathological change in which intense heat engenders wind internally

风中血脉 [fēng zhòng xuè mài]
wind attacking blood vessel: pathological change in which wind attacks a weakened blood vessel, causing deviated eye and mouth, hemiplegia, or numbness of limbs

湿郁肌表 [shī yù jī biǎo]
dampness stagnating in the superficies: pathological change characterized by stagnation of dampness in the superficial portion of the body, usually impeding the circulation of *qi* and blood, and causing a sensation of heaviness and aching of the limbs

湿蔽清阳 [shī bì qīng yáng]
dampness beclouding the head: pathological change that causes dizziness with a sensation as if the head were bound tight

湿邪困脾 [shī xié kùn pí]
dampness (pathogen) encumbering the spleen: pathological change that results in anorexia, epigastric distension, lassitude, and heaviness of limbs

湿郁化热 [shī yù huà rè]
stagnant dampness transforming into heat: pathological change that causes heat symptoms together with dampness syndrome/pattern

湿郁化火 [shī yù huà huǒ]
stagnant dampness transforming into fire: pathological change that causes fire symptoms together with dampness syndrome/pattern

湿热内蕴 [shī rè nèi yùn]
internal retention of dampness-heat: general term for the accumulation of dampness-heat in the *zang-fu* organs, especially in the stomach, spleen, liver, and gallbladder, causing persistent fever, heaviness of the body, lassitude, loss of appetite, abdominal distension, or jaundice

湿热下注 [shī rè xià zhù]
downpour of dampness-heat: pathological change that causes diarrhea with passage of mucus and blood in cases of dysentery, turbid urine in cases of urinary infection, morbid leukorrhea in cases of pelvic infection, etc.

湿毒流注 [shī dú liú zhù]
spilling of dampness-toxin: pathological change characterized by flow of dampness-toxin into muscles and skin, causing ulcer or festering sore on the shank

燥伤肺气 [zào shāng fèi qì]
dryness damaging lung *qi*: pathological change that may lead to dry cough, hemoptysis, diabetes, and even flaccidity

of the limbs due to inadequate distribution of body fluid to the muscles and tendons

燥干清窍 [zào gān qīng qiào]
dryness affecting the clear orifices: pathological change in which dryness-heat affects the upper part of the body and impairs the function of the sense organs

燥伤津液 [zào shāng jīn yè]
dryness damaging body fluid: pathological change that may result in upward adverse flow of stomach *qi* when the stomach is involved, constipation when the intestinal fluid is impaired, and diabetes when the kidney fluid is consumed

津枯肠燥 [jīn kū cháng zào]
fluid exhaustion with intestinal dryness: one of the mechanisms for constipation

燥气寒化 [zào qì hán huà]
dryness *qi* transforming into cold: pathological process characterized by transformation of a dryness syndrome/ pattern into a cold one, often occurring in patients with a yang-insufficient or yin-exuberant constitution

燥气化热 [zào qì huà rè]
dryness *qi* transforming into heat: pathological process characterized by transformation of a dryness syndrome/ pattern into one of heat, often occurring in patients with a yin-insufficient or yang-exuberant constitution

虚火上炎 [xū huǒ shàng yán]
deficiency fire flaming upward: pathological change occurring in cases of kidney yin deficiency, causing dry and sore throat, dizziness, restlessness, red eyes or oral ulcers

火伤血络 [huǒ shāng xuè luò]
fire damaging blood vessels: pathological change that causes hemoptysis, hematemesis, and epistaxis

寒热失调 [hán rè shī tiáo]
imbalance between cold and heat: general term for pathological changes of yin-yang imbalance with cold, heat or cold-and-heat manifestations

实寒 [shí hán]
excess cold: (1) pathological change characterized by excess of pathogenic cold; (2) abbreviation for excess cold syndrome/ pattern (实寒证 [shí hán zhèng])

实热 [shí rè]
excess heat:(1) pathological change characterized by excess of yang heat; (2) abbreviation for excess heat syndrome/ pattern (实热证 [shí rè zhèng])

实火 [shí huǒ]
excess fire: (1) pathological change characterized by fire of excess type; (2) abbreviation for excess fire syndrome/ pattern (实火证 [shí huǒ zhèng])

虚寒 [xū hán]
deficiency cold: (1) pathological change characterized by cold of deficiency type, usually resulting from yang deficiency; (2) abbreviation for deficiency cold syndrome/ pattern (虚寒证 [xū hán zhèng])

虚热 [xū rè]
(I) deficiency heat: (1) pathological change

characterized by coexistence of deficiency and heat due to yin-blood deficiency; (2) abbreviation for deficiency heat syndrome/pattern (虚热证 [xū rè zhèng]); **(II) fever of deficiency type:** fever caused by deficiency of yin, blood or *qi*

虚火 [xū huǒ]
deficiency fire: (1) pathological change in which consumption of yin leads to exuberance of yang with upsurging of fire; (2) pathological change in which excess of yin results in rejection of yang with pseudo-heat and pseudo-fire symptoms

寒热错杂 [hán rè cuò zá]
cold and heat in complexity: pathological change that causes complicated heat and cold conditions such as heat in the upper part of the body with cold in the lower, or cold in the exterior and heat in the interior of the body

上寒下热 [shàng hán xià rè]
upper cold and lower heat: (1) pathological change characterized by cold in the upper part of the body and heat in the lower part; (2) abbreviation for upper-cold and lower-heat syndrome/pattern (上寒下热证 [shàng hán xià rè zhèng])

上热下寒 [shàng rè xià hán]
upper heat and lower cold: (1) pathological change characterized by heat in the upper part of the body and cold in the lower part; (2) abbreviation for upper-heat and lower-cold syndrome/pattern (上热下寒证 [shàng rè xià hán zhèng])

寒邪外束 [hán xié wài shù]
cold pathogen fettering the exterior: pathological process that causes chills, general aching, headache, absence of sweating, and floating tense pulse

中寒 [zhōng hán]
cold in the middle (energizer): pathological change caused by deficiency of spleen and stomach yang, marked by abdominal pain relievable by warmth, intolerance of cold, cold limbs, loss of appetite, and loose bowels

寒从中生 [hán cóng zhōng shēng]
generation of cold from the interior: pathological process where an interior-cold syndrome results from yang deficiency of an internal organ

寒入血室 [hán rù xuè shì]
cold entering the blood chamber: pathological change in which pathogenic cold enters the uterus, congeals the liver meridian/channel and impedes blood flow

寒热真假 [hán rè zhēn jiǎ]
true or false cold and heat: appearance of cold or heat manifestations opposite to the true nature of the disease, attributable to repelling of either yin or yang, respectively

假寒 [jiǎ hán]
false cold; pseudo-cold: apparent cold symptoms in cases of heat syndromes/patterns

假热 [jiǎ rè]
false heat; pseudo-heat: apparent heat symptoms in cases of cold syndromes/patterns

真寒假热 [zhēn hán jiǎ rè]

true cold with false heat: (1) pathological change marked by excessive cold in the interior with pseudo-heat manifestations; (2) abbreviation for syndrome/pattern of true cold with false heat (真寒假热证 [zhēn hán jiǎ rè zhèng])

真热假寒 [zhēn rè jiǎ hán]
true heat with false cold: (1) pathological change marked by excessive heat in the interior with pseudo-cold manifestations; (2) abbreviation for syndrome/pattern of true heat with false cold (真热假寒证 [zhēn rè jiǎ hán zhèng])

化热 [huà rè]
transformation into heat: transformation of pathogenic factors such as wind, cold or dryness into heat, resulting in intolerance of heat, thirst, irritability, reddened tongue with yellow coating, and rapid pulse

热化 [rè huà]
heat transformation: transformation of another syndrome/pattern into one of heat in the course of disease

化火 [huà huǒ]
transformation into fire: pathological process characterized by transformation of intense heat into fire, producing such symptoms as persistent thirst, bloodshot eyes, flushed face, parched lips, dry and sore throat, hemoptysis, epistaxis, hematuria, and even impairment of consciousness or raving madness

胃热化火 [wèi rè huà huǒ]
transformation of stomach heat into fire: pathological change that causes the symptoms of stomach heat, usually accompanied by ulceration of the mouth

胃热消谷 [wèi rè xiāo gǔ]
stomach heat with accelerated digestion: pathological change in which stomach heat or fire induces abnormally rapid digestion

化风 [huà fēng]
transformation into wind: occurrence of wind symptoms such as dizziness, convulsions, or tremors in the course of a febrile disease

化燥 [huà zào]
transformation into dryness: transformation into a dryness syndrome/pattern due to consumption of body fluids, manifested by thirst, dry throat and lips, constipation and dry cough

燥化 [zào huà]
dryness transformation: transformation into a dryness syndrome/pattern in the course of disease

燥结 [zào jié]
dryness accumulation: pathological change characterized by lack of fluid in the intestines resulting in constipation

气虚 [qì xū]
***qi* deficiency:** (1) general term denoting the decline of *qi* activity, manifested by shortness of breath, weak voice, lassitude, listlessness and sweating upon mild exertion, mostly caused by overfatigue or protracted illness; (2) term particularly denoting deficiency of lung *qi*; (3) abbreviation for *qi* deficiency syndrome/pattern (气虚证 [qì xū zhèng])

气脱 [qì tuō]

***qi* collapse:** breakdown of vital energy, usually resulting from excessive sweating, severe diarrhea, massive bleeding, or excessive loss of semen

气机失调 [qì jī shī tiáo]

disorder of *qi* movement: a general term for disordered activity of *qi* in ascending, descending, exiting and entering that may cause various pathological changes such as stagnation of *qi*, reversed flow of *qi*, sinking of *qi*, blockage of *qi*, and collapse of *qi*

气机不利 [qì jī bù lì]

disturbance of *qi* movement: general term for disorder of *qi*, referring to dysfunction of the internal organs, especially functional derangement in sending things up or down, as manifested by hiccups, stuffy feeling in the chest, abdominal distension, or diarrhea

气机郁滞 [qì jī yù zhì]

depression and stagnation of *qi* movement: sluggish or stagnant flow of *qi* occurring in a certain part of the body or in an internal organ, usually causing local distension and pain and may lead to further pathological changes such as blood stasis or formation of phlegm and retained fluid

气郁 [qì yù]

***qi* depression:** (1) pathological change characterized by emotional depression with stagnation of *qi*; (2) abbreviation for *qi* depression syndrome/pattern (气郁证 [qì yù zhèng])

气滞 [qì zhì]

***qi* stagnation:** (1) pathological change characterized by impeded circulation of *qi* that leads to stagnation of *qi* movement and functional disorder of visceral organs, manifested as distension or pain in the affected part; (2) abbreviation for *qi* stagnation syndrome/pattern (气滞证 [qì zhì zhèng])

气郁化火 [qì yù huà huǒ]

depressed *qi* transforming into fire: pathological change of long-standing depression of *qi* that transforms into fire and leads to such symptoms as emotional depression, irritability, irascibility, distension and burning pain in the chest, and reddened tongue with yellow coating

气化不利 [qì huà bù lì]

disturbance of *qi* transformation; inhibited *qi* transformation: (1) general term for dysfunction of visceral organs, particularly referring to that of the triple energizer in water metabolism due to yang *qi* deficiency, leading to water-dampness retention or phlegm retention, also called failure of *qi* transformation (气化无权 [qì huà wú quán]); (2) in a narrow sense, denoting impaired fluid metabolism leading to water-dampness retention or phlegm retention, and also denoting disturbance in urine excretion due to dysfunction of the kidney and urinary bladder as the cause of edema and difficulty in urination

气化无权 [qì huà wú quán]

failure of *qi* transformation: synonymous with disturbance of *qi* transformation (气化不利 [qì huà bù lì])

水不化气 [shuǐ bù huà qì]

failure of water to transform into *qi*:

pathological change in which disturbance of *qi* transformation leads to disturbance of water metabolism or deficiency of yin fluid

气闭 [qì bì]
***qi* blockage:** pathological change in which blocked *qi* movement leads to functional disorders of *zang-fu* organs

气逆 [qì nì]
***qi* counterflow:** pathological change in which the movement of *qi* is impaired, resulting in upward counterflow. It often refers to functional disturbances of the liver, lung, and stomach. Upward counterflow of liver *qi* usually brings on such symptoms as vertigo, headache, tinnitus, deafness, pain in the chest and hypochondriac regions, and even fainting or hematemesis; upward counterflow of lung *qi* leads to dyspnea, asthma and cough; upward counterflow of stomach *qi* causes belching, hiccupping or vomiting.

气陷 [qì xiàn]
***qi* sinking:** pathological change of *qi* marked by failure in its lifting or holding function, often leading to prolapse of the uterus, prolapse of the anus or visceroptosis

升降失常 [shēng jiàng shī cháng]
disturbance in ascending and descending: general term referring to disturbance of ascending and descending movement of visceral *qi*, e.g., dysfunction of the spleen in sending up food essence and water, which causes diarrhea and abdominal distension, and dysfunction of the stomach in sending down food content, giving rise to nausea, vomiting, and regurgitation

下陷 [xià xiàn]
sinking: another expression for sinking of *qi*, usually due to deficiency of spleen *qi*, resulting in prolapse of visceral organs (cf. 中气下陷 [zhōng qì xià xiàn])

脾气下陷 [pí qì xià xiàn]
sinking of spleen *qi*: (1) pathological change characterized by weakness of the spleen with sinking of the middle *qi*, also known as sinking of the middle *qi* (中气下陷 [zhōng qì xià xiàn]) or spleen insufficiency with sinking of *qi* (脾虚气陷 [pí xū qì xiàn]); (2) abbreviation for spleen *qi* sinking syndrome/pattern (脾气下陷证 [pí qì xià xiàn zhèng])

中气下陷 [zhōng qì xià xiàn]
sinking of the middle *qi*: sinking of *qi* of the middle energizer, same as sinking of spleen *qi* (脾气下陷 [pí qì xià xiàn])

脾虚气陷 [pí xū qì xiàn]
spleen insufficiency with sinking of *qi*: same as sinking of spleen *qi* (脾气下陷 [pí qì xià xiàn])

内陷 [nèi xiàn]
inward invasion: a term referring to invasion of the interior of the body by pathogenic factors

寒凝气滞 [hán níng qì zhì]
***qi* stagnation due to congealing cold:** *qi* stagnation caused by cold with a congealing effect which impedes the flow of *qi*, often manifested clinically by spasms and pains

气虚不摄 [qì xū bù shè]
***qi* deficiency failing to control the blood:**

pathological change of *qi* deficiency in which *qi* is unable to keep the blood flowing within the vessels, resulting in bleeding

气不摄血 [qì bù shè xuè]
failure of *qi* to control the blood: synonymous with *qi* deficiency failing to control the blood (气虚不摄 [qì xū bù shè])

气虚血瘀 [qì xū xuè yū]
(I) *qi* deficiency and blood stasis: coexistence of *qi* deficiency and blood stasis; **(II) blood stasis due to *qi* deficiency:** pathological change of *qi* deficiency in which *qi* is insufficient to drive the blood flow, thereby forming blood stasis

气虚中满 [qì xū zhōng mǎn]
***qi* deficiency with abdominal fullness:** pathological change of *qi* deficiency in which *qi* is insufficient for normal transportation in the middle energizer, thereby causing sensation of abdominal fullness

气血失调 [qì xuè shī tiáo]
disharmony of *qi* and blood: pathological change marked by lack of normal coordination between *qi* and blood, e.g., *qi* in insufficiency leading to blood stasis instead of promoting blood flow under normal circumstances

血虚 [xuè xū]
blood deficiency: pathological change characterized by insufficiency of blood to nourish organs, tissues and meridians/channels, usually resulting from profuse bleeding or chronic hemorrhage, or impaired blood production due to diminished function of the internal organs, especially the spleen

血瘀 [xuè yū]
blood stasis: pathological change characterized by impediment or even stoppage of blood flow

血寒 [xuè hán]
blood cold: pathological change characterized by cold impeding the blood flow, leading to blood stasis

血热 [xuè rè]
(I) blood heat; fever at blood aspect: pathological change characterized by presence of heat in the blood aspect, causing frenetic blood flow; **(II) blood fever:** see P. 583

血脱 [xuè tuō]
blood collapse: critical pathological condition characterized by massive loss of blood

血不归经 [xuè bù guī jīng]
blood failing to stay in the vessels: basic mechanism of various hemorrhages

血不循经 [xuè bù xún jīng]
blood failing to circulate in the vessels: same as blood failing to stay in the vessels (血不归经 [xuè bù guī jīng])

血热妄行 [xuè rè wàng xíng]
heat enabling frenetic movement of blood: one of the mechanisms of bleeding

血不养筋 [xuè bù yǎng jīn]
failure of blood to nourish sinews/tendons: pathological change characterized by

insufficiency of liver blood with malnutrition of the sinews/tendons, leading to muscular contracture

气血两虚 [qì xuè liǎng xū]
deficiency of both *qi* and blood: (1) pathological change characterized by diminished supply of both *qi* and blood to the body, also called 气血两亏 [qì xuè liǎng kuī]; (2) abbreviation for syndrome/pattern of *qi*-blood dual deficiency (气血两虚证 [qì xuè liǎng xū zhèng])

气血两亏 [qì xuè liǎng kuī]
insufficiency of both *qi* and blood: same as deficiency of both *qi* and blood (气血两虚 [qì xuè liǎng xū])

气滞血瘀 [qì zhì xuè yū]
(I) *qi* stagnation and blood stasis: pathological change characterized by coexistence of *qi* stagnation and blood stasis; **(II) blood stasis due to *qi* stagnation:** pathological change in which long-standing or severe stagnation of *qi* leads to blood stasis, marked by aggravation of local pain with tenderness, and even formation of mass

气虚血瘀 [qì xū xuè yū]
(I) *qi* deficiency and blood stasis: pathological change characterized by coexistence of *qi* deficiency and blood stasis; **(II) blood stasis due to *qi* deficiency:** pathological change in which deficiency of *qi* leads to blood stasis

血脱气脱 [xuè tuō qì tuō]
blood loss with (*qi*) collapse: pathological change in which massive loss of blood leads to collapse, marked by pale complexion, cold extremities, profuse sweating, and thready and barely perceptible pulse, also called collapse following blood loss (气随血脱 [qì suí xuè tuō])

气随血脱 [qì suí xuè tuō]
(*qi*) collapse following blood loss: same as blood loss with (*qi*) collapse (血脱气脱 [xuè tuō qì tuō])扶

血随气陷 [xuè suí qì xiàn]
bleeding following sinking of *qi*: pathological change causing incessant bleeding such as uterine bleeding or bleeding per rectum, following sinking of *qi*

血随气逆 [xuè suí qì nì]
blood rush following counterflow of *qi*: pathological change in which upward counterflow of liver *qi* leads to flushing of the face, reddened eyes, vomiting of blood, or even syncope

脏腑病机 [zàng fǔ bìng jī]
pathogenesis of *zang-fu* organs: mechanism of origination and development of diseases of the visceral organs

肝气虚 [gān qì xū]
liver *qi* deficiency: (1) pathological change in which insufficiency of essential *qi* in the liver impaires the latter's function in smoothing the flow of *qi*, also called liver *qi* insufficiency (肝气不足 [gān qì bù zú]); (2) abbreviation for liver *qi* deficiency syndrome/pattern (肝气虚证 [gān qì xū zhèng])

肝气不足 [gān qì bù zú]
liver *qi* insufficiency: same as liver *qi* deficiency (肝气虚 [gān qì xū])

肝血虚 [gān xuè xū]
liver blood deficiency: (1) pathological change characterized by insufficient blood supply to nourish the liver, also called liver blood insufficiency (肝血不足 [gān xuè bù zú]); (2) abbreviation for liver blood deficiency syndrome/pattern (肝血虚证 [gān xuè xū zhèng])

肝血不足 [gān xuè bù zú]
liver blood insufficiency: same as liver blood deficiency (肝血虚 [gān xuè xū])

肝阴虚 [gān yīn xū]
liver yin deficiency: (1) pathological change attributed to lack of yin fluid to nourish and moisten the liver, also called liver yin insufficiency (肝阴不足 [gān yīn bù zú]); (2) abbreviation for liver yin deficiency syndrome/pattern (肝阴虚证 [gān yīn xū zhèng])

肝阴不足 [gān yīn bù zú]
liver yin insufficiency: same as liver yin deficiency (肝阴虚 [gān yīn xū])

肝阳虚 [gān yáng xū]
liver yang deficiency: pathological change of the liver that deficiency of yang *qi* gives rise to endogenous deficiency cold, impairing the liver's function of storing blood and smoothing the flow of *qi*, also called liver deficiency cold (肝虚寒 [gān xū hán])

肝虚寒 [gān xū hán]
liver deficiency cold: same as liver yang deficiency (肝阳虚 [gān yáng xū])

肝气不和 [gān qì bù hé]
disharmony of liver *qi*: pathological change of the liver in its smoothing and discharging function, either insufficient or excessive, causing irritability, hypochondriac, mammary or lower abdominal distension and pain, and irregular menstruation

肝气不舒 [gān qì bù shū]
constraint of liver *qi*: pathological change of the liver characterized by insufficiency of its smoothing and discharging function, usually manifested by irritability, irascibility, stuffy feeling in the chest, hypochondriac and lower abdominal distension and pain, and in women, distending pain of the breast and menstrual complaints

肝气郁结 [gān qì yù jié]
liver *qi* depression; liver *qi* stagnation: (1) pathological change often caused by emotional depression, characterized by stagnation of liver *qi* with impaired function of smoothing the *qi* flow, usually abbreviated as liver depression 肝郁 [gān yù]; (2) abbreviation for liver *qi* depression [stagnation] syndrome/pattern (肝气郁结证 [gān qì yù jié zhèng])

肝气横逆 [gān qì héng nì]
transverse counterflow of liver *qi*: pathological change in which hyperactive liver *qi* runs transversely, impairing the spleen and stomach

肝气犯胃 [gān qì fàn wèi]
liver *qi* invading the stomach: pathological change in which hyperactive *qi* running transversely, impairs the stomach function, and causes epigastric distension and pain, frequent sighing,

belching, acid regurgitation, or nausea and vomiting

肝气犯脾 [gān qì fàn pí]
liver *qi* invading the spleen: pathological change in which hyperactive *qi* running transversely, impairs the spleen function, and causes hypochondriac, epigastric and abdominal distension and pain, anorexia and diarrhea

肝气上逆 [gān qì shàng nì]
upward counterflow of liver *qi*: pathological change in which hyperactive liver *qi* running upward, attacks the upper portion of the body, and causes dizziness, headache, tinnitus, deafness, pain and distension of the chest and hypochondrium, and even hematemesis

肝阳上亢 [gān yáng shàng kàng]
ascendant hyperactivity of liver yang: (1) pathological change that occurs when liver yin is insufficient to counterbalance yang, resulting in stirring of liver yang mainly affecting the upper portion of the body; (2) abbreviation for syndrome/pattern of ascendant hyperactivity of liver yang (肝阳上亢证 [gān yáng shàng kàng zhèng])

肝阳亢盛 [gān yáng kàng shèng]
hyperactivity of liver yang: same as ascendant hyperactivity of liver yang (肝阳上亢 [gān yáng shàng kàng])

肝阳化火 [gān yáng huà huǒ]
liver yang transforming into fire: pathological change in which hyperactive liver yang transforms into fire, and causes such symptoms as dizziness, flushing of face, bitter taste in the mouth, irritability and irascibility

肝火炽盛 [gān huǒ chì shèng]
blazing liver fire: (1) pathological change characterized by exuberant fire in the liver meridian/channel that causes upward flow of *qi* and flaming of fire; (2) abbreviation for blazing liver fire syndrome/pattern (肝火炽盛证 [gān huǒ chì shèng zhèng])

肝火上炎 [gān huǒ shàng yán]
up-flaming of liver fire: (1) pathological change in which fire is generated from depressed liver *qi* and flames up along the liver meridian/channel, also called excess fire of the liver meridian/channel (肝经实火 [gān jīng shí huǒ]); (2) abbreviation for syndrome/pattern of up-flaming liver fire (肝火上炎证 [gān huǒ shàng yán zhèng])

肝经实火 [gān jīng shí huǒ]
excess fire in the liver meridian/channel: same as up-flaming of liver fire (肝火上炎 [gān huǒ shàng yán])

肝经风热 [gān jīng fēng rè]
wind-heat in the liver meridian/channel: (1) pathological change in which attack of pathogenic wind-heat on the liver meridian/channel causes head and eye troubles; (2) abbreviation for liver meridian/channel wind-heat syndrome/pattern (肝经风热证 [gān jīng fēng rè zhèng])

肝经郁热 [gān jīng yù rè]
stagnant heat in the liver meridian/channel: pathological change characterized by transformation of stagnant liver *qi* into heat, resulting in coexistence of stagnant

qi and exuberant heat in the liver meridian/channel

肝经湿热 [gān jīng shī rè]
dampness-heat in the liver meridian/channel: (1) pathological change in which pathogenic dampness-heat accumulated in the liver pours down along the liver meridian/channel; (2) abbreviation for liver meridian/channel dampness-heat syndrome/pattern (肝经湿热证[gān jīng shī rè zhèng])

心虚 [xīn xū]
heart deficiency: general term for deficiency conditions of the heart

心气虚 [xīn qì xū]
heart *qi* deficiency: (1) pathological change resulting from insufficiency of the heart *qi* with impaired blood-pumping function, chiefly manifested by palpitations, also called heart *qi* insufficiency (心气不足 [xīn qì bù zú]); (2) abbreviation for heart *qi* deficiency syndrome/pattern (心气虚证 [xīn qì xū zhèng])

心气不足 [xīn qì bù zú]
heart *qi* insufficiency: same as heart *qi* deficiency (心气虚 [xīn qì xū])

心气不宁 [xīn qì bù níng]
restlessness of heart *qi*: pathological change of the heart *qi* marked by a feeling of uneasiness, together with palpitations, susceptibility to fright, vexation, and insomnia

心气不固 [xīn qì bù gù]
insecurity of heart *qi*: pathological change of heart *qi* marked by floating of the mind, susceptibility to fright, forgetfulness, spontaneous sweating, or sweating upon mild exertion

心气不收 [xīn qì bù shōu]
non-contraction of heart *qi*: same as insecurity of heart *qi* (心气不固 [xīn qì bù gù])

心血虚 [xīn xuè xū]
heart blood deficiency: (1) pathological change resulting from insufficient supply of nourishing blood to the heart with impairment of mental activities such as abstraction, insomnia, and dream-disturbed sleep, as well as palpitations and thready weak pulse, also called insufficiency of heart blood (心血不足 [xīn xuè bù zú]); (2) abbreviation for heart blood deficiency syndrome/pattern (心血虚证 [xīn xuè xū zhèng])

心血不足 [xīn xuè bù zú]
insufficiency of heart blood: same as heart blood deficiency (心血虚 [xīn xuè xū])

心血瘀阻 [xīn xuè yū zǔ]
heart blood stasis (and obstruction): pathological change of the heart in which the blood flow in the heart vessels is impeded, causing a feeling of suffocation and precordial pain

心阴虚 [xīn yīn xū]
heart yin deficiency: (1) pathological change of the heart in which insufficient yin fails to suppress yang, resulting in relative preponderance of heart yang manifested by such symptoms as mental unsteadiness, insomnia, night sweats, and feverish sensation in the palms of the hands and soles of the feet, also called

insufficiency of heart yin (心阴不足 [xīn yīn bù zú]); (2) abbreviation for heart yin deficiency syndrome/pattern (心阴虚证 [xīn yīn xū zhèng])

心阴不足 [xīn yīn bù zú]
insufficiency of heart yin: same as heart yin deficiency (心阴虚 [xīn yīn xū])

心阳虚 [xīn yáng xū]
heart yang deficiency: (1) pathological change referring to the diminution of the heart function in controlling blood and vessels, and in governing mental activities associated with deficiency of yang *qi* that causes cold manifestations, also called decline of heart yang (心阳不振 [xīn yáng bù zhèn] or insufficiency of heart yang (心阳不足 [xīn yáng bù zú]); (2) abbreviation for heart yang deficiency syndrome/pattern (心阳虚证 [xīn yáng xū zhèng])

心阳不振 [xīn yáng bù zhèn]
decline of heart yang: synonymous with heart yang deficiency (心阳虚 [xīn yáng xū])

心阳不足 [xīn yáng bù zú]
insufficiency of heart yang: synonymous with heart yang deficiency (心阳虚 [xīn yáng xū])

心阳暴脱 [xīn yáng bào tuō]
sudden collapse of heart yang: pathological change in which sudden prostration of heart yang leads to mental derangement, abnormal blood flow and collapse

心营过耗 [xīn yíng guò hào]
over-consumption of heart nutrient: pathological change in which the nutrient in the heart blood is excessively consumed by heat, causing emaciation, night fever, and vexation

痰蒙心神 [tán méng xīn shén]
phlegm clouding the mind: (1) pathological change caused by phlegm which clouds the mind, chiefly manifested by impairment of consciousnessor even coma accompanied by phlegmatic sounds in the throat; (2) abbreviation for syndrome/pattern of phlegm clouding the mind (痰蒙心神证 [tán méng xīn shén zhèng])

痰迷心窍 [tán mí xīn qiào]
phlegm misting the heart orifices: synonym for phlegm clouding the mind (痰蒙心神 [tán méng xīn shén])

热伤神明 [rè shāng shén míng]
heat damaging the mind: pathological change marked by damage of the mental activity by heat, same as heat entering the pericardium (热入心包 [rè rù xīn bāo])

痰蒙心包 [tán méng xīn bāo]
phlegm clouding the pericardium: pathological change marked by mental confusion caused by phlegm

心神失养 [xīn shén shī yǎng]
impaired preservation of the mind: pathological change that may lead to palpitations, dysphoria, insomnia and amnesia

神不守舍 [shén bù shǒu shè]
failure of the mind to keep to its abode:

pathological change that may cause insomnia and mental derangement

心火亢盛 [xīn huǒ kàng shèng]
exuberance of heart fire: pathological change in which exuberant fire of the heart causes mental disturbance, damage to fluid, and even bleeding

心火上炎 [xīn huǒ shàng yán]
heart fire flaming upward: pathological change in which fire flares upward along the heart meridian/channel, causing oral or lingual erosion

心火内炽 [xīn huǒ nèi chì]
internal blazing of heart fire: pathological change in which intense heat disturbs the mental activity, causing vexation, insomnia, throbbing palpitation, restlessness, or even mania

心火内焚 [xīn huǒ nèi fén]
internal deflagration of heart fire: same as internal blazing of heart fire (心火内炽 [xīn huǒ nèi chì])

痰火扰心 [tán huǒ rǎo xīn]
phlegm-fire harassing the heart: pathological change in which phlegm and fire disturb the function of the heart, leading to mental derangement or mania

水气凌心 [shuǐ qì líng xīn]
retained fluid attacking the heart: (1) pathological change caused by retained fluid which leads to disorder of the heart; (2) abbreviation for syndrome/pattern of retained fluid attacking the heart (水气凌心证 [shuǐ qì líng xīn zhèng])

心脾两虚 [xīn pí liǎng xū]
deficiency in both the heart and spleen: (1) pathological change characterized by deficiency of both heart blood and spleen *qi*; (2) abbreviation for deficiency syndrome/pattern of both the heart and spleen (心脾两虚证 [xīn pí liǎng xū zhèng])

心肾不交 [xīn shèn bù jiāo]
heart-kidney non-interaction: (1) pathological change characterized by breakdown of the normal physiological coordination between the heart and the kidney with excess of heart yang and deficiency of kidney yin; (2) abbreviation for heart-kidney non-interaction syndrome/pattern (心肾不交证 [xīn shèn bù jiāo zhèng])

心移热于小肠 [xīn yí rè yú xiǎo cháng]
heart shifting heat to the small intestine: pathological change characterized by transmission of pathological fire of the heart to the small intestine, resulting in rough painful voidings of urine or even hematuria

小肠虚寒 [xiǎo cháng xū hán]
small intestinal deficiency cold: pathological change in which consumption of yang *qi* in the small intestine impairs the latter's function in receiving food content from the stomach and separating the usable substances from the unusable

小肠实热 [xiǎo cháng shí rè]
small intestinal excess heat: (1) pathological change ascribed to shifting of the heart fire to the small intestine; (2) abbreviation for small intestinal excess heat syndrome/pattern (小肠实热证 [xiǎo cháng shí rè zhèng])

肺虚 [fèi xū]
lung deficiency: general term for deficiency conditions of the lung

肺实 [fèi shí]
lung excess: general term for excess conditions of the lung

肺热 [fèi rè]
lung heat: general term for heat conditions of the lung

肺热炽盛 [fèi rè chì shèng]
intense lung heat: (1) pathological change characterized by excessive pathogenic heat accumulated in the lung, also called accumulation of pathogenic heat in the lung (邪热壅肺 [xié rè yōng fèi]); (2) abbreviation for intense lung heat syndrome/pattern (肺热炽盛证 [fèi rè chì shèng zhèng])

邪热壅肺 [xié rè yōng fèi]
accumulation of pathogenic heat in the lung: synonymous with intense lung heat (肺热炽盛 [fèi rè chì shèng])

肺火 [fèi huǒ]
lung fire: (1) pathological change referring to intense heat in the lung, either of deficiency type or of excess type; (2) abbreviation for lung fire syndrome/pattern (肺火证 [fèi huǒ zhèng])

肺燥 [fèi zào]
lung dryness: general term for dryness of the lung due to either deficiency of yin fluid or due to the attack of pathogenic dryness, manifested by dry cough, dryness of the nasal cavity and pharynx, sore throat, thirst, hoarseness, hemoptysis, etc.

阴虚肺燥 [yīn xū fèi zào]
yin deficiency with lung dryness: (1) pathological change characterized by deficiency of yin fluid and dryness of the lung; (2) abbreviation for syndrome/pattern of yin deficiency with lung dryness (阴虚肺燥证 [yīn xū fèi zào zhèng])

肺肾两虚 [fèi shèn liǎng xū]
deficiency in both the lung and kidney: general term for deficiency conditions of both the lung and the kidney, such as deficiency of lung-kidney *qi* and deficiency of lung-kidney yin

肺肾阴虚 [fèi shèn yīn xū]
lung-kidney yin deficiency: (1) pathological change characterized by deficiency of yin fluid of the lung and kidney with harassment of endogenous heat; (2) abbreviation for lung-kidney yin deficiency syndrome/pattern (肺肾阴虚证 [fèi shèn yīn xū zhèng])

肺肾气虚 [fèi shèn qì xū]
lung-kidney *qi* deficiency: (1) pathological change characterized by dual deficiency of the lung *qi* and kidney *qi*; (2) abbreviation for lung-kidney *qi* deficiency syndrome/pattern (肺肾气虚证 [fèi shèn qì xū zhèng])

肺肾阳虚 [fèi shèn yáng xū]
lung-kidney yang deficiency: (1) pathological change characterized by decline of kidney yang with flooding of cold-water into the lung; (2) abbreviation for lung-kidney yang deficiency syndrome/pattern (肺肾阳虚证 [fèi shèn yáng xū zhèng])

水寒射肺 [shuǐ hán shè fèi]
water-cold attacking the lung: synonym for lung-kidney yang deficiency (肺肾阳虚 [fèi shèn yáng xū])

肝寒 [gān hán]
liver cold: (1) pathological change characterized by cold due to insufficiency of liver yang, with symptoms such as depression, timidity, lassitude, cold limbs, and deep and thready pulse; (2) stagnation of cold in the liver meridian/channel (cf. 寒滞肝脉 [hán zhì gān mài])

肝热 [gān rè]
liver heat: general term for various heat syndromes/patterns of the liver such as liver fire and ascendant hyperactivity of liver yang

肝火 [gān huǒ]
liver fire: pathological change caused by emotional upset with retention of heat in the liver meridian/channel

肝风 [gān fēng]
liver wind: (1) any pathological change of the liver caused by pathogenic wind; (2) abbreviation for internal stirring of liver wind (肝风内动 [gān fēng nèi dòng])

肝风内动 [gān fēng nèi dòng]
internal stirring of liver wind: pathological change characterized by arising of liver wind due to exuberant yang, intense heat-fire, or deficiency of yin-blood, often referred to simply as liver wind (肝风 [gān fēng])

肝阳化风 [gān yáng huà fēng]
liver yang transforming into wind: (1) pathological change of hyperactive liver yang that leads to the production of wind; (2) abbreviation for syndrome/pattern of liver yang transforming into wind (肝阳化风证 [gān yáng huà fēng zhèng])

热极生风 [rè jí shēng fēng]
extreme heat producing wind; extreme heat engendering wind: (1) pathological change characterized by convulsions that arise when exuberant heat scorches the liver meridian/channel and deprives the sinews/tendons of nourishment; (2) abbreviation for syndrome/pattern of extreme heat producing wind (热极生风证 [rè jí shēng fēng zhèng])

阴虚风动 [yīn xū fēng dòng]
yin deficiency with stirring wind: (1) pathological change of yin deficiency which stirs up endogenous wind; (2) abbreviation for syndrome/pattern of yin deficiency with stirring wind (阴虚动风证 [yīn xū dòng fēng zhèng])

肝郁 [gān yù]
liver depression; liver stagnation: abbreviation for liver *qi* depression or liver *qi* stagnation (肝气郁结 [gān qì yù jié])

肝气犯胃 [gān qì fàn wèi]
liver *qi* invading the stomach: (1) pathological change of the stomach due to invasion of the hyperactive liver *qi*; (2) abbreviation for syndrome/pattern of liver *qi* invading the stomach (肝气犯胃证 [gān qì fàn wèi zhèng])

肝胃不和 [gān wèi bù hé]
liver-stomach disharmony: synonymous with liver *qi* invading the stomach (肝气犯胃 [gān qì fàn wèi])

肝气犯脾 [gān qì fàn pí]
liver *qi* invading the spleen: (1) pathological change of the spleen due to invasion of the hyperactive liver *qi*; (2) abbreviation for syndrome/pattern of liver *qi* invading the spleen (肝气犯脾证 [gān qì fàn pí zhèng])

肝脾不和 [gān pí bù hé]
liver-spleen disharmony: synonymous with liver *qi* invading the spleen (肝气犯脾 [gān qì fàn pí])

肝郁脾虚 [gān yù pí xū]
liver depression and spleen insufficiency; liver stagnation and spleen insufficiency: (1) pathological change characterized by depressed liver activity of smoothing *qi* flow together with diminished transporting and transforming function of the spleen; (2) abbreviation for syndrome/pattern of liver depression/stagnation and spleen insufficiency (肝郁脾虚证 [gān yù pí xū zhèng])

寒滞肝脉 [hán zhì gān mài]
cold stagnating in the liver meridian/channel: (1) pathological change characterized by attack of pathogenic cold which stagnates in the liver meridian; (2) abbreviation for syndrome/pattern of cold stagnating in the liver meridian/channel (寒滞肝脉证 [hán zhì gān mài zhèng])

肝肾阴虚 [gān shèn yīn xū]
liver-kidney yin deficiency: (1) pathological change characterized by deficiency of yin fluid in the liver and kidney with harassment of endogenous heat; (2) abbreviation for liver-kidney yin deficiency syndrome/pattern (肝肾阴虚证 [gān shèn yīn xū zhèng])

胆气虚 [dǎn qì xū]
gallbladder *qi* deficiency: (1) pathological change characterized by insufficiency of the gallbladder *qi* that makes the mind uneasy with feeling of fear; (2) abbreviation for gallbladder *qi* deficiency syndrome/pattern (胆气虚证 [dǎn qì xū zhèng])

胆虚气怯 [dǎn xū qì qiè]
gallbladder insufficiency with timidity: same as gallbladder *qi* deficiency (胆气虚 [dǎn qì xū])

肝胆湿热 [gān dǎn shī rè]
liver-gallbladder dampness-heat: (1) pathological change characterized by accumulation of dampness-heat in the liver and gallbladder that interferes with their normal functions in smoothing *qi* flow and bile excretion; (2) abbreviation for liver-gallbladder dampness-heat syndrome/pattern (肝胆湿热证 [gān dǎn shī rè zhèng])

胆热 [dǎn rè]
gallbladder heat: pathological change ascribed to attack on the gallbladder and gallbladder meridian/channel by pathogenic heat

脾虚 [pí xū]
spleen deficiency: general term for deficiency conditions of the spleen, such as spleen *qi* deficiency, spleen yang deficiency, and spleen yin deficiency

脾气虚 [pí qì xū]
spleen *qi* deficiency: (1) pathological change characterized by *qi* deficiency

with impaired transforming and transporting function of the spleen, also called spleen *qi* insufficiency (脾气不足 [pí qì bù zú]); (2) abbreviation for spleen *qi* deficiency syndrome/pattern (脾气虚证 [pí qì xū zhèng])

脾气不足 [pí qì bù zú]
spleen *qi* insufficiency: same as spleen *qi* deficiency (脾气虚 [pí qì xū])

脾阴虚 [pí yīn xū]
spleen yin deficiency: (1) pathological change ascribed to deficiency of fluid in the spleen; (2) abbreviation for spleen yin deficiency syndrome/pattern (脾阴虚证 [pí yīn xū zhèng])

脾阳虚 [pí yáng xū]
spleen yang deficiency: (1) pathological change characterized by decline of the spleen yang with diminished warming action, also called spleen yang insufficiency (脾阳不振 [pí yáng bù zhèn]); (2) abbreviation for spleen yang deficiency syndrome/pattern (脾阳虚证 [pí yáng xū zhèng])

脾阳不振 [pí yáng bù zhèn]
spleen yang insufficiency: same as spleen yang deficiency (脾阳虚 [pí yáng xū])

脾失健运 [pí shī jiàn yùn]
dysfunction of the spleen in transportation: dysfunction of the spleen in transporting and transforming nutrients and water, resulting in dyspepsia, diarrhea, emaciation, lassitude and even edema of the limbs

脾不统血 [pí bù tǒng xuè]
spleen failing to control blood: pathological change of the spleen that usually results in chronic hemorrhage

脾虚湿困 [pí xū shī kùn]
spleen deficiency with dampness encumbrance: (1) pathological change characterized by insufficiency of the spleen *qi* leading to dampness retention, which, in turn, further impairs the transporting and transforming function of the spleen; (2) abbreviation for syndrome/pattern of spleen deficiency with dampness encumbrance (脾虚湿困证 [pí xū shī kùn zhèng])

湿热蕴脾 [shī rè yùn pí]
accumulation of dampness-heat in the spleen: (1) pathological change characterized by dysfunction of the spleen in transportation due to accumulation of dampness and dampness-heat transformed from the former; (2) abbreviation for syndrome/pattern of dampness-heat accumulating in the spleen (湿热蕴脾证 [shī rè yùn pí zhèng])

寒湿困脾 [hán shī kùn pí]
cold-dampness encumbering the spleen: (1) pathological change ascribed to the attack of cold-dampness which impairs the function of the spleen; (2) abbreviation for syndrome/pattern of cold-dampness encumbering the spleen (寒湿困脾证 [hán shī kùn pí zhèng])

湿困脾阳 [shī kùn pí yáng]
dampness encumbering spleen yang: pathological change characterized by invasion of dampness which impairs the spleen yang, giving rise to clinical manifestations similar to those due to

cold-dampness encumbering the spleen (寒湿困脾 [hán shī kùn pí])

湿阻中焦 [shī zǔ zhōng jiāo]
dampness obstructing the middle energizer: pathological change referring to retention of pathogenic dampness in the spleen and stomach, impairing their normal movement and function

脾气不升 [pí qì bù shēng]
spleen *qi* failing to ascend: dysfunction of the spleen in sending up nutrients, usually due to spleen *qi* deficiency, retention of dampness or stagnation of food

脾虚生风 [pí xū shēng fēng]
spleen deficiency generating wind: (1) pathological change ascribed to spleen *qi* deficiency which weakens the function of transportation and transformation, leading to malnutrition of the sinews, and subsequently inducing endogenous wind symptoms such as tremors, twitches or even convulsions; (2) abbreviation for syndrome/pattern of spleen deficiency with stirring of wind (脾虚动风证 [pí xū dòng fēng zhèng])

脾虚生痰 [pí xū shēng tán]
spleen deficiency generating phlegm: (1) pathological change characterized by retention of water-dampness and subsequent phlegm formation ascribed to spleen *qi* deficiency; (2) abbreviation for syndrome/pattern of spleen deficiency with phlegm-dampness (脾虚痰湿证 [pí xū tán shī zhèng])

脾胃虚寒 [pí wèi xū hán]
spleen-stomach deficiency cold: (1) pathological change characterized by decline of yang *qi* of the spleen and stomach with diminished warming and transporting activities, also known as spleen-stomach yang deficiency (脾胃阳虚 [pí wèi yáng xū]); (2) abbreviation for syndrome/pattern of spleen-stomach deficiency cold (脾胃虚寒证 [pí wèi xū hán zhèng])

脾胃阳虚 [pí wèi yáng xū]
spleen-stomach yang deficiency: same as spleen-stomach deficiency cold (脾胃虚寒 [pí wèi xū hán])

脾胃湿热 [pí wèi shī rè]
spleen-stomach dampness-heat: (1) pathological change ascribed to accumulation of dampness-heat in the spleen and stomach, which impairs the latters' function, also known as middle energizer dampness-heat (中焦湿热 [zhōng jiāo shī rè]); (2) abbreviation for spleen-stomach dampness-heat syndrome/pattern (脾胃湿热证 [pí wèi shī rè zhèng])

中焦湿热 [zhōng jiāo shī rè]
middle energizer dampness-heat: same as spleen-stomach dampness-heat (脾胃湿热 [pí wèi shī rè])

脾肺两虚 [pí fèi liǎng xū]
deficiency in both the spleen and lung: (1) pathological change characterized by *qi* deficiency of both the spleen and lung, also called spleen-lung *qi* deficiency (脾肺气虚 [pí fèi qì xū]); (2) abbreviation for deficiency syndrome/pattern of both the spleen and lung (脾肺两虚证 [pí fèi liǎng xū zhèng])

脾肺气虚 [pí fèi qì xū]

spleen-lung *qi* deficiency: same as deficiency in both the spleen and lung (脾肺两虚 [pí fèi liǎng xū])

脾肾阳虚 [pí shèn yáng xū]
spleen-kidney yang deficiency: (1) pathological change characterized by insufficient yang-*qi* of the spleen and kidney with endogenous cold, also called spleen-kidney deficiency cold (脾肾虚寒 [pí shèn xū hán]); (2) abbreviation for spleen-kidney yang deficiency syndrome/pattern (脾肾阳虚证 [pí shèn yáng xū zhèng])

脾肾虚寒 [pí shèn xū hán]
spleen-kidney deficiency cold: synonymous with spleen-kidney yang deficiency (脾肾阳虚 [pí shèn yáng xū])

胃虚 [wèi xū]
stomach deficiency: general term for deficiency conditions of the stomach

胃气虚 [wèi qì xū]
stomach *qi* deficiency: (1) pathological change characterized by weakness of the stomach *qi* with impairment of appetite and digestion; (2) abbreviation for stomach *qi* deficiency syndrome (胃气虚证 [wèi qì xū zhèng])

胃阳虚 [wèi yáng xū]
stomach yang deficiency: (1) pathological change characterized by decline of the yang *qi* which fails to warm the stomach, also called stomach deficiency cold (胃虚寒 [wèi xū hán]); (2) abbreviation for stomach yang deficiency syndrome/pattern (胃阳虚证 [wèi yáng xū zhèng])

胃虚寒 [wèi xū hán]
stomach deficiency cold: synonymous with stomach yang deficiency (胃阳虚 [wèi yáng xū]), and cf. stomach cold (胃寒 [wèi hán])

胃实寒 [wèi shí hán]
stomach excess cold: cf. stomach cold (胃寒 [wèi hán])

胃寒 [wèi hán]
stomach cold: a pathological change due to deficiency of stomach yang or caused by direct attack of pathogenic cold, the former being stomach deficiency cold, while the latter stomach excess cold

胃阴虚 [wèi yīn xū]
stomach yin deficiency: (1) pathological change characterized by deficiency of fluid in the stomach impairing the harmonizing and descending activities, also called stomach yin insufficiency (胃阴不足 [wèi yīn bù zú]); (2) abbreviation for stomach yin deficiency syndrome/pattern (胃阴虚证 [wèi yīn xū zhèng])

胃阴不足 [wèi yīn bù zú]
stomach yin insufficiency: same as stomach yin deficiency (胃阴虚 [wèi yīn xū])

胃热 [wèi rè]
stomach heat: pathological change due to impairment of the stomach by pathogenic heat or caused by overeating of hot pungent food, mainly manifested by thirst, foul breath, hyperorexia, oliguria with dark urine, constipation, and even ulceration of the mouth or gingivitis, also called heat in the stomach (胃中热 [wèi zhōng rè])

胃中热 [wèi zhōng rè]
heat in the stomach: same as stomach heat (胃热 [wèi rè])

胃热壅盛 [wèi rè yōng shèng]
intense stomach heat: (1) pathological change due to flaring up of stomach fire, marked by dire thirst and preference for cold drinks, foul breath, oral ulcer, toothache and gingivitis, also called intense stomach fire (胃火炽盛 [wèi huǒ chì shèng]) or up-flaming of stomach fire (胃火上炎 [wèi huǒ shàng yán]); (2) accumulation of pathogenic heat in the stomach and intestines seen in cases of epidemic febrile disease, marked by high fever, constipation, abdominal pain, and even delirium

胃火 [wèi huǒ]
stomach fire: intense stomach heat or fire accumulated in the stomach

胃火炽盛 [wèi huǒ chì shèng]
intense stomach fire: cf. intense stomach heat (胃热壅盛 [wèi rè yōng shèng])

胃火上炎 [wèi huǒ shàng yán]
up-flaming of stomach fire: cf. intense stomach heat (胃热壅盛 [wèi rè yōng shèng])

胃热消［杀］谷 [wèi rè xiāo (shā) gǔ]
stomach heat with accelerated digestion: pathological change ascribed to stomach heat which gives rise to accelerated digestion and a tendency to get hungry quickly

胃气不和 [wèi qì bù hé]
stomach *qi* disharmony: general term referring to various functional disorders of the stomach, also called stomach disharmony (胃不和 [wèi bù hé])

胃不和 [wèi bù hé]
stomach disharmony: same as stomach *qi* disharmony (胃气不和 [wèi qì bù hé])

胃气不降 [wèi qì bù jiàng]
stomach *qi* failing to descend: dysfunction of the stomach in sending down its contents, causing such symptoms as anorexia, nausea, vomiting, belching, and stuffiness over the epigastric region

胃失和降 [wèi shī hé jiàng]
impairment of gastric harmony and down-sending: same as stomach *qi* failing to descend (胃气不降 [wèi qì bù jiàng])

胃气上逆 [wèi qì shàng nì]
upward counterflow of stomach *qi*: pathological change of the stomach function that causes belching, hiccup, regurgitation, and vomiting

中气不足 [zhōng qì bù zú]
insufficiency of middle *qi*: deficiency of *qi* in the middle energizer, leading to general weakness and diminished transporting and transforming function of the spleen and stomach

中阳不振 [zhōng yáng bù zhèn]
devitalized middle yang: weakened yang in the middle energizer (the spleen and stomach), resulting in dyspepsia, vomiting, diarrhea, cold limbs, and sallow face, often seen in cases of chronic dyspepsia and chronic dysentery

肺气虚 [fèi qì xū]

lung *qi* deficiency: (1) pathological change characterized by diminished function of the lung in governing *qi* and defending the exogenous pathogens, also called lung *qi* insufficiency (肺气不足 [fèi qì bù zú]); (2) abbreviation for lung *qi* deficiency syndrome/pattern (肺气虚证 [fèi qì xū zhèng])

肺气不足 [fèi qì bù zú]

lung *qi* insufficiency: same as lung *qi* deficiency (肺气虚 [fèi qì xū])

肺阴虚 [fèi yīn xū]

lung yin deficiency: (1) pathological change characterized by insufficient lung yin with endogenous heat, also called lung yin insufficiency (肺阴不足 [fèi yīn bù zú]); (2) abbreviation for lung yin deficiency syndrome/pattern (肺阴虚证 [fèi yīn xū zhèng])

肺阴不足 [fèi yīn bù zú]

lung yin insufficiency: same as lung yin deficiency (肺阴虚 [fèi yīn xū])

肺阳虚 [fèi yáng xū]

lung yang deficiency: (1) pathological change characterized by insufficient lung yang with endogenous cold and diminished function of the lung, also called deficiency-cold of lung *qi* (肺气虚寒 [fèi qì xū hán]); (2) abbreviation for lung yang deficiency syndrome/pattern (肺阳虚证 [fèi yáng xū zhèng])

肺气虚寒 [fèi qì xū hán]

deficiency-cold of lung *qi*: same as lung yang deficiency (肺阳虚 [fèi yáng xū])

肺气不利 [fèi qì bù lì]

dysfunction of lung *qi*: disturbance of the functional activities of the lung, especially referring to its function in maintaining water metabolism, giving rise to oliguria and edema together with respiratory symptoms

肺气不宣 [fèi qì bù xuān]

lung *qi* failing in dispersion: impaired function of the lung in dispersion, generally attributable to external pathogens invading the lung or fettering the exterior, and manifested by cough, hoarse voice, and nasal congestion

肺津不布 [fèi jīn bù bù]

lung failing to distribute fluid: failure of the lung to distribute essence and fluid, leading to production of sputum and causing cough and asthma

肺失清肃 [fèi shī qīng sù]

lung failing in purification: one of the common mechanisms of lung disease that gives rise to cough, dyspnea, expectoration of sputum, fullness sensation in the chest, etc.

肺气上逆 [fèi qì shàng nì]

upward counterflow of lung *qi*: one of the common mechanisms of lung disease that causes cough, dyspnea and asthma

风寒袭肺 [fēng hán xí fèi]

wind-cold attacking the lung: (1) pathological change often occurring when wind-cold pathogen attacks on the superficies of the body as well as the lung, impairing the normal flow of lung *qi*, also called wind-cold fettering the lung (风寒束肺 [fēng hán shù fèi]); (2) abbreviation for syndrome/pattern of wind-cold attacking the lung (风寒袭肺证 [fēng hán xí fèi zhèng])

风寒束肺 [fēng hán shù fèi]
wind-cold fettering the lung: synonymous with wind-cold attacking the lung (风寒袭肺 [fēng hán xí fèi])

风热犯肺 [fēng rè fàn fèi]
wind-heat invading the lung: (1) pathological change characterized by wind-heat invasion of the lung and the superficies; (2) abbreviation for syndrome/pattern of wind-heat invading the lung (风热犯肺证 [fēng rè fàn fèi zhèng])

痰湿阻肺 [tán shī zǔ fèi]
phlegm-dampness obstructing the lung: (1) pathological change characterized by accumulation of phlegm-dampness that obstructs the lung, also called phlegm-turbidity obstructing the lung (痰浊阻肺 [tán zhuó zǔ fèi]); (2) abbreviation for syndrome/pattern of phlegm-dampness obstructing the lung (痰湿阻肺证 [tán shī zǔ fèi zhèng])

痰浊阻肺 [tán zhuó zǔ fèi]
phlegm-turbidity obstructing the lung: synonymous with phlegm-dampness obstructing the lung (痰湿阻肺 [tán shī zǔ fèi])

痰热闭肺 [tán rè bì fèi]
phlegm-heat blocking the lung: (1) pathological change characterized by accumulation of phlegm-heat that blocks the passage of lung *qi*; (2) abbreviation for syndrome/pattern of phlegm-heat blocking the lung (痰热闭肺证 [tán rè bì fèi zhèng])

热伤肺络 [rè shāng fèi luò]
heat damaging lung vessels: pathological change characterized by pathogenic heat that damages lung vessels and causes bloody sputum or hemoptysis

肺络损伤 [fèi luò sǔn shāng]
damage to lung vessels: pathological change marked by expectoration of blood from the respiratory tract

大肠传导失职 [dà cháng chuán dǎo shī zhí]
dysfunction of the large intestine in conveyance: pathological change that may cause diarrhea or constipation

大肠寒结 [dà cháng hán jié]
large intestinal cold accumulation: (1) pathological change characterized by accumulation of cold in the interior with constipation; (2) abbreviation for large intestinal cold accumulation syndrome/pattern (大肠寒结证 [dà cháng hán jié zhèng])

大肠热结 [dà cháng rè jié]
large intestinal heat accumulation: (1) pathological change characterized by exuberant heat accumulated in the large intestine that causes dryness and constipation, also called heat accumulation with intestinal dryness (热结肠燥 [rè jié cháng zào]); (2) abbreviation for large intestinal heat accumulation syndrome/pattern (大肠热结证 [dà cháng rè jié zhèng])

热结肠燥 [rè jié cháng zào]
heat accumulation with intestinal

dryness: same as large intestinal heat accumulation (大肠热结 [dà cháng rè jié])

大肠津［液］亏 [dà cháng jīn (yè) kuī]
large intestinal fluid depletion: (1) pathological change ascribed to insufficient fluid in the large intestine; (2) abbreviation for large intestinal fluid insufficiency syndrome/pattern (大肠津[液]亏证 [dà cháng jīn (yè) kuī zhèng])

大肠湿热 [dà cháng shī rè]
large intestinal dampness-heat: (1) pathological change characterized by accumulation of dampness-heat in the large intestine; (2) abbreviation for large intestinal dampness-heat syndrome/pattern (大肠湿热证 [dà cháng shī rè zhèng])

大肠实热 [dà cháng shí rè]
excess heat in the large intestine (meridian/channel): pathological change of the large intestine meridian/channel in which excessive heat in the meridian/channel causes fever, flushed face, cough, dyspnea, and fullness sensation in the abdomen

大肠虚寒 [dà cháng xū hán]
large intestinal deficiency cold: (1) pathological change characterized by diarrhea of deficiency-cold type; (2) abbreviation for large intestinal deficiency cold syndrome/pattern (大肠虚寒证 [dà cháng xū hán zhèng])

肾虚 [shèn xū]
kidney deficiency: a general term for deficiency conditions of the kidney

肾亏 [shèn kuī]
kidney insufficiency: synonymous with kidney deficiency (肾虚 [shèn xū])

精髓空虚 [jīng suǐ kōng xū]
essence-marrow depletion: pathological change ascribed to kidney insufficiency with deprivation of essence and marrow, usually manifested by dizziness, amnesia, poor intelligence, and even dementia

肾阳衰微 [shèn yáng shuāi wēi]
debilitation of kidney yang: severe case of kidney yang deficiency (cf. 肾阳虚 [shèn yáng xū])

肾火偏亢 [shèn huǒ piān kàng]
hyperactive kidney fire: relative excess of kidney fire due to deficiency of kidney yin, marked by hyperaphrodisia, insomnia and dream-disturbed sleep, also called effulgent life gate fire (命门火旺 [mìng mén huǒ wàng])

命门火旺 [mìng mén huǒ wàng]
effulgent life gate fire: same as hyperactive kidney fire (肾火偏亢 [shèn huǒ piān kàng])

肾气虚 [shèn qì xū]
kidney *qi* deficiency: (1) pathological change characterized by weakness of the kidney function in managing growth, development, reproduction, water metabolism, etc., also called kidney *qi* insufficiency (肾气不足 [shèn qì bù zú]); (2) abbreviation for kidney *qi* deficiency syndrome/pattern (肾气虚证 [shèn qì xū zhèng])

肾气不足 [shèn qì bù zú]
kidney *qi* insufficiency: same as kidney *qi* deficiency (肾气虚 [shèn qì xū])

肾气不固 [shèn qì bù gù]
insecurity of kidney *qi*: (1) pathological change characterized by diminished storing and astringing function of the kidney, also called insecurity of the lower origin (下元不固 [xià yuán bù gù]); (2) abbreviation for kidney *qi* insecurity syndrome/pattern (肾气不固证 [shèn qì bù gù zhèng])

下元不固 [xià yuán bù gù]
insecurity of the lower origin: synonym for insecurity of kidney *qi* (肾气不固 [shèn qì bù gù])

肾精不足 [shèn jīng bù zú]
kidney essence insufficiency: pathological change of the kidney due to congenital weakness, old age, and malnutrition or after protracted illness, causing retarded growth and development in children, delayed sexual development in adolescents, hypogonadism and impotence in adults, as well as impaired mentality, weak legs and slow reflexes

肾阴虚 [shèn yīn xū]
kidney yin deficiency: (1) pathological change caused by consumption of fluid and essence of the kidney in chronic diseases or due to intemperance in sexual life, also called kidney yin insufficiency (肾阴不足 [shèn yīn bù zú]), genuine yin insufficiency (真阴不足 [zhēn yīn bù zú]), kidney water insufficiency (肾水不足 [shèn shuǐ bù zú]), or depletion of the lower origin (下元亏损 [xià yuán kuī sǔn]); (2) abbreviation for kidney yin deficiency syndrome/pattern (肾阴虚证 [shèn yīn xū zhèng])

肾阴不足 [shèn yīn bù zú]
kidney yin insufficiency: same as kidney yin deficiency (肾阴虚 [shèn yīn xū])

真阴不足 [zhēn yīn bù zú]
genuine yin insufficiency: same as kidney yin deficiency (肾阴虚 [shèn yīn xū])

肾水不足 [shèn shuǐ bù zú]
kidney water insufficiency: same as kidney yin deficiency (肾阴虚 [shèn yīn xū])

下元亏损 [xià yuán kuī sǔn]
depletion of the lower origin: same as kidney yin deficiency (肾阴虚 [shèn yīn xū])

封藏失职 [fēng cáng shī zhí]
dysfunction in essence storage: failure of the kidney to preserve essence and control urination and defecation, causing spermatorrhea, premature ejaculation, incontinence of urine, frequent urination at night, and diarrhea before dawn

相火妄动 [xiàng huǒ wàng dòng]
frenetic stirring of the ministerial fire: hyperactivity of ministerial fire of the liver and kidney, usually due to deficiency of yin and resulting in dizziness, headache, tinnitus and irritability if the liver is chiefly involved, and feverish feeling in the chest, palms of the hands and soles of the feet, aching lumbus, and hyperaphrodisia if the kidney is chiefly involved

肾阳虚 [shèn yáng xū]
kidney yang deficiency: (1) pathological change characterized by insufficiency of kidney yang with diminished warming

function, also called kidney yang insufficiency (肾阳不足 [shèn yáng bù zú]) or original yang insufficiency (元阳亏虚 [yuán yáng kuī xū]); (2) abbreviation for kidney yang deficiency syndrome/pattern (肾阳虚证 [shèn yáng xū zhèng])

肾阳不足 [shèn yáng bù zú]
kidney yang insufficiency: same as kidney yang deficiency (肾阳虚 [shèn yáng xū])

元阳亏虚 [yuán yáng kuī xū]
original yang insufficiency: same as kidney yang deficiency (肾阳虚 [shèn yáng xū])

肾不纳气 [shèn bù nà qì]
kidney failing to receive *qi*: (1) pathological change in which deficiency of kidney *qi* leads to dyspnea with prolonged expiration; (2) abbreviation for syndrome/pattern of kidney failing to receive *qi* (肾不纳气证 [shèn bù nà qì zhèng])

肾阳虚衰 [shèn yáng xū shuāi]
debilitation of kidney yang: pathological change occurring in a severe case of kidney yang deficiency, which causes chronic diarrhea especially diarrhea daily before dawn, cold sensation in the back, edema of the legs, lowered sexual ability, and frequent micturition at night, also called 肾阳衰微 [shèn yáng shuāi wēi]

肾阳衰微 [shèn yáng shuāi wēi]
debilitation of kidney yang: same as 肾阳虚衰 [shèn yáng xū shuāi]

命门火衰 [mìng mén huǒ shuāi]
debilitation of the life gate fire: synonymous with debilitation of kidney yang (肾阳虚衰 [shèn yáng xū shuāi])

肾虚水泛 [shèn xū shuǐ fàn]
kidney deficiency with water flooding: (1) pathological change characterized by deficiency of kidney *qi* with impaired water metabolism and resultant flooding of retained fluid, referring to the formation of edema; (2) abbreviation for syndrome/pattern of kidney deficiency with water flooding (肾虚水泛证 [shèn xū shuǐ fàn zhèng])

膀胱不利 [páng guāng bù lì]
inhibited bladder: dysfunction of the bladder in storing and discharging urine that may cause frequency and urgency of urination, dribbling of urine, anuria or enuresis and incontinence of urine

膀胱气闭 [páng guāng qì bì]
blockage of bladder *qi*: pathological change of the urinary bladder that often causes difficulty in urination

膀胱失约 [páng guāng shī yuē]
failure of bladder retention: impaired bladder function resulting in incontinence of urine

脬气不固 [pāo qì bù gù]
insecurity of bladder *qi*: pathological change marked by loss of control of urination, such as enuresis and incontinence of urine

热积［结］膀胱 [rè jī (jié) páng guāng]
heat accumulation (retention) in the bladder: (1) pathological change in which the pathogenic factor of an acute febrile

disease is transformed into heat and accumulated in the urinary bladder; (2) abbreviation for bladder heat accumulation [retention] syndrome/pattern (热积〔结〕膀胱证 [rè jī〔jié〕páng guāng zhèng])

膀胱湿热 [páng guāng shī rè]
bladder dampness-heat; dampness-heat in the bladder: (1) pathological change ascribed to the accumulation of dampness-heat in the urinary bladder; (2) abbreviation for bladder dampness-heat syndrome/pattern (膀胱湿热证 [páng guāng shī rè zhèng])

膀胱虚寒 [páng guāng xū hán]
bladder deficiency cold; deficiency cold in the bladder: (1) pathological change characterized by impaired activities of the urinary bladder with cold manifestations due to consumption of kidney yang; (2) abbreviation for bladder deficiency cold syndrome/pattern (膀胱虚寒证 [páng guāng xū hán zhèng])

冲任损伤 [chōng rèn sǔn shāng]
damage to the thoroughfare and conception vessels: pathological change in cases of gynecological diseases, usually caused by infection, intemperance in sexual activity or frequent pregnancy, resulting in dysmenorrhea, pain in the lower abdomen and back, uterine bleeding, or abortion

冲任失［不］调 [chōng rèn shī (bù) tiáo]
disharmony of the thoroughfare and conception vessels: pathological change characterized by disordered function of the thoroughfare and conception vessels

冲任不固 [chōng rèn bù gù]
insecurity of the thoroughfare and conception vessels: pathological change in cases of gynecological diseases marked by loss of control of menstruation or preservation of the fetus by the thoroughfare and conception vessels, usually causing uterine bleeding or abortion

经隧失职 [jīng suì shī zhí]
dysfunction of meridian/channel passages: pathological change of meridians/channels that causes impeded circulation of *qi* and blood

经气逆乱 [jīng qì nì luàn]
derangement of meridian/channel *qi*: pathological change of meridians/channels in which counterflowing of meridian/channel *qi* leads to disordered circulation of *qi* and blood

经气郁滞 [jīng qì yù zhì]
stagnation of meridian/channel *qi*: pathological change of meridians/channels in which stagnant meridian/channel *qi* impedes the flow of *qi* and blood in the corresponding *zang-fu* organs

经气虚损 [jīng qì xū sǔn]
consumption of meridian/channel *qi*: pathological change in which consumption of meridian/channel *qi* leads to insufficiency of *qi* and blood of the corresponding *zang-fu* organs

经气衰竭 [jīng qì shuāi jié]
exhaustion of meridian/channel *qi*: critical pathological change characterized by complete consumption of meridian/channel *qi*

六经病机 [liù jīng bìng jī]
pathogeneses of six meridians/channels: collective term for the pathogeneses of *taiyang* (greater yang) disease, *shaoyang* (lesser yang) disease, *yangming* (yang brightness) disease, *taiyin* (greater yin) disease, *shaoyin* (lesser yin) disease and *jueyin* (reverting yin) disease

太阳病机 [tài yáng bìng jī]
pathogenesis of *taiyang* (greater yang) disease: pathogenesis involving exogenous attack of wind-cold on the *taiyang* (greater yang) meridian/channeland its confrontation with healthy *qi* at the superficial part of the human body

阳明病机 [yáng míng bìng jī]
pathogenesis of *yangming* (yang brightness) disease: pathogenesis involving attack of exogenous pathogen to the *yangming* (yang brightness) meridian/channel, marked by high fever and dryness-heat in the stomach and intestines

阳明腑实 [yáng míng fǔ shí]
excessiveness in yang brightness *fu*-organ: (1) pathological change ascribed to accumulation of pathogenic heat in yang brightness *fu*-organs (the stomach and large intestine), which consumes fluid and causes fever and constipation; (2) abbreviation for yang brightness *fu*-organ syndrome/pattern (阳明腑证 [yáng míng fǔ zhèng])

阳明燥热 [yáng míng zào rè]
dryness-heat in yang brightness (*fu*-organs): pathological change ascribed to accumulation of pathogenic heat in yang brightness *fu*-organs (the stomach and large intestine), which consumes fluid and causes high fever, profuse sweating and dire thirst

阳明虚寒 [yáng míng xū hán]
deficiency-cold in yang brightness (*fu*-organs): pathological change ascribed to decline of stomach yang with accumulation of endogenous cold, which impairs the normal functioning of the stomach

少阳病机 [shào yáng bìng jī]
pathogenesis of *shaoyang* (lesser yang) disease: pathogenesis involving attack of exogenous pathogen to the *shaoyang* (lesser yang) meridian/channel and its confrontation with healthy *qi* at the interspace in between the exterior and interior parts of the body

太阴病机 [tài yīn bìng jī]
pathogenesis of *taiyin* (greater yin) disease: pathogenesis involving attack of pathogen to the *taiyin* (greater yin) meridian/channel, marked by debilitation of spleen yang with accumulation of endogenous cold-dampness

少阴病机 [shào yīn bìng jī]
pathogenesis of *shaoyin* (lesser yin) disease: pathogenesis involving attack of pathogen to the *shaoyin* (lesser yin) meridian/channel, impairing the heart and kidney, marked by either heart-kidney yin deficiency or heart-kidney yang deficiency

少阴寒化 [shào yīn hán huà]
cold transformation of lesser yin: decline of yang in lesser yin syndrome/pattern with transformation of the pathogen into yin cold in the interior

少阴热化 [shào yīn rè huà]
heat transformation of lesser yin: decline of yin with exuberance of yang in lesser yin syndrome/pattern with transformation of the pathogen into heat in the interior

厥阴病机 [jué yīn bìng jī]
pathogenesis of *jueyin* (reverting yin) disease: pathogenesis involving attack of pathogen to the *jueyin* (reverting yin) meridian/channel, marked by interweaving of cold and heat or yin and yang in a critical case

厥热胜复 [jué rè shèng fù]
interweaving of cold and heat: pathological change ascribed to attack of pathogen to the *jueyin* (reverting yin) meridian/channel, manifested by alternate chills and fever

循经传 [xún jīng chuán]
sequential meridian/channel transmission: transmission of a disease from one meridian/channel to another, in the order of greater yang, yang brightness, lesser yang, greater yin, lesser yin and reverting yin meridians/channels

越经传 [yuè jīng chuán]
skip-over meridian/channel transmission: transmission of a disease from one meridian/channel to another with skipping of one or more neighboring meridians/channels, e.g., transmission from greater yang meridian/channel to lesser yang meridian/channel with yang brightness meridian/channel skipped over

表里传 [biǎo lǐ chuán]
exterior-interior transmission: transmission of a disease between two exterior-interiorly related meridians/channels, e.g., greater yang and lesser yin, yang brightness and greater yin, lesser yang and reverting yin

传经 [chuán jīng]
meridian/channel transmission: transmission of a disease from one meridian/channel to another, with respective change of symptoms

传变 [chuán biàn]
transmission and change: development of a disease, particularly referring to a cold damage disease

不传 [bù chuán]
non-transmission: no further development of a cold damage disease

变证 [biàn zhèng]
deteriorated syndrome/pattern: deterioration of a case due to improper medication or weakened body resistance

直中 [zhí zhōng]
direct attack: attack of exogenous pathogen directly on the three yin meridians/channels instead of transmission from the yang meridians/channels

常用引文 Commonly Used Citations 

诸风掉眩，皆属于肝。
[zhū fēng diào xuàn, jiē shǔ yú gān]
All wind diseases marked by tremor and vertigo are ascribed to the liver.

诸寒收引，皆属于肾。
[zhū hán shōu yǐn, jiē shǔ yú shèn]
All cold diseases marked by astringency and contraction are ascribed to the kidney.

诸气膹郁，皆属于肺。
[zhū qì fèn yù, jiē shǔ yú fèi]
All *qi* disorders marked by dyspnea and oppression are ascribed to the lung.

诸湿肿满，皆属于脾。
[zhū shī zhǒng mǎn, jiē shǔ yú pí]
All dampness diseases maked by swelling and fullness are ascribed to the spleen.

诸热瞀瘛，皆属于火。
[zhū rè mào chì, jiē shǔ yú huǒ]
All heat diseases marked by impaired consciousness and convulsion are ascribed to fire.

诸痛痒疮，皆属于心。
[zhū tòng yǎng chuāng, jiē shǔ yú xīn]
All painful and itching sores are ascribed to the heart.

诸厥固泄，皆属于下。
[zhū jué gù xiè, jiē shǔ yú xià]
All cases of cold extremities, retention and incontinence of feces or urine are ascribed to the lower (energizer).

诸痿喘呕，皆属于上。
[zhū wěi chuǎn ǒu, jiē shǔ yú shàng]
All cases of flaccidity, panting and vomiting are ascribed to the upper (energizer).

诸禁鼓栗，如丧神守，皆属于火。
[zhū jìn gǔ lì, rú sàng shén shǒu, jiē shǔ yú huǒ]
All cases of trismus with shivering chills and delirium are ascribed to fire.

诸痉项强，皆属于湿。
[zhū jìng xiàng jiàng, jiē shǔ yú shī]
All cases of spasm and neck rigidity are ascribed to dampness.

诸逆冲上，皆属于火。
[zhū nì chōng shàng, jiē shǔ yú huǒ]
All disorders with upward perversion are ascribed to fire.

诸胀腹大，皆属于热。
[zhū zhàng fù dà, jiē shǔ yú rè]
All cases of abdominal distension and fullness are ascribed to heat.

诸躁狂越，皆属于火。
[zhū zào kuáng yuè, jiē shǔ yú huǒ]
All cases of mental agitation and mania are ascribed to fire.

诸暴强直，皆属于风。
[zhū bào jiàng zhí, jiē shǔ yú fēng]
All cases of sudden muscular spasm and

rigidity are ascribed to wind.

诸病有声，鼓之如鼓，皆属于热。

[zhū bìng yǒu shēng, gǔ zhī rú gǔ, jiē shǔ yú rè]

All diseases of abdominal distension like a drum with borborygmi are ascribed to heat.

诸病胕肿，疼酸惊骇，皆属于火。

[zhū bìng fù zhǒng, téng suān jīng hài, jiē shǔ yú huǒ]

All diseases marked by swelling, soreness and fright are ascribed to fire.

诸转反戾，水液混浊，皆属于热。

[zhū zhuǎn fǎn lì, shuǐ yè hún zhuó, jiē shǔ yú rè]

All cases of cramps, opisthotonos, and turbid urine are ascribed to heat.

诸病水液，澄澈清冷，皆属于寒。

[zhū bìng shuǐ yè, chéng chè qīng lěng, jiē shǔ yú hán]

All diseases marked by thin, clear and watery discharge are ascribed to cold.

诸呕吐酸，暴注下迫，皆属于热。

[zhū ǒu tù suān, bào zhù xià pò, jiē shǔ yú rè]

All cases of acid eructation and spouting diarrhea with tenesmus are ascribed to heat.

邪之所凑，其气必虚。

[xié zhī suǒ còu, qí qì bì xū]

Where there is invasion of pathogen, there is deficiency of (defense) *qi*.

阴盛［胜］则寒。

[yīn shèng zé hán]

Preponderance of yin gives rise to a cold syndrome/pattern.

阳盛［胜］则热。

[yáng shèng zé rè]

Exuberance of yang gives rise to a heat syndrome/pattern.

阳虚则外寒。

[yáng xū zé wài hán]

Deficiency of yang brings on external cold.

阴虚则内热。

[yīn xū zé nèi rè]

Deficiency of yin brings on internal heat.

湿盛则濡泻。

[shī shèng zé rú xiè]

Excessive dampness causes soggy diarrhea.

气虚则寒。

[qì xū zé hán]

Deficiency of *qi* brings on cold.

热盛则肿。

[rè shèng zé zhǒng]

Exuberant heat brings on swelling.

久热伤阴。

[jiǔ rè shāng yīn]

Long-standing heat injures yin.

风盛则动。

[fēng shèng zé dòng]

Fierce wind produces involuntary movement.

湿盛阳微。

[shī shèng yáng wēi]

Excessive dampness makes yang decline.

寒极生热。

[hán jí shēng rè]

Extreme cold leads to heat.

热极生寒。

[rè jí shēng hán]

Extreme heat leads to cold.

少火生气。

[shǎo huǒ shēng qì]

Mild fire supplements *qi*.

壮火食气。

[zhuàng huǒ shí qì]

Vigorous fire consumes *qi*.

气有余便是火。

[qì yǒu yú biàn shì huǒ]

***Qi* in excess will turn into fire.**

百病（皆）生于气。

[bǎi bìng (jiē) shēng yú qì]

All diseases originate in *qi* disorders.

荣气虚则不仁。

[róng qì xū zé bù rén]

Deficiency of nutrient *qi* leads to numbness.

卫气虚则不用。

[wèi qì xū zé bù yòng]

Deficiency of defense *qi* results in flaccidity.

温邪上受，首先犯肺。

[wēn xié shàng shòu, shǒu xiān fàn fèi]

Attack of warm pathogen on the upper body usually starts from the lung (respiratory tract).

诊断学
Diagnostics

诊断学 [zhěn duàn xué]
diagnostics: the science and practice of diagnosis

诊断 [zhěn duàn]
diagnosis: determination of the nature of a disease and the state of health of the patient based on information collected through inspection, inquiry and examination

症状 [zhèng zhuàng]
symptom: abnormal phenomenon or change of condition arising from and accompanying a disease, and constituting an indication or evidence of the disease. In modern usage, the term usually refers to subjective evidence of disease or physical disturbance described by the patient.

征候 [zhēng hòu]
sign: objective evidence or indication of disease, specially observed by the physician

疾病 [jí bìng]；疾 [jí]；病 [bìng]
disease; illness; sickness: condition of being out of health. In ancient texts, 疾 [jí] means a mild disease while 病 [bìng], a severe one, but at present there is no longer such a difference.

诊病 [zhěn bìng]
disease identification: determination of the category of a disease, also called disease differentiation (辨病 [biàn bìng])

辨病 [biàn bìng]
disease differentiation: act of distinguishing one category of disease from others, synonymous with disease identification (诊病 [zhěn bìng])

辨证 [biàn zhèng]
syndrome differentiation; pattern identification: determination of the location, cause and nature of a disease as well as the trend of its development at a certain period of a case in light of traditional Chinese medical theories

证型 [zhèng xíng]
syndrome/pattern type: one of the commonly encountered and typical syndromes/patterns with a well-established name

证候 [zhèng hòu]
syndrome/pattern manifestation: manifestation of a syndrome/pattern, including symptoms and signs

诊籍 [zhěn jí]
case record: traditional term for the record of a patient's medical history, diagnosis and treatment

诊法 Diagnostic Methods

诊法 [zhěn fǎ]

diagnostic method: method of examining a patient and collecting information for diagnosis

四诊 [sì zhěn]

four examinations: collective term for inspection, auscultation-olfaction, interrogation (history taking) and palpation (including pulse taking)

望诊 [wàng zhěn]

inspection: visual observation in the course of a medical examination, including inspection of vitality, complexion, expression, behavior, body surface, tongue, excreta, secretions, etc.

望神 [wàng shén]

inspection of vitality: inspection of the state and power of living, especially the general condition of mental and physical activities such as consciousness, thinking, facial expression, speech, and response to external stimuli

得神 [dé shén]

presence of vitality: one's general state marked by fullness of vigor, with lustrous eyes, resonant voice, radiant face, easy breathing, and nimble movements

少神 [shǎo shén]

lack of vitality: one's general state marked by indifference and listlessness, with dull eyes, reluctance to talk, and slow movements, also called insufficiency of vital *qi* (神气不足 [shén qì bù zú])

神气不足 [shén qì bù zú]

insufficiency of vital *qi*: synonym for lack of vitality (少神 [shǎo shén])

失神 [shī shén]

loss of vitality: one's general state marked by apathy and inertness, with dim eyes, incoherent speech, difficulty in movement and even impaired consciousness

假神 [jiǎ shén]

false vitality: transient spiritedness in a critical case, often indicating impending death with manifestation of divorced yang

回光返照 [huí guāng fǎn zhào]

"last radiance of the setting sun": metaphor for momentary recovery of consciousness just before death

神昏 [shén hūn]

clouded consciousness: a form of mental state with impairment of the cognitive function and reduced or no awareness of the environment

神志不清 [shén zhì bù qīng]

unconsciousness: synonym for clouded consciousness (神昏 [shén hūn])

昏蒙 [hūn mēng]

mental confusion: clouding of consciousness with sleepiness, but responsive to calling, also known as 神志昏愦 [shén zhì hūn kuì] or 神识昏溃 [shén shí hūn kuì]

神志昏愦［溃］[shén zhì hūn kuì]
mental confusion: same as 昏蒙 [hūn mēng]

不省人事 [bù xǐng rén shì]
loss of consciousness: a state of unconsciousness from which the patient cannot be aroused

循衣摸床 [xún yī mō chuáng]
floccillation: aimless semiconscious fumbling and picking at the bedclothes by a critically ill patient, also called 捻衣摸床 [niǎn yī mō chuáng]

捻衣摸床 [niǎn yī mō chuáng]
floccillation: same as 循衣摸床 [xún yī mō chuáng]

神乱 [shén luàn]
mental disorder: derangement of the mind and abnormal mentality

谵妄 [zhān wàng]
delirium: disturbance of consciousness characterized by confusion, disordered speech, and hallucination

躁狂 [zào kuáng]
mania: a type of mental disorder characterized by expansiveness, elation, agitation, hyperactivity and hyperexcitability

烦躁 [fán zào]
vexation and agitation: vexation followed by agitation, either due to yang deficiency or yin excess

躁烦 [zào fán]
agitated vexation: agitation followed by vexation, seen in a critical case of yin deficiency

心中懊侬 [xīn zhōng ào náo]
distress in the heart: distressing heat sensation in the heart and chest

心烦 [xīn fán]
vexation: the state of being vexed, often indicating depressed heat in the heart

望色 [wàng sè]
inspection of the complexion: observation of the patient's skin color, luster and appearance, particularly of the face

气色 [qì sè]
complexion: natural color, luster and appearance of the face

面色 [miàn sè]
(facial) complexion: color and luster of the face, synonymous with气色 [qì sè]

常色 [cháng sè]
normal complexion: normal color of the skin of the face

主色 [zhǔ sè]
individual's normal complexion: one's normal natural color of the skin of the face

客色 [kè sè]
varied normal complexion: climatically varied normal natural color of the skin of the face

病色 [bìng sè]
morbid complexion: abnormal color of the face caused by disease

善色 [shàn sè]
favorable complexion: complexion indicating a favorable prognosis

恶色 [è sè]
unfavorable complexion: complexion indicating an unfavorable prognosis

面黄肌瘦 [miàn huáng jī shòu]
sallow complexion with emaciation: complexion often seen in a chronically debilitated patient with consumption of *qi* and blood

面色淡白 [miàn sè dàn bái]
pale white complexion: a colorless complexion often indicating blood deficiency or loss of blood

面色苍白 [miàn sè cāng bái]
pale complexion: a white complexion with a hint of blue or grey, often caused by yang collapse or exuberance of cold

面色㿠白 [miàn sè huàng bái]
bright pale complexion: a white complexion with puffiness, often seen in yang deficiency

面色黎黑 [miàn sè lí hēi]
darkish complexion: dark discoloration of the face, a complexion indicating kidney insufficiency, cold syndrome/pattern, or blood stasis

面黑 [miàn hēi]
darkish complexion: abbreviation for 面色黎黑 [miàn sè lí hēi]

面色萎黄 [miàn sè wěi huáng]
sallow complexion: yellowish withered complexion, which usually occurs in cases of spleen *qi* deficiency

面红 [miàn hóng]
reddened complexion: a complexion redder than normal, indicating the presence of heat

面尘 [miàn chén]
dusty complexion: dark-gray complexion as if covered with dust, which indicates latent pathogens in excess syndromes/patterns, and consumption of liver and kidney yin in deficiency syndromes/patterns

面浮 [miàn fú]
puffy face: a soft swollen face, usually indicating a deficiency condition

五色 [wǔ sè]
five colors: blue (or green), red, yellow, white and black, which, according to the theory of the five elements/phases, correspond to the liver (wood), heart (fire), spleen (earth), lung (metal) and kidney (water), respectively

青色 [qīng sè]
bluish discoloration: cyanosis of the skin or complexion, usually due to stagnant blood circulation, seen in cold syndrome/pattern, severe pain, *qi* stagnation, blood stasis and convulsions

黄色 [huáng sè]
yellow discoloration: Yellow complexion suggests deficiency in the spleen or presence of dampness; yellow discoloration of the whole body surface including the sclera, i.e., jaundice, signifies the presence of dampness-heat if the color is bright yellow, and the presence of cold-dampness if the color is dark yellow.

萎黄 [wěi huáng]
sallowness: sallow color of the skin,

especially the face, which usually occurs in cases of spleen *qi* deficiency

赤色 [chì sè]
red discoloration: Reddening of the complexion usually indicates the presence of heat.

白色 [bái sè]
white discoloration: White complexion usually indicates cold or deficiency.

黑色 [hēi sè]
black discoloration: Black or dark gray complexion is often seen in severe and chronic cases of blood stasis, pains, and kidney yang deficiency.

五色主病 [wǔ sè zhǔ bìng]
diagnostic significance of the five colors: (1) The five colors – blue (or green), red, yellow, white, and black, indicate disorders of the liver, heart, spleen, lung and kidney, respectively. (2) Blue suggests wind, cold, pain, convulsions, or blood stasis; red indicates the presence of heat; yellow reveals dampness; white implies deficiency of *qi* and blood or presence of cold; black indicates pain, exhaustion or blood stasis.

真脏色 [zhēn zàng sè]
true visceral color; visceral exhaustion color: color reflected in the face indicating exhaustion of essence and *qi* of *zang*-organs with unfavorable prognosis

望形体 [wàng xíng tǐ]
inspection of the physique: method of detecting the nature of a disease by inspection of the patient's stature, constitution and body pattern

形气相得 [xíng qì xiāng dé]
equilibrium between physique and *qi*: physique, i.e., shape and appearance, of the patient's body in coordination with *qi* movement, usually indicating a favorable prognosis

形气相失 [xíng qì xiāng shī]
disequilibrium between physique and *qi*: loss or lack of balance between the physique and *qi* movement, e.g., a thin weak body suffering exuberant stomach fire characterized by polyphagia and irascibility, usually indicating an unfavorable prognosis

形胜气 [xíng shèng qì]
physique predominating *qi*: disequilibrium between physique and *qi* with the former predominating, e.g., an abese person suffering shortness of breath

气胜形 [qì shèng xíng]
***qi* predominating physique:** disequilibrium between physique and *qi* with the latter predominating, e.g., an emaciated person suffering dyspnea with rapid breathing

大骨枯槁 [dà gǔ kū gǎo]
cachexia with withering bones: general physical wasting and malnutrition with a bony appearance

大肉陷下 [dà ròu xiàn xià]
emaciation with sagging flesh: a wasted condition of the body marked by loss of a large amount of flesh

破䐃脱肉 [pò jùn tuō ròu]
loss of bulk and shedding of flesh: severe emaciation, a sign of debilitation of spleen *qi*

望姿态 [wàng zī tài]
inspection of the posture: identifying a patient's condition by inspecting his (her) posture, gestures, and movements

仰卧伸足 [yǎng wò shēn zú]
lying supine with the legs outstretched: posture often taken by a patient with excessive heat

踡［蜷］卧缩足 [quán wò suō zú]
lying on one's side with the knees drawn up: posture often taken by a patient with deficiency cold

手足蠕动 [shǒu zú rú dòng]
wriggling of the extremities: a type of involuntary movement of the extremities, usually indicating stirring of internal wind due to yin deficiency

手足颤动 [shǒu zú chàn dòng]
trembling of the extremities: a type of involuntary movement of the extremities, often due to blood deficiency involving the sinews/tendons or chronic alcoholism, but sometimes being a premonitory sign of convulsions

项强 [xiàng jiàng]
rigidity of the neck: stiffness or inflexibility of the back of the neck

角弓反张 [jiǎo gōng fǎn zhāng]
opisthotonus: form of spasm consisting of extreme hyperextension of the body, with the head and the heels bent backward and the body bowed forward

转筋 [zhuàn jīn]
(I) cramp: sudden, violent, involuntary contraction of a muscle or a group of muscles; **(II) systremma:** cramp occurring in the muscles of the calf of a leg, also called 抽筋 [chōu jīn]

抽筋 [chōu jīn]
cramp; systremma: same as 转筋 [zhuàn jīn]

拘挛 [jū luán]
contracture: condition of high resistance to passive stretch of a muscle

拘急 [jū jí]
contraction: shortening of a muscle or muscles with increased tonicity

筋惕肉瞤 [jīn tì ròu rún]
muscular twitching: short spastic muscular contractions

身瞤动 [shēn rún dòng]
twitching of the body: sudden rapid involuntary movement of the body

刚痉 [gāng jìng]
tonic convulsions: convulsions accompanied by rigidity of the neck and even opisthotonos, occurring in cases of febrile diseases

口㖞 [kǒu wāi]
wry mouth: deviation of the angle of the mouth to one side

口眼㖞斜 [kǒu yǎn wāi xié]
deviated eye and mouth: deviation of

one eye and the mouth to one side with the eye unable to close and salivation from the homolateral corner of the mouth, a sign indicating attack of wind-phlegm to meridian/channel

审苗窍 [shěn miáo qiào]
inspection of the signal orifices: inspection of the eyes, ears, nose, mouth and tongue which can indicate changes in the *zang-fu* organs

望目 [wàng mù]
inspection of the eye: inspection including observation of the luster, color, appearance, and motility of the eye, not only for diagnosing eye diseases, but also for determining the condition of *zang-fu* organs

察目 [chá mù]
examination of the eye: synonym for inspection of the eye (望目 [wàng mù])

目窠上微肿 [mù kē shàng wēi zhǒng]
puffiness of the eyelids: an early sign of edematous disease

目下有卧蚕 [mù xià yǒu wò cán]
"sleeping silkworm beneath the eye": swollen lower eyelids, a sign of edema due to spleen insufficiency

目胞浮肿 [mù bāo fú zhǒng]
edema of the eyelids: a sign of edema due to spleen insufficiency, as the eyelids pertain to the spleen

目下肿 [mù xià zhǒng]
edema under the eyes: synonym for "sleeping silkworm beneath the eye" (目下有卧蚕 [mù xià yǒu wò cán])

目窠肿 [mù kē zhǒng]
edema of the eye sockets: synonym for edema of the eyelids (目胞浮肿 [mù bāo fú zhǒng])

两眼无光 [liǎng yǎn wú guāng]
lusterless eyes: eyes without luster and sluggish in motion, often seen in a seriously ill person

神光耗散 [shén guāng hào sàn]
spiritless eyes: eyes without spirit, dull, clouded and inflexible in motion, often seen in a critically ill person

眼珠干涩 [yǎn zhū gān sè]
dryness and discomfort of the eyes: a condition of the eyes that lack secretion and tears, indicating consumption of body fluids in cases of febrile diseases

眼珠牵斜 [yǎn zhū qiān xié]
strabismus; squint: deviation of the eye which the patient cannot overcome

眼珠塌陷 [yǎn zhū tā xiàn]
sunken eyes: a sign indicating consumption of body fluids or deficiency of *qi* and blood

眼窝凹陷 [yǎn wō āo xiàn]
sunken eye sockets: same as sunken eyes (眼珠塌陷 [yǎn zhū tā xiàn])

眼球突出 [yǎn qiú tū chū]
protrusion of the eyeball; exophthalmos: a sign indicating obstruction of the lung by phlegm-turbidity if there is accompanying dyspnea, and indicating accumulation of phlegm and *qi* if there is accompanying goiter

瞪目直视 [dèng mù zhí shì]
staring straight ahead: looking fixedly straight ahead, a sign that indicates the patient is critically ill, particularly when there is loss of consciousness as well

横目斜视 [héng mù xié shì]
staring sideways: looking fixedly towards one side, a sign often occurring in cases of stirring-up of liver wind

两眼翻上 [liǎng yǎn fān shàng]
supraduction: upward rotation of the eyes around the horizontal axis

胞睑下垂 [bāo jiǎn xià chuí]
blepharoptosis: drooping of one or both upper eyelids

昏睡露睛 [hūn shuì lù jīng]
lethargic sleeping with the eyes open: a sign indicating failure of the spleen and stomach in children with consumption of body fluids due to severe vomiting and diarrhea

白睛色诊 [bái jīng sè zhěn]
inspection of the white of the eye: observing change in color of the white of the eye, e.g., redness in cases of lung fire or external contraction of wind-heat, and yellowness in cases of jaundice

白睛发黄 [bái jīng fā huáng]
yellow discoloration of the white of the eye: yellow pigmentation of the sclera, a major sign of jaundice

白睛红赤 [bái jīng hóng chì]
red discoloration of the white of the eye: congestion of the bulbar conjunctiva, a sign usually indicating attack of wind-heat to the eye(s)

望耳 [wàng ěr]
inspection of the ear: diagnostic method to detect not only local pathological changes but also the general condition of the internal organs, particularly that of the kidney and gallbladder

耳轮淡白 [ěr lún dàn bái]
pale helices: pale rims of the ears, frequently seen in cases of deficiency of *qi* and blood

耳轮红肿 [ěr lún hóng zhǒng]
red swollen helices: red and swollen rims of the ears, seen in cases of dampness-heat of the liver and gallbladder or attack of heat toxin

耳轮青黑 [ěr lún qīng hēi]
bluish dark helices: bluish dark rims of the ears, usually seen in cases of excessive interior cold or severe pain

耳轮干枯 [ěr lún gān kū]
withering of the helices: dried shriveled ears, a sign of extreme consumption of kidney yin

耳轮萎缩 [ěr lún wěi suō]
atrophy of the helices: wasting away of the ears, a sign indicating exhaustion of kidney *qi* in a critical case

耳轮甲错 [ěr lún jiǎ cuò]
scaly dry helices: dry ears as if covered with scales, a sign of blood stasis

望鼻 [wàng bí]
inspection of the nose: a diagnostic

method to detect the pathological changes of the lung, spleen, stomach, and other visceral organs, which involves the inspection of the color, form, structure and discharge of the nose

鼻翼煽动 [bí yì shān dòng]
flaring of the nares: a sign indicating dyspnea

鼻流清涕 [bí liú qīng tì]
thin nasal discharge: discharge of thin mucus from the nose, a symptom that usually occurs in cases of wind-cold

鼻流浊涕 [bí liú zhuó tì]
turbid nasal discharge: discharge of thick and turbid mucus from the nose, a symptom that usually occurs in cases of wind-heat

久流浊涕 [jiǔ liú zhuó tì]
chronic turbid nasal discharge: discharge of thick and turbid mucus from the nose for a long duration, a symptom that frequently appears in cases of nasal sinusitis

鼻不闻香臭 [bí bù wén xiāng chòu]
loss of smell: partial or total loss of the ability to smell

鼻色主病 [bí sè zhǔ bìng]
indications of the color of the nose: Blue, yellow, white, red and grey indicate abdominal pain, dampness-heat in the interior, loss of blood, heat in the spleen and lung, and retention of fluid, respectively.

鼻出血 [bí chū xuè]
nosebleed: bleeding from the nose

鼻衄 [bí nǜ]
epistaxis: bleeding from the nose, same as nosebleed (鼻出血 [bí chū xuè])

舌诊 [shé zhěn]
tongue diagnosis: diagnosis made according to the information obtained by inspection of the tongue

望舌 [wàng shé]
inspection of the tongue: one of the most important examinations for diagnosis, in which the tongue proper and its coating are carefully observed

舌象 [shé xiàng]
tongue manifestations: changes in the appearance of the tongue, including the color and form of the tongue proper as well as those of its coating

舌的分部 [shé de fēn bù]
partition of the tongue: The tongue is usually divided into the tip, middle, root and borders, revealing the physiological and pathological conditions of the heart and lung, spleen and stomach, kidney, and liver and gallbladder, respectively.

舌尖 [shé jiān]
tip of the tongue: the anterior end of the tongue, often reflecting the condition of the heart and lung

舌边 [shé biān]
margin of the tongue: the lateral edge of the tongue, often reflecting the condition of the liver and gallbladder

舌中 [shé zhōng]
middle of the tongue: the central part of

the tongue, often reflecting the condition of the spleen and stomach

舌心 [shé xīn]
center of the tongue: same as middle of the tongue (舌中 [shé zhōng])

舌根 [shé gēn]
root of the tongue: the part of the tongue that is attached basally to the bone, often reflecting the condition of the kidney

舌本 [shé běn]
base of the tongue: same as root of the tongue (舌根 [shé gēn])

舌体 [shé tǐ]
tongue body; tongue proper: the tongue itself, in contradistinction to the tongue coating

舌质 [shé zhì]
tongue texture: the muscular and vascular structure of the tongue

舌神 [shé shén]
tongue spirit: the general vitality of the tongue manifested in luxuriance or emaciation

荣枯老嫩 [róng kū lǎo nèn]
luxuriant, withered, tough and tender-soft: a collective term to describe four different states of the appearance of the tongue. A luxuriant tongue is moistened and fresh red in color; a withered tongue is dull, dark, dry and shriveled; a tough tongue is firm with a rough texture; a tender-soft tongue is delicate with a fine texture.

舌下脉络 [shé xià mài luò]
sublingual collateral vessel: the vein under the tongue on either side of the frenulum

舌色 [shé sè]
tongue color: color of the tongue body, which reflects the condition of *qi* and blood and functional state of the *zang-fu* organs

淡红舌 [dàn hóng shé]
light red tongue: tongue of normal color

淡白舌 [dàn bái shé]
pale tongue: tongue less red than normal, indicating *qi* and blood deficiency or yang deficiency, also called 舌淡 [shé dàn]

舌淡 [shé dàn]
pale tongue: same as 淡白舌 [dàn bái shé]

红舌 [hóng shé]
red tongue: tongue redder than normal, indicating the presence of heat

舌红 [shé hóng]
red tongue: same as 红舌 [hóng shé]

绛舌 [jiàng shé]
crimson tongue: tongue dark red in color, indicating the presence of intense heat, also called 舌绛 [shé jiàng]

舌绛 [shé jiàng]
crimson tongue: same as 绛舌 [jiàng shé]

紫舌 [zǐ shé]
purple tongue: tongue purple in color, indicating impaired circulation of *qi* and blood

青舌 [qīng shé]
blue tongue: tongue blue in color, indicating congealing cold with blood stasis

舌青紫 [shé qīng zǐ]
cyanosis of the tongue: bluish purple discoloration of the tongue due to blood stasis, penetration of toxic heat into nutrientblood, or *qi* stagnation with sluggish blood flow, also called cyanotic tongue (青紫舌 [qīng zǐ shé])

青紫舌 [qīng zǐ shé]
cyanotic tongue: same as cyanosis of the tongue (舌青紫 [shé qīng zǐ])

舌有瘀点 [shé yǒu yū diǎn]
tongue with purple spots: presence of purple spots on the tongue, a sign of blood stasis

舌有瘀斑 [shé yǒu yū bān]
tongue with ecchymosis: presence of black-and-blue or purple spot or area on the tongue, indicating blood stasis

舌形 [shé xíng]
form of the tongue: a collective term referring to the appearance or condition of the tongue, including the shape, luxuriance oremaciation, toughness or softness, thinness or thickness due to swelling of the tongue as well as the presence of spots, fissures and dental indentations

瘦薄舌 [shòu báo shé]
thin tongue: tongue thinner than normal, usually due to deficiency of *qi* and blood if the tongue is thin and pale, and due to yin deficiency if it is thin and red

胖大舌 [pàng dà shé]
enlarged tongue: tongue larger than normal, usually due to accumulation of fluid, often seen in cases of deficiency of *qi* or yang

舌胖 [shé pàng]
plump tongue: synonym for enlarged tongue (胖大舌 [pàng dà shé])

舌体胖大 [shé tǐ pàng dà]
plump tongue body: synonym for enlarged tongue (胖大舌 [pàng dà shé])

肿胀舌 [zhǒng zhàng shé]
swollen tongue: reddened tongue distended and larger than normal, often caused by exuberant fire of the heart and spleen or externally contracted dampness-heat, but sometimes by congenital vascular anomaly

齿痕舌 [chǐ hén shé]
tooth-marked tongue: tongue with dental indentations on its edges, seen in cases of retention of water-dampness when the tongue is enlarged as well, also called 舌有齿痕 [shé yǒu chǐ hén]

舌有齿痕 [shé yǒu chǐ hén]
tongue with teeth-marks: same as 齿痕舌 [chǐ hén shé]

点刺舌 [diǎn cì shé]
spotted tongue: tongue with red spots formed by swollen fungiform papillae, indicating the presence of exuberant heat

舌起芒刺 [shé qǐ máng cì]
prickles on the tongue: thorn-like protruding swollen fungiform papillae formed on the surface of the tongue

芒刺舌 [máng cì shé]
prickly tongue: tongue with thorn-like protrusions on its surface, indicating the presence of exuberant heat

裂纹舌 [liè wén shé]
fissured tongue: tongue with fissures on its surface, often indicating consumption of fluids or yin

舌裂 [shé liè]
fissure of the tongue: appearance of fissures on the surface of the tongue, cf. fissured tongue (裂纹舌 [liè wén shé])

舌肿 [shé zhǒng]
swelling of the tongue: abnormal enlargement of the tongue, usually red in color, cf. swollen tongue (肿胀舌 [zhǒng zhàng shé])

重舌 [chóng shé]
double tongue: hypertrophy of bilateral sublingual glands resembling a smaller tongue lying under the original one

舌态 [shé tài]
motility of the tongue: the ability of the tongue to move spontaneously

强硬舌 [jiàng yìng shé]
stiff tongue: tongue difficult to move freely, seen in cases of high fever with impairment of consciousness or loss of fluid, and also in cases of apoplexy, also known as 舌强 [shé jiàng]

舌强 [shé jiàng]
stiff tongue: same as 强硬舌 [jiàng yìng shé]

舌謇 [蹇] [shé jiǎn]
sluggish tongue: curling tongue, sluggish in motion with difficulty in speaking

颤动舌 [chàn dòng shé]
trembling tongue: tongue that involuntarily trembles as it moves, a sign of wind caused by deficiency of *qi* and blood, stirred up by extreme heat, or transformed from liver yang, also known as 舌战 [shé zhàn]

舌战 [shé zhàn]
trembling tongue: same as 颤动舌 [chàn dòng shé]

痿软舌 [wěi ruǎn shé]
flaccid tongue: tongue that is flabby and cannot move easily, seen in cases of impairment of yin or deficiency of *qi* and blood

舌痿 [shé wěi]
flaccid tongue: same as 痿软舌 [wěi ruǎn shé]

歪斜舌 [wāi xié shé]
deviated tongue: tongue that deviates to one side when extended, indicating the presence of liver wind with phlegm or obstruction of the meridian/channel by phlegm and stagnant blood

舌歪 [shé wāi]
deviated tongue: same as 歪斜舌 [wāi xié shé])

短缩舌 [duǎn suō shé]
contracted tongue: tongue that cannot be fully extended from the mouth and appears to be contracted, usually seen in critically

ill patients

舌短 [shé duǎn]
shortened tongue: synonym for contracted tongue (短缩舌 [duǎn suō shé])

舌卷囊缩 [shé juǎn náng suō]
curled tongue and retracted testicles: formation of the tongue into a curl and retraction of the testicles into the body, a sign that may occur in a critical case of febrile disease or the case of apoplexy

木舌 [mù shé]
wooden tongue: swollen, hard tongue resembling a piece of wood, seen in infantile glossitis

吐舌 [tǔ shé]
protruding tongue: tongue that extends out of the mouth with licking of the lips

弄舌 [nòng shé]
waggling tongue: tongue which moves from one side to the other when extended, or moves without stopping

吐弄舌 [tǔ nòng shé]
protruding and waggling of tongue: tongue that extends out of the mouth and moves from one side to the other without stopping, a sign seen in children with defective development of the brain, also in cases of febrile diseases with stirring-up of wind

舌苔 [shé tāi]
tongue coating; tongue fur: a layer of mosslike material covering the tongue, inspection of which can provide information about the nature, depth and location of the pathogenic factor, the strength and integrity of healthy *qi*, and the degree of fluid consumption

苔色 [tāi sè]
tongue coating/fur color: the color of tongue coating/fur, which reflects not only the heat or cold nature of the condition, but also the interior or exterior characteristics and degree of penetration of the disease

白苔 [bái tāi]
white (tongue) coating/fur: indication of the presence of cold, but thin white coating/fur often seen in persons of normal health

黄苔 [huáng tāi]
yellow (tongue) coating/fur: indication of the presence of heat

薄白苔 [báo bái tāi]
thin white (tongue) coating/fur: often seen in persons of normal health or at early stage of an exterior syndrome/pattern

薄黄苔 [báo huáng tāi]
thin yellow (tongue) coating: often seen in cases of exterior heat syndrome/pattern or early stage of interior heat

白腻苔 [bái nì tāi]
white greasy (tongue) coating/fur; white slimy (tongue) coating/fur: indication of accumulation of dampness-phlegm or retained food

黄腻苔 [huáng nì tāi]
yellow greasy (tongue) coating/fur; yellow slimy (tongue) coating/fur: tongue coating/fur indicating accumulation

of dampness-heat, phlegm-heat or retained food with heat

黑苔 [hēi tāi]
black (tongue) coating/fur: tongue coating/fur indicating either excessive cold if the coating/fur is moistened and the tongue proper pale, or extreme heat if the coating is dry and the tongue proper reddened

灰苔 [huī tāi]
gray (tongue) coating/fur: tongue coating/fur with similar clinical significance as black (tongue) coating/fur (黑苔 [hēi tāi])

染苔 [rǎn tāi]
stained (tongue) coating/fur: tongue coating/fur that is stained, often by food or medicine

薄苔 [báo tāi]
thin (tongue) coating/fur: tongue coating/fur, through which the surface of the underlying tongue proper is faintly visible

厚苔 [hòu tāi]
thick (tongue) coating/fur: tongue coating/fur, through which the underlying tongue proper's surface is not visible

润苔 [rùn tāi]
moist (tongue) coating/fur: tongue coating/fur that is moderately wet

燥苔 [zào tāi]
dry (tongue) coating/fur: tongue coating/fur that both looks and feels dry, indicating damage to body fluids

腐苔 [fǔ tāi]
curdy (tongue) coating/fur: tongue coating/fur consisting of coarse granules like bean dregs, capable of being wiped off, reflecting retention of food in the stomach

腻苔 [nì tāi]
greasy (tongue) coating/fur; slimy (tongue) coating/fur: dense, sticky, slimy tongue coating/fur, thick in the center, thin on the sides, and hard to wipe off, indicating the presence of phlegm-dampness or stagnancy of food

滑苔 [huá tāi]
slippery (tongue) coating/fur: moist tongue coating/fur with excessive fluid and an oily appearance, indicating the presence of dampness

糙苔 [cāo tāi]
rough coating/fur: very dry tongue coating/fur that both looks rough and feels rough when touched, indicating severe damage to body fluids

白砂苔 [bái shā tāi]
white sandy (tongue) coating/fur: white, thick and dry tongue coating/fur as rough as sand, indicating rapid transformation of heat into dryness with severe impairment of body fluids as the prelude to yellow coating

剥苔 [bō tāi]
peeling coating/fur: patchy tongue coating interspersed with furless areas

舌苔脱落 [shé tāi tuó luò]
peeling of the tongue coating/fur: complete or partial peeling of tongue coating/fur,

usually due to impairment of stomach *qi*, consumption of stomach yin, deficiency of *qi* and blood, or general debility

光剥舌 [guāng bō shé]
peeled tongue: tongue with its coating suddenly peeled, usually indicative of exhaustion of stomach yin and severe damage to stomach *qi*

镜面舌 [jìng miàn shé]
mirror tongue: completely peeled tongue resembling a mirror, indicating collapse of stomach *qi* or exhaustion of stomach yin

有根苔 [yǒu gēn tāi]
rooted (tongue) coating/fur: tongue coating/fur with root, closely attached to the surface of the tongue

无根苔 [wú gēn tāi]
rootless (tongue) coating/fur: tongue coating/fur without root, which can be easily wiped or scraped off

口唇干裂 [kǒu chún gān liè]
dry cracked lips: a sign of impairment of body fluids by dryness-heat or yin deficiency, also called cracked lips (唇裂 [chún liè])

唇裂 [chún liè]
cracked lips: same as dry cracked lips (口唇干裂 [kǒu chún gān liè])

口角流涎 [kǒu jiǎo liú xián]
drooling from the corner of the mouth: excessive flow of saliva from the corner of the mouth, often due to spleen dampness or stomach heat in children, or appearing in stroke patients with wry mouth

口唇糜烂 [kǒu chún mí làn]
erosion of the lips: a sign indicating upward streaming of accumulated heat in the spleen and stomach

口噤 [kǒu jìn]
lockjaw: inability to open the mouth, mainly caused by liver wind, and seen in cases of convulsive diseases and tetanus

口撮 [kǒu cuō]
pursed mouth: the mouth with puckered lips, like the mouth of a fish, a sign of infantile convulsions, also called 撮口 [cuō kǒu]

撮口 [cuō kǒu]
pursed mouth: same as 口撮 [kǒu cuō]

口僻 [kǒu pì]
wry mouth: deviation of the mouth, also known as 口㖞 [kǒu wāi]

口振 [kǒu zhèn]
trembling mouth: involuntary trembling of the lips, a sign of a violent struggle between healthy and pathogenic *qi*

口动 [kǒu dòng]
moving mouth: one that opens and closes frequently and involuntarily, signifying weakness of stomach *qi*

唇紫 [chún zǐ]
purple lips: lips having the mixed color of blue and red, a sign of blood stasis in patients with decline of heart yang and severe dyspnea, also called cyanotic lips (口唇青紫 [kǒu chún qīng zǐ])

口唇青紫 [kǒu chún qīng zǐ]
cyanotic lips: same as purple lips (唇紫 [chún zǐ])

望齿 [wàng chǐ]
inspection of the teeth: including the gums, not only for diagnosing local illness, but also for detecting diseases of internal organs, particularly disorders of the kidney and stomach, and impairment of body fluids

齿燥 [chǐ zào]
dry teeth: dry-looking, lusterless teeth, especially the two front teeth, a sign of excessive fire in the lung and stomach, with severe consumption of fluid in acute cases, or serious impairment of kidney yin in chronic cases

齿槁 [chǐ gǎo]
withered teeth: dry and old-looking teeth, a sign of exhaustion of kidney yin, seen in cases of febrile diseases at the late stage

齿焦 [chǐ jiāo]
parched teeth: extremely dry teeth, a sign of severe loss of fluid in critical cases

齿衄 [chǐ nǜ]
bleeding gums: bleeding from the gums irrelevant to trauma

齿摇 [chǐ yáo]
loose teeth: often suggesting kidney deficiency

齿龈肿痛 [chǐ yín zhǒng tòng]
painful gum swelling: often indicating excessive heat in the stomach

望痰 [wàng tán]
inspection of sputum: examination of the color, quality and quantity of the sputum to detect the conditions of the visceral organs and features of pathogenic factors

痰稀白 [tán xī bái]
thin white sputum: phlegm of cold nature

痰如泡沫 [tán rú pào mò]
frothy sputum: sputum with small bubbles on its surface, usually indicating the presence of cold

痰多 [tán duō]
profuse sputum: sputum produced in large amounts, usually indicating dampness, also known as abundant expectoration (痰盛 [tán shèng])

痰盛 [tán shèng]
abundant expectoration: same as profuse sputum (痰多 [tán duō])

痰黄 [tán huáng]
yellow sputum: phlegm of heat nature

咯血 [kǎ xuè]
hemoptysis: expectoration of blood or blood-stained sputum

咳血 [ké xuè]
coughing blood: bringing-up of blood or bloody sputum when coughing, synonymous with hemoptysis (咯血 [kǎ xuè])

血痰 [xuè tán]
bloody sputum: sputum containing blood, also known as blood-stained sputum (痰中带血 [tán zhōng dài xuè])

痰中带血 [tán zhōng dài xuè]
blood-stained sputum: same as 血痰 [xuè tán]

血丝痰 [xuè sī tán]
blood-streaked sputum: sputum containing blood streaks

望指纹 [wàng zhǐ wén]
inspection of finger venules: a diagnostic method for infants, in which the extension and color of the superficial venules on the palmar side of the index finger are examined and taken as reference for diagnosis, e.g., red venules with yellowish tint, faintly visible, not extending beyond the proximal segment of the finger indicating health; deep red venules suggesting the presence of heat; dark venules signifying blood stasis; purple and blue venules often occurring in conditions of convulsions and pain

三关 [sān guān]
three passes: collective term for the three segments of the index finger used for measuring the extension of the visible venules, i.e., "wind pass" (proximal segment), "*qi* pass" (middle segment) and "life pass" (distal segment). Venules only visible at "wind pass" usually indicate a mild disease. The farther the venules extend, the more serious the case.

风关 [fēng guān]
wind pass: the proximal segment of the index finger, a term in the inspection of finger venules

气关 [qì guān]
***qi* pass:** the middle segment of the index finger, a term in the inspection of finger venules

命关 [mìng guān]
life pass: the distal segment of the index finger, a term in the inspection of finger venules

透关射甲 [tòu guān shè jiǎ]
extension through the passes toward the nail: extension of visible venules through the wind, *qi* and life passes toward the nail, often indicating that the child is critically ill, also known as shooting through the passes to the nail (通关射甲 [tōng guān shè jiǎ])

通关射甲 [tōng guān shè jiǎ]
shooting through the passes to the nail: same as extension through the passes toward the nail (透关射甲 [tòu guān shè jiǎ])

望皮肤 [wàng pí fū]
inspection of the skin: an examination not only for skin diseases, but also for the condition of *qi*, blood and visceral organs

肿胀 [zhǒng zhàng]
swelling: abnormal protuberance or distension of a body part or area

水肿 [shuǐ zhǒng]
edema: an abnormal excess accumulation of fluid under the skin, often showing prolonged manifestation of the pits produced by pressure

脚肿 [jiǎo zhǒng]
swollen feet: edema of the lower extremities, a sign of yin edema

跗肿 [fū zhǒng]
instep edema: edema of the upper surface of the foot in front of the ankle joint

发黄 [fā huáng]
yellow discoloration: condition in which the skin and the whites of the eyes become abnormally yellow, usually indicating jaundice

黄胖 [huáng pàng]
yellow puffiness: yellow tinge of the skin with puffy face and ankle edema

斑 [bān]
macule: deep red or dark purple spot on the skin that is not elevated above the surface and does not fade under pressure

阳斑 [yáng bān]
yang macule: macula red-purple in color, accompanied by fever and other manifestations of excess heat, often occurring in cases of epidemic febrile diseases

阴斑 [yīn bān]
yin macule: macula dark purple in color, accompanied by pallor, cold limbs and other manifestations of deficiency cold, often due to spleen insufficiency or decline of yang

疹 [zhěn]
(I) rash: eruption on the skin; **(II) papule:** a small circumscribed, superficial, solid elevation of the skin, which fades upon pressure; **(III) measles**

斑疹 [bān zhěn]
maculo-papule; macule and papule: collective term for skin eruptions in a generalized disease

水疱 [shuǐ pào]
vesicle: small circumscribed epidermal elevation containing fluid

白痦 [bái pēi]
miliaria alba: skin eruption of fine white crystalline vesicles appearing on the neck and chest, and sometimes on the limbs, in the course of acute febrile diseases

晶痦 [jīng pēi]
miliaria crystalline; sudamina: fine white crystalline vesicles appearing on the skin surface due to the retention of sweat

肌肤甲错 [jī fū jiǎ cuò]
encrusted skin: dry, rough and scaly skin, usually indicating blood stasis

须发早白 [xū fà zǎo bái]
premature whitening of the hair: whitening of the hair happening before the proper age

闻诊 [wén zhěn]
auscultation and olfaction; listening and smelling examination: The Chinese character 闻 has dual meanings – hearing and smelling.

闻声音 [wén shēng yīn]
auscultation; listening to the sounds: listening to the patient's voice, sounds of breathing, coughing, vomiting, retching, etc., as a method to determine cold, heat, deficiency or excess nature of a disease

语声 [yǔ shēng]
voice: sounds made by a person speaking

语声重浊 [yǔ shēng zhòng zhuó]
deep turbid voice: change of voice due to nasal congestion in case of catching cold

声重 [shēng zhòng]
abbreviation for deep turbid voice (语声重浊 [yǔ shēng zhòng zhuó])

语声低微 [yǔ shēng dī wēi]
faint low voice: change of voice in a deficiency condition

嘶嗄 [sī shà]
hoarseness: rough and harsh voice

声嗄 [shēng shà]
hoarseness: same as 嘶嗄 [sī shà]

失音 [shī yīn]
loss of voice: failure to speak above a whisper

喑［瘖］[yīn]
aphonia: same as loss of voice (失音 [shī yīn])

谵语 [zhān yǔ]
delirious speech: disordered speech in delirium

郑声 [zhèng shēng]
unconscious murmuring: unconscious halting murmuring with frequent repetition, a sign of consumption of heart *qi* with mental confusion

独语 [dú yǔ]
soliloquy: talking during the absence of others, a sign of insufficient heart *qi* with mental derangement

错语 [cuò yǔ]
paraphrasia; paraphasia: a type of dysphasia in which the patient frequently employs wrong words or uses words in wrong and senseless combinations, and is aware of the mistakes after uttering them

呓语 [yì yǔ]
somniloquy: talking in one's sleep, often caused by heart fire, gallbladder heat or disharmonious stomach *qi*

狂言 [kuáng yán]
manic raving: mentally deranged wild talk with furious, incoherent and irrational utterances, seen in cases of mania

语言謇涩 [yǔ yán jiǎn sè]
sluggish speech: speech distorted by sluggish and discoordinated movements of the tongue

呼吸 [hū xī]
breathing; respiration: the process of drawing air into and expelling it from the lung

呼吸气粗 [hū xī qì cū]
heavy breathing: respiration with obvious breathing sound, often indicating an excess condition

呼吸气微 [hū xī qì wēi]
feeble breathing: very weak breathing, often indicating deficiency of lung and kidney *qi*

喘 [chuǎn]
dyspnea; panting: difficult or labored breathing

喘逆 [chuǎn nì]
dyspnea with reversed flow of *qi*: complex expression of dyspnea (喘 [chuǎn])

上气 [shàng qì]
(I) abnormal rising of *qi*: dyspnea with quick breaths due to obstruction of the airway which causes counterflow of air; **(II) upper *qi*:** *qi* of the upper portion of the body, including *qi* of the heart and lung

短气 [duǎn qì]
shortness of breath: panting with quick breaths, occurring both in deficiency and excess conditions

少气 [shǎo qì]
shortage of *qi*: synonymous with feeble breathing (呼吸气微 [hū xī qì wēi]), occurring only in a deficiency condition

咳逆上气 [ké nì shàng qì]
cough with reversed ascent of *qi*: cough and dyspnea with quick breaths due to obstruction of the airway by phlegm

不得偃卧 [bù dé yǎn wò]
inability to lie flat: dyspnea relieved by assuming an upright from a recumbent position

喘促 [chuǎn cù]
panting: labored breathing with short quick breaths, also called 喘急 [chuǎn jí]

喘急 [chuǎn jí]
panting: same as 喘促 [chuǎn cù]

喘鸣 [chuǎn míng]
wheezing dyspnea: difficult and labored breathing with a continuous sound in the airway, also called 哮 [xiào]

哮 [xiào]
wheezing: synonymous with wheezing dyspnea (喘鸣 [chuǎn míng])

痰鸣 [tán míng]
phlegm rale: abnormal breathing sound produced by the presence of phlegm in the airway

太息 [tài xī]
sighing: taking a deep breath and then letting it out audibly. Frequent sighing indicates stagnation of liver *qi*.

善太息 [shàn tài xī]
frequent sighing: cf. sighing (太息 [tài xī])

咳嗽 [ké sòu]
cough: (1) sudden noisy expulsion of air from the lung, resulting from failure of lung *qi* in descending, abnormal ascending or rushing up of lung *qi* or phlegm in the air passage; (2) disease in which cough is the main manifestation

咳声重浊 [ké shēng zhòng zhuó]
deep dull cough: cough that sounds heavy and harsh, indicating excess syndrome/pattern of the lung

咳声清脆 [ké shēng qīng cuì]
clear crisp cough: cough that indicates dryness-heat

咳声不扬 [ké shēng bù yáng]
muffled cough: indistinct cough, usually due to the presence of thick phlegm in the air passage, indicating heat syndrome/pattern of the lung

咳如犬吠 [ké rú quǎn fèi]

barking cough: sharp and harsh cough, specifically in cases of inflammation of the throat, particularly diphtheria

干咳 [gān ké]

dry cough: cough with little or no sputum, indicating lung dryness or yin deficiency

久咳 [jiǔ ké]

chronic cough: long-lasting or continually recurring cough, also called 久嗽 [jiǔ sòu]

久嗽 [jiǔ sòu]

chronic cough: synonym for 久咳 [jiǔ ké]

嗅气味 [xiù qì wèi]

smelling odors: one of the diagnostic methods with special attention to unusual smells from the secretions and excretions of a patient

腥臭气 [xīng chòu qì]

stink: offensive smell as given off from stools in cases of steatorrhea or from cancerous discharge

口气 [kǒu qì]

mouth odor; smell of breath: often referring to a bad breath smell

口臭 [kǒu chòu]

halitosis: fetid breath, often indicating stomach heat, dyspepsia, tooth decay or unclean oral cavity

口气臭秽 [kǒu qì chòu huì]

offensive breath smell: bad smell of breath that often indicates the presence of stomach heat

口气酸臭 [kǒu qì suān chòu]

sour breath: abnormal smell of breath that indicates dyspepsia

十问 [shí wèn]

ten questions: the ten questions recommended by Zhang Jie-bin (1563-1640) for a physician to ask of the patient while making a diagnosis: about (1) chills and fever; (2) perspiration; (3) head and body; (4) stool and urine; (5) food and drink; (6) chest and abdomen; (7) hearing; (8) thirst; (9) past illnesses; and (10) cause of present illness. In addition, inquiry should be made into the efficacy of medicine taken previously, about menstruation in the case of women, and history of smallpox and measles in the case of children.

问诊 [wèn zhěn]

inquiry: an important way of gaining information for diagnosis by inquiring of the patient the complaints and the history of the illness

问起病 [wèn qǐ bìng]

inquiry about the onset of illness: inquiry about the course of the illness, including the time of onset, predisposing factors, chief complaints, treatment and effects

问现证 [wèn xiàn zhèng]

inquiry about the present illness: cf. "ten questions" (十问 [shí wèn])

问寒热 [wèn hán rè]

inquiry about cold and heat: inquiring of the patient details of the sensations of cold and heat

恶热 [wù rè]

aversion to heat: strong dislike of heat, one of the manifestations of externally contracted febrile diseases, but sometimes also occurring in the case of internal injuries such as yin deficiency with endogenous heat or stomach fire

畏寒 [wèi hán]

intolerance of cold: sensation of cold which can be relieved by wearing more clothes or warming oneself near a source of heat

恶寒 [wù hán]

aversion to cold; chill: sensation of cold which cannot be relieved by warmth

憎寒 [zēng hán]

abhorrence of cold: strong aversion to cold

寒战 [hán zhàn]

rigor: tremor caused by a chill

战栗 [zhàn lì]

shiver: fit of trembling, often followed by high fever

恶风 [wù fēng]

aversion to wind: strong dislike of wind, a symptom often resulting from contraction of external pathogenic wind

恶寒发热 [wù hán fā rè]

aversion to cold with fever; chills and fever: simultaneous appearance of aversion to cold and fever

发热恶寒 [fā rè wù hán]

fever with chills: a common symptom of various externally contracted febrile diseases, in which chills usually precede fever, and disappear when the fever starts, but sometimes may persist together with the fever

但热不寒 [dàn rè bù hán]

fever without chills: elevation of the body temperature with no feeling of cold, a symptom usually caused by interior heat

但寒不热 [dàn hán bù rè]

chills without fever: feeling of cold with no fever, a symptom usually caused by interior cold, either of excess type or of deficiency type

寒热往来 [hán rè wǎng lái]

alternating chills and fever: condition in which fever and chills attack alternately

身热 [shēn rè]

generalized fever: elevation of the body temperature or feverish feeling all over the body

发热 [fā rè]

fever: elevation of the body temperature above the normal or subjective feeling of feverishness

壮热 [zhuàng rè]

high fever: remarkable elevation of the body temperature, usually persistent and without chills

灼热 [zhuó rè]

burning fever: high fever with a burning sensation or with the patient's skin hot to the touch

烦热 [fán rè]
vexing fever: fever accompanied by uneasiness and restlessness

微热 [wēi rè]
mild fever: low-grade fever, often occurring in certain cases of internal damage or at the late stage of warm diseases

潮热 [cháo rè]
tidal fever: fever with periodic rise and fall of the body temperature at fixed hours of the day, like the tide

日晡潮热 [rì bū cháo rè]
late afternoon (tidal) fever: fever more marked at 3-5 p.m.

午后潮热 [wǔ hòu cháo rè]
afternoon (tidal) fever: fever occurring in the afternoon

五心烦热 [wǔ xīn fán rè]
vexing heat in the chest, palms and soles: feeling of heat in the chest, the palms of the hands and soles of the feet accompanied by uneasiness and restlessness, a common symptom of the following conditions: (1) consumptive diseases with deficiency of yin or blood with exuberant endogenous fire, (2) persistent asthenic fire as a sequela of febrile diseases, and (3) stagnation of internal fire-heat

手足心热 [shǒu zú xīn rè]
feverish sensation in the palms and soles: cf. vexing heat in the chest, palms and soles (五心烦热 [wǔ xīn fán rè])

身热不扬 [shēn rè bù yáng]
submerged fever: fever which is not easily felt on the body surface and usually requires extended palpation by the physician, a sign of dampness-heat

问汗 [wèn hàn]
inquiry about sweating: asking about the patient's condition of sweating

多汗 [duō hàn]
(I) excessive sweating; hyperhidrosis: generalized or localized excessive sweating, not related to a hot environment or physical exertion; **(II) profuse sweating:** same as 大汗 [dà hàn]

自汗 [zì hàn]
spontaneous sweating: excessive sweating during the daytime with no apparent cause (such as hot weather, thick clothing, etc.) or upon the slightest physical exertion

盗汗 [dào hàn]
night sweats: sweating that occurs during sleep and ceases upon awakening, a symptom frequently occurring in cases of yin deficiency with endogenous heat

大汗 [dà hàn]
profuse sweating: sweating in large amounts which may cause excessive loss of body fluids, also known as 多汗 [duō hàn]

大汗淋漓 [dà hàn lín lí]
great dripping sweating: abnormal profuse sweating with continuous dripping

热汗 [rè hàn]
hot sweats: sweating in the case of a yang

syndrome/pattern, also called yang sweats (阳汗 [yáng hàn])

阳汗 [yáng hàn]
yang sweats: synonymous with hot sweats (热汗 [rè hàn])

冷汗 [lěng hàn]
cold sweats: profuse sweating accompanied by cold body and limbs and hardly perceivable pulse, a sign of exhaustion of yang

战汗 [zhàn hàn]
shivery sweating: sweating following shivering in the course of a febrile disease, indicating a violent struggle between healthy and pathogenic *qi*, which may lead either to subsidence of fever and then recovery, or to collapse

漏汗 [lòu hàn]
leaking sweating: abnormal incessant sweating

脱汗 [tuō hàn]
collapse sweating: profuse sweating associated with collapse

绝汗 [jué hàn]
expiry sweating: incessant profuse sweating of a patient in a moribund state

头汗 [tóu hàn]
sweating head: profuse sweating only on the head, face and neck

额汗 [é hàn]
sweating forehead: sweating most marked on the forehead

半身汗出 [bàn shēn hàn chū]
hemihidrosis: sweating only on the upper or lower, right or left half of the body, usually due to disharmony of *qi* and blood

半身无汗 [bàn shēn wú hàn]
hemilateral anhidrosis: abnormal absence of sweating on the upper or lower, right or left half of the body

手足汗 [shǒu zú hàn]
sweating hands and feet: excessive local sweating from the hands and feet

手足心汗 [shǒu zú xīn hàn]
sweating palms and soles: excessive sweating from the palms of the hands and soles of the feet, often indicating heat in the yin meridians/channels

心汗 [xīn hàn]
precordial sweating: excessive sweating in the precordial region

腋汗 [yè hàn]
armpit sweating: excessive local sweating in the armpit

阴汗 [yīn hàn]
(I) genital sweating: localized sweating in the genital region, particularly the scrotum; **(II) yin sweats:** another name for cold sweats (冷汗 [lěng hàn])

无汗 [wú hàn]
absence of sweating; anhidrosis: abnormal deficiency or absence of sweating

油汗 [yóu hàn]
oily sweat: sticky sweat like oil, also known as 汗出如油 [hàn chū rú yóu]

汗出如油 [hàn chū rú yóu]
oily sweat: same as 油汗[yóu hàn]

问头身 [wèn tóu shēn]
inquiry about the head and body: obtaining information through inquiry about the patient's head and body, especially headache and generalized pain

头痛 [tóu tòng]
headache: pain in the head

头项强痛 [tóu xiàng jiàng tòng]
headache and painful stiff neck: headache accompanied by rigidity and pain of the nape of the neck

头重 [tóu zhòng]
heavy-headedness: subjective feeling of heaviness in the head

头重脚轻 [tóu zhòng jiǎo qīng]
heavy head and light feet: subjective sensation whereby the head feels heavy and the feet light, accompanied by unsteady gait

头风 [tóu fēng]
head wind: chronic or recurrent headache, also called 脑风 [nǎo fēng]

脑风 [nǎo fēng]
brain wind: same as head wind (头风 [tóu fēng])

偏头痛 [piān tóu tòng]
hemilateral headache: pain on one side of the head

偏头风 [piān tóu fēng]
hemilateral head wind; migraine: recurrent unilateral severe headache

眩晕 [xuàn yūn]
(I) dizziness: sensation of unsteadiness with a feeling of movement within the head; **(II) vertigo:** illusory sense that either the environment or one's own body is revolving

瞑眩 [míng xuàn]
dimness of vision: temporary dimness of vision with vexation – a side-effect of drug therapy

眩冒 [xuàn mào]
dizziness with dimmed vision: sensation of unsteadiness with dimness of vision

掉眩 [diào xuàn]
dizziness with shaking: dizziness with shaking of the extremities – a symptom indicating the presence of liver wind

徇蒙招尤 [xùn méng zhāo yóu]
dizziness with dimmed vision and shaking: a symptom indicating disorder of the liver

健忘 [jiàn wàng]
forgetfulness: diminished ability to recall facts and events

胸痛 [xiōng tòng]
chest pain: pain in the chest

胁痛 [xié tòng]
hypochondriac pain: pain in the hypochondriac region, unilateral or bilateral

脘痛 [wǎn tòng]
epigastric pain: pain in the epigastric region

腹痛 [fù tòng]
abdominal pain: pain in the abdomen

身痛 [shēn tòng]
generalized pain: pain involving the whole body

身重 [shēn zhòng]
heavy body: subjective heaviness sensation of the body with difficulty in movement

身痒 [shēn yǎng]
generalized itching: itching all over the body

阴痒 [yīn yǎng]
pruritus vulvae: itching of the vulva

肌肤麻木 [jī fū má mù]
numbness of the skin: reduced sensibility to touch of the skin, also called insensitivity of the skin (肌肤不仁 [jī fū bù rén])

肌肤不仁 [jī fū bù rén]
insensitivity of the skin: synonymous with numbness of the skin (肌肤麻木 [jī fū má mù])

腰痛 [yāo tòng]
lumbar pain; lumbago: pain in the lumbar region

腰酸；腰痠 [yāo suān]
lumbar aching: continual dull pain and discomfort in the lumbar region, as distinct from lumbar pain which usually denotes more acute pain

背痛 [bèi tòng]
back pain: pain in the posterior part of the upper trunk

肩痛 [jiān tòng]
shoulder pain: pain in the shoulder

肩臂酸痛 [jiān bì suān tòng]
aching shoulder and arm: aching in the shoulder and arm, often due to contraction of pathogenic wind, cold and dampness

肩不举 [jiān bù jǔ]
inability to lift the shoulder and arm: a symptom often caused by attack of wind-dampness, injury or strain

痹痛 [bì tòng]
arthralgia: joint pain due to invasion of pathogenic wind, cold and/or dampness

乳房疼痛 [rǔ fáng téng tòng]
breast pain: pain in the breast, usually accompanied by feeling of distension

阴器痛 [yīn qì tòng]
genital pain: pain in the genitals

足跟痛 [zú gēn tòng]
heel pain: pain in either or both heels, worsened by standing and walking

胀痛 [zhàng tòng]
distending pain: pain accompanied by a distending sensation, a symptom caused by *qi* stagnation

闷痛 [mèn tòng]
stuffy pain: pain accompanied by feeling of stuffiness

刺痛 [cì tòng]
stabbing pain: sharp pain as if caused by a stab, usually due to blood stasis

酸［痠］痛 [suān tòng]
aching pain: continuous dull pain as the sensation produced by prolonged physical exertion

走窜痛 [zǒu cuàn tòng]
scurrying pain: pain which repeatedly changes its location, often occurring in the chest and abdomen

窜痛 [cuàn tòng]
scurrying pain: same as 走窜痛 [zǒu cuàn tòng]

游走痛 [yóu zǒu tòng]
wandering pain: pain in extremity joints with repeated changes of location

固定痛 [gù dìng tòng]
fixed pain: pain fixed in location, often due to blood stasis when it occurs in the chest and abdomen, and due to obstruction by cold-dampness when it occurs in the limbs and joints

痛无定处 [tòng wú dìng chù]
pain of unfixed location: pain whose location is not fixed

冷痛 [lěng tòng]
cold pain: pain accompanied by a cold sensation and relieved by warmth, often due to obstruction of collaterals by cold pathogen or insufficiency of yang *qi*

灼痛 [zhuó tòng]
burning pain: pain accompanied by a burning sensation, often due to attack of pathogenic fire

绞痛 [jiǎo tòng]
colicky pain: acute pain in the chest or abdomen, usually due to obstruction of *qi* movement by pathogenic cold or by a solid such as calculus

隐痛 [yǐn tòng]
dull pain: pain often continuous but not felt sharply

重痛 [zhòng tòng]
heavy pain: pain associated with a sensation of heaviness, frequently occurring when *qi* movement is obstructed by dampness

掣痛 [chè tòng]
pulling pain; dragging pain: pain in one part involving other parts along a meridian

空痛 [kōng tòng]
empty pain: pain associated with a sensation of emptiness, mostly occurring in the head or lower abdomen, often due to deficiency of *qi*, blood and essence

麻木 [má mù]
numbness: reduced sensitivity to touch

不仁 [bù rén]
insensitivity: loss of sensation to touch

问渴饮 [wèn kě yǐn]
inquiry about thirst and drink: asking the patient about his/her desire for drinks and condition of fluid intake

口渴 [kǒu kě]
thirst: feeling of dryness in the mouth

with a desire to drink water, a symptom often occurring in cases of dryness and heat syndromes/patterns

口渴引饮 [kǒu kě yǐn yǐn]
thirst with frequent drinking: a sign of consumption of body fluids

口渴喜冷 [kǒu kě xǐ lěng]
thirst with preference for cold drinks: sign of consumption of body fluids by excessive heat

口干 [kǒu gān]
dry mouth: lack of fluid in the mouth, usually but not necessarily associated with thirst, i.e., a desire to drink water

口干不欲饮 [kǒu gān bù yù yǐn]
dryness in the mouth with no desire to drink: symptom occurring in cases of spleen insufficiency with retention of dampness

烦渴 [fán kě]
vexing thirst: dire thirst with desire for voluminous drinking

问二便 [wèn èr biàn]
inquiry about stools and urine: obtaining information about change of stools and urine through inquiry

问大便 [wèn dà biàn]
inquiry about stools: inquiry about constipation, diarrhea, contents of stools, condition of defecation, etc.

大便秘结 [dà biàn bì jié]
constipation: abnormally delayed or infrequent evacuation of dry hardened feces, also called 不更衣 [bù gēng yī] as a euphemism

便秘 [biàn mì]
constipation: abbreviation for 大便秘结 [dà biàn mì jié]

不更衣 [bù gēng yī]
"no clothes-changing": an ancient euphemistic expression for constipation. It is so said because in ancient China *toilet* was called *clothes-changing room*, obselete in modern Chinese, similar to *bathroom* or *restroom* in modern English.

泄泻 [xiè xiè]
diarrhea: abnormally frequent discharge of loose or even watery stools

便溏 [biàn táng]
loose bowels: discharge of soft or semiliquid unformed stools

溏便 [táng biàn]
loose stool; sloppy stool: soft or semiliquid unformed stool

完谷不化 [wán gǔ bù huà]
undigested food (in stool): a condition in which the feces contain undigested food

溏结不调 [táng jié bù tiáo]
stools sometimes loose and sometimes bound: feces that vary greatly in consistency of their forms from time to time, a symptom often caused by disharmony of the liver and spleen

泻下不爽 [xiè xià bù shuǎng]
ungratifying diarrhea: diarrhea that leaves the patient with a feeling that the bowels

have not been satisfactorily emptied

脓血便 [nóng xuè biàn]
purulent and bloody stool: feces containing blood and pus, indicating dysentery

下利 [xià lì]
(I) diarrhea: frequent discharge of fluid stools; **(II) dysentery**

下利清谷 [xià lì qīng gǔ]
diarrhea with undigested food: frequent discharge of watery stools containing undigested food (particles)

下利［痢］脓血 [xià lì nóng xuè]
dysentery with purulent and bloody stools: a type of dysentery marked by expulsion of watery stools that contain pus, mucus and blood

注泄 [zhù xiè]
pouring diarrhea: serious diarrhea with a forceful discharge of watery stool, a classical designation of watery diarrhea (水泻 [shuǐ xiè])

泄注 [xiè zhù]
pouring diarrhea: same as 注泄[zhù xiè]

水泻 [shuǐ xiè]
watery diarrhea: popular designation for pouring diarrhea (注泄 [zhù xiè] or 泄注 [xiè zhù])

泄注赤白 [xiè zhù chì bái]
watery diarrhea with blood and mucus: a symptom indicating dysentery

里急后重 [lǐ jí hòu zhòng]
tenesmus: distressing but ineffectual urge to evacuate the bowels

上吐下泻 [shàng tù xià xiè]
simultaneous vomiting and diarrhea: a symptom often indicating damage to the spleen and stomach by pathogenic dampness or improper diet

问小便 [wèn xiǎo biàn]
inquiry about urine: inquiry about the volume of urine, frequency of urination, sensation during urinary discharge, etc.

多尿 [duō niào]
polyuria: discharge of excessive amount of urine

少尿 [shǎo niào]
oliguria: excretion of diminished amount of urine

小便频数 [xiǎo biàn pín shuò]
frequent urination: increased frequency of urination, also called 尿频 [niào pín]

尿频 [niào pín]
frequent urination: same as 小便频数 [xiǎo biàn pín shuò]

尿清长 [niào qīng cháng]
profuse clear urine: sign indicating the presence of cold in the body

小便清长 [xiǎo biàn qīng cháng]
long voiding of clear urine: synonymous with profuse clear urine (尿清长 [niào qīng cháng])

尿短赤 [niào duǎn chì]
scanty dark urine: sign of the presence of heat in the body

小便短赤 [xiǎo biàn duǎn chì]
short voiding of dark urine: synonymous with scanty dark urine (尿短赤 [niào duǎn chì])

小便黄赤 [xiǎo biàn huáng chì]
dark urine: dark-yellow or even reddish urine, usually indicating the presence of heat

尿赤 [niào chì]
deep-colored urine: synonymous with dark urine (小便黄赤 [xiǎo biàn huáng chì])

小便不利 [xiǎo biàn bù lì]
inhibited urination: (1) difficulty in urination; (2) deficient secretion of urine

小便涩痛 [xiǎo biàn sè tòng]
difficult painful urination: uneasy and painful voiding of urine, a major symptom of stranguria (淋证 [lín zhèng])

小便灼热 [xiǎo biàn zhuó rè]
burning sensation during urination: sign of the presence of heat in stranguria (淋证 [lín zhèng])

尿血 [niào xuè]
hematuria: presence of blood in urine

溲血 [sōu xuè]
hematuria: same as 尿血 [niào xuè]

小便失禁 [xiǎo biàn shī jìn]
urinary incontinence: failure of voluntary control of urination

小便淋漓 [xiǎo biàn lín lí]
dribbling urination: dribbling discharge of urine with inability to achieve a full stream

余沥不尽 [yú lì bù jìn]
dribbling after voiding: continued dribbling discharge of urine after voiding

遗尿 [yí niào]
enuresis: involuntary discharge of urine

失溲 [shī sōu]
enuresis: synonymous with 遗尿 [yí niào]

问胸腹 [wèn xiōng fù]
inquiry about the chest and abdomen: inquiry about discomfort in the chest and abdomen

心悸 [xīn jì]
palpitations: a subjective sensation of rapid and forceful beating of the heart

心下悸 [xīn xià jì]
palpitations below the heart: palpitations felt in the epigastric region below the xiphoid process

心动悸 [xīn dòng jì]
throbbing palpitations: palpitations with visible throbbing of the heart

心慌 [xīn huāng]
flusteredness: nervous agitated state accompanied by palpitations

怔忡 [zhēng chōng]
fearful throbbing; severe palpitations: throbbing palpitations that alarm the sufferer

心痛彻背 [xīn tòng chè bèi]
precordial pain radiating to the back: severe pain in the precordial region with radiation to the back

胃脘痛 [wèi wǎn tòng]
epigastric pain: pain in the epigastric region, also called 胃痛 [wèi tòng], 脘痛 [wǎn tòng], and 心下痛 [xīn xià tòng]

胃痛 [wèi tòng]
stomachache: synonymous with epigastric pain (胃脘痛 [wèi wǎn tòng])

脘痛 [wǎn tòng]
pain in the stomach: synonymous with epigastric pain (胃脘痛 [wèi wǎn tòng])

心下痛 [xīn xià tòng]
pain below the heart: synonymous with epigastric pain (胃脘痛 [wèi wǎn tòng])

恶心 [ě xīn]
nausea: unpleasant sensation with disgust for food and an urge to vomit

泛恶 [fàn ě]
slobbery nausea: an urge to vomit accompanied by outflow of saliva from the mouth

干呕 [gān ǒu]
retching: strong involuntary effort to vomit, but without bringing anything up from the stomach

反胃 [fǎn wèi]
(I) regurgitation: bringing the stomach contents up into the mouth, also called 胃反 [wèi fǎn]; **(II) dysphagia:** difficulty in swallowing with the food returning to the mouth

胃反 [wèi fǎn]
regurgitation: same as 反胃 [fǎn wèi]

吐血 [tù xuè]
spitting of blood: sending out blood from the mouth (with no regard to the source of bleeding), such as hematemesis and hemoptysis

呕血 [ǒu xuè]
hematemesis: vomiting of blood

呕吐清涎 [ǒu tù qīng xián]
vomiting of clear mucus: symptom indicating retention of phlegm that obstructs the descent of stomach *qi*

呕吐酸腐 [ǒu tù suān fǔ]
vomiting of sour fetid matter: symptom indicating retention of undigested food in the stomach

呕吐宿食 [ǒu tù sù shí]
vomiting of retained food: sign of retention of food contents in the stomach

朝食暮吐 [zhāo shí mù tù]
vomiting in the evening of food eaten in the morning: characteristic symptom of stomach reflux due to retention of undigested food with damage to the spleen, usually alternating with vomiting in the morning of food eaten the previous evening

暮食朝吐 [mù shí zhāo tù]
vomiting in the morning of food eaten the previous evening: characteristic symptom of stomach reflux due to retention of undigested food with damage to the spleen, usually alternating with vomiting in the evening of food eaten in the morning

食已即吐 [shí yǐ jí tù]
vomiting right after eating: symptom occurring in the course of obstruction of the stomach by heat, phlegm-*qi*, undigested food, or static blood

呃逆 [è nì]
hiccup; hiccough: sudden involuntary stopping of breath with a peculiar sound, often recurring at short intervals

嘈杂 [cáo zá]
gastric upset: stomach discomfort that resembles a vague ache but not real pain, seems to be in want of food but not actually hungry, and often makes the sufferer distressed

烧心 [shāo xīn]
heartburn: a burning discomfort in the lower part of the chest, usually caused by indigestion

吞酸 [tūn suān]
acid swallowing: swallowing of acid contents regurgitated from the stomach

反酸 [fǎn suān]
acid regurgitation: casting up of acid contents from the stomach

嗳气 [ài qì]
belching; eructation: casting up of gas from the stomach, accompanied by a prolonged sound

噫气 [ǎi qì]
belching: same as 嗳气 [ǎi qì]

嗳腐 [ǎi fǔ]
putrid belching: belching with an unpleasant smell, a symptom often caused by retention of undigested food in the stomach and intestines

纳呆 [nà dāi]
anorexia: loss of appetite

多食善饥 [duō shí shàn jī]
polyphagia with frequent hunger: excessive appetite with increased food intake and recurrent hunger sensation shortly after eating, symptom indicating exuberant stomach fire with increased digestion

消谷善饥 [xiāo gǔ shàn jī]
swift digestion with rapid hunger: synonymous with polyphagia with frequent hunger (多食善饥 [duō shí shàn jī])

饥不欲食 [jī bù yù shí]
no desire to eat despite hunger: symptom usually indicating deficiency of stomach yin with endogenous fire

饮食偏嗜 [yǐn shí piān shì]
dietary partiality: special desire for certain kind(s) of food

腹痛下坠 [fù tòng xià zhuì]
abdominal pain with tenesmus: abdominal pain accompanied by an urge to evacuate the bowels

肠鸣 [cháng míng]
borborygmus: rumbling sound made by the movement of gas through the intestines

腹鸣 [fù míng]
borborygmus: same as 肠鸣 [cháng míng]

腹中雷鸣 [fù zhōng léi míng]
thunderous borborygmus: loud rumbling sound caused by propulsion of gas through the intestines

中满 [zhōng mǎn]
middle fullness: (1) fullness sensation in the epigastric region; (2) abdominal distension

腹满 [fù mǎn]
abdominal fullness: subjective sensation of distension and fullness in the abdomen

腹胀 [fù zhàng]
abdominal distension: distended abdomen with subjective sensation of distension and fullness, cf. 腹满 [fù mǎn]

腹满旗胀 [fù mǎn chēn zhàng]
abdominal fullness and distension: subjective sensation of fullness and distension in the abdomen due to *qi* stagnation

小腹满 [xiǎo fù mǎn]
lower abdominal fullness: subjective feeling of abdominal distension and fullness in the lower abdomen

小腹不仁 [xiǎo fù bù rén]
lower abdominal numbness: loss of sensation in the lower abdomen

少腹拘急 [shào fù jū jí]
lower abdominal cramp: involuntary painful muscular contraction in the lower abdomen

少腹硬满 [shào fù yìng mǎn]
lower abdominal rigidity and fullness: abnormal stiffness and fullness of the lower abdomen, sign of accumulation of heat or retention of blood in the bladder

控睾 [kòng gāo]
referred testicular pain: lower abdominal pain referred to the testis, another name for hernia

腹中硬块 [fù zhōng yìng kuài]
hard mass in the abdomen: hard solid mass in the abdomen, usually caused by blood stasis

脐下悸 [qí xià jì]
throbbing below the umbilicus: rapid pulsation felt in the region below the umbilicus, also known as 脐下悸动 [qí xià jì dòng]

脐下悸动 [qí xià jì dòng]
throbbing below the umbilicus: same as 脐下悸 [qí xià jì]

问口味 [wèn kǒu wèi]
inquiry about taste in the mouth: inquiry about the taste experienced when the mouth is empty

口中和 [kǒu zhōng hé]
harmony in the mouth: normal taste in the mouth unaffected by illness

口淡 [kǒu dàn]
bland taste in the mouth: diminished sensitivity of taste with no apparent sense of flavor while and after eating, also called tastelessness in the mouth (口中无味 [kǒu zhōng wú wèi])

口中无味 [kǒu zhōng wú wèi]

tastelessness in the mouth: same as bland taste in the mouth (口淡 [kǒu dàn])

口甜 [kǒu tián]

sweet taste in the mouth: subjective sweet taste in the mouth, frequently caused by dampness-heat, either exogenous or endogenous, also called 口甘 [kǒu gān]

口甘 [kǒu gān]

sweet taste in the mouth: same as 口甜 [kǒu tián]

口苦 [kǒu kǔ]

bitter taste in the mouth: subjective bitter taste in the mouth, usually occurring in gallbladder disorders, particularly in cases of exuberant fire of the liver and gallbladder

口酸 [kǒu suān]

sour taste in the mouth: subjective sour taste in the mouth, usually attributed to indigestion

口咸 [kǒu xián]

salty taste in the mouth: subjective salty taste in the mouth, often due to deficiency in the kidney with flooding of water

口黏腻 [kǒu nián nì]

sticky slimy sensation in the mouth: unpleasant subjective sensation of stickiness and sliminess in the mouth, often caused by retained phlegm or stagnant food

口不仁 [kǒu bù rén]

numbness of the mouth: loss of normal sensation in the mouth and tongue, premonitory symptom of transformation of liver yang into wind or indicating overdose of medication

问睡眠 [wèn shuì mián]

inquiry about sleep: inquiry about sleep disorders

多梦 [duō mèng]

profuse dreaming; dreamfulness: condition in which sleep is frequently disturbed by dreams

失眠 [shī mián]

insomnia: prolonged and abnormal inability to obtain adequate sleep, also called 不寐 [bù mèi] or 不得眠 [bù dé mián]

不得眠 [bù dé mián]

inability to sleep: same as insomnia (失眠 [shī mián])

不寐 [bù mèi]

sleeplessness: same as insomnia (失眠 [shī mián])

嗜睡 [shì shuì]

somnolence: excessive sleepiness

嗜卧 [shì wò]

somnolence: same as 嗜睡 [shì shuì]

但欲寐 [dàn yù mèi]

desire only to sleep: ancient expression for somnolence (嗜睡 [shì shuì])

梦遗 [mèng yí]

dream emission; nocturnal emission: involuntary discharge of semen during sleep, accompanied by erotic dreams

滑精 [huá jīng]

spermatorrhea; spontaneous seminal

emission: involuntary and frequent discharge of semen without copulation

阳萎 [yáng wěi]
impotence: lack of copulative power in the male, manifested by failure to have or maintain an erection

早泄 [zǎo xiè]
premature ejaculation: ejaculation of semen consistently occurring prior to or immediately after the penis enters the vagina

胸闷 [xiōng mèn]
thoracic oppression: feeling of oppression in the chest

痞满 [pǐ mǎn]
stuffiness and fullness: sensation of stuffiness and fullness in the chest or epigastrium but without pain

胸痞 [xiōng pǐ]
thoracic stuffiness: sensation of stuffiness in the chest

心下痞 [xīn xià pǐ]
stuffiness below the heart; epigastric stuffiness: sensation of stuffiness and fullness below the heart and over the epigastrium, without rigidity and tenderness

心下硬 [xīn xià yìng]
rigidity below the heart; epigastric rigidity: abnormal muscular stiffness in the epigastric region, also called 心下坚 [xīn xià jiān]

心下坚 [xīn xià jiān]
rigidity below the heart: same as 心下硬 [xīn xià yìng]

心下痞硬 [xīn xià pǐ yìng]
stuffiness and rigidity below the heart; epigastric stuffiness and rigidity: sensation of stuffiness and fullness below the heart and over the epigastrium, with local rigidity

心下满 [xīn xià mǎn]
fullness below the heart; epigastric fullness: sensation of fullness in the epigastrium

心下逆满 [xīn xià nì mǎn]
counterflow fullness below the heart; epigastric fullness with counterflow: sensation of fullness in the epigastrium with reversed flow of *qi* marked by such symptoms as nausea and regurgitation

心下支结 [xīn xià zhī jié]
obstructive sensation below the heart: feeling of obstruction associated with vexation and distension in the epigastric region

心下急 [xīn xià jí]
distress below the heart: feeling of distress associated with slight pain and fullness in the epigastric region

下坠 [xià zhuì]
straining at stool; tenesmus: incessant but ineffectual desire for defecation

问妇女经带 [wèn fù nǚ jīng dài]
inquiry about menstruation and leukorrhea: inquiry about the condition of the periods, vaginal discharge, pregnancy and labor in women

月经 [yuè jīng]
menstruation: cyclic discharge of blood from the female genital tract, usually at approximately one-month intervals, also called 月信 [yuè xìn], 月事 [yuè shì] or 月水 [yuè shuǐ]

月信 [yuè xìn]
menstruation: same as 月经 [yuè jīng]

月事 [yuè shì]
menstruation: same as 月经 [yuè jīng]

月水 [yuè shuǐ]
menstruation: same as 月经 [yuè jīng]

月经过多 [yuè jīng guò duō]
hypermenorrhea; menorrhagia: excessive uterine bleeding occurring at regular intervals, also called 月水过多 [yuè shuǐ guò duō]

月水过多 [yuè shuǐ guò duō]
profuse menstruation: same as 月经过多 [yuè jīng guò duō]

月经过少 [yuè jīng guò shǎo]
scanty menstruation; hypomenorrhea: menstrual discharge of less than the normal amount occurring at regular intervals, the period of flow being shorter than the usual duration

月经提前 [yuè jīng tí qián]
advanced menstruation; early periods: periods that come one week or more ahead of due time, also called 月经先期 [yuè jīng xiān qī] or 经行先期 [jīng xíng xiān qī]

经行先期 [jīng xíng xiān qī]
early periods: same as 月经提前 [yuè jīng tí qián]

月经先期 [yuè jīng xiān qī]
early periods: same as 月经提前 [yuè jīng tí qián]

月经错后 [yuè jīng cuò hòu]
late periods: periods that come one week or more after the due time, also called 月经后期 [yuè jīng hòu qī] or 经行后期 [jīng xíng hòu qī]

月经后期 [yuè jīng hòu qī]
late periods: same as 月经错后 [yuè jīng cuò hòu]

经行后期 [jīng xíng hòu qī]
late periods: same as 月经错后 [yuè jīng cuò hòu]

经行先后无定期 [jīng xíng xiān hòu wú dìng qī]
irregular periods; irregular menstrual cycle: periods that come in an irregular cycle, more than one week early or late

经闭 [jīng bì]
amenorrhea; amenia: (1) no experience of menstruation in a women over the age of 18; (2) absence of menstruation for more than three months, not related to pregnancy, lactation or menopause; also called 闭经 [bì jīng]

闭经 [bì jīng]
amenorrhea: same as 经闭 [jīng bì]

经水断绝 [jīng shuǐ duàn jué]
menopause: (1) the natural cessation of menstruation occurring around the age of 50; (2) absence of menstruation for more than three months not due to pregnancy, lactation or menopause

经断 [jīng duàn]
menopause: abbreviation for 经水断绝 [jīng shuǐ duàn jué]

经绝 [jīng jué]
menopause: abbreviation for 经水断绝 [jīng shuǐ duàn jué]

经行腹痛 [jīng xíng fù tòng]
painful menstruation: lower abdominal pain occurring during or around menstruation, also called dysmenorrhea (痛经 [tòng jīng])

白带 [bái dài]
leukorrhea: whitish vaginal discharge: whitish discharge from the vagina

黄带 [huáng dài]
yellowish vaginal discharge: yellowish viscid discharge from the vagina

赤白带下 [chì bái dài xià]
reddish vaginal discharge: profuse leukorrhea mixed with reddish discharge

带下臭秽 [dài xià chòu huì]
fetid vaginal discharge: discharge from the vagina with foul smell, often indicating dampness-heat

切诊 [qiè zhěn]
palpation: examination of the surface of the body by feeling with a hand or fingers, including pulse taking

切脉 [qiè mài]
pulse taking: examination of pulsation of the blood vessels by feeling with the fingertips

脉象 [mài xiàng]
pulse manifestation; pulse condition: the condition of the pulse felt on examination

脉象主病 [mài xiàng zhǔ bìng]
pulse-to-disease correspondence: different types of pulse conditions indicating different diseases or syndromes/patterns, e.g., floating pulse indicating an exterior syndrome/pattern while sunken pulse indicating an interior syndrome/pattern

脉学 [mài xué]
study of the pulse; sphygmology: the sum of what is known regarding the pulse

脉诊 [mài zhěn]
pulse diagnosis: examination of the pulse for making diagnosis

寸、关、尺 [cùn、guān、chǐ]
***cun*, *guan*, *chi*; inch, bar and cubit:** the three sections over the radial artery considered when feeling the pulse. The bar (*guan*) is just over the eminent head of the radius at the wrist, where the tip of the physician's middle finger is placed; the inch (*cun*) is next to it on the distal side where the tip of the physician's index finger rests; and the cubit (*chi*) is on the proximal side where the tip of the physician's ring finger is placed.

举、按、寻 [jǔ、àn、xún]
touching, pressing and searching: the three manipulations in pulse taking. By touching is meant resting the fingers on the patient's wrist very lightly; by pressing is

meant feeling the pulse with proper force; and by searching is meant varying the force or moving the fingers to get a more distinct pulse reading.

举法 [jǔ fǎ]
touching: one of the manipulations in pulse taking, by which the physician's fingers contact the patient's wrist very lightly, cf. 举、按、寻 [jǔ、àn、xún]

按法 [àn fǎ]
pressing: one of the manipulations in pulse taking, by which the physician's fingers contact the patient's pulse with proper force, cf. 举、按、寻 [jǔ、àn、xún]

寻法 [xún fǎ]
searching: one of the manipulations in pulse taking, by which the physician examines the patient's pulse with different force on the fingers or by moving the fingers in different directions in order to get a distinct pulse reading, cf. 举、按、寻 [jǔ、àn、xún]

推法 [tuī fǎ]
pushing: pushing and moving the finger to examine the pulse

循法 [xún fǎ]
tracing: moving the examining finger along the radial artery to find out the pulse condition in detail

总按 [zǒng àn]
simultaneous palpation; pulse-taking with three fingers: taking the pulse of the three sections with three fingers simultaneously

单按 [dān àn]
individual palpation; pulse-taking with one finger: taking the pulse at each of the three sections individually

平息 [píng xī]
normal breathing: normal respiratory cycle of the physician, used as a unit for measuring the patient's pulse rate

三部九候 [sān bù jiǔ hóu]
three positions and nine pulse-takings: (1) taking the pulse on three portions of the body – the head, and the upper and lower limbs. At each portion, the pulses of the following arteries are examined: the temporal artery at point *Taiyang* (EX-HN5) for the state of the head, the auricular artery at point *Ermen* (TE21) for the ears, the buccal artery at points *Dicang* (ST4) and *Daying* (ST5) for the mouth and teeth, the radial artery at inch (*cun*) for the lung, and the ulnar artery at point *Shenmen* (HT7) for the heart. Also, the pulse at point *Hegu* (LI4) is examined for the chest, the pulse at points *Wuli* (LR10) and *Taichong* (LR3) for the liver, the pulse at points *Qimen* (LR14) and *Chongyang* (ST42) for the spleen and stomach, and the pulse at point *Taixi* (KI3) for the kidney – a method of general examination adopted in ancient times; (2) three sections of the radial artery at the wrist for pulse feeling designated as inch, bar and cubit, each of which is felt with light, moderate and heavy force to study the superficial, medium and deep pulses, respectively

寸口 [cùn kǒu]
***cunkou*; "inch opening":** the area of the wrist where the pulsation of radial artery

can be felt, also called 气口 [qì kǒu] or 脉口 [mài kǒu]

气口 [qì kǒu]
"*qi* opening": another name for "inch opening" or *cunkou* (寸口 [cùn kǒu])

脉口 [mài kǒu]
"vessel opening": another name for "inch opening" or *cunkou* (寸口 [cùn kǒu])

寸口脉 [cùn kǒu mài]
(I) wrist artery: the portion of the radial artery, the pulsation of which can be easily felt at the wrist; **(II) wrist pulse:** the pulsation of the radial artery felt at the wrist

趺阳脉 [fū yáng mài]
(I) anterior tibial artery: the artery, the pulsation of which can be easily felt at the instep close to the ankle joint; **(II) anterior tibial pulse:** the pulsation of the anterior tibial artery felt at the instep

人迎脉 [rén yíng mài]
(I) common carotid artery: the artery,the pulsation of which can be easily felt beside the laryngeal prominence; **(II) carotid pulse:** the pulsation of the carotid artery felt beside the laryngeal prominence

平脉 [píngmài]
normal pulse: the pulse of a healthy person, also called 常脉 [cháng mài]

常脉 [cháng mài]
normal pulse: same as 平脉[píng mài]

病脉 [bìng mài]
abnormal pulse; morbid pulse: pulse indicating pathological changes

二十八脉 [èr shí bā mài]
twenty-eight pulses: twenty-eight kinds of pulses, i.e., floating, sunken (deep), slow, rapid, slippery, choppy (unsmooth), feeble (vacuous), replete, long, short, surging, faint, tight, relaxed, wiry, hollow, tympanic (drumskin), firm, soggy, weak, scattered, thready (fine), hidden, stirred, skipping (irregularly rapid), bound (irregularly intermittent), regularly intermittent, and large

浮脉 [fú mài]
floating pulse: a pulse which can be felt by a light touch and growing faint on hard pressure, usually indicating an exterior syndrome/pattern

沉脉 [chén mài]
sunken pulse; deep pulse: a pulse which can only be felt while pressing hard, indicating that a disease is located in the interior of the body

伏脉 [fú mài]
hidden pulse: a pulse which can only be felt upon pressing to the bone, located even deeper than sunken pulse, seen in cases of syncope, shock, or severe pain

数脉 [shuò mài]
rapid pulse: a pulse with five or six beats to one cycle of the physician's respiration (more than 90 beats per minute), indicating the presence of heat

迟脉 [chí mài]
slow pulse: a pulse with less than four beats to one cycle of the physician's

respiration (less than 60 beats per minute), usually indicating a cold syndrome/pattern, but occasionally seen in cases of interior accumulation of heat

缓脉 [huǎn mài]
(I) moderate pulse: a pulse with a moderate rate, even rhythm and moderate tension, indicating a normal condition; **(II) relaxed pulse:** a pulse with diminished tension and moderate frequency, seen in cases of dampness or spleen insufficiency

虚脉 [xū mài]
(I) feeble pulse; vacuous pulse: a pulse feeble and void, indicating deficiency of *qi* and blood or consumption of body fluids; **(II) pulse of deficiency type:** collective term for various pulse conditions showing deficiency

实脉 [shí mài]
(I) replete pulse: a pulse felt to be vigorous and forceful upon both light and heavy pressure, indicating excess syndrome/pattern; **(II) pulse of excess type:** collective term for various pulse conditions indicating excess syndromes/patterns

洪脉 [hóng mài]
surging pulse: a pulse beating like dashing waves with forceful rising and gradual decline, usually indicating the presence of excess heat

细脉 [xì mài]
thready pulse; thin pulse; fine pulse: a pulse as thin as a silk thread, straight and soft, feeble yet always perceptible upon hard pressure, indicating deficiency of *qi* and blood, and seen in other kinds of deficiency conditions, but also in cases of sudden attack of cold or severe pain

微脉 [wēi mài]
faint pulse: a thready and soft pulse, scarcely perceptible, showing extreme exhaustion

弱脉 [ruò mài]
weak pulse: a deep, soft and thin pulse, seen in debilitated patients with deficiency of *qi* and blood

濡脉 [rú mài]
soggy pulse: a pulse which can be felt on light pressure like a thread floating on water, but growing faint upon hard pressure, seen in deficiency conditions or cases of retention of dampness, also called soft pulse (软脉 [ruǎn mài])

软脉 [ruǎn mài]
soft pulse: same as soggy pulse (濡脉 [rú mài])

滑脉 [huá mài]
slippery pulse: a pulse coming and going smoothly like beads rolling on a plate, seen in patients with phlegm and dampness or stagnation of food, but also in pregnant women and healthy persons

涩脉 [sè mài]
unsmooth pulse; choppy pulse: a pulse coming and going with a small, fine, slow joggling tempo like scraping bamboo with a knife, indicating sluggishness of blood circulation caused by deficiency of blood and essence or stagnancy of *qi* and blood

革脉 [gé mài]
tympanic pulse; drumskin pulse: a pulse feeling hard and hollow as if touching the surface of a drum, seen after loss of blood or spermatorrhea

牢脉 [láo mài]
firm pulse: a forceful and taut pulse, felt only by hard pressure, seen in cases of accumulation of yin cold and mass formation

长脉 [cháng mài]
long pulse: a pulse exceeding the span of *cun*, *guan* and *chi* sections, seen in cases of excess heat syndromes/patterns, but also in healthy persons

短脉 [duǎn mài]
short pulse: a pulse only felt at the *cun* or *guan* section, but not perceptible at *chi* section, indicating *qi* disorder

疾脉 [jí mài]
swift pulse; racing pulse: a hasty and swift pulse, 7-8 beats to one cycle of respiration (120-140 beats per minute), seen in severe cases of acute febrile diseases or consumptive conditions

促脉 [cù mài]
skipping pulse; irregular rapid pulse: a rapid pulse with irregular intermittence, seen in cases of excess heat, stagnation of *qi* and blood, retention of phlegm, or indigestion

代脉 [dài mài]
regularly intermittent pulse: a pulse pausing at regular intervals, indicating a decline of the visceral functions

结脉 [jié mài]
irregularly intermittent pulse; bound pulse: a pulse of moderate rate, pausing at irregular intervals, usually seen in cases of *qi* stagnation

紧脉 [jǐn mài]
tight pulse; tense pulse: a pulse feeling like a tightly stretched cord, usually indicating presence of pathogenic cold or pain

散脉 [sǎn mài]
scattered pulse: a pulse that feels diffused and feeble upon a light touch and faint upon hard pressure, indicating exhaustion of *qi* in cases of critical illness

弦脉 [xián mài]
wiry pulse, string-like pulse: a straight and long pulse, like a violin string, usually seen in cases of liver and gallbladder disorders or severe pain

芤脉 [kōu mài]
hollow pulse: a floating, large, soft, and hollow pulse, like a scallion stalk, formed by sudden decrease of circulating blood volume, seen in cases of massive loss of blood or severe vomiting and diarrhea

大脉 [dà mài]
large pulse: a broad pulse with a high wave which lifts the examiner's finger to a greater height than normal, either forceful (seen in cases of excess heat with undamaged body resistance) or weak (seen in cases of general debility)

动脉 [dòng mài]
(I) stirred pulse: a quick, jerky pulse,

feeling like a bouncing pea, seen in cases of fright or pregnancy; **(II) arterial pulsation:** pulsation of a blood vessel felt in any area of the body

七死脉 [qī sǐ mài]
seven moribund pulses: seven kinds of pulses indicating impending death, also known as 七怪脉 [qī guài mài]

七怪脉 [qī guài mài]
seven paradoxical pulses: same as 七死脉 [qī sǐ mài] and 七绝脉 [qī jué mài]

七绝脉 [qī jué mài]
seven moribund pulses: same as 七死脉 [qī sǐ mài] and 七怪脉 [qī guài mài]

雀啄脉 [què zhuó mài]
bird-pecking pulse: an abrupt, quick, arrhythmic pulse resembling the pecking of a bird, one of the seven pulses indicating impending death

鱼翔脉 [yú xiáng mài]
fish-swimming pulse: an extremely short pulse resembling a swimming fish with only its tail wagging, one of the seven pulses indicating impending death

虾游脉 [xiā yóu mài]
shrimp-darting pulse: a nearly imperceptible pulse with occasional darting beats, one of the seven pulses indicating impending death

釜沸脉 [fǔ fèi mài]
bubble-rising pulse: a markedly floating and rapid pulse like bubbles rising to the surface in boiling water, one of the seven pulses indicating impending death

屋漏脉 [wū lòu mài]
roof-leaking pulse: an extremely retarded and irregular pulse resembling water dripping from a roof crack, one of the seven pulses indicating impending death

弹石脉 [tán shí mài]
flicking stone pulse: a deep and solid pulse resembling flicking a stone with the finger tips, one of the seven pulses indicating impending death

解索脉 [jiě suǒ mài]
untwining rope pulse: a rhythmless pulse resembling the untwining of a rope, one of the seven pulses indicating impending death

喜脉 [xǐ mài]
pregnancy pulse: pulse indicating pregnancy

单一脉象 [dān yī mài xiàng]
single-featured pulse: pulse with only one distinct feature, such as slow pulse or slippery pulse

相兼脉象 [xiàng jiān mài xiàng]
multi-featured pulse: pulse with two or more distinct features, such as floating and tense pulse, or deep, fine and rapid pulse

反关脉 [fǎn guān mài]
pulse on the back of the wrist: an anatomic anomaly of the radial artery which causes the pulse beat to be felt on the dorsal aspect of the wrist

斜飞脉 [xié fēi mài]
oblique-running pulse: an anatomic anomaly of the radial artery which causes

the pulse beat to be felt running from the *chi* (cubit) section outward and slantwise to the back of the hand

脉从四时 [mài cóng sì shí]

congruity of pulse with the seasons: change of the pulse in response to the change of season, e.g., normal pulse being slightly taut in spring and somewhat full in summer, also called 脉应四时 [mài yìng sì shí]

脉应四时 [mài yìng sì shí]

congruity of pulse with the seasons: same as 脉从四时 [mài cóng sì shí]

脉逆四时 [mài nì sì shí]

incongruity of pulses with the seasons: failure of the pulse to vary with the change of the season, e.g., floating instead of taut in spring, and deep instead of full in summer, indicating inability of the body to adapt itself to the change of season

胃、神、根 [wèi、shén、gēn]

stomach *qi*, vitality, and root: the three qualities of a normal pulse: (1) regular, smooth and harmonious, indicating the presence of stomach *qi*; (2) with moderate but sufficient strength, indicating the presence of vitality; and (3) perceptible on deep palpation, indicating the presence of root

脉有胃气 [mài yǒu wèi qì]

pulse with stomach *qi*: a pulse beating smoothly with a regular rhythm, normal frequency, moderate force and appropriate volume, and situated at median depth (neither floating nor sunken), indicating adequacy of stomach *qi*

脉无胃气 [mài wú wèi qì]

pulse without stomach *qi*: a pulse that has lost its usual rhythm, frequency and evenness, indicating a critical lack of stomach *qi*

脉有神 [mài yǒu shén]

pulse with vitality: a pulse beating with moderate but sufficient strength

脉有根 [mài yǒu gēn]

pulse with root: a pulse that can be felt upon deep palpation

脉静 [mài jìng]

calmed pulse: pulse that becomes gentle and even in the course of an illness, usually indicating improvement of the condition

脉躁 [mài zào]

agitated pulse: pulse that becomes rapid and rushing, usually indicating deterioration of the condition

脉暴出 [mài bào chū]

sudden throbbing of a pulse: sudden throbbing of a hardly perceptible pulse, usually indicating a critical condition

脉阴阳俱浮 [mài yīn yáng jù fú]

floating pulse at both yin and yang: floating pulse felt at both inch (*cun*) and cubit (*chi*) sections, indicating an exterior syndrome/pattern

脉阴阳俱紧 [mài yīn yáng jù jǐn]

tense pulse at both yin and yang: tense pulse felt at both inch (*cun*) and cubit (*chi*) sections, indicating an exterior syndrome/pattern caused by cold

真脏脉 [zhēn zàng mài]
true visceral pulse; visceral exhaustion pulse: a pulse bereft of stomach *qi*, vitality and root, indicating exhaustion of *zang*-organs, often found in a critically ill patient

脉悬绝 [mài xuán jué]
extremely abnormal pulse: pulse very different from the normal, usually seen in severe cases

色脉合参 [sè mài hé cān]
comprehensive analysis of the pulse and complexion: making a diagnosis by reviewing the patient's pulse condition together with his/her complexion

四诊合参 [sì zhěn hé cān]
comprehensive analysis of the four examinations: making a diagnosis by analyzing the results of all the four examinations

脉症合参 [mài zhèng hé cān]
comprehensive analysis of the pulse and symptoms: making a diagnosis by reviewing the patient's pulse condition together with his/her symptoms

舍脉从症 [shě mài cóng zhèng]
precedence of symptoms over pulse: making a diagnosis on the basis of symptoms rather than pulse condition

舍症从脉 [shě zhèng cóng mài]
precedence of pulse over symptoms: making a diagnosis on the basis of pulse condition rather than symptoms

按诊 [àn zhěn]
palpation: examination of the body surface by touch with the hand or fingers

按尺肤 [àn chǐ fū]
palpation of the forearm: examination of the forearm with the hand for determining the texture of the skin, development of the muscles, and temperature of the extremities

按肌肤 [àn jī fū]
palpation of the skin: examination of a certain area of the skin with the hand for determining local temperature, moisture, pain, swelling and other local changes

按胸腹 [àn xiōng fù]
palpation of the chest and abdomen: examination of the chest and abdomen with the hand for determining location and extent of the affected region and pathological change of the viscera

按脘腹 [àn wǎn fù]
palpation of the epigastrium and abdomen: examination of the abdomen, including the epigastric region, with the hand for determining local temperature, consistency, distension, mass formation and tenderness

按手足 [àn shǒu zú]
palpation of the hands and feet: examination of the hands and feet chiefly for determining the cold or heat nature of a syndrome/pattern

按俞穴 [àn shù xué]
acupoint palpation: examination of acupoints with a finger to search for tender points which can reflect disease conditions in corresponding internal organs

拒按 [jù àn]

refusal of pressure: a condition in which pressing can aggravate discomfort or pain

喜按 [xǐ àn]

preference for pressing: a condition in which pressing can relieve discomfort or pain

常用引文 Commonly Used Citations

望而知之谓之神，闻而知之谓之圣，问而知之谓之工，切脉知之谓之巧。

[wàng ér zhī zhī wèi zhī shén, wén ér zhī zhī wèi zhī shèng, wèn ér zhī zhī wèi zhī gōng, qiè mài zhī zhī wèi zhī qiǎo]

It is wonderful to know by looking, it is wise to know by hearing and smelling, it is skillful to know by asking, and it is ingenious to know by pulse-taking: Diagnosis of a disease by looking, or hearing and smelling requires more intuitive and comprehensive ability on the part of a physician and thus one who can do this is considered to possess medical skills of the highest level, while achieving the same goal by asking or pulse-taking is considered exquisite and clever. (Nevertheless, one needs to do all four examinations to confirm the diagnostic result.)

欲知病色，必先知常色；欲知常色，必先知常色之变；欲知常色之变，必先知常色变中之变。

[yù zhī bìng sè, bì xiān zhī cháng sè; yù zhī cháng sè, bì xiān zhī cháng sè zhī biàn; yù zhī cháng sè zhī biàn, bì xiān zhī cháng sè biàn zhōng zhī biàn]

If you want to know what a sick complexion looks like, you must first know what the healthy one looks like; if you want to know what a healthy complexion looks like, you must first know the range of healthy complexions; if you want to know the range of healthy complexions, you must look into the details of all the possible varieties of a healthy complexion.

气由脏发，色随气华。

[qì yóu zàng fā, sè súi qì huá]

***Qi* originates from the *zang*-organs, and the complexion varies in accordance with the condition of *qi*.**

得神者昌。

[dé shén zhě chāng]

A patient with vitality is apt to recover from illness.

失神者亡。

[shī shén zhě wáng]

A patient losing vitality has a poor prognosis.

司外揣内。

[sī wài chuǎi nèi]

Inspection of the exterior leads to conjecture of the interior.

见微知著。

[jiàn wēi zhī zhù]

From the trivial details, one can figure out the big picture.

揆度奇恒。

[kúi duó qí héng]

One should assess both the generality and particularity.

肝脉弦。
[gān mài xián]
A wiry pulse indicates liver disorder.

心脉洪。
[xīn mài hóng]
A surging pulse often signals a heart disorder.

脾脉缓。
[pí mài huǎn]
A relaxed pulse suggests spleen insufficiency.

肺脉浮。
[fèi mài fú]
A floating pulse is frequently found in the case of lung disease.

肾脉沉。
[shèn mài chén]
A sunken pulse usually signifies kidney insufficiency.

春应中规。
[chūn yīng zhòng guī]
In spring, the pulse should be smooth like a circle.

夏应中矩。
[xià yīng zhòng jǔ]
In summer, the pulse should be full like a square.

秋应中衡。
[qiū yīng zhòng héng]
In autumn, the pulse should be floating like the beam of a steelyard.

冬应中权。
[dōng yīng zhòng quán]
In winter, the pulse should be sunken like the sliding weight of a steelyard.

辨证 Syndrome Differentiation (Pattern Identification)

辨证 [biàn zhèng]

syndrome differentiation; pattern identification: the process of overall analysis of clinical data to determine the location, cause and nature of a patient's disease, and achieve the diagnosis of syndrome or pattern

证 [zhèng]

syndrome; pattern: diagnostic conclusion of the pathological changes at a certain stage of a disease, including the location, cause and nature of the disease as well as the trend of development, also known as 证候 [zhèng hòu]

证候 [zhèng hòu]

(I) syndrome manifestation; pattern manifestation: symptoms and signs of syndrome/pattern; **(II) syndrome; pattern:** another term for 证 [zhèng] when a disyllabic word is needed

证型 [zhèng xíng]

syndrome type; pattern type: a common and typical syndrome or pattern with a standard name

八纲辨证 Eight-principle Syndrome Differentiation (Eight-principle Pattern Identification)

八纲 [bā gāng]

eight principles: guiding principles of syndrome differentiation (or pattern identification), viz., yin and yang, exterior and interior, cold and heat, deficiency (or insufficiency) and excess

八纲辨证 [bā gāng biàn zhèng]

eight-principle syndrome differentiation; eight-principle pattern identification: the process of diagnosing syndrome (or pattern) by analyzing the patient's condition according to the eight principles, i.e., differentiating the location of disease between exterior and interior, distinguishing the nature of disease between cold and heat, identifying the patient's condition as deficiency or excess, and generalizing the syndrome or pattern as yin or yang

阴阳辨证 [yīn yáng biàn zhèng]

yin-yang syndrome differentiation; yin-yang pattern identification: categorization of syndromes/patterns according to the yin-yang theory, e.g., interior, cold, and deficiency syndromes/patterns pertaining to yin, and exterior, heat, and excess syndromes/patterns pertaining to yang

阴证 [yīn zhèng]

yin syndrome/pattern: collective term for interior, cold and deficiency syndromes/patterns with inhibitory, hypofunctional, quiescent or dimmed manifestations, or inward and downward symptoms, as well as diseases caused by pathogenic factors of yin nature

阳证 [yáng zhèng]

yang syndrome/pattern: collective term

for exterior, heat and excess syndromes/patterns with excitatory, hyperfunctional, restless or bright manifestations, or outward and upward symptoms, as well as diseases caused by pathogenic factors of yang nature

表里 [biǎo lǐ]
exterior and interior: parts of the body, the exterior referring to the skin and body hair, subcutaneous tissues, muscles and superficial meridians/channels, and the interior referring to internal organs and bone marrow. An exogenous contraction only involving the exterior is usually milder than that penetrating into the interior.

表里辨证 [biǎo lǐ biàn zhèng]
exterior-interior syndrome differentiation; exterior-interior pattern identification: categorization of syndromes/patterns according to the location of a disease, in which exterior refers to the outer part of the body, and interior refers to the inner part of the body

表证 [biǎo zhèng]
exterior syndrome/pattern: general term for syndromes/patterns that occur chiefly at the early stage of exogenous contractions or acute infectious diseases invading the human body through the skin surface or respiratory tract, during which pathogenic factors only affect the exterior part of the body

里证 [lǐ zhèng]
interior syndrome/pattern: general term for syndromes/patterns that indicate the existence of disease in the *zang-fu* organs, *qi* and blood, or bone marrow

寒热 [hán rè]
(I) cold and heat: pair of principles for differentiating the nature of a disease; **(II) chills and fever**

寒热辨证 [hán rè biàn zhèng]
cold-heat syndrome differention; cold-heat pattern identification: categorization of syndromes/patterns according to the nature of a disease, in which cold refers to the presence of pathogenic cold or insufficient yang in the body, and heat refers to the presence of pathogenic heat or excessive yang in the body

寒证 [hán zhèng]
cold syndrome/pattern: general term for syndromes/patterns caused either by exogenous cold factors or by insufficient yang within the body

热证 [rè zhèng]
heat syndrome/pattern: general term for syndromes/patterns resulting either from yang prevalence or from yin deficiency

虚实 [xū shí]
deficiency and excess: pair of principles for determining the condition of the body's resistance to pathogenic factors. Deficiency denotes insufficiency of healthy *qi*, while excess indicates the presence of excessive pathogenic factors with intense body reaction or the accumulation of pathological products due to dysfunction of the internal organs.

虚实辨证 [xū shí biàn zhèng]
deficiency-excess syndrome differenti-

ation; deficiency-excess pattern identification: categorization of syndromes/patterns according to the condition of the body's resistance to pathogenic factors, in which deficiency refers to deficiency of healthy *qi* and excess refers to excessiveness of pathogenic *qi*

虚证 [xū zhèng]
deficiency syndrome/pattern: general term for syndromes/patterns caused by insufficiency of healthy *qi* (including yang *qi*, yin fluid, essence, blood, nutrients and defense *qi*)

实证 [shí zhèng]
excess syndrome/pattern: general term for syndromes/patterns caused by exogenous pathogenic factors or by accumulated pathological products due to dysfunction of the internal organs, such as phlegm, retained fluid, stagnant blood, and undigested food

表寒证 [biǎo hán zhèng]
exterior cold syndrome/pattern: a type of exterior syndrome/pattern in which the external part of the body is attacked by exogenous cold or wind, manifested by chills or aversion to cold or wind, headache, general aching or joint pains, thin and white tongue coating, and floating and tense pulse

表热证 [biǎo rè zhèng]
exterior heat syndrome/pattern: a type of exterior syndrome/pattern in which the external part of the body is attacked by exogenous wind-heat, manifested by mild aversion to wind, moderate fever, headache, slight thirst, thin white or thin yellowish tongue coating or red tip of the tongue, and floating rapid pulse

表虚证 [biǎo xū zhèng]
exterior deficiency syndrome/pattern: a type of exterior syndrome/pattern resulting from lowered superficial defense *qi*, and manifested by spontaneous sweating, intolerance of wind, and floating feeble pulse

表实证 [biǎo shí zhèng]
exterior excess syndrome/pattern: a type of exterior syndrome/pattern in which the external part of the body is attacked by exogenous pathogens, while defense *qi* is not yet damaged, manifested by lack of sweating and forceful or tight floating pulse in addition to the symptoms of an exterior syndrome/pattern

里寒证 [lǐ hán zhèng]
interior cold syndrome/pattern: a type of interior syndrome/pattern caused by either endogenous cold, i.e., deficiency of yang, or exogenous cold transmitted to the interior of the body, mainly manifested by intolerance of cold, pallor, cold limbs, pale tongue with white moistened coating, and deep, slow or fine pulse

里虚寒证 [lǐ xū hán zhèng]
interior deficiency cold syndrome/pattern: interior cold syndrome/pattern resulting from yang deficiency

里热证 [lǐ rè zhèng]
interior heat syndrome/pattern: a type of interior syndrome/pattern caused by pathogenic heat in the internal organs, especially in the stomach, intestines, lung, liver and gallbladder, mainly manifested

by fever, intolerance of heat, thirst, irritability, scanty and condensed urine, full, rapid and forceful or wiry pulse, and reddened tongue with yellow coating

里虚热证 [lǐ xū rè zhèng]
interior deficiency heat syndrome/pattern: interior heat syndrome resulting from yin deficiency

里实证 [lǐ shí zhèng]
interior excess syndrome/pattern: (1) syndrome/pattern caused by accumulated heat in the stomach and intestines after an attack of exogenous pathogenic factors; (2) syndrome/pattern caused by retention of phlegm, blood stasis, stagnation of undigested food or accumulation of parasitic worms

表寒里热证 [biǎo hán lǐ rè zhèng]
syndrome/pattern of exterior cold and interior heat: complicated condition seen either in cases of affection of exogenous cold and wind on the body with pre-existing internal heat, or in cases of transformation of exogenous cold into heat after having penetrated into the interior of the body while the pathogenic cold in the exterior of the body is still present. Its major symptomatic character is the coexistence of both exterior cold (chills and headache with no sweating) and interior heat (fever with irritability, thirst, scanty condensed urine, and constipation).

表热里寒证 [biǎo rè lǐ hán zhèng]
syndrome/pattern of exterior heat and interior cold: case of pre-existing deficiency-cold of the spleen and stomach complicated by contraction of wind-heat, with symptoms showing the coexistence of exterior heat (fever, headache, and intolerance of wind) and internal cold (cold limbs, loose bowels, etc.)

表虚里实证 [biǎo xū lǐ shí zhèng]
syndrome/pattern of exterior deficiency and interior excess: case in which symptoms of exterior deficiency such as intolerance of wind and spontaneous sweating exist together with symptoms of interior excess such as abdominal pain with tenderness and constipation

表实里虚证 [biǎo shí lǐ xū zhèng]
syndrome/pattern of exterior excess and interior deficiency: case in which symptoms of exterior excess such as chills, headache and general aching exist together with symptoms of interior deficiency such as anorexia, lassitude, palpitations, and shortness of breath, usually seen in cases of chronic disease complicated by new exogenous affliction

半表半里证 [bàn biǎo bàn lǐ zhèng]
half-exterior half-interior syndrome/pattern: variety of syndromes/patterns due to affliction of the region located between the exterior and interior of the body, marked by alternate fever and chills, fullness and choking feeling in the chest and costal region, bitter taste in the mouth, dry throat, nausea and loss of appetite, and wiry pulse. The syndrome/pattern of the *shaoyang* (lesser yang) meridian/channel belongs to this category.

上寒下热证 [shàng hán xià rè zhèng]
upper-cold and lower-heat syndrome/

pattern: case in which cold symptoms in the upper part of the body (e.g., aversion to cold, nausea, and vomiting) exist together with heat symptoms in the lower (e.g., constipation, scanty and condensed urine)

上热下寒证 [shàng rè xià hán zhèng]
upper-heat and lower-cold syndrome/pattern: case in which heat symptoms in the upper part of the body (e.g., acid regurgitation with annoying sensation of heat in the chest) appear simultaneously with cold symptoms in the lower (e.g., loose stools and abdominal pain which can be eased by warmth)

上虚下实证 [shàng xū xià shí zhèng]
upper-deficiency and lower-excess syndrome/pattern: case with deficiency of healthy *qi* in the upper and preponderance of pathogenic factors in the lower part of the body, e.g., case with cardiac palpitations due to heart insufficiency complicated by dampness-heat dysentery

上实下虚证 [shàng shí xià xū zhèng]
upper-excess and lower-deficiency syndrome/pattern: case with deficiency of healthy *qi* in the lower and preponderance of pathogenic factors in the upper part of the body, e.g., lumbago, weakened legs and nocturnal emission due to kidney insufficiency associated with dizziness, headache and irritability resulting from exuberant liver *qi*

虚寒证 [xū hán zhèng]
deficiency cold syndrome/pattern: cold syndrome/pattern caused by deficiency of yang, marked by intolerance of cold and epigastric or abdominal pain which can be relieved by heat and pressure, loose bowels, fine thready pulse, and profuse whitish and thin leukorrhea in women

虚热证 [xū rè zhèng]
deficiency heat syndrome/pattern: abbreviation for syndrome/pattern of yin deficiency with internal heat (阴虚内热证 [yīn xū nèi rè zhèng)])

阴虚内热证 [yīn xū nèi rè zhèng]
syndrome/pattern of yin deficiency with internal heat: syndrome/pattern of internal heat arising from yin deficiency, marked by persistent low-grade fever, night sweating, malar flush, thirst, short voiding of dark urine, dry and bound stools, reddened tongue lacking moisture, and rapid fine pulse

虚火证 [xū huǒ zhèng]
deficiency fire syndrome/pattern: abbreviation for syndrome/pattern of yin deficiency with effulgent fire (阴虚火旺证 [yīn xū huǒ wàng zhèng])

阴虚火旺证 [yīn xū huǒ wàng zhèng]
syndrome/pattern of yin deficiency with effulgent fire: syndrome/pattern of effulgent fire arising from yin deficiency, marked by vexation, insomnia, dry throat and mouth, night sweating, tidal fever, malar flush, dry and bound stools, short voiding of dark urine, or hemoptysis, epistaxis, reddened tongue lacking moisture, and rapid fine pulse

实寒证 [shí hán zhèng]
excess cold syndrome/pattern: syndrome/pattern caused by pathogenic cold

accumulated in the interior of the body, marked by aversion to cold, cold limbs, abdominal pain, constipation, absence of thirst, whitish thick or greasy coating on the tongue, and deep, wiry and forceful pulse

实热证 [shí rè zhèng]
excess heat syndrome/pattern: heat syndrome/pattern caused by excessive pathogenic factors while the body's resistance is still sufficient, marked by intense reactions such as high fever with restlessness, constipation, gigantic or slippery rapid pulse

实火证 [shí huǒ zhèng]
excess fire syndrome/pattern: fire syndrome/pattern caused by excessive pathogenic factors, usually marked by bloodshot eyes, bitterness in the mouth, thirst, irritability, constipation, reddened tongue with yellow coating, and gigantic rapid pulse

火热炽盛证 [huǒ rè chì shèng zhèng]
exuberant fire-heat syndrome/pattern: synonym for excess fire syndrome/pattern (实火证 [shí huǒ zhèng]) and excess heat syndrome/pattern (实热证 [shí rè zhèng])

阴虚证 [yīn xū zhèng]
yin deficiency syndrome/pattern: syndrome/pattern resulting from failure to restrain yang due to insufficiency of yin fluid, usually manifested by afternoon fever, night sweats, malar flush, vexatious heat sensation in the palms of the hands and soles of the feet, dryness of the mouth and throat, reddened tongue with scanty coating, and fine, rapid pulse

阴液亏虚证 [yīn yè kuī xū zhèng]
yin fluid insufficiency syndrome/pattern: a synonym for or a complex name of yin deficiency syndrome/pattern (阴虚证 [yīn xū zhèng])

阳虚证 [yáng xū zhèng]
yang deficiency syndrome/pattern: syndrome/pattern resulting from deficiency of yang *qi*, usually accompanied by cold symptoms, marked by pallor, intolerance of cold, cold extremities, loose bowels, pale tongue, and feeble pulse

亡阴证 [wáng yīn zhèng]
yin exhaustion syndrome/pattern: serious syndrome/pattern resulting from exhaustion of yin fluid, manifested by thirst and craving for cold drinks, flushed face, restlessness, dry tongue and thready, swift pulse

阴脱证 [yīn tuō zhèng]
yin collapse syndrome/pattern: synonym for yin exhaustion syndrome/pattern (亡阴证 [wáng yīn zhèng])

亡阳证 [wáng yáng zhèng]
yang exhaustion syndrome/pattern: serious syndrome/pattern resulting from exhaustion of yang *qi*, manifested by pallor, dripping of cold sweats, cold limbs, pale and moistened tongue, and hardly perceptible pulse

阳脱证 [yáng tuō zhèng]
yang collapse syndrome/pattern: synonym for yang exhaustion syndrome/pattern (亡阳证 [wáng yáng zhèng])

阴证似阳 [yīn zhèng sì yáng]
yin syndrome/pattern resembling yang:

yin syndrome/pattern that appears as a yang syndrome/pattern, e.g., an advanced case of yin deficiency showing pseudo-heat symptoms such as feeling hot and thirsty

阳证似阴 [yáng zhèng sì yīn]
yang syndrome/pattern resembling yin: yang syndrome/pattern that appears as a yin syndrome/pattern, e.g., a severe case of febrile disease showing pseudo-cold symptoms such as intolerance of cold and cold limbs

真寒假热证 [zhēn hán jiǎ rè zhèng]
syndrome/pattern of true cold with false heat: cold syndrome/pattern with pseudo-heat symptoms. The patient feels hot yet wishes to be thickly covered, feels thirsty yet drinks little, moves restlessly yet is mentally quiescent.

真热假寒证 [zhēn rè jiǎ hán zhèng]
syndrome/pattern of true heat with false cold: heat syndrome/pattern with pseudo-cold symptoms. The patient is intolerant of cold but dislikes being thickly covered, and has cold limbs though the chest and abdomen feel hot.

真实假虚证 [zhēn shí jiǎ xū zhèng]
syndrome/pattern of true excess with false deficiency: excess syndrome/pattern with pseudo-deficiency manifestations

真虚假实证 [zhēn xū jiǎ shí zhèng]
syndrome/pattern of true deficiency with false excess: deficiency syndrome/pattern with pseudo-excess manifestations

✦ 常用引文 Commonly Used Citations ✦

寒极似热。
[hán jí sì rè]
Extreme cold resembles heat.

热极似寒。
[rè jí sì hán]
Extreme heat resembles cold.

邪气盛则实。
[xié qì shèng zé shí]
Where the pathogenic *qi* is exuberant, there is excess.

精气夺则虚。
[jīng qì duó zé xū]
Where the essential *qi* is despoiled, there is deficiency.

大实如羸状。
[dà shí rú léi zhuàng]
Great excessiveness looks like debilitation.
cf. 真实假虚 [zhēn shí jiǎ xū]

至虚有盛候。
[zhì xū yǒu shèng hòu]
Extreme insufficiency presents signs of exuberance. cf. 真虚假实 [zhēn xū jiǎ shí]

六经辨证
Six-meridian / channel Syndrome Differentiation (Six-meridian / channel Pattern Identification)

六经辨证 [liù jīng biàn zhèng]
six-meridian/channel syndrome differentiation; six-meridian/channel pattern identification: differentiation of syndromes (or identification of patterns) in accordance with the theory of the six meridians/channels, applied to the diagnosis of acute febrile diseases at different stages, but also useful for syndrome differentiation (or pattern identification) of other diseases

六经病证 [liù jīng bìng zhèng]
syndromes of the six meridians/channels; disease patterns of the six meridians/channels: collective term for disease patterns or syndromes of *taiyang* (greater yang), *yangming* (yang brightness), *shaoyang* (lesser yang), *taiyin* (greater yin), *shaoyin* (lesser yin) and *jueyin* (reverting yin) meridians/channels

六经病 [liù jīng bìng]
diseases of the six meridians/channels: same as 六经病证 [liù jīng bìng zhèng]

太阳病证 [tài yáng bìng zhèng]
greater yang disease pattern; greater yang syndrome: disease pattern or syndrome characterized by attack of pathogenic wind-cold on the body's surface with struggle between healthy *qi* and the pathogenic factor(s) at the exterior portion of the body, also called greater yang disease (太阳病 [tài yáng bìng])

太阳病 [tài yáng bìng]
greater yang disease: same as greater yang disease pattern/syndrome (太阳病证 [tài yáng bìng zhèng])

太阳经证 [tài yáng jīng zhèng]
greater yang meridian/channel syndrome/pattern: one of the syndromes/patterns of the six meridians/channels due to attack of pathogenic wind-cold on the greater yang meridian/channel of the body's surface, usually seen in the initial stage of the contraction, marked by chills and fever, pain in the head and neck, and floating pulse, also known as greater yang meridian/channel disease (太阳经病 [tài yáng jīng bìng])

太阳经病 [tài yáng jīng bìng]
greater yang meridian/channel disease: same as greater yang meridian/channel syndrome/pattern (太阳经证 [tài yáng jīng zhèng]

太阳中风证 [tài yáng zhòng fēng zhèng]
greater yang wind attack syndrome/pattern: syndrome/pattern caused by pathogenic wind impacting the greater yang meridian/channel, chiefly manifested by fever, aversion to wind, sweating and floating relaxed pulse, also called greater yang wind attack (太阳中风 [tài yáng zhòng fēng])

太阳中风 [tài yáng zhòng fēng]
greater yang wind attack: same as greater yang wind attack syndrome/pattern 太阳中风证 [tài yáng zhòng fēng zhèng]

太阳伤寒证 [tài yáng shāng hán zhèng]
greater yang cold damage syndrome/

pattern: syndrome/pattern caused by pathogenic cold attacking the greater yang meridian/channel, chiefly manifested by fever, chills, absence of sweat and floating pulse, also called greater yang cold damage (太阳伤寒 [tài yáng shāng hán])

太阳伤寒 [tài yáng shāng hán]
greater yang cold damage: same as greater yang cold damage syndrome/pattern 太阳伤寒证 [tài yáng shāng hán zhèng]

太阳腑证 [tài yáng fǔ zhèng]
greater yang *fu*-organ syndrome/pattern: syndrome/pattern in which the urinary bladder (greater yang *fu*-organ) is attacked by pathogen in the case of an unrelieved greater yang meridian/channel syndrome/pattern, also known as greater yang *fu*-organ disease (太阳腑病 [tài yáng fǔ bìng])

太阳腑病 [tài yáng fǔ bìng]
greater yang *fu*-organ disease: same as greater yang *fu*-organ syndrome/pattern (太阳腑证 [tài yáng fǔ zhèng])

太阳蓄水证 [tài yáng xù shuǐ zhèng]
greater yang water accumulation syndrome/pattern: a type of greater yang *fu*-organ syndrome/pattern in which the pathogen penetrates and causes accumulation of water in the bladder, manifested by fever and chills, oliguria, lower abdominal fullness, vomiting immediately after drinking, and floating or floating and rapid pulse

太阳蓄血证 [tài yáng xù xuè zhèng]
greater yang blood accumulation syndrome/pattern: a type of greater yang *fu*-organ syndrome/pattern in which the pathogen combines with blood and accumulates in the lower abdomen, manifested by lower abdominal cramps or fullness with rigidity, polyuria, delirium, amnesia, dark stool, and sunken and choppy or sunken and irregularly intermittent pulse

阳明病证 [yáng míng bìng zhèng]
yang brightness disease pattern; yang brightness syndrome: disease pattern/syndrome marked by exuberant yang and dryness-heat in the stomach and intestines occurring in the course of a cold-induced febrile disease, also called yang brightness disease (阳明病[yáng míng bìng])

阳明病 [yáng míng bìng]
yang brightness disease: same as yang brightness disease pattern/syndrome阳明病证 [yáng míng bìng zhèng]

阳明经证 [yáng míng jīng zhèng]
yang brightness meridian/channel syndrome/pattern: syndrome/pattern caused by exuberant pathogenic heat flooding in yang brightness meridian/channel and spreading over the body but not yet inducing constipation, characteristically manifested by high fever without chills, profuse sweating, dire thirst, and full and gigantic pulse, also known as yang brightness meridian/channel disease (阳明经病 [yáng míng jīng bìng])

阳明经病 [yáng míng jīng bìng]
yang brightness meridian/channel disease: same as yang brightness meridian/channel syndrome/pattern (阳明经证 [yáng míng jīng zhèng])

阳明腑证 [yáng míng fǔ zhèng]
yang brightness *fu*-organ syndrome/pattern: syndrome/pattern caused by accumulation of pathogenic heat in the stomach and large intestine, manifested by tidal fever in the afternoon, abdominal pain and tenderness, constipation, deep and forceful pulse, or even delirium, also known as yang brightness *fu*-organ disease (阳明腑病 [yáng míng fǔ bìng])

阳明腑病 [yáng míng fǔ bìng]
yang brightness *fu*-organ disease: same as yang brightness *fu*-organ syndrome/pattern (阳明腑证 [yáng míng fǔ zhèng])

少阳病证 [shào yáng bìng zhèng]
lesser yang disease pattern; lesser yang syndrome: disease pattern or syndrome in which pathogenic heat exists between the exterior and interior of the body, marked by alternate fever and chills, fullness and choking feeling in the chest and hypochondriac region, dry throat, and wiry pulse, also called lesser yang disease (少阳病 [shào yáng bìng])

少阳病 [shào yáng bìng]
lesser yang disease: same as lesser yang disease pattern/syndrome (少阳病证 [shào yáng bìng zhèng)

太阴病证 [tài yīn bìng zhèng]
greater yin disease pattern/syndrome: disease pattern or syndrome characterized by decline of spleen yang with production of cold-dampness in the interior, and manifested by abdominal fullness and occasional abdominal pain, vomiting, diarrhea, anorexia, sunken and relaxed or weak pulse, also called greater yin disease (太阴病 [tài yīn bìng])

太阴病 [tài yīn bìng]
greater yin disease: same as greater yin disease pattern/syndrome (太阴病证 [tài yīn bìng zhèng])

少阴病证 [shào yīn bìng zhèng]
lesser yin disease pattern; lesser yin syndrome: disease pattern or syndrome occurring at the late state of a cold-induced disease marked by general decline of both yin and yang, also called lesser yin disease (少阴病 [shào yīn bìng])

少阴病 [shào yīn bìng]
lesser yin disease: same as lesser yin disease pattern/syndrome (少阴病证 [shào yīn bìng zhèng])

少阴寒化证 [shào yīn hán huà zhèng]
cold transformation syndrome/pattern of lesser yin: lesser yin syndrome/pattern with cold transformation of the pathogen which invades the heart and kidney, usually manifested as aversion to cold, cold limbs, sleepiness, lienteric diarrhea, pale tongue and deep faint pulse

少阴热化证 [shào yīn rè huà zhèng]
heat transformation syndrome/pattern of lesser yin: lesser yin syndrome/pattern with heat transformation of the pathogen, manifested by vexation, insomnia, dry mouth and throat, reddened tongue tip, and thready rapid pulse

厥阴病证 [jué yīn bìng zhèng]
reverting yin disease pattern; reverting yin syndrome: one of the disease patterns/syndromes of the six meridians/

channels occurring at the late stage of a cold-induced disease characterized by interweaving of cold and heat, or in more generalized terms – yin and yang, manifested by fever or burning sensation in the epigastrium with cold limbs, empty feeling in the stomach but no desire for eating, also called reverting yin disease (厥阴病 [jué yīn bìng])

厥阴病 [jué yīn bìng]
reverting yin disease: same as reverting yin disease pattern/syndrome (厥阴病证 [jué yīn bìng zhèng])

经证 [jīng zhèng]
meridian syndrome/pattern; channel syndrome/pattern: morbid condition of any of the three yang meridians/channels due to attack of pathogenic factors while the related *fu*-organ is not affected

腑证 [fǔ zhèng]
***fu*-organ syndrome/pattern:** morbid condition indicating that pathological changes of one or more yang meridians/channels have already affected the respective internal organs: the urinary bladder (greater yang), the stomach and large intestine (yang brightness), and the gallbladder (lesser yang)

并病 [bìng bìng]
overlapping of diseases: overlapping of two meridian/channel syndromes/patterns, in which they appear in succession and then coexist

二阳并病 [èr yáng bìng bìng]
overlapping of two yang diseases: overlapping of two yang meridian/channel syndromes/patterns, e.g., lesser yang syndrome/pattern (vomiting and fullness in the chest) appearing before the subsidence of greater yang syndrome/pattern (headache, chills, fever and joint pains)

合病 [hé bìng]
combination of diseases: occurrence of two or more meridian/channel diseases at the same time

太阳（与）少阳合病 [tài yáng (yǔ) shào yáng hé bìng]
combination of greater yang and lesser yang diseases: simultaneous occurrence of greater yang disease (headache and fever) and lesser yang disease (bitterness in the mouth, dry throat, and dizziness)

太阳（与）阳明合病 [tài yáng (yǔ) yáng míng hé bìng]
combination of greater yang and yang brightness diseases: simultaneous occurrence of greater yang disease (headache and neck rigidity) and yang brightness disease (fever and thirst)

阳明（与）少阳合病 [yáng míng (yǔ) shào yáng hé bìng]
combination of yang brightness and lesser yang diseases: simultaneous occurrence of yang brightness disease (fever and thirst) and lesser yang disease (bitterness in the mouth, dry throat, and fullness in the chest)

三阳合病 [sān yáng hé bìng]
triple combination of yang meridian/channel diseases: disease caused by transmission of the pathogenic heat

into yang brightness meridian/channel from both greater yang and lesser yang meridians/channels, resulting in a distinctive heat syndrome/pattern manifested by fever, thirst, perspiration, abdominal distension, utter loss of appetite, delirium, and incontinence of urine

顺传 [shùn chuán]
sequential transmission; normal transmission: transmission of a disease in the normal sequence, e.g., from the defense aspect to the *qi* aspect

逆传 [nì chuán]
adverse transmission: transmission of a disease not in the normal sequence, e.g., from the defense aspect directly to the nutrient and blood aspects, skipping the *qi* aspect

卫气营血辨证 Defense-*qi*-nutrient-blood Syndrome Differentiation (Defense-*qi*-nutrient-blood Pattern Identification)

卫气营血辨证 [wèi qì yíng xuè biàn zhèng]
defense-*qi*-nutrient-blood syndrome differentiation; defense-*qi*-nutrient-blood pattern identification: syndrome differentiation or pattern identification of epidemic febrile diseases in accordance with the theory of defense, *qi*, nutrient and blood, illustrating the stages of clinical course and explaining the corresponding pathological changes

卫分证 [wèi fèn zhèng]
defense aspect syndrome/pattern: initial stage of an epidemic febrile disease when only the superficial part of defensive *qi* is involved, marked by fever, slight aversion to wind and cold, headache, reddened tongue tip, and floating and rapid pulse

气分证 [qì fèn zhèng]
***qi* aspect syndrome/pattern:** second stage of an epidemic febrile disease showing invasion of pathogenic heat to yang brightness meridian/channel or the lung, gallbladder, spleen, stomach or large intestine, marked by high fever without chills, dire thirst, flushed face, dark urine, reddened tongue with yellow coating, and rapid forceful pulse

卫气同病证 [wèi qì tóng bìng zhèng]
syndrome/pattern of both defense and *qi* aspects: syndrome/pattern characterized by simultaneous involvement of the defense and *qi* aspects, manifested by high fever, slight aversion to wind and cold, thirst, irritability, reddened tongue with whitish or yellowish coating, and rapid floating pulse

卫营同病证 [wèi yíng tóng bìng zhèng]
syndrome/pattern of both defense and nutrient aspects: syndrome/pattern characterized by simultaneous involvement of the defense and nutrient aspects, manifested by high fever and chills with delirium, headache and general aching

营分证 [yíng fèn zhèng]
nutrient aspect syndrome/pattern: serious development of an epidemic febrile disease showing invasion of pathogenic

heat to the nutrient aspect including that of the heart (mind), marked by fever (higher at night), restlessness or delirium, faint skin rashes, and crimson tongue

血分证 [xuè fèn zhèng]
blood aspect syndrome/pattern: epidemic febrile disease at its severest stage, characterized by severe damage to yin blood, with various forms of bleeding such as hemoptysis, epistaxis, hematuria, hematochezia, in addition to high fever, coma, or convulsions

血热动血证 [xuè rè dòng xuè zhèng]
syndrome/pattern of blood heat stirring blood: syndrome/pattern marked by fever, thirst, vexing insomnia, crimson tongue, and various hemorrhagic disorders

血热风盛证 [xuè rè fēng shèng zhèng]
syndrome/pattern of blood heat with raging wind: syndrome/pattern marked by high fever, convulsions, opisthotonos, crimson tongue with dry yellow coating, and rapid wiry pulse

血热化燥证 [xuè rè huà zào zhèng]
syndrome/pattern of blood heat with dryness transformation: syndrome/pattern marked by dry mouth and throat, constipation, lassitude, fever (higher at night), thirst with not much desire to drink, crimson tongue with scanty coating, and rapid thready pulse

热入营血证 [rè rù yíng xuè zhèng]
syndrome/pattern of heat entering nutrient-blood: syndrome/pattern marked by fever (higher at night), vexing insomnia or impaired consciousness, barely visible skin rashes or bleeding, constipation, crimson tongue, and rapid thready pulse

气营两燔证 [qì yíng liǎng fán zhèng]
syndrome/pattern of dual blaze of *qi*-nutrient aspects: syndrome/pattern characterized by simultaneous existence of syndromes of *qi* and nutrient aspects, manifested by high fever, thirst, mental irritability, delirium and barely visible skin eruption

气血两燔证 [qì xuè liǎng fán zhèng]
syndrome/pattern of dual blaze of *qi*-blood aspects: syndrome/pattern characterized by simultaneous existence of syndromes of *qi* and blood aspects, manifested by high fever, thirst, delirium, skin eruptions, and various bleeding symptoms

热入［闭］心包证 [rè rù (bì) xīn bāo zhèng]
syndrome/pattern of heat entering the pericardium: syndrome/pattern marked by high fever, thirst, loss of consciousness or delirium, red face, coarse breath, reddened tongue with yellow coating, and slippery rapid pulse

热盛动血证 [rè shèng dòng xuè zhèng]
syndrome/pattern of exuberant heat with bleeding: syndrome/pattern marked by high fever, thirst, delirium, red face and eyes, hematochezia, hematuria, epistaxis, or distinct skin eruption, deep-red tongue with yellow coating and rapid surging pulse

余热未清证 [yú rè wèi qīng zhèng]
residual heat syndrome/pattern: syndrome/

pattern characterized by lingering of residual heat, and manifested by persistent low fever, irritability, thirst, constipation, deep-colored urine, reddened tongue lacking moisture, and rapid thready pulse

三焦辨证
Triple-energizer Syndrome Differentiation (Triple-energizer Pattern Identification)

三焦辨证 [sān jiāo biàn zhèng] **triple-energizer syndrome differentiation; triple-energizer pattern identification:** syndrome differentiation or pattern identification in accordance with the theory of the triple energizer

上焦病证 [shàng jiāo bìng zhèng] **upper-energizer syndrome/pattern:** syndrome/pattern due to invasion of pathogen to the lung meridian/channel at the early stage of epidemic febrile disease, marked by chills and fever, sweating, headache, and cough, or on the pericardium meridian/channel marked by delirium, and deep red tongue

中焦病证 [zhōng jiāo bìng zhèng] **middle-energizer syndrome/pattern:** syndrome/pattern due to invasion of pathogen to the stomach meridian/channel at the middle stage of epidemic febrile disease, marked by fever without chills, sweating, thirst, and full pulse, or on the spleen meridian/channel marked by continuous moderate fever, aching and heavy feeling in the body, stuffiness in the chest with nausea and vomiting, and greasy tongue coating

下焦病证 [xià jiāo bìng zhèng] **lower-energizer syndrome/pattern:** syndrome/pattern due to impairment of the kidney meridian/channel at the later stage of epidemic febrile disease, manifested by fever (more remarkable in the palms than on the back of hands), thirst, parched lips and restlessness, or due to impairment of the liver meridian/channel manifested by mental disorders, twitching or convulsion

三焦湿热证 [sān jiāo shī rè zhèng] **triple-energizer dampness-heat syndrome/pattern:** syndrome/pattern due to invasion of pathogenic dampness-heat involving all three energizers

上焦湿热证 [shàng jiāo shī rè zhèng] **upper-energizer dampness-heat syndrome/pattern:** syndrome/pattern occurring at the initial stage of a dampness-heat disease, generally manifested by chills, fever, no sweat, and soggy pulse, as well as the symptoms of the upper energizer such as heaviness in the head, oppression in the chest, and cough

中焦湿热证 [zhōng jiāo shī rè zhèng] **middle-energizer dampness-heat syndrome/pattern:** syndrome/pattern occurring at the middle stage of a dampness-heat disease, involving the spleen and stomach, manifested by submerged fever more marked in the afternoon, epigastric distension, nausea, loss of appetite, and dryness in the mouth with no desire to drink

下焦湿热证 [xià jiāo shī rè zhèng]
lower-energizer dampness-heat syndrome/pattern: syndrome/pattern due to invasion of pathogenic dampness-heat on the large intestine, bladder or genitalia, generally manifested by fever, lower abdominal pain, reddened tongue with yellow greasy coating, and rapid slippery pulse, associated with constipation or diarrhea, dysuria or anuria, or morbid leukorrhea

气血辨证
Qi-blood Syndrome Differentiation (*Qi*-blood Pattern Identification)

气血辨证 [qì xuè biàn zhèng]
***qi*-blood syndrome differentiation; *qi*-blood pattern identification:** differentiation of syndromes or identification of patterns according to the state of *qi* and blood

气虚证 [qì xū zhèng]
***qi* deficiency syndrome/pattern:** syndrome/pattern of insufficiency of genuine *qi* with diminished function of internal organs, marked by shortness of breath, lassitude, listlessness, spontaneous sweating, pale tongue, and pulse of deficiency type

气陷证 [qì xiàn zhèng]
***qi* sinking syndrome/pattern:** syndrome/pattern ascribed to failure in the lifting or holding function of *qi*, marked by shortage of *qi*, lassitude, prolapse of the anus, prolapse of the uterus or visceroptosis, pale tongue and weak pulse

气郁证 [qì yù zhèng]
***qi* depression syndrome/pattern:** syndrome/pattern marked by feeling of distension in the chest, pain in the hypochondriac region, irritability, irascibility, anorexia, and menstrual disorders in women

气滞证 [qì zhì zhèng]
***qi* stagnation syndrome/pattern:** syndrome/pattern resulting from stagnation of *qi*, marked by thoracic, hypochondriac, epigastric and abdominal distension or pain, on and off, often ameliorated by sighing or belching

气逆证 [qì nì zhèng]
***qi* counterflow syndrome/pattern:** syndrome/pattern featured by abnormal upward movement of *qi*, manifested by cough and dyspnea, or nausea, vomiting, hiccups, belching or even hematemesis, or feeling of gas ascending from the lower abdomen to the chest or throat

气闭证 [qì bì zhèng]
***qi* block syndrome/pattern:** syndrome/pattern ascribed to blockage of *qi* movement, manifested by colicky pain in the chest and abdomen with fecal retention and urinary block, or sudden loss of consciousness with trismus and contracture of limbs

气脱证 [qì tuō zhèng]
***qi* collapse syndrome/pattern:** critical syndrome/pattern ascribed to drastic discharge of *qi*, manifested by sudden appearance of profuse sweating, somber pale complexion, cyanotic lips, cold extremities, feeble breathing, hardly perceptible pulse, and even fainting or

loss of consciousness with incontinence of urine

气虚发热证 [qì xū fā rè zhèng]
syndrome/pattern of *qi* deficiency with fever: syndrome/pattern ascribed to *qi* deficiency, marked by a low persistent fever aggravated by physical exertion, associated with fatigue, lack of strength, shortness of breath, pale tongue and weak pulse

气虚湿阻［困］证 [qì xū shī zǔ (kùn) zhèng]
syndrome/pattern of *qi* deficiency with dampness obstruction: syndrome/pattern attributed to deficiency of healthy *qi* with retention of pathogenic dampness, manifested by listlessness, lassitude, reduced food intake, shortness of breath, heaviness in the head and body, abdominal distension, diarrhea, and soggy weak pulse

气虚水停证 [qì xū shuǐ tíng zhèng]
syndrome/pattern of *qi* deficiency with water retention: syndrome/pattern attributed to deficiency of healthy *qi* with retention of water in the body, manifested by shortness of breath, listlessness, lassitude, edema of the limbs, and reduced urine output

气虚气滞证 [qì xū qì zhì zhèng]
syndrome/pattern of *qi* deficiency and stagnation: syndrome/pattern attributed to deficiency of healthy *qi* together with stagnant *qi* movement, manifested by listlessness, shortness of breath, lassitude, feeling of distension and scurrying pain in the chest and abdomen

气虚外感证 [qì xū wài gǎn zhèng]
syndrome/pattern of *qi* deficiency with external contraction: syndrome/pattern of external contraction occurring in a person with *qi* deficiency, manifested by aversion to cold, fever, spontaneous sweating, headache, stuffy nose, feeble voice, lassitude, lack of strength, shortness of breath, and floating feeble pulse

气虚鼻窍失充证 [qì xū bí qiào shī chōng zhèng]
syndrome/pattern of *qi* deficiency with smell loss: syndrome/pattern marked by loss of sense of smell with nasal obstruction, clear discharge and frequent sneezing, pale swollen concha, associated with dizziness, lack of strength, shortness of breath, reluctance to speak, spontaneous sweating, aversion to wind, pale tongue and weak pulse

气虚耳窍失充证 [qì xū ěr qiào shī chōng zhèng]
syndrome/pattern of *qi* deficiency with hearing loss: syndrome/pattern marked by impairment of hearing with tinnitus like the sound of cicadas, associated with dizziness, lack of strength, shortness of breath, reluctance to speak, pale tongue and weak pulse

气阴两虚证 [qì yīn liǎng xū zhèng]
syndrome/pattern of deficiency of both *qi* and yin: syndrome/pattern marked by listlessness, lack of strength, shortness of breath, reluctance to speak, dry throat and mouth, vexing thirst, malar flush in the afternoon, short voidings of small amounts of urine, constipation, thin tongue with scanty dry coating, and rapid vacuous

pulse, also called *qi*-yin insufficiency syndrome/pattern (气阴亏虚证 [qì yīn kuī xū zhèng])

气阴亏虚证 [qì yīn kuī xū zhèng]
***qi*-yin insufficiency syndrome/pattern:** same as syndrome/pattern of deficiency of both *qi* and yin (气阴两虚证[qì yīn liǎng xū zhèng])

血虚证 [xuè xū zhèng]
blood deficiency syndrome/pattern: syndrome/pattern marked by pale or sallow complexion, pale lips and nails, dizziness, dimmed vision, palpitation, numbness of the extremities, and thready pulse

血脱证 [xuè tuō zhèng]
blood collapse syndrome/pattern: critical syndrome/pattern occurring in cases of acute massive bleeding, marked by pallor, dizziness, palpitations, faint and short breaths, cold extremities, pale tongue, and hollow or hardly perceptible pulse

血虚挟瘀证 [xuè xū xié yū zhèng]
syndrome/pattern of blood deficiency complicated by stasis: syndrome/pattern attributed to blood deficiency together with blood stasis, manifested by sallow or pale complexion, dizziness, blurred vision, palpitations, dream-disturbed sleep, stabbing pain fixed in location, scanty menstrual discharge in women with dark-purple blood with clots, dysmenorrhea or amenorrhea, purple tongue or purple spots on the tongue, and fine choppy pulse

血虚寒凝证 [xuè xū hán níng zhèng]
syndrome/pattern of blood deficiency and cold congealing: syndrome/pattern attributed to blood deficiency and cold congealing in combination, manifested by purplish complexion, dizziness, blurred vision, dark-purple lips and tongue, cold extremities and other localized cold feelings, pain and numbness; in women, late periods with scant menstrual discharge of dark blood or clots, and painful periods or amenorrhea

血虚外感证 [xuè xū wài gǎn zhèng]
syndrome/pattern of blood deficiency and external contraction: syndrome / pattern of external contraction occurring in a person with blood deficiency, manifested by fever, aversion to cold, scanty or no sweating, pale complexion, pale lips and nails, dizziness, palpitations, pale tongue, and floating pulse

血虚内热证 [xuè xū nèi rè zhèng]
syndrome/pattern of blood deficiency with internal heat: syndrome/pattern of internal heat arising from blood deficiency, marked by pale complexion, pale tongue and thready pulse accompanied by fever

血虚生［动］风证 [xuè xū shēng (dòng) fēng zhèng]
syndrome/pattern of blood deficiency generating wind: syndrome/pattern attributed to blood deficiency that deprives the sinews of nourishment, manifested by pale complexion, lips and nails, dizziness, blurred vision, numbness, itching, and tremor or involuntary movement of the limbs

血虚风燥证 [xuè xū fēng zào zhèng]
syndrome/pattern of blood deficiency

and wind-dryness: syndrome/pattern attributed to blood deficiency that deprives the skin of nourishment, manifested by dry, rough, itchy, shriveled skin with rhagades, withering and loss of hair, numbness of body surface, lusterless complexion, pale nails, dizziness and blurred vision, pale tongue and thready pulse, also called syndrome/pattern of blood deficiency with dryness of skin and generation of wind (血虚肤燥生风证 [xuè xū fū zào shēng fēng zhèng])

血虚肤燥生风证 [xuè xū fū zào shēng fēng zhèng]
syndrome/pattern of blood deficiency with dryness of skin and generation of wind: synonymous with syndrome/pattern of blood deficiency and wind-dryness (血虚风燥证 [xuè xū fēng zào zhèng])

血寒证 [xuè hán zhèng]
blood cold syndrome/pattern: syndrome/pattern ascribed to pathogenic cold obstructing *qi* movement and blood flow, manifested by aversion to cold, cold pain and numbness of the extremities, cyanotic lips and tongue, late periods and dark purple menstrual discharge in women with blood clots, white slippery tongue coating and slow sunken choppy pulse, also called blood cold congealing syndrome/pattern (血寒凝滞证 [xuè hán níng zhì zhèng])

血寒凝滞证 [xuè hán níng zhì zhèng]
blood cold congealing syndrome/pattern: another name for blood cold syndrome/pattern (血寒证 [xuè hán zhèng])

血热证 [xuè rè zhèng]
blood heat syndrome/pattern: synonym for blood aspect syndrome/pattern (血分证 [xuè fèn zhèng])

血瘀证 [xuè yū zhèng]
blood stasis syndrome/pattern: syndrome/pattern attributed to obstruction of blood flow by static blood, and marked by formation of painful and tender purple mass, or abdominal mass with stabbing pain and tenderness, or discharge of dark-purple blood with clots, purple tongue or purple spots on the tongue, and wiry choppy pulse, also called static blood obstruction syndrome/pattern (瘀血阻滞证 [yū xuè zǔ zhì zhèng])

瘀血阻滞证 [yū xuè zǔ zhì zhèng]
static blood obstruction syndrome/pattern: another name for blood stasis syndrome/pattern (血瘀证 [xuè yū zhèng])

瘀血犯头证 [yū xuè fàn tóu zhèng]
syndrome/pattern of static blood invading the head: syndrome/pattern ascribed to static blood obstructing the vessels of the head in cases of traumatic injury, manifested by persistent sharp pain in the head with fixed location, dizziness, forgetfulness, dim complexion, purple tongue or purple spots on the tongue, and wiry choppy pulse

血瘀舌下证 [xuè yū shé xià zhèng]
sublingual blood stasis syndrome/pattern: syndrome/pattern marked by the development of a dark purple mass under the tongue, associated with purple tongue or purple spots on the tongue, and impaired motility of the tongue

血瘀风燥证 [xuè yū fēng zào zhèng]
syndrome/pattern of blood stasis with

wind-dryness: syndrome/pattern ascribed to internally retained static blood leading to dryness and wind, manifested either by encrusted skin with desquamation and itching, or by vertigo and numbness of the limb, associated with purple tongue or purple spots on the tongue, and thready choppy pulse

血瘀水停证 [xuè yū shuǐ tíng zhèng]
syndrome/pattern of blood stasis with water retention: syndrome/pattern marked by formation of mass in the abdomen with stabbing pain, associated with enlarged and distended abdomen and inhibited urination, purple tongue or purple spots on the tongue, and choppy pulse

气血两虚证 [qì xuè liǎng xū zhèng]
syndrome/pattern of *qi*-blood dual deficiency: syndrome/pattern marked by listlessness, lack of strength, shortness of breath, pale or sallow complexion, dizziness, dimmed vision, pale lips and nails, palpitations, insomnia, pale tongue, and weak pulse

气滞血瘀证 [qì zhì xuè yū zhèng]
syndrome/pattern of *qi* stagnation and blood stasis: syndrome/pattern resulting from *qi* stagnation and blood stasis, marked by scurrying or stabbing pain in the thoracic, hypochondriac, epigastric or abdominal region with or without mass formation, purple tongue or purple-spotted tongue, and wiry and choppy pulse, also called *qi*-blood stagnation syndrome/pattern (气血瘀滞证 [qì xuè yū zhì zhèng])

气血瘀滞证 [qì xuè yū zhì zhèng]
***qi*-blood stagnation syndrome/pattern:** same as syndrome/pattern of *qi* stagnation and blood stasis (气滞血瘀证 [qì zhì xuè yū zhèng])

气虚血瘀证 [qì xū xuè yū zhèng]
syndrome/pattern of *qi* deficiency and blood stasis: syndrome/pattern marked by manifestations of blood stasis such as stabbing pain fixed in location together with listlessness, lassitude, shortness of breath and sweating upon mild exertion showing *qi* deficiency

气不摄［统］血证 [qì bù shè (tǒng) xuè zhèng]
syndrome/pattern of *qi* failing to control blood: syndrome/pattern of *qi* deficiency in which *qi* is unable to control blood, manifested by hematochezia, bleeding through the pores, gum bleeding, uterine bleeding or excessive menstrual discharge in women, listlessness, lack of strength, shortness of breath, reluctance to speak, lusterless complexion, pale tongue and weak pulse

气随血脱证 [qì suí xuè tuō zhèng]
syndrome/pattern of *qi* collapse following bleeding: critical syndrome/pattern attributed to acute massive bleeding, and manifested by pale complexion, reverse cold of limbs, profuse sweating, feeble breathing, and hardly perceptible pulse or vacuous rootless large pulse

气滞痰凝咽喉证 [qì zhì tán níng yān hóu zhèng]
syndrome/pattern of *qi* stagnation and phlegm coagulation in the throat: syndrome/pattern marked by depressed mood, sensation of the presence of a

foreign body in the throat, swelling of the pharyngeal mucus membrane, greasy tongue coating, and wiry slippery pulse

津液辨证
Body Fluid Syndrome Differentiation (Body Fluid Pattern Identification)

津液辨证 [jīn yè biàn zhèng]
body fluid syndrome differentiation; body fluid pattern identification: differentiation of syndromes or identification of patterns according to the condition of body fluids

津液亏虚证 [jīn yè kuī xū zhèng]
fluid deficiency syndrome/pattern: syndrome/pattern marked by dry mouth and throat, parched or cracked lips, thirst, oliguria, constipation, reddened tongue lacking moisture, and rapid thready weak pulse, also called 津液亏损证 [jīn yè kuī sǔn zhèng]

津液亏损证 [jīn yè kuī sǔn zhèng]
fluid deficiency syndrome/pattern: same as 津液亏虚证 [jīn yè kuī xū zhèng]

津亏证 [jīn kuī zhèng]
fluid inadequacy syndrome/pattern: mild case of fluid deficiency syndrome/pattern, also called fluid consumption syndrome/pattern (津伤证[jīn shāng zhèng])

津伤证 [jīn shāng zhèng]
fluid consumption syndrome/pattern: same as fluid inadequacy syndrome/pattern (津亏证 [jīn kuī zhèng])

液脱证 [yè tuō zhèng]
fluid collapse syndrome/pattern: severe case of fluid deficiency syndrome/pattern

津气亏虚证 [jīn qì kuī xū zhèng]
fluid-*qi* deficiency syndrome/pattern: syndrome/pattern due to deficiency of both fluid and *qi*, manifested by listlessness, shortness of breath, vexing thirst, dry skin, sunken eyeballs, reddened tongue with dry coating and thready weak pulse

肺燥津伤证 [fèi zào jīn shāng zhèng]
lung fluid depletion syndrome/pattern: syndrome/pattern marked by dryness of the nose and mouth, dry cough with hoarseness, and dry tongue coating

胃燥津亏证 [wèi zào jīn kuī zhèng]
stomach fluid depletion syndrome/pattern: syndrome/pattern marked by dry lips and mouth, retching, constipation, emaciation, and absence of tongue coating

肠燥津亏证 [cháng zào jīn kuī zhèng]
intestinal fluid depletion syndrome/pattern: syndrome/pattern marked by constipation, dry throat and fidgeting

津亏热结证 [jīn kuī rè jié zhèng]
syndrome/pattern of fluid depletion with retained heat: syndrome/pattern marked by fever, thirst, dry lips and tongue, oliguria, constipation, restlessness, reddened tongue with yellow coating, and rapid pulse

水饮内停证 [shuǐ yǐn nèi tíng zhèng]
syndrome/pattern of interior retention of water-fluid: syndrome/pattern due to accumulation and retention of fluid in the

interior of the body, marked by dizziness, stuffy thoracic and epigastric sensation, vomiting of clear fluid, slippery tongue coating, and wiry pulse

饮证 [yǐn zhèng]
fluid retention syndrome/pattern: abbreviation for syndrome/pattern of interior retention of water-fluid (水饮内停证 [shuǐ yǐn nèi tíng zhèng])

饮停心包证 [yǐn tíng xīn bāo zhèng]
pericardial fluid retention syndrome/pattern: syndrome/pattern marked by palpitations, orthopnea with fullness and stuffy sensation in the heart and chest, pale purplish tongue with white slippery coating, and hidden or weak pulse

饮停胸胁证 [yǐn tíng xiōng xié zhèng]
thoracic fluid retention syndrome/pattern: syndrome/pattern marked by fullness and stuffy sensation in the chest, cough, dyspnea, white slippery tongue coating, and wiry and slippery pulse

气滞水停证 [qì zhì shuǐ tíng zhèng]
syndrome/pattern of *qi* stagnation with water retention: syndrome/pattern of water retention due to *qi* stagnation, manifested by edema of the limbs, oliguria, heavy feeling in the head and body, distension, oppression and scurrying pain in the chest, epigastrium and abdomen, and pale tongue with white slippery coating

风水相搏证 [fēng shuǐ xiāng bó zhèng]
syndrome/pattern of wind-water combat: syndrome/pattern ascribed to pathogenic wind impacting the lung which causes dysfunction of the latter in regulating water passage leading to abnormal accumulation of water under the skin, manifested by acute onset of edema of the head and face, and then generalized edema, associated with aversion to wind, reduced amount of urine, and floating pulse

寒饮内停证 [hán yǐn nèi tíng zhèng]
syndrome/pattern of interior retention of cold-fluid: syndrome/pattern marked by aversion to cold with cold limbs, cough with frothy expectoration, or dizziness with palpitations and suffocating sensation, or epigastric stuffiness with vomiting of clear fluid, or costal and hypochondriac distension, plump tongue with white slippery coating, and wiry slippery pulse

寒饮停肺证 [hán yǐn tíng fèi zhèng]
syndrome/pattern of cold-fluid retention in the lung: syndrome/pattern marked by cough, dyspnea, wheezing or orthopnea, thin whitish sputum, white slippery tongue coating, and wiry pulse

寒饮停胃证 [hán yǐn tíng wèi zhèng]
syndrome/pattern of cold-fluid retention in the stomach: syndrome/pattern marked by epigastric distension with splashing sounds in the stomach, vomiting of clear fluid, white slippery tongue coating, and wiry pulse, also called syndrome/pattern of stomach cold with fluid retention (胃寒饮停证 [wèi hán yǐn tíng zhèng])

胃寒饮停证 [wèi hán yǐn tíng zhèng]
syndrome/pattern of stomach cold with fluid retention: same as syndrome/pattern of cold-fluid retention in the stomach (寒饮停胃证 [hán yǐn tíng wèi zhèng])

水停证 [shuǐ tíng zhèng]
water retention syndrome/pattern: syndrome/pattern marked by edema, oliguria, or accompanied by ascites, pale plump tongue with white slippery coating, and soggy and relaxed pulse, also called water-*qi* syndrome/pattern or edema syndrome/pattern (水气证 [shuǐ qì zhèng])

水气证 [shuǐ qì zhèng]
water-*qi* syndrome/pattern; edema syndrome/pattern: same as water retention syndrome/pattern (水停证 [shuǐ tíng zhèng])

痰证 [tán zhèng]
phlegm syndrome/pattern: syndrome/pattern caused by phlegm, often marked by cough, dyspnea with profuse expectoration, or by nausea, vomiting and dizziness, or by formation of local round masses, also called phlegm-turbidity syndrome/pattern (痰浊证 [tán zhuó zhèng])

痰浊证 [tán zhuó zhèng]
phlegm-turbidity syndrome: same as phlegm syndrome/pattern (痰证 [tán zhèng])

风痰证 [fēng tán zhèng]
wind-phlegm syndrome/pattern: syndrome/pattern due to either external wind with phlegm or liver wind with phlegm, marked by coughing with frothy expectoration, stuffy sensation in the chest, dizziness, headache, or phlegmatic sounds in the throat, wry eye and skewed mouth, white greasy tongue coating, and wiry slippery pulse

寒痰证 [hán tán zhèng]
cold-phlegm syndrome/pattern: syndrome/pattern marked by coughing with whitish expectoration, dyspnea or wheezing, aversion to cold with cool limbs, white greasy tongue coating, and wiry slippery or tense pulse

湿痰证 [shī tán zhèng]
dampness-phlegm syndrome/pattern: syndrome/pattern marked by coughing with profuse expectoration, heavy sensation in the limbs, stuffy feeling in the chest and stomach, reduced food intake, stickiness of the mouth, white greasy tongue coating, and wiry and slippery pulse

热痰证 [rè tán zhèng]
heat-phlegm syndrome/pattern: syndrome/pattern marked by coughing with yellowish expectoration, fever, thirst, reddened tongue with yellow greasy coating, and slippery and rapid pulse

燥痰证 [zào tán zhèng]
dryness-phlegm syndrome/pattern: syndrome/pattern marked by coughing with scanty sticky sputum difficult to spit out, or blood streaks in the sputum, chest pain with stuffy sensation, dry nose and mouth, tongue with scanty moisture but greasy coating, and choppy pulse

痰瘀互结证 [tán yū hù jié zhèng]
combined syndrome/pattern of phlegm and static blood: syndrome/pattern ascribed to turbid phlegm and static blood combining with each other, marked by formation of masses with stabbing pain, or numbness and atrophy of the limb, oppression in the chest with expectoration of profuse sputum or sputum with blood clots, purple tongue or purple spots on

the tongue with greasy coating, and wiry choppy pulse

瘀痰证 [yū tán zhèng]
syndrome/pattern of phlegm and static blood: abbreviation for combined syndrome/pattern of phlegm and static blood (痰瘀互结证 [tán yū hù jié zhèng])

痰浊犯头证 [tán zhuó fàn tóu zhèng]
syndrome/pattern of phlegm-turbidity invading the head: syndrome/pattern marked by headache and mental clouding, tinnitus, impaired hearing, blurred vision, stuffiness in the chest and epigastrium, vomiting of mucus, white slimy tongue coating and wiry slippery pulse

痰湿犯耳证 [tán shī fàn ěr zhèng]
syndrome/pattern of phlegm-dampness invading the ear: syndrome/pattern marked by distension and pressure in the ear, or dizziness, tinnitus, heaviness in the head and nausea, or purulent discharge from the ear and impaired hearing, associated with a visible fluid horizon through the tympanic membrane, slippery greasy tongue coating and wiry slippery pulse

痰核留结证 [tán hé liú jié zhèng]
syndrome/pattern of lingering phlegm nodules: syndrome/pattern marked by round, firm, slippery and movable lumps below the skin of the neck, without redness, hotness or pain

痰热内扰证 [tán rè nèi rǎo zhèng]
syndrome/pattern of internal harassment of phlegm-heat: syndrome/pattern ascribed to phlegm-heat in the interior disturbing the mental activities and *qi* movement, marked by vexation, insomnia, dream-disturbed sleep, associated with coughing with thick yellow expectoration, dyspnea, fever, thirst, reddened tongue with yellow greasy coating, and rapid slippery pulse

痰热内闭证 [tán rè nèi bì zhèng]
syndrome/pattern of internal block of phlegm-heat: syndrome/pattern ascribed to phlegm-heat in the interior blocking the mental activities, marked by impaired consciousness, and delirium or mania, associated with fullness, distension and scorching pain in the chest, coughing, panting or wheezing, expectoration of thick yellow sputum, fever, thirst, reddened tongue with yellow greasy coating and rapid slippery pulse

痰热动风证 [tán rè dòng fēng zhèng]
syndrome/pattern of phlegm-heat stirring wind: syndrome/pattern ascribed to exuberant phlegm-heat inducing liver wind, marked by convulsions or vertigo with nausea and vomiting, associated with fullness and oppression in the chest, cough, dyspnea and expectoration of thick sputum or rattling in the throat, reddened tongue with yellow greasy coating, and rapid slippery pulse

痰气互［郁］结证 [tán qì hù (yù) jié zhèng]
syndrome/pattern of combined phlegm and *qi*: syndrome/pattern marked by depressed mood, insomnia, dream-disturbed sleep, feeling of the presence of a foreign body in the throat which can be neither swallowed nor ejected, fullness and oppression in the chest, profuse

sputum, white and greasy tongue coating, and slippery wiry pulse

病因辨证
Disease-cause Syndrome Differentiation (Disease-cause Pattern Identification)

病因辨证 [bìng yīn biàn zhèng]
disease cause syndrome differentiation; disease cause pattern identification: diagnosis of syndrome or pattern via analysing and differentiating pathological conditions attributable to different kinds of causal factors

审证求因 [shěn zhèng qiú yīn]
cause seeking from symptoms: determining the cause of a disease according to the clinical manifestations

外风证 [wài fēng zhèng]
external wind syndrome/pattern: general term for syndromes/patterns caused by exogenous pathogenic wind alone or together with one or more of other pathogenic factors, such as dampness, heat, or pestilent toxin

风邪犯表证 [fēng xié fàn biǎo zhèng]
syndrome/pattern of wind pathogen invading the exterior: syndrome/pattern marked by aversion to wind, fever, sweating, and floating pulse, sometimes accompanied by skin itching and edema, or by coughing, sore throat and general aching, also called syndrome/pattern of external invasion of wind pathogen (风邪外袭证 [fēng xié wài xí zhèng])

风邪外袭证 [fēng xié wài xí zhèng]
syndrome/pattern of external invasion of wind pathogen: same as syndrome/pattern of wind pathogen invading the exterior (风邪犯表证 [fēng xié fàn biǎo zhèng])

风袭表疏证 [fēng xí biǎo shū zhèng]
syndrome/pattern of wind attacking the loose exterior: synonym for exterior deficiency syndrome/pattern (表虚证 [biǎo xū zhèng])

风中经络证 [fēng zhòng jīng luò zhèng]
syndrome/pattern of wind striking the meridians/channels: syndrome/pattern marked by numbness and itching of the skin, or sudden onset of wry eye and skewed mouth, also called syndrome/pattern of wind pathogen attacking the collaterals (风邪袭络证 [fēng xié xí luò zhèng])

风胜行痹证 [fēng shèng xíng bì zhèng]
syndrome/pattern of wind-prevailing migratory arthralgia: syndrome/pattern attributed to stagnation of pathogenic wind-cold-dampness (with predominance of wind) in sinews/tendons, bones and joints, and chiefly manifested by wandering arthralgia

风邪袭络证 [fēng xié xí luò zhèng]
syndrome/pattern of wind pathogen attacking the collaterals: same as syndrome/pattern of wind striking the meridians/channels (风中经络证 [fēng zhòng jīng luò zhèng])

风寒证 [fēng hán zhèng]
wind-cold syndrome/pattern: general term for various syndromes/patterns

caused by exogenous wind-cold

风寒表证 [fēng hán biǎo zhèng]
exterior wind-cold syndrome/pattern: syndrome/pattern marked by aversion to cold with mild fever, no sweating, general aching, or congested nose with watery discharge, dyspnea, thin white tongue coating, and floating and tense pulse

风寒袭表证 [fēng hán xí biǎo zhèng]
syndrome/pattern of wind-cold attacking the exterior: same as exterior wind-cold syndrome/pattern (风寒表证 [fēng hán biǎo zhèng])

风寒犯头证 [fēng hán fàn tóu zhèng]
syndrome/pattern of wind-cold invading the head: syndrome/pattern marked by headache with pain in the nape and back, aggravated by wind and cold, thin white tongue coating, and floating and tense pulse

风寒袭鼻证 [fēng hán xí bí zhèng]
syndrome/pattern of wind-cold attacking the nose: syndrome/pattern marked by stuffy runny nose or itchy nose with sneezing, and swollen nasal concha with pale mucous membrane and clear secretion, associated with aversion to wind and cold, thin white tongue coating and floating tight pulse

风寒袭喉［咽］证 [fēng hán xí hóu (yān) zhèng]
syndrome/pattern of wind-cold attacking the throat: syndrome/pattern marked by painful throat, associated with mild fever and aversion to cold, absence of sweating, thin white tongue coating and floating tight pulse

风寒袭肺证 [fēng hán xí fèi zhèng]
syndrome/pattern of wind-cold attacking the lung: syndrome/pattern marked by aversion to cold, no sweating, cough, dyspnea, whitish expectoration, whitish tongue coating, and floating and tense pulse

风寒袭络证 [fēng hán xí luò zhèng]
syndrome/pattern of wind-cold attacking the collaterals: synonym for syndrome/pattern of cold stagnating in the meridians/channels (寒滞经脉证 [hán zhì jīng mài zhèng])

风寒湿阻证 [fēng hán shī zǔ zhèng]
syndrome/pattern of obstruction by wind-cold-dampness: syndrome/pattern marked by joint pain, wandering or accompanied by sensation of heaviness

风热证 [fēng rè zhèng]
wind-heat syndrome/pattern: general term for various syndromes/patterns caused by exogenous wind-heat, also called syndrome/pattern of external invasion of wind-heat (风热外袭证 [fēng rè wài xí zhèng])

风热表证 [fēng rè biǎo zhèng]
wind-heat exterior syndrome/pattern: exterior syndrome/pattern marked by fever with slight aversion to wind and cold, headache, slight thirst or sore throat, reddened tongue tip and edges, yellowish thin tongue coating, and rapid floating pulse

风热外袭证 [fēng rè wài xí zhèng]
syndrome/pattern of external invasion of wind-heat: synonymous with wind-heat syndrome/pattern (风热证 [fēng rè zhèng])

风热犯肺证 [fēng rè fàn fèi zhèng]
syndrome/pattern of wind-heat invading the lung: syndrome/pattern marked by fever with mild aversion to wind and cold, general aching or sore throat, cough, dyspnea, reddened tip of the tongue with thin yellowish coating, and rapid floating pulse

风热闭肺证 [fēng rè bì fèi zhèng]
syndrome/pattern of wind-heat blocking the lung: syndrome/pattern marked by fever with aversion to wind, cough, dyspnea with coarse breath, pain and suffocating feeling in the chest, no sweating, reddened tongue, and rapid floating pulse

风热犯头证 [fēng rè fàn tóu zhèng]
syndrome/pattern of wind-heat invading the head: syndrome/pattern marked by headache with a distending sensation, fever or aversion to wind, thirst, flushing of face, reddened tongue tip and edges, thin and yellowish tongue coating, and rapid floating pulse

风热犯目证 [fēng rè fàn mù zhèng]
syndrome/pattern of wind-heat invading the eye: syndrome/pattern marked by reddened and painful eye with excessive gum excretion and tears, fever, and aversion to wind

风热犯鼻证 [fēng rè fàn bí zhèng]
syndrome/pattern of wind-heat invading the nose: syndrome/pattern marked by nasal obstruction and discharge, swollen conchae and congested mucous membrane with thick secretion, and impaired sense of smell, associated with fever and slight aversion to wind and cold, thin yellow tongue coating and floating rapid pulse

风热侵喉［咽］证 [fēng rè qīn hóu (yān) zhèng]
syndrome/pattern of wind-heat invading the throat: syndrome/pattern marked by painful swollen throat or enlarged congested tonsils, hoarseness of voice, fever with slight aversion to wind and cold, mild thirst, thin yellow tongue coating, and rapid floating pulse

风热犯耳证 [fēng rè fàn ěr zhèng]
syndrome/pattern of wind-heat invading the ear: syndrome/pattern marked by distension and obstruction in the ear, and congestion or depression of the tympanic membrane, associated with tinnitus, headache, fever with slight aversion to wind and cold, thin yellow tongue coating, and rapid floating pulse

风热攻目证 [fēng rè gōng mù zhèng]
syndrome/pattern of wind-heat attacking the eye: syndrome/pattern marked by reddened, swollen and painful eye with plenty of gum and lacrimination, associated with fever, aversion to wind and floating rapid pulse

风火攻目证 [fēng huǒ gōng mù zhèng]
syndrome/pattern of wind-fire attacking the eye: same as syndrome/pattern of wind-heat attacking the eye (风热攻目证 [fēng rè gōng mù zhèng])

风湿证 [fēng shī zhèng]
wind-dampness syndrome/pattern: exterior syndrome/pattern marked by chills and fever, aching joint(s), heaviness in the head as if tightly bound, and white greasy tongue coating, also called syndrome/pattern of wind-dampness attacking the

exterior (风湿袭表证 [fēng shī xí biǎo zhèng]), syndrome/pattern of external invasion of wind-dampness (风湿外袭证 [fēng shī wài xí zhèng]), or exterior dampness syndrome/pattern (表湿证 [biǎo shī zhèng])

风湿袭表证 [fēng shī xí biǎo zhèng]
syndrome/pattern of wind-dampness attacking the exterior: same as wind-dampness syndrome/pattern (风湿证 [fēng shī zhèng])

风湿外袭证 [fēng shī wài xí zhèng]
syndrome/pattern of external invasion of wind-dampness: same as wind-dampness syndrome/pattern (风湿证 [fēng shī zhèng])

风湿犯头证 [fēng shī fàn tóu zhèng]
syndrome/pattern of wind-dampness invading the head: syndrome/pattern marked by headache as if the head were tightly bound, slight aversion to wind and cold, feeling of heaviness in the body and limbs, stuffy sensation in the chest, anorexia, white slippery tongue coating, and soggy pulse

风湿凌目证 [fēng shī líng mù zhèng]
syndrome/pattern of wind-dampness invading the eye: syndrome/pattern marked by swelling of the eyelid, and reddened and itchy eye with lacrimination

风燥袭表证 [fēng zào xí biǎo zhèng]
syndrome/pattern of wind-dryness attacking the exterior: syndrome/pattern marked by mild fever, aversion to wind and cold, headache, no sweating, dry nose and throat, thirst, and floating pulse

实寒证 [shí hán zhèng]
excess-cold syndrome/pattern: general term for syndromes/patterns caused by excessive cold pathogen

寒滞胃肠证 [hán zhì wèi cháng zhèng]
syndrome/pattern of cold stagnating in the stomach and intestines: syndrome/pattern marked by severe epigastric and abdominal pain with cold sensation, alleviated by warmth, vomiting, watery diarrhea, aversion to cold with cool limbs, white tongue coating, and wiry tense pulse

寒滞心脉证 [hán zhì xīn mài zhèng]
syndrome/pattern of cold stagnating in the heart vessels: syndrome/pattern marked by pectoral pain aggravated by cold and alleviated by warmth, white tongue coating, and sunken and slow or tense pulse

寒凝血瘀证 [hán níng xuè yū zhèng]
syndrome/pattern of congealing cold with blood stasis: syndrome/pattern ascribed to pathogenic cold obstructing *qi* movement and blood flow, manifested by pain aggravated by cold and alleviated by warmth, cold and cyanotic extremities, delayed and painful periods in women with discharge of dark purple blood with clots, dark purple tongue with white coating, and sunken, slow and choppy pulse

寒凝胞宫证 [hán níng bāo gōng zhèng]
syndrome/pattern of cold congealing in the uterus: syndrome/pattern marked by cold and pain in the lower abdomen, dysmenorrhea or delayed periods with dark menstrual discharge, white tongue coating, and sunken and tense pulse

寒滞经脉证 [hán zhì jīng mài zhèng]
syndrome/pattern of cold stagnating in the meridians/channels: syndrome/pattern marked by aversion to cold, pain and cold feeling in the limbs with contracture or numbness and purple or pale discoloration of the skin, white tongue coating, and wiry and tense pulse

寒胜痛痹证 [hán shèng tòng bì zhèng]
syndrome/pattern of cold-dominant agonizing arthralgia: syndrome/pattern attributed to stagnation of pathogenic wind-cold-dampness, with predominace of cold, in sinews, bones and joints, and manifested by articular cold pain with fixed location

暑证 [shǔ zhèng]
summerheat syndrome/pattern: general term for fire- or heat-nature syndromes/patterns that only occur in the season of summer and are caused by summerheat

暑热证 [shǔ rè zhèng]
summerheat syndrome/pattern: syndrome/pattern ascribed to summerheat causing consumption of *qi* and fluid, marked by fever, thirst, listlessness, shortness of breath, irritability, dizziness, sweating, short voiding of deep-colored urine, and reddened tongue with dry yellow coating, also called syndrome/pattern of internal stagnation of summerheat (暑热内郁证 [shǔ rè nèi yù zhèng])

暑热内郁证 [shǔ rè nèi yù zhèng]
syndrome/pattern of internal stagnation of summerheat: another name for summerheat syndrome/pattern (暑热证 [shǔ rè zhèng])

暑热动风证 [shǔ rè dòng fēng zhèng]
syndrome/pattern of summerheat stirring wind: syndrome/pattern ascribed to intense summerheat inducing liver wind, marked by high fever, loss of consciousness, convulsions, opisthotonos and trismus

暑湿证 [shǔ shī zhèng]
summerheat-dampness syndrome/pattern: syndrome/pattern caused by summerheat and dampness in combination, marked by thirst, listlessness, lassitude, vexation with cumbersome limbs, reddened tongue with yellow greasy coating, and rapid slippery pulse, also called syndrome/pattern of internal accumulation of summerheat and dampness (暑湿内蕴证 [shǔ shī nèi yùn zhèng])

暑湿内蕴证 [shǔ shī nèi yùn zhèng]
syndrome/pattern of internal accumulation of summerheat and dampness: another name for summerheat-dampness syndrome/pattern (暑湿证 [shǔ shī zhèng])

暑湿袭表证 [shǔ shī xí biǎo zhèng]
syndrome/pattern of summerheat-dampness attacking the exterior: syndrome/pattern marked by fever, slight aversion to wind and cold, heavy sensation of the body, lassitude, thirst, reddened tongue with yellowish greasy coating, and rapid soggy pulse

暑伤津气证 [shǔ shāng jīn qì zhèng]
syndrome/pattern of summerheat impairing the fluid and *qi*: syndrome/pattern marked by fever, sweating, desire for voluminous drinks, vexation, flushed

face, lassitude, shortness of breath, scanty dark urine, reddened tongue with dry yellow coating, and big floating but weak pulse

暑闭气机证 [shǔ bì qì jī zhèng]
syndrome/pattern of summerheat blocking the *qi* activity: syndrome/pattern marked by sudden fainting with fever, cold limbs, dyspnea, and trismus

暑热闭神证 [shǔ rè bì shén zhèng]
syndrome/pattern of summerheat blocking the mental activity: syndrome/pattern marked by high fever, dire thirst, sudden fainting with loss of consciousness and trismus, and sunken and hidden pulse

湿证 [shī zhèng]
dampness syndrome/pattern: general term for syndromes/patterns caused by pathogenic dampness which may come from the external environment or may be derived from within the body owing to abnormal transportation and transformation of fluids

表湿证 [biǎo shī zhèng]
exterior dampness syndrome/pattern: synonymous with wind-dampness syndrome/pattern (风湿证 [fēng shī zhèng])

湿胜着痹证 [shī shèng zhuó bì zhèng]
syndrome/pattern of dampness-prevailing agonizing arthralgia: syndrome/pattern attributed to stagnation of pathogenic wind-cold-dampness, with predominance of dampness, in sinews, bones and joints, and manifested by arthralgia with fixed location, and heaviness and swelling of the joint(s)

寒湿内阻证 [hán shī nèi zǔ zhèng]
syndrome/pattern of internal obstruction of cold-dampness: syndrome/pattern attributed to pathogenic cold-dampness obstructing *qi* movement, marked by heaviness in the head and body, joint pain with inhibited bending and stretching, absence of sweat, or edema of the face and limbs, loose stools, oliguria, white and moistened tongue coating and slippery pulse, also called cold-dampness syndrome/pattern (寒湿证 [hán shī zhèng])

寒湿证 [hán shī zhèng]
cold-dampness syndrome/pattern: abbreviation for syndrome/pattern of internal obstruction of cold-dampness (寒湿内阻证[hán shī nèi zǔ zhèng])

湿热蒸口证 [shī rè zhēng kǒu zhèng]
syndrome/pattern of dampness-heat steaming the mouth: syndrome/pattern marked by redness, swelling and pain in the mucous membrane of the mouth, or ulceration in the oral cavity with discharge of fetid pus, or reddened, swollen and ulcerated lip with inflamed angular rhagades, reddened tongue with yellow greasy coating and rapid soggy pulse, also known as syndrome/pattern of dampness-heat steaming the lip (湿热蒸唇证 [shī rè zhēng chún zhèng])

湿热蒸唇证 [shī rè zhēng chún zhèng]
syndrome/pattern of dampness-heat steaming the lip: synonymous with syndrome/pattern of dampness-heat steaming the mouth (湿热蒸口证 [shī rè zhēng kǒu zhèng])

湿热蒸舌证 [shī rè zhēng shé zhèng]
syndrome/pattern of dampness-heat steaming the tongue: syndrome/pattern marked by a reddened, swollen and painful tongue, or with festering ulceration, and yellow greasy tongue coating

湿热蒸齿证 [shī rè zhēng chǐ zhèng]
syndrome/pattern of dampness-heat steaming the teeth: syndrome/pattern marked by toothache or dental caries with pain aggravated by heat, sweetness and sourness, or reddened swollen gums, fetid mouth odor, reddened tongue with yellow greasy coating, and rapid slippery pulse

湿热犯耳证 [shī rè fàn ěr zhèng]
syndrome/pattern of dampness-heat invading the ear: syndrome/pattern marked by redness, swelling, pain, erosion, exudation and incrustation of the meatus or auricle, or discharge of thick yellow pus from the ear, or distension in the ear with tinnitus, yellow greasy tongue coating and rapid slippery pulse

湿热阻痹证 [shī rè zǔ bì zhèng]
syndrome/pattern of dampness-heat obstructing arthralgia: syndrome/pattern attributed to stagnation of pathogenic dampness-heat in sinews, bones and joints, and manifested by scorching pain of the joint with local hotness, swelling, and heaviness, reddened tongue with yellow greasy coating, and rapid slippery pulse

湿热蕴脾证 [shī rè yùn pí zhèng]
syndrome/pattern of dampness-heat accumulating in the spleen: syndrome/pattern marked by abdominal distension, nausea, vomiting, anorexia, heavy sensation in the limbs, or jaundice, reddened tongue with yellow greasy coating, and rapid soggy pulse

湿热下注证 [shī rè xià zhù zhèng]
syndrome/pattern of down-pouring dampness-heat: syndrome/pattern marked by frequent and painful urination, or yellow fetid discharge from the vagina in women, or ulceration of the leg with purulent discharge

外燥证 [wài zào zhèng]
external dryness syndrome/pattern: general term for syndromes/patterns caused by climatic dryness commonly marked by dry skin, and dry nose, mouth and throat

内燥证 [nèi zào zhèng]
internal dryness syndrome/pattern: syndrome/pattern of dryness due to consumption of body fluids, marked by withered skin, dry throat, parched lips, thirst, oliguria, constipation, reddened tongue without coating, and rapid thready pulse

温燥证 [wēn zào zhèng]
warm-dryness syndrome/pattern: syndrome/pattern marked by fever with slight aversion to wind and cold, dry cough with scanty expectoration, fidgeting, thirst, dry skin, nose and throat, thin yellowish tongue coating, and rapid floating pulse

凉燥证 [liáng zào zhèng]
cool-dryness syndrome/pattern: syndrome/pattern marked by more chills than fever, headache, no sweating, dry nose, mouth and throat, coughing with

scanty expectoration, thin and dry whitish tongue coating, and floating and tense pulse

燥邪犯［伤］肺证 [zào xié fàn (shāng) fèi zhèng]
syndrome/pattern of dryness pathogen invading [damaging] the lung: syndrome/pattern marked by mild chills and fever, dry cough, no expectoration or scanty sputum with blood streaks, thirst, and tongue without moisture

燥结证 [zào jié zhèng]
dryness accumulation syndrome/pattern: syndrome/pattern marked by constipation due to deficiency of fluids in the intestines

燥干清窍证 [zào gān qīng qiào zhèng]
dry orifice syndrome/pattern: syndrome/pattern marked by dry nose, mouth and eyes with lack of nasal mucus, saliva and tears

实火证 [shí huǒ zhèng]
excess fire syndrome/pattern: general term for syndromes/patterns marked by fever, thirst with desire for cold drinks, flushed face, blood-shot eyes, constipation, scanty dark urine, reddened tongue with yellow coating, and rapid or surging pulse

火毒证 [huǒ dú zhèng]
fire toxin syndrome/pattern: syndrome/pattern marked by local redness, swelling and burning pain, followed by abscess formation and accompanied by fever, thirst, reddened tongue with yellow coating, and rapid pulse, also called heat toxin syndrome/pattern (热毒证 [rè dú zhèng])

热毒证 [rè dú zhèng]
heat toxin syndrome/pattern: synonym for fire toxin syndrome/pattern (火毒证 [huǒ dú zhèng)

热邪阻痹证 [rè xié zǔ bì zhèng]
syndrome/pattern of heat obstructing arthralgia: syndrome/pattern attributed to stagnation of pathogenic wind-dampness-heat, with predominance of heat, in sinews, bones and joints, and manifested by joint pain with local redness, swelling and scorching hotness

火毒内陷证 [huǒ dú nèi xiàn zhèng]
syndrome/pattern of inward invasion of fire toxin: syndrome/pattern attributed to fire-heat toxin penetrating into the *zang-fu* organs, usually manifested by high fever with thirst, delirium, constipation, dark-red complexion, deep-colored urine, crimson tongue with yellow coating, and rapid sunken pulse, also known as syndrome/pattern of inward invasion of heat toxin (热毒内陷证 [rè dú nèi xiàn zhèng])

热毒内陷证 [rè dú nèi xiàn zhèng]
syndrome/pattern of inward invasion of heat toxin: synonym for syndrome/pattern of inward invasion of fire toxin (火毒内陷证 [huǒ dú nèi xiàn zhèng])

毒火攻唇证 [dú huǒ gōng chún zhèng]
syndrome/pattern of toxic fire attacking the lip: syndrome/pattern marked by a red swollen lip with severe pain or local ulceration with discharge of fetid pus, high fever, thirst, reddened tongue with

yellow coating and rapid pulse, also called syndrome/pattern of toxic fire attacking the mouth (毒火攻口证 [dú huǒ gōng kǒu zhèng])

毒火攻口证 [dú huǒ gōng kǒu zhèng]
syndrome/pattern of toxic fire attacking the mouth: synonymous with syndrome/pattern of toxic fire attacking the lip (毒火攻唇证 [dú huǒ gōng chún zhèng])

热毒攻舌证 [rè dú gōng shé zhèng]
syndrome/pattern of heat toxin attacking the tongue: syndrome/pattern marked by redness, swelling and pain of the tongue or a part of the tongue with impaired lingual movement, fever, thirst and rapid forceful pulse, also called syndrome/pattern of fire toxin attacking the tongue (火毒攻舌证[huǒ dú gōng shé zhèng])

火毒攻舌证 [huǒ dú gōng shé zhèng]
syndrome/pattern of fire toxin attacking the tongue: same as syndrome/pattern of heat toxin attacking the tongue (热毒攻舌证 [rè dú gōng shé zhèng])

热毒攻喉证 [rè dú gōng hóu zhèng]
syndrome/pattern of heat toxin attacking the throat: syndrome/pattern marked by redness, swelling and pain of the throat with difficulty in swallowing or even ulceration and suppuration with fetid mouth odor, associated with high fever, thirst, reddened tongue with yellow coating and rapid forceful pulse, also known as syndrome/pattern of fire toxin attacking the throat (火毒攻喉证 [huǒ dú gōng hóu zhèng])

火毒攻喉证 [huǒ dú gōng hóu zhèng]
syndrome/pattern of fire toxin attacking the throat: same as syndrome/pattern of heat toxin attacking the throat (热毒攻喉证 [rè dú gōng hóu zhèng])

脓毒证 [nóng dú zhèng]
purulent toxin syndrome/pattern: syndrome/pattern marked by purulent discharge for an ulcerative lesion with fetid smell, accompanied by fever, thirst, curdy and greasy tongue coating, and rapid slippery pulse

风毒证 [fēng dú zhèng]
wind-toxin syndrome/pattern: syndrome/pattern due to attack of wind-toxin to the skin and flesh, manifested by sudden onset of edema, with itching and pain, or appearance of wheals, redness and swelling of the face, eyes, nose and mouth

食积证 [shí jī zhèng]
food retention syndrome/pattern: syndrome/pattern in children marked by epigastric and abdominal distension, vomiting of sour matter, anorexia, offensive odor from stools, and curdy and greasy tongue coating

乳食内积证 [rǔ shí nèi jī zhèng]
syndrome/pattern of interior retention of milk: food retention syndrome/pattern occurring in infancy

虫积证 [chóng jī zhèng]
worm accumulation syndrome/pattern: general term for syndromes/patterns caused by intestinal accumulation of parasitic worms, often marked by abdominal distension or pain, emaciation, lack of

strength, and sallow complexion

疫毒证 [yì dú zhèng]
pestilential toxin syndrome/pattern: general term for various syndromes/patterns caused by epidemic pathogens

脏腑辨证
Visceral Syndrome Differentiation (Visceral Pattern Identification)

脏腑辨证 [zàng fǔ biàn zhèng]
visceral syndrome differentiation; visceral pattern identification: differentiation of syndromes or identification of patterns according to the pathological changes of visceral organs

心病辨证 [xīn bìng biàn zhèng]
syndrome differentiation of heart diseases; pattern identification of heart diseases: syndrome differentiation or pattern identification in the diagnosis of heart diseases

心气（亏）虚证 [xīn qì (kuī) xū zhèng]
heart *qi* deficiency syndrome/pattern: deficiency syndrome/pattern of the heart marked by palpitations, shortness of breath, listlessness, spontaneous sweating, pallor, pale tongue, and weak or irregular pulse

心阳（亏）虚证 [xīn yáng (kuī) xū zhèng]
heart yang deficiency syndrome/pattern: deficiency syndrome/pattern of the heart marked by palpitations, dyspnea, oppressive feeling in the chest, aversion to cold with cold limbs, bright pale complexion, dark lips and tongue with white coating, and weak or irregular pulse

心阳虚脱证 [xīn yáng xū tuō zhèng]
heart yang collapse syndrome/pattern: syndrome/pattern occurring in a critically ill patient, marked by profuse sweating and cold skin, reversal cold of limbs, feeble breathing, palpitations, clouding of consciousness, pale complexion, and hardly perceptible pulse

心阳暴脱证 [xīn yáng bào tuō zhèng]
syndrome/pattern of sudden collapse of heart yang: acute critical syndrome/pattern marked by sudden occurrence of profuse cold sweat, reversal cold of limbs, feeble breathing, palpitations, clouding of consciousness, pale complexion, and hardly perceptible pulse

心血（亏）虚证 [xīn xuè (kuī) xū zhèng]
heart blood deficiency syndrome/pattern: deficiency syndrome/pattern of the heart marked by palpitations, dizziness, dream-disturbed sleep, forgetfulness, pale or sallow complexion, pale lips and tongue, and thready pulse

心气血两虚证 [xīn qì xuè liǎng xū zhèng]
syndrome/pattern of deficiency of both heart *qi* and heart blood: syndrome/pattern marked by palpitations, listnessness, lassitude, dizziness, forgetfulness, dream-disturbed sleep, pale complexion and tongue, and weak pulse

心血瘀阻证 [xīn xuè yū zǔ zhèng]
heart blood stasis syndrome/pattern: syndrome/pattern ascribed to impediment of the blood flow in the heart, marked

by stabbing pain in the precordial region referring to the shoulder, back or upper arm, associated with palpitations and feeling of oppression in the chest, cyanotic lips and tongue, and thready and choppy or irregular pulse, also called heart vessel obstruction syndrome/pattern (心脉痹阻证 [xīn mài bì zǔ zhèng])

心脉痹阻证 [xīn mài bì zǔ zhèng]
heart vessel obstruction syndrome/pattern: synonymous with heart blood stasis syndrome/pattern (心血瘀阻证 [xīn xuè yū zǔ zhèng])

心阴（亏）虚证 [xīn yīn (kuī) xū zhèng]
heart yin deficiency syndrome/pattern: deficiency syndrome/pattern of the heart marked by mental irritability, palpitations, insomnia, low fever, night sweating, malar flush, thirst, and thready rapid pulse

心火上炎证 [xīn huǒ shàng yán zhèng]
up-flaming heart-fire syndrome/pattern: syndrome/pattern of up-flaming fire from the heart meridian, marked by oral ulceration, mental irritability, insomnia, and red tip of the tongue

心火炽［亢］盛证 [xīn huǒ chì (kàng) shèng zhèng]
intense heart-fire syndrome/pattern: syndrome/pattern marked by fever, thirst, mental irritability, insomnia, palpitations, and in severe cases even delirium or mania

热扰心神证 [rè rǎo xīn shén zhèng]
syndrome/pattern of heat harassing the mind: syndrome/pattern marked by fever, thirst, palpitations, fidgeting, insomnia, dream-disturbed sleep or delirium, also called syndrome/pattern of fire harassing the mind (火扰心神证 [huǒ rǎo xīn shén zhèng])

火扰心神证 [huǒ rǎo xīn shén zhèng]
syndrome/pattern of fire harassing the mind: same as syndrome/pattern of heat harassing the mind (热扰心神证 [rè rǎo xīn shén zhèng])

痰火扰心证 [tán huǒ rǎo xīn zhèng]
syndrome/pattern of phlegm-fire harassing the heart: syndrome/pattern caused by phlegm-fire which disturbs the mind, marked by restlessness or raving accompanied by red tongue tip, yellow dense and greasy tongue coating, and slippery rapid pulse, also called syndrome/pattern of phlegm-fire harassing the mind (痰火扰神证 [tán huǒ rǎo shén zhèng])

痰火扰神证 [tán huǒ rǎo shén zhèng]
syndrome/pattern of phlegm-fire harassing the mind: same as syndrome/pattern of phlegm-fire harassing the heart 痰火扰心证 [tán huǒ rǎo xīn zhèng]

痰蒙心神证 [tán méng xīn shén zhèng]
syndrome/pattern of phlegm clouding the mind: syndrome/pattern marked by impairment of consciousness, psychotic depression, or even coma, accompanied by phlegmatic sound in the throat

瘀阻脑络证 [yū zǔ nǎo luò zhèng]
syndrome/pattern of static blood obstructing the brain collateral: syndrome/pattern marked by dizziness and persistent stabbing pain in the head with fixed location or loss of consciousness after traumatic injury to the head, dull

lusterless complexion, purple tongue or purple spots on the tongue, and thready choppy pulse

气闭神厥证 [qì bì shén jué zhèng]
syndrome/pattern of *qi* block with syncope: syndrome/pattern ascribed to emotional stimuli causing obstruction of *qi* movement in charge of mental activities, marked by fainting and aphasia or loss of consciousness, trismus, convulsions, and wiry or hidden pulse

水气凌心证 [shuǐ qì líng xīn zhèng]
syndrome/pattern of retained fluid attacking the heart: syndrome/pattern marked by palpitations and shortness of breath associated with general edema

心脾两虚证 [xīn pí liǎng xū zhèng]
deficiency syndrome/pattern of both the heart and spleen: syndrome/pattern marked by palpitations, amnesia, insomnia or dream-disturbed sleep, loss of appetite, abdominal distension, loose bowels, lassitude, sallow face and thready pulse

心肾不交证 [xīn shèn bù jiāo zhèng]
heart-kidney non-interaction syndrome/pattern: syndrome/pattern marked by fidgeting, insomnia, palpitations, dizziness, tinnitus, aching of the lower back and knees, and seminal emission

心移热小肠证 [xīn yí rè xiǎo cháng zhèng]
syndrome/pattern of transmission of heart heat to the small intestine: synonymous with small intestinal excess heat syndrome/pattern (小肠实热证 [xiǎo cháng shí rè zhèng])

心移热膀胱证 [xīn yí rè páng guāng zhèng]
syndrome/pattern of transmission of heart heat to the bladder: synonymous with small intestinal excess heat syndrome/pattern (小肠实热证 [xiǎo cháng shí rè zhèng])

小肠实热证 [xiǎo cháng shí rè zhèng]
small intestinal excess heat syndrome/pattern: syndrome/pattern marked by fidgeting, oral ulceration, dark urine and burning pain upon urination, abdominal distension, yellow coating of the tongue, and rapid slippery pulse, also called syndrome/pattern of transmission of heart heat to the small intestine (心移热小肠证 [xīn yí rè xiǎo cháng zhèng]) or syndrome/pattern of transmission of heart heat to the bladder (心移热膀胱证 [xīn yí rè páng guāng zhèng])

肺病辨证 [fèi bìng biàn zhèng]
syndrome differentiation of lung diseases; pattern identification of lung diseases: syndrome differentiation or pattern identification in the diagnosis of lung diseases

肺气虚证 [fèi qì xū zhèng]
lung *qi* deficiency syndrome/pattern: syndrome/pattern marked by pale complexion, shortness of breath, feeble voice, intolerance of wind, and spontaneous sweating

肺卫气虚（不固）证 [fèi wèi qì xū (bù gù) zhèng]
lung-defense *qi* deficiency syndrome: syndrome/pattern marked by aversion to wind, spontaneous sweating, vulnerability

to colds, shortness of breath, lack of strength, pale tongue and weak pulse

肺阴虚证 [fèi yīn xū zhèng]
lung yin deficiency syndrome/pattern: syndrome/pattern marked by unproductive cough, afternoon fever, night sweating, malar flush, dry throat, red and dry tongue, and thready and rapid pulse

肺虚热证 [fèi xū rè zhèng]
lung deficiency heat syndrome/pattern: synonymous with lung yin deficiency syndrome/pattern (肺阴虚证 [fèi yīn xū zhèng])

阴虚咽喉失濡证 [yīn xū yān hóu shī rú zhèng]
syndrome/pattern of yin deficiency with unmoistenable throat: syndrome/pattern attributed to lung yin deficiency, marked by a scorching feeling in the throat with itching, mild pain and hoarseness, or sensation of presence of a foreign body in the throat with dryness, slight redness or erosion, reddened tongue with scanty moisture and rapid thready pulse

肺阳虚证 [fèi yáng xū zhèng]
lung yang deficiency syndrome/pattern: syndrome/pattern marked by cough and dyspnea, expectoration of whitish thin sputum, cold limbs with intolerance of cold, whitish slippery tongue coating, and weak pulse

肺虚寒证 [fèi xū hán zhèng]
lung deficiency cold syndrome/pattern: synonymous with lung yang deficiency syndrome/pattern (肺阳虚证 [fèi yáng xū zhèng])

风寒袭肺证 [fēng hán xí fèi zhèng]
syndrome/pattern of wind-cold attacking the lung: syndrome/pattern marked by chills, stuffy nose, sneezing, profuse watery nasal discharge, thin sputum, thin white tongue coating, and floating tense pulse

风寒束肺证 [fēng hán shù fèi zhèng]
syndrome/pattern of wind-cold fettering the lung: synonymous with syndrome/pattern of wind-cold attacking the lung (风寒袭肺证 [fēng hán xí fèi zhèng])

风热犯肺证 [fēng rè fàn fèi zhèng]
syndrome/pattern of wind-heat invading the lung: syndrome/pattern marked by fever with mild chills, headache, sore throat, cough, reddened tip of the tongue with thin yellowish coating, and rapid floating pulse

痰湿阻肺证 [tán shī zǔ fèi zhèng]
syndrome/pattern of phlegm-dampness obstructing the lung: syndrome/pattern marked by coughing with expectoration of copious whitish thin sputum, feeling of stuffiness in the chest, whitish greasy coating of the tongue, and soggy pulse

痰浊阻肺证 [tán zhuó zǔ fèi zhèng]
syndrome/pattern of phlegm-turbidity obstructing the lung: synonymous with syndrome/pattern of phlegm-dampness obstructing the lung (痰湿阻肺证 [tán shī zǔ fèi zhèng])

寒痰阻肺证 [hán tán zǔ fèi zhèng]
syndrome/pattern of cold-phlegm obstructing the lung: syndrome/pattern marked by aversion to cold, cough, dyspnea, feeling of oppression in the

chest, expectoration of profuse amounts of whitish sputum, white slippery tongue coating, and tight pulse

痰热壅［蕴］肺证 [tán rè yōng (yùn) fèi zhèng]
syndrome/pattern of phlegm-heat accumulating in the lung: syndrome/pattern marked by fever, thirst, cough and dyspnea, expectoration of yellow thick sputm, reddened tongue with yellow greasy coating, and rapid slippery pulse

痰热闭肺证 [tán rè bì fèi zhèng]
syndrome/pattern of phlegm-heat blocking the lung: syndrome/pattern marked by fever, thirst, feeling of oppression and pain in the chest, cough and dyspnea with wheezing or nares flaring, reddened tongue with yellowish greasy coating, and rapid slippery pulse

肺热炽盛证 [fèi rè chì shèng zhèng]
intense lung heat syndrome/pattern: syndrome/pattern marked by fever, thirst, cough, dyspnea or chest pain, constipation, dark urine, reddened tongue with yellow coating, also called syndrome/pattern of accumulated pathogenic heat in the lung (邪热壅肺证 [xié rè yōng fèi zhèng])

邪热壅肺证 [xié rè yōng fèi zhèng]
syndrome/pattern of accumulated pathogenic heat in the lung: synonymous with intense lung heat syndrome/pattern (肺热炽盛证 [fèi rè chì shèng zhèng])

肺火证 [fèi huǒ zhèng]
lung fire syndrome/pattern: syndrome/pattern marked by fever, coughing with yellow sputum, or hemoptysis

阴虚肺燥证 [yīn xū fèi zào zhèng]
syndrome/pattern of yin deficiency with lung dryness: syndrome/pattern marked by dry cough, sore throat, hoarseness, blood-stained sputum, reddened tongue with scanty coating, and rapid thready pulse

暑伤肺络证 [shǔ shāng fèi luò zhèng]
syndrome/pattern of summerheat damaging the lung vessel: syndrome/pattern marked by fever, thirst, cough, expectoration of fresh blood, reddened tongue with yellow coating, and rapid weak pulse

热毒闭肺证 [rè dú bì fèi zhèng]
syndrome/pattern of heat toxin blocking the lung: syndrome/pattern marked by fever, reversal cold of the extremities, cough, dyspnea, feeling of pressure in the chest with coarse breath and nares flaring, reddened tongue with yellow coating, and rapid pulse

肺燥肠闭证 [fèi zào cháng bì zhèng]
syndrome/pattern of lung dryness with constipation: syndrome/pattern marked by cough, dyspnea, thirst, constipation, abdominal distension and fullness, yellow dry coating of the tongue, and sunken replete pulse

肺肾阴虚证 [fèi shèn yīn xū zhèng]
lung-kidney yin deficiency syndrome/pattern: syndrome/pattern marked by dry cough, shortness of breath, dry throat, afternoon fever, lumbago, night sweats, and nocturnal emission

肺肾气虚证 [fèi shèn qì xū zhèng]
lung-kidney *qi* deficiency syndrome/pattern: syndrome/pattern marked by dyspnea, asthma, shortness of breath, spontaneous sweating, and coughing with profuse sputum

肺肾阳虚证 [fèi shèn yáng xū zhèng]
lung-kidney yang deficiency syndrome/pattern: syndrome/pattern marked by cough, asthma, profuse white thin sputum, and whitish slippery tongue coating

水寒射肺证 [shuǐ hán shè fèi zhèng]
syndrome/pattern of water-cold attacking the lung: synonym for lung-kidney yang deficiency syndrome/pattern (肺肾阳虚证 [fèi shèn yáng xū zhèng])

脾病辨证 [pí bìng biàn zhèng]
syndrome differentiation of spleen diseases; pattern identification of spleen diseases: syndrome differentiation or pattern identification in the diagnosis of spleen diseases

脾虚证 [pí xū zhèng]
spleen deficiency syndrome/pattern: general term for deficiency syndromes/patterns of the spleen, such as spleen *qi* deficiency syndrome/pattern, spleen yang deficiency syndrome/pattern, and spleen yin deficiency syndrome/pattern

脾气虚证 [pí qì xū zhèng]
spleen *qi* deficiency syndrome/pattern: syndrome/pattern marked by dizziness, fatigue, sallow face, indigestion, abdominal distension, lassitude, anorexia, and loose bowels

脾阳虚证 [pí yáng xū zhèng]
spleen yang deficiency syndrome/pattern: syndrome/pattern attributed to insufficient yang *qi* to warm and activate the spleen, marked by cold limbs, coldness and pain in the abdomen, anorexia, abdominal fullness, chronic diarrhea, lassitude, emaciation, and edema, also called spleen deficiency cold syndrome/pattern (脾虚寒证[pí xū hán zhèng])

脾虚寒证 [pí xū hán zhèng]
spleen deficiency cold syndrome/pattern: another name for spleen yang deficiency syndrome/pattern (脾阳虚证 [pí yáng xū zhèng])

脾胃虚寒证 [pí wèi xū hán zhèng]
spleen-stomach deficiency cold syndrome/pattern: syndrome/pattern marked by coldness and pain in the stomach, accompanied by anorexia, abdominal fullness, belching, vomiting thin fluid, chronic diarrhea, lassitude and cold limbs, also known as spleen-stomach yang deficiency syndrome/pattern (脾胃阳虚证 [pí wèi yáng xū zhèng])

脾胃阳虚证 [pí wèi yáng xū zhèng]
spleen-stomach yang deficiency syndrome/pattern: same as spleen-stomach deficiency cold syndrome/pattern (脾胃虚寒证 [pí wèi xū hán zhèng])

脾阴虚证 [pí yīn xū zhèng]
spleen yin deficiency syndrome/pattern: syndrome/pattern marked by anorexia, dryness of the lips and mouth, reddened tongue with scanty coating, and especially constipation with abdominal distension

脾虚湿困证 [pí xū shī kùn zhèng] **syndrome/pattern of spleen deficiency with dampness encumbrance:** syndrome/pattern marked by epigastric distension, poor appetite, borborygmi, diarrhea, nausea, dryness in the mouth with no desire to drink, lassitude, and dense and slippery tongue coating

寒湿困脾证 [hán shī kùn pí zhèng] **syndrome/pattern of cold-dampness encumbering the spleen:** syndrome/pattern marked by epigastric and abdominal distension, stickiness and tastelessness in the mouth, nausea, loose bowels, heavy sensation of the head and body, or jaundice with dim yellow discoloration, pale plump tongue with white greasy coating, and soggy and relaxed pulse

湿困脾阳证 [shī kùn pí yáng zhèng] **syndrome/pattern of dampness encumbering spleen yang:** synonym for syndrome/pattern of cold-dampness encumbering the spleen (寒湿困脾证 [hán shī kùn pí zhèng])

湿阻中焦证 [shī zǔ zhōng jiāo zhèng] **syndrome/pattern of dampness obstructing the middle energizer:** syndrome/pattern marked by epigastric and abdominal distension, anorexia, lassitude, stickiness in the mouth, white thick greasy tongue coating, and relaxed pulse

脾气下陷证 [pí qì xià xiàn zhèng] **spleen *qi* sinking syndrome/pattern:** syndrome/pattern marked by bearing-down sensation in the epigastrium and abdomen, protracted diarrhea, even prolapse of the rectum or visceroptosis, also called middle *qi* sinking syndrome/pattern (中气下陷证 [zhōng qì xià xiàn zhèng]) or spleen deficiency syndrome/pattern with sinking of *qi* (脾虚气陷证 [pí xū qì xiàn zhèng])

中气下陷证 [zhōng qì xià xiàn zhèng] **middle *qi* sinking syndrome/pattern:** same as spleen *qi* sinking syndrome/pattern (脾气下陷证 [pí qì xià xiàn zhèng])

脾虚气陷证 [pí xū qì xiàn zhèng] **spleen deficiency syndrome/pattern with sinking of *qi*:** same as spleen *qi* sinking syndrome/pattern (脾气下陷证 [pí qì xià xiàn zhèng])

脾虚动风证 [pí xū dòng fēng zhèng] **syndrome/pattern of spleen deficiency with stirred wind:** syndrome/pattern ascribed to spleen deficiency leading to stirring of wind, marked by reduced food intake, abdominal distension, loose stools, lassitude, trembling or shaking of the limbs or even convulsions, pale complexion, pale tongue and weak pulse

脾虚痰湿证 [pí xū tán shī zhèng] **syndrome/pattern of spleen deficiency with phlegm-dampness:** syndrome/pattern ascribed to spleen deficiency leading to accumulation of phlegm-dampness, marked by reduced food intake, abdominal distension, loose stools, obesity, lassitude and sleepiness, pale and plump tongue with white greasy coating, and soggy pulse

脾胃湿热证 [pí wèi shī rè zhèng] **spleen-stomach dampness-heat syndrome/pattern:** syndrome/pattern marked by epigastric or abdominal distension, anorexia, nausea, vomiting, lassitude, heavy sensation of the body, or jaundice with bright yellow discoloration of the skin and the whites of the eyes, and yellow dense and greasy tongue coating

中焦湿热证 [zhōng jiāo shī rè zhèng]
middle-energizer dampness-heat syndrome/pattern: same as spleen-stomach dampness-heat syndrome/pattern (脾胃湿热证 [pí wèi shī rè zhèng])

脾肺两虚证 [pí fèi liǎng xū zhèng]
deficiency syndrome/pattern of both the spleen and lung: syndrome/pattern of *qi* deficiency in both the spleen and lung, marked by anorexia, loose stools, abdominal distension, feeble voice, shortness of breath, dyspnea and productive cough

脾肺气虚证 [pí fèi qì xū zhèng]
spleen-lung *qi* deficiency syndrome/pattern: same as deficiency syndrome/pattern of both the spleen and lung (脾肺两虚证 [pí fèi liǎng xū zhèng])

脾肾阳虚证 [pí shèn yáng xū zhèng]
spleen-kidney yang deficiency syndrome/pattern: syndrome/pattern marked by anasarca or chronic diarrhea before dawn together with aching of the loins, weakness of the knees and intolerance of cold

脾肾虚寒证 [pí shèn xū hán zhèng]
spleen-kidney deficiency cold syndrome/pattern: synonymous with spleen-kidney yang deficiency syndrome/pattern (脾肾阳虚证 [pí shèn yáng xū zhèng])

胃肠病辨证 [wèi cháng bìng biàn zhèng]
syndrome differentiation of gastro-intestinal diseases; pattern identification of gastro-intestinal diseases: syndrome differentiation or pattern identification in the diagnosis of the diseases of the stomach and intestines

胃气虚证 [wèi qì xū zhèng]
stomach *qi* deficiency syndrome/pattern: syndrome/pattern marked by dull epigastric pain relieved by pressure, anorexia, pale tongue, and weak pulse

胃阴虚证 [wèi yīn xū zhèng]
stomach yin deficiency syndrome/pattern: syndrome/pattern marked by dryness in the mouth, thirst, anorexia, constipation, retching, and reddened furless tongue

胃阳虚证 [wèi yáng xū zhèng]
stomach yang deficiency syndrome/pattern: syndrome/pattern marked by continuous epigastric pain, ameliorated by warmth and pressure, reduced food intake, stuffy sensation in the stomach, aversion to cold with cold limbs, pale tongue with whitish coating, and deep, slow and weak pulse

胃虚寒证 [wèi xū hán zhèng]
stomach deficiency cold syndrome/pattern: synonym for stomach yang deficiency syndrome/pattern (胃阳虚证 [wèi yáng xū zhèng])

胃实寒证 [wèi shí hán zhèng]
stomach excess cold syndrome/pattern: synonym for syndrome/pattern of cold pathogen invading the stomach (寒邪犯胃证 [hán xié fàn wèi zhèng])

寒邪犯胃证 [hán xié fàn wèi zhèng]
syndrome/pattern of cold pathogen invading the stomach: syndrome/pattern marked by acute epigastric pain with cold sensation, vomiting of watery fluid, aversion to cold with cold limbs, and whitish tongue coating

胃热壅盛证 [wèi rè yōng shèng zhèng]
intense stomach heat syndrome/pattern: syndrome/pattern marked by dire thirst and preference for cold drinks, foul breath, oral ulcer, toothache and gingivitis

胃火证 [wèi huǒ zhèng]
stomach fire syndrome: syndrome/pattern marked by dire thirst and preference for cold drinks, foul breath, oral ulcer, toothache and gingivitis

胃火炽盛证 [wèi huǒ chì shèng zhèng]
intense stomach fire syndrome/pattern: synonymous with intense stomach heat syndrome/pattern胃热壅盛证 [wèi rè yōng shèng zhèng]

大肠虚寒证 [dà cháng xū hán zhèng]
large intestinal deficiency cold syndrome/pattern: syndrome/pattern marked by diarrhea with watery stool, intolerance of cold, cold limbs, dull pain and cold feeling in the abdomen, and pale tongue with white moistened coating

大肠寒结证 [dà cháng hán jié zhèng]
large intestinal cold accumulation syndrome/pattern: syndrome/pattern marked by constipation with dull pain and cold feeling in the abdomen, and pale tongue with white moistened coating

大肠热结证 [dà cháng rè jié zhèng]
large intestinal heat accumulation syndrome/pattern: syndrome/pattern marked by constipation with abdominal pain and tenderness, yellow and dry coating of the tongue, deep and forceful pulse, also called syndrome/pattern of heat accumulation with intestinal dryness (热结肠燥证 [rè jié cháng zào zhèng])

热结肠燥证 [rè jié cháng zào zhèng]
syndrome/pattern of heat accumulatiom with intestinal dryness: same as large intestinal heat accumulation syndrome/pattern (大肠热结证 [dà cháng rè jié zhèng])

大肠津［液］亏证 [dà cháng jīn (yè) kuī zhèng]
large intestinal fluid insufficiency syndrome/pattern: syndrome/pattern marked by constipation or difficulty in defecation accompanied by dry throat, and red tongue with scanty coating

大肠湿热证 [dà cháng shī rè zhèng]
large intestinal dampness-heat syndrome/pattern: syndrome/pattern marked by discharge of purulent and bloody stools, abdominal pain, tenesmus, scanty dark urine, yellow and greasy tongue coating, and slippery and rapid pulse

肝胆病辨证 [gān dǎn bìng biàn zhèng]
syndrome differentiation of liver and gallbladder diseases; pattern identification of liver and gallbladder diseases: syndrome differentiation or pattern identification in the diagnosis of diseases of the liver and gallbladder

肝阴（亏）虚证 [gān yīn (kuī) xū zhèng]
liver yin deficiency syndrome/pattern: syndrome/pattern marked by dizziness, headache, blurred vision, dryness of the eye, insomnia, thirst, dry throat, scanty tongue coating, and thready pulse

肝血（亏）虚证 [gān xuè (kuī) xū zhèng]
liver blood deficiency syndrome/pattern: syndrome/pattern marked by sallow complexion, impaired vision, insomnia, scanty or absence of menstruation, and pale tongue and lips

肝气（亏）虚证 [gān qì (kuī) xū zhèng]
liver *qi* deficiency syndrome/pattern: syndrome/pattern marked by hypochondriac distension, emotional depression, fatigability, shortness of breath, dizziness, blurred vision, pale tongue, and weak pulse

肝阳（亏）虚证 [gān yáng (kuī) xū zhèng]
liver yang deficiency syndrome/pattern: syndrome/pattern marked by distension and oppression in the hypochondriac regions, intolerance of cold with cold limbs, dizziness with blurred vision, white moistened tongue coating, and sunken slow weak pulse, also called liver deficiency cold syndrome/pattern (肝虚寒证 [gān xū hán zhèng])

肝虚寒证 [gān xū hán zhèng]
liver deficiency cold syndrome/pattern: synonymous with liver yang deficiency syndrome/pattern (肝阳虚证 [gān yáng xū zhèng])

肝寒证 [gān hán zhèng]
liver cold syndrome/pattern: abbreviation for syndrome/pattern of cold stagnating in the liver meridian/channel (寒滞肝脉证 [hán zhì gān mài zhèng])

肝火证 [gān huǒ zhèng]
liver fire syndrome: abbreviation for blazing liver fire syndrome/pattern (肝火炽盛证 [gān huǒ chì shèng zhèng])

肝火炽盛证 [gān huǒ chì shèng zhèng]
blazing liver fire syndrome/pattern: syndrome/pattern marked by hypochondriac pain, dryness and bitterness in the mouth, vomiting of bitter fluid, irritability, insomnia or dream-disturbed sleep, flushing of face, blood-shot eyes, constipation, dark urine, reddened tongue with yellow coating, and rapid wiry pulse

肝火犯头证 [gān huǒ fàn tóu zhèng]
syndrome/pattern of liver fire invading the head: syndrome/pattern marked by severe headache, associated with flushed face, red eyes, irascibility, bitter taste in the mouth, reddened tongue with yellow coating, and rapid wiry pulse

肝火燔耳证 [gān huǒ fán ěr zhèng]
syndrome/pattern of liver fire blazing in the ear: syndrome/pattern marked by pain and distension in the ear, tinnitus, dizziness, congestion or perforation of the tympanic membrane, and discharge of pus and blood from the meatus, associated with bitter taste in the mouth, reddened tongue with yellow coating, and rapid wiry pulse

肝阳上亢证 [gān yáng shàng kàng zhèng]
syndrome/pattern of ascendant hyperactivity of liver yang: syndrome/pattern marked by dizziness, headache, flushed face, blurred

vision, tinnitus, bitter taste in the mouth, and wiry pulse

肝阳亢盛证 [gān yáng kàng shèng zhèng]
liver-yang hyperactivity syndrome: same as syndrome/pattern of ascendant hyperactivity of liver yang (肝阳上亢证 [gān yáng shàng kàng zhèng]

肝火上炎证 [gān huǒ shàng yán zhèng]
syndrome/pattern of up-flaming liver fire: syndrome/pattern marked by headache, dizziness, tinnitus with buzzing in the ears, impairment of hearing, blood-shot eyes, mental irritability, bitter taste in the mouth, yellow coating of the tongue, rapid wiry pulse, and in severe cases hematuria, hemoptysis or epistaxis

肝风内动证 [gān fēng nèi dòng zhèng]
syndrome/pattern of internal stirring of liver wind: syndrome/pattern marked by convulsion, tremor, or spasm

肝阳化风证 [gān yáng huà fēng zhèng]
syndrome/pattern of liver yang transforming into wind: syndrome/pattern marked by dizziness with tendency to fall or even sudden attack of syncope, shaking of the head, limb tremor, irritability, flushing of face, reddened tongue, and wiry pulse

热极生风证 [rè jí shēng fēng zhèng]
syndrome/pattern of extreme heat engendering wind: syndrome/pattern attributed to exuberant pathogenic heat, and marked by high fever with restlessness, convulsions, opisthotonos, and impaired consciousness

阴虚动风证 [yīn xū dòng fēng zhèng]
syndrome/pattern of yin deficiency with stirring wind: syndrome/pattern marked by twitching or wriggling of the extremities, accompanied by dizziness, tinnitus, malar flush, and dry reddened tongue

肝气郁结证 [gān qì yù jié zhèng]
liver *qi* depression syndrome/pattern; liver *qi* stagnation syndrome/pattern: syndrome/pattern marked by depression, frequent sighing, hypochondriac or lower abdominal distension or scurrying pain, distending pain of the breast and irregular menstruation in women, and wiry pulse, often abbreviated as liver depression [stagnation] syndrome/pattern (肝郁证 [gān yù zhèng])

肝郁证 [gān yù zhèng]
liver depression syndrome/pattern; liver stagnation syndrome/pattern: abbreviation for liver *qi* depression [stagnation] syndrome/pattern (肝气郁结证 [gān qì yù jié zhèng])

肝气犯胃证 [gān qì fàn wèi zhèng]
syndrome/pattern of liver *qi* invading the stomach: syndrome/pattern marked by dizziness, hypochondriac pain, irritability, epigastric distension and pain, anorexia, belching, nausea, vomiting, and wiry pulse

肝胃不和证 [gān wèi bù hé zhèng]
liver-stomach disharmony syndrome/pattern: synonym for syndrome/pattern of liver *qi* invading the stomach (肝气犯胃证 [gān qì fàn wèi zhèng])

肝气犯脾证 [gān qì fàn pí zhèng]
syndrome/pattern of liver *qi* invading

the spleen: syndrome/pattern marked by dizziness, hypochondriac pain, irritability, anorexia, abdominal pain and distension, diarrhea, borborygmi, and wiry pulse

肝脾不和证 [gān pí bù hé zhèng]
liver-spleen disharmony syndrome/pattern: synonym for syndrome/pattern of liver *qi* invading the spleen (肝气犯脾证 [gān qì fàn pí zhèng])

肝郁脾虚证 [gān yù pí xū zhèng]
syndrome/pattern of liver depression and spleen insufficiency; syndrome/pattern of liver stagnation and spleen insufficiency: syndrome/pattern marked by hypochondriac pain, abdominal distension, loose bowels, and lassitude

寒滞肝脉证 [hán zhì gān mài zhèng]
syndrome/pattern of cold stagnating in the liver meridian/channel: syndrome/pattern marked by spasmodic symptoms in the area related to the liver meridian/channel, such as stretching pain with cold sensation in the lower abdomen and testicles

肝经风热证 [gān jīng fēng rè zhèng]
syndrome/pattern of wind-heat in the liver meridian/channel: syndrome/pattern marked by fever with pain at the top of the head or ocular inflammation

肝经湿热证 [gān jīng shī rè zhèng]
syndrome/pattern of dampness-heat in the liver meridian/channel: syndrome/pattern marked by distending pain in the hypochondriac region, or itching and painful swollen genitalia, or distending pain in the ear with purulent discharge, reddened tongue with yellow greasy coating, and rapid slippery pulse

肝肾阴虚证 [gān shèn yīn xū zhèng]
liver-kidney yin deficiency syndrome/pattern: syndrome marked by dizziness, blurred vision, tinnitus, hypochondriac pain, aching of the loins and weakness of the knees and legs, malar flush, heat sensation in the palms of the hands and soles of the feet, red and dry tongue with scanty or no coating, and rapid thready pulse

胆气虚证 [dǎn qì xū zhèng]
gallbladder *qi* deficiency syndrome/pattern: syndrome/pattern marked by panic, suspicion, sighing, nervousness, irritability, lassitude, dizziness and insomnia

胆虚气怯证 [dǎn xū qì qiè zhèng]
syndrome of gallbladder insufficiency with timidity: same as gallbladder *qi* deficiency syndrome/pattern (胆气虚证 [dǎn qì xū zhèng])

肝胆湿热证 [gān dǎn shī rè zhèng]
liver-gallbladder dampness-heat syndrome/pattern: syndrome/pattern marked by fever and chills, jaundice, hypochondriac and abdominal pain, bitter taste in the mouth, nausea, and slippery and rapid pulse

胆热证 [dǎn rè zhèng]
gallbladder heat syndrome/pattern: syndrome/pattern marked by irritability, hypochondriac distension, bitterness in the mouth or ear pain, tinnitus, insomnia, reddened tongue with yellow coating

胆火证 [dǎn huǒ zhèng]
gallbladder fire syndrome/pattern: synonym for gallbladder heat syndrome/pattern (胆热证 [dǎn rè zhèng])

肾膀胱病辨证 [shèn páng guāng bìng biàn zhèng]
syndrome differentiation of kidney and bladder diseases; pattern identification of kidney and bladder diseases: syndrome differentiation or pattern identification in the diagnosis of diseases of the kidney and urinary bladder

肾虚证 [shèn xū zhèng]
kidney deficiency syndrome/pattern: any deficiency syndrome/pattern of the kidney, including deficiency of kidney *qi*, kidney yin and kidney yang

肾气（亏）虚证 [shèn qì (kuī) xū zhèng]
kidney *qi* deficiency syndrome/pattern: syndrome/pattern marked by dizziness, forgetfulness, tinnitus, backache, hyposexuality, and weak pulse

肾气不固证 [shèn qì bù gù zhèng]
kidney *qi* insecurity syndrome/pattern: syndrome/pattern marked by frequent urination, dribbling of urine after voiding, incontinence of urine or feces, nocturnal emission or premature ejaculation in males, continuous dribbling of menstrual discharge or liability to abortion in females, aching back and knees, and weak pulse

肾阴虚证 [shèn yīn xū zhèng]
kidney yin deficiency syndrome/pattern: syndrome/pattern marked by lumbago, lassitude, dizziness, tinnitus, nocturnal emission in men and oligmenorrhea in women, emaciation, dry throat, thirst, flushed cheeks, hot sensation in the palms of the hands and soles of the feet, afternoon fever, night sweating, reddened tongue with little or no coating, and thready and rapid pulse, also called genuine origin insufficiency syndrome/pattern (真元亏虚证 [zhēn yuán kuī xū zhèng]) or kidney-water insufficiency syndrome/pattern (肾水亏虚证 [shèn shuǐ kuī xū zhèng])

真元亏虚证 [zhēn yuán kuī xū zhèng]
genuine origin insufficiency syndrome/pattern: same as kidney yin deficiency syndrome/pattern (肾阴虚证 [shèn yīn xū zhèng])

肾水亏虚证 [shèn shuǐ kuī xū zhèng]
kidney-water insufficiency syndrome/pattern: same as kidney yin deficiency syndrome (肾阴虚证 [shèn yīn xū zhèng])

肾阴虚火旺证 [shèn yīn xū huǒ wàng zhèng]
syndrome/pattern of kidney yin deficiency with effulgent fire: syndrome/pattern marked by tidal fever, night sweating, malar flush, vexing heat in the chest, palms of the hands and soles of the feet, nocturnal emission, premature ejaculation, hypersexuality, lumbar pain, tinnitus, dark urine, reddened tongue with yellow coating lacking moisture, and rapid thready pulse

肾精亏虚证 [shèn jīng kuī xū zhèng]
kidney essence insufficiency syndrome/pattern: syndrome/pattern marked by retarded development in children, decreased reproductive function, premature senility, tinnitus, loss of hair,

loosening of teeth and forgetfulness in adults

肾阳虚证 [shèn yáng xū zhèng]
kidney yang deficiency syndrome/pattern: syndrome/pattern marked by aversion to cold, cold limbs, listlessness, weakness and soreness of the loins and knees, seminal emission or impotence in men and frigidity or infertility in women, nocturia, whitish tongue coating, and weak pulse at the cubit

肾虚水泛证 [shèn xū shuǐ fàn zhèng]
syndrome/pattern of kidney deficiency with water flooding: syndrome/pattern marked by edema, particularly of the lower extremities, accompanied by oliguria, tinnitus, aching of the back and knees, pale tongue with whitish slippery coating, and weak pulse

肾不纳气证 [shèn bù nà qì zhèng]
syndrome/pattern of the kidney failing to receive *qi*: syndrome/pattern marked by dyspnea with prolonged exhalation, asthenic cough, and feeble voice

肾经寒湿证 [shèn jīng hán shī zhèng]
kidney meridian/channel cold-dampness syndrome/pattern: syndrome/pattern marked by feeling of heaviness, cold and pain in the lumbus and knees with limitation of movement, intolerance of cold and cold limbs, white greasy tongue coating, and soggy relaxed pulse

热积［结］膀胱证 [rè jī (jié) páng guāng zhèng]
bladder heat accumulation [retention] syndrome/pattern: syndrome/pattern marked by distension and fullness of the lower abdomen, stranguria, frequent urination, and fever without chills

膀胱虚寒证 [páng guāng xū hán zhèng]
bladder deficiency cold syndrome/pattern: syndrome/pattern marked by frequent urination, incontinence of urine or dribbling of urine, cold feeling in the lower abdomen, whitish moist tongue coating, and weak pulse

胞宫虚寒证 [bāo gōng xū hán zhèng]
uterine deficiency-cold syndrome/pattern: syndrome/pattern marked by intolerance of cold with cold limbs, dull pain in the lower abdomen alleviated by warmth and pressure, pale-colored and thin menstrual discharge or clear thin leukorrhea, or infertility, or abortion, pale complexion, and pale tongue with white coating

寒凝胞宫证 [hán níng bāo gōng zhèng]
syndrome/pattern of cold congealing in the uterus: syndrome/pattern marked by cold and pain in the lower abdomen, dysmenorrhea or late periods with dark menstrual discharge, or thin whitish leukorrhea, white tongue coating, and sunken tight pulse

胞宫积热证 [bāo gōng jī rè zhèng]
syndrome/pattern of accumulated heat in the uterus: syndrome/pattern marked by scorching pain in the lower abdomen, early periods with profuse bright red menstrual discharge, or yellow thick and fetid leukorrhea, reddened tongue with yellow coating, and rapid pulse

胞宫湿热证 [bāo gōng shī rè zhèng]
uterine dampness-heat syndrome/pattern: syndrome/pattern marked by large amount of yellowish, thick, fetid leukorrhea, associated with pudental itching and erosion, reddened tongue with yellow greasy coating, and rapid slippery pulse

瘀阻胞宫证 [yū zǔ bāo gōng zhèng]
syndrome/pattern of static blood obstructing the uterus: syndrome/pattern marked by stabbing pain in the lower abdomen, fixed in location and tender to the touch, or accompanied by mass formation, or late periods with scanty discharge of dark purple blood or blood with clots, or cessation of menstruation, or excessive uterine bleeding, dark purple tongue or dark spots on the tongue, and wiry choppy pulse

热入血室证 [rè rù xuè shì zhèng]
syndrome/pattern of heat entering the blood chamber: syndrome/pattern attributed to penetration of pathogenic heat into the uterus, marked by scorching pain in the lower abdomen with tenderness, profuse menstrual discharge or abnormal stoppage of menses, associated with alternate fever and chills and delirium at night, deep red tongue with yellow coating, and rapid pulse

湿热阻滞精室证 [shī rè zǔ zhì jīng shì zhèng]
syndrome/pattern of dampness-heat obstructing the semen chamber: syndrome/pattern marked by heat and pain in the perineum, scrotal itching and erosion, seminal emission or pus in the seminal fluid, reddened tongue with yellow greasy coating, and rapid slippery pulse

痰阻精室证 [tán zǔ jīng shì zhèng]
syndrome/pattern of phlegm obstructing the semen chamber: syndrome/pattern marked by thin seminal fluid, impotence, lack of libido, obesity, lack of strength, pale tongue with white greasy coating, and slippery or soggy relaxed pulse, also called syndrome/pattern of phlegm-dampness obstructing the semen chamber (痰湿阻滞精室证 [tán shī zǔ zhì jīng shì zhèng])

痰湿阻滞精室证 [tán shī zǔ zhì jīng shì zhèng]
syndrome/pattern of phlegm-dampness obstructing the semen chamber: same as syndrome/pattern of phlegm obstructing the semen chamber (痰阻精室证 [tán zǔ jīng shì zhèng])

膀胱湿热证 [páng guāng shī rè zhèng]
bladder dampness-heat syndrome/pattern: syndrome/pattern marked by frequency and urgency of urination, stranguria, turbid urine or hematuria, reddened tongue with yellow greasy coating, and rapid pulse

三焦虚寒 [sān jiāo xū hán]
triple energizer deficiency cold; deficiency cold in the triple energizer: deficiency-cold syndrome/pattern occurring simultaneously in the upper, middle and lower energizers

上焦虚寒 [shàng jiāo xū hán]
upper energizer deficiency cold; deficiency cold in the upper energizer: deficiency-cold syndrome/pattern of the heart and lung with

such symptoms as listlessness and shortness of breath

中焦虚寒 [zhōng jiāo xū hán]
middle energizer deficiency cold; deficiency cold in the middle energizer: deficiency-cold syndrome/pattern of the spleen and stomach with such symptoms as diarrhea, abdominal pain and distension, also known as 脾胃虚寒 [pí wèi xū hán]

下焦虚寒 [xià jiāo xū hán]
lower energizer deficiency cold; deficiency cold in the lower energizer: deficiency-cold syndrome/pattern of the liver, kidney, intestines and urinary bladder with such symptoms as chronic diarrhea, incontinence of urine, and edema

三焦实热 [sān jiāo shí rè]
triple energizer excess heat; excess heat in the triple energizer: (1) heat of excess type in the triple energizer; (2) febrile disease with the pathogen penetrating into the *qi* aspect

上焦实热 [shàng jiāo shí rè]
upper energizer excess heat; excess heat in the upper energizer: excessive heat syndrome/pattern of the heart and lung with such symptoms as asthma, and stuffiness and fullness in the chest

中焦实热 [zhōng jiāo shí rè]
middle energizer excess heat; excess heat in the middle energizer: excess heat syndrome/pattern of the spleen and stomach with such symptoms as abdominal distension with nausea and constipation

下焦实热 [xià jiāo shí rè]
lower energizer excess heat; excess heat in the lower energizer: excess heat syndrome/pattern of the urinary bladder and large intestine with such symptoms as hematuria, burning sensation upon urination, or passage of purulent bloody stools

经络辨证
Meridian/Channel Syndrome Differentiation (Meridian/Channel Pattern Identification)

经络辨证 [jīng luò biàn zhèng]
meridian/channel syndrome differentiation; meridian/channel pattern identification: differentiation of syndromes or identification of patterns according to the pathological changes of the meridians/channels

冲任失［不］调证 [chōng rèn shī (bù) tiáo zhèng]
syndrome/pattern of thoroughfare-conception-vessel disorder: a syndrome/pattern marked by irregular menstruation and lower abdominal distension and pain

冲任不固证 [chōng rèn bù gù zhèng]
syndrome/pattern of insecurity of thoroughfare and conception vessels: a syndrome/pattern marked by continuous dribbling of menstrual discharge, profuse uterine bleeding or liability to abortion

带脉病证 [dài mài bìng zhèng]
belt vessel syndrome/pattern: syndrome/

pattern marked by pain around the waist, weakness of the lower limbs, and abnormal menstruation or leukorrhea

阴跷脉病证 [yīn qiāo mài bìng zhèng] **yin heel vessel syndrome/pattern:** syndrome/pattern marked by redness and pain of the eyes, muscular disability, lower abdominal pain, testicular pain in men and metrostaxis in women

阳跷脉病证 [yáng qiāo mài bìng zhèng] **yang heel vessel syndrome/pattern:** syndrome/pattern mainly marked by insomnia

阴维脉病证 [yīn wéi mài bìng zhèng] **yin link vessel syndrome/pattern:** syndrome/pattern marked by chest pain, hypochondriac distension, lumbar pain in men and vaginal pain in women

阳维脉病证 [yáng wéi mài bìng zhèng] **yang link vessel syndrome/pattern:** syndrome/pattern mainly marked by chills and fever accompanied by dizziness

治疗学
Therapeutics

治则 Therapeutic Principles

辨证施治 [biàn zhèng shī zhì]
syndrome differentiation and treatment; pattern identification and treatment: diagnosis and treatment based on overall analysis of symptoms and signs, including the cause, nature and location of the illness and the patient's physical condition, according to traditional Chinese medical theories, also known as 辨证论治 [biàn zhèng lùn zhì]

辨证论治 [biàn zhèng lùn zhì]
synonymous with 辨证施治 [biàn zhèng shī zhì]

审因施治 [shěn yīn shī zhì]
cause determination and treatment: diagnosis and treatment based on determination of the cause of the illness

审因论治 [shěn yīn lùn zhì]
synonymous with 审因施治 [shěn yīn shī zhì]

整体观念 [zhěng tǐ guān niàn]
concept of holism: viewing of the various parts of the human body as an organic whole, closely related to each other and to the external environment

因时制宜 [yīn shí zhì yí]
treatment according to time: therapeutic principle that the patient should be treated in accordance with the time of the year

因地制宜 [yīn dì zhì yí]
treatment according to place: therapeutic principle that the patient should be treated in accordance with the geographical location

因人制宜 [yīn rén zhì yí]
treatment according to individual: therapeutic principle that the patient should be treated in accordance with his or her age, constitution, mental attitude and life style

因时、因地、因人制宜 [yīn shí、yīn dì、yīn rén zhì yí]
treatment according to time, place and individual: comprehensive therapeutic principle based on the correspondence between nature and human that treatment should be determined on the basis of an overall consideration of the seasonal, geographical and personal conditions

同病异治 [tóng bìng yì zhì]
different treatments for the same disease: therapeutic principle that different methods of treatment should be applied to the same kind of disease in the light of different physical reactions and clinical manifestations (i.e., different syndromes/patterns)

异病同治 [yì bìng tóng zhì]
same treatment for different diseases: therapeutic principle that the same method of treatment should be applied to patients with different kinds of diseases if they are alike in clinical manifestations and pathogenesis (i.e., with the same syndrome/pattern)

治病求本 [zhì bìng qiú běn]
treating disease from the root: guiding therapeutic principle that the fundamental cause of the disease should be dealt with

标 [biāo]
tip; the incidental: referring to (1) manifestation of a disease in relation to its cause; (2) pathogenic factor in relation to body resistance; (3) complication or relapse of a disease in relation to its primary onset; (4) disease in the exterior in relation to one in the interior

本 [běn]
root; the radical: referring to (1) cause of a disease in relation to its manifestations; (2) body resistance in relation to pathogenic factors; (3) primary onset of a disease in relation to its complications; (4) disease in the interior in relation to one on the exterior

治本 [zhì běn]
treating the radical: treating the radical cause of a disease

治标 [zhì biāo]
treating the incidental: treating the manifestations of a disease

标本同治 [biāo běn tóng zhì]
treating the incidental and radical simultaneously: therapeutic principle applied to cases of severe illness with marked symptoms or complications, also called treating the incidental and radical together (标本兼治 [biāo běn jiān zhì])

标本兼治 [biāo běn jiān zhì]
treating the incidental and radical together: same as treating the incidental and radical simultaneously (标本同治 [biāo běn tóng zhì])

治未病 [zhì wèi bìng]
preventive treatment: (1) treatment of disease before its onset; (2) early treatment for prevention of complications

扶正 [fú zhèng]
reinforcing the healthy (*qi*): general term for treating disease by strengthening the healthy *qi* of the patient's body

祛邪 [qū xié]
eliminating the pathogenic (factors): general term for treating disease by removing the pathogenic factors from the patient's body

扶正祛邪 [fú zhèng qū xié]
reinforcing the healthy and eliminating the pathogenic: two general therapeutic principles – to strengthen the patient's resistance (healthy *qi*) and to dispel the invading pathogenic factors, which can be applied separately or in combination according to the particular condition of the case

扶正兼祛邪 [fú zhèng jiān qū xié]
reinforcing the healthy with elimination of the pathogenic: therapeutic principle that reinforcement of healthy *qi* is primary and dispelling the pathogenic factors is auxiliary, indicated for complicated cases of deficiency and excess with predominance of healthy *qi* deficiency

祛邪兼扶正 [qū xié jiān fú zhèng]
eliminating the pathogenic with reinforcement of the healthy: therapeutic principle that elimination of the pathogenic factors is primary and strengthening healthy *qi* is auxiliary, indicated for complicated cases of deficiency and excess with predominance of excess of pathogenic factors

扶正固本 [fú zhèng gù běn]
reinforcing the healthy and strengthening the base: (1) reinforcing the body resistance and improving the constitution; (2) restoring the normal functioning of the body to improve the constitution

扶正培本 [fú zhèng péi běn]
same as 扶正固本 [fú zhèng gù běn]

攻补兼施 [gōng bǔ jiān shī]
simultaneous elimination and reinforcement: therapeutic principle in which combined methods may be applied so that elimination of pathogenic factors and reinforcement of the healthy *qi* occur at the same time, suitable for patients with a weak constitution suffering from an excess syndrome/pattern

先攻后补 [xiān gōng hòu bǔ]
elimination followed by reinforcement: therapeutic principle in which elimination of the pathogenic factors precedes reinforcement of the healthy *qi*, suitable for cases in which, although the healthy *qi* is insufficient, excess of pathogenic factors predominates and any form of reinforcement therapy at the early stage may aggravate the disease

先补后攻 [xiān bǔ hòu gōng]
reinforcement followed by elimination: therapeutic principle marked by reinforcing the healthy *qi* first and then eliminating the pathogenic factors, suitable for debilitated patients who are incapable of withstanding the required elimination therapy

寓攻于补 [yù gōng yú bǔ]
reinforcemnt for elimination: one of the therapeutic principles for a complicated case of deficiency and excess that reinforcing therapy is applied for the purpose of eliminating the pathogenic factors

寓补于攻 [yù bǔ yú gōng]
elimination for reinforcement: one of the therapeutic principles for a complicated case of deficiency and excess that eliminating therapy is applied for the purpose of reinforcing the healthy *qi*

正治 [zhèng zhì]
routine treatment: use of medicines opposite in nature to the disease, e.g., treating heat syndrome with medicines cold in nature

反治 [fǎn zhì]
paradoxical treatment: use of medicines similar in nature to the disease, e.g., treating pseudo-heat syndrome with medicines hot in nature

逆治 [nì zhì]
counteracting treatment: same as routine treatment (正治 [zhèng zhì])

从治 [cóng zhì]
coacting treatment: same as paradoxical treatment (反治 [fǎn zhì])

反佐 [fǎn zuǒ]

use of corrigents: use of medicinals with property opposite to that of the principal ingredient in order to favorably modify the action of the latter which might be too powerful or harsh

阴病治阳 [yīn bìng zhì yáng]

treating yang for yin diseases: (1) Since chronic diseases of cold nature (pertaining to yin) are apt to damage yang, it is necessary to invigorate yang during the treatment. (2) Diseases with symptoms of the yin meridians/channels are often treated by needling the points on the yang meridians/channels, e.g., needling *Dazhu* (BL 11) and *Fengmen* (BL 12) (points of the foot greater yang meridian/channel) to treat cough after catching cold, a manifestation of pathological changes in the lung meridian/channel of hand greater yin.

阳病治阴 [yáng bìng zhì yīn]

treating yin for yang diseases: (1) A febrile disease (pertaining to yang) is apt to injure yin (vital essence and fluids), and should be treated with the method of replenishing yin in protracted cases. (2) Diseases with symptoms of the yang meridians/channels may be treated by needling points on the yin meridians/channels, e.g., needling *Neiguan* (PC 6) (a point on the hand reverting yin meridian) to treat vomiting, a manifestation of pathological changes in the stomach meridian/channel of foot yang brightness.

上病下取，下病上取 [shàng bìng xià qǔ, xià bìng shàng qǔ]

treating the lower for the upper, and treating the upper for the lower: (1) In acupuncture, the points on the lower part of the body are needled when the symptoms appear in the upper part, and vice versa, e.g., needling *Taichong* (LR 3) on the foot to treat dizziness, needling *Baihui* (GV 20) on the top of the head to treat prolapse of the rectum. (2) In medication, medicinals acting on the lower part of the body are often administered while the symptoms appear in the upper part, and vice versa, e.g., using rhubarb to induce catharsis for treating dizziness due to excessive fire, and using medicinals to clear up the lung for inducing diuresis.

左病右取，右病左取 [zuǒ bìng yòu qǔ, yòu bìng zuǒ qǔ]

treating diseases of the left with points on the right, and vice versa: treating diseases on one side of the body by needling points on the opposite side

寒因寒用 [hán yīn hán yòng]

cooling for the cold: treating pseudo-cold symptoms with medicines cool or cold in nature

热因热用 [rè yīn rè yòng]

heating for the hot: treating pseudo-heat symptoms with medicines warm or hot in nature

塞因塞用 [sāi yīn sāi yòng]

filling for the stuffed: treating a stuffed condition such as abdominal distension or constipation with tonics if it is caused by insufficient functioning of the spleen

通因通用 [tōng yīn tōng yòng]

purging for the diarrhetic: an unusual treatment, e.g., purgation in treating diarrhea caused by food stagnation

常用引文 Commonly Used Citations

治病必求其本。

[zhì bìng bì qiú qí běn]

Disease should be treated from its root.

治标不如治本。

[zhì biāo bù rú zhì běn]

Radical treatment is better than symptomatic relief.

急则治标。

[jí zé zhì biāo]

In emergency cases treat the acute symptoms.

缓则治本。

[huǎn zé zhì běn]

In non-acute cases treat the root of the disease.

小大不利治其标；小大利治其本。

[xiǎo dà bù lì zhì qí biāo; xiǎo dà lì zhì qí běn]

If the patient has difficulty in urination or defecation, treat the tip (give symptomatic relief) **first; otherwise, treat the root** (give radical treatment).

间者并行，甚者独行。

[jiān zhě bìn xíng, shèn zhě dú xíng]

If the illness is mild, treat the root and tip; if the illness is serious, treat the root or tip.

上工治未病。

[shàng gōng zhì wèi bìng]

An expert doctor treats a disease before it occurs. Preventive treatment is better than curative treatment.

治寒以热。

[zhì hán yǐ rè]

Treat cold with heat.

治热以寒。

[zhì rè yǐ hán]

Treat heat with cold.

实则泻之。

[shí zé xiè zhī]

In a case of excess, purge or reduce it.

虚则补之。

[xū zé bǔ zhī]

In a case of deficiency, reinforce or tonify it.

寒者热之。

[hán zhě rè zhī]

Treat cold with heat.

热者寒之。

[rè zhě hán zhī]

Treat heat with cold.

客者除之。

[kè zhě chú zhī]

Remove what is intruding.

逸者行之。

[yì zhě xíng zhī]

Activate what flows sluggishly.

留者攻之。

[liú zhě gōng zhī]

Attack what is lingering.

燥者濡之。
[zào zhě rú zhī]
Moisten what is dry.

急者缓之。
[jí zhě huǎn zhī]
Relieve what goes into spasm.

散者收之。
[sàn zhě shōu zhī]
Consolidate what has come loose.

劳者温之。
[láo zhě wēn zhī]
Give warming tonics to the debilitated.

坚者削之。
[jiān zhě xiāo zhī]
Disintegrate what has turned into a hard mass.

结者散之。
[jié zhě sàn zhī]
Dissipate what are bound together.

下者举之。
[xià zhě jǔ zhī]
Lift what prolapses.

高者抑之。
[gāo zhě yì zhī]
Suppress what goes perversely upward.

惊者平之。
[jīng zhě píng zhī]
Calm one who takes fright.

微者逆之。
[wēi zhě nì zhī]
Treat mild and simple cases by counteracting principle (with drugs opposite in nature to that of the disease). For example, cold syndromes should be treated with drugs warm or hot in nature, and heat syndromes with drugs cool or cold in nature.

甚者从之。
[shèn zhě cóng zhī]
Treat complicated cases by co-acting principle (with drugs similar in nature to the pseudo-symptoms). For example, in treating a febrile case with pseudo-cold symptoms, drugs of cold nature should be used.

木郁达之。
[mù yù dá zhī]
Mollify the liver (wood) if it is depressed.

火郁发之。
[huǒ yù fā zhī]
Expel fire if it is accumulated.

土郁夺之。
[tǔ yù duó zhī]
Remove dampness if it is accumulated in the spleen (earth).

金郁泻之。
[jīn yù xiè zhī]
Purge the lung (metal) if it is obstructed.

水郁折之。
[shuǐ yù zhé zhī]
Drain the kidney if water is retained.

形不足者温之以气。
[xīng bù zú zhě wēn zhī yǐ qì]

Treat patients with a flabby appearance with warming drugs to reinforce *qi*.

精不足者补之以味。

[jīng bù zú zhě bǔ zhī yǐ wèi]

Treat patients deficient in essence with a nutritious diet or drug rich in flavor.

其高者因而越之。

[qí gāo zhě yīn ér yuè zhī]

Troubles in the upper portion may be treated by way of emesis.

其下者引而竭之。

[qí xià zhě yǐn ér jié zhī]

Troubles in the lower portion may be treated by way of diuresis or purgation.

其在皮者汗而发之。

[qí zài pí zhě hàn ér fā zhī]

When pathogens reside at the superficies, expel them by way of diaphoresis.

寒之而热者取之阴。

[hán zhī ér rè zhě qǔ zhī yīn]

If a heat disease becomes worse after being treated with cold-natured medicines, turn to replenishing yin.

热之而寒者取之阳。

[rè zhī ér hán zhě qǔ zhī yáng]

If a cold disease becomes worse after being treated with hot-natured medicines, turn to invigorating yang.

壮水之主，以制阳光。

[zhuàng shuǐ zhī zhǔ, yǐ zhì yáng guāng]

Enrich the governor of water to restrain the brilliance of yang. If exuberance of yang is caused by deficiency of yin, treatment should be targeted at replenishing yin instead of suppressing yang directly.

益火之源，以消阴翳。

[yì huǒ zhī yuán, yǐ xiāo yīn yì]

Supply the source of fire to disperse the shroud of yin. For example, warming tonics to invigorate the life gate fire are used to treat cold symptoms such as general debility with aversion to cold, aching and creeping chills in the back, impotence, and frequent urination at night.

虚者补其母，实者泻其子。

[xū zhě bǔ qí mǔ, shí zhě xiè qí zǐ]

In cases of insufficiency, tonify the "mother" organ, while in cases of excessiveness, purge the "child" organ. For example, insufficiency of the liver is usually treated by way of tonifying the kidney, while excessiveness of the liver is treated by way of dispelling the fire from the heart.

无犯胃气。

[wú fàn wèi qì]

No medication should impair stomach *qi*.

有胃气则生，无胃气则死。

[yǒu wèi qì zé shēng, wú wèi qì zé sǐ]

So long as stomach *qi* remains, hope of life exists. When stomach *qi* disappears, death follows.

毋逆天时，是谓至治。

[wù nì tiān shí, shì wèi zhì zhì]

No violation of the relations between the weather of the four seasons and the human body is the best principle of treatment.

治法 Therapeutic Methods

三法 [sān fǎ]
three therapeutic methods: collective term for diaphoresis, emesis and purgation

八法 [bā fǎ]
eight therapeutic methods: collective term for diaphoresis, emesis, purgation, harmonization, warming, heat clearing, tonification, and resolution

汗法 [hàn fǎ]
diaphoretic method: one of the eight therapeutic methods used for relieving exterior syndromes, also called releasing the exterior (解表[jiě biǎo])

解表 [jiě biǎo]
releasing the exterior: general term for the methods of dispelling pathogenic factors from the exterior portion of the body, commonly used in the treatment of exterior syndromes/patterns

辛温解表 [xīn wēn jiě biǎo]
releasing the exterior with pungent-warm (medicinals): method of using medicinals pungent in flavor and warm in nature for treating wind-cold exterior syndrome/pattern

辛凉解表 [xīn liáng jiě biǎo]
releasing the exterior with pungent-cool (medicinals): method of using medicinals pungent in flavor and cool in nature for treating wind-heat exterior syndrome/pattern

疏散风热 [shū sàn fēng rè]
dispersing wind-heat: synonymous with releasing the exterior with pungent-cool (medicinals) (辛凉解表 [xīn liáng jiě biǎo])

辛凉清热 [xīn liáng qīng rè]
clearing heat with pungent-cool (medicinals): method of using medicinals pungent in flavor and cool in nature to release the exterior and clearing heat for treating a febrile disease at both the defense and *qi* aspects, also known as releasing the exterior and clearing heat (解表清热 [jiě biǎo qīng rè])

解表清热 [jiě biǎo qīng rè]
releasing the exterior and clearing heat: synonymous with clearing heat with pungent-cool (medicinals) (辛凉清热 [xīn liáng qīng rè])

发汗解表 [fā hàn jiě biǎo]
inducing sweating to release the exterior: method for treating exterior syndromes/patterns by using diaphoretics

解表清肺 [jiě biǎo qīng fèi]
releasing the exterior and clearing the lung: method for treating attack of wind-heat to the lung

解肌 [jiě jī]
releasing the flesh: general term for the methods of dispelling pathogens from the superficial flesh

解肌清热 [jiě jī qīng rè]
releasing the flesh and clearing heat: method of clearing heat accumulated in the superficial flesh

解肌发表 [jiě jī fā biǎo]
releasing the flesh to relieve the exterior: method of dispelling pathogenic factors from the superficial flesh and other exterior portions of the body

解肌透疹 [jiě jī tòu zhěn]
releasing the flesh to promote eruption: method of dispersing pathogens in the superficial flesh to promote skin eruption, chiefly used in the treatment of measles and rubella

解毒透疹 [jiě dú tòu zhě]
removing toxins to promote eruption: method of applying toxin-removing and pathogen-dispelling medicinals to promote skin eruption in the treatment of measles and rubella

疏风 [shū fēng]
dispersing wind: therapeutic method of dispersing external wind for releasing exterior syndromes/patterns

散寒 [sàn hán]
dissipating cold: therapeutic method of dissipating external cold pathogen

疏风散寒 [shū fēng sàn hán]
dispersing wind and dissipating cold: method of using medicinals pungent in flavor and warm in nature for relieving an exterior syndrome/pattern of wind-cold

疏风解表 [shū fēng jiě biǎo]
dispersing wind and releasing the exterior: method for treating an exterior syndrome/pattern caused by exogenous pathogenic wind

疏风解肌 [shū fēng jiě jī]
dispersing wind and releasing the flesh: method for treating attack of pathogenic wind to the superficial flesh

疏风清热 [shū fēng qīng rè]
dispersing wind and clearing heat: combined use of exterior-releasing and heat-clearing medicinals for treating contraction of external wind with interior heat, also known as dispersing wind and discharging heat (疏风泄热 [shū fēng xiè rè])

疏风泄热 [shū fēng xiè rè]
dispersing wind and discharging heat: same as dispersing wind and clearing heat (疏风清热 [shū fēng qīng rè])

疏风清肺 [shū fēng qīng fèi]
dispersing wind and clearing the lung: method of dispelling wind and heat from the lung meridian/channel

疏风透疹 [shū fēng tòu zhěn]
dispersing wind to promote eruption: method of using wind-dispersing medicinals to promote eruption in cases of measles and rubella, also called releasing the exterior to promote eruption (解表透疹 [jiě biǎo tòu zhěn])

解表透疹 [jiě biǎo tòu zhěn]
releasing the exterior to promote eruption: synonymous with dispersing wind to promote eruption (疏风透疹 [shū fēng tòu zhěn])

疏风宣肺 [shū fēng xuān fèi]
dispersing wind and ventilating the lung: method for treating attack to the lung by pathogenic wind

疏风消肿 [shū fēng xiāo zhǒng]
dispersing wind to alleviate edema: method for treating edema caused by pathogenic wind

疏风和营 [shū fēng hé yíng]
dispersing wind and harmonizing the nutrient (aspect): method for treating disharmony between the nutrient and defensive aspects caused by attack of pathogenic wind to the exterior of the body

疏风止痒 [shū fēng zhǐ yǎng]
dispersing wind to relieve itching: method for relieving itching caused by wind toxin

疏表润燥 [shū biǎo rùn zào]
releasing the exterior and moistening dryness: method of using exterior-releasing and dryness-moistening medicinals in the treatment of wind-dryness attacking the exterior

祛风 [qū fēng]
dispelling wind: method of expelling pathogenic wind from the body surface, meridians/channels, flesh and joints, used for treating external contraction at the early stage with exterior syndrome/pattern, and also for rheumatic or rheumatoid arthritis

祛风解表 [qū fēng jiě biǎo]
dispelling wind and releasing the exterior: method of dispelling wind from the body surface in the treatment of exterior syndrome caused by exogenous wind

祛风散寒 [qū fēng sàn hán]
dispelling wind and dissipating cold: common method for treating exterior syndrome/pattern of wind-cold, also known as dispersing wind and dissipating cold (疏风散寒 [shū fēng sàn hán])

祛风清热 [qū fēng qīng rè]
dispelling wind and clearing heat: common method for treating exterior syndrome/pattern of wind-heat, also known as dispersing wind and clearing heat (疏风清热 [shū fēng qīng rè])

祛风除湿 [qū fēng chú shī]
dispelling wind and removing dampness: method for treating wind-dampness contraction such as rheumatism

祛风化痰 [qū fēng huà tán]
dispelling wind and resolving phlegm: method for treating wind-phlegm syndrome/pattern

祛风止痛 [qū fēng zhǐ tòng]
dispelling wind to relieve pain: therapeutic method for relieving pain caused by attack of pathogenic wind

祛风除湿止痛 [qū fēng chú shī zhǐ tòng]
dispelling wind and removing dampness to relieve pain: common method for relieving pain caused by contraction of wind-dampness, e.g., rheumatic pains

祛风解痉 [qū fēng jiě jìng]
dispelling wind and relieving spasm: method for treating spasms due to pathogenic wind attacking the meridians/channels

祛风通络 [qū fēng tōng luò]
dispelling wind and unblocking collaterals: method for treating pathogenic wind attack to collateral meridians

祛风止痒 [qū fēng zhǐ yǎng]
dispelling wind to relieve itching: same as dispersing wind to relieve itching (疏风止痒 [shū fēng zhǐ yǎng])

祛风行水 [qū fēng xíng shuǐ]
dispelling wind and promoting diuresis: method for treating wind edema

养血祛风 [yǎng xuè qū fēng]
nourishing blood and dispelling wind: method for treating endogenous wind due to liver blood deficiency

宣肺 [xuān fèi]
ventilating the lung: method for treating affection of the lung by exogenous pathogens that leads to such functional disturbances as cough, dyspnea or edema, also called 宣白 [xuān bái]

宣白 [xuān bái]
same as 宣肺 [xuān fèi]

化痰宣肺 [huà tán xuān fèi]
resolving phlegm to ventilate the lung: method of resolving retained phlegm to restore the normal ventilation of the lung for treating phlegm-turbidity obstructing the lung

宣肺化痰 [xuān fèi huà tán]
ventilating the lung and resolving phlegm: combined use of exterior-releasing medicinals (to ventilate the lung) and phlegm-resolving medicinals (to relieve cough), for treating wind-cold cough with profuse expectoration

宣肺化饮 [xuān fèi huà yǐn]
ventilating the lung and resolving retained fluid: method of removing retained fluid and phlegm to unblock the lung

宣肺止咳 [xuān fèi zhǐ ké]
ventilating the lung to relieve cough: method of regulating *qi* to facilitate free movement of air in the lung for relieving cough

宣肺平喘 [xuān fèi píng chuǎn]
ventilating the lung to relieve dyspnea: method of regulating *qi* to facilitate free movement of air in the lung for relieving dyspnea

宣肺止咳平喘 [xuān fèi zhǐ ké píng chuǎn]
ventilating the lung to relieve cough and dyspnea: method of regulating *qi* to facilitate free movement of air in the lung for treating cough and dyspnea

宣肺降气 [xuān fèi jiàng qì]
ventilating the lung and directing *qi* downward: method for treating impairment of the dispersing and descending function of the lung caused by pathogenic *qi*

透表 [tòu biǎo]
expelling pathogens through the exterior: method of expelling pathogenic factors from

the body in the treatment of acute febrile disease at the early stage with exterior syndrome/pattern of wind-heat

透表清热 [tòu biǎo qīng rè]
expelling pathogens through the exterior and clearing heat: method of using exterior-releasing and heat-clearing therapies in combination to relieve a febrile disease involving both the defense and *qi* aspects

透疹 [tòu zhěn]
promoting eruption: method of using pungent and cool-natured medicinals with the effect of expelling the pathogens from the exterior part of the body through skin eruption in order to prevent complications in the treatment of measles and rubella

透斑 [tòu bān]
promoting eruption of macules: method of applying medicinals to expel heat from the blood for treating acute febrile disease with indistinct maculation

透邪 [tòu xié]
expelling pathogens: method of driving pathogens out of the body, usually used in the treatment of an exterior syndrome/pattern, also known as 达邪 ([dá xié])

达邪 [dá xié]
expelling pathogens: same as 透邪 [tòu xié]

透泄 [tòu xiè]
expelling through the exterior and removing from the interior: method of using medicinals pungent in flavor and cool in nature to eliminate pathogenic heat of the exterior portion of the body, together with medicinals bitter in taste and cold in nature to remove pathogenic heat of the interior

调和营卫 [tiáo hé yíng wèi]
harmonizing the nutrient and defense: method for relieving exterior syndrome/pattern associated with spontaneous sweating due to disharmony between the nutrient and defense

开鬼门 [kāi guǐ mén]
opening the "ghost gates"; opening sweat pores: method of inducing perspiration

发汗禁例 [fā hàn jìn lì]
contraindications of diaphoresis: cases in which diaphoresis is contraindicated, such as heat due to deficiency of yin, external cold due to deficiency of yang, and hemorrhagic diseases

辛开苦泄 [xīn kāi kǔ xiè]
dispersion with the pungent and purgation with the bitter: (1) method of using pungent medicinals to disperse pathogenic factors from the exterior together with bitter medicinals to relieve interior heat; (2) method of using pungent medicinals to remove phlegm-dampness in the chest and bitter medicinals to remove dampness-heat

开泄 [kāi xiè]
dispersion and purgation: abbreviation for dispersion with the pungent and purgation with the bitter (辛开苦泄 [xīn kāi kǔ xiè])

扶正解表 [fú zhèng jiě biǎo]
reinforcing healthy *qi* and releasing the exterior: combined use of exterior-releasing medicinals and tonics for treating exterior syndrome/pattern occurring in a deficiency condition

滋阴解表 [zī yīn jiě biǎo]
replenishing yin and releasing the exterior: method of using both yin-tonifying and exterior-releasing medicinals to expel exogenous pathogenic factors from the exterior portion of the body in patients with yin deficiency

养阴解表 [yǎng yīn jiě biǎo]
nourishing yin and releasing the exterior: same as replenishing yin and releasing the exterior (滋阴解表 [zī yīn jiě biǎo])

助阳解表 [zhù yáng jiě biǎo]
supporting yang and releasing the exterior: method of using both yang-tonifying and exterior-releasing medicinals to expel exogenous pathogenic factors from the exterior portion of the body in patients with yang deficiency

益气解表 [yì qì jiě biǎo]
replenishing *qi* and releasing the exterior: therapeutic method of using both *qi*-tonifying and exterior-releasing medicinals to expel exogenous pathogenic factors from the exterior portion of the body in patients with *qi* deficiency

养血解表 [yǎng xuè jiě biǎo]
nourishing blood and releasing the exterior: therapeutic method of using both blood-tonifying and exterior-releasing medicinals to expel exogenous pathogenic factors from the exterior portion of the body in patients with blood deficiency

化饮解表 [huà yǐn jiě biǎo]
resolving retained fluid and releasing the exterior: method for treating a complex syndrome/pattern of wind-cold in the exterior and retained fluid in the interior

表里双解 [biǎo lǐ shuāng jiě]
releasing both the exterior and interior: treatment entailing dispelling pathogenic factors from both the exterior and the interior, indicated for a disease involving both the exterior and interior of the body

逆流挽舟 [nì liú wǎn zhōu]
"rowing upstream": metaphor referring to the treatment of dysentery at its initial stage with exterior syndrome by using exterior-releasing and dampness-expelling medicinals to drive the pathogen outward, i.e., in the opposite direction to the inward penetration of the pathogen

清法 [qīng fǎ]
(heat-)clearing method: one of the eight principal therapeutic methods whereby medicinals of cool or cold nature are used to treat fire or heat syndromes/patterns, also called 清热法 [qīng rè fǎ]

清热法 [qīng rè fǎ]
heat-clearing therapy: general term for therapeutic methods for treating various kinds of heat syndromes, also abbreviated as clearing method (清法[qīng fǎ])

苦寒清热 [kǔ hán qīng rè]

clearing heat with bitter-cold: common therapeutic method for relieving internal heat by using medicinals bitter in taste and cold in nature, also called purging heat with bitter-cold (苦寒泄热 [kǔ hán xiè rè])

苦寒泄热 [kǔ hán xiè rè]
purging heat with bitter-cold: another term for clearing heat with bitter-cold (苦寒清热 [kǔ hán qīng rè])

苦寒泻火 [kǔ hán xiè huǒ]
discharging fire with bitter-cold: therapeutic method of using bitter-cold medicinals to discharge fire

苦寒清气 [kǔ hán qīng qì]
clearing *qi* with bitter-cold: method of clearing heat from the *qi* aspect with medicinals bitter in taste and cold in nature, usually used in the treatment of acute febrile diseases with *qi*-aspect syndrome

清热生津 [qīng rè shēng jīn]
clearing heat and promoting fluid production: therapeutic method of using sweet-cool heat-clearing medicinals together with medicinals that promote fluid production for treating fire or heat syndromes/patterns with damage to body fluids, also called purging heat to preserve fluids (泄热存津 [xiè rè cún jīn])

泄热存津 [xiè rè cún jīn]
purging heat to preserve fluids: synonymous with clearing heat and promoting fluid production (清热生津 [qīng rè shēng jīn])

除烦止渴 [chú fán zhǐ kě]
relieving vexation and thirst: therapeutic method for relieving vexing thirst in heat syndromes/patterns

清热解毒 [qīng rè jiě dú]
clearing heat and resolving toxins: common method of using heat-clearing and toxin-resolving medicinals for treating acute infectious diseases and pyogenic inflammations

清热泻火 [qīng rè xiè huǒ]
clearing heat and purging fire: method for treating exuberant fire and heat

清热祛湿 [qīng rè qū shī]
clearing heat and dispelling dampness: therapeutic method of using heat-clearing medicinals together with dampness-dispelling medicinals for treating accumulation of dampness-heat

清热除湿 [qīng rè chú shī]
clearing heat and removing dampness: same as clearing heat and dispelling dampness (清热祛湿 [qīng rè qū shī])

清热利湿 [qīng rè lì shī]
clearing heat and draining dampness: method of using heat-clearing medicinals together with diuretics to clear heat and remove dampness through diuresis for treating accumulation of dampness-heat in the lower energizer

清热燥湿 [qīng rè zào shī]
clearing heat and drying dampness: therapeutic method of using heat-clearing and dampness-drying medicinals for relieving accumulation of dampness-heat

清热消食 [qīng rè xiāo shí]
clearing heat and promoting digestion: combined use of heat-clearing medicinals and digestants for treating food stagnation with stomach heat

清热导滞 [qīng rè dǎo zhì]
clearing heat and relieving (food) stagnation: method of using heat-clearing medicinals and digestants for treating food stagnation with stomach heat or undigested food retained in the stomach and intestines

清热明目 [qīng rè míng mù]
clearing heat to improve vision: method of using heat-clearing, fire-purging and toxin-resolving medicinals for treating eye diseases of heat nature, also known as clearing the liver to improve vision 清肝明目 [qīng gān míng mù]

清热和胃 [qīng rè hé wèi]
clearing heat and harmonizing the stomach: method for treating exuberance of stomach fire

清热和中 [qīng rè hé zhōng]
clearing heat and harmonizing the middle: same as clearing heat and harmonizing the stomach (清热和胃[qīng rè hé wèi])

清热止呕 [qīng rè zhǐ ǒu]
clearing heat to stop vomiting: method for treating vomiting caused by exuberant heat in the stomach

清热止泻 [qīng rè zhǐ xiè]
clearing heat to stop diarrhea: method for treating diarrhea due to retention of heat in the intestines, also known as clearing the intestines to stop diarrhea (清肠止泻 [qīng cháng zhǐ xiè]

清热止痢 [qīng rè zhǐ lì]
clearing heat to relieve dysentery: method for treating dysentery due to retention of heat in the intestines, also known as clearing the intestines to relieve dysentery (清肠止痢 [qīng cháng zhǐ lì])

清热解暑 [qīng rè jiě shǔ]
clearing summerheat: basic method for treating summerheat

清暑热 [qīng shǔ rè]
clearing summerheat: same as 清热解暑 [qīng rè jiě shǔ]

清暑化湿 [qīng shǔ huà shī]
clearing summerheat and resolving dampness: combined use of summerheat-clearing medicinals and dampness-resolving medicinals for treating summerheat dampness syndrome/pattern, also called dispelling summerheat and resolving dampness (祛暑化湿 [qū shǔ huà shī])

祛暑化湿 [qū shǔ huà shī]
dispelling summerheat and resolving dampness: same as clearing summerheat and draining dampness (清暑化湿 [qīng shǔ huà shī])

清暑利湿 [qīng shǔ lì shī]
clearing summerheat and draining-dampness: basic method for treating summerheat-dampness

清营 [qīng yíng]
clearing the nutrient aspect: common

method for treating acute febrile disease involving the nutrient (*ying*) aspect

清营泄热 [qīng yíng xiè rè]
clearing the nutrient aspect and purging heat: same as clearing the nutrient aspect (清营 [qīng yíng])

清营透疹 [qīng yíng tòu zhěn]
clearing the nutrient aspect and promoting eruption: combined method of clearing the nutrient aspect of heat and promoting skin eruption for treating pathogenic heat entering the nutrient aspect

清热凉血 [qīng rè liáng xuè]
clearing heat and cooling blood: method of removing heat from blood for treating acute febrile diseases and other diseases with exuberant heat in the blood aspect, also abbreviated as cooling blood (凉血 [liáng xuè])

凉血 [liáng xuè]
cooling blood: abbreviation for clearing heat and cooling blood (清热凉血 [qīng rè liáng xuè])

凉血解毒 [liáng xuè jiě dú]
cooling blood and removing toxins: method of removing heat toxins from blood for treating infections from toxins in the nutrient and blood aspects

清热开窍 [qīng rè kāi qiào]
clearing heat to open the orifices; clearing heat to induce resuscitation: method for treating impaired consciousness in cases of acute febrile diseases

清脏腑热 [qīng zàng fǔ rè]
clearing *zang-fu* organ heat: general term for clearing heat from *zang-fu* organs

清肝 [qīng gān]
clearing the liver: method of clearing the liver of heat or fire

清肝泻火 [qīng gān xiè huǒ]
clearing the liver and purging fire: method for treating excessive fire in the liver, also abbreviated as purging the liver (泻肝 [xiè gān]), or known as clearing liver fire (清肝火 [qīng gān huǒ])

泻肝 [xiè gān]
purging the liver: abbreviation for clearing the liver and purging fire (清肝泻火 [qīng gān xiè huǒ]), also known as clearing liver fire (清肝火 [qīng gān huǒ])

清肝火 [qīng gān huǒ]
clearing liver fire: synonym for clearing the liver and purging fire (清肝泻火 [qīng gān xiè huǒ]), or purging the liver (泻肝 [xiè gān])

清肝明目 [qīng gān míng mù]
clearing the liver to improve vision: synonym for clearing heat to improve vision (清热明目 [qīng rè míng mù])

清心 [qīng xīn]
clearing the heart: method of clearing exuberant heat or fire from the heart or pericardium

清宫 [qīng gōng]
clearing the pericardium: method of clearing pathogenic heat from the pericardium

清心火 [qīng xīn huǒ]
clearing heart fire: method of clearing the heart of pathogenic fire for treating exuberant heart fire syndrome/pattern

清心泻火 [qīng xīn xiè huǒ]
clearing the heart and purging fire: method for treating exuberant heart fire syndrome/pattern

清心安神 [qīng xīn ān shén]
clearing the heart and calming the mind: method of clearing the heart fire and inducing tranquilization for treating mental disturbance caused by heat

清心开窍 [qīn xīn kāi qiào]
clearing the heart to open the orifices; clearing the heart to restore consciousness: method for treating contraction of exuberant heat or fire in the heart with impaired consciousness

泻心火 [xiè xīn huǒ]
purging heart fire: method for treating contraction of exuberant fire in the heart

泻心 [xiè xīn]
purging the heart: method of using heat-clearing and purgative medicinals for treating contraction of excessive heat or pathogenic fire in the heart and stomach

清肺热 [qīng fèi rè]
clearing lung heat: method for treating contraction of excessive heat in the lung, also known as clearing the lung (清肺 [qīng fèi])

清肺火 [qīng fèi huǒ]
clearing lung fire: method for treating-contraction of exuberant fire in the lung, also known as clearing the lung (清肺 [qīng fèi])

清肺 [qīng fèi]
clearing the lung: same as clearing lung heat (清肺热 [qīng fèi rè]) or clearing lung fire (清肺火 [qīng fèi huǒ])

清肺润燥 [qīng fèi rùn zào]
clearing the lung and moistening dryness: method for treating contraction of dryness-heat in the lung

清肺化痰 [qīng fèi huà tán]
clearing the lung and resolving phlegm: method of combined use of heat-clearing and phlegm-resolving medicinals for treating contraction of heat-phlegm in the lung

清肺止咳 [qīng fèi zhǐ ké]
clearing the lung to relieve cough: method for treating cough due to exuberant heat in the lung

清肺止喘 [qīng fèi zhǐ chuǎn]
clearing the lung to relieve dyspnea: method for treating dyspnea due to exuberant heat in the lung

清肺利咽 [qīng fèi lì yān]
clearing the lung to soothe the throat: method for treating sore throat due to exuberant heat in the lung

清热泻肺 [qīng rè xiè fèi]
clearing heat and purging the lung: method for treating contraction of exuberant lung heat, also abbreviated as purging the lung (泻肺 [xiè fèi])

泻肺 [xiè fèi]
purging the lung: abbreviation for clearing heat and purging the lung (清热泻肺 [qīng rè xiè fèi])

泻肺平喘 [xiè fèi píng chuǎn]
purging the lung to relieve dyspnea: method for treating dyspnea caused by accumulation of pathogens in the lung

清胃热 [qīng wèi rè]
clearing stomach heat: method for treating contraction of excessive heat in the stomach, also known as clearing the stomach and purging heat (清胃泄热 [qīng wèi xiè rè]), and abbreviated as clearing the stomach (清胃 [qīng wèi])

清胃火 [qīng wèi huǒ]
clearing stomach fire: method for treating contraction of exuberant fire in the stomach, also known as clearing the stomach and purging fire 清胃泄火([qīng wèi xiè huǒ]), and abbreviated as clearing the stomach (清胃 [qīng wèi])

清胃泄热 [qīng wèi xiè rè]
clearing the stomach and purging heat: synonymous with clearing stomach heat (清胃热 [qīng wèi rè])

清胃泄火 [qīng wèi xiè huǒ]
clearing the stomach and purging fire: synonymous with clearing stomach fire (清胃火[qīng wèi huǒ])

清胃 [qīng wèi]
clearing the stomach: abbreviation for clearing the stomach and purging heat (清胃泄热 [qīng wèi xiè rè]) or clearing the stomach and purging fire (清胃泄火 [qīng wèi xiè huǒ])

清肠止泻 [qīng cháng zhǐ xiè]
clearing the intestines to stop diarrhea: same as clearing heat to stop diarrhea (清热止泻 [qīng rè zhǐ xiè])

清肠止痢 [qīng cháng zhǐ lì]
clearing the intestines to relieve dysentery: same as clearing heat to relieve dysentery (清热止痢 [qīng rè zhǐ lì])

清肠润燥 [qīng cháng rùn zào]
clearing the intestines and moistening dryness: method for treating constipation due to excessive heat in the intestines

清泄相火 [qīng xiè xiàng huǒ]
clearing and purging ministerial fire: method for treating preponderance of ministerial fire, also known as clearing ministerial fire (清相火 [qīng xiàng huǒ])

清相火 [qīng xiàng huǒ]
clearing ministerial fire: synonymous with clearing and purging ministerial fire (清泄相火 [qīng xiè xiàng huǒ])

凉血散瘀 [liáng xuè sàn yū]
cooling the blood and dissipating stasis: method for treating blood heat with blood stasis

凉血止痢 [liáng xuè zhǐ lì]
cooling the blood to treat dysentery: method for treating dysentery with bloody stools caused by heat in the blood

下法 [xià fǎ]
purgative method: one of the eight principal therapeutic methods used to relieve constipation, remove stagnant food or static blood, and expel internal heat or

excessive fluid through the bowels, also known as purgation (泻下 [xiè xià], 攻下 [gōng xià], and 通下 [tōng xià])

泻下 [xiè xià]
purgation: synonymous with purgation method (下法 [xià fǎ])

攻下 [gōng xià]
purgation: same as 泻下 [xiè xià]

通下 [tōng xià]
purgation: same as 泻下 [xiè xià]

通里 [tōng lǐ]
unblocking the interior: another expression for purgative method (下法 [xià fǎ])

寒下 [hán xià]
cold purgation: method of inducing purgation with cold-natured medicinals to remove excessive heat in the interior, manifested by constipation and abdominal distension with fever and thirst, as occurring in cases of dampness-heat dysentery, or indigestion with stagnant undigested food

温下 [wēn xià]
warm purgation: method of inducing purgation with warm-natured medicinals for treating stagnation of food or accumulation of pathogenic factors marked by cold syndrome/pattern, e.g., constipation and abdominal pain with cold extremities and white tongue coating

温下寒积 [wēn xià hán jī]
warm purgation of cold accumulation: method of using yang-warming medicinals with cathartics for treating constipation due to cold congealment in cases of yang deficiency

缓下 [huǎn xià]
laxation: therapeutic method of using medicinals with mild action for relieving constipation

润下 [rùn xià]
lubricant laxation: method of inducing laxation with lubricants for treating constipation due to intestinal dryness, also called moistening the intestines (润肠 [rùn cháng])

润肠 [rùn cháng]
moistening the intestines: synonymous with lubricant laxation (润下 [rùn xià])

通便 [tōng biàn]
relaxing the bowels: therapeutic method for relieving constipation

峻下 [jùn xià]
drastic purgation: therapeutic method of using medicinals with drastic action to induce purgation, also called emergency purgation (急下[jí xià])

急下 [jí xià]
emergency purgation: synonymous with drastic purgation (峻下 [jùn xià])

急下存阴 [jí xià cún yīn]
emergency purgation to preserve yin: therapeutic method of using drastic cathartics to purge excessive heat to prevent further loss of fluid, for treating persistent high fever and impairment of body fluid, also known as emergency

purgation to preserve fluid (急下存津 [jí xià cún jīn])

急下存津 [jī xià cún jīn]
emergency purgation to preserve fluid: same as emergency purgation to preserve yin (急下存阴 [jí xià cún yīn])

润肠通便 [rùn cháng tōng biàn]
moistening the intestines to relax the bowels: method of using moistening medicinals for treating constipation due to intestinal dryness, also called moistening dryness to relax the bowels (润燥通便 [rùn zào tōng biàn]) or increasing fluid to induce laxation (增液通下 [zēng yè tōng xià])

润燥通便 [rùn zào tōng biàn]
moistening dryness to relax the bowels: same as moistening the intestines to relax the bowels (润肠通便 [rùn cháng tōng biàn])

增液通下 [zēng yè tōng xià]
increasing fluid to induce laxation: synonymous with moistening the intestines to relax the bowels (润肠通便 [rùn cháng tōng biàn])

通腑泄热 [tōng fǔ xiè rè]
relaxing the bowels and purging heat: therapeutic method of removing internal heat by catharsis, also abbreviated as relaxing and purging (通泄 [tōng xiè])

通泄 [tōng xiè]
relaxing and purging: abbreviation for relaxing the bowels and purging heat (通腑泄热 [tōng fǔ xiè rè])

逐水 [zhú shuǐ]
expelling water; hydragogue therapy: therapeutic method of producing copious watery discharges, especially from the bowels

泻下逐水 [xiè xià zhú shuǐ]
expelling water by catharsis: method of using hydrogogues to eliminate water retention, also known as expelling retained water (攻逐水饮 [gōng zhú shuǐ yǐn]) or expelling retained water (泻水逐饮 [xiè shuǐ zhú yǐn])

攻逐水饮 [gōng zhú shuǐ yǐn]
expelling retained water: synonymous with expelling water by catharsis (泻下逐水 [xiè xià zhú shuǐ])

泻水逐饮 [xiè shuǐ zhú yǐn]
expelling retained water: same as 攻逐水饮 [gōng zhú shuǐ yǐn]

泻下逐饮 [xiè xià zhú yǐn]
expelling retained fluid by catharsis: method of using hydrogogues to eliminate retained fluid

轻下 [qīng xià]
mild purgation: method of using mild laxative medicinals to induce bowel movement

釜底抽薪 [fǔ dǐ chōu xīn]
"removing firewood from under the cauldron": metaphorical expression for the method of clearing heat or fire by way of purgation

去菀陈莝 [qù yù chén cuò]
eliminating the stale and the stagnant:

ancient term for the elimination of retained water and stagnant blood

攻下逐瘀 [gōng xià zhú yū]
eliminating stagnant blood by catharsis: method of using purgatives together with stasis-resolving medicinals for treating blood stasis

误下 [wù xià]
erroneous administration of purgatives: administration of purgatives in the case where purgation is contraindicated

和法 [hé fǎ]
harmonizing method: therapeutic method involving administration of medicinals with regulatory or intermediary action to restore normal correlation among the internal organs or to eliminate pathogenic factors from the portion connecting the exterior and interior of the body, also known as 和解法 [hé jiě fǎ]

和解法 [hé jiě fǎ]
harmonizing method: same as 和法 [hé fǎ]

和解表里 [hé jiě biǎo lǐ]
harmonizing the exterior and interior: method for treating mild cases of dual exterior-interior syndrome/pattern

和解少阳 [hé jiě shào yáng]
harmonizing *shaoyang* meridian/channel; harmonizing lesser yang meridian/channel: method of using medicinals to combat the pathogenic factors lingering at *shaoyang* or lesser yang meridian/channel and at the same time to strengthen the body resistance, for treating *shaoyang* disease or lesser yang disease (cf. 少阳病 [shào yáng bìng])

开达膜［募］原 [kāi dá mó (mù) yuán]
dredging the pleurodiaphragmatic space: method for treating a disease believed to be located in the pleurodiaphragmatic space marked by irregular spells of alternate fever and chills occurring one to three times a day, associated with tightness in the chest, nausea, headache, irritability, and taut and rapid pulse

和胃 [hé wèi]
harmonizing the stomach: method for treating dysfunction of the stomach with such symptoms as epigastric distension and distress, anorexia, belching, or nausea, also known as harmonizing the middle (和中 [hé zhōng])

和中 [hé zhōng]
harmonizing the middle: another name for harmonizing the stomach (和胃 [hé wèi])

理中 [lǐ zhōng]
regulating the middle: method to regulate the spleen and stomach in deficiency-cold conditions

理气和胃 [lǐ qì hé wèi]
regulating *qi* and harmonizing the stomach: method of regulating *qi* and removing stagnation to restore the normal function of the stomach, for treating stomach *qi* stagnation

调和脾胃 [tiáo hé pí wèi]
harmonizing the spleen and stomach: method to regulate spleen and stomach

qi activity, for treating disharmony of the spleen and stomach

调和肝胃 [tiáo hé gān wèi]
harmonizing the liver and stomach: method of soothing the liver and harmonizing the stomach for treating dysfunction of the stomach caused by perverted flow of liver *qi*

调和肝脾 [tiáo hé gān pí]
harmonizing the liver and spleen: method of soothing the liver, invigorating the spleen and regulating *qi* activity for treating liver *qi* stagnation with spleen insufficiency

交通心肾 [jiāo tōng xīn shèn]
coordinating the heart and kidney: method to nourish kidney yin, astringe kidney yang, reduce heart fire and calm the mind for treating pathological changes due to breakdown of the normal coordination between the heart and the kidney

调和气血 [tiáo hé qì xuè]
harmonizing *qi* and blood: method of using *qi*-regulating and blood-activating medicinals for treating disharmony of *qi* and blood, also called regulating *qi* and blood (调理气血 [tiáo lǐ qì xuè]), or regulating *qi* and harmonizing blood (理气和血 [lǐ qì hé xuè])

调理气血 [tiáo lǐ qì xuè]
regulating *qi* and blood: same as harmonizing *qi* and blood (调和气血 [tiáo hé qì xuè]) or regulating *qi* and harmonizing blood (理气和血 [lǐ qì hé xuè])

理气和血 [lǐ qì hé xuè]
regulating *qi* and harmonizing blood: synonymous with harmonizing *qi* and blood (调和气血 [tiáo hé qì xuè]) or regulating *qi* and blood (调理气血 [tiáo lǐ qì xuè])

和血熄风 [hé xuè xī fēng]
harmonizing blood to extinguish wind: method to tonify liver blood for treating syndrome/pattern of blood deficiency with stirring wind, also known as nourishing blood to extinguish wind (养血熄风 [yǎng xuè xī fēng])

养血熄风 [yǎng xuè xī fēng]
nourishing blood to extinguish wind: synonymous with harmonizing blood to extinguish wind (和血熄风 [hé xuè xī fēng])

和血调经 [hé xuè tiáo jīng]
harmonizing blood to regulate menstruation: method to activate blood and regulate *qi* for treating menstrual disorders due to disharmony of *qi* and blood

和血安胎 [hé xuè ān tāi]
harmonizing blood to prevent abortion: method to activate blood and regulate *qi* for preventing abortion caused by disharmony of *qi* and blood

和血止痛 [hé xuè zhǐ tòng]
harmonizing blood to relieve pain: method to normalize the blood flow for relieving pain

和营 [hé yíng]
harmonizing the nutrient: therapeutic method to regulate the nutrient aspect

和营止痛 [hé yíng zhǐ tòng]
harmonizing the nutrient to relieve pain: method to regulate the nutrient and blood for relieving pain due to disturbed nutrient-blood flow

和营活血 [hé yíng huó xuè]
harmonizing the nutrient and activating blood: therapeutic method of using blood-tonifying and nutrient-harmonizing medicinals in combination with blood-activating and stasis-resolving medicinals for treating blood deficiency complicated by blood stasis

和营生新 [hé yíng shēng xīn]
harmonizing the nutrient to promote regeneration: method to regulate the nutrient and blood and facilitate blood flow to promote tissue regeneration for treating unhealed wounds

温法 [wēn fǎ]
warming method: one of the eight principal therapeutic methods in which interior-warming medicinals are used for treating cold syndromes/patterns, also known as cold-dispelling method (祛寒法 [qū hán fǎ])

祛寒法 [qū hán fǎ]
cold-dispelling method: therapeutic method of using interior-warming medicinals to dispel internal cold, also called warming method (温法 [wēn fǎ])

温阳 [wēn yáng]
warming yang: general term for the therapeutic methods to warm and unblock yang *qi*

温里 [wēn lǐ]
warming the interior: general term for the methods for treating interior-cold syndromes/patterns

温肝 [wēn gān]
warming the liver: method for treating pain with cold sensation in the lower abdomen along the liver meridian/channel

温心阳 [wēn xīn yáng]
warming heart yang: method for treating yang deficiency of the heart

回阳救逆 [huí yáng jiù nì]
restoring yang from collapse: method for treating yang exhaustion with cold limbs (collapse)

回阳 [huí yáng]
restoring yang: synonymous with restoring yang from collapse (回阳救逆 [huí yáng jiù nì])

救脱 [jiù tuō]
saving from collapse: emergency treatment of collapse

救阳 [jiù yáng]
rescuing yang: same as restoring yang from collapse (回阳救逆 [huí yáng jiù nì])

通阳 [tōng yáng]
unblocking yang: method of using medicinals warm or hot in nature to remove blockage of yang *qi* caused by accumulation of cold-dampness, phlegm or stagnant blood, so as to normalize the flow of yang *qi*

宣痹通阳 [xuān bì tōng yáng]
removing impediment and unblocking yang: method of removing impediment to normalize the flow of yang *qi*, as in the treatment of angina pectoris

通脉 [tōng mài]
invigorating the pulse: method to warm up and restore the normal flow of yang *qi* to stimulate the pulse beat

温中 [wēn zhōng]
warming the middle: method of using warming tonics to dispel cold and harmonize the middle energizer for treating yang deficiency of the spleen and stomach

温脾 [wēn pí]
warming the spleen: method of using warming tonics for treating deficiency-cold of the spleen, also known as warming the middle (温中 [wēn zhōng])

温胃 [wēn wèi]
warming the stomach: method of using medicinals warm or hot in nature for treating stomach cold

温中祛寒 [wēn zhōng qū hán]
warming the middle and dispelling cold: method of using medicinals warm or hot in nature for treating deficiency-cold of the middle energizer (i.e., the spleen and stomach), also called warming the middle and dissipating cold (温中散寒 [wēn zhōng sàn hán])

温中散寒 [wēn zhōng sàn hán]
warming the middle and dissipating cold: same as warming the middle and dispelling cold (温中祛寒 [wēn zhōng qū hán])

温中行气 [wēn zhōng xíng qì]
warming the middle and moving *qi*: method for treating abdominal distension or pain due to cold in the spleen and stomach with *qi* stagnation

温中和胃 [wēn zhōng hé wèi]
warming the middle and harmonizing the stomach: method to warm yang and invigorate the stomach for treating stomach yang deficiency

温补胃阳 [wēn bǔ wèi yáng]
warming and tonifying stomach yang: synonymous with warming the middle and harmonizing the stomach (温中和胃 [wēn zhōng hé wèi])

温胃降逆 [wēn wèi jiàng nì]
warming the stomach to suppress upward counterflow of *qi*: method for treating vomiting, retching or hiccups due to deficiency-cold of the stomach

温胃止呕 [wēn wèi zhǐ ǒu]
warming the stomach to stop vomiting: method for treating vomiting due to cold in the stomach, also called warming the middle to stop vomiting (温中止呕 [wēn zhōng zhǐ ǒu] or 温中止吐 [wēn zhōng zhǐ tù])

温中止呕 [wēn zhōng zhǐ ǒu]
warming the middle to stop vomiting: synonymous with warming the stomach to stop vomiting (温胃止呕 [wēn wèi zhǐ ǒu])

温中止吐 [wēn zhōng zhǐ tù]
warming the middle to stop vomiting: same as 温中止呕 [wēn zhōng zhǐ ǒu]

温中止泻 [wēn zhōng zhǐ xiè]
warming the middle to stop diarrhea: method of treating diarrhea due to deficiency-cold of the spleen

温中止痛 [wēn zhōng zhǐ tòng]
warming the middle to relieve pain: method of treating abdominal pain due to deficiency-cold of the spleen and stomach

温肺 [wēn fèi]
warming the lung: method of using warming tonics for treating cold syndromes/patterns of the lung

温肺散寒 [wēn fèi sàn hán]
warming the lung and dissipating cold: method of using warm-tonifying medicinals for treating deficiency-cold of the lung

温肺化痰 [wēn fèi huà tán]
warming the lung and resolving phlegm: method for treating accumulation of cold-phlegm in the lung

温肺化饮 [wēn fèi huà yǐn]
warming the lung and resolving retained fluid: method of using warming and fluid-resolving medicinals for treating retention of cold fluid in the lung

温肾 [wēn shèn]
warming the kidney: method of using warming tonics to invigorate kidney yang, also known as warming kidney yang (温肾阳 [wēn shèn yáng])

温肾阳 [wēn shèn yáng]
warming kidney yang: same as warming the kidney (温肾 [wēn shèn])

温补肾阳 [wēn bǔ shèn yáng]
warming and tonifying kidney yang: therapeutic method to warm yang and tonify the kidney for treating kidney yang deficiency

温肾纳气 [wēn shèn nà qì]
warming the kidney to improve *qi* reception: method to warm kidney yang for improving the respiration, particularly for relieving dyspnea in cases of chronic asthma

纳气平喘 [nà qì píng chuàn]
improving *qi* reception to relieve asthma: method to improve the kidney's function in reception of *qi* for relieving dyspnea

温肾缩尿 [wēn shèn suō niào]
warming the kidney to reduce urination: method of using kidney-warming tonics for treating frequent micturition or enuresis

温肾止泻 [wēn shèn zhǐ xiè]
warming the kidney to stop diarrhea: method of using kidney-warming tonics for relieving chronic diarrhea caused by kidney yang deficiency

温肾壮阳 [wēn shèn zhuàng yáng]
warming the kidney to invigorate yang: method to promote virility in the treatment of sexual impotence

温肾化痰 [wēn shèn huà tán]
warming the kidney to resolve phlegm:

method for treating kidney yang deficiency with cold phlegm

温肾化饮 [wēn shèn huà yǐn]
warming the kidney to resolve retained fluid: method for treating kidney yang deficiency with retained fluid

温补脾肾 [wēn bǔ pí shèn]
warming and tonifying the spleen and kidney: method for treating yang deficiency of the spleen and kidney

温经 [wēn jīng]
warming the meridians/channels: method to warm and unblock the meridians/channels

暖宫 [nuǎn gōng]
warming the uterus: method for treating cold congealing in the uterus

温经祛寒 [wēn jīng qū hán]
warming the meridians/channels and dispelling cold: method of using yang-warming, cold-dispelling and meridian/channel-opening medicinals for treating syndrome/pattern of cold congealing in the meridian/channel, also known as warming the meridians/channels and dissipating cold (温经散寒 [wēn jīng sàn hán])

温经散寒 [wēn jīng sàn hán]
warming the meridians/channels and dissipating cold: synonymous with warming the meridians/channels and dispelling cold (温经祛寒 [wēn jīng qū hán])

温经通阳 [wēn jīng tōng yáng]
warming the meridians/channels and unblocking yang: method for treating stagnation of cold in the meridians/channels

温经回阳 [wēn jīng huí yáng]
warming the meridians/channels and restoring yang: method to warm and tonify yang *qi* in the meridians/channels for treating impending collapse, also called warming the meridians/channels and supporting yang (温经扶阳 [wēn jīng fú yáng])

温经扶阳 [wēn jīng fú yáng]
warming the meridians/channels and supporting yang: same as warming the meridians/channels and restoring yang (温经回阳 [wēn jīng huí yáng])

温经暖宫 [wēn jīng nuǎn gōng]
warming the meridians/channels and the uterus: method for treating cold congealing in the uterus

温经通络 [wēn jīng tōng luò]
warming and unblocking the meridians/channels and collaterals: method of using warming medicinals to free the flow of *qi* and blood in the meridians/channels and collaterals for relieving cold stagnation

温经行滞 [wēn jīng xíng zhì]
warming the meridians/channels to move stagnation: combined use of meridian/channel-warming medicinals and stasis-resolving medicinals for treating congealing cold with blood stasis

温经活血 [wēn jīng huó xuè]
warming the meridians/channels and activating blood: combined use of meridian/

channel-warming and blood-activating medicinals for treating cold congealing in the meridians/channels with sluggish blood flow

温经养血 [wēn jīng yǎng xuè]
warming the meridians/channels and nourishing blood: method of combined use of meridian/channel-warming medicinals and blood-nourishing medicinals for treating syndrome/pattern of blood deficiency with congealing cold

温经止痛 [wēn jīng zhǐ tòng]
warming the meridians/channels to relieve pain: method for relieving pain caused by cold stagnation in the meridians/channels

甘温除热 [gān wēn chú rè]
relieving fever with sweet-warm: method of using medicinals sweet in taste and warm in nature for treating fever caused by deficiency of *qi*

温里散寒 [wēn lǐ sàn hán]
warming the interior and dissipating cold: method for treating interior-cold syndromes/patterns

温里祛寒 [wēn lǐ qū hán]
warming the interior and dispelling cold: synonymous with warming the interior and dissipating cold (温里散寒 [wēn lǐ sàn hán])

苦温平燥 [kǔ wēn píng zào]
relieving dryness with bitter-warm: method of using medicinals bitter in taste and warm in nature for treating exterior syndrome/pattern due to cold and dryness

苦温燥湿 [kǔ wēn zào shī]
drying dampness with bitter-warm: method of using medicinals bitter in taste and warm in nature for treating dampness syndrome/pattern

补法 [bǔ fǎ]
(I) tonification; tonifying method: general term for the methods of using tonics to treat various deficiency syndromes/patterns, one of the eight principal therapeutic methods; **(II) reinforcement:** reinforcing method in acupuncture

补气 [bǔ qì]
tonifying *qi*: therapeutic method of using *qi* tonifying medicinals for treating *qi* deficiency, also known as replenishing *qi* (益气 [yì qì])

益气 [yì qì]
replenishing *qi*: synonymous with tonifying *qi* (补气 [bǔ qì])

补气固表 [bǔ qì gù biǎo]
tonifying *qi* to strengthen the superficies: method for treating spontaneous sweating and aversion to wind due to superficial *qi* deficiency

补益心气 [bǔ yì xīn qì]
tonifying and replenishing heart *qi*: method for treating deficiency of heart *qi*, also known as tonifying the heart and replenishing *qi* (补心益气 [bǔ xīn yì qì])

补心益气 [bǔ xīn yì qì]
tonifying the heart and replenishing *qi*: same as tonifying and replenishing heart *qi* (补益心气 [bǔ yì xīn qì])

健脾 [jiàn pí]
invigorating the spleen: method of invigorating the transporting and transformingfunctions of the spleen

补脾 [bǔ pí]
tonifying the spleen: method of using tonics for treating diminished functional activities of the spleen, also known as banking up earth (培土 [péi tǔ])

培土 [péi tǔ]
banking up earth: synonymous with tonifying the spleen (补脾 [bǔ pí])

运脾 [yùn pí]
activating the spleen: method chiefly involving combined use of medicinals to dispel dampness and tonics to activate functions of the spleen for treating accumulation of dampness in the spleen marked by indigestion with nausea, abdominal distension, diarrhea, white greasy coating of the tongue, and soft pulse

醒脾 [xǐng pí]
enlivening the spleen: method of using tonics for treating dyspepsia due to diminished functions of the spleen marked by anorexia, dull abdominal pain, loose bowels, pale tongue and feeble pulse

健脾和胃 [jiàn pí hé wèi]
invigorating the spleen and harmonizing the stomach: method of using spleen tonics and stomachics for treating diminished functions of the spleen and stomach

健脾消食 [jiàn pí xiāo shí]
invigorating the spleen to promote digestion: method for treating indigestion due to spleen insufficiency

健脾化湿 [jiàn pí huà shī]
invigorating the spleen to resolve dampness: method chiefly involving the use of spleen tonics for treating stagnancy of dampness due to spleen insufficiency, also called invigorating the spleen to dispel dampness (健脾祛湿 [jiàn pí qū shī])

健脾祛湿 [jiàn pí qū shī]
invigorating the spleen to dispel dampness: same as 健脾化湿 [jiàn pí huà shī]

健脾利湿 [jiàn pí lì shī]
invigorating the spleen and draining dampness: method of using spleen tonics in combination with dampness-draining medicinals for treating spleen insufficiency with dampness retention or disturbance of the spleen by dampness

健脾利水 [jiàn pí lì shuǐ]
invigorating the spleen and inducing diuresis: combined use of spleen *qi* tonics and diuretics for treating spleen insufficiency with edema

健脾化痰 [jiàn pí huà tán]
invigorating the spleen to resolve phlegm: method chiefly involving the use of spleen tonics for treating retention of phlegm due to spleen insufficiency

健脾止泻 [jiàn pí zhǐ xiè]
invigorating the spleen to arrest diarrhea: method chiefly involving the use of spleen tonics for treating chronic diarrhea due to spleen insufficiency

健脾止带 [jiàn pí zhǐ dài]
invigorating the spleen to arrest leukorrhea: method for treating leukorrhea due to spleen insufficiency with excessive dampness

健脾补肺 [jiàn pí bǔ fèi]
invigorating the spleen and tonifying the lung: method for treating deficiency in both the spleen and lung

健脾益气 [jiàn pí yì qì]
invigorating the spleen and replenishing *qi*: method for treating spleen *qi* deficiency, also known as tonifying the spleen and replenishing *qi* (补脾益气 [bǔ pí yì qì])

补脾益气 [bǔ pí yì qì]
tonifying the spleen and replenishing *qi*: synonymous with invigorating the spleen and replenishing *qi* (健脾益气 [jiàn pí yì qì])

补益中气 [bǔ yì zhōng qì]
replenishing the middle qi: method of replenishing *qi*, invigorating the spleen and harmonizing the stomach, for treating *qi* deficiency of the spleen and stomach, also called tonifying the middle and replenishing *qi* (补中益气 [bǔ zhōng yì qì])

补中益气 [bǔ zhōng yì qì]
tonifying the middle and replenishing *qi*: synonymous with tonifying the spleen and replenishing *qi* (补脾益气 [bǔ pí yì qì])

健脾养血 [jiàn pí yǎng xuè]
invigorating the spleen and nourishing the blood: method for treating spleen insufficiency with blood deficiency

温补脾胃 [wēn bǔ pí wèi]
warming and tonifying the spleen and stomach: method for treating yang deficiency of the spleen and stomach

健胃 [jiàn wèi]
invigorating the stomach: method for invigorating the stomach function and promoting digestion

开胃 [kāi wèi]
improving the appetite: method to stimulate the desire for food

健胃止呕 [jiàn wèi zhǐ ǒu]
invigorating the stomach to stop vomiting: use of stomachics to arrest vomiting

升提中气 [shēng tí zhōng qì]
elevating the middle *qi*: method to invigorate the functions of the spleen in sending *qi* and nutrients upward for treating chronic diarrhea, visceroptosis, and prolapse of the rectum or uterus, also known as raising the middle *qi* (升举中气 [shēng jǔ zhōng qì])

升举中气 [shēng jǔ zhōng qì]
raising the middle *qi*: same as elevating the middle *qi* (升提中气 [shēng tí zhōng qì])

升阳举陷 [shēng yáng jǔ xiàn]
elevating yang to cure drooping: method for treating spleen insufficiency with drooping symptoms such as protracted diarrhea, prolapse of the rectum or uterus, also abbreviated as elevating yang (升阳 [shēng yáng])

升阳 [shēng yáng]
elevating yang: abbreviation for elevating yang to cure drooping (升阳举陷 [shēng yáng jǔ xiàn])

补脾益肺 [bǔ pí yì fèi]
tonifying the spleen to replenish the lung: method to tonify the spleen for treating chronic consumptive diseases of the lung, also known as banking up earth to benefit metal (培土生金 [péi tǔ shēng jīn])

培土生金 [péi tǔ shēng jīn]
banking up earth to benefit metal: metaphoric expression for tonifying the spleen to replenish the lung (补脾益肺 [bǔ pí yì fèi])

培土抑木 [péi tǔ yì mù]
banking up earth and supressing wood: method for treating dysfunction of the spleen due to stagnation of liver *qi*

补肺 [bǔ fèi]
tonifying the lung: a general term for using tonics to treat deficiency syndromes/patterns of the lung

补益肺气 [bǔ yì fèi qì]
replenishing lung *qi*: method for treating lung *qi* deficiency

补肺益气 [bǔ fèi yì qì]
tonifying the lung and replenishing *qi*: synonymous with replenishing lung *qi* (补益肺气 [bǔ yì fèi qì])

补血 [bǔ xuè]
tonifying blood: use of blood tonics for treating deficiency of blood, also called nourishing blood (养血 [yǎng xuè])

养血 [yǎng xuè]
nourishing blood: synonymous with tonifying blood (补血 [bǔ xuè])

补气生血 [bǔ qì shēng xuè]
tonifying *qi* and generating blood: method for treating deficiency of both *qi* and blood primarily due to *qi* deficiency

补养心血 [bǔ yǎng xīn xuè]
nourishing heart blood: method for treating deficiency of heart blood with giddiness, pallor, palpitations, insomnia, and forgetfulness

补益心脾 [bǔ yì xīn pí]
tonifying the heart and spleen: method for treating deficiency of both the heart blood and spleen *qi*

补益气血 [bǔ yì qì xuè]
tonifying *qi* and blood: therapeutic method for treating deficiency of both *qi* and blood, also known as tonifying *qi* and nourishing blood (补气养血 [bǔ qì yǎng xuè])

补气养血 [bǔ qì yǎng xuè]
tonifying *qi* and nourishing blood: same as tonifying *qi* and blood (补益气血 [bǔ yì qì xuè])

补阴 [bǔ yīn]
tonifying yin: general method of using tonics for treating yin deficiency, also called nourishing yin (养阴 [yǎng yīn] or 育阴 [yù yīn]), replenishing yin (滋阴 [zī yīn] or 益阴 [yì yīn])

养阴 [yǎng yīn]
nourishing yin: same as tonifying yin (补阴 [bǔ yīn])

育阴 [yù yīn]
nourishing yin: same as tonifying yin (补阴 [bǔ yīn])

滋阴 [zī yīn]
replenishing yin: same as tonifying yin (补阴 [bǔ yīn])

益阴 [yì yīn]
replenishing yin: same as tonifying yin (补阴 [bǔ yīn])

酸甘化阴 [suān gān huà yīn]
transformation of the sour-sweet into yin: method to replenish yin with medicinals sour and sweet in taste

补肝阴 [bǔ gān yīn]
tonifying liver yin: method for treating liver yin deficiency, also called nourishing liver yin (养肝阴 [yǎng gān yīn])

养肝阴 [yǎng gān yīn]
nourishing liver yin: synonymous with 补肝阴 [bǔ gān yīn]

滋养肝肾 [zī yǎng gān shèn]
nourishing the liver and kidney: (1) method to reinforce liver yin by replenishing kidney essence; (2) method of using tonics for treating yin deficiency of both the liver and kidney, also called tonifying the liver and kidney (补益肝肾 [bǔ yì gān shèn]) or replenishing water and moistening wood (滋水涵木 [zī shuǐ hán mù])

补益肝肾 [bǔ yì gān shèn]
tonifying the liver and kidney: same as nourishing the liver and kidney (滋养肝肾 [zī yǎng gān shèn])

滋水涵木 [zī shuǐ hán mù]
(I) replenishing water to moisten wood: method to nourish kidney yin (pertaining to water) for treating liver yin deficiency (pertaining to wood); **(II) replenishing water and moistening wood:** synonymous with nourishing the liver and kidney (滋养肝肾 [zī yǎng gān shèn])

补养心阴 [bǔ yǎng xīn yīn]
nourishing heart yin: method for treating heart yin deficiency marked by palpitations, insomnia or dream-disturbed sleep, also abbreviated as 补心阴 [bǔ xīn yīn], 养心阴 [yǎng xīn yīn] (tonifying heart yin) or simply 养心 [yǎng xīn] (nourishing the heart)

补心阴 [bǔ xīn yīn]
tonifying heart yin: synonymous with nourishing heart yin (补养心阴 [bǔ yǎng xīn yīn])

养心阴 [yǎng xīn yīn]
nourishing heart yin: same as 补养心阴 [bǔ yǎng xīn yīn]

养心 [yǎng xīn]
nourishing the heart: abbreviation for

nourishing heart yin (补养心阴 [bǔ yǎng xīn yīn])

滋养胃阴 [zī yǎng wèi yīn]
nourishing stomach yin: using tonics for treating stomach yin deficiency, also abbreviated as 养胃阴 [yǎng wèi yīn] or 补胃阴 [bǔ wèi yīn] (tonifying stomach yin) or simply 养胃 [yǎng wèi] (nourishing the stomach)

养胃阴 [yǎng wèi yīn]
nourishing stomach yin: same as滋养胃阴 [zī yǎng wèi yīn]

补胃阴 [bǔ wèi yīn]
tonifying stomach yin: synonymous with nourishing stomach yin (滋养胃阴 [zī yǎng wèi yīn])

养胃 [yǎng wèi]
nourishing the stomach: abbreviation for nourishing stomach yin (滋养胃阴 [zī yǎng wèi yīn])

养胃生津 [yǎng wèi shēng jīn]
nourishing the stomach to produce fluid: method for treating deficiency of stomach yin fluid

补养肺阴 [bǔ yǎng fèi yīn]
replenishing lung yin: using tonics for treating lung yin deficiency marked by dry throat and unproductive cough, also abbreviated as 补肺阴 [bǔ fèi yīn] (tonifying lung yin) or 养肺阴 [yǎng fèi yīn]

补肺阴 [bǔ fèi yīn]
tonifying lung yin: synonymous with replenishing lung yin (补养肺阴 [bǔ yǎng fèi yīn])

养肺阴 [yǎng fèi yīn]
nourishing lung yin: synonymous with replenishing lung yin 补养肺阴 [bǔ yǎng fèi yīn]

滋阴润肺 [zī yīn rùn fèi]
replenishing yin to moisten the lung: method of using yin tonics for treating dryness of the lung

滋补肺肾 [zī bǔ fèi shèn]
nourishing the lung and kidney: method for treating yin deficiency of both the lung and kidney

补肾 [bǔ shèn]
tonifying the kidney: general term for treating deficiency syndromes/patterns of the kidney

补益肾气 [bǔ yì shèn qì]
replenishing kidney *qi*: method for treating kidney *qi* deficiency, also known as tonifying the kidney and replenishing *qi* (补肾益气 [bǔ shèn yì qì])

补肾益气 [bǔ shèn yì qì]
tonifying the kidney and replenishing *qi*: synonymous with replenishing kidney *qi* (补益肾气 [bǔ yì shèn qì])

滋补肾阴 [zī bǔ shèn yīn]
replenishing kidney yin: method for treating kidney yin deficiency, also abbreviated as 补肾阴[bǔ shèn yīn] (tonifying kidney yin), 滋肾阴 [zī shèn yīn] or simply 滋肾 [zī shèn] (replenishing the kidney)

补肾阴 [bǔ shèn yīn]
tonifying kidney yin: synonymous with replenishing kidney yin (滋补肾阴 [zī bǔ shèn yīn])

滋肾阴 [zī shèn yīn]
replenishing kidney yin: same as 滋补肾阴 [zī bǔ shèn yīn]

滋肾 [zī shèn]
replenishing the kidney: abbreviation for replenishing kidney yin (滋补肾阴 [zī bǔ shèn yīn])

补肾固精 [bǔ shèn gù jīng]
tonifying the kidney to arrest emission: method for treating kidney insufficiency manifested by seminal emission or spermatorrhea

滋阴补血 [zī yīn bǔ xuè]
replenishing yin and tonifying blood: method of using yin tonics together with blood tonics for treating yin-blood deficiency

滋阴润燥 [zī yīn rùn zào]
replenishing yin to moisten dryness: method to replenish yin, clear heat and promote fluid production for treating yin deficiency with internal dryness

滋阴利水 [zī yīn lì shuǐ]
replenishing yin and inducing diuresis: using yin-replenishing medicinals combined with diuretics to treat edema complicated with yin deficiency

滋阴清热 [zī yīn qīng rè]
replenishing yin and clearing heat: method for treating yin deficiency with endogenous heat

滋阴降火 [zī yīn jiàng huǒ]
replenishing yin and reducing fire: method for treating yin deficiency with exuberant fire

滋阴凉血 [zī yīn liáng xuè]
replenishing yin and cooling the blood: combined use of yin-replenishing and blood-cooling medicinals for treating syndromes/patterns of blood heat with damage to yin or those of yin deficiency with blood heat

滋阴抑阳 [zī yīn yì yáng]
replenishing yin to suppress yang: method of supplementing yin fluid to suppress excessive yang *qi* for treating yin deficiency with exuberant yang

壮水制阳 [zhuàng shuǐ zhì yáng]
supplementing water to inhibit yang: synonymous with replenishing yin to suppress yang (滋阴抑阳[zī yīn yì yáng])

补阳 [bǔ yáng]
tonifying yang: general term for using tonics for treating yang deficiency of the heart, spleen and kidney, also called reinforcing yang (扶阳 [fú yáng]), supporting yang (助阳 [zhù yáng]), or invigorating yang (壮阳 [zhuàng yáng])

扶阳 [fú yāng]
reinforcing yang: synonymous with tonifying yang (补阳 [bǔ yáng])

助阳 [zhù yáng]
supporting yang: synonymous with tonifying yang (补阳 [bǔ yáng])

壮阳 [zhuàng yáng]
invigorating yang: synonym for tonifying yang (补阳 [bǔ yáng]), especially referring to promotion of virility in the treatment of sexual impotence

补火壮阳 [bǔ huǒ zhuàng yáng]
supplementing fire and invigorating yang: therapeutic method to supplement the fire of the life gate to invigorate yang

补肾助阳 [bǔ shèn zhù yáng]
tonifying the kidney and supporting yang: method for treating kidney yang deficiency

温补命门 [wēn bǔ mìng mén]
warming and tonifying the life gate: using warming tonics to invigorate the vital function of the kidney, used in the treatment of declining fire of the life gate manifested by aversion to cold, chronic diarrhea before dawn or sexual impotence

引火归原 [yǐn huǒ guī yuán]
conducting fire back to its origin: therapeutic method to lead ascending fire down to the kidney, used in the treatment of declining fire of the life gate with floating of asthenic yang

补肾纳气 [bǔ shèn nà qì]
tonifying the kidney to improve inspiration: method of using kidney tonics for treating dyspnea and cough due to *qi* deficiency of the lung and kidney, also called tonifying the kidney and reinforcing the lung (补肾益肺 [bǔ shèn yì fèi])

补肾益肺 [bǔ shèn yì fèi]
tonifying the kidney and reinforcing the lung: synonym for tonifying the kidney to improve inspiration (补肾纳气 [bǔ shèn nà qì])

补火生土 [bǔ huǒ shēng tǔ]
reinforcing fire to generate earth: using kidney yang-strengthening tonics to warm and tonify the spleen for treating spleen deficiency-cold syndrome/pattern

补肾健骨 [bǔ shèn jiàn gǔ]
tonifying the kidney to strengthen the bones: method of using kidney tonics for treating weakness of the bones

强筋健骨 [qiáng jīn jiàn gǔ]
strengthening the muscles and bones: method for treating weak muscles and bones in the debilitated or after injury

消法 [xiāo fǎ]
resolution; resolving method: one of the eight principal therapeutic methods of using digestants or resolvents to remove retained food and mass due to stagnation of *qi* and blood

消食 [xiāo shí]
promoting digestion: general term for the methods of using digestants for treating food stagnation

消食化滞 [xiāo shí huà zhì]
promoting digestion and resolving (food) stagnation: synonymous with promoting digestion and removing food stagnation 消食导滞 [xiāo shí dǎo zhì]

消食导滞 [xiāo shí dǎo zhì]
promoting digestion and removing (food) stagnation: method for treating

dyspepsia caused by improper diet or overeating, also abbreviated as 消导 [xiāo dǎo]

消导 [xiāo dǎo]
abbreviation for 消食导滞 [xiāo shí dǎo zhì]

消食和胃 [xiāo shí hé wèi]
promoting digestion to harmonize the stomach: method of promoting digestion to harmonize the stomach for treating food stagnation in the stomach and intestines, also called promoting digestion to harmonize the middle (energizer) (消食和中 [xiāo shí hé zhōng])

消食和中 [xiāo shí hé zhōng]
promoting digestion to harmonize the middle (energizer): synonymous with promoting digestion to harmonize the stomach (消食和胃 [xiāo shí hé wèi])

消积 [xiāo jī]
removing accumulation: therapeutic method to relieve accumulation of *qi* or undigested food

消积除胀 [xiāo jī chú zhàng]
removing accumulation and relieving distension: therapeutic method for relieving epigastric or abdominal distension caused by stagnation of *qi* or accumulation of undigested food, also known as 消食下气 [xiāo shí xià qì]

消食下气 [xiāo shí xià qì]
promoting digestion and relieving distension: synonymous with removing accumulation and relieving distension消积除胀 [xiāo jī chú zhàng]

消痞 [xiāo pǐ]
(I) eliminating mass: therapeutic method for eliminating mass in the hypochondriac region; **(II) relieving stuffiness:** method for treating stuffiness in the chest and epigastrium caused by stagnancy of phlegm and food

消胀 [xiāo zhàng]
relieving distension: method for treating abdominal distension and flatulence

消肿 [xiāo zhǒng]
relieving swelling: therapeutic method to induce detumescence or promote subsidence of swelling

消肿退红 [xiāo zhǒng tuì hóng]
relieving swelling and redness: method for treating inflammation with local swelling and redness

理气 [lǐ qì]
regulating *qi*: general term for treating disordered flow of *qi*, including stagnant flow and counterflow

行气 [xíng qì]
moving *qi*: method to relieve stagnation of *qi*, also called disinhibiting *qi* (利气 [lì qì]) or freeing *qi* (通气 [tōng qì])

利气 [lì qì]
disinhibiting *qi*: same as moving *qi* (行气 [xīng qì])

通气 [tōng qì]
freeing *qi*: same as moving *qi* (行气 [xíng qì])

理气止痛 [lǐ qì zhǐ tòng]

regulating *qi* to relieve pain: method for relieving pain attributed to *qi* stagnation

行气止痛 [xíng qì zhǐ tòng]
moving *qi* to relieve pain: synonymous with regulating *qi* to relieve pain (理气止痛 [lǐ qì zhǐ tòng])

行气宽胸 [xíng qì kuān xiōng]
moving *qi* to soothe the chest: method to promote the flow of *qi* for relieving stuffiness in the chest

行气宽中 [xíng qì kuān zhōng]
moving *qi* to soothe the middle: method to promote the flow of *qi* for alleviating stagnancy in the spleen and stomach, also known as moving *qi* to relieve stuffiness (行气消痞 [xíng qì xiāo pǐ]) or regulating *qi* to relieve stuffiness (理气消痞 [lǐ qì xiāo pǐ])

行气消痞 [xíng qì xiāo pǐ]
moving *qi* to relieve stuffiness: synonymous with moving *qi* to soothe the middle (行气宽中 [xíng qì kuān zhōng])

理气消痞 [lǐ qì xiāo pǐ]
regulating *qi* to relieve stuffiness: same as moving *qi* to relieve stuffiness (行气消痞 [xíng qì xiāo pǐ])

行气化痰 [xíng qì huà tán]
moving *qi* and resolving phlegm: combined use of *qi*-regulating and phlegm-resolving medicinals for treating syndrome/pattern of *qi* stagnation with congealing phlegm

理气化痰 [lǐ qì huà tán]
regulating *qi* and resolving phlegm: same as moving *qi* and resolving phlegm (行气化痰 [xíng qì huà tán])

降气化痰 [jiàng qì huà tán]
directing *qi* downward and resolving phlegm: combined use of *qi*-descending and phlegm-resolving medicinals for treating reversed flow of *qi* due to phlegm obstruction, also called directing *qi* downward and eliminating phlegm (下气消痰 [xià qì xiāo tán])

下气消痰 [xià qì xiāo tán]
directing *qi* downward and eliminating phlegm: same as directing *qi* downward and resolving phlegm (降气化痰 [jiàng qì huà tán])

理气健脾 [lǐ qì jiàn pí]
regulating *qi* and invigorating the spleen: therapeutic method to restore diminished transporting function of the spleen in syndromes/patterns of spleen *qi* stagnation, spleen *qi* deficiency, and spleen insufficiency with *qi* stagnation

行气活血 [xíng qì huó xuè]
moving *qi* and activating blood; moving *qi* to activate blood: therapeutic method for relieving *qi* stagnation with blood stasis, also called regulating *qi* and activating blood or regulating *qi* to activate blood (理气活血 [lǐ qì huó xuè])

理气活血 [lǐ qì huó xuè]
regulating *qi* and activating blood; regulating *qi* to activate blood: same as moving *qi* and activating blood or moving *qi* to activate blood (行气活血 [xíng qì huó xuè])

行气通络 [xíng qì tōng luò]
moving *qi* to unblock collaterals: therapeutic method for relieving obstruction of the collaterals by stagnant *qi*

顺气 [shùn qì]
arranging *qi*: therapeutic method to let *qi* flow in its normal direction and tracks, synonymous with suppressing upward perversion of *qi* (降逆下气 [jiàng nì xià qì])

宽胸 [kuān xiōng]
soothing the chest: measure for relieving chest stuffiness

宽胸散结 [kuān xiōng sàn jié]
soothing the chest and dissipating stagnation: method for treating angina pectoris with chest stuffiness

宽中散结 [kuān zhōng sàn jié]
soothing the middle and dissipating stagnation: therapeutic method for relieving stagnation in the middle energizer

降逆下气 [jiàng nì xià qì]
suppressing upward perversion of *qi* (and directing qi downward): method for treating upward perverted flow of *qi* in the lung and stomach manifested as cough, asthma, hiccupping or vomiting, also abbreviated as directing *qi* downward (降气 [jiàng qì] or 下气 [xià qì])

降气 [jiàng qì]
directing *qi* downward: synonymous with suppressing upward perversion of *qi* (降逆下气 [jiàng nì xià qì])

下气 [xià qì]
directing *qi* downward: abbreviation for suppressing upward perversion of *qi* (降逆下气 [jiàng nì xià qì])

降气平喘 [jiàng qì píng chuǎn]
directing *qi* downward to relieve dyspnea: method for treating dyspnea, also called 降逆平喘 [jiàng nì píng chuǎn]

降逆平喘 [jiàng nì píng chuǎn]
suppressing upward perversion of *qi* to relieve dyspnea: same as directing *qi* downward to relieve dyspnea (降气平喘 [jiàng qì píng chuǎn])

降逆止咳平喘 [jiàng nì zhǐ ké píng chuǎn]
suppressing upward perversion of *qi* to relieve cough and dyspnea: method for treating cough and dyspnea

降逆止呕 [jiàng nì zhǐ ǒu]
suppressing upward perversion of *qi* to stop vomiting: method to move *qi* downward and harmonize the stomach for treating vomiting

降逆止呃 [jiàng nì zhǐ è]
suppressing upward perversion of *qi* to stop hiccupping: therapeutic method for hiccupping, also called directing *qi* downward to stop hiccupping (降气止呃 [jiàng qì zhǐ è])

降气止呃 [jiàng qì zhǐ è]
directing *qi* downward to stop hiccupping: same as suppressing upward perversion of *qi* to stop hiccupping (降逆止呃 [jiàng nì zhǐ è])

调气 [tiáo qì]

adjusting *qi*: (1) regulating the flow of *qi* in the meridians; (2) adjusting the flow of *qi* in order to guarantee its smoothness, a term for promoting the natural flow of *qi* in general, and keeping it going downward in particular

破气 [pò qì]

breaking stagnant *qi*: drastic measure to relieve stagnation of *qi*

疏肝 [shū gān]

soothing the liver: method to restore the normal functioning of a depressed liver

疏肝养血 [shū gān yǎng xuè]

soothing the liver and nourishing blood: combined use of liver-soothing and blood-nourishing medicinals for treating liver depression with blood deficiency

疏肝理气 [shū gān lǐ qì]

soothing the liver and regulating *qi*: method for treating liver *qi* depression syndrome/pattern, also known as soothing the liver and relieving depression (疏肝解郁 [shū gān jiě yù])

疏肝解郁 [shū gān jiě yù]

soothing the liver and relieving depression: synonymous with soothing the liver and regulating *qi* (疏肝理气 [shū gān lǐ qì])

疏肝和胃 [shū gān hé wèi]

soothing the liver and harmonizing the stomach: method to regulate *qi* activity of the liver and stomach for treating liver-stomach *qi* stagnation and liver-stomach disharmony

疏肝理脾 [shū gān lǐ pí]

soothing the liver and regulating the spleen: method to regulate the activities of the liver and spleen to restore their normal coordination for treating liver stagnation with spleen insufficiency

疏肝和脾 [shū gān hé pí]

soothing the liver and harmonizing the spleen: synonymous with soothing the liver and regulating the spleen (疏肝理脾 [shū gān lǐ pí])

疏肝健脾 [shū gān jiàn pí]

soothing the liver and invigorating the spleen: method to regulate liver *qi* and strengthen spleen *qi* to harmonize the liver and spleen for treating depressed liver with spleen insufficiency

理气解郁 [lǐ qì jiě yù]

regulating *qi* and relieving depression: method for treating *qi* depression syndrome/pattern

理气导滞 [lǐ qì dǎo zhì]

regulating *qi* and removing stagnation: general method for treating *qi* stagnation syndrome/pattern

理气消胀 [lǐ qì xiāo zhàng]

regulating *qi* to relieve distension: method for treating abdominal distension caused by *qi* stagnation

理气化湿 [lǐ qì huà shī]

regulating *qi* and resolving dampness: using *qi*-regulating medicinals together with dampness-resolving aromatics for treating dampness retention with *qi* stagnation

理气化瘀 [lǐ qì huà yū]
regulating *qi* and resolving blood stasis: using *qi*-regulating medicinals together with stasis-resolving medicinals for treating syndrome/pattern of *qi* stagnation and blood stasis

理气止痛 [lǐ qì zhǐ tòng]
regulating *qi* to relieve pain: method for treating painful conditions due to *qi* stagnation

理气通经 [lǐ qì tōng jīng]
regulating *qi* to promote menstrual discharge: method for treating amenorrhea due to *qi* stagnation

理气安胎 [lǐ qì ān tāi]
regulating *qi* to quiet the fetus: method for preventing abortion due to *qi* stagnation

理血 [lǐ xuè]
regulating blood: collective term for various methods for treating blood disorders, including tonification of blood, removal of heat from blood, promotion of blood flow, as well as resolution of stasis and stoppage of bleeding

活血 [huó xuè]
activating blood: general term for promoting blood flow in the treatment of blood stasis

活血行气 [huó xuè xíng qì]
activating blood and moving *qi*: method for treating blood stasis with *qi* stagnation

活血化瘀 [huó xuè huà yū]
activating blood and resolving stasis: general term for various therapeutic methods with blood-activating and stasis-resolving effect indicated in the treatment of blood stasis, also known as activating blood and dispelling stasis (活血祛瘀 [huó xuè qū yū])

活血祛瘀 [huó xuè qū yū]
activating blood and dispelling stasis: synonymous with activating blood and resolving stasis (活血化瘀 [huó xuè huà yū])

活血调经 [huó xuè tiáo jīng]
activating blood to regulate menstruation: therapeutic method to activate blood and regulate *qi* for treating irregular menstruation due to disharmony of *qi* and blood

活血通经 [huó xuè tōng jīng]
activating blood to stimulate menstruation: method of using blood-activating medicinals for treating amenorrhea

活血通络 [huó xuè tōng luò]
activating blood to unblock collaterals: method of using blood-activating medicinals for treating blood stasis in collateral meridians/channels

活血止痛 [huó xuè zhǐ tòng]
activating blood to relieve pain: method for treating painful conditions caused by blood stasis

祛瘀活血 [qū yū huó xuè]
dispelling stasis to activate blood: method to eliminate stasis to promote blood flow

祛瘀消肿 [qū yū xiāo zhǒng]
dispelling stasis to reduce swelling: method for treating hematoma and the like

祛瘀通络 [qū yū tōng luò]

dispelling stasis to unblock collaterals: method for treating obstruction of the collateral meridians/channels due to stagnant blood

祛瘀生新 [qū yū shēng xīn]

dispelling stasis to promote regeneration: method to activate blood and remove stasis to promote blood regeneration for treating blood stasis complicated with blood deficiency

破血祛瘀 [pò xuè qū yū]

breaking and dispelling blood stasis: method of using drastic medicinals for treating blood stasis, also known as breaking and expelling blood stasis (破血逐瘀 [pò xuè zhú yū]), and abbreviated as breaking blood stasis (破血 [pò xuè] or 破瘀 [pò yū])

破血逐瘀 [pò xuè zhú yū]

breaking and expelling blood stasis: synonymous with breaking and dispelling blood stasis (破血祛瘀 [pò xuè qū yū])

破血 [pò xuè]

breaking blood stasis: abbreviation for breaking and dispelling blood stasis (破血祛瘀 [pò xuè qū yū])

破瘀 [pò yū]

breaking blood stasis: abbreviation for breaking and dispelling blood stasis (破血祛瘀 [pò xuè qū yū])

破瘀消癥 [pò yū xiāo zhēng]

breaking blood stasis and eliminating masses: method of using blood-activating and stasis-removing medicinals to eliminate stagnant blood and masses in the abdomen

破瘀生新 [pò yū shēng xīn]

breaking blood stasis and promoting regeneration: method of using drastic stasis-removing medicinals to eliminate stagnant blood and promote tissue regeneration

舒筋通络 [shū jīn tōng luò]

relaxing tendons and unblocking collaterals: method for treating blockage of meridian/channel *qi* with muscle contraction, also known as relaxing tendons and activating collaterals (舒筋活络 [shū jīn huó luò]) or relaxing tendons and harmonizing collaterals (舒筋和络 [shū jīn hé luò])

舒筋活络 [shū jīn huó luò]

relaxing tendons and activating collaterals: synonymous with relaxing tendons and unblocking collaterals (舒筋通络 [shū jīn tōng luò])

舒筋和络 [shū jīn hé luò]

relaxing tendons and harmonizing collaterals: synonymous with relaxing tendons and unblocking collaterals (舒筋通络 [shū jīn tōng luò])

舒筋止痛 [shū jīn zhǐ tòng]

relaxing tendons to relieve pain: method for treating painful conditions caused by muscle contraction

止血 [zhǐ xuè]

stopping bleeding; hemostasis: general term for stopping the escape of blood from vessels

清热止血 [qīng rè zhǐ xuè]
clearing heat to stop bleeding: method of using heat-clearing hemostatics for treating bleeding due to exuberant heat

凉血止血 [liáng xuè zhǐ xuè]
cooling the blood to stop bleeding: method of using blood-cooling hemostatics for treating bleeding due to heat in the blood

补气摄血 [bǔ qì shè xuè]
replenishing *qi* to arrest bleeding: method of using *qi* tonics for treating chronic hemorrhage due to *qi* deficiency, also known as replenishing *qi* to stop bleeding (补气止血 [bǔ qì zhǐ xuè])

补气止血 [bǔ qì zhǐ xuè]
replenishing *qi* to stop bleeding: same as replenishing *qi* to arrest bleeding (补气摄血 [bǔ qì shè xuè])

祛瘀止血 [qū yū zhǐ xuè]
dispelling stasis to stop bleeding: method for treating bleeding related to blood stasis

祛痰 [qū tán]
dispelling phlegm: general term for therapeutic methods for treating phlegm syndromes/patterns

化痰 [huà tán]
resolving phlegm: one of the therapeutic methods to dispel phlegm whereby phlegm is disintegrated and dissolved

温化寒痰 [wēn huà hán tán]
warming and resolving cold-phlegm: method to warm yang, dispel cold and resolve phlegm for treating cold-phlegm syndrome/pattern

清化热痰 [qīng huà rè tán]
clearing and resolving heat-phlegm: method to clear heat and resolve phlegm for treating heat-phlegm syndrome/pattern

清热化痰 [qīng rè huà tán]
clearing heat and resolving phlegm: method of combined use of heat-clearing and phlegm-dispelling medicinals for treating heat-phlegm syndrome/pattern

润肺化痰 [rùn fèi huà tán]
moistening the lung and resolving phlegm: method for treating dryness-phlegm affection in the lung, also known as moistening dryness and resolving phlegm (润燥化痰[rùn zào huà tán])

润燥化痰 [rùn zào huà tán]
moistening dryness and resolving phlegm: synonymous with moistening the lung and resolving phlegm (润肺化痰 [rùn fèi huà tán]), also known as moistening and resolving dryness-phlegm (润化燥痰 [rùn huà zào tán])

润化燥痰 [rùn huà zào tán]
moistening and resolving dryness-phlegm: same as moistening dryness and resolving phlegm (润燥化痰 [rùn zào huà tán])

燥湿化痰 [zào shī huà tán]
drying dampness and resolving phlegm: method for treating dampness-phlegm syndromes/patterns

祛寒化痰 [qū hán huà tán]
dispelling cold and resolving phlegm:

method of combined use of cold-dispersing and phlegm-dispelling medicinals for treating cold-phlegm syndrome/pattern

治风化痰 [zhì fēng huà tán]
treating wind and resolving phlegm: method of combined use of wind-dispelling and phlegm-resolving medicinals for treating wind-phlegm syndrome/pattern

熄 [息] 风化痰 [xī fēng huà tán]
extinguishing wind and resolving phlegm: method of combined use of wind-extinguishing and phlegm-resolving medicinals for treating wind-phlegm syndrome/pattern

涤痰 [dí tán]
flushing phlegm away: method of using drastic expectorants to expel phlegm for treating stubborn phlegm syndromes/patterns

豁痰 [huò tán]
eliminating phlegm: method to eliminate phlegm for resuscitation used in the treatment of impaired consciousness, e.g., loss of consciousness in cases of apoplexy

化饮 [huà yǐn]
resolving retained fluid: general term for methods to dispel retained fluid

散寒化饮 [sàn hán huà yǐn]
dissipating cold and resolving retained fluid: method of using pungent-warm medicinals for treating syndrome/pattern of interior retention of cold-fluid

化饮宁心 [huà yǐn níng xīn]
resolving retained fluid to calm the heart: method for treating syndrome/pattern of retained fluid in the pericardium marked by palpitations and orthopnea with fullness and stuffy sensation in the heart and chest

化饮宽胸 [huà yǐn kuān xiōng]
resolving retained fluid to soothe the chest: method for treating syndrome/pattern of retained fluid in the chest marked by fullness and stuffy sensation in the chest, cough and dyspnea

祛湿 [qū shī]
dispelling dampness: general term for various methods for treating dampness syndromes/patterns, including resolving dampness by using aromatics, drying dampness by using medicinals bitter in taste and cold in nature, and draining dampness through diuresis

化湿 [huà shī]
resolving dampness: one of the therapeutic methods to dispel dampness, especially that lodging in the upper energizer or exterior portion of the body, by using aromatics

芳香化湿 [fāng xiāng huà shī]
resolving dampness with aromatics: method of using aromatics for treating dampness syndromes/patterns

芳香化浊 [fāng xiāng huà zhuó]
resolving turbidity with aromatics: method of using aromatics for treating dampness-turbidity syndromes/patterns

清热化湿 [qīng rè huà shī]
clearing heat and resolving dampness:

method of using heat-clearing and dampness-resolving medicinals for treating dampness-heat in the upper or middle portions of the body

燥湿 [zào shī]
drying dampness: one of the therapeutic methods to dispel dampness, especially that lodging in the middle energizer (spleen and stomach) by using medicinals bitter in taste

苦温燥湿 [kǔ wēn zào shī]
drying dampness with bitter-warmth: method of using medicinals bitter in taste and warm in nature for treating cold-dampness syndrome/pattern

苦寒燥湿 [kǔ hán zào shī]
drying dampness with bitter-cold: method of using medicinals bitter in taste and cold in nature for treating dampness-heat syndrome/pattern

燥湿健脾 [zào shī jiàn pí]
drying dampness to invigorate the spleen: therapeutic method of using pungent drying medicinals to eliminate dampness for the purpose of invigorating the spleen, indicated in the treatment of dampness disturbing the spleen

利湿 [lì shī]
draining dampness: method of using diuretics to dispel dampness, especially that lodging in the lower energizer

利尿 [lì niào]
inducing diuresis: method to increase urine excretion, also known as 利水 [lì shuǐ]

利水 [lì shuǐ]
inducing diuresis: same as 利尿 [lì niào]

清热利湿 [qīng rè lì shī]
clearing heat and draining dampness: combined use of heat-clearing medicinals and diuretics to clear heat and remove dampness through diuresis for treating accumulation of dampness-heat in the lower portion of the body

淡渗利湿 [dàn shèn lì shī]
draining dampness with bland diuretics: one of the common methods for treating diarrhea with watery stools, and edema with oliguria, also known as dispelling dampness with bland diuretics (淡渗祛湿 [dàn shèn qū shī]), and abbreviated as draining dampness (渗湿 [shèn shī])

淡渗祛湿 [dàn shèn qū shī]
dispelling dampness with bland diuretics: synonymous with draining dampness with bland diuretics (淡渗利湿 [dàn shèn lì shī])

渗湿 [shèn shī]
draining dampness: abbreviation for draining dampness with bland diuretics (淡渗利湿 [dàn shèn lì shī])

利水渗湿 [lì shuǐ shèn shī]
inducing diuresis to drain dampness: therapeutic method of using diuretics to get rid of dampness, also called inducing diuresis to expel dampness (利水除湿 [lì shuǐ chú shī])

利水除湿 [lì shuǐ chú shī]
inducing diuresis to expel dampness: synonymous with inducing diuresis to

drain dampness (利水渗湿 [lì shuǐ shèn shī])

利水消肿 [lì shuǐ xiāo zhǒng]
inducing diuresis to alleviate edema: method of using diuretics for treating edema

温阳利湿 [wēn yáng lì shī]
warming yang to drain dampness: combined use of warming medicinals and diuretics to remove dampness, usually used in the treatment of cold-dampness syndrome/pattern

温阳利水 [wēn yáng lì shuǐ]
warming yang to induce diuresis: method of combined use of yang-invigorating medicinals and diuretics for treating water retention due to yang deficiency of the spleen and kidney, also known as warming yang to promote urination (温阳行水 [wēn yáng xíng shuǐ])

温阳行水 [wēn yáng xíng shuǐ]
warming yang to promote urination: same as warming yang to induce diuresis (温阳利水 [wēn yáng lì shuǐ])

温肾利水 [wēn shèn lì shuǐ]
warming the kidney to induce diuresis: method for treating edema due to kidney yang deficiency

利小便，实大便 [lì xiǎo biàn, shí dà biàn]
treating diarrhea with diuretics: method of using spleen tonics to promote diuresis for treating diarrhea

洁净府 [jié jìng fǔ]
"cleaning the bladder": an ancient term for the treatment of edema by inducing diuresis

固涩 [gù sè]
astringency; arresting discharge: therapeutic method of using styptic or astringent agents for treating spontaneous sweating, seminal emission, chronic diarrhea, or hemorrhage, also called 收涩 [shōu sè]

收涩 [shōu sè]
arresting discharge: same as astringency (固涩 [gù sè])

敛汗 [liǎn hàn]
arresting sweating: method for treating excessive or abnormal sweating, also known as checking sweating (止汗 [zhǐ hàn])

止汗 [zhǐ hàn]
checking sweating: same as arresting sweating (敛汗 [liǎn hàn])

敛汗固表 [liǎn hàn gù biǎo]
arresting sweating and consolidating the superficies: method for treating defense *qi* deficiency with spontaneous sweating, also called consolidating the superficies and checking sweating (固表止汗 [gù biǎo zhǐ hàn])

固表止汗 [gù biǎo zhǐ hàn]
consolidating the superficies and checking sweating: synonymous with arresting sweating and consolidating the superficies (敛汗固表 [liǎn hàn gù biǎo])

敛汗固脱 [liǎn hàn gù tuō]
arresting sweating to prevent collapse:

method to strengthen the superficies and arrest sweating used in the treatment of incessant profuse sweating with impending collapse

敛肺 [liǎn fèi]
astringing the lung: method of using astringents and tonics for treating deficiency syndromes/patterns of the lung with chronic persistent cough

敛肺止咳 [liǎn fèi zhǐ ké]
astringing the lung to stop coughing: method of using astringents for treating persistent unproductive cough due to lung insufficiency

敛肺平喘 [liǎn fèi píng chuǎn]
astringing the lung to relieve dyspnea: method of using astringents for treating dyspnea due to lung insufficiency

敛气 [liǎn qì]
astringing *qi*: method of using astringents for treating consumption of *qi*

敛阴 [liǎn yīn]
astringing yin: method of using astringents to replenish and preserve yin fluid for treating consumption of yin

固精 [gù jīng]
arresting emission: abbreviation for strengthening the kidney to arrest emission (固肾涩精 [gù shèn sè jīng]), also known as checking emission (涩精 [sè jīng])

涩精 [sè jīng]
checking emission: same as arresting emission (固精 [gù jīng])

固肾 [gù shèn]
strengthening the kidney: therapeutic method for treating insecurity of kidney *qi*

固肾涩精 [gù shèn sè jīng]
strengthening the kidney to arrest emission: method of using kidney tonics in combination with astringents for treating seminal emission due to insecurity of kidney *qi*

固肾缩尿 [gù shèn suō niào]
strengthening the kidney to reduce urination: method for treating frequent urination or enuresis due to kidney *qi* insufficiency

固经止血 [gù jīng zhǐ xuè]
astringing menstruation and stopping bleeding: method for treating excessive menstrual discharge

固崩止血 [gù bēng zhǐ xuè]
arresting blood flooding: method for treating profuse uterine bleeding

固冲止血 [gù chōng zhǐ xuè]
astringing the thoroughfare vessel to stop bleeding: method to astringe the thoroughfare and conception vessels for treating abnormal uterine bleeding or excessive menstrual flow

固肾止带 [gù shèn zhǐ dài]
strengthening the kidney to check leukorrhagia: method for treating excessive leukorrhea due to kidney insufficiency

涩精止遗 [sè jīng zhǐ yí]
astringing semen and checking emission: method of using astringents for treating

seminal emission or spermatorrhea

固崩止带 [gù bēng zhǐ dài]
arresting metrorrhagia and leukorrhagia: astringing method for treating abnormal uterine bleeding or excessive leukorrhea

涩肠止泻 [sè cháng zhǐ xiè]
astringing the intestines to check diarrhea: method of using astringents for treating chronic diarrhea

涩肠止痢 [sè cháng zhǐ lì]
astringing the intestines to check dysentery: method of using astringents for treating chronic dysentery

固冲止带 [gù chōng zhǐ dài]
strengthening the thoroughfare vessel and stopping leukorrhagia: method for treating leukorrhagia due to kidney insufficiency with insecurity of the thoroughfare and conception vessels

润燥 [rùn zào]
moistening (dryness): general term for measures to relieve dryness

甘寒润燥 [gān hán rùn zào]
moistening (dryness) with sweet-cold: method of using sweet-tasting and cold-natured medicinals for treating deficiency of fluid in the lung and kidney

养阴润燥 [yǎng yīn rùn zào]
nourishing yin to moisten dryness: method for treating yin deficiency with endogenous dryness

养血润燥 [yǎng xuè rùn zào]
nourishing blood to moisten dryness: method for treating blood deficiency with endogenous dryness

养血润肠 [yǎng xuè rùn cháng]
nourishing blood to moisten the intestines: method for treating constipation due to blood deficiency with dryness of the intestines

润肠通便 [rùn cháng tōng biàn]
moistening the intestines to relieve constipation: method of combined use of moistening medicinals and laxatives for relieving constipation due to intestinal dryness

润肺 [rùn fèi]
moistening the lung: therapeutic method of using medicines with moistening action for relieving dryness syndrome/pattern of the lung

养阴润肺 [yǎng yīn rùn fèi]
nourishing yin to moisten the lung: method for treating dryness syndrome/pattern of the lung due to yin deficiency

清燥润肺 [qīng zào rùn fèi]
clearing dryness to moisten the lung: method for treating dryness-heat damaging the lung or lung yin deficiency with heat syndrome/pattern, also called clearing the lung and moistening dryness (清肺润燥 [qīng fèi rùn zào])

清肺润燥 [qīng fèi rùn zào]
clearing the lung and moistening dryness: same as clearing dryness to moisten the lung (清燥润肺 [qīng zào rùn fèi])

润肺生津 [rùn fèi shēng jīn]
moistening the lung and engendering fluid: method for treating lung yin deficiency with dryness

润肺止咳 [rùn fèi zhǐ ké]
moistening the lung to relieve cough: method for treating cough due to lung yin deficiency with dryness

止咳化痰 [zhǐ ké huà tán]
relieving cough and resolving phlegm: method for symptomatic relief of cough with expectoration

生津 [shēng jīn]
engendering fluid: general term for therapeutic methods to replenish body fluid

甘寒生津 [gān hán shēng jīn]
engendering fluid with sweet-cold: method of using medicinals sweet in taste and cold in nature to replenish body fluid

益气生津 [yì qì shēng jīn]
replenishing *qi* and engendering fluid: method of using tonics for treating a prostrated state with deficiency of *qi* and fluid after profuse sweating

安神 [ān shén]
calming the mind: general term for tranquilizing measures

安神定志 [ān shén dìng zhì]
calming and stabilizing the mind: method for treating palpitations and insomnia due to heart insufficiency

益气安神 [yì qì ān shén]
replenishing *qi* to calm the mind: method for treating palpitations, insomnia and forgetfulness due to heart *qi* deficiency

益肾宁神 [yì shèn níng shén]
replenishing the kidney to calm the mind: method for treating palpitations and insomnia caused by frightening or disharmony between the heart and kidney, also known as tonifying the kidney to calm the mind (补肾安神 [bǔ shèn ān shén])

补肾安神 [bǔ shèn ān shén]
tonifying the kidney to calm the mind: same as replenishing the kidney to calm the mind (益肾宁神 [yì shèn níng shén])

养心安神 [yǎng xīn ān shén]
nourishing the heart to calm the mind: method of using heart-blood tonics and tranquilizing medicinals for treating palpitations, insomnia, dream-disturbed sleep and forgetfulness due to heart insufficiency

镇惊安神 [zhèn jīng ān shén]
settling fright and calming the mind: therapeutic method involving the use of settling tranquilizers to relieve mental uneasiness caused by fright, abbreviated as settling fright (镇惊 [zhèn jīng]), also known as settling the heart and calming the mind (镇心安神 [zhèn xīn ān shén])

镇心安神 [zhèn xīn ān shén]
settling the heart and calming the mind: same as settling fright and calming the mind (镇惊安神 [zhèn jīng ān shén])

镇惊 [zhèn jīng]
settling fright: abbreviation for settling

fright and calming the mind (镇惊安神 [zhèn jīng ān shén])

重镇安神 [zhòng zhèn ān shén]
calming the mind with heavy settling (medicinals): method for treating insomnia and excitement due to exuberant heart yang, also known as inducing sedation and calming the mind (镇静安神 [zhèn jìng ān shén])

镇静安神 [zhèn jìng ān shén]
inducing sedation and calming the mind: synonymous with 重镇安神[zhòng zhèn ān shén]

潜阳 [qián yáng]
subduing yang: method of using weighty agents to suppress exuberant yang for treating adverse upsurge of liver yang due to deficiency of yin

潜阳熄风 [qián yáng xī fēng]
subduing yang and extinguishing wind: method for treating transformation of liver yang into wind

滋阴潜阳 [zī yīn qián yáng]
nourishing yin and subduing yang: method of combined use of yang-suppressing and yin-nourishing medicinals for treating exuberance of liver yang due to yin deficiency

柔肝 [róu gān]
emolliating the liver: method for treating liver yin deficiency or liver blood insufficiency, also called nourishing the liver (养肝 [yǎng gān])

养肝 [yǎng gān]
nourishing the liver: therapeutic method for nourishing liver yin or blood, synonymous with emolliating the liver (柔肝 [róu gān])

养血柔肝 [yǎng xuè róu gān]
nourishing blood and emolliating the liver: therapeutic method for nourishing liver blood

平肝 [píng gān]
pacifying the liver: general term for methods for treating hyperactivity of the liver

平肝潜阳 [píng gān qián yáng]
pacifying the liver and subduing yang: method of using weighty agents such as shells, metals or minerals for treating hyperactivity of the liver, also called settling the liver and subduing yang (镇肝潜阳 [zhèn gān qián yáng])

镇肝潜阳 [zhèn gān qián yáng]
settling the liver and subduing yang: synonymous with pacifying the liver and subduing yang (平肝潜阳 [píng gān qián yáng]), abbreviated as settling and subduing (镇潜 [zhèn qián])

镇潜 [zhèn qián]
settling and subduing: abbreviation for settling the liver and subduing yang (镇肝潜阳 [zhèn gān qián yáng])

熄 [息] 风 [xī fēng]
extinguishing wind: method of using sedatives to relieve endogenous wind syndrome/pattern, indicated in the treatment of vertigo, tremor, convulsions, epilepsy, etc.

熄[息]风解痉 [xī fēng jiě jìng]
extinguishing wind to relieve convulsions: method for relieving involuntary muscle contractions in syndrome/pattern of internal stirring of liver wind, also called extinguishing wind to arrest convulsions (息风定痉 [xī fēng dìng jìng])

熄[息]风定痉 [xī fēng dìng jìng]
extinguishing wind to arrest convulsions: synonymous with extinguishing wind to relieve convulsions (息风解痉 [xī fēng jiě jìng])

熄[息]风定痫 [xī fēng dìng xián]
extinguishing wind to arrest epilepsy: method for treating epilepsy caused by wind-phlegm

滋阴熄[息]风 [zī yīn xī fēng]
nourishing yin to extinguish wind: method for treating endogenous wind due to serious impairment of yin fluid at the late stage of a febrile disease

平肝熄[息]风 [píng gān xī fēng]
pacifying the liver to extinguish wind: method for treating endogenous wind caused by hyperactivity of the liver, also called settling the liver to extinguish wind (镇肝熄风 [zhèn gān xī fēng])

镇肝熄[息]风 [zhèn gān xī fēng]
settling the liver to extinguish wind: same as pacifying the liver to extinguish wind (平肝熄风 [píng gān xī fēng])

凉肝熄[息]风 [liáng gān xī fēng]
cooling the liver to extinguish wind: method to clear and purge the liver of fire to extinguish liver wind

清热熄[息]风 [qīng rè xī fēng]
clearing heat to extinguish wind: method for treating convulsions due to high fever

养血熄[息]风 [yǎng xuè xī fēng]
nourishing blood to extinguish wind: method for treating endogenous wind caused by blood deficiency, with such symptoms as dizziness and involuntary movement of the limbs

开窍 [kāi qiào]
opening the orifices; inducing resuscitation: therapeutic method of bringing an unconscious person back to consciousness, also called arousing from unconsciousness (醒神 [xǐng shén]) and arousing the brain (醒脑 [xǐng nǎo])

醒神 [xǐng shén]
arousing from unconsciousness: synonymous with opening the orifices or inducing resuscitation (开窍 [kāi qiào])

醒脑 [xǐng nǎo]
arousing the brain: synonymous with opening the orifices or inducing resuscitation (开窍 [kāi qiào])

芳香开窍 [fāng xiāng kāi qiào]
inducing resuscitation with aromatics: emergency treatment for loss of consciousness in cases of apoplexy, epilepsy or high fever, involving administering aromatic medicinals

清热开窍 [qīng rè kāi qiào]
clearing heat to induce resuscitation: method for treating impaired consciousness in cases of acute febrile diseases

化痰开窍 [huà tán kāi qiào]
resolving phlegm to induce resuscitation: method of using phlegm-resolving medicinals for treating phlegm syncope and phlegm misting the heart orifices

清热化痰开窍 [qīng rè huà tán kāi qiào]
clearing heat and resolving phlegm to induce resuscitation: method of using heat-clearing and phlegm-resolving medicinals for relieving convulsions and coma due to high fever

豁痰开窍 [huò tán kāi qiào]
eliminating phlegm to induce resuscitation: method for treating impairment of consciousness in cases of apoplexy or psychosis

豁痰醒脑 [huò tán xǐng nǎo]
eliminating phlegm to arouse the brain: method to eliminate phlegm for resuscitation used in the treatment of loss of consciousness

吐法 [tù fǎ]
emetic method; emesis: one of the eight principal therapeutic methods used to expel noxious substances (such as retained phlegm, undigested food or toxic substances) by using emetics or mechanical stimulation to induce vomiting

探吐 [tàn tù]
mechanical induction of vomiting: method of inducing vomiting with mechanical stimulation of the soft palate or throat

涌吐禁例 [yǒng tù jìn lì]
contraindications for emesis: conditions that make emetic therapy inadvisable, e.g., insufficiency of the spleen and stomach, hemorrhagic diseases, old age, and debility

止痛 [zhǐ tòng]
relieving pain: any therapeutic measure that relieves pain

止痒 [zhǐ yǎng]
relieving itching: any therapeutic measure that has an antipruritic effect

燥湿止痒 [zào shī zhǐ yǎng]
drying dampness and relieving itching: therapeutic method to remove exudate and alleviate itching as used in the treatment of eczema

润燥止痒 [rùn zào zhǐ yǎng]
moistening dryness to relieve itching: therapeutic method to tonify blood, nourish yin, dispel wind and moisten dryness for relieving itching in cases of blood deficiency with wind-dryness

止呕 [zhǐ ǒu]
arresting vomiting: any therapeutic measure that has an anti-emetic effect

止呃 [zhǐ è]
stopping hiccups: any therapeutic measure that can give relief in cases of hiccups

止渴 [zhǐ kě]
quenching thirst: any therapeutic measure that has an antidiptic effect

止晕 [zhǐ yūn]
relieving fainting: any therapeutic measure that can give relief in cases of dizziness, vertigo, and even fainting

止痉 [zhǐ jìng]
relieving spasm; arresting convulsion: any therapeutic measure that relieves spasms or arrests convulsions

止遗尿 [zhǐ yí niào]
arresting enuresis: method for checking involuntary discharge of urine

安胎 [ān tāi]
preventing miscarriage: preventive and therapeutic measure for threatened miscarriage and habitual abortion

催生 [cuī shēng]
expediting child delivery: method of speeding up child delivery by strengthening the parturient's *qi*

催乳 [cuī rǔ]
stimulating lactation: method of starting or promoting the secretion to yield mammary milk

通乳 [tōng rǔ]
freeing milk flow: method for treating galactostasis

下乳 [xià rǔ]
promoting lactation: method for treating lack of lactation

回乳 [huí rǔ]
terminating lactation: method of bringing lactation to a halt, also called 断乳 [duàn rǔ]

断乳 [duàn rǔ]
(I) terminating lactation: same as 回乳 [huí rǔ]; **(II) weaning:** stopping feeding a baby with its mother's milk and starting feeding it with ordinary food

通经 [tōng jīng]
(I) stimulating menstrual discharge: any method that can stimulate menstruation, used in the treatment of amenorrhea; **(II) unblocking the meridian/channel:** removing obstruction in the meridian/channel

通经活络 [tōng jīng huó luò]
unblocking meridians/channels and activating collaterals: therapeutic method of removing obstruction in the meridians/channels and collaterals

通利血脉 [tōng lì xuè mài]
unblocking and promoting blood flow: therapeutic method of improving blood flow in the vessels

通络止痛 [tōng luò zhǐ tòng]
unblocking collaterals to relieve pain: method for treating painful condition caused by blockage of collateral meridians/channels

通经止痛 [tōng jīng zhǐ tòng]
unblocking meridians/channels to relieve pain: method for treating painful condition caused by blockage of meridian/channel *qi*

调经 [tiáo jīng]
regulating menstruation: general term referring to methods for treating irregular menstruation

通淋 [tōng lín]
relieving stranguria: any therapeutic method for treating stranguria

通利关节 [tōng lì guān jié]
easing joint movement: therapeutic method for relieving arthralgia and improving joint movement

退黄 [tuì huáng]
eliminating jaundice: therapeutic method for treating jaundice

内消 [nèi xiāo]
elimination from within: therapeutic method for curing a sore before it undergoes suppuration, usually by way of oral administration of antiphlogistics

内托 [nèi tuō]
expulsion from within: therapeutic method of supporting healthy *qi* and promoting pus discharge for preventing inward penetration of the pathogenic toxin, usually by way of oral administation of tonics, also called expulsion method (托法 [tuō fǎ])

托法 [tuō fǎ]
expulsion method: synonymous with expulsion from within (内托 [nèi tuō])

托毒 [tuō dú]
expelling toxins: method of expelling toxins from within in the treatment of boils and sores

托疮 [tuō chuāng]
expelling pus from sores: method of expelling pus in the treatment of boils, sores and abscesses

排脓 [pái nóng]
evacuating pus: method of promoting pus discharge

清热排脓 [qīng rè pái nóng]
clearing heat and evacuating pus: therapeutic method of removing heat toxin and draining pus from an abscess

排脓消肿 [pái nóng xiāo zhǒng]
evacuating pus and eliminating swelling: method for treating abscesses in external diseases

排脓托毒 [pái nóng tuō dú]
evacuating pus and expelling toxins: therapeutic method of evacuating pus and expelling toxins from the body

托里排脓 [tuō lǐ pái nóng]
evacuating pus from within: method of expelling toxins from within to evacuate pus, usually by way of oral administration of tonics

拔毒 [bá dú]
drawing out toxins: therapeutic method of removing toxins from inflammatory lesions

提脓拔毒 [tí nóng bá dú]
drawing out pus and toxins: method used in the treatment of suppurative external diseases

化腐 [huà fǔ]
resolving putridity: method of using corrosive medicinals for treating external diseases, especially wounds and sores

去腐肉 [qù fǔ ròu]
removing necrotic tissue: synonymous with resolving putridity (化腐 [huà fǔ])

提脓去腐 [tí nóng qù fǔ]
drawing out pus and removing putridity:

therapeutic method of promoting pus discharge and removing putridity in the treatment of embedded sores

蚀疮去腐 [shí chuāng qù fǔ]
corroding wounds and removing putridity: therapeutic method of eliminating putrid material in the treatment of wounds and sores

生肌 [shēng jī]
(I) promoting tissue regeneration: promoting the renewal, regrowth or restoration of the tissue after injury; **(II) promoting granulation:** promoting the process of granule formation (as of a wound)

生肌敛疮 [shēng jī liǎn chuāng]
promoting tissue regeneration and wound healing: therapeutic method of promoting the healing of wounds or ulcers on the body surface

生肌收口 [shēng jī shōu kǒu]
promoting tissue regeneration and closing the wound: therapeutic method of promoting the growth of new tissues for treating wounds, usually by using medicinals

煨脓长肉 [wēi nóng zhǎng ròu]
promoting suppuration to regenerate flesh: method of using pus-discharging medicinals to promote the growth of granulation tissue and healing of a wound

溃坚 [kuì jiān]
promoting rupture: method for treating an abscess by using suppurants

攻溃 [gōng kuì]
promoting suppuration: method for treating ulcers and boils, usually by using suppurants

攻毒 [gōng dú]
counteracting toxins: removal of toxic properties from a poison

以毒攻毒 [yǐ dú gōng dú]
combatting poison with poison: any therapeutic measure to treat malignant or poisoning diseases with poisonous medicinals or medicinals with high toxicity, e.g., chaulmoogra for treating leprosy, gamboge for treating a carbuncle

解毒 [jiě dú]
removing toxins; detoxication: (1) measure to lessen the virulence of pathogenic organism, as in the treatment of pyogenic inflammation; (2) method of neutralizing the toxic property of poisons, e.g., venom

解酒毒 [jiě jiǔ dú]
removing alcoholic toxins: therapeutic method of relieving alcoholism

解毒消肿 [jiě dú xiāo zhǒng]
removing toxins and promoting subsidence of swelling: therapeutic method for treating abscesses and sores

消痈散结 [xiāo yōng sàn jié]
dispersing abscesses and nodules: therapeutic method of dissolving abscesses and nodules before suppuration

消痈散疖 [xiāo yōng sàn jiē]
dispersing abscesses and boils: therapeutic method of dissolving abscesses and boils before suppuration

消肿止痛 [xiāo zhǒng zhǐ tòng]
dispersing swelling to relieve pain: therapeutic method of dispersing inflammatory swelling for relieving pain

止血行瘀 [zhǐ xuè xíng yū]
arresting bleeding and removing ecchymosis: method for treating traumatic injuries with bleeding and ecchymosis

止血敛疮 [zhǐ xuè liǎn chuāng]
arresting bleeding and closing sores: method for treating open sores with bleeding

止血收口 [zhǐ xuè shōu kǒu]
arresting bleeding and closing cut: method for treating incisions

通鼻 [tōng bí]
relieving stuffy nose: any therapeutic method that relieves nasal obstruction

通鼻窍 [tōng bí qiào]
relieving stuffy nose: same as 通鼻 [tōng bí]

利咽 [lì yān]
relieving sore throat: any therapeutic method that relieves a sore throat

消骨鲠 [xiāo gǔ gěng]
dissolving fish bone: method for treating fishbone stuck in the throat or esophagus

摄唾 [shè tuò]
constraining spittle: therapeutic method of checking excessive salivation

乌须发 [wū xū fà]
blackening the hair and beard: method for treating premature graying of the hair and beard

明目 [míng mù]
improving the eyesight: any therapeutic method that can ameliorate impaired vision

退翳明目 [tuì yì míng mù]
removing nebula to improve vision: method for treating nebula, also known as removing nebula (退目翳 [tuì mù yì])

退目翳 [tuì mù yì]
removing nebula: synonymous with removing nebula to improve vision (退翳明目 [tuì yì míng mù])

聪耳 [cōng ěr]
improving the hearing; improving auditory acuity: method for treating impaired hearing

截疟 [jié nüè]
interrupting malaria: method for preventing attack of malaria

安蛔 [ān huí]
quieting ascaris: method used in the treatment of ascariasis, usually for relieving abdominal pain or biliary colic caused by ascaris

安蛔定痛 [ān huí dìng tòng]
quieting ascaris to relieve pain: method for treating abdominal pain due to intestinal or biliary ascariasis

驱虫 [qū chóng]
expelling worms: method for treating intestinal parasites

驱虫消积 [qū chóng xiāo jī]
expelling intestinal worms and dissipating

accumulation: therapeutic method for dissipating the accumulation of intestinal parasites, especially ascarides, usually by oral administration of anthelmintic agents

杀虫 [shā chóng]
killing worms: method for destroying intestinal parasites

化石 [huà shí]
dissolving calculi: therapeutic method for treating biliary or urinary calculi by way of dissolution

排石 [pái shí]
expelling calculi: method for treating biliary or urinary calculi by way of expulsion of the calculi from the biliary duct or urinary tract

外治 [wài zhì]
external treatment: treatment applied on the body surface or given from outside, also called external therapy (外治法 [wài zhì fǎ])

外治法 [wài zhì fǎ]
external therapy: same as external treatment (外治 [wài zhì])

外敷 [wài fū]
external application: putting or spreading medicine on the skin, abbreviated as 敷 [fū]

敷 [fū]
abbreviation for 外敷 [wài fū]

罨 [yǎn]
compression: therapeutic measure involving local application of a folded towel or piece of cloth soaked in hot or cold water or medicated solution

冷罨 [lěng yǎn]
cold compression: therapeutic measure involving local application of a folded towel or piece of cloth soaked in cold water

热罨 [rè yǎn]
hot compression: therapeutic measure involving local application of a folded towel or piece of cloth soaked in hot water

熨法 [yùn fǎ]
hot compression with rubbing: therapeutic measure involving pressing and rubbing the diseased area with hot medical substances wrapped in cloth

熏蒸 [xūn zhēng]
fuming and steaming: therapy involving fumes from a burning roll of medicated paper or vapor from boiling medicinal ingredients

吸入 [xī rù]
inhalation: treatment of a disease by inhaling fumes or vapor

热烘 [rè hōng]
warming over fire: therapeutic method involving heating the diseased area after applying medical ointment, indicated in the treatment of skin diseases with dryness and itching, such as tinea manuum, chronic eczema and neurodermatitis

烙法 [lào fǎ]
cauterization: application of a searing iron to destroy diseased tissue

溻浴 [tā yù]
medicated immersion: therapeutic method involving immersing a certain part of or the whole body in a medicated solution

膏摩 [gāo mó]
rubbing with ointment: method for treating arthralgia or skin diseases whereby ointment is applied and rubbed into the skin

发泡 [fā pào]
vesiculation: skin stimulation with medicinals to cause blister formation as a therapeutic method

点眼 [diǎn yǎn]
eye dropping: dropping medicated solution into the conjunctival sac

搐鼻 [chù bí]
insufflating into the nose: inhaling powdered medicine into the nostrils

含漱 [hán shù]
gargling: method of treatment involving holding a liquid in the mouth and throat and agitating it with a stream of air from the lung, also called washing by gargling 漱涤 [shù dí]

漱涤 [shù dí]
washing by gargling: same as gargling (含漱 [hán shù])

吹药 [chuī yào]
insufflation into the throat: blowing powdered medicine into the throat or inner part of the mouth for therapeutic purposes

扑粉 [pū fěn]
application of medicinal powder: therapeutic method involving applying powdered medicine on the skin

导便 [dǎo biàn]
inducing defecation: method of opening the bowels with an enema or suppository, also called 导法 [dǎo fǎ]

导法 [dǎo fǎ]
same as 导便 [dǎo biàn]

塞法 [sāi fǎ]
insertion method: therapeutic method involving inserting medicinal powder packed in cotton, gauze or suppositories into the nostril, vagina or rectum

枯痔法 [kū zhì fǎ]
necrotizing therapy for hemorrhoids: method for curing hemorrhoids involving local application or injection of necrotizing agents

结扎疗法 [jié zā liáo fǎ]
ligation therapy: therapeutic method whereby hemorrhoids or warts are necrotized via ligation with a medicated silk thread or rubber band, and removed gradually

挂线疗法 [guà xiàn liáo fǎ]
threaded ligation therapy: therapeutic method whereby anal fistula is ligated in the pathway with a medicated silk thread or rubber band. This method makes use of the tensile strength of the thread or band to cause degeneration of tissue so as to eventually open the fistula.

药捻疗法 [yào niǎn liáo fǎ]

medicated spill therapy: method for treating abscesses or sores whereby a piece of twisted paper enveloping or coated with medicinal powder is applied at the diseased site, also called medicated thread therapy (药线疗法 [yào xiàn liáo fǎ])

药线疗法 [yào xiàn liáo fǎ]

medicated thread therapy: same as medicated spill therapy (药捻疗法 [yào niǎn liáo fǎ])

熏洗疗法 [xūn xǐ liáo fǎ]

fuming-washing therapy: therapeutic method involving fuming the diseased area with the vapor of a boiling decoction and then washing the area with the decoction

拔罐疗法 [bá guàn liáo fǎ]

cupping therapy: therapeutic method whereby a vacuumized cup or small jar is sucked onto the skin to cause local congestion

膏摩疗法 [gāo mó liáo fǎ]

massage therapy with ointment: a massage therapy whereby medicated ointment is applied to the area to be treated before manipulation

食疗 [shí liáo]

diet therapy: therapeutic use of diet and food based on the tastes and actions of different foodstuffs, also called 食治 [shí zhì]

食治 [shí zhì]

same as 食疗 [shí liáo]

中药学 Chinese Pharmaceutics

中药学 [zhōng yào xué]
Chinese pharmaceutics: the branch of health sciences dealing with the preparation, dispensing, and proper utilization of Chinese medicinals

本草 [běn cǎo]
materia medica: traditional name for Chinese pharmaceutics

中药 [zhōng yào]
Chinese medicinals; Chinese drugs: usually referring to those recorded in Chinese materia medica

草药 [cǎo yào]
herbal medicinals; herbal drugs: usually referring to those not recorded in Chinese materia medica or only used in folk medicine. A clear-cut differentiation between herbal medicinals in folk medicine and regular traditional medicinals (Chinese medicinals) is difficult to make, and so they are often collectively called Chinese herbal medicinals (中草药 [zhōng cǎo yào]).

中草药 [zhōng cǎo yào]
Chinese herbal medicinals: cf. Chinese medicinals (中药 [zhōng yào]) and herbal medicinals (草药 [cǎo yào])

药材 [yào cái]
medicinal substance, materia medica: crude natural medicinal for processing

道地药材 [dào dì yào cái]
geo-authentic materia medica: quality medicinal substance or raw material collected from the traditional or original place, as recorded in the Chinese Pharmacopoeia

中药的炮制、性能和剂型
Processing, Properties and Dosage Forms of Chinese Medicinals/Drugs

药材炮制 [yào cái páo zhì]
processing of medicinal substances: treatment of crude medicinals by way of cleansing, cutting, soaking, drying, calcining, baking, steaming, simmering, carbonizing, roasting, etc., for fulfilling therapeutic, dispensing or manufacturing requirements and assuring the safety and efficacy of the final dosage

炮制 [páo zhì]
processing (of materia medica): general term for preparative treatment of an individual herb or medicinal substance before its medical use

炮炙 [páo zhì]
processing (of materia medica): a term synonymous with 炮制 [páo zhì], but properly limited to processing with heat

修治 [xiū zhì]
(I) processing (of materia medica): ancient term for 炮制 [páo zhì]; **(II) primary processing:** elementary procedures for the preparation of a medicinal herb,

including purification, crushing, slicing, etc.

修事 [xiū shì]
ancient term for processing of materia medica (炮制 [páo zhì])

水制 [shuǐ zhì]
water processing: processing by utilizing water, including washing, bleaching, soaking, refining with water, etc.

火制 [huǒ zhì]
fire processing: processing by utilizing heat or fire, including stir-baking, baking, calcining, etc.

水火共制 [shuǐ huǒ gòng zhì]
water-fire processing: processing by utilizing water in combination with heat or fire, including simmering, steaming, blanching, quenching, etc.

洗 [xǐ]
washing: process of cleansing by immersing in or applying water

泡 [pào]
maceration; soaking: process of softening a medicinal substance by immersing it in water, usually before peeling or cutting

润 [rùn]
moistening: process of softening a medicinal substance with a small amount of liquid, such as water, wine or ginger juice

漂 [piǎo]
rinsing: washing a medicinal substance quickly with water running continuously, either whole or in portions, to remove toxic components, unpleasant odors or unwanted mineral salt

切片 [qiē piàn]
slicing: refinement by cutting previously cleansed and softened medicinal substance into slices

水飞 [shuǐ fēi]
elutriation; refining with water: removing impurities from a powdered medicinal and at the same time obtaining finer powder by mixing it with water in a tank and allowing the supernatant turbid fluid to settle in another tank and then collecting the deposit

煅 [duàn]
calcination: burning a medicinal substance on a fire to make it crispy

煅淬 [duàn cuì]
calcining and quenching: burning a medicinal substance till red hot and then dipping it quickly into a specified liquid to make it crispy

制炭 [zhì tàn]
carbonization: heating a vegetable medicinal substance in an airtight container or by stir-baking over a strong fire till its outer part is charred while its inner part becomes yellowish-brown, so that its original property is retained

烘焙 [hōng bèi]
baking: drying a medicinal substance over a slow fire

煨 [wēi]
roasting (in hot ashes): baking a medicinal

substance wrapped in wet paper or coated with dough in hot ashes till the paper or coat turns black

炒 [chǎo]
stir-baking: baking a medicinal substance in a pan with constant stirring

清炒 [qīng chǎo]
stir-baking without adjuvant: baking a medicinal substance in a pan with constant stirring free of any adjuvant

加辅料炒 [jiā fǔ liào chǎo]
stir-baking with adjuvant: baking a medicinal substance in a pan with constant stirring, together with earth, bran, or rice as an adjuvant

炙 [zhì]
stir-baking with fluid adjuvant: baking, with constant stirring, a medicinal substance with wine, vinegar, salt water, honey, or ginger juice, until the latter is infiltrated into the former, for property alteration, therapeutic effect enhancement or side effect reduction of the medicinal substance

蜜炙 [mì zhì]
stir-baking with honey: baking a medicinal substance in a pan with constant stirring, together with honey as an adjuvant

酒炙 [jiǔ zhì]
stir-baking with wine: baking a medicinal substance in a pan with constant stirring, together with wine as an adjuvant,

姜炙 [jiāng zhì]
stir-baking with ginger: baking a medicinal substance in a pan with constant stirring, together with ginger juice as an adjuvant

醋炙 [cù zhì]
stir-baking with vinegar: baking a medicinal substance in a pan with constant stirring, together with vinegar as an adjuvant

微炒 [wēi chǎo]
stir-baking to dryness: baking a medicinal substance in a pan over a slow fire, with constant stirring, to make it dry

炒爆 [chǎo bào]
stir-baking to cracking: baking a medicinal substance (usually seeds) in a pan, with constant stirring, till it cracks

炒黄 [chǎo huáng]
stir-baking to yellowish: baking a medicinal substance in a pan, with constant stirring, till it turns yellowish and gives off a scent

炒焦 [chǎo jiāo]
stir-baking to brown: baking a medicinal substance in a pan, with constant stirring, till it turns brown

炒炭 [chǎo tàn]
stir-baking to charcoal: baking a medicinal substance in a pan, with constant stirring, till it partly turns to charcoal

炮 [páo]
stir-baking at a high temperature: baking a medicinal substance, with constant stirring (usually together with hot sand) at a high temperature for a short time, so as to reduce its violent action

蒸 [zhēng]
steaming: preparing a medicinal substance thoroughly mixed with a fluid adjuvant by exposing it to steam or vapor in a suitable container

炖 [dùn]
simmering in a bath: preparing a medicinal substance thoroughly mixed with fluid adjuvant by putting it into an airtight container, and then heating the container in a water bath or with steam until the fluid adjuvant is well absorbed

熬 [áo]
simmering: concentrating fluid adjuvant by boiling the medicinal substance slowly and gently

煮 [zhǔ]
boiling: heating a medicinal substance with boiling water or other fluid adjuvant

燀 [shàn]
blanching: putting certain seeds in boiling water, and stirring for a short time until the shrunken testa is extended, then transfering the seeds into cold water and removing the testa

淬 [cuì]
quenching: cooling a red-hot substance rapidly by placing it in cold water in order to make it crispy

烧存性 [shāo cún xìng]
burning with the original property retained: burning a vegetable medicinal substance till its outer part is charred while its inner part becomes tawny, so that its original property is retained while some others are modified

去油 [qù yóu]
defatting: removing fat or oil from medicinal substances (such as croton seeds) to reduce their toxicity

去火毒 [qù huǒ dú]
removal of fire toxin: the process of eliminating the irritating quality of newly prepared plaster base by placing it in a shady and cool place or in water for a period of time before using it

制霜 [zhì shuāng]
frosting: making defatted vegetable medicinal substances (usually seeds) into frost-like powder or re-crystallizing the mineral substances into fine particles

发酵 [fā jiào]
fermentation: making a medicinal substance undergo fermenting process

发芽 [fā yá]
sprouting: making a medicinal substance, either vegetable or seed, start to shoot or bud, respectively

药味 [yào wèi]
(I) medicinal ingredients (in a prescription); **(II) taste or flavor of a medicinal**, representing the basic action of a medicinal

气味 [qì wèi]
property and flavor: the property and flavor of a medicinal that represent the main effects of the latter

性味 [xìng wèi]
property and flavor: same as 气味 [qì wèi]

药性 [yào xìng]
medicinal properties: the basic properties of a medicinal, including its nature, taste, meridian/channel tropism, acting direction, and toxicity

四性 [sì xìng]
four properties: collective term for the basic properties of medicinals, i.e., cold, hot, warm or cool, classified according to their therapeutic effects, e.g., medicinals effective for treating heat syndromes/patterns being endowed with cold or cool property, while those effective for cold syndromes/patterns, with warm or hot property

四气 [sì qì]
four natures: collective term for the basic natures of medicinals: same as the four properties (四性 [sì xìng])

五味 [wǔ wèi]
five tastes (flavors): collective term for the tastes of medicinals, i.e., pungent, sweet, sour, bitter or salty, and sometimes including tasteless, representing the basic action of a medicinal, e.g., most medicinals with a dispersing action being pungent, astringents being sour, tonics being sweet, and vice versa

归经 [guī jīng]
meridian/channel tropism: classification of medicinals according to the meridian(s)/channel(s) on which their therapeutic action is manifested, e.g., *Radix Platycodi*, *FlosFarfarae* and *Radix Asteris* being grouped under the lung meridian/channel owing to their antitussive effect in cases of lung diseases

升降浮沉 [shēng jiàng fú chén]
ascending, descending, floating and sinking: collective term for the directions of medicinal actions. The ascending and floating medicinals have an upward and outward effect and are used for activating vitality and inducing sweating and dispelling cold, while the descending and sinking medicinals, having a downward and inward effect, are used for tranquillizing, inducing contraction, relieving cough, arresting emesis, and promoting diuresis or purgation.

大毒、常毒、小毒、无毒 [dà dú、cháng dú、xiǎo dú、wú dú]
extremely poisonous, moderately poisonous, slightly poisonous and non-poisonous (medicinals): classification of medicinals according to their toxicity

三品 [sān pǐn]
three grades of medicinals: ancient classification of medicinals chiefly based upon their toxicity, by which medicinals are grouped into top-grade, medium-grade and inferior-grade varieties

上品 [shàng pǐn]
top-grade medicinal: medicinal that is non-toxic, possesses a rejuvenating effect and can be taken frequently and for a long period of time without harm to the patient

中品 [zhōng pǐn]
medium-grade medicinal: medicinal that has no or only slightly toxic effect and is effective for treating diseases of deficiency condition

下品 [xià pǐn]
inferior-grade medicinal: medicinal that is effective for expelling pathogens, but is toxic and should not be taken for a long period of time

五味所入 [wǔ wèi suǒ rù]
what the different tastes act on: collective term for the locations of drug action in relation to tastes of medicinals, derived from an ancient hypothesis in Chinese pharmacology based upon the theory of the five elements/phases, meaning that medicinals of different tastes act on different viscera selectively

剂量 [jì liàng]
dosage: the measured quantity of a medicinal to be taken by the patient

剂型 [jì xíng]
preparation form; dosage form: form of a prepared medicine, e.g., decoction, pill, tablet, powder or granule

丸剂 [wán jì]
pill: a solid globular mass, coated or uncoated, made of finely powdered medicinals with a suitable excipient or binder, often abbreviated as 丸 [wán]

丸 [wán]
pill: abbreviation for 丸剂 [wán jì]

水丸 [shuǐ wán]
watered pill: a small globular medicated mass, in which water is used as a binder

蜜丸 [mì wán]
honeyed pill: a globular medicated mass, in which processed honey is used as a binder

蜡丸 [là wán]
(I) waxed pill: a globular medicated mass, in which beeswax is used as a binder; **(II) wax-coated pill:** a globular medicated mass covered with a layer of wax

糊丸 [hú wán]
pasted pill: a small globular medicated mass, in which rice-paste or flour-paste is used as a binder

浓缩丸 [nóng suō wán]
concentrated pill: a small globular medicated mass, in which part of the medicinal is made into an extract and used as a binder

微丸 [wēi wán]
minute pellet: a very small globular medicated mass with a diameter less than 2.5 mm

滴丸 [dī wán]
dripping pill: a small globular pill of medicinal extract mixed with a ground substance, formed by dripping into an insoluble liquor condensate

泡腾片 [pào téng piàn]
effervescent tablet: tablet designed to dissolve in contact with water or another liquid, releasing carbon dioxide in the process

散剂 [sǎn jì]
powder: medicated preparation in the form of discrete fine particles, for internal administration or topical application, often abbreviated as 散 [sǎn]

散 [sǎn]
powder: abbreviation for 散剂 [sǎn jì]

膏剂 [gāo jì]
paste: general term for soft extract, ointment and adhesive plaster, often abbreviated as 膏 [gāo]

膏 [gāo]
paste: abbreviation for 膏剂 [gāo jì]

煎膏 [jiān gāo]
soft extract: medicated preparation for oral administration, usually made by concentrating a decoction to a syrupy consistency with the addition of sugar or honey, also known as 膏滋 [gāo zī]

膏滋 [gāo zī]
soft extract: same as 煎膏 [jiān gāo]

软膏 [ruǎn gāo]
ointment: an unguent for application to the skin

乳膏 [rǔ gāo]
cream: ointment with emulsifying base

膏药 [gāo yào]
adhesive plaster: medicated dressing that consists of a film (as of cloth or paper) spread with a medicated substance

丹剂 [dān jì]
pellet: medicated preparation in the form of small particles, usually made from minerals by sublimation, mainly for topical application, but some also for internal administration, often abbreviated as 丹 [dān]

丹 [dān]
pellet: abbreviation for 丹剂 [dān jì]

露剂 [lù jì]
distillate: a liquid product of herbal medicine, usually aromatic, condensed from vapor during distillation, often abbreviated as 露 [lù]

露 [lù]
distillate: abbreviation for 露剂 [lù jì]

糖浆 [táng jiāng]
syrup: a thick sticky liquid consisting of a concentrated aqueous solution of sugar with the addition of medicinal substance

锭剂 [dìng jì]
pastil; lozenge: ingot-shaped tablet of medicine, prepared according to specified method and used internally or externally

锭 [dìng]
pastil; lozenge: abbreviation for 锭剂 [dìng jì]

药酒 [yào jiǔ]
medicinal wine; medicated wine: wine or spirit in which medicinal substances have been steeped, also called 酒剂 [jiǔ jì]

酒剂 [jiǔ jì]
medicinal wine; medicated wine: same as 药酒 [yào jiǔ]

酒醴 [jiǔ lǐ]
ancient term for medicinal wine (药酒 [yào jiǔ])

汤药 [tāng yào]
(medicinal) decoction: liquid medicine

prepared by boiling the ingredients in water, and taken after the dregs are removed, also called 汤剂 [tāng jì]

汤剂 [tāng jì]
decoction: same as 汤药 [tāng yào]

饮 [yǐn]
cold decoction: decoction to be taken cold

饮片 [yǐn piàn]
medicinal slices: herbs in small pieces or slices, mostly after appropriate processing

药面 [yào miàn]
medicinal powder: medicinal made into powder

茶剂 [chá jì]
medicated tea: medicinals in coarse powder form or made into small cakes, taken as tea after being infused with boiling water or boiled in water, often abbreviated as tea (茶 [chá])

茶 [chá]
(medicated) tea: abbreviation for 茶剂 [chá jì]

曲 [qū]
leaven: powdered medicinal mixed with wheat flour and beaten into cakes for fermentation, usually used as a stomachic

胶 [jiāo]
glue: solid lumps for internal administration after melting, prepared by extracting substance from animal skin, bone, shell or horn with water, concentrating the extracted liquid to a thick gelatinoid consistency, drying and cutting into lumps

片剂 [piàn jì]
tablet: small, flattened pellet of compressed powdered medicinal or extract of medicinal with starch as a formative agent, often abbreviated as 片 [piàn]

片 [piàn]
tablet: abbreviation for 片剂 [piàn jì]

冲剂 [chōng jì]
infusion granules: granules made of medicinal extract, usually with sugar as a corrigent, to be dissolved in boiling water before being taken

冲服剂 [chōng fú jì]
infusion granules: same as 冲剂 [chōng jì]

颗粒剂 [kē lì jì]
granules: small particles of medicine made of medicinal extract, to be dissolved in water for oral administration

胶囊剂 [jiāo náng jì]
capsule: a medicinal preparation for oral use consisting of a gelatin shell and its contents

栓剂 [shuān jì]
suppository: a readily meltable solid cone or cylinder of medicated material for insertion into a body passage or cavity such as the rectum or vagina

溶化 [róng huà]
dissolution: dissolving a medicinal with water into a decoction before taking

烊化 [yáng huà]
melting: melting a medicinal (such as honey or ass-hide glue) in hot water or decoction before taking

煎药法 [jiān yào fǎ]
method of making a decoction: method including mixing the ingredients of a prescription with an adequate amount of water, boiling them for a certain period of time and removing the dregs from the liquid before taking

文火 [wénhuǒ]
mild fire: fire used for making the decoctions which need a longer period of boiling, such as tonics, also called slow fire (慢火 [màn huǒ])

慢火 [màn huǒ]
slow fire: same as 文火 [wén huǒ]

武火 [wǔ huǒ]
strong fire: fire used for making decoctions that only allow a short period of boiling, such as pungent diaphoretics, also called 急火 [jí huǒ]

急火 [jí huǒ]
strong fire: same as 武火 [wǔ huǒ]

先煎 [xiān jiān]
to be decocted first: While making a decoction, certain medicinals (chiefly minerals and shells with active constituents difficult to extract) should be boiled before other ingredients are added.

后下 [hòu xià]
to be decocted later: Medicinals with active constituents ready to diffuse or evaporate should be added when the decocting is almost complete.

包煎 [bāo jiān]
to be decocted with wrapping; wrap-decoct: Downy or powdered medicinals or medicinals containing much mucilage are usually wrapped with a piece of cloth or gauze when the decoction is made.

另煎 [lìng jiān]
to be decocted separately: Some expensive medicinals, e.g., ginseng, should be decocted separately in order to avoid adsorption of its extract by the dregs of other ingredients.

别煮 [bié zhǔ]
to be decocted separately: same as 另煎 [lìng jiān]

单煎 [dān jiān]
to be decocted alone: synonym for "to be decocted separately" (另煎 [lìng jiān])

服药法 [fú yào fǎ]
administration: method of taking medicines

冲服 [chōng fú]
to be taken infused: take medicine (usually an aromatic or powdered medicinal) after pouring hot water or hot decoction of other medicinals over it while stirring

调服 [tiáo fú]
to be taken after mixing: take medicine (usually a powdered medicinal) after mixing it with liquid such as a portion of hot decoction of other medicinals, water, and wine

吞服 [tūn fú]
to be swallowed: take medicine through the throat into the stomach without chewing

送服 [sòng fú]
to be taken with fluid: take medicine (usually medicinal pills or powder) by swallowing it together with warm water (in most cases), dilute decoction of fresh ginger for warming medicinals, mint solution for heat-clearing medicinals, dilute salt water for tonics, etc.

噙化 [qín huà]
to be dissolved in the mouth: take medicine (usually pills or pastilles) by dissolving it in the mouth and then swallowing the residue or spitting it out

食远服 [shí yuǎn fú]
to be taken midway between meals: take medicine at a long interval between meals

临睡前服 [lín shuì qián fú]
to be taken before bed-time: take medicine (usually tranquilizers) before going to bed at night

空腹服 [kōng fù fú]
to be taken on an empty stomach: take medicine in the morning before breakfast

平旦服 [píng dàn fú]
to be taken in the early morning: take medicine at 4—5 a.m.

顿服 [dùn fú]
to be taken at a draught: take medicine in one single dose

频服 [pín fú]
to be taken frequently: take medicine (usually a decoction) in small portions at frequent intervals

温服 [wēn fú]
to be taken warm: take a decoction neither hot nor cold

热服 [rè fú]
to be taken hot: A decoction with ingredients hot in nature for treating a cold syndrome may give better results if taken hot.

冷服 [lěng fú]
to be taken cold: A decoction with ingredients cold in nature for treating a heat syndrome may give better results if taken cold.

妊娠禁忌药 [rèn shēn jìn jì yào]
medicinals contraindicated during pregnancy: medicinals the administration of which is prohibited during pregnancy

服药食忌 [fú yào shí jì]
dietary prohibitions during medication: species of food that are not allowed to be taken during the medicinal treatment period

食忌 [shí jì]
dietary prohibitions: abbreviation for dietary prohibitions during medication (服药食忌 [fú yào shí jì])

忌口 [jì kǒu]
food taboo: food prohibited from the patient's diet

常用引文 Commonly Used Citations

苦入心。
[kǔ rù xīn]
Medicinals bitter in taste act on the heart.

酸入肝。
[suān rù gān]
Medicinals sour in taste act on the liver.

甘入脾。
[gān rù pí]
Medicinals sweet in taste act on the spleen.

辛入肺。
[xīn rù fèi]
Medicinals pungent in taste act on the lung.

咸入肾。
[xián rù shèn]
Medicinals salty in taste act on the kidney.

辛散，酸收，甘缓，苦坚，咸软。
[xīn sǎn, suān shōu, gān huǎn, kǔ jiān, xián ruǎn]
The pungent induce dispersion, the sour contraction, the sweet moderation, the bitter hardening, and the salty softening: A pungent medicinal causes dispersion, a sour medicinal is usually astringent, a sweet medicinal has a moderating effect, a bitter medicinal promotes firmness, and a salty medicinal softens hard masses.

治热以寒，温而行之。
[zhì rè yǐ hán, wēn ér xíng zhī]
Treat a heat syndrome/pattern with cold-natured medicinals, which should be taken warm.

治寒以热，凉而行之。
[zhì hán yǐ rè, liáng ér xíng zhī]
Treat a cold syndrome/pattern with hot-natured medicinals, which should be taken cool.

用温远温，用热远热，用凉远凉，用寒远寒。
[yòng wēn yuǎn wēn, yòng rè yuǎn rè, yòng liáng yuǎn liáng, yòng hán yuǎn hán]
The warm is applied away from the warm, the hot away from the hot, the cool away from the cool, and the cold away from the cold: Avoid using warm-natured medicinals in a warm environment, hot-natured medicinals in a hot environment, cool-natured medicinals in a cool environment, and cold-natured medicinals in a cold environment.

诸寒之而热者取之阴，热之而寒者取之阳。
[zhū hán zhī ér rè zhě qǔ zhī yīn, rè zhī ér hán zhě qǔ zhī yáng]
If the use of cold-natured medicinals worsens the heat symptoms, nourish yin; if the use of hot-natured medicinals worsens cold symptoms, invigorate yang: If a patient who suffers from heat syndrome shows more heat symptoms after being treated with cold-natured

medicinals, he or she should be treated by the principle of nourishing yin. If a patient who suffers from cold syndrome shows more cold symptoms after being treated with hot-natured medicinals, he or she should be treated by invigorating yang.

有毒无毒，所治为主。
[yǒu dú wú dú, suǒ zhì wéi zhǔ]
Toxic or non-toxic, medicinal treatments are chosen case by case: The selection of a medicine with higher or lower toxicity is case dependent.

大毒治病，十去其六。
[dà dú zhì bìng, shí qù qí liù]
A medicine with great toxicity should be discontinued when the disease is 60% cured.

常毒治病，十去其七。
[cháng dú zhì bìng, shí qù qí qī]
A medicine with moderate toxicity should be discontinued when the disease is 70% cured.

小毒治病，十去其八。
[xiǎo dú zhì bìng, shí qù qí bā]
A medicine with low toxicity should be discontinued when the disease is 80% cured.

无毒治病，十去其九。
[wú dú zhì bìng, shí qù qí jiǔ]
A medicine without any toxicity should be discontinued when the disease is 90% cured.

有故无殒，亦无殒也。
[yǒu gù wú yǔn, yì wú yǔn yě]
If there is enough reason, a toxic medicine can also be used without harm.

因其轻而扬之。
[yīn qí qīng ér yáng zhī]
If the pathogen is in the exterior, use pungent diaphoretics to disperse it.

因其重而减之。
[yīn qí zhòng ér jiǎn zhī]
If the pathogen is in the interior, use purgatives to eliminate it.

因其衰而彰之。
[yīn qí shuāi ér zhāng zhī]
If healthy *qi* is debilitated, use tonics to fortify it.

血实宜决之。
[xuè shí yí jué zhī]
Excess syndrome of the blood should be treated with eliminating therapy.

气虚宜掣引之。
[qì xū yí zhì yǐn zhī]
Deficiency syndrome of *qi* should be treated with lifting therapy.

其高者，因而越之。
[qí gāo zhě, yīn ér yuè zhī]
If the pathogenic factors are accumulated in the upper (above the diaphragm), **use emetics.**

其下者，引而竭之。
[qí xià zhě, yǐn ér jié zhī]
If the pathogenic factors are accumulated in the lower (in the intestines), **use purgatives.**

中满者，泻之于内。
[zhōng mǎn zhě, xiè zhī yú nèi]

For treating accumulation in the middle energizer with abdominal fullness, use digestives and carminatives.

上燥治气。[shàng zào zhì qì]
For relieving dryness in the upper (chiefly referring to the upper respiratory tract)**, treat *qi*.** Here, *qi* refers to the lung which dominates *qi*.

中燥增液。[zhōng zào zēng yè]
For relieving dryness in the middle (referring to the spleen and stomach), **supplement with fluids.** It is so said because dryness of the spleen and stomach is marked by abnormal depletion of body fluids.

下燥治血。[xià zào zhì xuè]
For relieving dryness in the lower (referring to the liver and kidney), **treat the blood.** It is so said because impairment of the liver and kidney is bound to consume blood and essence, for the liver stores blood and the kidney stores essence.

轻可去实。[qīng kě qù shí]
Lightweight medicinals cure excess syndromes: Lightweight medicinals such as *Herba Ephedrae* and *Radix Puerariae* are effectively used to treat exterior excess syndrome in the initial stage of a wind-warm disease.

重可去怯。[zhòng kě qù qiè]
Weighty medicinals (referring to settling tranqilizers) **cure timidity.**

热可制寒。[rè kě zhì hán]
Hot-natured medicinals cure cold syndromes.

涩可固脱。[sè kě gù tuō]
Astringent medicinals cure abnormal discharges (e.g., excessive or spontaneous sweating, and seminal emission) **or prolapses** (e.g., prolapse of the anus or rectum).

中药的分类
Classification of Chinese Medicinals/Drugs

解表药 [jiě biǎo yào]
exterior-releasing medicinal/drug; superficies-releasing medicinal/drug: agent or substance that has the effect of dispelling exogenous pathogenic factors from the superficial or exterior aspect of the body, usually through sweating

发汗解表药 [fā hàn jiě biǎo yào]
diaphoretic exterior-releasing medicinal/drug: agent or substance that releases the exterior syndrome/pattern through sweating

发表药 [fā biǎo yào]
exterior-effusing medicinal/drug: synonym for exterior-releasing medicinal/drug (解表药 [jiě biǎo yào])

发散风寒药 [fā sàn fēng hán yào]
wind-cold dispersing medicinal/drug: agent or substance that has the effect of dispersing wind and cold in the treatment of an exterior syndrome/pattern

发散风热药 [fā sàn fēng rè yào]
wind-heat dispersing medicinal/drug: agent or substance that has the effect of

dispersing wind and heat in the treatment of an exterior syndrome/pattern

辛温解表药 [xīn wēn jiě biǎo yào]
pungent-warm exterior-releasing medicinal/drug: agent or substance pungent in flavor and warm in nature, such as *HerbaEphedrae* or *Ramulus Cinnamomi*, which is usually used for treating wind-cold exterior syndrome/pattern

辛凉解表药 [xīn liáng jiě biǎo yào]
pungent-cool exterior-releasing medicinal/drug: agent or substance pungent in flavor and cool in nature, such as *Herba Menthae* or *Flos Chrysanthemi*, which is usually used for treating wind-heat exterior syndrome/pattern

清热药 [qīng rè yào]
heat-clearing medicinal/drug: agent or substance cold or cool in nature, which has the effect of clearing up internal heat in cases of externally contracted febrile diseases with high fever and dire thirst, dampness-heat dysentery, eruptive epidemic warm diseases, boils, sores and abscesses, or fever in cases of yin deficiency

清热泻火药 [qīng rè xiè huǒ yào]
heat-clearing and fire-purging medicinal/drug: agent or substance that has the effect of clearing up heat in the *qi* aspect manifested by high fever, dire thirst, dry yellow tongue coating and rapid surging pulse, or purging fire of the internal organs such as heart fire, liver fire, etc.

清热凉血药 [qīng rè liáng xuè yào]
heat-clearing and blood-cooling medicinal/drug: agent or substance that has the effect of eliminating pathological heat from the nutrient and blood aspects in cases of warm diseases marked by fever accompanied by delirium, eruptions and bleeding, and also in cases of bleeding due to heat in the blood

清热燥湿药 [qīng rè zào shī yào]
heat-clearing and dampness-drying medicinal/drug: agent or substance, bitter in taste and cold in nature that is effective for eliminating heat and dampness, usually used in the treatment of diseases caused by dampness-heat, such as acute jaundice, acute dysentery, urinary infection, eczema, boils and abscesses

清热解毒药 [qīng rè jiě dú yào]
heat-clearing and toxicity-relieving medicinal/drug: agent or substance that counteracts heat toxins or fire toxins, mainly indicated in the treatment of boils, sores, abscesses, erysipelas, epidemic infectious diseases, mumps, dysentery, insect or snakebites, and burns

清虚热药 [qīng xū rè yào]
deficiency-heat-clearing medicinal/drug: agent or substance that clears the heat in deficiency conditions, often indicated in the treatment of heat due to yin deficiency marked by afternoon fever with heat sensation in the palms of the hands and soles of the feet, night sweats, and reddened tongue with scanty coating, but also used in the late stage of a warm disease with residual heat

泻下药 [xiè xià yào]
purgative (medicinal/drug): agent or substance that promotes defecation or even causes diarrhea, not only for relieving constipation, but also for driving stagnant matter, excessive heat and retained fluid out of the body

攻下药 [gōng xià yào]
offensive purgative (medicinal/drug): agent or substance, usually bitter in taste and cold in nature, that has a potent purgative effect for moving the bowels and driving away excessive heat and stagnant matter

温下药 [wēn xià yào]
warming purgative (medicinal/drug): agent or substance warm in nature, which relieves constipation caused by excessive cold stagnation

润下药 [rùn xià yào]
laxative (medicinal/drug): agent or substance that lubricates the intestinal tract to facilitate defecation for relieving constipation in the aged with fluid deficiency, in cases of febrile diseases with fluid impairment and in those of postpartum blood deficiency

峻下逐水药 [jùn xià zhú shuǐ yào]
drastic hydragogue: cathartic that causes copious water discharge for reducing accumulated fluid in anasarca, ascites and pleural effusion

祛风湿药 [qū fēng shī yào]
wind-dampness-dispelling medicinal/drug; antirheumatic: agent or substance that dispels wind and dampness, mainly for relieving rheumatism and related conditions

祛风湿散寒药 [qū fēng shī sàn hán yào]
wind-dampness-dispelling and cold-dispersing medicinal/drug: agent or substance that dispels wind-dampness, disperses cold, soothes the tendons and unblocks the collateral meridians/channels, indicated in cases of wind-dampness (rheumatic or rheumatoid) arthralgia of cold type

祛风湿清热药 [qū fēng shī qīng rè yào]
wind-dampness-dispelling and heat-clearing medicinal/drug: agent or substance that dispels wind-dampness, unblocks the collateral meridians/channels, clears heat, reduces swelling and alleviates pain, suitable for treating wind-dampness (rheumatic or rheumatoid) arthralgia of heat type with redness, swelling, hotness and pain in the joints

祛风湿强筋骨药 [qū fēng shī qiáng jīn gǔ yào]
wind-dampness-dispelling and tendon-bone-strengthening medicinal/drug: agent or substance that dispels wind-dampness, tonifies the liver and kidney and strengthens the tendons and bones, mainly used in the treatment of chronic arthralgia with aching back and weak legs

化湿药 [huà shī yào]
dampness-resolving medicinal/drug: agent or substance with fragrant odor, and warming and drying functions, that resolves dampness and invigorates the spleen, also called aromatic dampness-

resolving medicinal/drug (芳香化湿药 [fāng xiāng huà shī yào])

芳香化湿药 [fāng xiāng huà shī yào]
aromatic dampness-resolving medicinal/drug: aromatic agent or substance effective for resolving dampness, often used in the treatment of dampness syndrome marked by anorexia, lassitude, nausea and vomiting, distension in the chest and abdomen, greasy tongue coating and slippery pulse, found in cases of febrile diseases or in those of other miscellaneous diseases

利水渗湿药 [lì shuǐ shèn shī yào]
dampness-draining diuretic (medicinal/drug): agent or substance that increases urine excretion and water discharge for treating internal retention of dampness

利湿药 [lì shī yào]
dampness-draining medicinal/drug: synonym for dampness-draining diuretic (利水渗湿药 [lì shuǐ shèn shī yào])

利水消肿药 [lì shuǐ xiāo zhǒng yào]
edema-alleviating diuretic (medicinal/drug): agent or substance that increases urine excretion for treating edema with oliguria, diarrhea, and retained fluid

利尿通淋药 [lì niào tōng lín yào]
stranguria-relieving diuretic (medicinal/drug): agent or substance that increases urine excretion and relieves stranguria, mainly indicated in the treatment of dampness-heat in the lower energizer with painful discharge of urine

通淋药 [tōng lín yào]
stranguria-relieving medicinal/drug: agent or substance that relieves various kinds of stranguria, including dampness-heat stranguria and urolithiasis

利湿退黄药 [lì shī tuì huáng yào]
dampness-draining anti-icteric (medicinal/drug): agent or substance that drains dampness and relieves icterus, indicated in the treatment of dampness-heat jaundice

利胆退黄药 [lì dǎn tuì huáng yào]
bile-draining anti-icteric (medicinal/drug): agent or substance that promotes increased flow of bile to relieve jaundice

利尿逐水药 [lì niào zhú shuǐ yào]
diuretic hydragogue (medicinal/drug): agent or substance that causes copious discharge of water through catharsis and at the same time increases urine excretion

温里药 [wēn lǐ yào]
interior-warming medicinal/drug: agent or substance that warms the interior and expels internal cold, also called cold-expelling medicinal/drug (祛寒药 [qū hán yào])

祛寒药 [qū hán yào]
cold-dispelling medicinal/drug: synonym for interior-warming medicinal/drug (温里药 [wēn lǐ yào])

理气药 [lǐ qì yào]
***qi*-regulating medicinal/drug:** agent or substance that regulates the movement of *qi* to treat *qi* stagnation or adverse *qi* flow, also called *qi*-moving medicinal/drug (行气药 [xíng qì yào])

行气药 [xíng qì yào]
***qi*-moving medicinal/drug:** agent or substance that restores the normal movement of *qi*, a synonym for *qi*-regulating medicinal/drug (理气药 [lǐ qì yào])

消食药 [xiāo shí yào]
digestant (medicinal/drug): agent or substance that aids digestion to eliminate accumulated undigested food, also called digestant and evacuant medicinal/drug (消导药 [xiāo dǎo yào])

消导药 [xiāo dǎo yào]
digestant and evacuant medicinal/drug: the full name of digestant (medicinal/drug) (消食药 [xiāo shí yào])

理血药 [lǐ xuè yào]
blood-regulating medicinal/drug: agent or substance that has the effects of regulating blood (including arresting bleeding, activating circulation, etc.) and tonifying blood

止血药 [zhǐ xuè yào]
hemostatic (medicinal/drug): agent or substance that arrests bleeding, either internal or external

凉血止血药 [liáng xuè zhǐ xuè yào]
blood-cooling hemostatic (medicinal/drug): agent or substance that arrests bleeding by clearing the blood of heat, indicated in the treatment of blood-heat hemorrhage

化瘀止血药 [huà yū zhǐ xuè yào]
stasis-resolving hemostatic (medicinal/drug): agent or substance that arrests bleeding and at the same time removes stagnant blood which may cause further bleeding

收敛止血药 [shōu liǎn zhǐ xuè yào]
astringent hemostatic (medicinal/drug): agent or substance that arrests bleeding by its astringent action, indicated in various types of hemorrhage, but not in those associated with excessive pathogens or blood stasis

温经止血药 [wēn jīng zhǐ xuè yào]
meridian-warming hemostatic (medicinal/drug); channel-warming hemostatic (medicinal/drug): agent or substance, warm or hot in nature, that arrests bleeding by warming the internal organs, replenishing spleen yang and strengthening the thoroughfare vessel, effective for treating hemorrhage due to failure of the spleen to control blood or insecurity of the thoroughfare vessel

活血化瘀药 [huó xuè huà yū yào]
blood-activating and stasis-resolving medicinal/drug: agent or substance that promotes blood flow and removes stagnant blood, also called blood-activating and stasis-dispelling medicinal/drug (活血祛瘀药 [huó xuè qū yū yào]), or blood-activating medicinal/drug (活血药 [huó xuè yào]) and stasis-resolving medicinal/drug (化瘀药 [huà yū yào]) for short

活血祛瘀药 [huó xuè qū yū yào]
blood-activating and stasis-dispelling medicinal/drug: synonym for blood-activating and stasis-resolving medicinal/drug (活血化瘀药 [huó xuè huà yū yào])

活血药 [huó xuè yào]

blood-activating medicinal/drug: agent or substance used in the treatment of retarded or static blood flow

化瘀药 [huà yū yào]

stasis-resolving medicinal/drug: agent or substance used in the treatment of blood stasis

活血止痛药 [huó xuè zhǐ tòng yào]

blood-activating analgesic (medicinal/ drug): agent or substance that activates blood, moves *qi* and relieves pain, indicated in the treatment of painful conditions caused by stagnation of *qi* and blood

活血行气药 [huó xuè xíng qì yào]

blood-activating and *qi*-moving medicinal/ drug: agent or substance that activates blood and promotes the flow of *qi*, used primarily in cases of stagnation of *qi* and blood

活血调经药 [huó xuè tiáo jīng yào]

blood-activating and menstruation-regulating medicinal/drug: agent or substance that activates blood and regulates menstruation for treating menstrual disorders, dysmenorrhea, amenorrhea and postpartum blood stagnation

活血疗伤药 [huó xuè liáo shāng yào]

blood-activating and trauma-curing medicinal/drug: agent or substance that activates blood, reduces swelling, arrests bleeding and promotes the healing of wounds or fractures

破血消癥药 [pò xuè xiāo zhēng yào]

blood-stasis-breaking and mass-eliminating medicinal/drug: agent or substance that, acting drastically, breaks up static blood and eliminates mass

化痰止咳平喘药 [huà tán zhǐ ké píng chuǎn yào]

phlegm-resolving, cough-stopping and asthma-relieving medicinal/drug; expectorant, antitussive and antiasthmatic: agent or substance that resolves phlegm, stops coughing and relieves asthma or dyspnea

化痰药 [huà tán yào]

phlegm-resolving medicinal/drug: agent or substance that resolves phlegm, either warm in nature and drying in action for treating disorders of cold-phlegm, or cold or cool in nature for treating disorders of heat-phlegm

温化寒痰药 [wēn huà hán tán yào]

warming phlegm-resolving medicinal/ drug: agent or substance warm in nature, such as *RhizomaPinelliae*, used in treating disorders of cold-phlegm or phlegm-dampness

清化热痰药 [qīng huà rè tán yào]

cooling phlegm-resolving medicinal/ drug: agent or substance cold in nature, such as *Bulbus Fritillariae Thunbergii*, used in treating disorders of phlegm-heat

止咳平喘药 [zhǐ ké píng chuǎn yào]

antitussive and antasthmatic (medicinal/ drug): agent or substance that relieves cough and asthma (or dyspnea), usually by ventilating, clearing or moistening the lung, or directing lung *qi* to move downward, astringing lung *qi* or resolving phlegm

安神药 [ān shén yào]
tranquilizer, tranquilizing medicinal/drug: agent or substance that calms the mind and relieves mental tension

重镇安神药 [zhòng zhèn ān shén yào]
settling tranquilizer; settling tranquilizing medicinal/drug: agent or substance, mostly a mineral, fossil bone or shell, that induces tranquilization associated with its settling action

养心安神药 [yǎng xīn ān shén yào]
heart-nourishing tranquilizer; heart-nourishing tranquilizing medicinal/drug: agent or substance that nourishes the heart to calm the mind

平肝息 [熄] 风药 [píng gān xī fēng yào]
liver-pacifying and wind-extinguishing medicinal/drug: agent or substance that pacifies the liver, suppresses exuberant yang, extinguishes endogenous wind and controls spasms or tremors

平肝抑阳药 [píng gān yì yáng yào]
liver-pacifying and yang-suppressing medicinal/drug: agent or substance that pacifies the liver and suppresses exuberant yang for the treatment of headache, dizziness, tinnitus and blurred vision

熄 [息] 风止痉药 [xī fēng zhǐ jìng yào]
wind-extinguishing and spasm-controlling medicinal/drug: agent or substance that extinguishes endogenous wind and stops spasms or tremors

芳香开窍药 [fāng xiāng kāi qiào yào]
aromatic stimulant; aromatic orifice-opening medicinal/drug: agent or substance, fragrant in flavor, with a resuscitating effect, used for emergency treatment of impairment or loss of consciousness, also called stimulant or orifice-opening medicinal/drug (开窍药 [kāi qiào yào]) for short

开窍药 [kāi qiào yào]
stimulant; orifice-opening medicinal/drug: synonym for aromatic stimulant or aromatic orifice-opening medicinal/drug (芳香开窍药 [fāng xiāng kāi qiào yào])

补益药 [bǔ yì yào]
tonic; tonifying and replenishing medicinal/drug: agent or substance that strengthens or supplements what is insufficient or weakened in the body, also called 补养药 [bǔ yǎng yào]

补养药 [bǔ yǎng yào]
tonic; tonifying and nourishing medicinal/drug: synonym for tonifying and replenishing medicinal/drug (补益药 [bǔ yì yào])

补气药 [bǔ qì yào]
***qi* tonic; *qi*-tonifying medicinal/drug:** agent or substance that tonifies *qi*, used in treating *qi* deficiency

补阳药 [bǔ yáng yào]
yang tonic; yang-tonifying medicinal/drug: agent or substance that tonifies yang-*qi*, used in treating yang deficiency

补肾阳药 [bǔ shèn yáng yào]
kidney-yang tonic: agent or substance

that tonifies kidney yang, used in treating kidney yang deficiency

补血药 [bǔ xuè yào]
blood tonic; blood-tonifying medicinal/drug: agent or substance that tonifies blood in treating blood deficiency of the heart and liver, marked by pallor, dizziness, tinnitus, palpitations, insomnia, oligomenorrhea or amenorrhea, also called blood-nourishing medicinal/drug (养血药 [yǎng xuè yào])

养血药 [yǎng xuè yào]
blood-nourishing medicinal/drug: synonym for blood tonic or blood-tonifying medicinal/drug (补血药 [bǔ xuè yào])

柔肝药 [róu gān yào]
liver-emolliating medicinal/drug: agent or substance that replenishes the liver blood or yin in treating deficiency of liver blood or yin with dizziness, tinnitus, insomnia, and blurred vision

补阴药 [bǔ yīn yào]
yin tonic; yin-tonifying medicinal/drug: agent or substance that tonifies the yin of the heart, lung, stomach, liver, or kidney

养阴药 [yǎng yīn yào]
yin-nourishing medicinal/drug: synonym for yin tonic or yin-tonifying medicinal/drug (补阴药 [bǔ yīn yào])

滋阴药 [zī yīn yào]
yin-replenishing medicinal/drug: synonym for yin tonic or yin-tonifying medicinal/drug (补阴药 [bǔ yīn yào])

收涩药 [shōu sè yào]
discharge-arresting medicinal/drug: agent or substance that arrests discharges such as sweat, diarrhea, urine, blood, leukorrhea, and semen

固涩药 [gù sè yào]
astringent (medicinal/drug): synonym for discharge-arresting medicinal/drug (收涩药 [shōu sè yào])

固表止汗药 [gù biǎo zhǐ hàn yào]
superficies-consolidating anhidrotic: agent or substance that arrests excessive sweating by consolidating the superficies

敛汗固表药 [liǎn hàn gù biǎo yào]
sweating-arresting and superficies-strengthening medicinal/drug: agent or substance that consolidates the superficies by arresting excessive sweating

敛肺涩肠药 [liǎn fèi sè cháng yào]
lung-intestine astringent (medicinal/drug): agent or substance that relieves cough and asthma, and arrests chronic diarrhea

涌吐药 [yǒng tù yào]
emetic (medicinal/drug): agent or substance that induces vomiting

催吐药 [cuī tù yào]
emetic (medicinal/drug): same as 涌吐药 [yǒng tù yào]

驱虫药 [qū chóng yào]
anthelmintic; worm-expelling medicinal/drug: agent or substance that expels or even kills intestinal parasitic worms

常用的中药
Commonly Used Chinese Medicinals/Drugs

解表药
Exterior-releasing Medicinals/Drugs

辛温解表药
Pungent-warm Exterior-releasing Medicinals / Drugs

麻黄 [má huáng]

***Herba Ephedrae*; Ephedra:** dried herbaceous stem of *Ephedra sinica* Stapf, *Ephedra equisetina* Bunge or *Ephedra intermedia* Schrenk et C.A. Meyer (family Ephedraceae), used (1) to induce sweating for releasing the superficies in wind-cold contraction, (2) to relieve asthma, and (3) to induce diuresis for relieving edema caused by wind

桂枝 [guì zhī]

***Ramulus Cinnamomi*; Cassia Twig:** dried young stem of *Cinnamomum cassia* Presl. (family Lauraceae), used (1) to induce sweating for releasing the muscles in wind-cold contraction, (2) to warm and unblock the meridians/channels to relieve various pains due to cold and congealing blood, and (3) to stimulate menstrual discharge for treating amenorrhea

生姜 [shēng jiāng]

***Rhizoma Zingiberis Recens*; Fresh Ginger:** fresh rhizome of *Zingiber officinale* (Willd.) Rosc. (family Zingiberaceae), used (1) to induce sweating for releasing the superficies in cases of wind-cold contraction, (2) to warm the middle energizer for arresting vomiting

防风 [fáng fēng]

***Radix Saposhnikoviae*; Divaricate Saposhnikovia Root:** dried root of *Saposhnikovia divaricata* (Turcz.) Schischk. (family Umbelliferae), used (1) to release the superficies in cases of exterior syndromes, (2) to dispel wind in cases of urticaria, (3) to dispel wind-dampness and alleviate pain in cases of rheumatalgia, and (4) to relieve spasms in cases of tetanus

白芷 [bái zhǐ]

***Radix Angelicae Dahuricae*; Dahurian Angelica Root:** dried root of *Angelica dahurica* (Fisch. ex Hoffm.) Benth. et Hook. f. or *Angelica dahurica* var. *formosana* (Boiss.) Shan et Yuan (family Umbelliferae), used (1) to release the superficies, dispel wind and alleviate pain in cases of frontal headache and stuffy nose in cases of colds, rheumatalgia and toothache, (2) to eliminate dampness for suppressing leukorrhagia, and (3) to discharge pus and reduce swelling for the treatment of boils, sores, abscesses, rhinitis and nasosinusitis

荆芥 [jīng jiè]

***Herba Schizonepetae*; Fineleaf Schizonepeta Herb:** dried aerial part of *Schizonepeta tenuifolia* Briq. (family Labiatae), used (1) to release the superficies and dispel wind in cases of wind-cold contraction, (2) to promote eruption for treating measles, and (3) to dispel wind for treating urticaria

荆芥穗 [jīng jiè suì]
***Spica Schizonepetae*; Fineleaf Schizonepeta Spike:** seed-bearing part of schizonepeta used in a similar way to *Herba Schizonepetae*, fineleaf schizonepeta herb, with stronger action

荆芥炭 [jīng jiè tàn]
***Herba Schizonepetae Carbonisata*; Carbonized Fineleaf Schizonepeta Herb:** carbonized schizonepeta used as a hemostatic for treating functional uterine bleeding and hematochezia.

紫苏叶 [zǐ sū yè]
***Folium Perillae*; Perilla Leaf:** dried leaf of *Perilla frutescens* (L.) Britt. (family Labiatae), used (1) to induce sweating in cases of wind-cold contraction, (2) to arrest vomiting, and (3) as an antidote to fish or crab poisoning

香薷 [xiāng rú]
***Herba Elshotziae*; Elsholtzia Herb:** dried aerial part of *Elsholtzia splendens* Nakai ex F. Maekawa (family Labiatae), used (1) to induce sweating and resolve dampness in cases of colds in summer, and (2) to cause diuresis for relieving edema

细辛 [xì xīn]
***Herba Asari*; Manchurian Wild Ginger:** dried entire plant of *Asarum heterotropoides* var. *mandshuricum* (Maxim.) Kitagawa, *Asarum sieboldii* Miq. var. *seoulense* Nakai (family Aristolochiaceae), used (1) to dispel wind and disperse cold for treating colds, (2) to relieve nasal congestion and alleviate pain for treating nasosinusitis, headache, toothache or rheumatic pain, and (3) to warm the lung and resolve retained fluid for treating cough with copious thin expectoration

藁本 [gǎo běn]
***Rhizoma Ligustici*; Chinese Lovage:** dried rhizome and root of *Ligustrum sinense* Oliver or *Ligustrum jeholense* Nakai et Kitagawa (family Umbelliferae), used to relieve pain in the vertex of the head in cases of wind-cold contraction and rheumatic arthralgia

辛夷 [xīn yí]
***Flos Magnoliae*; Biond Magnolia Flower:** dried flower bud of *Magnoliabiondii* Pamp., *Magnoliadenudata* Desr. or *Magnolia sprengeri* Pamp. (family Magnoliaceae), used for treating stuffy nose and nasal discharge in cases of rhinitis and nasosinusitis

苍耳子 [cāng ěr zǐ]
***Fructus Xanthii*; Siberian Cocklebur Fruit:** dried ripe fruit of *Xanthium sibiricum* Patrin. (family Compositae), used to dispel wind, eliminate dampness, relieve nasal congestion and alleviate pain for the treatment of wind-cold contraction of stuffy nose, rhinitis, nasosinusitis, urticaria with pruritus, and rheumatism

鹅不食草 [é bù shí cǎo]
***Herba Centipedae*; Small Centipeda Herb:** dried entire plant of *Centipeda minima* (L.) A. Braum et Aschers (family Compositae), used (1) to disperse cold and relieve nasal congestion for the treatment of colds with acute rhinitis, and (2) to arrest cough

辛凉解表药
Pungent-cool Exterior-releasing Medicinals/Drugs

柴胡 [chái hú]

***Radix Bupleuri*; Chinese Thorowax Root:** dried root of *Bupleurum chinense* DC. or *Bupleurum scorzonerifolium* Willd.(family Umbelliferae), used (1) to reduce fever for relieving alternate spells of chills and fever, (2) to relieve liver *qi* stagnation for alleviating hypochondriac and thoracic pains, and (3) to lift spleen *qi* for correcting visceroptosis

薄荷 [bò he]

***Herba Menthae*; Peppermint:** dried aerial part of *Mentha haplocalyx* Briq. (family Labiatae), used (1) to dispel wind and heat in the treatment of wind-heat contraction, (2) to clear the head and eyes for relieving headache and conjunctivitis, (3) to promote eruption in the treatment of measles, and (4) to soothe the liver for alleviating hypochondriac and thoracic pain

桑叶 [sāng yè]

***Folium Mori*; Mulberry Leaf:** dried leaf of White Mulberry, *Morus alba* L. (family Moraceae), used (1) to dispel wind and heat in the treatment of wind-heat contraction, (2) to pacify the liver and brighten the eyes for relieving hyperactivity of the liver with headache and acute conjunctivitis, and (3) to clear and moisten the lung for arresting dry cough

菊花 [jú huā]

***Flos Chrysanthemi*; Chrysanthemum Flower:** dried flower-head of *Chrysanthemum morifolium* Ramat.(family Compositae), used (1) to dispel wind and heat in the treatment of wind-heat contraction with fever and headache, (2) to pacify the liver and brighten the eyes for treating acute conjunctivitis, and dizziness due to hyperactive liver yang, and (3) to clear heat and counteract toxins for treating boils and sores

葛根 [gě gēn]

***Radix Puerariae*; Kudzuvine Root:** dried root of *Pueraria lobata* (Willd.) Ohwi or *Pueraria thomsonii* Benth. (family Leguminosae), used (1) to reduce heat in cases of exterior syndromes with fever and painful stiffness of the back and nape, (2) to relieve thirst in febrile diseases and diabetes mellitus, (3) to arrest diarrhea due to spleen insufficiency, and (4) to promote eruption in cases of measles

牛蒡子 [niú bàng zǐ]

***Fructus Arctii*; Burdock Fruit:** dried ripe fruit of great burdock, *Arctium lappa* L. (family Compositae), used (1) to dispel wind and heat in the treatment of wind-heat contraction, (2) to promote eruption in cases of measles, and (3) to counteract toxins and reduce swelling in cases of boils, sores, mumps and erysipelas

蔓荆子 [màn jīng zǐ]

***Fructus Viticis*; Shrub Chaste-tree Fruit:** dried ripe fruit of the simple-leaved chaste tree, *Vitex simplicifolia* Cham. or three-leaved chaste tree, *Vitex trifolia* L. (family Verbenaceae), used for treating wind-heat contraction with fever and headache, acute conjunctivitis, blurred vision, and dizziness

蝉蜕 [chán tuì]

***Periostracum Cicadae*; Cicada Slough:** slough shed by the nymph of *Cryptotympana pustulata* Fabr. (family Cicadidae), used (1) to dispel wind and heat in the treatment of wind-heat contraction, (2) to promote eruption in cases of measles and relieve itching in cases of urticaria, (3) to remove the nebula and improve eyesight, and (4) to relieve spasms in infantile convulsions and tetanus

蝉衣 [chán yī]

same as 蝉蜕 [chán tuì]

升麻 [shēng má]

***Rhizoma Cimicifugae*; Largetrifoliolious Bugbane Rhizome:** dried rhizome of *Cimicifuga heracleifolia* Kom., *Cimicifuga dahurica* (Turcz.) Maxim. or *Cimicifuga foetida* L. (family Ranunculaceae), used (1) to promote eruption in the treatment of measles, (2) to clear heat and counteract toxins for treating sore throat and stomatitis, and (3) to restore normal position of the viscera in cases of splanchnoptosis

淡豆豉 [dàn dòu chǐ]

***Semen Sojae Preparatum*; Fermented Soybean:** fermented preparation of the ripe seed of *Glycine max* (L.) Merr. (family Leguminosae), used in the early stage of febrile diseases to relieve exterior syndromes/patterns and in the late stage to relieve fidgetiness and insomnia

西河柳 [xī hé liǔ]

***Cacumen Tamaricis*; Chinese Tamarisk Twig:** dried young green twig of *Tamarix chinensis* Lour. (familyTamaricaceae), used in cases of measles to promote eruption, and also in cases of rheumatism to relieve arthralgia

浮萍 [fú píng]

***Herba Spirodelae*; Common Ducksmeat Herb:** dried entire plant of *Spirodela polyrrhiza* (L.) Schneid. (family Lemnaceae), used (1) to promote eruption in cases of measles, (2) to relieve itching in cases of urticaria, and (3) to induce diuresis in cases of edema

常山 [cháng shān]

***Radix Dichroae*; Antifeverile Dichroa Root:** dried root of *Dichroa febrifuga* Lour. (family Saxifragaceae), used for treating malaria

止咳化痰平喘药
Antitussives, Expectorants and Antiasthmatics

温化寒痰药
Medicinals/Drugs for Resolving Cold-phlegm

半夏 [bàn xià]

***Rhizoma Pinelliae*; Pinellia Tuber:** dried tuber of *Pinellia ternata* (Thunb.) Breit. (family Araceae), used as (1) an expectorant for relieving cough with profuse thin phlegm, and (2) antiemetic for relieving nausea, vomiting and morning sickness

天南星 [tiān nán xīng]

***Rhizoma Arisaematis*; Jack-in-the-Pulpit Tuber:** dried tuber of *Arisaema erubescens* (Wall.) Schott., *Arisaema*

heterophyllum Bl. or *Arisaema amurense* Maxim. (family Araceae), used as (1) an expectorant for relieving cough with profuse phlegm, and (2) an anticonvulsive for relieving epilepsy or tetanus

胆南星 [dǎn nán xīng]
***Aridaema cum Bile*; Bile Arisaema:** finely powdered *Rhizoma Arisaematis* prepared with the bile of ox, sheep or pig, used to remove heat and resolve phlegm, and to calm the mind for treating cough with yellowish sticky expectoration, stroke, mania, and epilepsy

白芥子 [bái jiè zǐ]
***Semen Sinapis Albae*; White Mustard Seed:** ripe seed of *Brassica alba* (L.) Boiss. (family Cruciferae), used to warm the lung and resolve phlegm for treating cough with profuse expectoration and stuffy feeling in the chest, and also in cases of cold abscess and pleural fluid retention

白附子 [bái fù zǐ]
***Rhizoma Typhonii*; Giant Typhonium Tuber:** dried tuber of *Typhonium giganteum* Engl. (family Araceae), used as (1) an expectorant for relieving cough with profuse phlegm, and (2) an anticonvulsive for relieving epilepsy or tetanus

旋覆花 [xuán fù huā]
***Flos Inulae*; Inula Flower:** dried flower-head of *Inula japonica* Thunb. or *Inula britannica* L. (family Compositae), used as (1) an expectorant for relieving cough and dyspnea with excessive phlegm, and (2) an antiemetic for relieving belching and vomiting

金沸草 [jīn fèi cǎo]
***Herba Inulae*; Inula Herb:** dried aerial part of *Inula japonica* Thunb. or *Inula britannica* L. (family Compositae), used as an expectorant for relieving cough and dyspnea with excessive phlegm

紫菀 [zǐ wǎn]
***Radix Asteris*; Tartarian Aster Root:** dried root and rhizome of *Aster tataricus* L.f. (family Compositae), used as an expectorant and antitussive for relieving cough with profuse phlegm as well as phthisical cough

桔梗 [jié gěng]
***Radix Platycodi*; Platycodon Root:** dried root of *Platycodon grandiflorum* (Jacq.) A.DC. (family Campanulaceae), used to resolve phlegm, soothe the throat and evacuate pus for treating cough with much phlegm, lung abscess with purulent expectoration, painful swelling of the throat and hoarse voice

清化热痰药
Medicinals/Drugs for Resolving Heat-phlegm

瓜蒌 [guā lóu]
***Fructus Trichosanthis*; Snakegourd Fruit:** dried ripe fruit of *Trichosanthes kirilowii* Maxim. or *Trichosanthesrosthornii* Harms (family Cucurbitaceae), used (1) to clear heat and resolve phlegm for relieving cough and dyspnea caused by heat-phlegm, (2) to soothe the chest in cases of angina pectoris, (3) to reduce swelling in the treatment of lung abscess, appendicitis and mastitis, and (4) to moisten the intestines for opening the bowels

天花粉 [tiān huā fěn]

***Radix Trichosanthis*; Snake-gourd Root:** dried root of *Trichosanthes kirilowii* Maxim. or *Trichosanthes rosthornii* Harms (family Cucurbitaceae), used to clear heat, promote fluid production, moisten the lung, counteract toxins and reduce swelling for relieving thirst in cases of febrile diseases and diabetes, and treating boils, sores and abscesses

天竺黄 [tiān zhú huáng]

***Concretio Silicea Bambusae*; Tabashir:** dried masses of secretion in the stem of *Bambusatextilis* McClure or *Schizostachyum chinense* Rendle (family Gramineae), used to clear heat and cleanse phlegm from the heart for the treatment of impaired consciousness in cases of high fever and stroke, and also for the treatment of infantile convulsions

竹茹 [zhú rú]

***Caulis Bambusae in Taeniam*; Bamboo Shavings:** dried shavings of the stem of *Bambusa tuldoides* Munro, *Sinocalamus beecheyanus* (Munro) McClure var. *pubescens* P.F. Li or *Phyllostachys nigra* var. *henonis* Stapf (family Gramineae), used to clear heat, resolve phlegm, induce tranquilization and arrest vomiting for relieving cough or insomnia due to phlegm-heat, and vomiting due to stomach heat

南沙参 [nán shā shēn]

***Radix Adenophorae*; Fourleaf Ladybell Root:** dried root of *Adenophora tetraphylla* (Thunb.) Fisch. or *Adenophora stricta* Miq. (family Campanulaceae), used to nourish yin, clear the lung, resolve phlegm and replenish *qi* for relieving cough in cases of lung yin deficiency, and deficiency of *qi* and fluid in the late stage of a febrile disease

海藻 [hǎi zǎo]

***Sargassum*; Seaweed:** dried thallus of seaweed, *Sargassum pallidum* (Turn.) C. Ag. or *Sargassum fusiforme* (Harv.) Setch. (family Sargassaceae), used (1) to eliminate phlegm and soften hard masses for treating goiter, scrofula and swelling of the testis, and (2) to induce diuresis for treating edema

昆布 [kūn bù]

***Thallus Laminariae seu Eckloniae*; Kelp or Tangle:** dried thallus of Japanese sea tangle, *Laminaria japonica* Aresch. or *Ecklonia kurome* Okam. (family Laminariaceae), used together with seaweed to eliminate phlegm, soften hard masses and induce diuresis

前胡 [qián hú]

***Radix Peucedani*; Hogfennel Root:** dried root of *Peucedanum praeruptorum* Dunn or *Peucedanum decursivum* Maxim. (family Umbelliferae), used to check the adverse up-flow of *qi*, resolve phlegm for relieving cough and dyspnea with copious or yellow sticky expectoration

山慈菇 [shān cí gū]

***Pseudobulbus Cremastrae seu Pleiones*; Appendiculate Cremastra Pseudobulb; Common Pleione Pseudobulb:** dried ripe pseudobulb of *Cremastra appendiculata* (D. Don) Makino, *Pleione bulbocodioides* (Franch.) Rolfe or *Pleione yunnanensis* Rolfe (family Orchidaceae), used to clear heat for treating boils, sores, scrofula, and snake bite

黄药子 [huáng yào zǐ]
***Rhizoma Dioscoreae Bulbiferae*; Airpotato Yam:** dried rhizome of *Dioscorea bulbifera* L. (family Dioscoreaceae), used as a blood-cooling hemostatic for arresting various kinds of bleeding, and to counteract toxins for treating boils and sores

金礞石 [jīn méng shí]
***Lapis Micae Aureus*; Mica-schist:** gold-colored mineral mica-schist, usually made into pills or powders to purge phlegm and arrest convulsions in the treatment of cough and dyspnea with sticky sputum, epilepsy and mania

止咳药 Antitussives

苦杏仁 [kǔ xìng rén]
***Semen Armeniacae Amarum*; Bitter Apricot Seed:** dried ripe seed or kernel of *Prunus armeniaca* L.var. *ansu* Maxim., *Prunus sibirica* L., *Prunus mandshurica* (Maxim.) Koehne or *Prunus armeniaca* L. (family Rosaceae), used to relieve cough and dyspnea with profuse expectoration, and also to relieve constipation

白前 [bái qián]
***Rhizoma Cynanchi Stauntonii*; Willowleaf Swallowwort Rhizome:** dried rhizome and root of *Cynanchum stauntonii* (Decne.) Schltr. ex Lévl. or *Cynanchum glaucescens* (Decne.) Hand.-Mazz. (family Asclepiadaceae), used for treating cough and dyspnea with profuse phlegm

枇杷叶 [pí pa yè]
***Folium Eriobotryae*; Loquat Leaf:** dried leaf of *Eriobotrya japonica* (Thunb.) Lindl. (family Rosaceae), used (1) to clear the lung and resolve phlegm to arrest coughing in cases of lung heat, and (2) to arrest vomiting in cases of stomach heat

白果 [bái guǒ]
***Semen Ginkgo*; Ginkgo Seed:** dried ripe seed of maiden-hair tree, *Ginkgo biloba* L. (family Ginkgoaceae), used (1) as an antitussive and anti-asthmatic for treating prolonged cough or asthma with profuse expectoration, (2) to suppress leukorrhagia, and (3) to reduce urination in cases of enuresis and frequent micturition

罗汉果 [luó hàn guǒ]
***Fructus Momordicae*; Grosvenor Momordica Fruit:** dried fruit of *Momordica grosvenori* Swingle (family Cucurbitaceae), used (1) to clear heat and moisten the lung for treating dry cough, sore throat and hoarseness of voice due to heat in the lung, and (2) to relax the bowels for treating constipation

沙棘 [shā jí]
***Fructus Hippophae*; Seabuckthorn Fruit:** dried ripe fruit of *Hippophae rhamnoides* L. (family Elaeagnaceae), used (1) as an antitussive and expectorant for treating cough with profuse phlegm, (2) as a stomachic for dyspepsia and abdominal pain due to undigested food, and (3) to promote blood circulation and remove stasis for treating traumatic wounds and amenorrhea

款冬花 [kuǎn dōng huā]
***Flos Farfarae*; Common Coltsfoot Flower:** dried flower-bud of *Tussilago farfara* L. (family Compositae), used for treating

chronic cough with profuse expectoration and hemoptysis in cases of consumptive diseases

百部 [bǎi bù]

***Radix Stemonae*; Stemona Root:** steamed and dried tuberous root of *Stemona sessilifolia* (Miq.) Miq., *Stemona japonica* (Bl.) Miq. or *Stemona tuberosa* Lour. (family Stemonaceae), used to moisten the lung and relieve acute and chronic cough, and externally to kill trichomonads and lice

浙贝母 [zhè bèi mǔ]

***Bulbus Fritillariae Thunbergii*; Thunbery Fritillary Bulb:** dried bulb of *Fritillaria thunbergii* Miq. (family Liliaceae), used (1) to clear heat and resolve phlegm in cases of cough with thick expectoration, and (2) to reduce nodulation in cases of mastitis and scrofula

伊贝母 [yī bèi mǔ]

***Bulbus Fritillariae Pallidiflorae*; Sinkiang Fritillary Bulb:** dried bulb of *Fritillaria walujewii* Regel or *Fritillaria pallidiflora* Schrenk (family Liliaceae), used as thunbery fritillary bulb (浙贝母 [zhè bèi mǔ])

川贝母 [chuān bèi mǔ]

***Bulbus Fritillarie Cirrhosae*; Tendrilleaf Fritillary Bulb:** dried bulb of *Fritillaria cirrhosa* D. Don, *Fritillariaunibracteata* Hsiao et K.C. Hsia, *Fritillaria przewalskii* Maxim. or *Fritillaria delavayi* Franch. (family Liliaceae), used (1) to clear heat, resolve phlegm, moisten the lung for relieving dry cough due to lung heat and chronic cough with bloody sputum in cases of phthisis, and (2) to dissipate nodulation for treating boils, sores, mastitis and lung abscess

平贝母 [píng bèi mǔ]

***Bulbus Fritillarie Ussuriensis*; Ussuri Fritillary Bulb:** dried bulb of *Fritillaria ussuriensis* Maxim. (family Liliaceae), used to clear the lung of heat, arrest cough and resolve phlegm for treating cough with expectoration of sticky and blood-streaked sputum

罂粟壳 [yīng sù qiào]

***Pericarpium Papaveris*; Poppy Capsule:** dried pericarp of the ripe fruit of *Papaver somniferum* L. (family Papaveraceae) with the seeds removed, used as an antitussive, antidiarrheal and analgesic for treating chronic cough, chronic diarrhea and abdominal pain

满山红 [mǎn shān hóng]

***Folium Rhododendri Daurici*; Dahurian Rhododendron Leaf:** dried leaf of *Rhododendron dauricum* L. (Family Ericaceae), used as an antitussive and expectorant for relieving acute and chronic bronchitis

百合 [bǎi hé]

***Bulbus Lilii*; Lily Bulb:** dried scale leaf of the bulb of *Lilium lancifolium* Thunb., *Lilium brownii* F.E. Brown var. *viridulum* Baker or *Lilium pumilum* DC. (family Liliaceae), used (1) to nourish lung yin and arrest cough in cases of consumptive diseases, and (2) to clear the heart and induce tranquilization for ameliorating insomnia and fidgetiness in the late stage of febrile diseases with residual heat

桑白皮 [sāng bái pí]
***Cortex Mori*; White Mulberry Root-bark:** dried root-bark, deprived of the external brown corky part, of *Morus alba* L. (familyMoraceae), used (1) to purge the lung and relieve dyspnea for treating lung heat with cough and dyspnea, and (2) to induce diuresis for treating edema

木蝴蝶 [mù hú dié]
***Semen Oroxyli*; Indian Trumpetflower Seed:** dried ripe seed of *Oroxylum indicum* (L.) Vent. (family Bignoniaceae), used to clear the lung of heat, and soothe the throat for treating cough, sore throat, and hoarseness of voice in cases of wind-heat contractions

暴马子皮 [bào mǎ zǐ pí]
***Cortex Syringae*; Manchurian Lilac Bark:** dried stem-bark of *Syringa reticulata* (Bl.) Hara var. *mandshurica* (Maxim.) Hara (family Oleaceae), used as an antipyretic, antitussive, and diuretic for treating acute or chronic bronchitis, asthma and cardiac edema

胖大海 [pàng dà hǎi]
***Semen Sterculiae Lychnophorae*; Boat-fruited Sterculia Seed:** dried ripe seed of *Sterculia lychnophora* Hance (family-Sterculiaceae), used (1) to clear the lung of heat for relieving sore throat, hoarseness and cough, and (2) to moisten the intestines for relieving constipation

平喘药 Antiasthmatics

洋金花 [yáng jīn huā]
***Flos Daturae*; Datura Flower:** dried flower of *Datura metel* L. (family Solanaceae), used to relieve cough, asthma, gastralgia, rheumatalgia, and epilepsy

葶苈子 [tíng lì zǐ]
***Semen Lepidii seu Descurainiae*; Pepperweed Seed; Tansy Mustard Seed:** dried ripe seed of *Lepidium apetalum* Willd. or Descurainia sophia (L.) Webb ex Prantl. (family Cruciferae), used (1) to purge the lung for relieving cough and dyspnea with excessive phlegm, and (2) to induce diuresis for treating edema

马兜铃 [mǎ dōu líng]
***Fructus Aristolochiae*; Dutchmanspipe Fruit:** dried ripe fruit of *Aristolochia contorta* Bge. or *Aristolochia debilis* Sieb. et Zucc. (family Aristolochiaceae), used (1) to clear the lung and resolve phlegm for relieving cough and dyspnea due to heat in the lung, and (2) to remove heat from the large intestine for treating hemorrhoids

紫苏子 [zǐ sū zǐ]
***Fructus Perillae*; Perilla Fruit:** dried ripe fruit of *Perilla frutescens* (L.) Britt. (family labiatiae), used as an antitussive, antiasthmatic, and expectorant for treating chronic bronchitis with thin white phlegm and stuffy feeling in the chest, and also as an aperient for relieving constipation, often simplified as 苏子 [sū zǐ]

苏子 [sū zǐ]
simplified term for 紫苏子 [zǐ sū zǐ]

天仙子 [tiān xiān zǐ]
***Semen Hyoscyami*; Henbane Seed:** dried seed of *Hyoscyamus niger* L. (family Solanaceae), used (1) to relieve cough and

labored breathing in cases of bronchial asthma, (2) to relieve gastralgia, and (3) to induce tranquilization

莨若子 [làng dàng zǐ]
same as 天仙子 [tiān xiān zǐ]

华山参 [huà shān shēn]
***Radix Physochlainae*; Funneled Physochlaina Root:** dried root of funnel-shaped physochlaina, *Physochlaina infundibularis* Kuang (family Solanaceae), used to relieve cough and dyspnea, and induce tranquilization

热参 [rè shēn]
same as 华山参 [huà shān shēn]

芸香草 [yún xiāng cǎo]
***Herba Cymbopogonis*; Lemongrass:** dried aerial part of *Cymbopogon distans* (Nees) A. Camus (family Gramineae), used to relieve cough and dyspnea

清热药
Heat-clearing Medicinals/Drugs

清热泻火药
Heat-clearing and Fire-purging Medicinal/Drugs

石膏 [shí gāo]
***Gypsum Fibrosum*; Gypsum:** soft mineral chiefly composed of hydrated calcium sulfate ($CaSO_4 \cdot 2H_2O$), used to clear heat and purge fire for relieving (1) high fever with fidgetiness and thirst in cases of warm diseases, (2) heat in the lung with cough and dyspnea, and (3) heat in the stomach with toothache and painful swelling of the gums, also externally to promote healing of wounds and ulcers

知母 [zhī mǔ]
***Rhizoma Anemarrhenae*; Common Anemarrhena Rhizome:** dried rhizome of *Anemarrhena asphodeloides* Bge. (family Liliaceae), used (1) to clear heat and purge fire for relieving high fever with dire thirst in cases of warm diseases, and cough due to heat in the lung, and (2) to nourish yin and moisten the intestines for treating low fever in cases of yin deficiency, diabetes, and constipation

决明子 [jué míng zǐ]
***Semen Cassiae*; Cassia Seed:** dried ripe seed of *Cassia obtusifolia* L. or *Cassia tora* L. (family Leguminosae), used (1) to clear the liver and brighten the eye for treating acute inflammation of the eye, (2) to moisten the intestines for relieving constipation, and nowadays (3) for reducing high blood pressure and blood cholesterol

青葙子 [qīng xiāng zǐ]
***Semen Celosiae*; Feather Cockscomb Seed:** dried ripe seed of *Celosia argentea* L. (family Amaranthaceae), used to clear the liver of heat, improve vision and remove nebula for treating acute conjunctivitis, blurred vision due to nebula, and dizziness due to hyperactivity of the liver

谷精草 [gǔ jīng cǎo]
***Flos Eriocauli*; Pipewort Flower:** dried flower-head with stalk of *Eriocaulon buergerianum* Koern. (family Eriocaulaceae), used to dispel wind and

heat for treating acute conjunctivitis, nebula, and headache

密蒙花 [mì méng huā]
***Flos Buddlejae*; Pale Butterfly-bush Flower:** dried flower-bud and inflorescenceof *Buddleja officinalis* Maxim. (family Loganiaceae), used to clear the liver of heat and remove nebula for treating acute conjunctivitis with lacrimation and photophobia, and blurred vision due to nebula

木贼 [mù zéi]
***Herba Equiseti Hiemalis*; Common Scouring Rush Herb:** dried aerial part of *Equisetum hiemale* L. (family Equisetaceae), used in ophthalmology for treating acute infections and removing nebula

淡竹叶 [dàn zhú yè]
***Herba Lophatheri*; Lophatherum Herb:** dried stem and leaf of *Lophatherum gracile* Brongn. (family Gramineae), used for relieving fidgetiness and thirst in cases of febrile diseases, and dysuria with painful urination, also called竹叶 [zhú yè]

竹叶 [zhú yè]
another name for *Herba Lophatheri*, Lophatherum Herb (淡竹叶 [dàn zhú yè])

莲子心 [lián zǐ xīn]
***Plumula Nelumbinis*; Lotus Plumule:** dried plumule and radicle in the ripe seed of *Nelumbo nucifera* Gartn. (family Nymphaeaceae), used (1) to clear the heart and induce tranquilization for treating delirium in cases of acute febrile diseases, insomnia, and nocturnal emission, and (2) to arrest seminal discharge and bleeding in cases of seminal emission and hematemesis due to blood heat

芦根 [lú gēn]
***Rhizoma Phragmitis*; Reed Rhizome:** fresh or dried rhizome of *Phragmites communis* (L.) Trin. (family Gramineae), used (1) to clear heat and promote fluid production in cases of high fever with thirst, (2) to evacuate pus for treating lung abscess, and (3) to arrest vomiting in cases of stomach heat

罗布麻叶 [luó bù má yè]
***Folium Apocyni Veneti*; Dogbane Leaf:** dried leaf of red dogbane, *Apocynum venetum* L. (family Apocynaceae), used for suppressing hyperactive liver yang, clearing heat and inducing diuresis

夏枯草 [xià kū cǎo]
***Spica Prunellae*; Common Selfheal Fruit-Spike:** dried fruit-spike of *Prunella vulgaris* L. (family Labiatae), used (1) to clear liver fire for treating acute conjunctivitis, headache, and dizziness, and (2) to dissipate nodulation for treating acute mastitis, mumps, scrofula, and goiter

清热凉血药
Heat-clearing and Blood-cooling Medicinals/Drugs

犀角 [xī jiǎo]
***Cornu Rhinoceri*; Rhinoceros Horn:** horn of Asiatic rhinoceros, *Rhinoceros unicornis* L., *Rhinoceros sondaicus* Desmarest or *Rhinoceros sumatrensis* Cuvier (family Rhinocerotidae), used in ancient times for treating febrile diseases with heat entering

the nutrient and blood aspects manifested by delirium, maculation and high fever, and arresting bleeding by clearing heat and cooling blood, but nowadays replaced by buffalo horn

水牛角 [shuǐ niú jiǎo]
***Cornu Bubali*; Buffalo Horn:** horn of *Bubalus bubalis* L. (family Bovidae), used similarly to rhinoceros horn (犀角 [xī jiǎo])

地黄 [dì huáng]
***Radix Rehmanniae*; Rehmannia Root:** fresh or dried tuberous root of *Rehmannia glutinosa* Libosch (family Scrophulariaceae), used to clear heat, cool blood, nourish yin and promote fluid production for the treatment of heat entering the nutrient and blood aspects in cases of febrile diseases, bleeding due to blood heat, and thirst in cases of diabetes

生地 [shēng dì]
another name for unprocessed rehmannia root (地黄 [dì huáng])

赤芍 [chì sháo]
***Radix Paeoniae Rubra*; Red Peony Root:** dried root of *Paeonia lactiflora* Pall. or *Paeonia veitchii* Lynch (family Ranunculaceae), used to remove stagnant blood and dispel heat from the blood for treating epidemic febrile diseases with eruptions, pain due to blood stasis, dysmenorrhea, amenorrhea, traumatic injuries, boils and sores

牡丹皮 [mǔ dān pí]
***Cortex Moutan*; Tree Peony Bark:** dried root-bark of *Paeonia suffruticosa* Andr. (family Ranunculaceae), used (1) to clear heat and cool the blood for treating febrile diseases with eruptions and bleeding, and (2) to activate blood flow and eliminate stasis for treating amenorrhea, dysmenorrhea, traumatic injuries, boils, sores and appendicitis

玄参 [xuán shēn]
***Radix Scrophulariae*; Figwort Root:** dried root of *Scrophularia ningpoensis* Hemsl. (family Scrophulariaceae), used to clear heat, cool the blood, replenish yin and counteract toxins for the treatment of warm disease at the nutrient level with high fever and delirium or skin eruption, also for treating inflammation of the throat, boils and sores

紫草 [zǐ cǎo]
***Radix Arnebiae seu Lithospermi*; Arnebia Root or Gromwell Root:** dried root of *Arnebia euchroma* (Royle) Johnst. or*Lithospermum erythrorhizon* Sieb. et Zucc. (family Boraginaceae), used for promoting eruption in cases of measles, and externally for treating burns, frostbite, dermatitis and eczema

地骨皮 [dì gǔ pí]
***Cortex Lycii*; Chinese Wolfberry Bark:** dried root-bark of *Lycium chinense* Mill. or *Lycium barbarum* L. (family Solanaceae), used for treating chronic fever and hemoptysis in cases of consumptive diseases, and also for diabetes

银柴胡 [yín chái hú]
***Radix Stellariae*; Starwort Root:** dried root of *Stellaria dichotoma* L. var. *lanceolata* Bge. (family Caryophyllaceae), used for clearing heat of deficiency type

and malnutritional fever in children

青蒿 [qīng hāo]
***Herba Artemisiae Annuae*; Sweet Wormwood Herb:** dried aerial part of *Artemisia annua* L. (family Compositae), used to clear heat of deficiency type for relieving consumptive fever and also for combating malaria

白薇 [bái wēi]
***Radix Cynanchi Atrati*; Blackened Swallowwort Root:** dried root and rhizome of *Cynanchum atratum* Bge. or *Cynanchum versicolor* Bge. (family Asclepiadaceae), used (1) to clear heat and cool blood for fever in cases of consumptive diseases or cases due to yin deficiency, (2) to induce diuresis in cases of heat stranguria and bloody stranguria, and (3) to counteract toxins for boils and sores

白茅根 [bái máo gēn]
***Rhizoma Imperatae*; Lalang Grass Rhizome:** dried rhizome of *Imperata cylindrica* Beauv. var. *major* (Nees) C.E. Hubb. (family Gramineae), used to cool the blood, arrest bleeding, clear heat and induce diuresis for treating epistaxis and hematuria due to blood heat, edema, jaundice, and stranguria associated with heat

清热燥湿药

Heat-clearing and Dampness-drying Medicinals/Drugs

黄芩 [huáng qín]
***Radix Scutellariae*; Baical Skullcap Root:** dried root of *Scutellaria baicalensis* Georgi (family Labiatae), used (1) to clear heat and dry dampness for treating dampness-warmth and dampness-heat diseases, (2) to clear the lung of heat for relieving cough in cases of lung heat, (3) to purge fire and counteract toxins for treating boils, sores, painful swelling of the throat, (4) to cool blood for arresting hematemesis, epistaxis, abnormal uterine bleeding, and (5) to prevent miscarriage in cases of threatened abortion

黄连 [huáng lián]
***Rhizoma Coptidis*; Golden Thread:** dried rhizome of *Coptis chinensis* Franch., *Coptis deltoidea* C.Y. Cheng et Hsiao or *Coptis teeta* Wall. (family Ranunculaceae), used to clear heat, dry dampness, purge fire and counteract toxins for treating dysentery, high fever with restlessness, boils, sores, abscess, and externally for relieving eczema

黄柏 [huáng bǎi]
***Cortex Phellodendri*; Amur Cork-tree:** dried bark of Chinese corktree, *Phellodendron chinense* Schneid. or Amur Corktree, *Phellodendron amurense* Rupr. (family Rutaceae), used (1) to clear heat and dry dampness in cases of acute dysentery, jaundice, morbid leukorrhea, and heat stranguria, (2) to purge fire and counteract toxins for treating boils, sores and ulcers, and (3) to relieve fever in cases of yin deficiency with night sweats

三颗针 [sān kē zhēn]
***Radix Berberidis*; Barberry Root:** dried root of *Berberis soulieana* Schneid, *Berberis wilsonae* Hemsl., *Berberis poiretii* Schneid. or *Berberis vernae* Schneid. (family Berberidaceae), used in a

similar way to golden thread (黄连 [huáng lián])

龙胆 [lóng dǎn]
***Radix Gentianae*; Chinese Gentian:** dried root and rhizome of *Gentiana manshurica* Kitag., *Gentiana scabra* Bge., *Gentiana triflora* Pall. or *Gentiana ringescens* Franch. (family Gentianaceae), used to clear heat, dry dampness, and purge the liver and gallbladder of fire for treating (1) dampness-heat in the liver and gallbladder with morbid leukorrhea, jaundice, or eczema, (2) liver fire with headache, hypochondriac pain, deafness, or convulsions

龙胆草 [lóng dǎn cǎo]
the full name of Chinese gentian (龙胆 [lóng dǎn])

苦参 [kǔ shēn]
***Radix Sophorae Flavescentis*; Light-yellow Sophora Root:** dried root of *Sophora flavescens* Ait. (family Leguminosae), used to clear heat, dry dampness, kill parasitic worms and induce diuresis for treating acute dysentery, jaundice, morbid leucorrhoea, and externally for treating eczema and scabies

秦皮 [qín pí]
***Cortex Fraxini*; Ash Bark:** dried branch bark or trunk bark of *Fraxinus rhynchophylla* Hance, *Fraxinus chinensis* Roxb., or *Fraxinus stylosa* Lingelsh. (family Oleaceae), used for treating acute dysentery and inflammation of the eye

胡黄连 [hú huáng lián]
***Rhizoma Picrorhizae*; Figwortflower Picrorhiza Rhizome:** dried rhizome of *Picrorhiza scrophulariiflora* Pennell (family Scrophulariaceae), used (1) to remove dampness-heat for treating acute dysentery and jaundice, and (2) to relieve consumptive fever in cases of phthisis and infantile malnutrition

鸡骨草 [jī gǔ cǎo]
***Herba Abri*; Canton Love-pea Vine:** dried entire plant of *Abrus cantoniensis* Hance (family Leguminosae), used to clear heat, remove dampness, soothe the liver and alleviate pain for treating hepatitis and epigastric pain

白鲜皮 [bái xiān pí]
***Cortex Dictamni*; Dittany Root-bark:** dried root-bark of *Dictamnus dasycarpus* Turcz. (family Rutaceae), used internally or externally for treating skin diseases with excessive secretion and itching

鸦胆子 [yā dǎn zǐ]
***Fructus Bruceae*; Java Brucea Fruit:** dried ripe fruit of *Brucea javanica* (L.) Merr. (family Simarubaceae), used for treating amebic dysentery and malaria, also used externally for treating warts, clavus and trichomonas vaginitis

白头翁 [bái tóu wēng]
***Radix Pulsatillae*; Chinese Pulsatilla Root:** dried root of *Pulsatilla chinensis* (Bge.) Regel (family Ranunculaceae), used for treating bacterial and amebic dysentery, and externally for treating trichomonas vaginitis

椿皮 [chūn pí]
***Cortex Ailanthi*; Tree-of-heaven Bark:**

dried root bark or stem bark of *Ailanthus altissima* (Mill.) Swingle (family Simarubaceae), used for treating diarrhea, chronic dysentery, abnormal uterine bleeding and leukorrhea

椿根白皮 [chūn gēn bái pí]
same as 椿皮 [chūn pí]

茵陈 [yīn chén]
***Herba Artemisiae Scopariae*; Virgate Wormwood Herb:** dried young shoot or flowering top of *Artemisia scoparia* Waldst. et Kit. or *Artemisia capillaris* Thunb. (family Compositae), used to eliminate dampness-heat in the liver and gallbladder for treating jaundice and also for treating eczema

茵陈蒿 [yīn chén hāo]
same as 茵陈 [yīn chén]

垂盆草 [chuí pén cǎo]
***Herba Sedi*; Stringy Stonecrop Herb:** fresh or dried entire plant of *Sedum sarmentosum* Bunge (family Crassulaceae), used to remove dampness-heat and counteract toxins for treating acute and chronic hepatitis, jaundice, boils and sores

土茯苓 [tǔ fú líng]
***Rhizoma Smilacis Glabrae*; Glabrous Greenbrier Rhizome:** dried rhizome of *Smilax glabra* Roxb. (family Libiaceae), used to counteract toxins and eliminate dampness for treating syphilis, morbid leukorrhea, and heat stranguria

马齿苋 [mǎ chǐ xiàn]
***Herba Portulacae*; Purslane Herb:** dried aerial part of *Portulaca oleracea* L. (family Portulacaceae), used for treating dysentery with bloody stools, and externally for treating boils and sores, eczema, erysipelas, and snake- and insect-bite

地锦草 [dì jǐn cǎo]
***Herba Euphorbiae Humifusae*; Creeping Euphorhia:** dried whole plant of *Euphorbia humifusa* Willd. or *Euphorbia maculate* L. (family Euphorbiaccae), used to remove toxic heat and arrest bleeding for treating dysentery, boils, hemoptysis, hematuria, and abnormal uterine bleeding

黄栌 [huáng lú]
***Folium et Ramulus Cotini*; Smoketree Twig:** dried leaf and branch of *Cotinus coggygria* Scop. var. *cinera* Engl. (familyAnacardiaceae), used for treating hepatitis with jaundice, dysentery, and eczema with pruritus

拳参 [quán shēn]
***Rhizoma Bistortae*; Bistort Rhizome:** dried rhizome of *Polygonum bistorta* L. (family Polygonaceae), used (1) to clear heat and counteract toxins for treating dysentery, boils and sores, (2) to arrest bleeding for hematemesis, epistaxis, hemorrhoidal bleeding, and (3) externally for treating snake-bite

虎杖 [hǔ zhàng]
***Rhizoma Polygoni Cuspidati*; Giant Knotweed Rhizome:** dried rhizome of giant or Japanese knotweed, *Polygonum cuspidatum* Sieb. et Zucc. (family Polygonaceae), used (1) to clear heat, counteract toxins, and promote bile flow in cases of hepatitis, jaundice, dysentery, bladder dampness-heat, and lung heat

with cough, (2) to activate blood flow and remove stasis for treating amenorrhea and traumatic injuries, and (3) externally for treating burns and venomous snake-bite

翻白草 [fān bái cǎo]
***Herba Potentillae Discoloris*; Diverse-color Cinquefoil:** dried entire plant of *Potentilla discolor* Bge. (family Rosaceae), used for treating enteritis, dysentery, pharyngitis, and gastro-intestinal bleeding

栀子 [zhī zǐ]
***Fructus Gardeniae*; Cape-jasmine Fruit:** dried ripe fruit of *Gardenia jasminoides* Ellis (family Rubiaceae), used (1) to purge fire and calm the mind in cases of fever with fidgetiness and insomnia, (2) to clear dampness-heat from the liver and gallbladder in cases of acute icteric hepatitis, and to cool blood and counteract toxins in cases of bleeding, sores and ulcers

清热解毒药
Heat-clearing and Toxin-counteracting Medicinals / Drugs

金银花 [jīn yín huā]
***Flos Lonicerae*; Honeysuckle Flower:** dried flower-bud of *Lonicera japonica* Thunb., *Lonicera hypoglauca* Miq., *Lonicera confusa* DC. or *Lonicera dasystyla* Rehd. (family Caprifoliaceae), used to clear heat, counteract toxins, and disperse wind-heat for treating (1) boils, sores and abscesses, (2) wind-heat contractions and warm diseases at the early stage, and (3) toxin-heat dysentery

银花 [yín huā]
another name for *Flos Lonicerae* or Honeysuckle Flower (金银花 [jīn yín huā])

忍冬藤 [rěn dōng téng]
***Caulis Lonicerae*; Honeysuckle Stem:** dried stem and branch of *Lonicera japonica* Thunb. (family Caprifoliaceae), with actions similar to those of honeysuckle flower (金银花 [jīn yín huā]), but more frequently used to clear heat from the meridians/channels and collaterals for treating acute rheumatic arthritis

金银藤 [jīn yín téng]
another name for *Caulis Lonicerae* or Honeysuckle Stem (忍冬藤 [rěn dōng téng])

连翘 [lián qiào]
***Fructus Forsythiae*; Weeping Forsythia Fruit:** dried fruit of weeping forsythia, *Forsythia suspensa* (Thunb.) Vahl (family Oleaceae), often used together with honeysuckle flower (1) to clear heat, counteract toxins and dissipate nodulation in cases of boils, sores and abscesses, and (2) to disperse wind-heat for treating wind-heat contractions and warm diseases at the early stage

板蓝根 [bǎn lán gēn]
***Radix Isatidis*; Isatis Root:** dried root of *Isatis indigotica* Fort. (family Cruciferae), used to clear heat, counteract toxins and cool the blood in the treatment of warm diseases with fever, headache and sore throat, eruptive epidemic diseases, mumps, boils, sores, and erysipelas

大青叶 [dà qīng yè]
***Folium Isatidis*; Dyers Woad Leaf:** dried leaf of *Isatis indigotica* Fort. (family Cruciferae), used to clear heat, counteract toxins and cool the blood for treating warm diseases affecting the nutrient and blood aspects with eruption, and also for treating mumps, painful swollen throat, and erysipelas

蓼大青叶 [liǎo dà qīng yè]
***Folium Polygoni Tinctorii*; Indigoplant Leaf:** dried leaf of *Polygonumtinctorium* Ait. (family Polygonaceae), used as dyers woad leaf (大青叶 [dà qīng yè]) with stronger effect

青黛 [qīng dài]
***Indigo Naturalis*; Natural Indigo:** deep blue powder prepared from the leaves of *Baphicacanthus cusia* (Nees) Bremek. (family Acanthaceae), *Polygonum tinctorium* Ait. (family Polygonaceae) or *Isatisindigotica* Fort. (family Cruciferae), used chiefly for treating eruptive epidemic diseases and high fever in children, and externally for treating oral ulcers, mumps, and skin infections

蒲公英 [pú gōng yīng]
***Herba Taraxaci*; Dandelion:** dried entire plant of *Taraxacum mongolicum* Hand.-Mazz., *Taraxacum sinicum* Kitag. or several other *Taraxacum*species (family Compositae), used for treating boils, sores and other pyogenic infections

野菊花 [yě jú huā]
***Flos Chrysanthemi Indici*; Wild Chrysanthemum Flower:** dried flower-head of *Chrysanthemum indicum* L. (family Compositae), used to clear heat and counteract toxins for treating boils, sores, carbuncles, erysipelas, acute conjunctivitis, and also externally for treating eczema and skin itching

紫花地丁 [zǐ huā dì dīng]
***Herba Violae*; Tokyo Violet Herb:** the dried herb of *Viola yedoensis* Makino (family Violaceae), used to clear heat and counteract toxins for treating acute pyogenic infections such as boils, sores and abscesses, and also for treating venomous snake-bite

鱼腥草 [yú xīng cǎo]
***Herba Houttuyniae*; Heartleaf Houttuynia Herb:** dried aerial part of *Houttuynia cordata* Thunb. (family Saururaceae), used to clear heat, counteract toxins, evacuate pus and relieve stranguria for treating lung abscesses with purulent expectoration, cough in cases of lung heat, boils and sores, dampness-heat stranguria, and acute dysentery

重楼 [chóng lóu]
***Rhizoma Paridis*; Paris Rhizome:** dried rhizome of *Paris polyphylla* Smith var. *yunnanensis* (Franch.) Hand.-Mazz. or *Paris polyphylla* Smith var. *chinensis* (Franch.) Hara (family Liliaceae), used for treating acute pyogenic inflammations, and also used as an anticonvulsive in the treatment of infantile convulsion

蚤休 [zǎo xiū]
another name for *Rhizoma Paridis*, Paris Rhizome (重楼 [chóng lóu])

败酱草 [bài jiàng cǎo]
Herba Patriniae; **Patrinia:** dried entire plant of *Patrinia scabiosaefolia* Fisch. or *Patrinia villosa* Juss. (family Valerianaceae), used for clearing heat, counteracting toxins, evacuating pus, dispelling blood stasis and relieving pain in the treatment of lung abscess, acute appendicitis, boils, sores, ulcers, and postpartum abdominal pain

鸭跖草 [yā zhí cǎo]
Herba Commelinae; **Common Dayflower Herb:** dried aerial part of *Commelina communis* L. (family Commelianceae), used (1) to clear heat and counteract toxins for treating warm diseases, boils, sores, and painful swelling of the throat, and (2) to induce diuresis for treating edema and heat stranguria

穿心莲 [chuān xīn lián]
Herba Andrographitis; **Common Andrographis Herb:** dried aerial part of *Andrographis paniculata* (Burm. f.) Nees (family Acanthaceae), used to clear heat, counteract toxins, dry dampness and reduce swelling for treating wind-heat contractions, warm diseases at the early stage, heat in the lung with cough and dyspnea, lung abscess, dampness-heat dysentery, and painful swelling of the throat

白花蛇舌草 [bái huā shé shé cǎo]
Herba Oldenlandiae; **Oldenlandia:** dried entire plant of *Oldenlandia diffusa* (Willd.) Roxb., *Oldenlandia corymbosa* L. and other related species (family Rubiaceae), used to clear heat, counteract toxins, remove dampness, and relieve stranguria for treating boils, sores, abscesses, venomous snake bite, and heat stranguria

漏芦 [lòu lú]
Radix Rhapontici; **Uniflower Swisscentaury Root:** dried root of *Rhaponticum uniflorum* (L.) DC. (family Compositae), used (1) to clear heat and counteract toxins for treating mastitis, and (2) to promote lactation in cases of galactostasis

龙葵 [lóng kuí]
Herba Solani Nigri; **Black Nightshade Herb:** dried aerial part of *Solanum nigrum* L. (family Solanaceae), used for treating cancer of the stomach and esophagus

半枝莲 [bàn zhī lián]
Herba Scutellariae Barbatae; **Barbated Skullcap Herb:** dried entire plant of *Scutellaria barbata* D. Don (family Labiatae), used for treating boils and sores, cirrhosis of the liver with ascites, and snake- and insect-bite

半边莲 [bàn biān lián]
Herba Lobeliae Chinensis; **Chinese Lobelia Herb:** dried entire plant of *Lobelia chinensis* Lour. (family Campanulaceae), used to clear heat, counteract toxins and induce diuresis for treating anasarca, ascites, boils, and snake- and insect-bite

白蔹 [bái liǎn]
Radix Ampelopsis; **Japanese Ampelopsis Root:** dried root tuber of *Ampelopsis Japonica* (Thunb.) Makino (family Vitaceae), used to remove toxic heat and reduce nodules for treating carbuncles, deep-rooted boils, scrofula, scalds and burns

土牛膝 [tǔ niú xī]
***Radix Achyranthis Asperae*; Native Achyranthes Root:** dried root of *Achyranthes aspera* L. and other related species (family Amaranthaceae), used for treating sore throat and diphtheria

山豆根 [shān dòu gēn]
***Radix Sophorae Tonkinensis*; Vietnamese Sophora Root:** dried root and rhizome of *Sophora tonkinensis* Gapnep. (family Leguminosae), used for treating sore throat and gingivitis

广豆根 [guǎng dòu gēn]
same as 山豆根 [shān dòu gēn]

北豆根 [běi dòu gēn]
***Rhizoma Menispermi*; Asiatic Moonseed Rhizome:** dried rhizome of *Menispermum dauricum* DC. (family Menispermaceae), used in a similar way to Vietnamese sophora root (山豆根 [shān dòu gēn])

射干 [shè gān]
***Rhizoma Belamcandae*; Blackberrylily Rhizome:** dried rhizome of *Belamcanda chinensis* (L.) DC. (family Iridaceae), used in the relief of painful swelling of the throat, cough and dyspnea with profuse expectoration

马勃 [mǎ bó]
***Lasiosphaera seu Calvatia*; Puff-ball:** dried sporophore of *Lasiosphaera fenzlii* Reich., *Calvatia gigantea* (Batsch ex Pers.) Lloyd or *Calvatia lilacina* (Mont. et Berk.) Lloyd (family Lycoperdaceae), used to clear heat, counteract toxins, soothe the throat and arrest bleeding for relieving painful swelling of the throat and hoarseness of voice in cases of wind-heat contractions or fire in the lung, and also for treating epistaxis, hematemesis and traumatic bleeding

青果 [qīng guǒ]
***Fructus Canarii*; Chinese White Olive:** dried ripe fruit of *Canarium album* Raeusch. (family Burseraceae), used for relieving sore throat and hoarseness in phonation

锦灯笼 [jǐn dēng lóng]
***Calyx seu Fructus Physalis*; Franchet Groundcherry Fruit:** dried persistent calyx or with the fruit of winter cherry, *Physalis alkekengi* L. var. franchetii (Mast.) Makino (family Solanaceae), used chiefly for treating sore throat

酸浆 [suān jiāng]
another name for *Calyx seu Fructus Physalis*, Franchet Groundcherry Fruit (锦灯笼 [jǐn dēng lóng])

葎草 [lǜ cǎo]
***Herba Humuli Scandentis*; Climbing Hop Herb:** dried aerial part of *Humulus scandens* (Lour.) Merr. (family Moraceae), used for treating enteritis, dysentery, acute urinary infection, and also as a tranquilizer in cases of insomnia

祛风湿药
Wind-dampness-dispelling Medicinals/Drugs (Antirheumatics)

羌活 [qiāng huó]
***Rhizoma seu Radix Notopterygii*; Notopterygium Rhizome or Root:** dried rhizome or root of *Notopterygium incisum*

Ting ex H.T. Chang or *Notopterygium forbesii* Boiss. (family Umbelliferae), used to dispel wind, cold and dampness for treating wind-cold contraction, and wind-cold-dampness (rheumatic or rheumatoid) arthralgia, especially that of the upper part of the body

独活 [dú huó]
***Radix Angelicae Pubescentis*; Doubleteeth Pubescent Angelica Root:** dried root of *Angelica pubescens* Maxim. f. biserrata Shan et Yuan (family Umbelliferae), used to dispel wind-dampness, relieve arthralgia and release the superficies for treating wind-cold-dampness (rheumatic or rheumatoid) arthralgia, especially that of the lower part of the body, and contraction of wind-cold with dampness

威灵仙 [wēi líng xiān]
***Radix Clematidis*; Chinese Clematis Root:** dried root and rhizome of *Clematis chinensis* Osbeck, *Clematis hexapetala* Pall. or *Clematis manshurica* Rupr. (family Ranunculaceae), used (1) to dispel wind-dampness and unblock the collateral meridian/channel for treating wind-dampness (rheumatic or rheumatoid) arthralgia, and (2) for dissolving fish bone stuck in the throat

川乌 [chuān wū]
***Radix Aconiti*; Mother Root of Common Monkshood:** dried parent root of *Aconitum carmichaeli* Debx. (family Ranunculaceae), used to dispel wind-dampess and disperse cold to relieve pain in cases of serious rheumatalgia, and cold pain in the abdomen. For internal use, the prepared root is usually employed.

制川乌 [zhì chuān wū]
***Radix Aconiti Preparata*; Prepared Mother Root of Common Monkshood:** cf *Radix Aconiti*, Mother Root of Common Monkshood (川乌 [chuān wū])

草乌 [cǎo wū]
***Radix Aconiti Kusnezoffii*; Wild Aconite Root, Kusnezoff Monkshood Root:** dried tuberous root of *Aconitum kusnezoffii* Reichb. (family Ranunculaceae), used in a similar way to mother root of common monkshood (川乌 [chuān wū]), but usually in smaller doses

秦艽 [qín jiāo]
***Radix Gentianae Macrophyllae*; Large-leaf Gentian Root:** dried root of *Gentiana macrophylla* Pall., *Gentiana straminea* Maxim.,*Gentiana dahurica* Fisch. (family Gentianaceae), used (1) to dispel wind-dampness, relieve arthralgia and clear consumptive heat for treating wind-dampness (rheumatic or rheumatoid) pain, and also for relieving fever in phthisis, and (2) to remove dampness-heat for treating jaundice

木瓜 [mù guā]
***Fructus Chaenomelis*; Common Flowering-quince Fruit:** dried ripe fruit of *Chaenomeles speciosa* (Sweet) Nakai (family Rosaceae), used (1) to soothe the tendons and unblock collateral meridians/channels for treating wind-dampness (rheumatoid) arthralgia with contracture, and (2) to dispel dampness and harmonize the stomach for treating vomiting and diarrhea with systremma

豨莶草 [xī xiān cǎo]
***Herba Siegesbeckiae*; Siegesbeckia**

Herb: dried aerial part of *Siegesbeckia orientalis* L., *Siegesbeckia pubescens* Makino or *Siegesbeckia glabrescens* Makino (family Compositae), used (1) to dispel wind-dampness and unblock collateral meridians/channels for treating wind-dampness (rheumatic or rheumatoid) arthralgia, and (2) to clear heat and counteract toxins for treating boils, sores, abscesses and ulcers

桑枝 [sāng zhī]
***Ramulus Mori*; Mulberry Twig:** dried young twig of *Morus alba* L. (family Moraceae), used as an antirheumatic for treating arthralgia and shoulder pain

海风藤 [hǎi fēng téng]
***Caulis Piperis Kadsurae*; Kadsura Pepper Stem:** dried stem of *Piper kadsura* (Choisy) Ohwi. (family Piperaceae), used to dispel wind-dampness, unblock the meridian/channel, disperse cold and alleviate pain in cases of rheumatalgia of joints with muscular contracture and traumatic pain

络石藤 [luò shí téng]
***Caulis Trachelospermi*; Chinese Starjasmine Stem:** dried stem with leaf of *Trachelospermum jasminoides* (Lindl.) Lem. (family Apocynaceae), used to dispel wind-dampness, unblock the meridian/channel, cool the blood and reduce swelling in the treatment of rheumatalgia of the joints with muscular contracture, as well as sore throat

千年健 [qiān nián jiàn]
***Rhizoma Homalomenae*; Obscured Homalomena Rhizome:** dried rhizome of *Homalomena occulta* (Lour.) Schott (family Araceae), used to dispel wind-dampness, strengthen the tendons and bones, and alleviate rheumatic pain for treating rheumatoid arthritis with cold sensation and pain in the back and knees, and contracture of the lower limbs

蕲蛇 [qí shé]
***Agkistrodon*; Long-noded Pit Viper:** dried body of *Agkistrodon acutus* (Guenther) (family Viperidae), used to unblock the meridians/channels for relieving chronic and stubborn rheumatalgia, and to relieve spasm for treating hemiplegia, convulsion and tetanus

金钱白花蛇 [jīn qián bái huā shé]
***Bungarus Parvus*; Coin-like White-banded Snake:** dried body of a young *Bungarus multicinctus* Blyth (family Elapidae), used in a similar way to the long-noded pit viper (蕲蛇 [qí shé])

乌梢蛇 [wū shāo shé]
***Zaocys*; Black-tailed Snake:** dried body of *Zaocys dhumnades* (Cantor) (family Colubridae), used to dispel wind, unblock the meridian/channel, and relieve convulsion and spasm for treating chronic and stubborn rheumatalgia, hemiplegia in cases of stroke, convulsions and tetanus

蛇蜕 [shé tuì]
***Periostracum Serpentis*; Snake Slough:** dried epidermal membrane of *Elaphe taeniura* Cope or *Elaphe carinata* (family Colabridae), used to arrest convulsion, counteract toxicity, and clear corneal opacity of the eye, for

treating infantile convulsion, nebula, inflammation of the throat, boils, and cutaneous itching

马钱子 [mǎ qián zǐ]
***Semen Strychni*; Nux Vomica:** dried ripe seed of *Strychnos nux-vomica L. or Strychnos pierriana* A.W. Hill (family Loganiaceae), used to promote the flow of *qi* and blood in collateral meridians/channels, alleviate pain and reduce swelling in cases of rheumatoid arthritis, sequelae of infantile paralysis, and traumatic injuries with pain

五加皮 [wǔ jiā pí]
***Cortex Acanthopanacis*; Slenderstyle Acanthopanax Bark:** dried root-bark of *Acanthopanax gracilistylus* W. W. Smith (family Araliaceae), used to dispel wind-dampness, strengthen the tendons and bones, and induce diuresis in the treatment of rheumatic conditions and edema

海桐皮 [hǎi tóng pí]
***Cortex Erythrinae*; Coral-bean Bark:** dried bark of *Erythrina variegata* L. var. *orientalis* (L.) Merr. or *Erythrina arborescens* Roxb. (family Leguminosae), used to dispel wind-dampness, unblock the collateral meridians/channels and relieve itching in cases of rheumatalgia, and also externally for treating neurodermatitis and chronic eczema

丝瓜络 [sī guā luò]
***Retinervus Luffae Fructus*; Luffa Vegetable Sponge:** dried vascular bundles of the ripe fruit of *Luffa cylindrica* (L.) Roem. (family Cucurbitaceae), used to dispel wind, unblock collateral meridians/channels, and counteract toxins for treating rheumatalgia with muscular contracture, and also for treating mastitis

伸筋草 [shēn jīn cǎo]
***Herba Lycopodii*; Common Club-moss Herb:** dried entire plant of *Lycopodium japonicum* Thunb. (family Lycopodiaceae), used to dispel wind-dampness and relieve contracture in cases of arthralgia with stiffness

老鹳草 [lǎo guàn cǎo]
***Herba Erodii seu Geranii*; Heron's Bill or Wilford Ganesbill Herb:** dried aerial part of *Erodium stephanianum* Willd. or *Geranium wilfordii* Maxim. (family Geraniaceae), used to dispel wind-dampness, unblock collateral meridians/channels and arrest dysenteric diarrhea in cases of rheumatalgia with muscular contracture, and also for treating enteritis and dysentery

臭梧桐叶 [chòu wú tóng yè]
***Folium Liriodendra Tracheotomy*; Glory Bower Leaf:** dried leaf of *Clerodendrum trichotomum* Thunb. (family Verbenaceae), used to dispel wind-dampness and reduce high blood pressure in cases of rheumatism and hypertension

穿山龙 [chuān shān lóng]
***Rhizoma Dioscoreae Nipponicae*; Japanese Yam:** dried rhizome of *Dioscorea nipponica Makino* (family Dioscoreaceae), used to dispel wind-dampness, activate blood flow, unblock collateral meridians/channels and resolve phlegm in the treatment of rheumatalgia, sprain,

traumatic pain, and chronic cough with expectoration

穿地龙 [chuān dì lóng]

same as 穿山龙 [chuān shān lóng]

徐长卿 [xú cháng qīng]

***Radix Cynanchi Paniculati*; Paniculate Swallowwort Root:** dried root and rhizome of *Cynanchum paniculatum* (Bge.) Kitag. (family Asclepiadaceae), used to unblock collateral meridians/channels, and alleviate pain and itching, for treating rheumatalgia, toothache, lumbago, traumatic injuries, dysmenorrhea, and eczema

青风藤 [qīng fēng téng]

***Caulis Sinomenii*; Orientvine Stem:** dried lianoid stem of *Sinomenium acutum* (Thunb.) Rehd. et Wils. or *Sinomenium acutum*var. *cinereum* Rehd. et Wils. (family Menispermaceae), used to dispel wind-dampness and alleviate pain in cases of rheumatic arthritis with articular swelling and pain

香加皮 [xiāng jiā pí]

***Cortex Periplocae*; Chinese Silkvine Bark:** dried root-bark of *Periploca sepium* Bge. (family Asclepiadaceae), used to dispel wind-dampness for treating rheumatic arthritis, and induce diuresis for treating edema

防己 [fáng jǐ]

***Radix Stephaniae Tetrandrae*; Fourstamen Stephania Root:** dried root of *Stephania tetrandra* S. Moore (family Menispermaceae), used to dispel wind-dampness, and induce diuresis in cases of rheumatic arthritis, edema and oliguria

温里药
Interior-warming Medicinals/Drugs

附子 [fù zǐ]

***Radix Aconiti Lateralis Preparata*; Prepared Daughter Root of Common Monkshood:** prepared daughter root of *Aconitum carmichaeli* Debx. (family Ranunculaceae), used (1) to restore heart yang for the relief of collapse and shock, (2) to dispel cold for treating deficiency-cold conditions such as gastralgia and abdominal pain with cold sensation, and also for treating cold rheumatalgia with severe pain, and (3) to reinforce the kidney and spleen for treating edema, chronic diarrhea, and impotence

肉桂 [ròu guì]

***Cortex Cinnamomi*; Cassia Bark:** dried stem bark of *Cinnamomum cassia* Presl. (family Lauraceae), used (1) to warm the kidney in the treatment of impotence and chronic diarrhea with coldness of the limbs, (2) to dispel cold for alleviating epigastric and abdominal pain due to cold attack or deficiency-cold, and (3) to promote menstruation in cases of amenorrhea and dysmenorrhea

干姜 [gān jiāng]

***Rhizoma Zingiberis*; Dried Ginger:** the dried rhizome of *Zingiber officinale* (Willd.) Rosc. (family Zingiberaceae), used (1) to warm the spleen and stomach for the relief of nausea, vomiting, abdominal pain and diarrhea due to deficiency-cold of the spleen and stomach, and (2) to warm the lung for treating chronic cough with thin, white and foamy expectoration

炮姜 [páo jiāng]

***Rhizoma Zingiberis Preparata*; Prepared Dried Ginger:** dried ginger scalded with hot sand until it turns brownish, used to warm the meridian/channel to arrest bleeding and warm the middle energizer to relieve pain, for treating hematemesis, hematochezia and abnormal uterine bleeding of deficiency-cold pattern, and abdominal pain and diarrhea due to spleen yang deficiency

高良姜 [gāo liáng jiāng]

***Rhizoma Alpiniae Officinarum*; Lesser Galangal Rhizome:** dried rhizome of *Alpinia officinarum* Hance (family Zingiberaceae), used to warm the stomach for relieving gastralgia and vomiting due to cold

花椒 [huā jiāo]

***Pericarpium Zanthoxy*; Prickly-ash Peel:** dried ripe pericarp of *Zanthoxylum schinifolium* Sieb. et Zucc. or *Zanthoxylum bungeanum* Maxim. (family Rutaceae), used (1) to warm the stomach for treating gastralgia and dyspepsia due to cold, (2) as an ascaricide, and (3) externally for treating eczema and pruritus

荜澄茄 [bì chéng qié]

***Fructus Litseae*; Mountain Spicy Fruit:** dried ripe fruit of *Litsea cubeba* (Lour.) Pers. (family Lauraceae), used to warm the stomach for relieving vomiting, and epigastric and abdominal pain due to cold

吴茱萸 [wú zhū yú]

***Fructus Evodiae*; Evodia Fruit:** dried nearly mature fruit of *Evodia rutaecarpa* (Juss.) Benth., *Evodia rutaecarpa* var. *officinalis* (Dode) Huang or *Evodia rutaecarpa* var. *bodinieri* (Dode) Huang (family Rutaceae), used to warm the stomach and relieve pain in cases of gastralgia, abdominal pain, acid regurgitation and vomiting

丁香 [dīng xiāng]

***Flos Caryophylli*; Cloves:** dried flower-bud of *Eugenia caryophyllata* Thunb. (family Myrtaceae), used (1) to warm the stomach for the relief of vomiting and hiccups due to cold, and (2) to warm the kidney for treating impotence

小茴香 [xiǎo huí xiāng]

***Fructus Foeniculi*; Fennel Fruit:** the dried fruit of *Foeniculum vulgare* Mill. (family Umbelliferae), used to dispel cold, regulate *qi* flow and relieve pain for treating cold pain in the lower abdomen and distending pain in the testis

胡椒 [hú jiāo]

***Fructus Piperis*; Pepper Fruit:** dried ripe fruit of *Piper nigrum* L. (family Piperaceae), used to dispel cold from the stomach and eliminate phlegm, for treating vomiting, diarrhea and abdominal pain due to cold in the stomach, and also for treating epilepsy induced by phlegm

艾叶 [ài yè]

***Folium Artemisiae Argyi*; Argyi Leaf; Argyi Wormwood Leaf:** dried leaf of *Artemisia argyi* Levl. et Vant. (family Compositae), used to warm the uterus and stop bleeding in cases of functional uterine bleeding, sterility and dysmenorrhea

荜拔 [bì bō]

***Fructus Piperis Longi*; Long Pepper:** dried nearly ripe or ripe fruit-spike of *Piper longum* L. (family Piperaceae), used to warm the stomach for treating cold and pain in the stomach

芳香化湿药
Fragrant Dampness-resolving Medicinals/Drugs

广藿香 [guǎng huò xiāng]

***Herba Pogostemonis*; Cablin Patchouli Herb:** dried aerial part of *Pogostemon cablin* (Blanco) Benth. (family Labiatae), used to resolve dampness for treating nausea, vomiting and diarrhea, especially in cases of summer contractions

藿香 [huò xiāng]

***Herba Agastachis*; Agastache:** dried aerial part of *Agastache rugosus* (Fisch. et Mey.) O. Ktze. (family Labiatae), used in a similar way to cablin patchouli herb (广藿香 [guǎng huò xiāng])

佩兰 [pèi lán]

***Herba Eupatorii*; Fortune Eupatorium Herb:** aerial part of *Eupatorium fortunei* Turcz. (family Compositae), used to resolve dampness for relieving nausea, vomiting and abdominal distension, especially in cases of contraction of summer dampness

苍术 [cāng zhú]

***Rhizoma Atractylodis*; Atractylodes Rhizome:** dried rhizome of *Atractylodes lancea* (Thunb.) DC. or *Atractylodes chinensis* (DC.) Koidz. (family Compositae), used (1) to eliminate dampness and invigorate the spleen for treating dampness accumulation in the spleen and stomach, (2) to dispel wind-dampness for treating rheumatic arthritis, and (3) to improve vision in cases of night blindness

豆蔻 [dòu kòu]

***Fructus Amomi Rotundus*; Round Cardamom Fruit:** dried ripe fruit of *Amomum kravanh* Pirre ex Gagnep. or *Amomum compactum* Soland ex Maton (family Zingiberaceae), used to resolve dampness, move *qi*, and warm the middle energizer for relieving epigastric and abdominal distension, nausea, vomiting due to accumulation of cold-dampness or stagnation of *qi* in the spleen and stomach

白豆蔻 [bái dòu kòu]

same as 豆蔻 [dòu kòu]

蔻仁 [kòu rén]

***Semen Amomi Rotundus*; Round Cardamom Seed:** seed of round cardamom fruit freshly removed from the pericarp, which is stronger in activity than the fruit

砂仁 [shā rén]

***Fructus Amomi*; Spiny Amomum Fruit:** dried ripe fruit of *Amomum villosum* Lour., *Amomum villosum* var. *xanthioides* T.L. Wu et Senjen or *Amomum longiligulare* T.L. Wu (family Zingiberaceae), used (1) to resolve dampness for treating dampness accumulation in the spleen and stomach, (2) to warm the middle energizer for treating vomiting and diarrhea due to deficiency-cold of the spleen and stomach, and (3) to prevent miscarriage in cases of threatened abortion

草豆蔻 [cǎo dòu kòu]
***Semen Alpiniae Katsumadai*; Katsumada Galangal Seed:** dried seed of *Alpinia katsumadai* Hayata (family Zingiberaceae), used to dry dampness, move *qi*, and warm the middle energizer for relieving gastralgia, vomiting, diarrhea due to accumulation of cold-dampness or *qi* stagnation in the spleen and stomach

草果 [cǎo guǒ]
***Fructus Tsaoko*; *Tsaoko*; *Caoguo*:** dried ripe fruit of *Amomum tsao-ko* Crevost et Lemaire (family Zingiberaceae), used (1) to remove dampness and warm the stomach in cases of epigastric distension, vomiting and abdominal pain, and (2) for treating malaria

荷叶 [hé yè]
***Folium Nelumbinis*; Lotus Leaf:** dried leaf of *Nelumbo nucifera* Gaertn. (family Nymphaecaceae), used (1) to resolve summer-dampness for treating diarrhea caused by summer-dampness, (2) to arrest bleeding by reducing heat in the blood for treating various hemorrhagic conditions, and (3) to resolve dampness for treating edema and inducing loss of body weight

利尿逐水药
Diuretics and Hydragogues

利尿渗湿药 Diuretics

茯苓 [fú líng]
***Poria*; Indian Bread:** dried sclerotium of the fungus, *Poria cocos* (Schw.) Wolf (family Polyporaceae), used (1) as a diuretic in cases of edema and oliguria, (2) to invigorate the spleen for treating anorexia and diarrhea, and (3) to induce tranquilization for treating palpitations and insomnia

猪苓 [zhū líng]
***Polyporus*; *Chuling*; Umbellate Polypore:** dried sclerotium of the fungus, *Polyporus umbellatus* (Pers.) Fries (family Polyporaceae), used as a diuretic for treating edema and oliguria, and also to filter out dampness for treating leukorrhagia

泽泻 [zé xiè]
***Rhizoma Alismatis*; Water-plantain Rhizome:** dried tuber of *Alisma orientalis* (Sam.) Juzep. (family Alismaceae), used (1) to promote urine excretion in cases of oliguria and edema, (2) to filter out dampness in cases of diarrhea and leukorrhea, and (3) to purge heat in cases of bladder dampness-heat

车前子 [chē qián zǐ]
***Semen Plantaginis*; Plantain Seed:** dried ripe seed of *Plantago asiatica* L. or *Plantago depressa* Willd. (family Plantaginaceae), used (1) to induce diuresis and filter out dampness for treating watery diarrhea, edema, and stranguria, (2) to clear the liver and improve vision in cases of eye diseases, and (3) to clear the lung and resolve phlegm in cases of cough with profuse phlegm

车前草 [chē qián cǎo]
***Herba Plantaginis*; Plantain Herb:** dried entire plant of *Plantago asiatica* L. or *Plantago depressa* Willd. (family Plantaginaceae), used (1) to induce diuresis in cases of edema, oliguria and stranguria,

and (2) to clear heat and counteract toxin in cases of sores, carbuncles, dysentery, and acute pulmonary and urinary infections

滑石 [huá shí]
***Talcum*; Talc:** very soft mineral composed mainly of hydrous magnesium silicate, used to induce diuresis, clear summerheat and dispel dampness in the treatment of summer contractions, watery diarrhea, oliguria and urinary infection, and also externally for treating eczema and miliaria

薏苡仁 [yì yǐ rén]
***Semen Coicis*; Coix Seed; Job's-tears Seed:** dried ripe kernel obtained by removing the hard husk and seed coat of *Coix lacryma-jobi* L. var. *ma-yuen* (Roman.) Stapf (family Graminae), used (1) to invigorate the spleen and dispel dampness for treating diarrhea and edema, (2) to clear heat and discharge pus for treating lung abscess and acute appendicitis, and (3) for treating verruca plana

冬瓜皮 [dōng guā pí]
***Exocarpium Benincasae*; Chinese Wax-gourd Peel:** dried exocarp of *Benincasa hispida* (Thunb.) Cogn. (family Cucurbitaceae), used to induce diuresis for treating oliguria and edema

青木香 [qīng mù xiāng]
***Radix Aristolochiae*; Dutchmanspipe Root:** dried root of *Aristolochia debilis* Sieb. et Zucc. (family Aristolochiaceae), used (1) to move *qi* and alleviate pain for treating thoracic, epigastric, hypochondriac and abdominal distension and pain, and (2) to counteract toxins and reduce swelling for treating boils, sores, eczema, and venomous snake-bite

大腹皮 [dà fù pí]
***Pericarpium Arecae*; Areca Peel:** dried pericarp of *Areca catechu* L. (family Palmae), used to induce diuresis and remove stagnant *qi* for relieving abdominal distension and edema

木通 [mù tōng]
***Caulis Aristolochiae Manshuriensis*; Manchurian Dutchmanspipe Stem** (关木通 [guān mù tōng]) or ***Caulis Clematidis Armandii*, Armand Clematis Stem** (川木通 [chuān mù tōng]) (see below)

关木通 [guān mù tōng]
***Caulis Aristolochiae Manshuriensis*; Manchurian Dutchmanspipe Stem:** dried stem of *Aristolochia manshuriensis* Kom. (family Aristolochiaceae), used in a similar way to 川木通 [chuān mù tōng], but with nephrotropic toxicity

川木通 [chuān mù tōng]
***Caulis Clematidis Armandii*; Armand Clematis Stem:** dried stem of *Clematis armandii* Franch. or *Clematis montana* Buch.-Ham. (family Ranunculaceae), used (1) to induce diuresis and relieve stranguria in cases of bladder dampness-heat, and (2) as an emmenagogue and galactogogue in cases of amenorrhea and inadequate lactation, respectively

通草 [tōng cǎo]
***Medulla Tetrapanacis*; Ricepaper-plant Pith:** stem pith of *Tetrapanax papyriferus*

(Hook.) K. Koch (family Araliaceae), used (1) to clear heat and remove dampness in cases of stranguria and oliguria, and (2) to promote milk secretion in cases of inadequate lactation

萹蓄 [biān xù]
***Herba Polygoni Avicularis*; Common Knotgrass Herb:** dried aerial part of *Polygonum aviculare* L. (family Polygonaceae), used (1) to promote diuresis and eliminate dampness-heat in cases of stranguria with turbid urine and morbid leukorrhea, and (2) to dispel wind-dampness in cases of arthralgia

瞿麦 [qú mài]
***Herba Dianthi*; Liliac Pink Herb:** dried aerial part of *Dianthus superbus* L. or *Dianthus chinensis* L. (family Caryophyllaceae), used to promote diuresis and eliminate dampness-heat for treating heat stranguria and blood stranguria, and (2) as an emmenagogue for treating amenorrhea

苘麻子 [qǐng má zǐ]
***Semen Abutili*; Chingma Abutilon Seed:** dried ripe seed of *Abutilon theophrastii* Medic. (family Malvaceae), used to remove dampness-heat and counteract toxins for treating dysentery, heat stranguria, boils and sores

冬葵果 [dōng kuí guǒ]
***Fructus Malvae*; Cluster Mallow Fruit:** dried ripe fruit of *Malva verticillata* L. (family Malvaceae), used to clear heat and induce diuresis for treating stranguria, oliguria and edema

萆薢 [bì xiè]
***Rhizoma Dioscoreae Septemlobae*; Seven-lobed Yam Rhizome** (绵萆薢 [mián bì xiè]) or ***Rhizoma Dioscoreae Hypoglaucae*, Hypoglaucous Yam Rhizome** (粉萆薢 [fěn bì xiè])

绵萆薢 [mián bì xiè]
***Rhizoma Dioscoreae Septemlobae*; Seven-lobed Yam Rhizome:** dried rhizome of *Dioscorea septemloba* Thunb. or *Dioscorea futschauensis* Uline (family Dioscoreaceae), used (1) to eliminate dampness-turbidity in cases of chyluria and stranguria with turbid urine, and (2) to dispel wind-dampness in cases of rheumatic arthritis

粉萆薢 [fěn bì xiè]
***Rhizoma Dioscoreae Hypoglaucae*; Hypoglaucous Yam Rhizome:** dried rhizome of *Dioscorea hypoglauca* Palib. (family Dioscoreaceae), used in a similar way to 绵萆薢 [mián bì xiè]

地肤子 [dì fū zǐ]
***Fructus Kochiae*; Belvedere Fruit:** dried ripe fruit of *Kochia scoparia* (L.) Schrad. (family Chenopodiaceae), used (1) to clear dampness-heat in cases of bladder dampness-heat with stranguria, and (2) to relieve itching in cases of urticaria, eczema, and pruritus

金钱草 [jīn qián cǎo]
***Herba Lysimachiae*; Christina Loosestrife:** dried entire plant of *Lysimachia christinae* Hance (family Primulaceae), used (1) as a cholagogue, lithagogue and diuretic for treating acute jaundice, biliary and urinary calculi, respectively, and (2) to relieve

toxicity and reduce swelling in cases of boils and venomous snake-bite

海金沙 [hǎi jīn shā]
***Spora Lygodii*; Japanese Climbing-fern Spores:** spores of *Lygodium japonicum* (Thunb.) Sw. (family Ligodiaceae), used to eliminate dampness-heat and as lithagogue for treating bladder dampness-heat and urinary calculi

赤小豆 [chì xiǎo dòu]
***Semen Phaseoli*; Rice Bean:** dried ripe seed of *Phaseolus calcaratus* Roxb. or *Phaseolus angularis* Wight (family Leguminosae), used to induce diuresis, counteract toxins and promote the drainage of pus in cases of boils, sores and abscesses

石韦 [shí wěi]
***Folium Pyrrosiae*; Shearer's Pyrrosia Leaf:** dried leaf of *Pyrrosia sheareri* (Bak.) Ching, *Pyrrosia lingua* (Thunb.) Farwell or *Pyrrosia petiolosa* (Christ) Ching (family Polypodiaceae), used (1) to induce diuresis and relieve dysuria for treating bladder dampness-heat, and (2) to clear the lung for relieving cough and dyspnea

葫芦 [hú lu]
***Pericarpium Lagenariae*; Calabash Gourd:** dried pericarp of *Lagenaria siceraria* (Molina) Standl. var. *depressa* (Ser.) Hara (family Cucurbitaceae), a diuretic for treating severe edema and ascites

抽葫芦 [chōu hú lu]
same as 葫芦 [hú lu]

蝼蛄 [lóu gū]
***Gryllotalpa*; Mole Cricket:** dried body of *Gyllotalpa africana* Palisot et Beaurois (family Gryllotalpidae), a diuretic for treating severe edema, ascites and retention of urine

路路通 [lù lù tōng]
***Fructus Liquidambaris*; Beautiful Sweetgum Fruit:** dried strobile (cone) of *Liquidambar formosana* Hance (family Hamamelidaceae), used (1) to induce diuresis for treating edema, (2) to dispel wind-dampness in cases of arthralgia, and (3) to promote menstrual discharge in cases of amenorrhea

玉米须 [yù mǐ xū]
***Stigma Maydis*; Corn Stigma:** dried styles and stigmata of Indian Corn, *Zea mays* L. (family Gramineae), used (1) to induce diuresis for treating edema, (2) to promote bile discharge in cases of jaundice, and (3) to reduce high blood pressure in cases of hypertension

灯心草 [dēng xīn cǎo]
***Medulla Junci*; Common Rush:** dried pith of *Juncus effusus* L. (family Juncaceae), used (1) to induce diuresis for treating heat stranguria, and (2) to calm the mind for relieving fidgetiness and insomnia

逐水药
Hydragogues or Drastic Purgatives

牵牛子 [qiān niú zǐ]
***Semen Pharbitidis*; Pharbitis Seed:** dried ripe seed of *Pharbitis nil* (L.) Choisy or *Pharbitis purpurea* (L.) Voigt (family

Convolvulaceae), used as a hydragogue for treating edema and oliguria, and as an anthelmintic in cases of ascariasis

黑丑 [hēi chǒu]
Black Pharbitis Seed: pharbitis seed with grayish black surface (cf. Pharbitis Seed 牵牛子 [qiān niú zǐ])

白丑 [bái chǒu]
White Pharbitis Seed: pharbitis seed with pale yellowish surface (cf. Pharbitis Seed 牵牛子 [qiān niú zǐ])

黑白丑 [hēi bái chǒu]
Black and White Pharbitis Seed: black and white pharbitis seeds mixed in equal quantities (cf. Pharbitis Seed 牵牛子 [qiān niú zǐ])

商陆 [shāng lù]
***Radix Phytolaccae*; Pokeberry Root:** dried root of *Phytolacca acinosa* Roxb. or *Phytolacca americana* L. (family Phytolaccaceae), used as diuretic and hydragogue for treating edema and ascites, also used externally for treating boils and sores

巴豆霜 [bā dòu shuāng]
***Semen Crotonis Pulveratum*; Defatted Croton Seed Powder:** partly defatted and powdered seed of *Croton tiglium* L. (family Euphorbiaceae), used as a drastic purgative for treating constipation with abdominal distension and pain due to accumulation of cold and stagnation of food

甘遂 [gān suì]
***Radix Euphorbiae Kansui*; Kansui Root:** dried tuberous root of *Euphorbia kansui* T.N. Liou ex T. P. Wang (family Euphorbiaceae), used as hydragogue and purgative for treating hydrothorax and ascites with oliguria and constipation

芫花 [yuán huā]
***Flos Genkwa*; Lilac Daphne Flower Bud:** dried flower-bud of *Daphne genkwa* Sieb. et Zucc. (family Thymelaeaceae), used as a hydragogue and purgative for treating severe edema, hydrothorax and ascites with oliguria and constipation, and externally for treating scabies and frostbite

黄芫花 [huáng yuán huā]
***Folium et Flos Wikstroemiae Chamaedaphnis*; Chamaedaphne Leaf and Flower; Yellow Genkwa Leaf and Flower:** leaf and flower-bud of *Wikstroemia chamaedaphne* Meisn. (family Thymeleaceae), used in a similar way to 芫花 [yuán huā], and also for treating acute and chronic hepatitis, schizophrenia, and epilepsy

京大戟 [jīng dà jǐ]
***Radix Euphorbiae Pekinensis*; Peking Euphorbia Root:** dried root of *Euphorbia pekinensis* Rupr. (family Euphorbiaceae), used as a hydragogue and purgative for treating severe edema, hydrothorax and ascites with oliguria and constipation, also used externally for treating scrofula

龙虎草 [lóng hǔ cǎo]
another name for *Radix Euphorbiae Pekinensis* or Peking Euphorbia Root (京大戟 [jīng dà jǐ])

狼毒 [láng dú]
***Radix Euphorbiae Ebractealatae*; Unbracteolated Euphorbia Root:** dried root

of *Euphobia ebracteolata* Hayata or *Euphorbia fischeriana* Steud. (family Euphorbiaceae), used as a drastic purgative to remove stagnant food, and as an anthelmintic for treating intestinal parasites, also used for treating scrofula

理气药
Qi-regulating Medicinals/Drugs

陈皮 [chén pí]
***Pericarpium Citri Reticulatae*; Dried Tangerine Peel:** dried ripe pericarp of *Citrus reticulata* Blanco and its cultivated varieties (family Rutaceae), used to regulate *qi*, invigorate the spleen, dry dampness, and resolve phlegm in the treatment of *qi* stagnation in the spleen and stomach, and cough with profuse phlegm

青皮 [qīng pí]
***Pericarpium Citri Reticulatae Viride*; Green Tangerine Peel:** dried green unripe exocarp of *Citrus reticulata* Blanco and its cultivated varieties (family Rutaceae), used to regulate *qi*, soothe the liver, and remove stagnation for treating liver *qi* stagnation and food retention

橘核 [jú hé]
***Semen Citri Reticulatae*; Tangerine Seed:** dried ripe seed of *Citrus reticulata* Blanco and its cultivated varieties (family Rutaceae), used to regulate *qi*, dissipate nodulation and alleviate pain for treating hernial pain, nodules in the breast, and swelling and pain of the testis

橘红 [jú hóng]
***Exocarpium Citri Rubrum*; Red Tangerine Peel:** dried exocarp of *Citrus reticulata* Blanco and its cultivated varieties (family Rutaceae), used in the same way as dried tangerine peel (陈皮 [chén pí]), but with stronger action

枳实 [zhǐ shí]
***Fructus Aurantii Immaturus*; Immature Orange Fruit:** dried small immature fruit of *Citrus aurantium* L. and its cultivated varieties or *Citrus sinensis* Osbeck with a diameter under 2.5 cm (family Rutaceae), used to break down the stuffed *qi*, resolve phlegm and remove accumulation for treating dyspepsia, constipation and abdominal distension due to food stagnation, and served in large doses for treating visceroptosis

枳壳 [zhǐ qiào]
***Fructus Aurantii*; Orange Fruit:** dried immature fruit of *Citrus aurantium* L. and its cultivated varieties with a diameter of 3-5 cm (family Rutaceae), used in the same way as immature orange fruit (枳实 [zhǐ shí]), but with a milder effect

厚朴 [hòu pò]
***Cortex Magnoliae Officinalis*; Medicinal Magnolia Bark:** dried stem bark, root bark or branch bark of *Magnolia officinalis* Rehd. et Wils. or *Magnolia officinalis* var. *biloba* Rehd. et Wils. (family Magnoliaceae), used (1) to promote the flow of *qi* for relieving abdominal distension and pain due to food stagnation, (2) to invigorate the spleen by drying dampness for treating vomiting and diarrhea due to dyspepsia, and (3) to relieve cough and dyspnea with profuse phlegm

紫苏梗 [zǐ sū gěng]
***Caulis Perillae*; Perilla Stem:** dried stem of *Perilla frutescens* (L.) Britt. (family Labiatae), used to regulate the flow of *qi*, relieve pain and calm the fetus for treating stuffiness in the chest, epigastric pain, eructation, vomiting, and threatened abortion

木香 [mù xiāng]
***Radix Aucklandiae*; Common Aucklandia Root:** dried root of *Aucklandia lappa* Decne. (family Compositae), used to move *qi* and alleviate pain for relieving abdominal distension and pain due to *qi* stagnation, tenesmus in cases of dysentery, and liver *qi* depression with hypochondriac pain and jaundice

香附 [xiāng fù]
***Rhizoma Cyperi*; Nutgrass Galingale Rhizome:** dried tuber of *Cyperus rotundus* L. (family Cyperaceae), used to soothe liver *qi*, regulate menstruation and alleviate pain for treating chest and abdominal distension with pain, amenorrhea and dysmenorrhea

乌药 [wū yào]
***Radix Linderae*; Combined Spicebush Root:** dried tuberous root of *Lindera aggregata* (Sims) Kosterm. (family Lauraceae), used to move *qi*, alleviate pain, warm the kidney and disperse cold for relieving distension and pain of the lower abdomen, frequent micturition and enuresis

香橼 [xiāng yuán]
***Fructus Citri*; Citron Fruit:** dried ripe fruit of *Citrus medica* L. or *Citrus wilsonii* Tanaka (family Rutaceae), used to soothe the liver, regulate *qi*, and resolve phlegm for treating gastric distension with pain, and fullness sensation in the chest, as well as cough with profuse phlegm

佛手 [fó shǒu]
***Fructus Citri Sarcodactylis*; Finger Citron:** dried fruit of *Citrus medica* L. var. *sarcodactylis* Swingle (family Rutaceae), used to soothe the liver, regulate *qi*, harmonize the middle energizer, resolve dampness and phlegm for treating *qi* stagnation of the liver or disharmony between the spleen and stomach, as well as chronic cough with profuse expectoration

薤白 [xiè bái]
***Bulbus Allii Macrostemoni*; Longstamen Onion:** dried bulb of *Allium macrostemon* Bge. (family Liliaceae), used to unblock the meridians/channels, regulate yang *qi* and remove stagnation in the treatment of angina pectoris with stuffiness sensation in the chest, and also for treating tenesmus in cases of dysentery.

甘松 [gān sōng]
***Radix et Rhizoma Nardostachyos*; Nardus Root; Spikenard Root:** dried rhizome and root of *Nardostachys chinensis* Batal. or *Nardostachys jatamansi* DC. (family Valerianaceae), used to move *qi*, alleviate pain and invigorate the spleen for treating epigastric and abdominal pain and anorexia due to stagnation of *qi*

檀香 [tán xiāng]
***Lignum Santali Albi*; Sandalwood:** heartwood of trunk of *Santalum album*

L. (family Santalaceae), used to move *qi*, alleviate pain, disperse cold and regulate the stomach function, for treating angina pectoris and gastralgia due to cold

降香 [jiàng xiāng]
***Lignum Dalbergiae Odoriferae*; Rosewood:** heartwood of trunk and root of *Dalbergia odorifera* T. Chen (family Leguminosae), used to regulate *qi*, resolve blood stasis, and alleviate pain for treating angina pectoris, abdominal distension with pain, and various traumatic painful swellings

沉香 [chén xiāng]
***Lignum Aquilariae Resinatum*; Chinese Eagle Wood:** resinous wood of *Aquilaris sinensis* (Lour.) Gilg (family Thymelaeaceae), used to move *qi* for alleviating pain, to warm the middle energizer for arresting vomiting, and to improve inhalation for relieving dyspnea

娑罗子 [suō luó zǐ]
***Semen Aesculi*; Buckeye Seed:** dried ripe seed of *Aesculus chinensis* Bge., *Aesculus chinensis* var. *chekiangensis* (Hu et Fang) Fang or *Aesculus wilsonii* Rehd. (family Hippocastanaceae), used to regulate *qi*, harmonize the stomach and alleviate pain for relieving distension and stuffiness in the chest and abdomen, and especially gastralgia

荔枝核 [lì zhī hé]
***Semen Litchi*; Lychee Seed:** dried ripe seed of *Litchi chinensis* Sonn. (family Sapindaceae), used to move *qi*, dissipate nodulation, disperse cold and alleviate pain for treating hernial pain, dysmenorrhea, lower abdominal distension with pain, and swelling and pain of the testis

梅花 [méi huā]
***Flos Mume*; Plum Flower:** dried flower-bud of *Prunus mume* (Sieb.) Zieb. et Zucc. (family Rosaceae), used to regulate *qi*, ease the mind and resolve phlegm for treating depression, fidgetiness, hypochondriac and epigastric pain, and globus hystericus

绿萼梅 [lǜ è méi]
same as 梅花 [méi huā]

九香虫 [jiǔ xiāng chóng]
***Aspongopus*; Stink-bug:** dried body of *Aspongopus chinensis* Dallas (family Pentatomidae), used (1) to regulate *qi* and alleviate pain for treating epigastric distension and pain, and (2) to invigorate the kidney for treating impotence and lumbago

化橘红 [huà jú hóng]
***Exocarpium Citri Grandis*; Pummelo Peel:** the dried exocarp of unripe *Citrus grandis* (family Rutaceae), used to dispel cold, eliminate dampness and phlegm, and arrest emesis and nausea for treating cough with profuse expectoration in cases of colds, nausea, vomiting and epigastric distension caused by improper diet

厚朴花 [hòu pò huā]
***Flos Magnoliae Officinalis*; Officinal Magnolia Flower:** dried flower bud of *Magnolia Officinalis* Rehd. et Wils. (family Magnoliaceae), used to regulate the flow of *qi* and eliminate dampness for treating feeling of stuffiness and distension in the chest and epigastrium with loss of appetite

柿蒂 [shì dì]

***Calyx Kaki*; Persimmon Calyx:** dried persistent calyx of *Diospyros kaki* L. f. (family Ebenaceae), used to direct *qi* to move downward for stopping hiccups

刀豆 [dāo dòu]

***Semen Canavaliae*; Jack Bean:** dried ripe seed of *Canavalia gladiata* (Jacq.) DC. (family Leguminosae), used to warm the stomach and check its upward adverse movement for treating hiccuping and vomiting of deficiency-cold pattern

川楝子 [chuān liàn zǐ]

***Fructus Toosendan*; Szechwan Chinaberry:** dried ripe fruit of *Melia toosendan* Sieb. et Zucc. (family Meliaceae), used to move *qi* for relieving hypochondriac, epigastric and abdominal pain, and (2) to kill parasitic worms in cases of enterobiasis and scabies

理血药

Blood-regulating Medicinals/Drugs

止血药 Hemostatics

仙鹤草 [xiān hè cǎo]

***Herba Agrimoniae*; Hairvein Agrimonia Herb:** dried aerial part of *Agrimonia pilosa* Ledeb. (family Rosaceae), used (1) as an astringent hemostatic for treating various kinds of bleeding including bloody dysentery, (2) to counteract toxins and reduce swelling for treating boils and sores, and (3) for treating malaria.

三七 [sān qī]

***Radix Notoginseng*; Sanchi:** dried root of *Panax notoginseng* (Burk.) F.H. Chen (family Araliaceae), used to resolve stasis, stop bleeding, activate blood and alleviate pain for treating various kinds of external and internal hemorrhages, blood stasis and pain in cases of traumatic injuries, and angina pectoris

白及 [bái jí]

***Rhizoma Bletillae*; Common Bletilla Tuber:** steamed and dried tuber of *Bletilla striata* (Thunb.) Reichb. f. (family Orchidaceae), used (1) as a hemostatic for treating hemoptysis, hematemesis and traumatic bleeding, and (2) to reduce swelling and promote regeneration for treating boils and burns

大蓟 [dà jì]

***Herba seu Radix Cirsii Japonici*; Japanese Thistle:** dried aerial part or root of *Cirsium japonicum* DC. (family Compositae), used as a hemostatic for treating hematemesis and hematuria due to blood heat, also used for treating hepatitis and hypertension

小蓟 [xiǎo jì]

***Herba Cirsii*; Field Thistle:** dried aerial part of *Cirsium setosum* (Willd.) (family Compositae), used (1) to cool the blood and stop bleeding, chiefly for treating hematuria, (2) to dissipate stasis and counteract toxins for treating boils, and (3) as an antihypertensive

茜草 [qiàn cǎo]

***Radix Rubiae*; Indian Madder Root:** dried root and rhizome of Indian Madder, *Rubia cordifolia* L. (family Rubiaceae), used to cool the blood, resolve stasis and stop bleeding in cases of epistaxis, metrorrhagia and traumatic bleeding

地榆 [dì yú]
***Radix Sanguisorbae*; Garden Burnet Root:** dried root of *Sanguisorba officinalis* L. or *Sanguisorba officinalis* var. *longifolia* (Bert.) Yu et Li (family Rosaceae), used (1) as a blood-cooling hemostatic for treating various kinds of hemorrhages such as hematemesis, hemoptysis, epistaxis, hematochezia, metrorrhagia, and (2) as an important agent for treating burns

槐花 [huái huā]
***Flos Sophorae*; Pagodatree Flower:** dried flower of *Sophora japonica* L. (family Leguminosae), used (1) to cool the blood and stop bleeding for treating various hemorrhages due to blood heat, particularly hemorrhoidal bleeding, (2) to clear liver fire for treating up-flaming of liver fire with headache and also for treating hypertension

槐米 [huái mǐ]
***Flos Sophorae Immaturus*; Pagodatree Flower-bud:** used in the same way as the flower, but with a stronger action

槐角 [huái jiǎo]
***Fructus Sophorae*; Japanese Pagodatree Pod:** dried ripe fruit of *Sophora japonica* L. (family Leguminosae), used as pagodatree flower (槐花 [huái huā]), chiefly for treating hemorrhoidal bleeding

侧柏叶 [cè bǎi yè]
***Cacumen Platycladi*; Chinese Arborvitae Twig and Leaf:** dried twig and leaf of *Platycladus orientalis* (L.) Franco (family Cupressaceae), used in the same way as a blood-cooling hemostatic for treating epistaxis, hemoptysis, hematemesis, hematochezia and metrorrhagia, also used for treating premature graying of hair

苎麻根 [zhù má gēn]
***Radix Boehmeriae*; Ramie Root:** dried root of *Boehmeria nivea* (L.) Gaud. (family Urticaceae), used to arrest bleeding and prevent miscarriage for the treatment of bleeding in cases of threatened abortion and menorrhagia

血余炭 [xuè yú tàn]
***Crinis Carbonisatus*; Carbonized Hair:** used to arrest bleeding and remove blood stasis for treating various kinds of hemorrhage

棕榈炭 [zōng lǘ tàn]
***Petiolus Trachycarpi Carbonisatus*; Carbonized Windmillpalm Petiole:** carbonized petiole of *Trachycarpus fortunei* H. Wendl. (family Palmae), used as astringent hemostatic for treating hematemesis, epistaxis, hematochezia, and menorrhagia

花蕊石 [huā ruǐ shí]
***Ophicalcitum*; Ophicalcite:** marble containing green serpentine, used as an astringent hemostatic for treating hemoptysis and hematemesis, and externally for treating incised wounds

荠菜 [jì cài]
***Herba Capsellae*; Shepherd's Purse:** dried entire plant of *Capsella bursa-pastoris* (L.) Medic. (family Cruciferae), used (1) as a blood-cooling hemostatic for treating menorrhagia, postpartum hemorrhage and hematuria, and (2) as a diuretic for treating nephritic edema and hypertension

瓦松 [wǎ sōng]
***Herba Orostachyos*; Roof Stonecrop:** dried aerial part of *Orostachys fimbriatus* (Turcz.) Berg. (family Crassalaceae), used as a hemostatic mainly for treating hematochezia and hematemesis, and externally for treating skin ulcers

藕节 [ǒu jié]
***Nodus Nelumbinis Rhizomatis*; Lotus Rhizome Node:** dried node of the rhizome of *Nelumbo nucifera* Gaertn. (family Nymphaeaceae), used to cool the blood, arrest bleeding and remove blood stasis for treating nasal bleeding, hemoptysis, hematuria and abnormal uterine bleeding

墨旱莲 [mò hàn lián]
***Herba Ecliptae*; *Eclipta*; Yerbadetajo Herb:** aerial part of *Eclipta prostrata* L. (family Compositae), used (1) as a blood-cooling hemostatic for treating various hemorrhages due to excessive heat in the blood, and (2) as a tonic to nourish the liver and kidney in the treatment of dizziness, tinnitus, premature graying of hair, and aching and weakness in the back and legs

牛西西 [niú xī xī]
***Radix Rumecis Patientiae*; Patient Dock Root:** dried root of *Rumex patientia* L. (family Polygonaceae), used as a blood-cooling hemostatic for treating various types of hemorrhage due to excessive heat in the blood

活血化瘀药

Blood-activating and Stasis-resolving Medicinals / Drugs

川芎 [chuān xiōng]
***Rhizome Chuanxiong*; Szechwan Lovage Rhizome:** dried rhizome of *Ligusticum chuanxiong* Hort. (family Umbelliferae), used (1) to activate blood flow and promote the flow of *qi* for treating irregular menstruation, dysmenorrhea, amenorrhea and coronary heart disease, and (2) to dispel wind and alleviate pain for relieving headache and rheumatalgia

红花 [hóng huā]
***Flos Carthami*; Safflower:** dried flower of *Carthamus tinctorius* L. (family Compositae), used to activate blood flow, eliminate stasis and alleviate pain for treating amenorrhea, chest pain, abdominal mass, and traumatic injuries

西红花 [xī hóng huā]
***Stigma Croci*; *Crocus*; Saffron:** dried stigma of *Crocus sativus* L. (family Iridaceae), used in the same way as 红花 [hóng huā], with a stronger effect

番红花 [fān hóng huā]
another name for *Stigma Croci*, *Crocus* or Saffron (西红花 [xī hóng huā])

藏红花 [zàng hóng huā]
another name for *Stigma Croci*, *Crocus* or Saffron (西红花 [xī hóng huā])

桃仁 [táo rén]
***Semen Persicae*; Peach Seed:** dried ripe seed of *Prunus persica* (L.) Batsch or *Prunus davidiana* (Carr.) Franch. (family Rosaceae), used (1) to promote blood flow and remove stasis for treating amenorrhea,

dysmenorrhea, abdominal masses, and traumatic injuries, and (2) as an aperient for treating constipation in the aged and debilitated

川牛膝 [chuān niú xī]

***Radix Cyathulae*; Medicinal Cyathula Root:** dried root of *Cyathula officinalis* Kuan (family Amaranthaceae), used (1) to promote blood flow for treating amenorrhea, dysmenorrhea, and traumatic injuries, (2) to tonify the liver and kidney and strengthen the tendons and bones for treating lumbago and aching joints, and (3) to direct fire and blood to move downward for treating headache, epistaxis and hematemesis

丹参 [dān shēn]

***Radix Salviae Miltiorrhizae*; Danshen Root:** dried root and rhizome of *Salvia miltiorrhiza* Bge. (family Labiatae), used (1) to promote blood flow and to remove blood stasis for treating dysmenorrhea, amenorrhea, and abdominal masses due to blood stagnation, as well as ischemic apoplexy and coronary heart disease, (2) to remove heat from the blood for treating boils and sores, and (3) to induce tranquilization for treating palpitation and insomnia

郁金 [yù jīn]

***Radix Curcumae*; Turmeric Root Tuber:** steamed and dried tuberous root of *Curcuma wenyujin* Y. H. Chen et C. Ling, *Curuma longa* L., *Curcuma kwangsiensis* S. G. Lee et C. F. Liang, or *Curcuma phaeocaulis* Val. (family Zingiberaceae), used (1) to activate blood flow and move *qi* for relieving pain in the chest, abdomen or costal regions due to *qi* stagnation and blood stasis, (2) to cool the blood for treating various types of hemorrhages due to upward perversion of *qi* and fire, (3) to calm the mind in the treatment of delirium, mania and epilepsy, and (4) as a cholagogue for treating jaundice

姜黄 [jiāng huáng]

***Rhizoma Curcumae Longae*; Turmeric:** steamed and dried rhizome of *Curcuma longa* L. (family Zingiberaceae), used to activate blood flow, move *qi*, unblock meridians/channels and relieve pain in cases of rheumatalgia, dysmenorrhea, epigastric, abdominal and costal pains, and traumatic injuries

片姜黄 [piàn jiāng huáng]

***Rhizoma Wenyujin Concisa*; Wenyujin Concise Rhizome:** dried rhizome of *Curcuma wenyujin* Y.H. Chen et C. Ling (family Zingiberaceae), used to resolve blood stasis and relieve pain in cases of dysmenorrhea, rheumatalgia, shoulder pain, and traumatic injuries

莪术 [é zhú]

***Rhizoma Curcumae*; Zedoary Rhizome:** steamed and dried rhizome of *Curcuma zedoaria* Rosc., *Curcuma phaeocaulis* Valeton, or *Curcuma kwangsiensis* S. G. Lee et C.F. Liang or *Curcuma wenyujin* Y.H. Chen et C. Ling (family Zingiberaceae), used to relieve pain caused by retention of food and activate blood flow and remove blood stasis for treating abdominal mass and amenorrhea, also used as an anticancer agent, especially for treating cervical cancer of the uterus

温莪术 [wēn é zhú]
specific name for the rhizome of *Curcuma wenyujin* Y.H. Chen et C. Ling (family Zingiberaceae) (cf. 莪术 [é zhú])

水红花子 [shuǐ hóng huā zǐ]
***Fructus Polygoni Orientalis*; Prince's-feather Fruit:** dried ripe fruit of *Polygonum orientalis* L. (family Polygonaceae), used to eliminate blood stasis in the treatment of abdominal pain, and relieve epigastric pain due to food stagnation

鸡血藤 [jī xuè téng]
***Caulis Spatholobi*; Suberect Spatholobus Stem:** dried lianoid stem of *Spatholobus suberectus* Dunn (family Leguminosae), used to move and tonify the blood, regulate menstruation and unblock collateral meridians/channels for treating menstrual disorders due to blood deficiency complicated by blood stasis, inflammation of peripheral vessels or thrombosis, numbness of the body and limbs, and also effective for leucopenia

月季花 [yuè jì huā]
***Flos Rosae Chinensis*; Chinese Rose Flower:** dried flower of *Rosa chinensis* Jacq. (family Rosaceae), used to promote blood flow and regulate menstruation for treating menstrual disorders and dysmenorrhea

凌霄花 [líng xiāo huā]
***Flos Campsis*; Trumpetcreeper Flower:** dried flower of *Campsis grandiflora* (Thunb.) or *Campsis radicans* (L.) (family Bignoneaceae), used to promote blood flow and eliminate stasis, to remove heat from blood and dispel wind, for treating amenorrhea with abdominal mass formation, breast swelling after childbirth, itching of the skin, and acne

延胡索 [yán hú suǒ]
***Rhizoma Corydalis*; *Yanhusuo*:** steamed and dried tuber of *Corydalis turtschaninovii* Bess (family Papaveraceae), used to activate blood flow and move *qi* for relieving pain in the chest and abdomen, dysmenorrhea and traumatic pain

元胡 [yuán hú]
another name for *Rhizoma Corydalis*, *Yanhusuo* (延胡索 [yán hú suǒ])

五灵脂 [wǔ líng zhī]
***Faeces Trogopterorum*; Trogopterus Dung:** dried faeces of *Trogopterus xanthipes* Milne-Edwards (family Petauristidae), used to relieve pain by eliminating blood stasis mainly for treating gastric and abdominal pain, and dysmenorrhea

卷柏 [juǎn bǎi]
***Herba Selaginellae*; Spikemoss:** dried herb of *Selaginella tamariscina* (family Selaginellaceae), used to promote blood flow and stimulate menstrual discharge for treating amenorrhea and dysmenorrhea

蒲黄 [pú huáng]
***Pollen Typhae*; Cat-tail Pollen:** dried pollen of *Typha angustifolia* L., *Typhaorientalis* Presl. or related species (family Typhaceae), used to promote blood flow and relieve pain by eliminating blood stasis for treating dysmenorrhea, postpartum abdominal pain and gastralgia

蒲黄炭 [pú huáng tàn]
***Pollen Typhae Carbonisatum*; Carbonized Cat-tail Pollen:** used as a stasis-removing hemostatic

穿山甲 [chuān shān jiǎ]
***Squama Manitis*; Pangolin Scale:** scale of the anteater, *Manis pentadactyla* L. (family Manidae), used (1) as an emmenagogue and galactagogue for amenorrhea and deficiency of lactation, respectively, and (2) to reduce swelling and dispel pus for treating acute suppurative inflammations

皂角刺 [zào jiǎo cì]
***Spina Gleditsiae*; Chinese Honeylocust Spine:** dried spine of *Gleditsia sinensis* Lam. (family Leguminosae), used (1) to reduce swelling and dispel pus for treating acute suppurative inflammations with the effect of promoting local rupture, and (2) as an antipruritic in the treatment of skin diseases

两面针 [liǎng miàn zhēn]
***Radix Zanthoxyli*; Shinyleaf Pricklyash Root:** dried root of *Zanthoxylum nitidum* (Roxb.) DC. (family Rutaceae), used to promote *qi* flow, eliminate blood stasis, relieve pain, and dispel wind, for treating traumatic injury, rheumatic arthralgia, toothache, stomachache, venomous snake-bite, and by way of topical application for treating burns and scalds

王不留行 [wáng bù liú xíng]
***Semen Vaccariae*; Cow-herb Seed:** dried ripe seed of *Vaccaria segetalis* (Neck.) Garcke (family Caryophyllaceae), used (1) as an emmenagogue and galactagogue for treating amenorrhea and lack of lactation, respectively, and (2) as a stranguria-relieving diuretic for treating urinary calculus

水蛭 [shuǐ zhì]
***Hirudo*; Leech:** dried body of *Whitmania pigra* Whitman, *Whitmania acranulata* Whitman or *Hirudo nipponica* Whitman (family Hirudinidae), used to break down stasis and reduce swellings for treating severe cases of blood stasis, such as hematoma, amenorrhea, gynecological mass, and contusions

虻虫 [méng chóng]
***Tabanus*; Gadfly:** dried female insect of *Tabanus bivittatus* Matsum. (family Tabanidae), used to break down stasis and reduce swellings for treating severe cases of blood stasis, such as amenorrhea and gynecological mass

䗪虫 [zhè chóng]
***Eupolyphaga seu Steleophaga*; Ground Beetle:** dried female insect of *Eupolyphaga sinensis* Walk. or *Steleophaga plancyi* (Bol.) (family Corydiidae), used (1) to break down stasis for treating amenorrhea and gynecological mass, and (2) to promote the healing of bone fracture

土鳖虫 [tǔ biē chóng]
another name for *Eupolyphaga seu Steleophaga*, Ground Beetle (䗪虫 [zhè chóng])

苏木 [sū mù]
***Lignum Sappan*; Sappan Wood:** dried heart wood of *Caesalpinia sappan* L. (family Leguminosae), used to activate blood flow and remove stasis, mainly for

treating contused wounds, dysmenorrhea and amenorrhea

益母草 [yì mǔ cǎo]
***Herba Leonuri*; Motherwort Herb:** dried aerial part of *Leonurus heterophyllus* Sweet (family Labiatae), used (1) to activate blood flow and regulate the menstrual discharge for treating menstrual disorders, and (2) as a diuretic for treating nephritic edema

坤草 [kūn cǎo]
another name for *Herba Leonuri* or Motherwort Herb (益母草 [yì mǔ cǎo])

茺蔚子 [chōng wèi zǐ]
***Fructus Leonuri*; Motherwort Fruit:** dried ripe fruit of *Leonurus heterophyllus* Sweet (family Labiatae), used (1) to activate blood flow and regulate menstrual discharge for treating menstrual disorders, and (2) to clear the eye of opacity for treating inflammation of the eye with formation of corneal opacity

马鞭草 [mǎ biān cǎo]
***Herba Verbenae*; European Verbena Herb:** dried aerial part of *Verbena officinalis* L. (family Verbenaceae), used (1) to activate blood flow and promote menstrual flow for treating amenorrhea and dysmenorrhea, (2) to counteract toxins for treating boils and other types of suppurative inflammations, and (3) as an antimalarial agent for treating malarial splenomegaly

三棱 [sān léng]
***Rhizoma Sparganii*; Common Burreed Tuber:** peeled and dried tuber of *Sparganium stoloniferum* Buch.-Ham. (family Sparganiaceae), used to break down blood stasis and eliminate masses for treating dysmenorrhea, amenorrhea and abdominal mass

泽兰 [zé lán]
***Herba Lycopi*; Bugleweed Herb:** dried aerial part of *Lycopus lucidus* Turcz. var. *hirtus* Regel (family Labiatae), used (1) to activate blood flow, remove stasis and regulate menstruation for treating irregular menstruation and postpartum abdominal pain, (2) to reduce swelling for treating traumatic injuries, boils and sores, and (3) to induce diuresis for treating edema and ascites

毛冬青 [máo dōng qīng]
***Radix Ilicis Pubescentis*; Pubescent Holly Root:** dried root of *Ilex pubescens* Hook. et Arn. (family Aquifoliaceae), used (1) to activate blood flow and unblock the meridians/channels and collaterals for treating thromboangitis obliterans and angina pectoris, (2) to clear heat and counteract toxins for treating inflammations such as acute tonsillitis, and (3) as an antitussive and expectorant for treating acute bronchitis

乳香 [rǔ xiāng]
***Olibanum*; Frankincense:** gum-resin obtained from *Boswellia carterii* Birdwood and possibly other species of *Boswellia* (family Burseraceae), used to relieve pain and swelling in cases of traumatic injuries by activating the local blood flow

没药 [mò yào]
***Myrrha*; Myrrh:** gum-resin obtained

from the stem of *Commphora molmol* Engler and probably other species (family Burseraceae), used for the relief of pain and swelling in cases of traumatic injury

自然铜 [zì rán tóng]
***Pyritum*; Pyrite:** yellow mineral, iron disulphide, cube-like crystals, used for promoting the healing of fractures and relieving traumatic pain

芳香开窍药
Aromatic Stimulants

冰片 [bīng piàn]
***Borneolum*; Borneol:** crystalline organic compound obtained synthetically or from *Dryobalanops aromatica* Gaertn. f., used (1) as an aromatic stimulant for treating loss of consciousness and convulsions due to high fever, and (2) topically to clear heat and alleviate pain for treating pharyngitis, tonsillitis, laryngitis, and stomatitis

牛黄 [niú huáng]
***Calculus Bovis*; Cow-Bezoar:** dried gallstone of domestic cattle, *Bos taurus domesticus* Gmelin (family Bovidae), used to arrest convulsions, resolve phlegm, restore consciousness, clear heat and counteract toxins for treating delirium and convulsions in cases of acute febrile diseases, infantile convulsion, inflammation of the pharynx, larynx and mouth, boils and sores

石菖蒲 [shí chāng pú]
***Rhizoma Acori Tatarinowii*; Grass-leaved Sweetflag Rhizome:** dried rhizome of *Acorus tatarinowii* Schott. (family Araceae), used (1) as an aromatic stimulant for treating impaired consciousness, insanity and epilepsy, and (2) to resolve dampness and harmonize the stomach for treating accumulation of dampness in the middle energizer with anorexia, epigastric stuffiness and abdominal distension

苏合香 [sū hé xiāng]
***Styrax*; Storax:** purified, semi-fluid, viscid balsam obtained from the trunk of *Liquidamber orientalis* Miller (family Hamamelidaceae), used as an aromatic stimulant for treating loss of consciousness due to apoplexy, and also for relieving angina pectoris

麝香 [shè xiāng]
***Moschus*; Musk:** dried secretion obtained from the musk sac of adult male musk deer, *Muschus berezovskii* Flerov, *Moschus sifanicus* Przewalski or *Moschus moschiferus* L. (family Cervidae), used (1) as an aromatic stimulant for treating loss of consciousness in cases of high fever and apoplexy, (2) to activate blood flow and alleviate pain for treating painful swellings of boils, carbuncles and thromboangitis obliterans, and (3) to expedite child delivery in cases of difficult labor and detention of afterbirth

安息香 [ān xī xiāng]
***Benzoinum*; Benzoin:** dried resin obtained from Tokin Snowbell, *Styrax tonkenensis* (Pierre) Craib ex Hart. (family Styracaceae), used (1) as an aromatic stimulant for restoring consciousness in cases of apoplexy, and (2) to activate the flow of *qi* and blood for relieving pain of the chest and abdomen

安神药 Tranquilizers

朱砂 [zhū shā]

***Cinnabaris*; Cinnabar:** mineral composed of red mercuric sulphide, used (1) as a settling tranquilizer for treating palpitation, insomnia, infantile convulsion and epilepsy, and (2) as a detoxicant for treating boils and carbuncles

琥珀 [hǔ pò]

***Succinum*; Amber:** yellowish or brownish fossil resin, used as (1) a sedative for treating insomnia, dream-disturbed sleep, palpitation and convulsion, and (2) as a diuretic and hemostatic for treating urodynia and hematuria due to acute urinary infection and urinary calculus

磁石 [cí shí]

***Magnetitum*; Magnetite:** magnetic iron ore composed mainly of ferriferrous oxide (Fe_3O_4), used as a settling tranquilizer and anti-asthmatic for treating tinnitus, palpitation, insomnia, epilepsy, mania, and asthma.

酸枣仁 [suān zǎo rén]

***Semen Ziziphi Spinosae*; Spine Date Seed:** dried ripe seed of *Ziziphus jujuba* Mill. var. *spinosa* (Bunge) Hu ex H. F. Chou (family Rhamnaceae), used (1) as a tranquilizer for treating fidgetiness, insomnia and palpitation, and (2) to arrest excessive sweating in cases of spontaneous perspiration and night sweats

远志 [yuǎn zhì]

***Radix Polygalae*; Thin-leaf Milkwort Root:** dried root of *Polygala tenuifolia* Willd. or *Polygala sibirica* L. (family Polygalaceae), used (1) as a tranquilizer in cases of palpitation and insomnia due to disharmony of the heart and kidney, (2) as an expectorant in cases of acute or chronic cough with profuse sputum, (3) to expel phlegm for treating epilepsy and mania due to obstruction of the heart orifice by phlegm, and (4) to reduce swelling in cases of boils and sores

合欢皮 [hé huān pí]

***Cortex Albiziae*; Silktree Albizia Bark:** dried bark of *Albizia julibrissin* Durazz. (family Leguminosae), used (1) as a tranquilizer for treating palpitation and insomnia due to anxiety, and (2) to activate blood flow for relieving pain in cases of traumatic swellings, boils or sores

合欢花 [hé huān huā]

***Flos Albiziae*; Albizia Flower:** dried flower-head of *Albizia julibrissin* Durazz. (family Leguminosae), used as a tranquilizer for treating fidgetiness and insomnia

首乌藤 [shǒu wū téng]

***Caulis Polygoni Multiflori*; Fleeceflower Stem:** dried lianoid stem of *Polygonum multiflorum* Thunb. (family Polygonaceae), used (1) as a heart-nourishing tranquilizer for treating insomnia and dream-disturbed sleep, and (2) to activate collateral blood flow for treating aching limbs

夜交藤 [yè jiāo téng]

another name for *Caulis Polygoni Multiflori* or Fleeceflower Stem (首乌藤 [shǒu wū téng])

灵芝 [líng zhī]

***Ganoderma Lucidum*; Lucid Ganoderma:** dried fructifications of the fungus, *Ganoderma lucidum* (Leyss. ex Fr.) Karst. (family Polyporaceae), used (1) as a tranquilizer for treating dizziness and insomnia, and (2) as a tonic for treating weakness or debility

缬草 [xié cǎo]

***Rhizoma Valerianae*; Valerian Rhizome:** dried rhizome of *Valeriana officinalis* L. (family Valerianaceae), used (1) as a tranquilizer for treating insomnia, and (2) to regulate the flow of *qi* for relieving abdominal distension and pain

珍珠 [zhēn zhū]

***Margarita*; Pearl:** lustrous concretion found in certain bivalve shell-fish, e.g., *Pteria martensii* (Dunker) (family Pteriidae), *Hyriopsis cumingii* (Lea), *Cristaria plicata* (Leach) (family Unionidae), used (1) as a settling tranquilizer and anticonvulsive agent for treating convulsion due to high fever or infantile convulsion, (2) externally to hasten the healing of wounds.

珍珠母 [zhēn zhū mǔ]

***Concha Margaritifera Usta*; Nacre:** calcined shell of certain pearl-yielding shell-fish, *Hyriopsis cumingii* (Lea), *Cristaria plicata* (Leach) (family Unionidae) or *Pteria martensii* (Dunker) (family Pteriidae), used (1) as a settling tranquilizer for treating palpitation, insomnia, and mania, and (2) to pacify the liver and subdue the exuberant yang for relieving headache and dizziness

柏子仁 [bǎi zǐ rén]

***Semen Platycladi*; Chinese Arborvitae Seed:** kernel of dried ripe seed of *Platycladus orientalis* (L.) Franco (family Cupressaceae), used (1) to nourish the heart and relieve mental strain for treating palpitation and insomnia in cases of heart blood deficiency, and (2) as an aperient for relieving constipation in debilitated patients

茯神 [fú shén]

***Poria cum Radice Pino*; Indian Bread with Pine:** *poria* with a piece of pine root embedded in it, used as a tranquilizer for treating palpitation and insomnia

紫贝齿 [zǐ bèi chǐ]

***Concha Mauritiae*; Purple Cowry Shell:** dried shell of *Mauritia (Arabica) arabica* (L.) (family Cypaeidae), used as a settling tranquilizer for treating palpitation and infantile convulsion

龙骨 [lóng gǔ]

***Os Draconis*; Dragon's Bone:** fossil bone of a large ancient mammal, such as *Stegodon orientalis* or *Rhinocerus sinensis*, used (1) as a settling tranquilizer for treating palpitation, insomnia, and dream-disturbed sleep, (2) to pacify the liver and subdue the exuberant yang for relieving dizziness or vertigo, and (3) to arrest discharge for treating enuresis, seminal emission, spermatorrhea and leukorrhagia, and (4) externally for adsorbing exudate in cases of skin diseases

龙齿 [lóng chǐ]

***Dens Draconis*; Dragon's Teeth:** fossil teeth from a large ancient mammal, such as *Stegodon orientalis* or *Rhinocerus sinensis*, used in a similar way to *Os Draconis* or Dragon's Bone 龙骨 [lóng gǔ], with a stronger action

牡蛎 [mǔ lì]
***Concha Ostreae*; Oyster Shell:** shell of *Ostrea gigas* Thunb., *Ostrea talienwhanensis* Crosse or *Ostrea rivularis* Gould (family Ostreidae), used (1) as a settling tranquilizer for treating headache, dizziness, palpitation and insomnia, and (2) to soften and disperse hard lumps in cases of scrofula

平肝熄风药
Liver-pacifying and Wind-extinguishing Medicinals/Drugs

天麻 [tiān má]
***Rhizoma Gastrodiae*; Gastrodia Tuber:** dried tuber of *Gastrodia elata* Bl. (family Orchidaceae), used (1) to extinguish wind and relieve spasm for treating convulsion and hemiplegia in cases of apoplexy, (2) to pacify the liver and subdue the exuberant yang for relieving headache, dizziness and vertigo, and (3) for relieving rheumatalgia

钩藤 [gōu téng]
***Ramulus Uncariae cum Uncis*; Gambir Plant:** dried hook-bearing stem branch of *Uncaria rhynchophylla* (Miq.) Jack., *Uncaria macrophylla* Wall., *Uncaria hirsuta* Havil., *Uncaria sinensis* (Oliv.) Havil. or *Uncaria sessilifructus* Roxb. (family Rubiaceae), used to extinguish wind, relieve spasm, clear heat and pacify the liver for treating convulsions due to high fever, and headache, dizziness and vertigo due to liver heat

全蝎 [quán xiē]
***Scorpio*; Scorpion:** boiled and dried body of *Buthus martensii* Karsch (family Buthidae), used to subdue endogenous wind for treating various kinds of tics, convulsion, tetanus and sequelae of cerebrovascular accidents

全虫 [quán chóng]
same as 全蝎 [quán xiē]

蜈蚣 [wú gōng]
***Scolopendra*; Centipede:** dried body of *Scolopendra subspinipes mutilans* L. Koch (family Scolopendridae), used (1) to extinguish wind for relieving spasm in cases of tics, convulsion, tetanus and facial paralysis, (2) to unblock collateral meridians/channels for alleviating pain in cases of stubborn arthralgia and intractable migraine, and (3) as a detoxicant for treating scrofula and venomous snake-bite

僵蚕 [jiāng cán]
***Bombyx Batryticatus*; Stiff Silkworm:** dried body of the 4-5th stage larva of *Bombyx mori* L., dead and stiffened due to *Beauveria bassiana* fungus infection, used (1) to extinguish endogenous wind for relieving convulsions, (2) to resolve phlegm and dissipate nodulation for treating scrofula, and (3) to dispel exogenous wind in the case of wind-heat contraction manifested by headache, sore throat, hoarseness of voice or urticaria

白僵蚕 [bái jiāng cán]
same as 僵蚕 [jiāng cán]

羚羊角 [líng yáng jiǎo]
***Cornu Saigae Tataricae*; Antelope**

Horn: horn of *Saiga tatarica* L. (family Bovidae), used to pacify the liver, extinguish wind, clear heat, and counteract toxins for treating (1) liver wind with impaired consciousness and convulsions, (2) liver fire with headache, dizziness and acute conjunctivitis, and (3) high fever with delirium

地龙 [dì lóng]

***Lumbricus*; Earthworm:** dried body of *Pheretima aspergillum* (Perrier) or *Allolobophora caliginosa* (Savigny) *trapezoides* (Ant. Duges) (family Megascolecidae), used to clear heat, extinguish wind, unblock collateral meridians/channels, relieve asthma, and induce diuresis, for treating convulsion due to high fever, rheumatalgia, hemiplegia, bronchial asthma, and dysuria due to accumulated heat in the bladder

赭石 [zhě shí]

***Haematitum*; Hematite:** dark-brown-colored iron ore mainly composed of ferric oxide (Fe_2O_3), used (1) to pacify the liver and subdue exuberant yang for treating up-rising of liver yang with headache, vertigo and tinnitus, (2) to suppress the reversed upward flow of *qi* for relieving belching, nausea, vomiting and asthma, and (3) as a blood-cooling hemostatic in cases of hematemesis and epistaxis

代赭石 [dài zhě shí]

synonym for 赭石 [zhě shí]

石决明 [shí jué míng]

***Concha Haliotidis*; Sea-ear Shell:** shell of *Haliotis diversicolor* Reeve, *Haliotis discus hanai* Ino or *Haliotis ovina* Gmelin, *Haliotis ruber* (Leach), *Haliotis asinina* L. or *Haliotis Laevigata* (Donovan) (family Haliotidae), used (1) to pacify the liver and subdue exuberant yang for treating up-rising of liver yang with headache and vertigo, and (2) to clear liver heat for improving vision in cases of glaucoma and cataract

蒺藜 [jí lí]

***Fructus Tribuli*; Puncture-vine Caltrop Fruit:** dried fruit of *Tribulus terrestris* L. (family Zygophylaceae), used (1) to pacify and soothe the liver for treating headache, vertigo, thoracic and hypochondriac pain, and mastitis due to depressed liver *qi*, (2) to improve vision in cases of conjunctivitis and nebula, and (3) to dispel wind in cases of urticaria and pruritus

刺蒺藜 [cì jí lí]

same as *Fructus Tribuli* or Puncture-vine Caltrop Fruit (蒺藜 [jí lí])

玳瑁 [dài mào]

***Carapax Eretmochelydis*; Hawksbill Shell:** carapace of the hawksbill turtle, *Eretmochelys imbricata* (L.) (family Chelonidae), used to extinguish wind, clear heat and counteract toxins for treating convulsion and delirium in cases of febrile diseases

熊胆 [xióng dǎn]

***Fel Ursi*; Bear Gall:** dried gall-bladder of the bear, *Selenarctos thibetanus* Cuvier or *Ursus arctos* L. (family Ursidae), used (1) to extinguish wind, clear heat, and counteract toxins for treating febrile convulsions and epilepsy, and externally for treating boils, sores and hemorrhoidal swelling, (2) to clear the liver for improving vision in cases of conjunctivitis and nebula

补养药 Tonics

补气药
Qi Tonics (Medicinals/Drugs for Replenishing *Qi*)

人参 [rén shēn]
***Radix Ginseng*; Ginseng:** dried root of *Panax ginseng* C. A. Mey. (family Araliaceae), used (1) to powerfully replenish *qi* and to promote fluid production for treating prostration, general weakness, diabetes mellitus, impotence or frigidity, heart failure, and cardiogenic shock, (2) to tonify the spleen and lung for treating anorexia, cough and shortness of breath, and (3) as a tranquilizer for treating cardiac palpitation and insomnia

党参 [dǎng shēn]
***Radix Codonopsis*; Tangshen:** dried root of *Codonopsis pilosula* (Franch.) Nannf., *Codonopsis pilosula* var. *modesta* (Nannf.) L.T. Shen or *Codonopsis tangshen* Oliv. (family Campanulaceae), used to replenish *qi*, promote fluid production and nourish the blood for treating (1) deficiency of the middle *qi* with general debility, anorexia, lassitude and loose stools, and (2) deficiency of both *qi* and yin with shortness of breath, pallor, dizziness and palpitations

太子参 [tài zǐ shēn]
***Radix Pseudostellariae*; Heterophylly Falsestarwort Root:** dried tuberous root of *seudostellaria heterophylla* (Miq.) Pax ex Pax et Hoffm. (family Caryophyllaceae), used in a similar way to *Radix Codonopsis* or Tangshen (党参 [dǎng shēn]), less active as a tonic, but more active in promoting the production of body fluids

孩儿参 [hái ér shēn]
another name for *Radix Pseudostellariae* or Heterophylly Falsestarwort Root (太子参[tài zǐ shēn])

黄芪 [huáng qí]
***Radix Astragali*; Milkvetch Root:** dried root of *Astragalus membranaceus* (Fisch.) Bge. or *Astragalus membranaceus* var. *mongholicus* (Bge.) Hsiao (family Leguminosae), used (1) to replenish *qi* for treating general weakness, anorexia and loose stools, prolapse of uterus or anus, spontaneous sweating, and chronic nephritis with edema and proteinuria, and (2) to dispel pus and accelerate the healing of chronic ulcers

红芪 [hóng qí]
***Radix Hedysari*; Sweetvetch Root:** dried root of *Hedysarum polybotrys* Hand.-Mazz. (family Leguminosae), used as a substitute for *Radix Astragali* or Milkvetch Root (黄芪 [huáng qí])

甘草 [gān cǎo]
***Radix Glycyrrhizae*; Licorice Root:** dried root and rhizome of *Glycyrrhiza uralensis* Fisch., *Glycyrrhiza inflata* Bat. or *Glycyrrhiza glabra* L. (family Leguminosae), used (1) to replenish *qi* and tonify the heart for treating arrythmia in cases of deficiency of heart *qi*, (2) to tonify the spleen for treating lassitude, anorexia

and loose bowels in cases of spleen insufficiency, (3) to relieve epigastric colic and spastic pain of the limbs, (4) to dispel phlegm and arrest cough, (5) to clear heat and counteract toxins for treating sore throat, boils, sores and drug poisoning, and most frequently (6) for modulating other ingredients in a prescription

炙甘草 [zhì gān cǎo]
***Radix Glycyrrhizae Preparata*; Prepared Licorice Root:** processed *Radix Glycyrrhizae*, Licorice Root by stir-baking with honey, used to tonify the spleen and heart, particularly for treating arrhythmia

刺五加 [cì wǔ jiā]
***Radix Acanthopanacis Senticosi*; Thorny Acathopanax Root:** dried root and rhizome of *Acanthopanax senticosus* (Rupr. et Maxim.) Harms (family Aralicaceae), used to replenish *qi*, strengthen the spleen, tonify the kidney, and induce tranquilization for treating general weakness, anorexia, aching back and knees, insomnia, and dream-disturbed sleep

白术 [bái zhú]
***Rhizoma Atractylodis Macrocephalae*; Largehead Atractylodes Rhizome:** dried rhizome of *Atractylodes macrocephala* Koidz. (family Compositae), used (1) to replenish *qi*, invigorate the spleen for treating general weakness, anorexia, dyspepsia and chronic diarrhea, (2) to arrest excessive sweating, and (3) to calm the fetus for treating threatened abortion

山药 [shān yào]
***Rhizoma Dioscoreae*; Common Yam Rhizome:** dried rhizome of *Dioscorea opposita* Thunb. (family Dioscoreaceae), used to replenish *qi* and yin, tonify the spleen, lung and kidney for treating (1) weakness of the spleen and stomach with poor appetite and chronic diarrhea, (2) lung insufficiency with chronic cough, (3) insecurity of the kidney with nocturnal emission, polyuria and leukorrhagia, and (4) yin deficiency in cases of diabetes

白扁豆 [bái biǎn dòu]
***Semen Lablab Album*; White Hyacinth Bean:** dried ripe seed of *Dolichos lablab* L. (family Leguminosae), used to strengthen the spleen and resolve dampness for treating (1) weakness of the spleen and stomach with anorexia, loose stools, and leukorrhagia, and (2) vomiting and diarrhea due to summer dampness

大枣 [dà zǎo]
***Fructus Jujubae*; Jujube; Chinese Date:** dried ripe fruit of *Ziziphus jujuba* Mill. (family Rhamnaceae), used to replenish the middle *qi*, nourish the blood and induce tranquilization, and also used to moderate drug actions of other ingredients in a prescription

黄精 [huáng jīng]
***Rhizoma Polygonati*; Solomonseal Rhizome:** steamed and dried rhizome of *Polygonatum sibiricum* Red., *Polygonatum kingianum* Coll. et Hemsl. or *Polygonatum cyrtonema* Hua (family Liliaceae), used (1) to replenish spleen *qi* for treating general debility and poor appetite, and (2) to nourish lung yin for treating chronic dry cough in cases of phthisis

饴糖 [yí táng]

***Extractum Malti*; Malt Extract:** amber or yellowish brown, viscous liquid, with an agreeable odor and a sweet taste, prepared from malted grains of barley, *Hordeum vulgare* L. or malted grains of wheat, *Triticum aestivum* L., used as a tonic to replenish the middle *qi* for treating general weakness, also used as an antitussive for treating chronic cough

补血药

Blood Tonics (Medicinals/Drugs for Nourishing the Blood)

当归 [dāng guī]

***Radix Angelicae Sinensis*; Chinese Angelica:** dried root of *Angelica sinensis* (Oliv.) Diels (family Umbelliferae), used (1) to nourish the blood for treating blood deficiency of the heart and liver, (2) activate the blood flow and regulate menstruation for treating menstrual disorders, and (3) as an emollient and laxative for treating chronic constipation in the aged and debilitated

白芍 [bái sháo]

***Radix Paeoniae Alba*; White Peony Root:** peeled and dried root of *Paeonia lactiflora* Pall. (family Ranunculaceae), used (1) to nourish the blood and regulate menstruation for treating menstrual disorders, (2) to pacify the liver for alleviating pain such as headache, hypochondriac pain, and spastic pain of the limbs, and (3) to arrest excessive sweating

阿胶 [ē jiāo]

***Colla Corii Asini*; Ass-hide Glue:** solid glue prepared from the skin of an ass, *Equus asinus* L. (family Equidae), used (1) to nourish the blood for treating blood deficiency, (2) to arrest bleeding for treating all kinds of hemorrhages, and (3) to nourish yin for treating insomnia and dry cough

紫河车 [zǐ hé chē]

***Placenta Hominis*; Human Placenta:** dried human placenta, used to replenish *qi*, nourish the blood and supplement essence for treating deficiency of *qi* and blood, general weakness, sterility, impotence, chronic cough and asthma

龙眼肉 [lóng yǎn ròu]

***Arillus Longan*; Longan Aril:** dried aril of *Dimocarpus longan* Lour. (family Sapindaceae), used to nourish the blood and induce tranquilization for treating palpitations, dizziness and insomnia

熟地黄 [shú dì huáng]

***Radix Rehmanniae Praeparata*; Prepared Rehmannia Root:** steamed and dried tuberous root of *Rehmannia glutinosa* Libosch. (family Scrophulariaceae), used as (1) the main tonic for treating blood deficiency with pallor, dizziness, palpitations, menstrual disorders, and (2) an important kidney-yin tonic for treating chronic tidal fever, night sweats, lumbago, nocturnal emission, and diabetes

补阴药

Yin Tonics (Medicinals/Drugs for Replenishing Yin)

西洋参 [xī yáng shēn]
***Radix Panacis Quinquefolii*; American Ginseng:** dried root of *Panax quinquefolium* L. (family Araliaceae), used to replenish *qi*, nourish yin, reduce internal heat and promote fluid production, for treating (1) yin deficiency with exuberant fire with cough and blood-streaked sputum, and (2) impairment of both *qi* and yin in cases of febrile diseases with fidgetiness and thirst

石斛 [shí hú]
***Herba Dendrobii*; Dendrobium:** fresh or dried stem of *Dendrobium loddigesii* Rolfe., *Dendrobium chrysanthum* Wall., *Dendrobium fimbriatum* var. *oculatum* Hook., *Dendrobium candidum* Wall. ex Lindl. or *Dendrobium nobile* Lindl. (family Orchidaceae), used to replenish stomach yin, clear heat, and promote fluid production for treating chronic febrile diseases with thirst and dry mouth, deficiency of stomach yin with epigastric distress and pain, and also for improving vision in cases of cataracts

玉竹 [yù zhú]
***Rhizoma Polygonati Odorati*; Fragrant Solomonseal Rhizome:** steamed and dried rhizome of *Polygonatum odoratum* (Will.) Druce (family Liliaceae), used to nourish yin and promote fluid production for treating dipsosis, dry throat and dry cough in cases of febrile diseases and diabetes

麦冬 [mài dōng]
***Radix Ophiopogonis*; Dwarf Lilyturf Root:** dried tuberous root of *Ophiopogon japonicus* (Thunb.) Ker-Gawl. (family Liliaceae), used (1) to replenish and promote fluid production for treating dipsosis, dry throat, dry cough and bloody sputum in cases of acute febrile diseases and yin deficiency of the lung and stomach, and (2) to calm the mind for treating fidgetiness and insomnia

麦门冬 [mài mén dōng]
synonym for 麦冬[mài dōng]

天冬 [tiān dōng]
***Radix Asparagi*; Asparagus Root:** steamed, peeled and dried tuberous root of *Asparagus cochinchinensis* (Lour.) Merr. (family Liliaceae), used to replenish yin and promote fluid production for treating dipsosis, dry throat, cough with sticky phlegm, bloody sputum and constipation

天门冬 [tiān mén dōng]
synonym for 天冬 [tiān dōng]

北沙参 [běi shā shēn]
***Radix Glehniae*; Coastal Glehia Root:** dried root of *Glehnialittoralis* Fr. Schmidt ex Miq. (family Umbelliferae), used to replenish yin of the lung and stomach and promote fluid production for treating dipsosis, dry throat and dry cough

枸杞子 [gǒu qǐ zǐ]
***Fructus Lycii*; Barbary Wolfberry Fruit:** dried ripe fruit of *Lycium barbarum* L. (family Solanaceae), used to replenish liver and kidney yin for treating aching back and legs, impotence and nocturnal emission, vertigo and weakened eyesight

山茱萸 [shān zhū yú]
***Fructus Corni*; Asiatic Cornelian Cherry Fruit:** dried ripe sarcocarp of *Cornus*

officinalis Sieb. et Zucc. (family Cornaceae), used (1) to replenish liver and kidney yin for treating aching back, weakened knees, vertigo and impotence, and (2) to arrest discharge for treating nocturnal emission, enuresis, abnormal uterine bleeding, and excessive perspiration

何首乌 [hé shǒu wū]

***Radix Polygoni Multiflori*; Fleeceflower Root:** dried tuberous root of *Polygonum multiflorum* Thunb. (family Polygonaceae), used as a laxative for relieving constipation and also as an antimalarial agent

首乌 [shǒu wū]

synonym for 何首乌 [hé shǒu wū]

制何首乌 [zhì hé shǒu wū]

***Radix Polygoni Multiflori Preparata*; Prepared Fleeceflower Root:** fleeceflower root processed with black bean juice, used to replenish liver and kidney yin and nourish the blood for treating blood deficiency of the liver and essence deficiency of the kidney with dizziness, tinnitus, aching back and knees, and early graying of the hair

牛膝 [niú xī]

***Radix Achyranthis Bidentatae*; Twoteethed Achyranthes Root:** dried root of *Achyranthes bidentata* Bl. (family Amaranthaceae), used (1) to nourish the liver and kidney and to strengthen the sinews and bones for treating aching back and knees, and asthenia of the lower limbs, (2) to activate blood flow for treating amenorrhea, dysmenorrhea and irregualr menstruation, as well as traumatic injuries, (3) to direct fire or blood to move downward in the treatment of headache and dizziness due to up-rising of liver-yang, and epistaxis and hemoptysis due to up-flaming of fire

怀牛膝 [huái niú xī]

synonym for 牛膝 [niú xī]

沙苑子 [shā yuàn zǐ]

***Semen Astragali Complanati*; Flatstem Milkvetch Seed:** dried ripe seed of *Astragalus complanatus* R. Br. (family Leguminosae), used to replenish liver and kidney yin for treating dizziness, blurred vision, seminal emission, premature ejaculation, impotence, frequent micturition and leukorrhagia

潼蒺藜 [tóng jí lí]

synonym for 沙苑子 [shā yuàn zǐ]

女贞子 [nǔ zhēn zǐ]

***Fructus Ligustri Lucidi*; Glossy Privet Fruit:** dried ripe fruit of *Ligustrum lucidum* Ait. (family Oleaceae), used to replenish liver and kidney yin, darken the hair and improve the eyesight for treating early graying of the hair, dim eyesight, lumbago and low fever in cases of yin deficiency

桑寄生 [sāng jì shēng]

***Ramulus Taxilli*; Mulberry Mistletoe:** dried leaf-bearing stem and branch of *Taxillus chinensis* (DC.) Danser (family Loranthaceae), used (1) to replenish liver and kidney yin, strengthen the sinews and bones and dispel wind-dampness for treating arthralgia with aching back and limbs, and (2) to nourish the blood and prevent miscarriage for treating menorrhagia and threatened abortion

鹿衔草 [lù xián cǎo]
***Herba Pyrolae*; Pyrola Herb:** dried entire plant of *Pyrola calliantha* H. Andres or *Pyrola decorata* H. Andres (family Pyrolaceae), used to replenish kidney yin, strengthen the sinews and bones, dispel wind-dampness, and arrest bleeding for treating lumbago, rheumatism, menorrhagia, hemoptysis and epistaxis

龟甲 [guī jiǎ]
***Carapax et Plastrum Testudinis*; Tortoise Shell:** carapace and plastron of fresh-water tortoise, *Chinemys reevesii* (Gray) (family Testudinidae), used to replenish liver and kidney yin and subdue hyperactive liver yang, for treating vertigo, chronic tidal fever, night sweats, dry mouth and throat, and aching back and knees with asthenia, osteomalacia and rickets

龟板 [guī bǎn]
***Plastrum Testudinis*; Tortoise Plastron:** ventral shell of fresh-water tortoise with the same uses as *carapax et plastrum testudinis*, tortoise shell (龟甲 [guī jiǎ])

鳖甲 [biē jiǎ]
***Carapax Trionycis*; Turtle Shell:** dorsal shell of the soft-shelled turtle, *Trionyx sinensis* Wiegmann (family Trionychidae), used to replenish yin, subdue exuberant yang, and soften and resolve hard lumps for treating (1) chronic tidal fever and night sweats in cases of yin deficiency, and (2) splenomegaly in cases of chronic malaria

桑椹 [sāng shèn]
***Fructus Mori*; Mulberry Fruit:** dried fruit-spike of *Morus alba* L. (family Moraceae), used (1) to replenish yin and nourish the blood for treating dizziness, tinnitus, blurred vision in cases of deficiency of yin and blood, and (2) to promote fluid production for relieving dipsosis in cases of diabetes

黑芝麻 [hēi zhī má]
***Semen Sesami Nigrum*; Black Sesame:** dried ripe seed of Sesamum indicum L. (family Pedaliaceae), used (1) to tonify the liver and kidney and replenish essence and blood for treating dizziness, blurred vision, premature graying of hair and beard, and (2) to relax the bowels for treating constipation

补阳药
Yang Tonics (Medicinals / Drugs for Reinforcing Yang)

鹿茸 [lù róng]
***Cornu Cervi Pantotrichum*; Hairy Deer-horn:** hairy, unossified young horn of male sika deer, *Cervus nippon* Temminck or red deer, *Cervus elaphus* L. (family Cervidae), used to reinforce the kidney yang and strengthen the bones and muscles for treating intolerance of cold, loss of strength, impotence, spontaneous seminal emission, leukorrhagia and other symptoms of yang deficiency in cases of chronic diseases

鹿角 [lù jiǎo]
***Cornu Cervi*; *Antler*; Deer-horn:** ossified horn of male red deer, *Cervus elaphus* L. or sika deer *Cervas nippon* Temminck (family Cervidae), used in a similar way to hairy deer-horn (鹿茸 [lù róng]), but less

active, also used to remove blood stasis for treating traumatic wounds

鹿角胶 [lù jiǎo jiāo]
***Colla Cornus Cervi*; Deer-horn Gelatin:** gelatin prepared from decoction of deer-horn, with a kidney-nourishing action superior to that of deer-horn (鹿角 [lù jiǎo]), and additional effects of nourishing the blood and stopping bleeding

鹿角霜 [lù jiǎo shuāng]
***Cornu Cervi Degelatinatum*; Degelatinated Deer-horn:** by-product in the preparation of deer-horn gelatin (dried residual deer-horn left after decoction) with an action similar but inferior to that of deer-horn (鹿角 [lù jiǎo])

肉苁蓉 [ròu cōng róng]
***Herba Cistanchis*; Desert-living Cistanche:** dried fleshy stem with scales of *Cistanche deserticola* Y.C. Ma (family Orobanchaceae), used (1) to reinforce kidney yang for treating impotence and premature ejaculation, and (2) as a mild laxative for treating chronic constipation in the aged

大芸 [dà yún]
synonym for 肉苁蓉 [ròu cōng róng]

益智仁 [yì zhì rén]
***Semen Alpiniae Oxyphyllae*; Sharpleaf Galangal Seed:** dried ripe seed of *Alpinia oxyphylla* Miq. (family Zingiberaceae), used to warm the spleen and kidney for treating (1) chronic diarrhea with cold pain in the abdomen, and (2) enuresis, frequent micturition, and seminal emission

仙茅 [xiān máo]
***Rhizoma Curculiginis*; Common Curculigo Rhizome:** dried rhizome of *Curculigo orchioides* Gaertn. (family Amaryllidaceae), used to warm the kidney, reinforce yang, strengthen the tendons and bones, and dispel cold-dampness for treating aching back and knees with intolerance of cold, impotence, enuresis, stubborn arthralgia, and chronic diarrhea

淫羊藿 [yín yáng huò]
***Herba Epimedii*; Epimedium Herb:** dried aerial part of *Epimedium brevicornum* Maxim., *Epimedium sagittatum* (Sieb. et Zucc.) Maxim., *Epimedium koreanum* Nakai, *Epimedium pubescens* Maxim. or *Epimedium wushanense* T. S. Ying (family Berberidaceae), used (1) to replenish kidney yang for treating impotence, sterility and frequent micturition, and (2) to strengthen the tendons and bones, and dispel wind-dampness for treating rheumatalgia, contracture and numbness

仙灵脾 [xiān líng pí]
synonym for 淫羊藿 [yín yáng huò]

核桃仁 [hé táo rén]
***Semen Juglandis*; English Walnut Seed:** dried ripe seed of *Juglans regia* L. (family Juglandeceae), used to tonify the kidney and lung for treating aching back and knees, cough and dyspnea of deficiency-cold type, seminal emission and impotence

锁阳 [suǒ yáng]
***Herba Cynomorii*; Songaria Cynomorium Herb:** dried fleshy stem of *Cynomorium songaricum* Rupr. (family Cynomoriaceae), used (1) to reinforce kidney yang for

treating impotence, and seminal emission, and (2) as a mild laxative for treating chronic constipation in the aged

巴戟天 [bā jǐ tiān]

***Radix Morindae Officinalis*; Morinda Root:** dried root of *Morinda officinalis* How (family Rubiaceae), used to reinforce kidney yang for treating impotence and premature ejaculation in men, and frigidity in women

葫芦巴 [hú lú bā]

***Semen Trigonellae*; Common Fenugreek Seed:** dried ripe seed of *Trigonella foenum-graecum* L. (family Leguminosae), used to warm the kidney, disperse cold and relieve pain for treating cold pain in the testis, hernial pain, and weakness and edema of the legs due to cold-dampness

补骨脂 [bǔ gǔ zhī]

***Fructus Psoraleae*; Malaytea Scurfpea Fruit:** dried ripe fruit of *Psoralea corylifolia* L. (family Leguminosae), used to warm the kidney and spleen and reinforce yang for treating impotence, nocturnal emission, frequent micturition, chronic asthma due to kidney insufficiency, and diarrhea occurring daily just before dawn due to deficiency of spleen and kidney yang

菟丝子 [tù sī zǐ]

***Semen Cuscutae*; Dodder Seed:** dried ripe seed of *Cuscuta chinensis* Lam. (family Convolvulaceae), used to tonify the liver and kidney, improve vision and prevent miscarriage for treating nocturnal emission, impotence, enuresis, diabetes, decreased eyesight and threatened abortion

杜仲 [dù zhòng]

***Cortex Eucommiae*; Eucommia Bark:** dried stem-bark of *Eucommia ulmoides* Oliv. (family Eucommiaceae), used to tonify the liver and kidney, strengthen the tendons and bones, and prevent miscarriages, for treating aching back and knees, impotence, frequent micturition, threatened abortion and nowadays for treating hypertension

狗脊 [gǒu jǐ]

***Rhizoma Cibotii*; Cibot Rhizome:** dried rhizome of *Cibotum barometz* (L.) J. Sm. (family Dicksoniaceae), used to tonify the liver and kidney, strengthen the back and knees and dispel wind-dampness, for treating insecurity of the kidney with enuresis and leukorrhagia, aching back and knees, rheumatic pain in the back, and strained lumbar muscles

续断 [xù duàn]

***Radix Dipsaci*; Himalayan Teasel Root:** dried root of *Dipsacus asperoides* C.Y. Cheng et T.M.Ai (family Dipsacaceae), used (1) to tonify the liver and kidney and strengthen the tendons and bones for treating aching back and joints, and rheumatic pain in the lumbar region, (2) to improve the healing of fractures, and (3) to stop bleeding and prevent miscarriage, for treating functional uterine bleeding and threatened abortion

骨碎补 [gǔ suì bǔ]

***Rhizoma Drynariae*; Fortune's Drynaria Rhizome:** dried rhizome of *Drynaria fortunei* (Kunze) J. Sm. or *Drynaria baronii* (Christ) Diels (family Polypodiaceae), used (1) to tonify the kidney for treating lumbago, impaired hearing, and tinnitus, (2) to promote the healing of traumatic injuries and bone fracture, and (3) externally for treating alopecia areata and vitiligo

韭菜子 [jiǔ cài zǐ]
***Semen Allii Tuberosi*; Tuber Onion Seed:** dried ripe seed of Allium tuberosum Rotti (family Liliaceae), used to tonify the liver and kidney, promote virility and arrest spontaneous emission for treating impotence, nocturnal emission, aching lumbus and knees, and morbid leukorrhea, also called 韭子 [jiǔ zǐ]

韭子 [jiǔ zǐ]
abbreviation for 韭菜子 [jiǔ cài zǐ]

冬虫夏草 [dōng chóng xià cǎo]
***Cordyceps*; Chinese Caterpillar Fungus:** dried body of stroma of the fungus, *Cordyceps sinensis* (Berk.) Sacc. (family Hypocreaceae) growing on the larva of certain insect (family Hepialidae) and the dead caterpillar, used to reinforce kidney yang and tonify the lung for treating impotence, nocturnal emission, night sweats, chronic cough with hemoptysis in cases of phthisis

蛤蚧 [gé jiè]
***Gecko*; Tokay Gecko:** dried body, with the viscera removed, of a lizard, *Gekko gecko* L. (family Geckonidae), used to reinforce kidney yang and replenish lung *qi* for treating chronic asthma

海马 [hǎi mǎ]
***Hippocampus*; Sea-Horse:** dried body of *Hippocampus kelloggi* Jordan et Snyder, *H.histrix* Kaup, *H.* kuda Bleeker, *H.trimaculatus* Leach or *H. japonicus* Kaup. (family Syngnathidae), used (1) to tonify kidney yang for treating impotence and frigidity, (2) to reduce swelling of abdominal masses and traumatic wounds, and (3) externally for treating boils and sores

固涩药
Astringents and Hemostatics

浮小麦 [fú xiǎo mài]
***Fructus Tritici Levis*; Light Wheat:** dried light grains of *Triticum aestivum* L. (family Graminae), used as an antihidrotic agent for treating spontaneous sweating or night sweats

麻黄根 [má huáng gēn]
***Radix Ephedrae*; Ephedra Root:** dried root and rhizome of *Ephedra sinica* Stapf. or *Ephedra intermedia* Schrenk et C.A. Mey (family Ephedraceae), used as an anhidrotic agent for treating spontaneous perspiration and night sweats

五倍子 [wǔ bèi zǐ]
***Galla Chinensis*; Chinese Gall:** gall produced mainly by aphides of *Melaphis chinensis* (Bell) Baker on the leaf of various Sumac, *Rhus chinensis* Mill., *Rhuspotaninii* Maxim., *Rhus punjabensis* Stew. var. *sinica* (Diels) Rehd. et Wils. (family Anacardiaceae), used (1) as an astringent for treating persistent cough, night sweats, chronic diarrhea, bloody stool and, enuresis, and (2) externally for treating burns, traumatic bleeding, hemorrhoids and oral ulcers

诃子 [hē zǐ]

***Fructus Chebulae*; Terminalia Fruit:** dried ripe fruit of *Terminalia chebula* Retz. or *Terminalia chebula* var. *tomentella* Kurt. (family Combretaceae), used as an antidiarrhetic and antitussive agent for treating chronic diarrhea or dysentery, persistent cough and hoarse voice

石榴皮 [shí liú pí]

***Pericarpium Granati*; Pomegranate Rind:** dried pericarp of *Punica granatum* L. (family Punicaceae), used (1) as an antidiarrhetic for treating chronic diarrhea or dysentery, and (2) as an anthelmintic for treating intestinal taeniasis and ascariasis

赤石脂 [chì shí zhī]

***Halloysitum Rubrum*; Red Halloysite:** mineral, hydrated aluminum silicate, red in color due to the presence of iron oxides, used as an antidiarrhetic and hemostatic for treating chronic diarrhea, menorrhagia and leukorrhagia

莲子 [lián zǐ]

***Semen Nelumbinis*; Lotus Seed:** dried ripe seed of *Nelumbo nucifera* Gaertn. (family Nymphaeaceae), used as an astringent for treating chronic diarrhea, spontaneous emission and leukorrhagia

莲须 [lián xū]

***Stamen Nelumbinis*; Lotus Stamen:** dried stamen of Lotus, *Nelumbo nucifera* Gaertn. (family Nymphaeaceae), used as an astringent to consolidate kidney *qi* for treating seminal emission and leukorrhagia

芡实 [qiàn shí]

***Semen Euryales*; Gordon Euryale Seed:** dried kernel of ripe seed of *Euryale ferox* Salisb. (family Nymphaeaceae), used as an astringent for treating chronic diarrhea, spontaneous emission, enuresis, and leukorrhagia

禹余粮 [yǔ yú liáng]

***Limonitum*; Limonite:** brownish iron ore, mainly composed of basic iron oxide [FeO(OH)], used as an astringent for treating chronic diarrhea or dysentery, menorrhagia and leukorrhagia

禹粮石 [yǔ liáng shí]

synonym for 禹余粮 [yǔ yú liáng]

伏龙肝 [fú lónggān]

***Terra Flava Usta*; Calcined Yellow Earth:** calcined clean yellow earth in small lumps, used as (1) an anti-emetic for treating nausea and vomiting due to chronic stomach diseases or pregnancy, (2) an antidiarrhetic for treating chronic diarrhea, and (3) a hemostatic for treating bleeding due to failure of the spleen to control the blood

乌梅 [wū méi]

***Fructus Mume*; Smoked Plum:** dried nearly ripe fruit of Japanese Apricot, *Prunus Mume* (Sieb.) Sieb. et Zucc. (family Rosaceae), used as an antidiarrhetic, antitussive, antidiptic and anthelmintic agent for treating chronic diarrhea, persistent cough, morbid thirst and ascariasis

肉豆蔻 [ròu dòu kòu]

***Semen Myristicae*; Nutmeg:** dried kernel of *Myristica fragrans* Houtt. (family Myristicaceae), used as an antidiarrhetic agent by warming the spleen and stomach for treating chronic diarrhea

肉果 [ròu guǒ]
synonym for 肉豆蔻 [ròu dòu kòu]

罂粟壳 [yīng sù qiào]
***Pericarpium Papaveris*; Poppy Capsule:** dried ripe capsule of Opium Poppy, *Papaver somniferum* L. (family Papaveraceae), used as an antidiarrhetic, antitussive and analgesic agent for treating chronic diarrhea, persistent cough and abdominal pain

米壳 [mǐ qiào]
synonym for 罂粟壳 [yīng sù qiào]

五味子 [wǔ wèi zǐ]
***Fructus Schisandrae*; Chinese Magnoliavine Fruit:** dried ripe fruit of *Schisandra chinensis* (Turcz.) Baill. or *Schisandra sphenanthera* Rehd. et Wils. (family Magnoliaceae), used as (1) an astringent for treating dry cough, asthma, night sweats, seminal emission and chronic diarrhea, and (2) a tranquilizer for palpitations and insomnia

桑螵蛸 [sāng piāo xiāo]
***Oötheca Mantidis*; Mantid Egg Capsule:** dried egg capsule of a praying mantis, *Tenodera sinensis* Saussure, *Statilja maculata* (Thunb.) or *Hierodula patellifera* (Serville) (family Mantidae), used as an astringent for treating frequent micturition, enuresis, seminal emission and leukorrhagia

海螵蛸 [hǎi piāo xiāo]
***Os Sepiae*; Cuttlebone:** dried internal shell of *Sepiella maindroni* de Rochebrune or *Sepia esculenta* Hoyle (family Sepiadae), used as a hemostatic and antacid agent for treating hematemesis, bloody stools, menorrhagia, acid regurgitation and leukorrhagia

乌贼骨 [wū zéi gǔ]
synonym for 海螵蛸 [hǎi piāo xiāo]

瓦楞子 [wǎ léng zǐ]
***Concha Arcae*; Arc Shell:** shell of *Arca subcrenata* Lischke, *Arca granosa* L. or *Arca inflata* Reeve (family Arcidae), used to eliminate phlegm and soften hard lumps for treating scrofula and goiter

煅瓦楞 [duàn wǎ léng]
***Concha Arcae Usta*; Calcined Arc Shell:** calcined shell of *Arca subcrenata* Lischke, *Arca granosa* L. or *Arca inflata* Reeve (family Arcidae), used as an antacid agent for treating acid regurgitation

煅龙骨 [duàn lóng gǔ]
***Os Draconis Ustum*; Calcined Dragon's Bone:** calcined fossil bone of large ancient mammals, such as *Stegodon orientalis* and *Rhinocerus sinensis*, used as an astringent for treating seminal emission, night sweats, leukorrhagia and uterine bleeding

煅牡蛎 [duàn mǔ lì]
***Concha Ostreae Usta*; Calcined Oyster Shell:** calcined shell of *Ostrea gigas* Thunb., *Ostrea talienwhanensis* Crosse or *Ostrea rivularis* Gould (family Ostreidae), used as an astringent and antacid for treating excessive sweating, seminal emission, leukorrhagia and acid regurgitation

金樱子 [jīn yīng zǐ]

***Fructus Rosae Laevigatae*; Cherokee Rose Fruit:** dried ripe fruit of Cherokee Rose, *Rosa laevigata* Mickx. (family Rosaceae), used as an astringent for treating seminal emission, enuresis, frequent micturition and chronic diarrhea

覆盆子 [fù pén zǐ]

***Fructus Rubi*; Palmleaf Raspberry Fruit:** steamed and dried fruit of *Rubus chingii* Hu (family Rosaceae), used as an astringent for treating frequent micturition, enuresis and seminal emission

消导药
Digestives and Evacuants

山楂 [shān zhā]

***Fructus Crataegi*; Hawthorn Fruit:** dried ripe fruit of Large Chinese Hawthorn, *Crataegus pinnatifida* Bge. var. *major* N.E. Br. or Chinese Hawthorn, *Crataegus pinnatifida* Bge. (family Rosaceae), used (1) to improve digestion and relieve food stagnation for treating dyspepsia and stagnation of fatty food, and (2) to activate blood flow for treating amenorrhea and postpartum abdominal pain due to blood stasis

焦山楂 [jiāo shān zhā]

***Fructus Crataegi Preparatus*; Charred Hawthorn Fruit:** hawthorn fruit stir-baked to a brown color, used to improve digestion and relieve food stagnation for treating dyspepsia and stagnation of fatty food

麦芽 [mài yá]

***Fructus Hordei Germinatus*; Germinated Barley:** dried germinated grain of barley, *Hordeum vulgare* L. (family Graminae), used (1) to improve digestion for treating dyspepsia, and (2) to inhibit milk secretion for stopping lactation

焦麦芽 [jiāo mài yá]

***Fructus Hordei Germinatus Preparatus*; Charred Germinated Barley:** germinated grain of barley stir-baked to a brown color, used to improve digestion for treating dyspepsia induced by cereal food and infantile lactodyspepsia

稻芽 [dào yá]

***Fructus Oryzae Germinatus*; Rice-grain Sprout:** dried germinated grains of rice, *Oryza sativa* L. (family Graminae), used to improve digestion for treating poor appetite and dyspepsia

谷芽 [gǔ yá]

***Fructus Setariae Germinatus*; Millet Sprout:** dried germinated grains of millet, *Setaria italica* (L.) Beauv. (family Graminae), used in the same way as rice-grain sprout (稻芽 [dào yá]) to improve digestion for treating poor appetite and dyspepsia

粟芽 [sù yá]

synonym for 谷芽 [gǔ yá]

神曲 [shén qū]

***Massa Fermentata Medicinalis*; Medicated Leaven:** dried mass of a fermented mixture of wheat flour, fresh aerial parts of *Artemisia annua*, *Xanthium sibiricum*, and *Polygonum hydropiper*, used to improve digestion for treating dyspepsia and abdominal distension due to food stagnation

焦三仙 [jiāo sān xiān]

Charred Triplet: mixture consisting of equal parts of charred medicated leaven, charred hawthorn fruit and charred germinated barley, stronger in effect for improving digestion than each of them alone

鸡内金 [jī nèi jīn]

***Endothelium Corneum Gigeriae Galli*; Chicken's Gizzard-skin:** dried lining membrane of the gizzard of common fowl, *Gallus gallus domesticus* Briss. (family Phasianidae), used to improve appetite and digestion for treating poor appetite and dyspepsia

莱菔子 [lái fú zǐ]

***Semen Raphani*; Radish Seed:** dried ripe seed of garden radish, *Raphanus sativus* L. (family Cruciferae), used (1) to improve digestion and direct *qi* to move downward for treating food stagnation with abdominal distension and pain, and (2) to resolve phlegm for treating cough and dyspnea with profuse expectoration

泻下药
Purgatives

蜂蜜 [fēng mì]

***Mel*; Honey:** saccharine fluid made by the hive-bee, *Apis cerana* Fabr. or *Apis mellifera* L. (family Apidae), used as an antitussive for dry cough, and as an aperient for constipation in the aged

郁李仁 [yù lǐ rén]

***Semen Pruni*; Chinese Dwarf Cherry Seed:** dried ripe seed of *Prunus humilis* Bge., *Prunus japonica* Thunb. or *Prunus pedunculata* Maxim. (family Rosaceae), used as an aperient for treating constipation, and a diuretic for relieving edema

火麻仁 [huǒ má rén]

***Fructus Cannabis*; Hemp Seed:** dried ripe fruit of *Cannabis sativa* L. (family Moraceae), used as aperient for treating constipation in the debilitated or aged

大黄 [dà huáng]

***Radix et Rhizoma Rhei*; Rhubarb:** dried root and rhizome of *Rheum palmatum* L., *Rheum tanguticum* Maxim. ex Balf. or *Rheum officinale* Baill. (family Polygonaceae), used to induce catharsis, clear heat, purge fire, arrest bleeding, counteract toxins, and remove blood stasis for treating (1) constipation with gastrointestinal accumulation, (2) warm diseases with high fever, delirium and constipation, (3) postpartum abdominal pain and amenorrhea due to blood stasis, (4) hemoptysis, hematemesis and epistaxis associated with excessive heat in the blood, and (5) externally for treating burns, boils and sores

番泻叶 [fān xiè yè]

***Folium Sennae*; Senna Leaf:** dried leaf of *Cassia angustifolia* Vahl or *Cassia acutifolia* Delile (family Leguminosae), used as a purgative for treating constipation, especially habitual constipation

芒硝 [máng xiāo]

***Natrii Sulfas*; Sodium Sulfate; Glauber's Salt:** crystalline hydrated sodium sulfate, usually made from natural sources, used (1) as a purgative for treating constipation, and (2) externally to soften hard mass for treating acute mastitis

玄明粉 [xuán míng fěn]
***Natrii Sulfas Exsiccatus*; Exsiccated Sodium Sulfate:** white powder composed of sodium sulfate, used as a purgative for treating constipation

芦荟 [lú huì]
***Aloe*; Aloes:** dried leaf juice of *Aloe barbadensis* Mill., *Aloe ferox* Mill. or related species (family Liliaceae), used (1) as a purgative for treating constipation, (2) to clear the liver for treating liver fire with dizziness, headache and irritability, and (3) to kill intestinal parasitic worms

驱虫药
Anthelmintics

苦楝皮 [kǔ liàn pí]
***Cortex Meliae*; Szechwan Chinaberry Bark:** dried stem- or root-bark of *Melia toosendan* Sieb. et Zucc. or *Melia azedarach* L. (family Meliaceae), used as an antiparasitic for treating helminths, and externally for treating scabies

使君子 [shǐ jūn zǐ]
***Fructus Quisqualis*; Rangoon-creeper Fruit:** dried ripe fruit of *Rangoon* Creeper, *Quisqualis indica* L. (family Combretaceae), used as an anthelmintic for treating ascariasis, enterobiasis and infantile malnutrition associated with intestinal parasitosis

槟榔 [bīng láng]
***Semen Arecae*; Areca Seed:** dried ripe seed of Betel Palm, *Areca catechu* L. (family Palmae), used (1) to expel helminths for treating ascariasis, fasciolopsiasis, ancylostomiasis, oxyuriasis andparticularly taeniasis, (2) to remove undigested food for relieving abdominal distension and diarrhea with tenesmus in cases of food stagnation, (3) to induce diuresis for treating edema, and (4) to arrest malarial episodes

南瓜子 [nán guā zǐ]
***Semen Cucurbitae*; Pumpkin Seed:** dried seed of *Cucurbita moschata* Duch. (family Cucurbitaceae), used as an anthelmintic for treating taeniasis, schistosomiasis and clonorchiasis

榧子 [fěi zǐ]
***Semen Torreyae*; Grand Torreya Seed:** dried ripe seed of Chinese Torreya, *Torreya grandis* Fort. (family Taxaceae), used as an anthelmintic and laxative for treating taeniasis, enterobiasis, ancylostomiasis, ascariasis and fasciolopsiasis

雷丸 [léi wán]
***Omphalia*; Thunder Ball:** dried sclerotium of *Omphalia lapidescens* Schroet. (family Polyporaceae), used as an anthelmintic for treating taeniasis, ancylostomiasis, and ascariasis

鹤虱 [hè shī]
***Fructus Carpesii*; Common Carpesium Fruit:** dried ripe fruit of *Carpesium abrotanoides* L. (family Compositae), used as an anthelmintic for treating ascariasis, enterobiasis and taeniasis

北鹤虱 [běi hè shī]
same as 鹤虱 [hè shī]

南鹤虱 [nán hè shī]

***Fructus Carotae*; Carrot Fruit:** dried ripe fruit of *Daucus carota* L. (family Umbelliferae), used (1) to kill parasitic worms in cases of ascariasis, oxyuriasis and taeniasis, and (2) to remove undigested food for treating food stagnation

鹤草芽 [hè cǎo yá]

***Gemma Agrimoniae*; Agrimonia Bud:** dried bud, with a short piece of rhizome attached, of *Agrimonia pilosa* Ledeb. (family Rosaceae), used as an anthelmintic for treating taeniasis

外用药
Medicinals/Drugs for External Use

硫黄 [liú huáng]

***Sulfur*; Sulfur:** obtained from natural sources after purification, used (1) externally as antiparasitic for treating scabies, and (2) internally to reinforce yang for treating impotence and chronic asthma

雄黄 [xióng huáng]

***Realgar*; Realgar:** mineral, orange to reddish in color, mainly composed of arsenic disulfide (As_2S_2), used externally as a detoxicant and antiparasitic agent for treating snake and insect bites, boils, and scabies

信石 [xìn shí]

***Arsenicum Trioxidum*; Arsenic Trioxide:** used (1) externally as a caustic to remove dead tissue for treating boils, ulcers, scrofula and hemorrhoids, and (2) internally in minute quantities as an expectorant and antiasthmatic agent for treating asthma with thin and frothy phlegm

白砒 [bái pī]

synonym for 信石 [xìn shí]

轻粉 [qīng fěn]

***Calomelas*; Calomel:** crystalline mercurous chloride (Hg_2Cl_2), used (1) externally as an antiparasitic for treating scabies, tinea, neurodermatitis and eczematous lesions, and (2) internally, in small quantities, to remove phlegm and cause purgation

甘汞 [gān gǒng]

synonym for 轻粉 [qīng fěn]

白矾 [bái fán]

***Alumen*; Alum:** crystalline mineral salt, hydrated potassium aluminum sulfate, used (1) externally to kill parasites, arrest discharges and relieve itching in cases of scabies, tinea, neurodermatitis and eczematous lesions, and (2) internally to dispel wind-phlegm for treating epilepsy and mania

明矾 [míng fán]

synonym for 白矾 [bái fán]

枯矾 [kū fán]

***Alumen Ustum*; Calcined Alumen:** calcined potassium aluminum sulfate, used to arrest discharges, promote the healing of ulcers, stop bleeding, and cause cauterization, (1) externally for treating eczema, excessive leukorrhea with pudendal itching, and nasal polyp, and (2) internally as an astringent for treating chronic diarrhea and bloody stools

炉甘石 [lú gān shí]
***Calamina*; Calamine:** calcined and elutriated powder of smithsonite, mainly composed of zinc carbonate ($ZnCO_3$) with a pink tint due to the presence of a small amount of ferric oxide, used externally as an astringent for treating chronic ulcers, eczema, conjunctivitis and keratitis

血竭 [xuè jié]
***Sanguis Draconis*; Dragon's Blood:** red resin secreted from the fruit of *Daemonorops draco* Bl. (family Palmae), used to eliminate blood stasis, relieve pain and promote healing in cases of traumatic injuries

硇砂 [náo shā]
***Sal Purpureum*; Purple Rock Salt; *Sal Ammoniacum*; Sal Ammoniac:** mineral salt-containing ammonium chloride, used (1) externally for treating nebula and pterygium, and (2) internally for treating cancer of the esophagus

紫硇砂 [zǐ náo shā]
***Sal Purpureum*; Purple Rock Salt:** purple-colored rock salt (cf. 硇砂[náo shā])

白硇砂 [bái náo shā]
***Sal Ammoniacum*; Sal Ammoniac:** colorless crystalline mineral salt mainly containing ammonium chloride (cf. 硇砂 [náo shā])

硼砂 [péng shā]
***Borax*; Borax:** colorless crystalline mineral salt, hydrated sodium tetraborate, used (1) externally as a gargle for treating oral ulcers and acute tonsillitis, and (2) internally as an expectorant

蛇床子 [shé chuáng zǐ]
***Fructus Cnidii*; Common Cnidium Fruit:** dried ripe fruit of *Cnidium monnieri* (L.) Cuss. (family Umbelliferae), used (1) externally as an astringent and antiparasitic for treating eczema, pruritus vulvae and trichomonas vaginitis, and (2) internally to warm the kidney and promote virility for treating impotence

土荆皮 [tǔ jīng pí]
***Cortex Pseudolaricis*; Golden Larch Bark:** dried root bark of *Pseudolarix kaempferi* Gord. (family Pinaceae), used to kill parasites and relieve itching for treating scabies and tinea

巴豆 [bā dòu]
***Semen Crotonis*; Croton Seed:** dried ripe seed of *Croton tiglium* L. (family Euphorbiaceae), used externally for treating scabies, tinea, and warts (cf. 巴豆霜 [bā dòu shuāng])

千金子 [qiān jīn zǐ]
***Semen Euphorbiae*; Caper Euphorbia Seed:** dried ripe seed of *Euphorbialathyris* L. (family Euphorbiaceae), used to induce drastic purgation for treating edema, and eliminate blood stasis for treating amenorrhea and abdominal mass

斑蝥 [bān máo]
***Mylabris*; Mylabris; Blister Beetle:** dried body of *Mylabris phalerata* Pall. or *Mylabris cichorii* L. (family Meloidae), used (1) externally as a rubefacient, irritant and caustic to promote local blood flow, remove dead tissue and accelerate

the healing of wounds for treating psoriasis, neurodermatitis, chronic ulcers and scrofula, and (2) internally in small quantities for treating swelling of the lymph glands, and rabies

蟾酥 [chán sū]
***Venenum Bufonis*; Toad Venom:** dried secretion of the skin glands of the toad, *Bufo bufo gargarizans* Cantor or *Bufo melanostictus* Schneider (family Bufonidae), used as a detoxicant, discutient and anodyne, applied externally and taken internally for treating boils, sores, ulcers, tumors, chronic osteomyelitis, and sore throat

蜂房 [fēng fáng]
***Nidus Vespae*; Wasp's Nest:** nest of wasps or hornets, *Polistes olivaceus* (DeGeer), *Polistes japonicus* Sauss. or *Parapolybia varia* Fabr. (family Vespidae), used (1) externally for treating tinea, (2) as a gargle for treating painful swelling of the gums, and (3) internally for treating convulsions, urticaria and chronic cough

儿茶 [ér chá]
***Catechu*; Cutch; Black Catechu:** dry extract prepared from the peeled stem and branches of *Acacia catechu* (L.) Willd. (family Leguminosae), used externally as an astringent for treating chronic ulcer, eczema, and traumatic bleeding

方剂 Formulas

方剂 [fāng jì]
formula; prescription; recipe: direction of the preparation (including ingredients and doses) and administration of a remedy, also called 方 [fāng] for short

方 [fāng]
abbreviation for 方剂 [fāng jì]

药方 [yào fāng]
prescription: popular name for formula (方剂 [fāng jì]), usually referring to a written direction for preparation and administration of a medicine

单方 [dān fāng]
simple formula/prescription: formula or prescription consisting of one or two medicinal substances for treating a particular illness in uncomplicated condition

奇方 [jī fāng]
odd-numbered formula/prescription: (1) formula or prescription with ingredients odd in number; (2) formula or prescription with one single ingredient

偶方 [ǒu fāng]
even-numbered formula/prescription: (1) formula or prescription with ingredients even in number; (2) formula or prescription with two ingredients

复方 [fù fāng]
compound formula/prescription: formula or prescription formed by (1) two or more set formulae; (2) one set formula with additional ingredients

成方 [chéng fāng]
set formula: formula that has already been set and recorded

验方 [yàn fāng]
proven formula: formula that has been proven effective in the treatment of a certain morbid condition

良方 [liáng fāng]
effective formula: formula that often shows good results in the treatment of a certain morbid condition

秘方 [mì fāng]
secret formula: formula that is kept unknown to others, also called 禁方 [jìn fāng]

禁方 [jìn fāng]
secret formula: formula that is not allowed to be told to others

祖传秘方 [zǔ chuán mì fāng]
secret formula handed down in a family

偏方 [piān fāng]
special but irregular recipe: simple recipe that has not been recorded in regular formularies but has special effect in treating a certain illness

土方 [tǔ fāng]
folk recipe/formula: simple empirical recipe/formula used by the people living in a certain area

土法 [tǔ fǎ]
folk treatment: simple empirical method of treatment used by the people living in a certain area

经方 [jīng fāng]
classical formula: (1) formula recorded in *the Inner Classic* or Zhang Zhongjing's works; (2) formula recorded in Zhang Zhongjing's works

时方 [shí fāng]
updated formula: formula introduced by physicians after the time of the noted physician Zhang Zhongjing

大方 [dà fāng]
major formula; heavy formula: (1) formula or prescription consisting of a number of ingredients with strong actions; (2) large dosage of medicine given at one time for a strong action; and (3) formula or prescription for treating a serious disease or a disease of the lower energizer

小方 [xiǎo fāng]
minor formula; mild formula: (1) formula or prescription consisting of only a few ingredients with mild actions; (2) small dosage of medicine; or (3) formula or prescription for treating an uncomplicated disease or a disease of the upper energizer

缓方 [huǎn fāng]
slow-acting formula: formula or prescription composed of ingredients that act slowly or counteract each other to moderate the overall effect, and indicated in the treatment of cases of chronic debilitation

急方 [jí fāng]
quick-acting formula: formula or prescription employed for immediate effect in the treatment of emergency or critical cases

配方 [pèi fāng]
dispensing a prescription: preparing a medicine according to the prescription

汤头 [tāng tóu]
decoction formula: formula for the preparation of a decoction

汤头歌 [tāng tóu gē]
formulae in rhyme: docoction formulae put into rhyme for ease of remembrance

方剂配伍 [fāng jì pèi wǔ]
ingredient combination in formula/prescription: combination of various ingredients in formula or prescription, selected in accordance with medicinal compatibility rules and for producing the desired therapeutic effect in unison, and in the meantime minizing toxic or side effects

君臣佐使 [jūn chén zuǒ shǐ]
sovereign, minister, adjuvant and courier; chief, associate, assistant and guide: four different roles which the ingredients in formula or prescription play

君药 [jūn yào]
sovereign ingredient; chief ingredient: ingredient that produces the principal curative action

臣药 [chén yào]
minister ingredient; associated ingredient: ingredient that helps strengthen the principal action

佐药 [zuǒ yào]
adjuvant ingredient; assistant ingredient: ingredient that relieves secondary symptoms or tempers the action of the principal ingredient when the latter is too potent

使药 [shǐ yào]
courier ingredient; guide ingredient: ingredient that directs action to the affected meridian/channel or site

主辅佐引 [zhǔ fǔ zuǒ yǐn]
principal, adjuvant, auxiliary and conductant: alternative descriptions for sovereign, minister, adjuvant and courier, or chief, associate, assistant and guide (君臣佐使[jūn chén zuǒ shǐ])

引经报使 [yǐn jīng bào shǐ]
directing to the affected meridian/channel or site: action of a conductant ingredient in directing other ingredients to work on the affected meridian/channel or site, e.g., *Radix Bupleuri* directing to the lesser yang meridian/channel, *Radix Platycodi* to the throat, and *Radix Cyathulae* to the lower extremities

药引子 [yào yǐn zi]
"medicinal guide"; extra conductant ingredient: extra ingredient in formula or prescription, used to strengthen the efficacy of the whole recipe by directing the latter's action to the affected site

反佐 [fǎn zuǒ]
using a corrigent: adding a conductant ingredient opposite in nature to the other ingredients, e.g., adding an ingredient cold in nature to a recipe hot in nature, or an ingredient hot in nature to a recipe cold in nature

相须 [xiāng xū]
reinforcing relationship; mutual reinforcement: compatibility rule in which two ingredients with similar

properties used in combination may reinforce each other's action

相使 [xiāng shǐ]
assisting relationship: compatibility rule in which two or more ingredients in a prescription may be used in combination, one being the principal substance while the other or others play a subsidiary role to reinforce the action of the former

相畏 [xiāng wèi]
restraining relationship: compatibility rule in which toxic or side effects of one ingredient may be neutralized by another, e.g., the side effects of pinella tuber being restrained by fresh ginger (半夏畏生姜 [bàn xià wèi shēng jiāng])

相恶 [xiāng wù]
inhibiting relationship; counteracting: compatibility rule in which the efficacy of one ingredient may be weakened or counteracted by another

相杀 [xiāng shā]
suppressing relationship; neutralizing: compatibility rule in which the property of one ingredient may neutralize the toxicity of another, e.g., fresh ginger suppressing the side effects of pinella tuber (生姜杀半夏 [shēng jiāng shā bàn xià])

相反 [xiāng fǎn]
antagonizing relationship; incompatibility: compatibility rule in which the property of one ingredient may enhance the side effects of another if used together

十八反 [shí bā fǎn]
eighteen antagonisms: incompatible medicinals which, if given in combination, have serious side effects: *Radix Glycyrrhizae* being antagonistic to *Radix Euphorbiae Pekinensis*, *Flos Genkwa*, *Radix Euphorbiae Kansui*, and *Sargassum*; *Radix Aconiti* being antagonistic to *Bulbus Fritillariae*, *Fructus Trichosanthis*, *Rhizoma Pinelliae*, *Radix Ampelopsis* and *Rhizoma Bletillae*; and *Radix Veratri Nigri* being antagonistic to *Radix Ginseng*, *Radix Salviae Miltiorrhizae*, *Radix Adenophorae*, *Radix Sophorae Flavescentis*, *Radix Scrophulariae*, *Herba Asari* and *Radix Paeoniae*

十九畏 [shí jiǔ wèi]
nineteen incompatibilities: medicinals of restraining pairs which, if used in combination, one may restrain or neutralize the other's action: sulfur restraining crude sodium sulfate; mercury restraining arsenic trioxide; *Radix Euphorbiae Ebracteolatae* restraining litharge; *Semen Crotonis* restraining *Semen Pharbitidis*; *Flos Caryophylli* restraining *Radix Curcumae*; crystalline sodium sulfate restraining *Rhizoma Sparganii*; *Radix Aconiti* and *Radix Aconiti Kuznezoffi* restraining *Cornu Rhinoceri*; *Radix Ginseng* restraining *Faeces Trogopterorum*; and *Cortex Cinnamomi* restraining *Halloysitum Rubrum*

十剂 [shí jì]
ten categories of formulae: collective term for obstruction-removing, dispelling, tonifying, purgative, light, heavy, lubricating, astringent, desiccating, and moistening formulae

通剂 [tōng jì]
obstruction-removing formula: formula

used in treating stasis or obstruction, e.g., amenorrhea, galactostasis and arthralgia due to obstruction of *qi* and blood in the collateral meridians/channels

宣剂 [xuān jì]
dispersing formula: formula indicated for removing stasis, reducing phlegm, and inducing emesis

补剂 [bǔ jì]
tonifying formula: formula used in the treatment of various deficiency conditions and boosting health

泄剂 [xiè jì]
purgative formula: formula used not only for relieving constipation, but also for removing excessive heat, eliminating accumulated cold, and purging retained fluid

轻剂 [qīng jì]
light (diaphoretic) formula: formula composed of light dispersing ingredients to release the superficies from exogenous pathogens

重剂 [zhòng jì]
heavy formula: formula that contains weighty medicinals/drugs with tranquilizing action

滑剂 [huá jì]
lubricating formula: formula that relieves dysuria and aids discharge of calculi

涩剂 [sè jì]
astringent formula: formula that arrests discharge, often used for treating excessive sweating, seminal emission, and protracted diarrhea

燥剂 [zào jì]
desiccating formula: formula that has the effect of removing pathogenic dampness, often used for treating edema and retention of excessive fluid and phlegm

湿剂 [shī jì]
moistening formula: formula that has the effect of replenishing body fluid

十二剂 [shí èr jì]
twelve categories of formulae: the ten categories of formulae plus cooling and warming formulae

寒剂 [hán jì]
cooling formula: formula with medicinals/drugs cool or cold in nature (as the chief ingredients), used in treating heat syndromes/patterns

热剂 [rè jì]
warming formula: formula with medicinals/drugs warm or hot in nature (as the chief ingredients), used in treating cold syndromes/patterns

十四剂 [shí sì jì]
fourteen categories of formulae: the twelve categories of formulae plus elevating formula and depressant formula

升剂 [shēng jì]
elevating formula: formula with elevating effect for treating prolapse of the rectum, prolapse of the uterus, and other kinds of visceroptosis

降剂 [jiàng jì]
depressant formula: formula with the effect of suppressing the reversed upward

flow of *qi*, air or gas, for treating cough, hiccups, belching and vomiting

解表剂 [jiě biǎo jì]
exterior-releasing formula: formula to dispel pathogenic factors from the superficies of the body for treating exterior syndrome/pattern

辛温解表剂 [xīn wēn jiě biǎo jì]
pungent-warm exterior-releasing formula: formula mainly consisting of ingredients pungent in flavor and warm in nature to dispel pathogenic factors from the superficies of the body for treating exterior syndrome/pattern of wind-cold contraction

麻黄汤 [má huáng tāng]
***Mahuang* Decoction; Ephedra Decoction:** formula composed of *Herba Ephedrae* (麻黄), *Ramulus Cinnamomi* (桂枝), *Semen Armeniacae Amarum* (苦杏仁) and *Radix Glycyrrhizae* (甘草), used as a diaphoretic and antasthmatic for treating exterior excess syndrome/pattern of wind-cold contraction

桂枝汤 [guì zhī tāng]
***Guizhi* Decoction; Cassia-twig Decoction:** formula composed of *Ramulus Cinnamomi* (桂枝), *Radix Paeoniae Alba* (白芍), *Rhizoma ZingiberisRecens* (生姜), *Radix Glycyrrhizae* (甘草), and *Fructus Ziziphi Jujubae* (大枣), used to expel exogenous pathogenic factors from the superficial muscles and rectify derangement of the nutrient and defensive aspects for treating exterior deficiency syndrome/pattern of wind-cold contraction

九味羌活汤 [jiǔ wèi qiāng huó tāng]
***Jiuwei Qianghuo* Decoction; Nine-ingredient Decoction with Notopterygium:** formula composed of *Rhizoma seu Radix Notopterygii* (羌活), *Radix Saposhnikoviae* (防风), *Rhizoma Atractylodis* (苍术), *Rhizoma Chuanxiong* (川芎), *Herba Asari* (细辛), *Radix Angelicae Dahuricae* (白芷), *Radix Rehmanniae* (生地黄), and *Radix Glycyrrhizae* (甘草), used to induce sweating, dispel dampness and clear internal heat for treating external contraction of wind-cold-dampness complicated by contraction of internal heat

香薷散 [xiāng rú sǎn]
***Xiangru* Powder; Elshotzia Powder:** formula composed of *Herba Elshotziae* (香薷), *Semen Lablab Album* (白扁豆), and *Cortex Magnoliae Officinalis* (厚朴), used to dispel summerheat, release the exterior, resolve dampness and harmonize the middle engergizer for treating colds in summer

小青龙汤 [xiǎo qīng lóng tāng]
***Xiao Qinglong* Decoction; Minor Decoction of Blue Dragon:** decoction composed of *Herba Ephedrae* (麻黄), *Ramulus Cinnamomi* (桂枝), *Herba Asari* (细辛), *Rhizoma Zingiberis* (干姜), *Rhizoma Pinelliae Praeparata* (制半夏), *Fructus Schisandrae* (五味子), *Radix Paeoniae Alba* (白芍), and *Radix Glycyrrhizae* (甘草), used to release the exterior, disperse cold, warm the lung and resolve retained fluid in the treatment of cold in the exterior and retained fluid in the interior

止嗽散 [zhǐ sòu sǎn]
***Zhisou* Powder; Antitussive Powder:** formula composed of *Radix Platycodi*

(桔梗), *Herba Schizonepetae* (荆芥), *Radix Asteris* (紫菀), *Radix Stemonae* (百部), *Rhizoma Cynanchi Stauntonii* (白前), *Radix Glycyrrhizae* (甘草), and *Pericarpium Citri Reticulatae* (陈皮), used to disperse wind and stop coughing in the treatment of wind attack of the lung

辛凉解表剂 [xīn liáng jiě biǎo jì]
pungent-cool exterior-releasing formula: formula mainly consisting of ingredients pungent in flavor and cool in nature to disperse wind-heat in the treatment of exterior syndrome/pattern of wind-heat contraction or warm diseases at the early stage

辛凉平剂 [xīn liáng píng jì]
moderate pungent-cool formula: formula composed of pungent cool ingredients to relieve wind-heat exterior syndrome/pattern via a moderate action, e.g., lonicera-forsythia powder

辛凉轻剂 [xīn liáng qīng jì]
mild pungent-cool formula: formula composed of pungent cool ingredients to relieve wind-heat exterior syndrome/pattern via a mild action, e.g., morus-chrysanthemum decoction

辛凉重剂 [xīn liáng zhòng jì]
drastic pungent-cool formula: formula composed of pungent cool ingredients to relieve wind-heat exterior syndrome/pattern via a drastic action

银翘散 [yín qiào sǎn]
***Yin Qiao Powder*; Lonicera-Forsythia Powder:** formula composed of *Flos Lonicerae* (金银花), *Fructus Forsythiae* (连翘), *Fructus Arctii* (牛蒡子), *Herba Menthae* (薄荷), *Herba Schizonepetae* (荆芥), *Semen Sojae Praeparatum* (豆豉), *Radix Platycodi* (桔梗), *Radix Glycyrrhizae* (甘草), *Herba Lophatheri* (淡竹叶), and *Rhizoma Phragmitis* (芦根), used as an exterior-releasing, heat-clearing and toxin-counteracting remedy for treating warm diseases at the early stage

桑菊饮 [sāng jú yǐn]
***Sang Ju Yin*; Morus-Chrysanthemum Decoction:** formula composed of *Folimu Mori* (桑叶), *Flos Chrysanthemi* (菊花), *Herba Menthae* (薄荷), *Semen ArmeniacaeAmarum* (苦杏仁), *Radix Platycodi* (桔梗), *Radix Glycyrrhizae* (甘草), *HerbaLophatheri* (淡竹叶) and *Rhizoma Phragmitis* (芦根), used to disperse wind, clear heat and stop coughing in the treatment of wind-warmth diseases at the early stage

麻杏石甘汤 [má xìng shí gān tāng]
***Ma Xing Shi Gan* Decoction; Decoction of Ephedra, Apricot Kernel, Gypsum and Liquorice:** formula composed of *Herba Ephedrae* (麻黄), *Semen Armeniacae Amarum* (苦杏仁), *Gypsum Fibrosum* (石膏), and *Radix Glycyrrhizae* (甘草), used to ventilate the lung and clear the lung of heat for treating lung heat contraction with cough and dyspnea complicated by exterior syndrome/pattern

柴葛解肌汤 [chái gě jiě jī tāng]
***Chai Ge Jieji* Decoction; Bupleurum-Pueraria Muscle-releasing Decoction:** formula composed of *Radix Bupleuri* (柴胡), *Radix Puerariae* (葛根), *Radix Glycyrrhizae* (甘草), *Radix Scutellariae*

(黄芩), *Rhizoma seu Radix Notopterygii* (羌活), *Radix Angelicae Dahuricae* (白芷), and *Radix Platycodi* (桔梗), used to release the flesh and clear heat for treating wind-cold contraction with heat transformation

升麻葛根汤 [shēng má gě gēn tāng]
***Shengma Gegen* Decoction; Cimicifuga-Pueraria Decoction:** formula composed of *Rhizoma Cimicifugae* (升麻), *Radix Puerariae* (葛根), *Radix Paeoniae* (芍药), and *Radix Glycyrrhizae* (甘草), used to release the flesh and promote eruption for treating measles at the early stage

扶正解表剂 [fú zhèng jiě biǎo jì]
healthy-*qi*-reinforcing exterior-releasing formula: formula to relieve exterior syndrome/pattern in patients with weak constitution

败毒散 [bài dú sǎn]
***Baidu* Powder; Antiphlogistic Powder:** formula composed of *Radix Bupleuri* (柴胡), *Radix Peucedani* (前胡), *Radix Chuanxiong* (川芎), *Fructus Aurantii* (枳壳), *Rhizoma seu Radix Notopterygii* (羌活), *Radix Angelicae Pubescentis* (独活), *Radix Platycodi* (桔梗), *Poria* (茯苓), *Radix Ginseng* (人参), and *Radix Glycyrrhizae* (甘草), used to disperse cold, remove dampness, replenish *qi* and release the exterior for treating external contraction in patients with *qi* deficiency

荆防败毒散 [jīng fáng bài dú sǎn]
***Jingfang Baidu* Powder; Schizonepeta-Saposhnikovia Antiphlogistic Powder:** formula composed of *Herba Schizonepetae* (荆芥), *Radix Saposhnikoviae* (防风), *Rhizoma seu Radix Notopterygii* (羌活), *Radix Angelicae Pubescentis* (独活), *Radix Chuanxiong* (川芎), *Radix Platycodi* (桔梗), *Fructus Aurantii* (枳壳), *Poria* (茯苓), *Radix Glycyrrhizae* (甘草), and *Herba Menthae* (薄荷), used to induce sweating, release the exterior, and dispel wind and dampness in the treatment of external contraction of wind, cold and dampness

参苏饮 [shēn sū yǐn]
***Shen Su Yin*; Ginseng-Perilla Decoction:** formula composed of *Radix Ginseng* (人参), *Folium Perillae* (紫苏叶), *Radix Puerariae* (葛根), *Radix Platycodi* (桔梗), *Rhizoma Pinelliae* (半夏), *Radix Peucedani* (前胡), *Poria* (茯苓), *Radix Aucklandiae* (木香), *Fructus Aurantii* (枳壳), *Pericarpium Citri Reticulatae* (陈皮), and *Radix Glycyrrhizae Preparata* (炙甘草), used to replenish *qi*, release the exterior, regulate *qi* and resolve phlegm for treating wind-cold contraction in patients with weak constitution and phlegm-fluid in the interior

加减葳蕤汤 [jiā jiǎn wēi ruí tāng]
***Jiajian Weirui* Decoction; Modified Solomon's Seal Decoction:** formula composed of *Rhizoma Polygoni odorati* (葳蕤), *Radix Platycodi* (桔梗), *Radix Cynanchi Atrati* (白薇), *Semen Sojae Preparatum* (淡豆豉), *Herba Menthae* (薄荷), and *Radix Glycyrrhizae Preparata* (炙甘草), used to nourish yin and release the exterior in the treatment of wind-heat contraction in patients with yin deficiency

泻下剂 [xiè xià jì]
purgative formula: formula used for

relieving constipation and purging various kinds of pathogenic factors from the interior of the body

寒下剂 [hán xià jì]

cold purgative formula: formula indicated in the treatment of interior accumulation and stagnation of heat

大承气汤 [dà chéng qì tāng]

***Da Chengqi* Decoction; Drastic Purgative Decoction:** formula composed of *Radix et Rhizoma Rhei* (大黄), *Natrii Sulfas* (芒硝), *Fructus Aurantii Immaturus* (枳实), and *Cortex Magnoliae Officinalis* (厚朴), used to purge the bowels drastically of accumulated heat in the treatment of excess *fu*-syndrome/pattern of yang brightness, fecal impaction with watery discharge, and excessive internal heat with heat syncope, convulsions or mania

小承气汤 [xiǎo chéng qì tāng]

***Xiao Chengqi* Decoction; Mild Purgative Decoction:** formula composed of *Radix et Rhizoma Rhei* (大黄), *Fructus Aurantii Immaturus* (枳实), and *Cortex Magnoliae Officinalis* (厚朴), used to gently purge the bowels of accumulated heat

大黄牡丹汤 [dà huáng mǔ dān tāng]

***Dahuang Mudan* Decoction; Rhubarb-Peony Decoction:** formula composed of *Radix et Rhizoma Rhei* (大黄), *Cortex Moutan* (牡丹皮), *Semen Persicae* (桃仁), *Semen Benincasae Hispidae* (冬瓜子), and *Natrii Sulfas* (芒硝), used to purge heat, break down stasis and dissipate swelling for treating appendicitis at the early stage

温下剂 [wēn xià jì]

warm purgative formula: formula used for treating interior accumulation and stagnation of excess cold

大黄附子汤 [dà huáng fù zǐ tāng]

***Dahuang Fuzi* Decoction; Rhubarb-Aconite Decoction:** formula composed of *Radix et Rhizoma Rhei* (大黄), *Radix Aconiti Lateralis Preparata* (附子), and *Herba Asari* (细辛), used to warm the interior, disperse cold, move the bowels and alleviate pain for treating abdominal pain due to accumulated cold

温脾汤 [wēn pí tāng]

***Wenpi* Decoction; Spleen-warming Decoction:** formula composed of *Radix et Rhizoma Rhei* (大黄), *Radix Angelicae Sinensis* (当归), *Rhizoma Zingiberis* (干姜), *Radix Aconiti Lateralis Preparata* (附子), *Radix Ginseng* (人参), *Natrii Sulfas* (芒硝) and *Radix Glycyrrhizae* (甘草), used to dispel the accumulated cold and warm-tonify the spleen for relieving abdominal pain due to cold accumulation

润下剂 [rùn xià jì]

lubricant laxative formula: formula indicated in the treatment of constipation due to insufficiency of intestinal fluid

五仁丸 [wǔ rén wán]

***Wuren* Pill; Five-seed Pill:** formula composed of *Semen Persicae* (桃仁), *Semen Armenicae* (杏仁), *Semen Platycladi* (柏子仁), *Semen Pini Tabulaeformis* (松子仁), *Semen Pruni* (郁李仁), and *Pericarpium Citri Reticulatae* (陈皮), used to moisten the intestines and move the bowels for relieving constipation due to consumption of fluid

麻子仁丸 [má zǐ rén wán]

***Maziren* Pill; Hemp-seed Pill:** formula composed of *Fructus Cannabis* (麻子仁), *Radix Paeoniae* (芍药), *Fructus Aurantii Immaturus* (枳实), *Radix et Rhizoma Rhei* (大黄), and *Semen Armenicae* (杏仁), used to moisten the intestines, purge heat, promote *qi* flow and move the bowels for treating splenic constipation

脾约丸 [pí yuē wán]

another name for hemp-seed pill (麻子仁丸 [má zǐ rén wán])

逐水剂 [zhú shuǐ jì]

hydragogue formula: formula to expel retained fluid drastically, indicated in the treatment of accumulation and retention of water in the interior (excess syndrome/pattern)

十枣汤 [shí zǎo tāng]

***Shizao* Decoction; Ten-Dates Decoction:** formula composed of *Radix Euphorbiae Kansui* (甘遂), *Flos Genkwa* (芫花) and *Radix Euphorbiae* (大戟) together with ten pieces of date, used to expel retained fluid in cases of anasarca or pleural fluid retention

和解剂 [hé jiě jì]

harmonizing formula: formula that regulates the correlation of viscera, meridians/channels, *qi* and blood, so as to remove pathogenic factors and restore normal functions

和解少阳剂 [hé jiě shào yáng jì]

***shaoyang*-harmonizing formula; lesser-yang-harmonizing formula:** formula useful in the treatment of contraction of cold pathogen in the *shaoyang* (lesser yang) meridian/channel, marked by alternate chills and fever, discomfort in the chest and hypochondriac region, loss of appetite, fidgetiness, nausea, dryness of the throat and bitterness in the mouth, dizziness and wiry pulse

小柴胡汤 [xiǎo chái hú tāng]

***Xiao Chaihu* Decoction; Minor/Mild Bupleurum Decoction:** formula composed of *Radix Bupleuri* (柴胡), *Radix Scutellariae* (黄芩), *Fructus Ziziphi Jujubae* (大枣), *Rhizoma Zingiberis Recens* (生姜), *Rhizoma Pinelliae Praeparata* (制半夏), *Radix Glycyrrhizae* (甘草), and *Radix Codonopsis Pilosulae* (党参), used to harmonize the *shaoyang* (lesser yang) meridian/channel in the treatment of *shaoyang* (lesser yang) syndrome/pattern in cases of cold damage diseases and in gynecological cases of heat in the blood chamber

蒿芩清胆汤 [hāo qín qīng dǎn tāng]

***Hao Qin Qingdan* Decoction; Arteminsia-Scutellaria Gallbladder-clearing Decoction:** formula composed of *Herba Artemisiae Annuae* (青蒿), *Caulis Bambusae in Taeniam* (竹茹), *Rhizoma Pinelliae Praeparata* (制半夏), *Radix Scutellariae* (黄芩), *Fructus Aurantii* (枳壳), *Pericarpium Citri Reticulatae* (陈皮), and jasper powder (碧玉散), used to clear the gallbladder, remove dampness, harmonize the stomach and resolve phlegm for treating *shaoyang* (lesser yang) dampness-heat syndrome/pattern

调和肝脾剂 [tiáo hé gān pí jì]

liver-spleen harmonizing formula:

formula indicated in the treatment of disharmony between the liver and spleen

四逆散 [sì nì sǎn]
***Sini* Powder; Counterflow-relieving Powder:** formula composed of *Radix Bupleuri* (柴胡), *Radix Paeoniae Alba* (白芍), *Fructus Aurantii Immaturus* (枳实), and *Radix Glycyrrhizae* (甘草), principal formula for restoring the normal function of depressed liver in which there is stagnancy of *qi* in the interior with coldness in the extremities, accompanied by costal or abdominal pain and menstrual complaints in women

逍遥散 [xiāo yáo sǎn]
***Xiaoyao* Powder; Carefree Powder:** formula composed of *Radix Bupleuri* (柴胡), *Radix Angelicae Sinensis* (当归), *Radix Paeoniae Alba* (白芍), *Rhizoma Atractylodis Macrocephalae* (白术), *Poria* (茯苓), *Radix Glycyrrhizae* (甘草), *Rhizoma Zingiberis Praeparata* (煨生姜), and *Herba Menthae* (薄荷), used to soothe the liver, relieve depression, nourish the blood and strengthen the spleen for treating the syndrome with depressed liver, deficient blood and weakened spleen

痛泻要方 [tòng xiè yào fāng]
***Tongxie Yaofang*; Important Formula for Painful Diarrhea:** formula composed of *Rhizoma Atractylodis Macrocephalae* (白术), *Radix Paeoniae Alba* (白芍), *Pericarpium Citri Reticulatae* (陈皮), and *Radix Saposhnikoviae* (防风), used to tonify the spleen, mollify the liver, and dispel dampness for stopping diarrhea associated with abdominal pain

调和寒热剂 [tiáo hé hán rè jì]
cold-heat harmonizing formula: formula indicated in the treatment of binding of cold and heat in the middle energizer, marked by epigastric stuffiness, nausea, vomiting, borborygmi and diarrhea

半夏泻心汤 [bàn xià xiè xīn tāng]
***Banxia Xiexin* Decoction; Pinellia Heart-purging Decoction:** formula composed of *Rhizoma Pinelliae Praeparata* (制半夏), *Radix Scutellariae* (黄芩), *Rhizoma Coptidis* (黄连), *Rhizoma Zingiberis* (干姜), *Radix Ginseng* (人参), *Fructus Ziziphi Jujubae* (大枣), and *Radix Glycyrrhizae* (甘草), used to regulate cold and heat, and eliminate epigastric stuffiness

表里双解剂 [biǎo lǐ shuāng jiě jì]
exterior-interior releasing formula: formula that releases the exterior and interior simultaneously

大柴胡汤 [dà chái hú tāng]
***Da Chaihu* Decoction; Major Bupleurum Decoction:** formula composed of *Radix Bupleuri* (柴胡), *Radix Scutellariae* (黄芩), *Radix Paeoniae Alba* (白芍), *Rhizoma Pinelliae Praeparata* (制半夏), *Radix et Rhizoma Rhei* (大黄), *FructusAurantii Immaturus* (枳实), *Fructus Ziziphi Jujubae* (大枣), and *Rhizoma Zingiberis Recens* (生姜), used to treat combined syndrome/pattern of *shaoyang* (lesser yang) and *yangming* (yang brightness) meridians/channels

防风通圣散 [fáng fēng tōng shèng sǎn]
***Fangfeng Tongsheng* Powder; Miraculous Powder of Saposhnikovia:** formula composed of *Radix Saposhnikoviae* (防

风), *Fructus Forsythiae* (连翘), *Herba Ephedrae* (麻黄), *Fructus Gardeniae* (栀子), *Radix et Rhizoma Rhei* (大黄), *Gypsum Fibrosum* (石膏), *Radix Scutellariae* (黄芩), *Radix Paeoniae Alba* (白芍), *Rhizoma Chuanxiong* (川芎), etc., used to disperse wind, release the exterior, clear heat and move the bowels for treating wind-heat contraction with excessive nature in both the exterior and interior

葛根黄芩黄连汤 [gě gēn huáng qín huáng lián tāng]
***Gegen Huangqin Huanglian* Decoction; Pueraria-Scutellaria-Coptis Decoction:** formula composed of *Radix Puerariae* (葛根), *Radix Scutellariae* (黄芩), *Rhizoma Coptidis* (黄连), and *Radix Glycyrrhizae* (甘草), used to release the exterior and clear the interior for treating dysentery with fever

清热剂 [qīng rè jì]
heat-clearing formula: any formula that is mainly composed of heat-clearing ingredients and used for clearing heat, purging fire, cooling the blood, or counteracting toxins

清气分热剂 [qīng qì fēn rè jì]
***qi*-aspect heat-clearing formula:** formula for treating febrile diseases affecting the *qi* aspect, marked by high fever, profuse sweating, dire thirst and gigantic surging pulse

白虎汤 [bái hǔ tāng]
***Baihu* Decoction; White Tiger Decoction:** formula composed of *Gypsum Fibrosum* (石膏), *Rhizoma Anemarrhenae* (知母), *Radix Glycyrrhizae* (甘草), and *Semen Oryzae Nonglutinosae* (粳米), used to clear heat at the *qi* aspect with high fever, dire thirst, sweating and gigantic surging pulse

竹叶石膏汤 [zhú yè shí gāo tāng]
***Zhuye Shigao* Decoction; Laphatherum-Gypsum Decoction:** classical formula composed of *Herba Laphatheri* (淡竹叶), *Gypsum Fibrosum* (石膏), *Radix Ophiopogonis* (麦冬), *Rhizoma Pinelliae* (半夏), *Radix Ginseng* (人参) or *Radix CodonopsisPilosulae* (党参), *Semen Oryzae Nonglutinosae* (粳米), and *Radix Glycyrrhizae* (甘草), used to clear heat, promote fluid production, replenish *qi*, and harmonize the stomach for treating febrile diseases at the stage of restoration with lingering heat and impaired *qi* and body fluid

清营凉血剂 [qīng yíng liáng xuè jì]
nutrient-blood-aspect heat-clearing formula: formula used in the treatment of febrile diseases with heat entering the nutrient or blood aspect

清营汤 [qīng yíng tāng]
***Qingying* Decoction; Nutrient-clearing Decoction:** formula composed of *Cornu Bubali* (水牛角), *Radix Rehmanniae* (生地黄), *Radix Scrophularlae* (元参), *Radix Ophiopogonis* (麦冬), *Herba Lophatheri* (竹叶), *Radix Salviae Miltiorrhizae* (丹参), *Rhizoma Coptidis* (黄连), *Flos Lonicerae* (银花), and *Fructus Forsythiae* (连翘), used for treating febrile diseases with heat entering the nutrient aspect

犀角地黄汤 [xī jiǎo dì huáng tāng]
***Xijiao Dihuang* Decoction; Decoction**

of Rhinoceros Horn and Rehmannia: formula composed of *Cornu Bubali* (水牛角), *Radix Rehmanniae* (生地黄), *Radix Paeoniae Rubra* (赤芍), and *Cortex Moutan* (牡丹皮), used for treating febrile diseases with heat entering the blood aspect

清热解毒剂 [qīng rè jiě dú jì]
heat-clearing toxin-counteracting formula: formula indicated in the treatment of epidemic pestilence, toxic warm diseases, boils, sores, and abscesses

黄连解毒汤 [huáng lián jiě dú tāng]
Huanglian Jiedu **Decoction; Detoxicant Coptis Decoction:** formula composed of *Rhizoma Coptidis* (黄连), *Radix Scutellariae* (黄芩), *Cortex Phellodendri* (黄柏) and *Fructus Gardeniae* (栀子), used to purge fire and counteract toxins for treating various pyogenic infections

普济消毒饮 [pǔ jì xiāo dú yǐn]
Puji Xiaodu **Decoction; Universal Antitoxic Decoction:** formula composed of *Radix Scutellariae* (黄芩), *Rhizoma Coptidis* (黄连), *Radix Scrophularlae* (元参), *Radix Bupleuri* (柴胡), *Fructus Forsythiae* (连翘), *Radix Platycodi* (桔梗), *Radix Isatidis* (板蓝根), *Lasiosphaera seu Calvatia* (马勃), *Rhizoma Cimicifugae* (升麻), *Herba Menthae* (薄荷), etc., mainly used for treating facial erysipelas

清脏腑热剂 [qīng zàng fǔ rè jì]
zang-fu **heat-clearing formula:** formula that clears heat from a certain *zang-fu* organ

导赤散 [dǎo chì sǎn]
Daochi **Powder; Redness-removing Powder:** formula composed of *Radix Rehmanniae* (生地黄), *Herba Lophatheri* (竹叶), *Caulis Aristolochiae* (木通), and *Radix Glycyrrhizae* (甘草), used to clear the heart, induce diuresis and nourish yin for treating fire syndrome/pattern of the heart meridian/channel, marked by oral ulceration or passage of reddened urine with pain

清胃散 [qīng wèi sǎn]
Qingwei **Powder; Stomach-clearing Powder:** formula composed of *RhizomaCoptidis* (黄连), *Radix Angelicae Sinensis* (当归), *Radix Rehmanniae* (生地黄), *Rhizoma Cimicifugae* (升麻), and *Cortex Moutan* (丹皮), used to clear the stomach and cool the blood for relieving toothache due to stomach fire

龙胆泻肝汤 [lóng dǎn xiè gān tāng]
Longdan Xiegan **Decoction; Gentian Liver-purging Decoction:** formula composed of *Radix Gentianae* (龙胆), *Radix Scutellariae* (黄芩), *Fructus Gardeniae* (栀子), *Rhizoma Alismatis* (泽泻), *Caulis Aritolochiae Manshuriensis* (关木通), *Semen Plantaginis* (车前子), *Radix Angelicae Sinensis* (当归), *Radix Rehmanniae* (生地黄), *Radix Bupleuri* (柴胡), and *Radix Glycyrrhizae* (甘草), used to clear the liver and gallbladder fire and purge dampness-heat from the lower energizer

泻白散 [xiè bái sǎn]
Xiebai **Powder; Lung-purging Powder:** formula composed of *Cortex Lycii* (地骨皮), *Cortex Mori* (桑白皮), and *Radix Glycyrrhizae* (甘草), used to clear and purge the lung of heat for treating lung

heat contraction with cough and dyspnea, also called 泻肺散 [xiè fèi sǎn]

泻肺散 [xiè fèi sǎn]
synonym for 泻白散[xiè bái sǎn]

白头翁汤 [bái tóu wēng tāng]
***Baitouweng* Decoction; Pulsatilla Decoction:** formula composed of *Radix Pulsatillae* (白头翁), *Rhizoma Coptidis* (黄连), *Cortex Phellodendri* (黄柏), and *Cortex Fraxini* (秦皮), used to clear heat, counteract toxins and cool the blood for treating heat-toxic dysentery

清热祛暑剂 [qīng rè qū shǔ jì]
summerheat-clearing formula: formula that clears summerheat for treating heat syndromes/patterns occurring in summer

六一散 [liù yī sǎn]
***Liu Yi* Powder; Six-to-one Powder:** formula composed of *Talcum* (滑石) and *Radix Glycyrrhizae* (甘草) at a ratio of six to one in weight, used for relieving summerheat with dampness

清虚热剂 [qīng xū rè jì]
deficiency-heat-clearing formula: formula indicated in the treatment of febrile diseases at the late stage with lingering pathogens and impaired yin fluid

青蒿鳖甲汤 [qīng hāo biē jiǎ tāng]
***Qinghao Biejia* Decoction; *Chinghao* and Turtle Shell Decoction:** formula composed of *Herba Artemisiae Chinghao* (青蒿), *Carapax Trionycis* (鳖甲), *Radix Rehmanniae* (生地黄), *Rhizoma Anemarrhenae* (知母) and *Cortex Moutan* (牡丹皮), used to nourish yin and expel heat in the treatment of warm diseases at the late stage when the pathogens are concealed in the yin aspect

清骨散 [qīng gǔ sǎn]
***Qinggu* Powder; Bone-clearing Powder:** formula composed of *Radix Stellariae* (银柴胡), *Radix Gentianae Macrophyllae* (秦艽), *Rhizoma Picrorhizae* (胡黄连), *Herba Artemisiae Chinghao* (青蒿), *Carapax Trionycis* (鳖甲), *Cortex Lycii* (地骨皮), *Herba Artemisiae Chinghao* (青蒿), *Rhizoma Anemarrhenae* (知母), and *Radix Glycyrrhizae* (甘草), used to clear deficiency-heat for treating consumptive fever

温里剂 [wēn lǐ jì]
interior-warming formula: warming formula used for treating interior cold contractions

温中祛寒剂 [wēn zhōng qū hán jì]
center-warming cold-dispelling formula: formula that warms the middle energizer and dispels pathogenic cold for treating deficiency-cold of the spleen and stomach

理中汤 [lǐ zhōng tāng]
***Lizhong* Decoction; Center-regulating Decoction:** formula composed of *Radix Codonopsis Pilosulae* (党参), *Rhizoma Zingiberis* (干姜), *Rhizoma Atractylodis Macrocephalae* (白术), and *Radix Glycyrrhizae Praeparata* (炙甘草), used to warm the middle energizer, disperse cold, replenish *qi* and strengthen the spleen for treating deficiency-cold of the spleen and stomach

小建中汤 [xiǎo jiàn zhōng tāng]
***Xiao Jianzhong* Decoction; Minor Center-constructing Decoction:** formula composed of *Radix Paeoniae Alba* (白芍), *Ramulus Cinnamomi* (桂枝), *Radix Glycyrrhizae Praeparata* (炙甘草), *Rhizoma Zingiberis Recens* (生姜), *Fructus Ziziphi Jujubae* (大枣), and malt extract (饴糖), used to warm and tonify the middle energizer and relieve spasmodic pains for treating abdominal pain in deficiency conditions

吴茱萸汤 [wú zhū yú tāng]
***Wuzhuyu* Decoction; Evodia Decoction:** formula composed of *Fructus Evodiae* (吴茱萸), *Radix Ginseng* (人参), *Fructus Ziziphi Jujubae* (大枣), and *Rhizoma Zingiberis Recens* (生姜), used for arresting deficiency-cold vomiting

回阳救逆剂 [huí yáng jiù nì jì]
yang-restoring emergency formula: formula for emergency treatment of failure of yang *qi* with exuberant yin cold or even repelling of yang

祛寒剂 [qū hán jì]
cold-dispelling formula: formula composed chiefly of medicinals warm or hot in nature and indicated in the treatment of cold syndrome/pattern

四逆汤 [sì nì tāng]
***Sini* Decoction; Cold-extremities Decoction:** formula composed of *Radix Aconiti Lateralis Praeparata* (制附子), *Rhizoma Zingiberis* (干姜), and *Radix Glycyrrhizae Praeparata* (炙甘草), used to restore yang from collapse or shock with cold limbs

温经散寒剂 [wēn jīng sàn hán jì]
meridian/channel-warming cold-dispersing formula: formula that warms the meridians/channels and disperses pathogenic cold for treating blood congealing in the meridians/channels

当归四逆汤 [dāng guī sì nì tāng]
***Danggui Sini* Decoction; Angelica Cold-extremities Decoction:** formula composed of *Radix Angelicae Sinensis* (当归), *Ramulus Cinnamomi* (桂枝), *Radix Paeoniae* (芍药), *Herba Asari* (细辛), *Radix Glycyrrhizae Praeparata* (炙甘草), *Medulla Tetrapanacis* (通草), and *Fructus Ziziphi Jujubae* (大枣), used to warm the meridians/channels, disperse cold, nourish the blood and unblock the vessels for treating blood deficiency with syncope

黄芪桂枝五物汤 [huáng qí guì zhī wǔ wù tāng]
***Huangqi Guizhi Wuwu* Decoction; Five-ingredient Decoction with Milkvetch and Cassia Twig:** formula composed of *Radix Astragali* (黄芪), *Radix Paeoniae* (芍药), *Ramulus Cinnamomi* (桂枝), *Rhizoma Zingiberis Recens* (生姜), and *Fructus Ziziphi Jujubae* (大枣), used to replenish *qi*, warm the meridians/channels, harmonize the blood and remove blockage for treating numbness

阳和汤 [yáng hé tāng]
***Yanghe* Decoction; Yang-harmonizing Decoction:** formula composed of *Rhizoma Rehmanniae Praeparata* (熟地黄), *Cortex Cinnamomi* (肉桂), *Herba Ephedrae* (麻黄), *Semen Sinapis Albae* (白芥子), *Rhizoma Zingiberis Carbonisatum* (姜炭), and *Radix Glycyrrhizae* (甘草), used to

warm yang, tonify the blood, disperse cold and remove stagnation for treating yin cellulitis (cellulitis with pain and swelling but without local hotness or reddening of the skin)

补益剂 [bǔ yì jì]
tonifying formula: any formula that reinforces yang, replenishes *qi*, nourishes the blood or supplements yin in deficiency conditions

补气剂 [bǔ qì jì]
***qi*-tonifying formula:** formula for replenishing *qi*, mainly indicated in cases of deficiency of the lung *qi* or spleen *qi*

四君子汤 [sì jūn zǐ tāng]
***Sijunzi* Decoction; Decoction of Four Noble Ingredients:** basic formula composed of *Radix Ginseng* (人参) or *Radix Codonopsis Pilosulae* (党参), *Poria* (茯苓), *Rhizoma Atractylodis Macrocephalae* (白术), and *Radix Glycyrrhizae Praeparata* (炙甘草), used to replenish *qi* and strengthen the spleen for treating *qi* deficiency of the spleen and stomach

参苓白术散 [shēn líng bǎi zhú sǎn]
***Shenling Baizhu* Powder; Ginseng-Poria-Atractylodes Powder:** formula composed of *Radix Ginseng* (人参), *Poria* (茯苓), *Rhizoma Atractylodis Macrocephalae* (白术), *Rhizoma Dioscoreae* (山药), *Semen Nelumbinis* (莲子), *Fructus Amomi* (砂仁), etc., used to replenish *qi*, strengthen the spleen, drain dampness and arrest diarrhea for treating spleen insufficiency complicated by dampness

补中益气汤 [bǔ zhōng yì qì tāng]
***Buzhong Yiqi* Decoction; Center-tonifying *Qi*-replenishing Decoction:** formula composed of *Radix Astragali* (黄芪), *Radix Ginseng* (人参) or *Radix Codonopsis Pilosulae* (党参), *Radix Angelicae Sinensis* (当归), *Pericarpium Citri Reticulatae* (陈皮), *Radix Glycyrrhizae* (甘草), *Rhizoma Atractylodis Macrocephalae* (白术), *Rhizoma Cimicifugae* (升麻), and *Radix Bupleuri* (柴胡), used to tonify the middle energizer, replenish *qi* and elevate yang for treating deficiency of spleen and stomach *qi*, sinking of *qi*, and fever in cases of *qi* deficiency

玉屏风散 [yù píng fēng sǎn]
***Yupingfeng* Powder; Jade-screen Powder:** formula composed of *Radix Astragali* (黄芪), *Rhizoma Atractylodis Macrocephalae* (白术), and *Radix Saposhnikoviae* (防风), used to replenish *qi*, consolidate the superficies and suppress perspiration for treating superficial deficiency with spontaneous sweating

补血剂 [bǔ xuè jì]
blood-tonifying formula: formula suitable for treating blood deficiency

四物汤 [sì wù tāng]
***Siwu* Decoction; Four-Medicinal Decoction:** formula composed of *Radix Rehmanniae Praeparata* (熟地黄), *Radix Paeoniae Alba* (白芍), *Radix Angelicae Sinensis* (当归), and *Rhizoma Chuanxiong* (川芎), used to tonify and harmonize the blood for treating deficiency and stagnation of nutrient-blood

当归补血汤 [dāng guī bǔ xuè tāng]
***Danggui Buxue* Decoction; Angelica Blood-tonifying Decoction:** formula composed of *Radix Angelicae Sinensis* (当归) and *Radix Astragali* (黄芪), used to replenish *qi* and promote blood production for treating blood deficiency with fever

归脾汤 [guī pí tāng]
***Guipi* Decoction; Spleen-restoring Decoction:** formula composed of *Radix Codonopsis Pilosulae* (党参), *Rhizoma Atractylodis Macrocephalae* (白术), *Radix Astragali* (黄芪), *Poria cum Radice Pino* (茯神), *Radix Glycyrrhizae Praeparata* (炙甘草), *Radix Angelicae Sinensis* (当归), *Semen Ziziphi Spinosae* (酸枣仁), *Arillus Longan* (龙眼肉), *Radix Polygalae* (远志), *Radix Aucklandiae* (木香), *Rhizoma Zingiberis Recens* (生姜), and *Fructus Ziziphi Jujubae* (大枣), used to replenish *qi*, tonify the blood, strengthen the spleen and nourish the heart, for treating deficiency of spleen *qi* and heart blood, and failure of the spleen to control the blood

气血双补剂 [qì xuè shuāng bǔ jì]
***qi*-blood tonifying formula:** formula to tonify both *qi* and blood for treating dual *qi*-blood deficiency

八珍汤 [bā zhēn tāng]
***Bazhen* Decoction, Eight-treasure Decoction:** formula composed of *Radix Ginseng* (人参) or *Radix Codonopsis Pilosulae* (党参), *Rhizoma Atractylodis Macrocephalae* (白术), *Poria* (茯苓), *Radix Glycyrrhizae* (甘草), *Radix Angelicae Sinensis* (当归), *Radix Paeoniae Alba* (白芍), *Rhizoma Chuanxiong* (川芎), and *Rhizoma Rehmanniae Praeparata* (熟地黄), used to replenish *qi* and tonify the blood in the treatment of dual *qi*-blood deficiency

十全大补汤 [shí quán dà bǔ tāng]
***Shiquan* Dabu Decoction; All-inclusive Grand Tonic Decoction:** formula composed of *Radix Ginseng* (人参) or *Radix Codonopsis Pilosulae* (党参), *Rhizoma Atractylodis Macrocephalae* (白术), *Poria* (茯苓), *Radix Glycyrrhizae* (甘草), *Radix Angelicae Sinensis* (当归), *Radix Paeoniae Alba* (白芍), *Rhizoma Chuanxiong* (川芎), *Rhizoma Rehmanniae Praeparata* (熟地黄), *Cortex Cinnamomi* (肉桂), and *Radix Astragali* (黄芪), used to warm and tonify *qi* and blood in cases of general debility with dual *qi*-blood deficiency

补阴剂 [bǔ yīn jì]
yin-replenishing formula: formula indicated in the treatment of yin deficiency

六味地黄汤 [liù wèi dì huáng tāng]
***Liuwei Dihuang* Decoction; Six-ingredient Rehmannia Decoction:** formula composed of *Radix Rehmanniae Praeparata* (熟地黄), *Fructus Corni* (山茱萸), *Rhizoma Dioscoreae* (山药), *Rhizoma Alismatis* (泽泻), *Poria* (茯苓), and *Cortex Moutan* (牡丹皮), used to nourish and tonify the liver and kidney in the treatment of kidney yin deficiency

左归丸 [zuǒ guī wán]
***Zuo Gui* Pill; Yin-restoring Pill:** formula composed of *Radix Rehmanniae Praeparata* (熟地黄), *Rhizoma Dioscoreae* (山药), *Fructus Corni* (山茱萸), *Fructus*

Lycii (枸杞子), *Semen Cuscuta* (菟丝子), *Radix Cyathulae* (川牛膝), *Colla Cornus Cervi* (鹿角胶), and *Colla Plastri Testudinis* (龟板胶), used to nourish yin and tonify the kidney for treating kidney yin deficiency

一贯煎 [yī guàn jiān]
***Yiguan* Decoction; Ever-effective Decoction:** formula composed of *Radix Glehniae* (沙参), *Radix Ophiopogonis* (麦冬), *Radix Rehmanniae* (生地黄), *Radix Angelicae Sinensis* (当归), *Fructus Lycii* (枸杞子) and *Fructus Toosendan* (川楝子), used to nourish yin and soothe the liver for treating yin deficiency of the liver and kidney with restraint of liver *qi*

补阳剂 [bǔ yáng jì]
yang-tonifying formula: formula used for treating deficiency of yang *qi*

肾气丸 [shèn qì wán]
***Shenqi* Pill; Kidney *Qi* Pill:** formula composed of *Radix Aconiti Lateralis Praeparata* (附子), *Cortex Cinnamomi* (肉桂), *Radix Rehmanniae Praeparata* (熟地黄), *Fructus Corni* (山茱萸), *Rhizoma Dioscoreae* (山药), *Rhizoma Alismatis* (泽泻), *Poria* (茯苓), and *Cortex Moutan* (牡丹皮), used to tonify the kidney and reinforce yang for treating kidney yang deficiency

金匮肾气丸 [jīn guì shèn qì wán]
***Jingui Shenqi* Pill; Golden-chamber Kidney *Qi* pill:** another name for *Shenqi* Pill or Kidney *Qi* Pill (肾气丸 [shèn qì wán])

右归丸 [yòu guī wán]
***You Gui* Pill; Yang-restoring Pill:** formula composed of *Radix Rehmanniae Praeparata* (熟地黄), *Fructus Corni* (山茱萸), *Rhizoma Dioscoreae* (山药), *Fructus Lycii* (枸杞子), *Semen Cuscuta* (菟丝子), *Colla Cornus Cervi* (鹿角胶), *Cortex Eucommiae* (杜仲), *Cortex Cinnamomi* (肉桂), *Radix Angelicae Sinensis* (当归), and *Radix Aconiti Lateralis Preparata* (附子), used to warm and tonify kidney yang for treating kidney yang deficiency with decline of the life fire

阴阳并补剂 [yīn yáng bìng bǔ jì]
simultaneous yin-yang tonifying formula: formula that tonifies yin and yang simultaneously, suitable for treating deficiency of both yin and yang

龟鹿二仙胶 [guī lù èr xiān jiāo]
***Gui Lu Erxian* Glue; Two-elixir Glue of Tortoise Plastron and Deer Horn:** formula composed of *Cornu Cervi* (鹿角), *Plastron Testudinis* (龟板), *Radix Ginseng* (人参), and *Fructus Lycii* (枸杞子), used to nourish yin, supplement essence, replenish *qi* and invigorate yang

二仙汤 [èr xiān tāng]
***Erxian* Decoction; Two-elixir Decoction:** formula composed of *Rhizoma Curculiginis* (仙茅), *Herba Epimedii* (仙灵脾), *Radix Morindae Officinalis* (巴戟天), *Radix Angelicae Sinensis* (当归), *Cortex Phellodendri* (黄柏) and *Rhizoma Anemarrhenae* (知母), used to tonify both yin and yang of the kidney for treating menopausal syndrome and hypertension

固涩剂 [gù sè jì]
astringent formula: formula that arrests

discharges, including excessive perspiration, persistent diarrhea, seminal emission, incontinence of urine, profuse uterine bleeding, and leukorrhea

固表止汗剂 [gù biǎo zhǐ hàn jì]
superficies-consolidating sweating-arresting formula: formula that consolidates the superficies and arrests excessive sweating, for strengthening the superficial body resistance

牡蛎散 [mǔ lì sǎn]
***Muli* Powder; Ostrea Powder:** formula composed of *Radix Astragali* (黄芪), *Radix Ephedrae* (麻黄根), and *Concha Ostreae* (牡蛎), used to replenish *qi*, consolidate the superficies and astringe yin for arresting spontaneous sweating and night sweats

敛肺止咳剂 [liǎn fèi zhǐ ké jì]
lung-astringing antitussive formula: formula to stop coughing by astringing the lung

涩肠固脱剂 [sè cháng gù tuō jì]
intestine-astringing antidiarrheal formula: formula to suppress protracted diarrhea by astringing the intestines

四神丸 [sì shén wán]
***Sishen* Pill; Four-miracle Pill:** formula composed of *Fructus Psoraleae* (补骨脂), *Fructus Schisandrae* (五味子), *Semen Myristicae* (肉豆蔻), and *Fructus Evodiae* (吴茱萸), used to warm the kidney and spleen, and astringe the intestines for relieving diarrhea occurring daily before dawn

涩精止遗剂 [sè jīng zhǐ yí jì]
semen-astringing enuresis-arresting formula: astringent formula to arrest seminal emission or involuntary discharge of urine

固精丸 [gù jīng wán]
***Gujing* Pill; Semen-securing Pill:** formula composed of *Semen Astragali Complanati* (潼蒺藜), *Semen Euryales* (芡实), *Stamen Nelumbinis* (莲须), *Os Draconis Usta* (煅龙骨), and *Concha Ostreae Usta* (煅牡蛎), used for treating nocturnal and spontaneous emission due to kidney insufficiency, also called *Jinsuo Gujing* Pill or Golden-lock Semen-securing Pill (金锁固精丸 [jīn suǒ gù jīng wán])

金锁固精丸 [jīn suǒ gù jīng wán]
***Jinsuo Gujing* Pill; Golden-lock Semen-securing Pill:** another name for *Gujing* Pill or Semen-securing Pill (固精丸[gù jīng wán])

缩泉丸 [suō quán wán]
***Suoquan* Pill; Stream-reducing Pill:** formula composed of *Radix Linderae* (乌药) and *Semen Alpiniae Oxyphyllae* (益智仁), used to warm the kidney, dispel cold, reduce urination and arrest involuntary discharge of urine in cases of deficiency-cold of the bladder

理气剂 [lǐ qì jì]
***qi*-regulating formula:** formula to regulate and normalize the flow of *qi*

行气剂 [xíng qì jì]
***qi*-moving formula:** formula to facilitate the smooth movement of *qi*, indicated in

relieving stagnation or retardation of *qi* flow

瓜蒌薤白半夏汤 [guā lóu xiè bái bàn xià tāng]

***Gualou Xiebai Banxia* Decoction; Trichosanthes-Allium-Pinellia Decoction:** formula composed of *Fructus Trichosanthis* (瓜蒌), *Bulbus Allii Macrostemi* (薤白), *Spiritus* (白酒), and *Rhizoma Pinelliae Praeparata* (制半夏), used for relieving chest pain due to *qi* obstruction with phlegm, such as angina pectoris

半夏厚朴汤 [bàn xià hòu pò tāng]

***Banxia Houpo* Decoction; Pinellia-Magnolia Decoction:** classical formula composed of *Rhizoma Pinelliae Praeparata* (制半夏), *Cortex Magnoliae Officinalis* (厚朴), *Poria* (茯苓), *Rhizoma Zingiberis Recens* (生姜), and *Folium Perillae* (紫苏叶), used to move *qi*, dissipate nodulation and resolve phlegm in the treatment of globus hystericus

良附丸 [liáng fù wán]

***Liang Fu* Pill; Alpinia-Cyperus Pill:** formula composed of *Rhizoma Alpiniae Officinarum* (高良姜) and *Rhizoma Cyperi* (香附), used to move *qi*, soothe the liver and dispel cold for relieving epigastric, hypochondriac and abdominal pain due to cold-induced *qi* congealment

金铃子散 [jīn líng zǐ sǎn]

***Jinlingzi* Powder; Toosendan Powder:** formula composed of *Fructus Toosendan* (金铃子) and *Rhizoma Corydalis* (玄胡索), used to soothe the liver, purge heat, activate the blood and alleviate pain, for treating fire transformation in depressed liver

暖肝煎 [nuǎn gān jiān]

***Nuangan* Decoction; Liver-warming Decoction:** formula composed of *Radix Angelicae Sinensis* (当归), *Fructus Lycii* (枸杞子), *Fructus Foeniculi* (小茴香), *Cortex Cinnamomi* (肉桂), *Radix Linderae* (乌药), *Lignum Aquilariae Resinatum* (沉香), and *Poria* (茯苓), used to warm and tonify the liver and kidney, move *qi* and alleviate pain for treating deficiency-cold of the liver and kidney with testicular or lower abdominal pain

加味乌药汤 [jiā wèi wū yào tāng]

***Jiawei Wuyao* Decoction; Supplemented Lindera Decoction:** formula composed of *Radix Linderae* (乌药), *Fructus Amomi* (砂仁), *Rhizoma Corydalis* (延胡索), *Rhizoma Cyperi* (香附), *Radix Aucklandiae* (木香), and *Radix Glycyrrhizae* (甘草), used to move *qi*, activate the blood, regulate menstruation and alleviate pain for treating dysmenorrhea

降气剂 [jiàng qì jì]

***qi*-descending formula:** formula that brings down the reverse upward flow of *qi*, usually for relieving asthma or vomiting

定喘汤 [dìng chuǎn tāng]

***Dingchuan* Decoction; Asthma-arresting Decoction:** formula composed of *Semen Ginkgo* (白果), *Herba Ephedrae* (麻黄), *Cortex Mori Radicis* (桑白皮), *Fructus Perillae* (苏子), *Semen Armenizacae Amarum* (苦杏仁), *Radix Scutellariae* (黄芩), *Flos Farfarae* (款冬花), *Phizoma Pinelliae Preparata* (制半夏), and *Radix Glycyrrhizae* (甘草), used for relieving asthma with heat and phlegm

旋复代赭汤 [xuán fù dài zhě tāng]
Xuanfu Daizhe **Decoction; Inula-Haematite Decoction:** formula composed of *Flos Inulae* (旋复花), *Haematitum* (赭石), *Rhizoma Zingiberis Recens* (生姜), *Rhizoma Pinelliae Praeparata* (制半夏), *Radix Glycyrrhizae Praeparata* (炙甘草), *Fructus Ziziphi Jujubae* (大枣), and *Radix Codonopsis Pilosulae* (党参), used to relieve nausea and arrest vomiting due to dysfunction of the stomach with retention of phlegm

丁香柿蒂汤 [dīng xiāng shì dì tāng]
Dingxiang Shidi **Decoction; Decoction of Cloves and Persimon Calyx:** formula composed of *Flos Caryophylli* (丁香), *Calyx Kaki* (柿蒂), *Radix Ginseng* (人参), and *Rhizoma Zingiberis Recens* (生姜), used to warm the middle energizer, replenish *qi*, and suppress the reversed upward flow of *qi* for stopping deficiency-cold hiccups

橘皮竹茹汤 [jú pí zhú rú tāng]
Jupi Zhuru **Decoction; Decoction of Tangerine Peel and Bamboo Shavings:** formula composed of *Pericarpium Citri Reticulatae* (橘皮), *Caulis Bambusae* in *Taeniam* (竹茹)，*Rhizoma Zingiberis Recens* (生姜), *Radix Glycyrrhizae* (甘草), *Radix Ginseng* (人参), and *Fructus Ziziphi Jujubae* (大枣), used to suppress the reversed upward flow of *qi* for stopping stomach-heat hiccups

理血剂 [lǐ xuè jì]
blood-regulating formula: any formula that regulates the blood, including blood-tonifying formula, blood-activating and stasis-removing formula, and hemostatic formula

活血祛瘀剂 [huó xuè qū yū jì]
blood-activating and stasis-removing formula: formula that activates the blood flow and removes blood stasis, indicated in the treatment of various conditions of blood aggregation and stagnation

血府逐瘀汤 [xuè fǔ zhú yū tāng]
Xuefu Zhuyu **Decoction; Thoracic Stasis-expelling Decoction:** formula composed of *Radix Angelicae Sinensis* (当归), *Radix Paeoniae Rubra* (赤芍), *Radix Rehmanniae* (生地黄), *Rhizoma Ligustici Chuanxiong* (川芎), *SemenPersicae* (桃仁), *Flos Carthami* (红花), *Radix Bupleuri* (柴胡), *FructusAurantii* (枳壳), *Radix Platycodi* (桔梗), *Radix Glycyrrhizae* (甘草), and *Radix Achyranthis Bidentatae* (牛膝), used to activate the blood, remove stasis, move *qi* and alleviate pain for treating blood stasis in the chest

补阳还五汤 [bǔ yáng huán wǔ tāng]
Buyang Huanwu **Decoction; Yang-tonifying Five-tenths-restoring Decoction:** formula composed of *Radix Astragali* (黄芪), *Radix Angelicae Sinensis* (当归), *Radix Paeoniae Rubra* (赤芍), *Rhizoma Chuanxiong* (川芎), *Semen Persicae* (桃仁), *Flos Carthami* (红花), and *Lumbricus* (地龙), used to supplement *qi*, activate the blood and unblock collateral meridians/channels for treating post-apoplectic hemiplegia

生化汤 [shēng huà tāng]
Shenghua **Decoction; Generation and Resolution Decoction:** formula composed of *Radix Angelicae Sinensis* (当归), *Rhizoma Chuanxiong* (川芎), *Semen Persicae* (桃仁), *Rhizoma Zingiberis Praeparata* (炮

姜), and *Radix Glycyrrhizae Praeparata* (炙甘草), used to resolve blood stasis, generate new blood, warm the meridians/channels and alleviate pain for treating retaining of lochia and lower abdominal pain after childbirth

止血剂 [zhǐ xuè jì]
styptic formula: formula to arrest bleeding

小蓟饮子 [xiǎo jì yǐn zi]
***Xiaoji* Decoction; Cirsium Decoction:** formula composed of *Radix Rehmanniae* (生地黄), *Herba Cirsii* (小蓟), *Pulvis Talci* (滑石), *Caulis Aristolochiae Manshuriensis* (木通), *Pollen Typhae Carbonizatum* (炒蒲黄), *Nodus Nelumbinis Rhizomatis* (藕节), *Herba Lophatheri* (淡竹叶), *RadixAngelicae Sinensis* (当归), *Fructus Gardeniae* (栀子), and *Radix Glycyrrhizae* (甘草), used to cool the blood, arrest bleeding, induce diuresis and relieve stranguria for treating hematuria and bloody stranguria

黄土汤 [huáng tǔ tāng]
***Huangtu* Decoction; Oven-earth Decoction:** formula composed of *Radix Glycyrrhizae* (甘草), *Radix Rehmanniae* (地黄), *Rhizoma Atractylodis Macrocephalae* (白术), *Radix Aconiti Lateralis Praeparata* (附子), *Radix Scutellariae* (黄芩), and *Terra Flava Usta* (灶心土), used for treating hematochezia in cases of yang deficiency

治风剂 [zhì fēng jì]
wind-treating formula: formula that dispels or extinguishes pathogenic wind, either exogenous or endogenous

疏散外风剂 [shū sàn wài fēng jì]
exogenous-wind-dispersing formula: formula that disperses exogenous wind, used for treating various external wind contractions

独活寄生汤 [dú huó jì shēng tāng]
***Duhuo Jisheng* Decoction; Pubescent Angelica and Loranthus Decoction:** formula composed of *Radix Angelicae Pubescentis* (独活), *Ramulus Taxilli* (桑寄生), *Rhizoma Chuanxiong* (川芎), *Herba Asari* (细辛), *Radix Gentianae Macrophyllae* (秦艽), *Radix Saposhnikoviae* (防风), *Radix Achyranthis Bidentatae* (牛膝), *Cortex Eucommiae* (杜仲), *Radix Angelicae sinensis* (当归), *Radix Paeoniae Alba* (白芍), *Radix Rehmanniae Praeparata* (熟地黄), *Poria* (茯苓), *Radix Codonopsis Pilosulae* (党参), *Ramulus Cinnamomi* (桂枝), and *Radix Glycyrrhizae* (甘草), used to dispel wind-dampness, tonify the liver and kidney, replenish *qi* and blood, and relieve arthralgia for treating chronic rheumatic or rheumatoid troubles

牵正散 [qiān zhèng sǎn]
***Qianzheng* Powder; Pulling-aright Powder:** formula composed of *Rhizoma Typhonii* (白附子), *Bombyx Batryticatus* (白僵蚕), and *Scorpio* (全蝎), used for treating facial paralysis

平熄内风剂 [píng xī nèi fēng jì]
endogenous-wind-extinguishing formula: formula used for treating endogenous wind, also called wind-extinguishing formula (熄风剂 [xī fēng jì]) for short

熄风剂 [xī fēng jì]
wind-extinguishing formula: abbreviation for endogenous-wind-extinguishing formula (平熄内风剂 [píng xī nèi fēng jì])

天麻钩藤饮 [tiān má gōu téng yǐn]
***Tianma Gouteng* Decoction; Gastrodia-Uncaria Decoction:** formula composed of *Rhizoma Gastrodiae* (天麻), *Ramulus Uncariae cum Uncis* (钩藤), *Concha Hallotidis* (生石决明), *Ramulus Taxilli* (桑寄生), *Cortex Eucommiae* (杜仲), *Fructus Gardeniae* (栀子), *Radix Astragali* (黄芪), *Radix Achyranthis Bidentatae* (牛膝), *Herba Leonuri* (益母草), *Poria cum Radice Pino* (茯神), and *Caulis Polygoni Multiflori* (首乌藤), used to pacify the liver, extinguish wind, clear heat, activate the blood and tonify the liver and kidney for treating exuberant liver yang with embarrassing wind

治燥剂 [zhì zào jì]
dryness-treating formula: formula that relieves dryness syndromes/patterns, either exogenous or endogenous

轻宣外燥剂 [qīng xuān wài zào jì]
exogenous-dryness-dispersing formula: formula used for treating externally contracted cool dryness or warm dryness

杏苏散 [xìng sū sǎn]
***Xing Su* Powder; Apricot-seed and Perilla-leaf Powder:** formula composed of *Semen Armeniacae Amarum* (苦杏仁), *Folium Perillae* (紫苏叶), *Rhizoma Pinelliae* (半夏), *Radix Peucedani* (前胡), *Radix Platycodi* (桔梗), *Poria* (茯苓), *Fructus Aurantii* (枳壳), *Pericarpium Citri Reticulatae* (陈皮), *Radix Glycyrrhizae* (甘草), *Rhizoma Zingiberis Recens* (生姜), and *Fructus Ziziphi Jujubae* (大枣), used for treating externally contracted cool-dryness

清燥救肺汤 [qīng zào jiù fèi tāng]
***Qingzao Jiufei* Decoction; Dryness-clearing Lung-saving Decoction:** formula composed of *Folium Mori* (桑叶), *Gypsum Fibrosum* (石膏), *Radix Glycyrrhizae* (甘草), *Radix Ginseng* (人参), *Colla Corii Asini* (阿胶), *Radix Ophiopogonis* (麦冬), *Semen Armeniacae Amarum* (杏仁), and *Folium Eriobotryae* (枇杷叶), used to clear dryness and moisten the lung for treating warm-dryness damage to the lung

滋阴润燥剂 [zī yīn rùn zào jì]
yin-replenishing moistening formula: formula used for treating internal dryness due to fluid consumption in the *zang-fu* organs

麦门冬汤 [mài mén dōng tāng]
***Maimendong* Decoction; Ophiopogon Decoction:** formula composed of *Radix Ophiopogonis* (麦冬), *Rhizoma Pinelliae* (半夏), *Radix Ginseng* (人参), *Radix Glycyrrhizae* (甘草), *Fructus Ziziphi Jujubae* (大枣), and non-glutinous rice, used to moisten the lung for treating lung atrophy

养阴清肺汤 [yǎng yīn qīng fèi tāng]
***Yangyin Qingfei* Decoction; Yin-nourishing and Lung-clearing Decoction:** formula composed of *Radix Rehmanniae* (生地黄), *Radix Ophiopogonis* (麦冬), *Radix Scrophulariae* (玄参), *Cortex Moutan* (牡丹皮), *Bulbus Fritillariae Cirrhosae* (川贝母), *Radix Glycyrrhizae* (甘草), *Herba Menthae* (薄荷), and *Radix Paeoniae Alba* (白芍), used to nourish yin,

clear the lung, counteract toxins and soothe the throat, particularly suitable for treating diphtheria

祛湿剂 [qū shī jì]
dampness-dispelling formula: formula to resolve dampness, remove water and relieve stranguria, for treating water-dampness ailments

化湿和胃剂 [huà shī hé wèi jì]
dampness-resolving stomach-pacifying formula: formula for relieving internal accumulation of dampness-turbidity in cases of disharmony of the spleen and stomach

平胃散 [píng wèi sǎn]
***Pingwei* Powder; Stomach-pacifying Powder:** formula composed of *Rhizoma Atractylodis* (苍术), *Cortex MagnoliaeOfficinalis* (厚朴), *Pericarpium Citri Reticulatae* (陈皮), and *Radix Glycyrrhizae* (甘草), used to dry dampness, invigorate the spleen and harmonize the stomach for treating dampness stagnation in the spleen and stomach

藿香正气散 [huò xiāng zhèng qì sǎn]
***Huoxiang Zhengqi* Powder; Health-restoring Agastache Powder:** formula composed of *Herba Agastachis* (藿香), *Folium Perillae* (紫苏叶), *Radix AngelicaeDahuricae* (白芷), *Pericarpium Arecae* (大腹皮), *Poria* (茯苓), *Rhizoma AtractylodisMacrocephalae* (白术) or *Rhizoma Atractylodis* (苍术), *Pericarpium CitriReticulatae* (陈皮), *Massa Pinelliae Fermentata* (半夏曲), *Cortex Magnoliae Officinalis* (厚朴), *Radix Platycodi* (桔梗), and *Radix Glycyrrhizae* (甘草), used for treating wind-cold contraction with internal stagnation of dampness

清热祛湿剂 [qīng rè qū shī jì]
heat-clearing dampness-dispelling formula: formula used for treating dampness-heat, externally contracted, internally exuberant or downward pouring

茵陈蒿汤 [yīn chén hāo tāng]
***Yinchenhao* Decoction; Oriental Wormwood Decoction:** formula composed of *Herba Artemisiae Scopariae* (茵陈), *Fructus Gardeniae* (栀子), and *Radix et Rhizoma Rhei* (大黄), used to clear heat, remove dampness and relieve icterus for treating dampness-heat jaundice

五苓散 [wǔ líng sǎn]
***Wuling* Powder; Powder of Five Medicinals with Poria:** formula composed of *Poria* (茯苓), *Polypolus umbellatus* (猪苓), *Rhizoma Atractylodis Macrocephalae* (白术), *Rhizoma Alismatis* (泽泻), and *Ramulus Cinna-momi* (桂枝), commonly used to induce diuresis for treating various kinds of edema and oliguria

消食剂 [xiāo shí jì]
digestant formula: formula to promote digestion and remove stagnant food

保和丸 [bǎo hé wán]
***Baohe* Pill; Lenitive Pill:** formula composed of *Fructus Crataegi* (山楂), *Massa Fermentata Medicinalis* (神曲), *Semen Raphani* (莱菔子), *Poria* (茯苓), *Pericarpium Citri Reticulatae* (陈皮), *Rhizoma Pinelliae* (半夏), and *Fructus Forsythiae* (连翘), used to remove

stagnant food and harmonize the stomach for treating dyspepsia

祛痰剂 [qū tán jì]
phlegm-dispelling formula: formula used for dispelling or dissipating phlegm

二陈汤 [èr chén tāng]
***Erchen* Decoction; Decoction of Two Old Drugs:** formula composed of *Pericarpium Citri Reticulatae* (陈皮), *Rhizoma Pinelliae Praeparata* (制半夏), *Poria* (茯苓), and *Radix Glycyrrhizae Praeparata* (炙甘草), used to dry internal dampness, regulate the functions of the spleen and stomach for resolving phlegm in cases of dampness-phlegm syndromes/patterns

真武汤 [zhēn wǔ tāng]
***Zhenwu* Decoction:** formula composed of *Poria* (茯苓), *Rhizoma Atractylodis Macrocephalae* (白术), *Radix Paeoniae Alba* (白芍), *Rhizoma Zingiberis Recens* (生姜), and *Radix Aconiti Lateralis Praeparata* (制附子), used to invigorate the kidney and spleen for relieving water retention in cases of edema and prolonged diarrhea (*Zhenwu* supposedly being the god who controls water)

八正散 [bā zhèng sǎn]
***Bazheng* Powder; Eight-ingredient Rectification Powder:** formula composed of *Semen Plantaginis* (车前子), *Caulis Aristolochiae Manshuriensis* (关木通), *Herba Dianthi* (瞿麦), *Herba Polygoni Avicularis* (萹蓄), *Pulvis Talci* (滑石), *Radix Glycyrrhizae* (甘草), *Fructus Gardeniae* (栀子), *Radix et RhizomaRhei Praeparata* (熟大黄), and *Medulla Junci* (灯芯草), used to promote urination for clearing pathogenic heat and dispelling dampness in cases of dampness-heat stranguria

安神剂 [ān shén jì]
sedative or tranquilizing formula: formula that causes sedation or tranquilization

重镇安神剂 [zhòng zhèn ān shén jì]
settling tranquilizing formula: formula that causes sedation by using heavy mineral and shell medicinals, indicated for treating exuberant heart yang or fire, manifested by insomnia, fidgetiness, palpitations or even epilepsy

朱砂安神丸 [zhū shā ān shén wán]
***Zhusha Anshen* Pill; Cinnabar Tranquilizing Pill:** formula composed of *Cinnabaris* (朱砂), *Rhizoma Coptidis* (黄连), *Radix Glycyrrhizae Preparata* (炙甘草), *Radix Angelicae Sinensis* (当归), and *Radix Rehmanniae* (生地黄), used in the treatment of exuberant heart fire with deficiency of yin-blood marked by insomnia, fidgetiness and palpitations

磁朱丸 [cí zhū wán]
***Ci Zhu* Pill; Cinnabar-Magnetite Pill:** formula composed of *Cinnabaris* (朱砂) and *Magnetitum* (磁石), used for treating disharmony between the heart and kidney with insomnia, palpitations, and also for treating epilepsy

补养安神剂 [bǔ yǎng ān shén jì]
tonifying tranquilizing formula: tranquilizing formula used for treating blood deficiency of the heart and liver marked by insomnia, palpitations, fidgetiness and forgetfulness

酸枣仁汤 [suān zǎo rén tāng]

***Suanzaoren* Decoction; Spiny Jujube Seed Decoction:** formula composed of *Semen Ziziphi Spinosae* (酸枣仁), *Rhizoma Anemarrhenae* (知母), *Poria* (茯苓), *Rhizoma Chuanxiong* (川芎), and *Radix Glycyrrhizae Praeparata* (炙甘草), used to nourish the blood, clear heat and induce tranquilization for treating insomnia with fidgetiness

甘麦大枣汤 [gān mài dà zǎo tāng]

***Gan Mai Dazao* Decoction; Decoction of Liquorice, Wheat and Jujube:** formula composed of *Radix Glycyrrhizae Praeparata* (炙甘草), *Fructus Ziziphi Jujubae* (大枣), and *Fructus Tritici Levis* (浮小麦), used as a tranquilizer especially for treating hysteria

成药 Patent Medicines/Drugs

感冒清热冲剂 [gǎn mào qīng rè chōng jì]

***Ganmao Qingre* Granules; Antipyretic Granules for Colds:** granules for infusion prepared from *Spica Schizonepetae* (荆芥穗), *Herba Menthae* (薄荷), *Radix Saposhnikoviae* (防风), *Radix Bupleuri* (柴胡), *Folium Perillae* (紫苏叶), *Radix Puerariae* (葛根), *Radix Platycodi* (桔梗), *Semen Armeniacae Amarum* (苦杏仁), *Radix Angelicae Dahuricae* (白芷), *Herba Corydalis Bungeanae* (苦地丁), and *Rhizoma Phragmitis* (芦根), used for treating colds with headache, fever, chills, general aching, stuffed and running nose and cough

感冒退热冲剂 [gǎn mào tuì rè chōng jì]

***Ganmao Tuire* Granules; Antiphlogistic Granules for Flu:** granules for infusion prepared from *Folium Isatidis* (大青叶), *Radix Isatidis* (板蓝根), *Fructus Forsythiae* (连翘), and *Rhizoma Bistortae* (拳参), used for treating upper respiratory infection, acute tonsilitis and pharyngitis

小儿感冒冲剂 [xiǎo ér gǎn mào chōng jì]

***Xiao'er Ganmao* Granules; Children's Colds Granules:** granules for infusion prepared from *Herba Pogostemonis* (广藿香), *Flos Chrysanthemi* (菊花), *Fructus Forsythiae* (连翘), *Folium Isatidis* (大青叶), *Radix Isatidis* (板蓝根), *Radix Rehmanniae* (生地黄), *Cortex Lycii* (地骨皮), *Radix Cynanchi Atrati* (白薇), *Herba Menthae* (薄荷), and *Gypsum Fibrosum* (生石膏), used to remove heat and induce diaphoresis for colds and influenza with fever in children

板蓝根冲剂 [bǎn lán gēn chōng jì]

***Banlangen* Granules; Isatis-root Granules:** granules for infusion prepared from *Radix Isatidis* (板蓝根), used for treating tonsilitis, mumps and sore throat, also for preventing and treating infectious hepatitis and measles

银翘解毒丸［片］ [yín qiào jiě dú wán/piàn]

***Yinqiao Jiedu* Pills [Tablets]; Detoxicant Pills [Tablets] of Lonicera and Forshythia:** pills [tablets] prepared from *Flos Lonicerae* (金银花), *Fructus Forsythiae* (连翘), *Herba Menthae* (薄荷), *Radix Platycodi* (桔梗), *Fructus Arctii* (牛蒡子), *Herba Schizonepetae* (荆芥), etc., used to expel toxic heat from the exterior of the body, for treating wind-heat contraction with chills and fever, headache, and sore throat

防风通圣丸 [fáng fēng tōng shèng wán]

***Fangfeng Tongsheng* Pills; Miraculous Saposhnikovia Pills:** pills prepared from *Radix Saposhnikoviae* (防风), *Fructus Forsythiae* (连翘), *Herba Ephedrae* (麻黄), *Fructus Gardeniae* (栀子), *Radix et Rhizoma Rhei* (大黄), *Gypsum Fibrosum* (石膏), *Radix Scutellariae* (黄芩), *Radix Paeoniae Alba* (白芍), *Rhizoma Chuanxiong* (川芎), etc., used for treating wind-heat contraction characterized by headache, sore throat, fullness in the chest, constipation, skin eruption or ulcers

通宣理肺丸［片］[tōng xuān lǐ fèi wán/piàn]

***Tongxuan Lifei* Pills [Tablets]; Lung-ventilating Pills [Tablets]:** pills [tablets] prepared from *Folium Perillae* (紫苏叶), *Herba Ephedrae* (麻黄), *Semen Armeniacae Amarum* (苦杏仁), *Radix Peucedani* (前胡), *Radix Platycodi* (桔梗), *Radix Scutellariae* (黄芩), *Pericarpium Citri Reticulatae* (陈皮), *Rhizoma Pinelliae* (半夏), etc., used for treating cough, stuffed nose and headache in cases of wind-cold contraction

二母宁嗽丸［片］[èr mǔ níng sòu wán/piàn]

***Ermu Ningsou* Pills [Tablets]; Cough Pills [Tablets] with Anemarrhena and Fritillary:** pills [tablets] prepared from *Rhizoma Anemarrhenae* (知母), *Bulbus Fritillariae Cirrhosae* (川贝母), *Cortex Mori* (桑白皮), *Semen Trichosanthis* (瓜蒌仁), *Gypsum Fibrosum* (石膏), *Fructus Gardeniae* (栀子), *Pericarpium Citri Reticulatae* (陈皮), *Poria* (茯苓), etc., used to clear the lung of heat for relieving cough with yellow sputum

复方川贝精片 [fù fāng chuān bèi jīng piàn]

***Fufang Chuanbeijing* Tablets; Compound Tablets of Fritillary Extract:** tablets prepared from *Bulbus Fritillariae Cirrhosae* (川贝母), *Herba Ephedrae* (麻黄), *Radix Glycyrrhizae* (甘草), *Fructus Schisandrae* (五味子), *Pericarpium Citri Reticulatae* (陈皮), etc., used for relieving cough and asthma due to wind-cold contraction

川贝枇杷糖浆 [chuān bèi pí pá táng jiāng]

***Chuanbei Pipa* Syrup; Fritillary-Loquat Syrup:** syrup prepared from *Extractum Bulbus Fritillariae Cirrhosae Liquidum* (川贝母流浸膏), *Folium Eriobotryae* (枇杷叶), *Radix Platycodi* (桔梗) and *Mentholum* (薄荷脑), used to clear the lung of heat and resolve phlegm for treating cough in cases of bronchitis

蛇胆川贝散 [shé dǎn chuān bèi sǎn]

***Shedan Chuanbei* Powder; Snake-bile and Tendrilled-Fritillary Powder:** powder prepared from *Fel Serpentis Liquidum*(蛇胆汁) and *Bulbus Fritilleriae Cirrhosae* (川贝), used to remove heat from the lung, arrest cough and eliminate phlegm for treating bronchitis

蛇胆陈皮散 [shé dǎn chén pí sǎn]

***Shedan Chenpi* Powder; Snake-bile and Tangerine-peel Powder:** powder prepared from *Fel Serpentis Liquidum* (蛇胆汁) and *Pericarpium Citri Reticulatae* (陈皮), used to relieve cough, resolve phlegm and promote digestion for treating cough and expectoration with nausea and vomiting in cases of colds

橘红丸［片］[jú hóng wán/piàn]
***Juhong* Pills [Tablets]; Red Tangerine Pills [Tablets]:** pills [tablets] prepared from *Exocarpium Citri Rubrum* (橘红), *Flos Farfarae* (款冬花), *Poria* (茯苓), *Radix Asteris* (紫菀), *Semen Trichosanthis* (瓜蒌仁), *Gypsum Fibrosum* (生石膏), etc., used to remove pathogenic heat from the lung and resolve phlegm for relieving cough and dyspnea with sticky or yellow sputum in cases of acute or chronic bronchitis

定喘丸 [dìng chuǎn wán]
***Dingchuan* Pills; Antasthmatic Pills:** pills prepared from *Fructus Perillae* (紫苏子), *Semen Armeniacae Amarum* (苦杏仁), *Bulbus Fritillariae Cirrhosae* (川贝母), *Radix Astragali* (黄芪), *Colla Corii Asini* (阿胶), *Flos Farfarae* (款冬花), etc., used to replenish and regulate lung *qi* for relieving cough and asthma in chronic cases

气管炎丸 [qì guǎn yán wán]
Bronchitis Pills: pills prepared from *Herba Ephedrae* (麻黄), *Flos Farfarae* (款冬花), *Semen Armeniacae Amarum* (苦杏仁), *Bulbus Fritillariae Cirrhosae* (川贝母), etc., used to expel phlegm and relieve cough and dyspnea for treating chronic bronchitis

养阴清肺膏 [yǎng yīn qīng fèi gāo]
***Yangyin Qingfei* Extract; Yin-nourishing Lung-clearing Extract:** extract prepared from *Radix Rehmanniae* (生地), *Radix Ophiopogonis* (麦冬), *Radix Scrophulariae* (玄参), *Bulbus Fritillariae Cirrhosae* (川贝母), *Radix Paeoniae Alba* (白芍), *Cortex Moutan* (牡丹皮), *Herba Menthe* (薄荷), and *Radix Glycyrrhizae* (甘草), used for treating lung-yin deficiency characterized by dryness and pain in the throat, and dry cough with scanty expectoration or bloody sputum

玉屏风口服液 [yù píng fēng kǒu fú yè]
***Yupingfeng* Oral Liquid; Jade-screen Liquid:** an oral liquid prepared from *Radix Astragali* (黄芪), *Radix Saposhnikoviae* (防风), and *Rhizoma Atractylodis Macrocephalae* (白术), used to replenish *qi*, strengthen superficial resistance and arrest excessive sweating, for treating spontaneous sweating and liability to colds

双黄连口服液 [shuāng huáng lián kǒu fú yè]
***Shuanghuanlian* Oral Liquid; Lonicera-Scutellaria-Forsythia Oral Liquid:** an oral liquid prepared from *Flos Lonicerae* (金银花), *Radix Scutellariae* (黄芩) and *Fructus Forsythiae* (连翘), used to disperse wind, release the exterior, clear heat and resolve toxins for treating wind-heat affliction with fever and sore throat

银黄口服液 [yín huáng kǒu fú yè]
***Yinhuang* Oral Liquid; Lonicera-Scutellariae Oral Liquid:** an oral liquid prepared from *Flos Lonicerae* (金银花) and *Radix Scutellariae* (黄芩), used to clear wind-heat and soothe the throat for treating acute and chronic tonsilitis and pharyngitis

西黄丸 [xī huáng wán]

Xihuang **Pill; Bezoar Pill:** a pill prepared from *Calculus Bovis* (牛黄), *Olibanum* (乳香) and *Myrrha* (没药), used to clear heat, resolve toxins, relieve swelling and disperse nodules for treating scrofula, pyogenic infection, and cancer

三黄片 [sān huáng piàn]

Sanhuang **Tablets; Rhubarb-Scutellaria-Coptis Tablets:** tablets prepared from *Radix et Rhizoma Rhei* (大黄), *Radix Scutellariae* (黄芩) and *Rhizoma Coptidis* (黄连), used to clear heat, resolve toxins and purge the bowels, for treating intense heat in the triple energizer manifested by inflammation of the conjunctiva, sores in the mouth and nose, painful throat, bleeding gum, fidgetiness, thirst, deep-colored urine and constipation

清开灵注射液 [qīng kāi líng zhù shè yè]

Qingkailing **Injection:** injection prepared from *Concha Margaritifera Usta* (珍珠母), Hyodesoxycholic Acid (猪去氧胆酸), *Fructus Gardeniae* (栀子), *Pulvis Cornus Bubali* (水牛角粉), *Radix Isatidis* (板蓝根), Baicalin (黄芩苷) and *Flos Lonicerae* (金银花), used to clear heat and toxins, resolve phlegm, unblock the collaterals and induce resuscitation for treating loss of consciousness in stroke and febrile diseases

牛黄上清丸 [niú huáng shàng qīng wán]

Niuhuang Shangqing **Pills; Bezoar Pills for Clearing the Upper:** pills prepared from *Calculus Bovis* (牛黄), *Rhizoma Coptidis* (黄连), *Radix et Rhizoma Rhei* (大黄), *Radix Scutellariae* (黄芩), *Fructus Forsythiae* (连翘), *Fructus Gardeniae* (栀子), *Gypsum Fibrosum* (生石膏), *Flos Chrysanthemi* (菊花), etc., used to clear toxic heat particularly in the upper part of the body characterized by headache, dizziness, inflammation of the eyes, tinnitus, ulceration of the mouth and tongue, swelling and pain in the gums, and constipation

牛黄解毒丸［片］ [niú huáng jiě dú wán/piàn]

Niuhuang Jiedu **Pills [Tablets]; Bezoar Detoxicant Pills [Tablets]:** pills [tablets] prepared from *Radix Scutellariae* (黄芩), *Rhizoma Coptidis* (黄连), *Cortex Phellodendri* (黄柏), *Radix et Rhizoma Rhei* (大黄), *Fructus Forsythiae* (连翘), *Flos Lonicerae* (金银花), *Calculus Bovis* (牛黄), etc., used to clear toxic heat for treating intense heat or fire in the liver and stomach, characterized by headache and dizziness, inflammed eyes, tinnitus, oral ulcers, periodontitis, and constipation

牛黄清心丸［片］ [niú huáng qīng xīn wán/piàn]

Niuhuang Qingxin **Pills [Tablets]; Bezoar Sedative Pills [Tablets]:** pills [tablets] prepared from *Calculus Bovis* (牛黄), *Moschus* (麝香), *Corni Rhinoceri* (犀角), *Cornu Saigae Tataricae* (羚羊角), *Cinnabaris* (朱砂), etc., used to clear pathogenic heat from the heart and induce sedation, for treating excessive heat in the heart meridian/channel characterized by vertigo, irritability, delirium, and even convulsions

牛黄降压丸 [niú huáng jiàng yā wán]

Niuhuang Jiangya **Pills; Bezoar Antihypertensive Pills:** pills prepared from

Calculus Bovis (牛黄), *Cornu Saigae Tataricae* (羚羊角), *Magarita* (珍珠), *Borneolum Syntheticum* (冰片), *Radix Astragali* (黄芪), *Radix Curcumae* (郁金), *Radix PaeoniaeAlba* (白芍), etc., used to induce sedation and reduce high blood pressure for treating hypertension

血脂宁丸 [xuè zhī níng wán]
***Xuezhining* Pills; Blood-lipid Lowering Pills:** pills prepared from *Fructus Crataegi* (山楂), *Radix Polygoni Multiflori* (何首乌), *Folium Nelumbinis* (荷叶), etc., used to lower the blood lipids, soften the blood vessels, and increase the coronary blood circulation for treating hyperlipemia and arrhythmia

脑立清 [nǎo lì qīng]
***Nao Li Qing*; Head-clearing Pills:** pills prepared from *Haematitum* (赭石), *Rhizoma Pinelliae* (半夏), *Radix AchyranthisBidentatae* (牛膝), *Concha Margaritifera Usta* (珍珠母), etc., used to quench fire in the liver for treating hypertension due to deficiency of liver yin with exuberance of yang, characterized by dizziness, tinnitus and insomnia

补心丹 [pǔ xīn dān]
***Buxin* Pills; Mind-tonic Pills:** pills prepared from *Poria* (茯苓), *Radix Ginseng* (人参), *Radix Ophiopogonis* (麦冬), *Semen Zizyphi Spinosae* (酸枣仁), *Semen Boitae* (柏子仁), *Radix Polygalae* (远志), *Radix Angelica Sinensis* (当归), etc., used to nourish heart blood so as to calm the mind, for treating heart blood deficiency with restlessness, insomnia, and forgetfulness

朱砂安神丸 [zhū shā ān shén wán]
***Zhusha Anshen* Pills; Cinnabar Sedative Pills:** pills prepared from *Cinnabaris* (朱砂), *Dens Draconis* (龙齿), *Radix Angelicae Sinensis* (当归), *Rhizoma Coptidis* (黄连), *Semen Zizyphi Spinosae* (酸枣仁), *Radix Rehmanniae Preparata* (熟地黄), etc., used to calm the mind for treating fidgetiness and insomnia, forgetfulness, palpitations and shortness of breath due to deficiency of *qi* and blood in the heart

柏子养心丸 [bǎi zǐ yǎng xīn wán]
***Baizi Yangxin* Pills; Mind-tonic Pills of Arborvitae Seed:** pills prepared from *Semen Biotae* (柏子仁), *Radix Ginseng* (人参), *Radix Astragali* (黄芪), *Semen Zizyphi Spinosae* (酸枣仁), *Radix Angelicae Sinensis* (当归), *Fructus Schizandrae* (五味子), *Radix Polygalae* (远志), etc., used for relieving anxiety and mental strain, also for treating palpitations, insomnia and amnesia

安神补心丸 [ān shén bǔ xīn wán]
***Anshen Buxin* Pills; Heart-tonifying Tranquilizing Pills:** pills prepared from *Radix Salviae Miltiorrhizae* (丹参), *Fructus Schizandrae* (五味子), *Rhizoma Acori Tatarinowii* (石菖蒲) and Decoctum Tranquilizici Concentratum, used to nourish the heart and calm the nerves for treating palpitations, insomnia, dizziness and tinnitus

败酱片 [bài jiàng piàn]
***Baijiang* Tablets; Dahurican Patrinia Tablets:** tablets prepared from extract of *Rhizoma et Radix Patriniae Scabiosaefoliae* (黄花败酱), used as a sedative for treating

insomnia in cases of neurasthenia and psychoses

麻仁丸 [má rén wán]

***Maren* Pills; Cannabis-seed Pills:** pills prepared from *Semen Cannabis* (火麻仁), *Radix et Rhizoma Rhei* (大黄), *Semen Armeniacae Amarum* (苦杏仁), *Cortex Magnoliae Officinalis* (厚朴), *Fructus Aruantii Immaturus* (枳实) and *Radix Paeoniae Alba* (白芍), used for relieving constipation due to deficiency of fluids and constipation in the aged and debilitated persons

麻仁润肠丸 [má rén rùn cháng wán]

***Maren Runchang* Pills; Cannabis Laxative Pills:** pills prepared from *Semen Cannabis* (火麻仁), *Semen Armeniacae Amarum* (苦杏仁), *Radix et Rhizoma Rhei* (大黄), *Radix Aucklandiae* (木香), *Pericarpium Citri Reticulatae* (橘皮) and *Radix Paeoniae Alba* (白芍), used to purge the bowels for treating stagnation of heat in the stomach and intestines manifested by constipation and distension in the abdomen

香连丸 [xiāng lián wán]

***Xianglian* Pills; Aucklandia-Coptis Pills:** pills prepared from *Rhizoma Coptidis* (黄连) and *Radix Aucklandiae* (木香), used to eliminate dampness-heat, promote the flow of *qi* and relieve pain, for treating dysentery with tenesmus, abdominal pain and diarrhea

舒肝丸 [shū gān wán]

***Shugan* Pills; Liver-soothing Pills:** pills prepared from *Cortex Magnoliae Officinalis* (厚朴), *Rhizoma Curcumae Longae* (姜黄), *Lignum Aquilariae Resinatum* (沉香), *Fructus Galangae* (红豆蔻), *Radix Bupleuri* (柴胡), *Rhizoma Corydalis* (元胡), etc., used for removing stagnancy of liver *qi* manifested by depression, pain and fullness over the hypochondriac and epigastric regions, eructation, and acid regurgitation

逍遥丸 [xiāo yáo wán]

***Xiaoyao* Pills; Carefree Pills:** formula composed of *Radix Bupleuri* (柴胡), *Radix Angelicae Sinensis* (当归), *Radix Paeoniae Alba* (白芍), *Rhizoma Atractylodis Macrocephalae* (白术), *Poria* (茯苓), *Radix Glycyrrhizae* (甘草), *Rhizoma Zingiberis Preparata* (煨生姜) and *Herba Menthae* (薄荷), used to soothe the liver, invigorate the spleen, nourish the blood and regulate menstruation for treating depressed liver *qi* characterized by hypochondriac distension and pain, dizziness, impaired appetite and menstrual disorders

加味逍遥丸 [jiā wèi xiāo yáo wán]

***Jiawei Xiaoyao* Pills; Modified Carefree Pills:** pills prepared from*Radix Bupleuri* (柴胡), *Radix Angelicae Sinensis* (当归), *Radix Paeoniae Alba* (白芍), *Rhizoma Atractylodis Macrocephalae* (白术), *Poria* (茯苓), *Radix Glycyrrhizae* (甘草), *Rhizoma Zingiberis Preparata* (煨生姜), *Cortex Moutan* (牡丹皮), *Fructus Gardeniae* (栀子), and *Herba Menthae* (薄荷), used to remove stagnant liver *qi*, clear heat, and invigorate the spleen and stomach, for treating stagnation of the liver and disharmony between the liver and stomach, characterized by distension and pain in the hypochondriac region, dizziness, anorexia, menoxenia, and abdominal distension and pain

木香顺气丸 [mù xiāng shùn qì wán]
***Muxiang Shunqi* Pills; Aucklandia Carminative Pills:** pills prepared from *Radix Aucklandiae* (木香), *Pericarpium Citri Reticulatae Viride* (青皮), *Cortex Magnoliae Officinalis* (厚朴), *Radix Linderae* (乌药), *Radix et Rhizoma Rhei* (大黄), *Semen Pharbitidis* (牵牛子), etc., used to relieve stagnancy of food and gas, for treating indigestion with flatulence and constipation

大山楂丸 [dà shān zhā wán]
***Dashanzha* Pills; Large Haw Pills:** pills prepared from *Fructus Crataegi* (山楂), *Massa FermentataMedicinalis* (六神曲), and *Fructus Hordei Germinatus* (麦芽), used to promote the appetite and digestion for treating indigestion with anorexia and epigastric distension

启脾丸 [qǐ pí wán]
***Qipi* Pills; Spleen-activating Pills:** pills prepared from *Radix Genseng* (人参), *Rhizoma Atractylodis Macrocephalae* (白术), *Poria* (茯苓), *Radix Glycyrrhizae* (甘草), *Pericarpium Citri Reticulatae* (陈皮), *Rhizoma Dioscoreae* (山药), *Semen Nelumbinis* (莲子), *Fructus Crataegi* (山楂), *Massa Medicata Fermentata* (六神曲), *Fructus Hordei Germinatus* (麦芽), and *Rhizoma Alismatis* (泽泻), used for treating spleen insufficiency characterized by dyspepsia, abdominal distension and loose bowels

附子理中丸 [fù zǐ lǐ zhōng wán]
***Fuzi Lizhong* Pills; Aconite Middle-regulating Pills:** pills prepared from *Radix Aconiti Lateralis Preparata* (附子), *Radix Codonopsis Pilosulae* (党参), *Rhizoma Atractylodis Macrocephalae* (白术), *Rhizoma Zingiberis* (干姜), and *Radix Glycyrrhizae* (甘草), used to warm and invigorate the spleen and stomach for treating deficiency-cold of the spleen and stomach with epigastric pain accompanied by cold sensation, vomiting, diarrhea and cold limbs

气滞胃痛颗粒 [qì zhì wèi tòng kē lì]
***Qizhi Weitong* Granules; *Qi*-stagnant Gastralgia Relieving Granules:** granules prepared from *Radix Bupleuri* (柴胡), *Rhizoma Cyperi* (香附), *Radix Paeoniae Alba* (白芍) and *Rhizoma Corydalis* (延胡索), used to soothe liver *qi*, harmonize the stomach and relieve pain for treating stomach troubles with epigastric pain and distension due to depressed liver *qi*

越鞠丸 [yuè jū wán]
***Yueju* Pills; Distension-relieving Pills:** pills prepared from *Rhizoma Cyperi* (香附), *Rhizoma Ligustici Chuanxiong* (川芎), *Fructus Gardeniae* (栀子), *Rhizoma Atractylodis* (苍术) and *Massa Fermentata Medicinalis* (神曲), used to regulate *qi* and relieve distension for treating stomach diseases manifested by epigastric and abdominal stuffiness and distension, anorexia, belching and acid regurgitation

香砂养胃丸 [xiāng shā yǎng wèi wán]
***Xiangsha Yangwei* Pills; Cyperus-Amomum Stomach-nourishing Pills:** pills prepared from *Rhizoma Cypri* (香附), *Fructus Amomi* (砂仁), Radix *Aucklandiae* (木香), *Rhizoma Atractylodis*

Macrocephalae (白术), *Pericarpium Citri Reticulatae* (陈皮), *Cortex Magnoliae Officinalis* (厚朴), etc., used for treating dyspepsia due to weakness of the stomach characterized by epigastric distension, vomiting, belching and acid regurgitation

香砂六君丸 [xiāng shā liù jūn wán]
***Xiangsha Liujun* Pills; Cyperus-Amomum Six-noble Pills:** pills prepared from *Radix Codonopsis Pilosulae* (党参), *Poria* (茯苓), *Rhizoma Atractylodis Macrocephalae* (白术), *Radix Glycyrrhizae* (甘草), *Pericarpium Citri Reticulatae* (陈皮), *Rhizoma Pinelliae* (半夏), *Radix Aucklandiae* (木香), and *Fructus Amomi* (砂仁), used to invigorate the spleen and regulate the stomach for treating dyspepsia, belching, anorexia, epigastric and abdominal distension, and loose bowels

参苓白术丸 [shēn líng bái zhú wán]
***Shenling Baizhu* Pills; Ginseng-Poria-Atractylodes Pills:** pills prepared from *Radix Ginseng* (人参), *Poria* (茯苓), *Rhizoma Atractylodis Macrocephalae* (白术), *Rhizoma Dioscoreae* (山药), *Semen Nelumbinis* (莲子), *Fructus Amomi* (砂仁), etc., used for the treating diminished function of the spleen and stomach characterized by loss of appetite, abdominal distension, diarrhea and lassitude

人参健脾丸 [rén shēn jiàn pí wán]
***Renshen Jianpi* Pills; Ginseng Spleen-strengthening Pills:** pills prepared from *Radix Ginseng* (人参), *Poria* (茯苓), *Rhizoma Dioscoreae* (山药), *Radix Astragali* (黄芪), *Rhizoma Atractylodis Macrocephalae* (白术), *Pericarpium Citri Reticulatae* (陈皮), etc., used for treating diminished function of the spleen and stomach characterized by emaciation, general weakness, loss of appetite, and alternate diarrhea and constipation

八珍丸 [bā zhēn wán]
***Bazhen* Pills; Eight-treasure Pills:** pills prepared from *Radix Ginseng* (人参) or *Radix Codonopsis Pilosulae* (党参), *Rhizoma Atractylodis Macrocephalae* (白术), *Poria* (茯苓), *Radix Glycyrrhizae* (甘草), *Radix Angelicae Sinensis* (当归), *Radix Paeoniae Alba* (白芍), *Rhizoma Chuanxiong* (川芎), and *Rhizoma Rehmanniae Preparata* (熟地黄), used to improve the function of the spleen and stomach, reinforce *qi* and nourish the blood for treating general debility, loss of appetite, lassitude, etc.

十全大补丸 [shí quán dà bǔ wán]
***Shiquan Dabu* Pills; All-inclusive Grand Tonic Pills:** pills prepared from *Radix Ginseng* (人参) or *Radix Codonopsis Pilosulae* (党参), *Rhizoma Atractylodis Macrocephalae* (白术), *Poria* (茯苓), *Radix Glycyrrhizae* (甘草), *Radix Angelicae Sinensis* (当归), *Radix Paeoniae Alba* (白芍), *Rhizoma Chuanxiong* (川芎), *Rhizoma Rehmanniae Preparata* (熟地黄), *Cortex Cinnamomi* (肉桂), and *Radix Astragali* (黄芪), used to replenish both *qi* and blood for treating general debility after illness

补中益气丸 [bǔ zhōng yì qì wán]
***Buzhong Yiqi* Pills; Middle-reinforcing *Qi*-replenishing Pills:** pills prepared from *Radix Astragali* (黄芪), *Radix*

Ginseng (人参) or *Radix Codonopsis Pilosulae* (党参), *Radix Astragali* (黄芪), *Rhizoma Atractylodis Macrocephalae* (白术), *Radix Angelicae Sinensis* (当归), *Pericarpium Citri Reticulatae* (陈皮), *Radix Glycyrrhizae* (甘草), *Rhizoma Atractylodis Macrocephalae* (白术), *Rhizoma Cimicifugae* (升麻), and *Radix Bupleuri* (柴胡), used to reinforce spleen *qi* for treating general debility, lassitude and somnolence, prolonged diarrhea, uterine bleeding, sometimes accompanied by prolapse of the rectum or uterus

生脉饮 [shēng mài yǐn]
***Shengmai* Drink; Pulse-activating Drink:** solution prepared from *Radix Ginseng* (人参), *Radix Ophiopogonis* (麦冬), and *Fructus Schisandrae* (五味子), used to replenish *qi* and yin, for treating cardiac palpitations, shortness of breath, faint pulse and spontaneous sweating

大补阴丸 [dà bǔ yīn wán]
***Dabuyin* Pills; Large Yin-nourishing Pills:** pills prepared from *Radix Rehmanniae Preparata* (熟地黄), *Rhizoma Anemarrheanae* (知母), *Cortex Phellodendri* (黄柏), *Carapax et Plastrum Testudinis* (龟板), and *Medulla Spinalis Suis* (猪脊髓), used to nourish yin and reduce fire, for treating yin deficiency manifested by afternoon fever, night sweats, cough, hemoptysis, tinnitus, and seminal emission

河车大造丸 [hé chē dà zào wán]
***Heche Dazao* Pills; Restorative Placenta Pills:** pills prepared from *Placenta Hominis* (紫河车), *Radix Ophiopogonis* (麦冬), *Radix Asparagi* (天冬), *Cortex Eucommiae* (杜仲), *Plastrum Testudinis* (龟板), *Rhizoma Rehmanniae Preparata* (熟地黄), etc., used to nourish kidney essence for treating general debility, night sweats, nocturnal emission, lassitude, tidal fever and maldevelopment

五子衍宗丸 [wǔ zǐ yǎn zōng wán]
***Wuzi Yanzong* Pills; Pills of Five Kinds of Seeds for Offsprings:** pills prepared from *Fructus Lycii* (枸杞子), *Semen Cuscutae* (菟丝子), *Fructus Rubi* (复盆子), *Fructus Schisandrae* (五味子), and *Semen Plantaginis* (车前子), used to replenish kidney essence for treating dribbling of urine after micturition, seminal emission, premature ejaculation, impotence and sterility

六味地黄丸 [liù wèi dì huáng wán]
***Liuwei Dihuang* Pills; Six-ingredient Rehmannia Pills:** pills prepared from *Radix Rehmanniae Preparata* (熟地黄), *Fructus Corni* (山茱萸), *Rhizoma Dioscoreae* (山药), *Rhizoma Alismatis* (泽泻), *Poria* (茯苓), and *Cortex Moutan* (牡丹皮), used to replenish kidney yin for treating yin deficiency characterized by dizziness, tinnitus, aching and limpness of the loins and knees, and night sweats, and also used for treating diabetes

地黄丸 [dì huáng wán]
***Dihuang* Pills; Rehmannia Pills:** another name for *Liuwei Dihuang* Pills or Six-ingredient Rehmannia Pills (六味地黄丸 [liù wèi dì huáng wán])

杞菊地黄丸 [qǐ jú dì huáng wán]
***Qiju Dihuang* Pills; Wolfberry-Chrysanthemum Rehmannia Pills:**

pills prepared from *Fructus Lycii* (枸杞子), *Flos Chrysanthemi* (菊花), *Radix Rehmanniae Preparata* (熟地黄), *Fructus Corni* (山茱萸), *Rhizoma Dioscoreae* (山药), *Rhizoma Alismatis* (泽泻), *Poria* (茯苓), and *Cortex Moutan* (牡丹皮), used to nourish liver and kidney yin for treating yin deficiency of the liver and kidney with dizziness, tinnitus and blurred vision

知柏地黄丸 [zhī bǎi dì huáng wán]
***Zhibai Dihuang* Pills; Amenarrhena-Phellodendron Rehmannia Pills:** pills prepared from *Rhizoma Anemarrheanae* (知母), *Cortex Phellodendri* (黄柏), *Radix Rehmanniae Preparata* (熟地黄), *Fructus Corni* (山茱萸), *Rhizoma Dioscoreae* (山药), *Rhizoma Alismatis* (泽泻), *Poria* (茯苓), and *Cortex Moutan* (牡丹皮), used to nourish yin and reduce fire, for treating yin deficiency with up-flaming of fire characterized by daily recurring fever, night sweats, dry mouth, sore throat and tinnitus

麦味地黄丸 [mài wèi dì huáng wán]
***Maiwei Dihuang* Pills; Lilyturf-Magnoliavine Rehmannia Pills:** pills prepared from *Radix Ophiopogonis* (麦冬), *Fructus Schisandrae* (五味子), *Radix Rehmanniae Preparata* (熟地黄), *Fructus Corni* (山茱萸), *Rhizoma Dioscoreae* (山药), *Rhizoma Alismatis* (泽泻), *Poria* (茯苓), and *Cortex Moutan* (牡丹皮), used (1) to nourish kidney and lung yin for treating yin deficiency of the lung and kidney characterized by recurring fever, night sweats, dry throat, hemoptysis, dizziness, and tinnitus, and (2) for treating diabetes

桂附地黄丸 [guì fù dì huáng wán]
***Guifu Dihuang* Pills; Cassia-Aconite Rehmannia Pills:** pills prepared from *Cortex Cinnamomi* (肉桂), *Radix Aconiti Lateralis Preparata* (附子), *Radix Rehmanniae Preparata* (熟地黄), *Fructus Corni* (山茱萸), *Rhizoma Dioscoreae* (山药), *Rhizoma Alismatis* (泽泻), *Poria* (茯苓), and *Cortex Moutan* (牡丹皮), used (1) to reinforce kidney yang for treating kidney yang deficiency charaterized by cold sensation in the loins and knees, edema of the legs, and oliguria, and (2) for treating diabetes

龟龄集 [guī líng jí]
***Guilingji* Capsules; Longevity Capsules:** granules in capsules prepared from *Radix Ginseng* (人参), *Cornu Cervi Pantotrichum* (鹿茸), *Hippocampus* (海马), *Herba Epimedii* (淫羊藿), sparrow's brain (雀脑), etc., used to invigorate kidney yang for treating impotence, sterility, amnesia, and mental debility

全鹿丸 [quán lù wán]
***Quanlu* Pills; Deer Tonic Pills:** pills prepared from *Radix Ginseng* (人参), *Cornu Cervi Pantotrichum* (鹿茸), *Herba Cynomorii* (锁阳), *Radix Morindae Officinalis* (巴戟天), *Radix Angelicae Sinensis* (当归), *Lignum Aquilariae Resinatum* (沉香), *Rhizoma Rehmanniae Preparata* (熟地黄), etc., used (1) as a tonic for treating kidney insufficiency characterized by asthenia, lassitude, amnesia, insomnia, night sweats, and spontaneous emission, and (2) for treating metrorrhagia, leukorrhagia and miscarriage

参茸卫生丸 [shēn róng wèi shēng wán] ***Shenrong Weisheng*** **Pills; Ginseng-Antler Life-preserving Pills:** pills prepared from *Radix Ginseng* (人参), *Cornu Cervi Pantotrichum* (鹿茸), *Semen Nelumbinis* (莲子), *Semen Zizyphi Spinosae* (酸枣仁), *Herba Cynomorii* (锁阳), *Radix Morindae Officinalis* (巴戟天), *Fructus Lycii* (枸杞子), etc., used to replenish *qi* and blood, nourish essence of both the liver and the kidney, and invigorate the functions of the spleen and stomach, for treating deficiency of *qi* and blood and kidney insufficiency with lassitude, fatigue, poor appetite, spermatorrhea, anemia, early graying of the hair, etc.

人参养荣丸 [rén shēn yǎng róng wán] ***Renshen Yangrong*** **Pills; Ginseng Nutritive Pills:** pills prepared from *Radix Ginseng* (人参), *Rhizoma Atractylodis Macrocephalae* (白术), *Poria* (茯苓), *Radix Glycyrrhizae* (甘草), *Radix Angelicae Sinensis* (当归), *Radix Rehmanniae Preparata* (熟地黄), *Radix Paeoniae Alba* (白芍), *Radix Astragali* (黄芪), *Pericarpium Citri Reticulatae* (陈皮), *Radix Polygalae* (远志), *Cortex Cinnamomi* (肉桂), and *Fructus Schisandrae* (五味子), used to warm and tonify *qi* and blood for treating deficiency syndrome/pattern of both the heart and spleen with insufficiency of *qi* and blood characterized by emaciation, lassitude, anorexia, and loose stools, and also for weakness during convalescence

参茸固本片 [shēn róng gù běn piàn] ***Shenrong Guben*** **Tablets; Ginseng-Antler Restorative Tablets:** tablets prepared from *Radix Angelicae Sinensis* (当归), *Rhizoma Dioscoreae* (山药), *Poria* (茯苓), *Fructus Corni* (山茱萸), *Cortex Eucommiae* (杜仲), *Fructus Lycii* (枸杞子), *Radix Rehmanniae Preparata* (熟地黄), *Fructus Cuscutae* (菟丝子), *Radix Ginseng* (人参), *Cornu Cervi Pantotrichum* (鹿茸), etc., used to tonify *qi* and blood for treating various kinds of deficiency syndromes/patterns with tinnitus, dizziness, and lassitude

参附注射液 [shēn fù zhù shè yè] ***Shenfu*** **Injection; Ginseng-Aconite Injection:** injection prepared from *Radix Ginseng* (人参) and *Radix Aconiti Lateralis Preparata* (附子), used to replenish *qi* and warm yang for treating yang deficiency or *qi* deficiency syndrome/pattern in various chronic diseases as well as in the course of radiotherapy or chemotherapy for cancer

再造丸 [zài zào wán] ***Zaizao*** **Pills; Restorative Pills:** pills prepared from *Agkistrodon* (蕲蛇) deprived of head, scales and bones, *Scorpio* (全蝎), *Pulvis Cornus Bubali Concentratus* (水牛角浓缩粉), *Calculus Bovis* (牛黄), *Rhizoma Gastrodiae* (天麻), *Radix Ginseng* (人参), *Moschus* (麝香), etc., used to dispel wind-phlegm and promote blood flow for treating apoplectic coma and hemiplegia

人参再造丸 [rén shēn zài zào wán] ***Renshen Zaizao*** **Pills; Ginseng Restorative Pills:** synonym for *Zaizao* Pills or Restorative Pills (再造丸 [zài zào wán])

紫雪 [zǐ xuě]

***Zixue* Powder; Purple Snowy Powder:** powder prepared from *Pulvis Cornus Bubali Concentratus* (水牛角浓缩粉), *Cornu Saigae Tataricae* (羚羊角), *Moschus* (麝香), *Lignum Aquilariae Resinatum* (沉香), *Gypsum Fibrosum* (石膏), etc., used to clear pathogenic heat, relieve convulsions and promote the restoration of consciousness, for treating high fever with restlessness, delirium and convulsions

安宫牛黄丸 [ān gōng niú huáng wán]

***Angong Niuhuang* Pills; Bezoar Resurrection Pills:** pills prepared from *Calculus Bovis* (牛黄), *Pulvis Cornus Bubali Concentratus* (水牛角浓缩粉), *Margarita* (珍珠), *Moschus* (麝香), *Fructus Gardeniae* (栀子), etc., used for eliminating toxic heat and bringing the patient back to consciousness from coma, and relieving convulsions due to high fever or cerebral hemorrhage

苏合香丸 [sū hé xiāng wán]

***Suhexiang* Pills; Storax Pills:** pills prepared from *Styrax* (苏合香), *Benzoinum* (安息香), *Borneolum Syntheticum* (冰片), *Cornu Bubali* (水牛角), *Moschus* (麝香), *Lignum Santali Albi* (檀香), *Lignum Aquilariae Resinatum* (沉香), *Flos Caryophylli* (丁香), *Rhizoma Cyperi* (香附), *Radix Aucklandiae* (木香), *Olibanum* (乳香), etc., used (1) to promote the restoration of consciousness as an aromatic stimulant, to promote the flow of *qi* and relieve pain for emergency treatment of apoplexy and heatstroke with loss of consciousness, and (2) for treating precordial and epigastric pain due to *qi* stagnation

小活络丸 [丹] [xiǎo huó luò wán/dān]

***Xiaohuoluo* Pills: Collateral-activating Pills (mild recipe):** pills prepared from *Radix Aconiti Preparata* (制川乌), *Radix Aconiti Kusnezoffii Preparata* (制草乌), *Arisaema cum Bile* (胆南星), *Olibanum* (乳香), *Myrrha* (没药), and *Lumbricus* (地龙), used to dispel wind and dampness, and invigorate blood flow in collaterals for relieving rheumatic pain, numbness and difficulty in movement of joints

大活络丸 [丹] [dà huó luò wán/dān]

***Dahuoluo* Pills: Collateral-activating Pills (heavy recipe):** pills prepared from *Agkistrodon* (蕲蛇), *Zaocys* (乌梢蛇), *Rhizoma Gastrodiae* (天麻), *Radix Ginseng* (人参), *Calculus Bovis* (牛黄), *Moschus* (麝香), *Pulvis Cornus Bubali Concentratus* (水牛角浓缩粉), *Lumbricus* (地龙), *Sanguis Draconis* (血竭), etc., used to dispel wind and dampness, activate blood flow in collateral meridians/channels, relax the contracture of the limbs for treating apoplectic paralysis and traumatic injury

木瓜丸 [mù guā wán]

***Mugua* Pills; Chaenomeles Pills:** pills prepared from *Fructus Chaenomelis* (木瓜), *Radix Angelicae* (当归), *Rhizoma Chuanxiong* (川芎), *Radix Angelicae Dahuricae* (白芷), *Radix Clematis* (威灵仙), *Rhizoma Ciboti* (狗脊), *Radix Achyranthis Bidentatae* (牛膝), *Caulis Statholobi* (鸡血藤), *Caulis Piperis Kadsurae* (海风藤), *Radix Ginseng* (人参), *Radix Aconiti Preparata* (制川乌) and *Radix Aconiti Kusnezoffii Preparata* (制草乌), used to dispel wind-cold, remove obstruction from collateral meridians/

channels and relieve pain for treating rheumatic and rheumatoid arthritis

豨莶丸 [xī xiān wán]

Xixian **Pills; Siegesbeckia Pills:** pills prepared from *Herba Siegesbeckiae* (豨莶草), used to relieve rheumatic conditions, and to improve the motility of joints, for treating rheumatic arthralgia with aching and weakness of the loins and knees, and numbness of the limbs

国公酒 [guó gōng jiǔ]

Guogong **Wine:** medicinal wine prepared from *Radix Angelicae Sinensis* (当归), *Rhizoma Chuanxiong* (川芎), *Radix Angelicae Pubescentis* (独活), *Radix Achyranthis Bidentatae* (牛膝), *Fructus Citri Sarcodactylis* (佛手), *Rhizoma Polygonati Odorati* (玉竹), *Pericarpium Citri Reticulatae* (陈皮), etc., used to relieve muscular contracture in cases of rheumatoid arthritis

尪痹颗粒 [wāng bì kē lì]

Wangbi **Granules; Lameness Granules:** granules prepared from *Radix Rehmanniae* (地黄), *Radix Dipsaci* (续断), *Rhizoma Drynariae* (骨碎补), *Rhizoma Ciboti* (狗脊), *Herba Epimedii* (淫羊藿), *Radix Angelicae Pubescentis* (独活), *Ramulus Cinnamomi* (桂枝), *Radix Saposhnikoviae* (防风), *Radix Clematis* (威灵仙), *Flos Carthami* (红花), *Herba Lycopodii* (伸筋草), etc., used to tonify the liver and kidney, strengthen the sinews and bones, dispel wind-dampness and unblock the meridians/channels and collaterals for treating rheumatoid arthritis with local swelling, stiffness, deformity and impaired movement

天麻丸 [tiān má wán]

Tianma **Pills; Gastrodia Pills:** pills prepared from *Rhizoma Gastrodiae* (天麻), *Rhizoma seu Radix Notopterygii* (羌活), *Radix Angelicae Pubescentis* (独活), *Cortex Eucommiae* (杜仲), *Radix Aconiti Lateralis Preparata* (附子), *Radix Angelicae Sinensis* (当归), *Radix Rehmanniae* (地黄) and *Radix Scrophulariae* (玄参), used to nourish the blood, unblock the collaterals to promote blood flow and soothe the sinews to relieve pain for treating rheumatalgia due to deficiency of liver blood and kidney yin

冠心苏合丸 [guàn xīn sū hé wán]

Guanxin Suhe **Pills; Coronary Storax Pills:** pills prepared from *Styrax* (苏合香), *Borneolum* (冰片), *Olibanum* (乳香), *Lignum Santali Albi* (檀香), and *Radix Aristolochiae* (青木香), used to regulate the flow of *qi* in the chest and relieve pain for treating angina pectoris with stuffy sensation in the chest

复方丹参片 [fù fāng dān shēn piàn]

Fufang Danshen **Tablets; Compound Salvia Tablets:** tablets prepared from *Salviae Miltiorrhzae* (丹参), *Radix Notoginseng* (三七), and *Borneolum* (冰片), used to activate blood flow and eliminate blood stasis for treating angina pectoris

元胡止痛片 [yuán hú zhǐ tòng piàn]

Yuanhu Zhitong **Tablets; Corydalis Analgesic Tablets:** tablets prepared from *Rhizoma Corydalis* (元胡) and *Radix Angelicae Dahuricae* (白芷), used to regulate *qi*, activate blood and relieve pain, for treating gastralgia, headache, hypochondriac pain and dysmenorrhea due to *qi* stagnation and blood stasis

速效救心丸 [sù xiào jiù xīn wán]
***Suxiao Jiuxin* Pills; Quick-acting Heart-saving Pills:** pills prepared from *Rhizoma Chuanxiong* (川芎) and *Borneolum Syntheticum* (冰片), used to move *qi*, activate blood, resolve stasis and relieve pain for treating angina pectoris

华佗再造丸 [huà tuó zài zào wán]
***Huatuo Zaizao* Pills; Restorative Pills:** pills prepared from *Rhizoma Chuanxiong* (川芎)，*Borneolum Syntheticum* (冰片)，*Fructus Evodiae* (吴茱萸), etc., used to resolve static blood and phlegm from the collaterals for treating stroke with paralysis and contracture of the limbs, deviated eye and mouth, and blurred speech

川芎嗪注射液 [chuān xiōng qín zhù shè yè]
Ligustrazine Injection: injection containing ligustrazine, used to activate the flow of *qi* and blood, dispel wind and relieve pain, for treating ischemic stroke, hypertension, coronary heart disease, and migraine

当归丸 [dāng guī wán]
***Danggui* Pills; Chinese Angelica Pills:** pills prepared from *Radix Angelicae Sinensis* (当归), used to activate blood flow and tonify the blood for treating menstrual disturbance such as infrequent menstruation and dysmenorrhea

乌鸡白凤丸 [wū jī bái fèng wán]
***Wuji Baifeng* Pills; White Phoenix Pills:** pills prepared from white-feathered chicken with dark skin (乌鸡), *Radix Ginseng* (人参), *Radix Angelicae Sinensis* (当归), *Rhizoma Cyperi* (香附), *Radix Rehmanniae* (地黄), *Radix Astragali* (黄芪), *Colla Cornus Cervi* (鹿角胶), etc., used for treating menstrual disturbances and morbid leukorrhea due to deficiency of *qi* and blood

艾附暖宫丸 [ài fù nuǎn gōng wán]
***Aifu Nuangong* Pills; Argyi-Cyperus Uterus-warming Pills:** pills prepared from *Folium Artemisiae Argyi* (艾叶), *Rhizoma Cyperi* (香附), *Fructus Evodiae* (吴茱萸), *Cortex Cinnamomi* (肉桂), *Radix Angelicae Sinensis* (当归), *Rhizoma Chuanxiong* (川芎), *Radix Astragali* (黄芪), etc., used to replenish *qi*, warm the uterus and regulate menstruation, for treating menstrual disorders of deficiency-cold type

痛经丸 [tòng jīng wán]
***Tongjing* Pills; Dysmenorrhea Pills:** pills prepared from *Radix Angelicae Sinensis* (当归), *Radix Paeoniae Alba* (白芍), *Rhizoma Chuanxiong* (川芎), *Radix Rehmanniae Preparatae* (熟地黄), *Rhizoma Cyperi* (香附), *Radix Aucklandiae* (木香), *Rhizoma Corydalis* (元胡), *Rizoma Zingiberis* (炮姜), *Cortex Cinnamomi* (肉桂), *Radix Salviae Miltiorrhizae* (丹参), *Flos Carthami* (红花), *Herba Leonuri* (益母草), etc., used to promote blood flow, disperse cold, regulate menstruation and relieve pain in cases of dysmenorrhea

八珍益母丸 [bā zhēn yì mǔ wán]
***Bazhen Yimu* Pills; Eight-precious Motherwort Pills:** pills prepared from *Herba Leonuri* (益母草), *Radix Codonopsis Pilosulae* (党参), *Rhizoma Atractylodis Macrocephalae* (白术), *Poria* (茯苓), *Radix Glycyrrhizae* (甘草), *Radix Angelicae Sinensis* (当归), *Radix Paeoniae Alba* (白芍), *Rhizoma Chuanxiong* (川芎), and *Rhizoma Rehmanniae Preparata* (熟地黄), used to replenish *qi* and blood and to regulate menstruation, for treating deficiency of *qi* and blood in women with general weakness and menstrual disorders

益母草膏 [yì mǔ cǎo gāo]
Concentrated *Yimucao* Decoction; Concentrated Motherwort Decoction: concentrated decoction prepared from *Herba Leonuri* (益母草), used to activate the blood flow and regulate menstruation for treating menstrual disorders due to blood stasis, and prolonged discharge of lochia after childbirth

妇科十味片 [fù kē shí wèi piàn]
***Fuke Shiwei* Tablets; Ten-ingredient Gynecological Tables:** tablets prepared from *Radix Codonopsis Pilosulae* (党参), *Rhizoma Atractylodis Macrocephalae* (白术), *Radix Angelicae Sinensis* (当归), *Radix Rehmanniae* (地黄), *Fructus Zizyphi Jujubae* (大枣), *Rhizoma Cyperi* (香附), *Poria* (茯苓), *Rhizoma Chuanxiong* (川芎), *Radix Paeoniae Alba* (白芍), and *Radix Glycyrrhizae* (甘草), used to replenish *qi* and blood for regulating menstrual disturbances

更年安 [gēng nián ān]
***Gengnian'an* Tablets; Climacteric Peace Tablets:** pills prepared from *Radix Rehmanniae Preparata* (熟地黄), *Radix Polygoni Multiflori* (何首乌), *Rhizoma Alismatis* (泽泻), *Poria* (茯苓), *Fructus Schisandrae* (五味子), *Concha Margaritifera Usta* (珍珠母), *Radix Scrophulariae* (玄参), *Fructus Tritici Levis* (浮小麦), etc., used to nourish yin, remove heat, ease the mind and induce tranquilization for treating menopausal syndrome characterized by afternoon fever, excessive sweating, dizziness, tinnitus, insomnia and unsteady blood pressure

小金丸［丹］[xiǎo jīn wán/dān]
***Xiaojin* Pills; Minor Panacea:** pills prepared from *Moschus* (麝香), *Olibanum* (乳香), *Radix Angelicae Sinensis* (当归), *Radix Aconiti Kusnezoffii Preparata* (制草乌), etc., used to promote blood flow, remove blood stasis and reduce swelling for treating traumatic wounds, also for treating scrofula, carbuncle, cutaneous abscesses and ulcers

六神丸 [liù shén wán]
***Liushen* Pills; Miraculous Pills of Six Ingredients:** pills prepared from *Calculus Bovis* (牛黄), *Moschus* (麝香), *Margarita* (珍珠), *Borneol* (冰片), *Camphora* (樟脑), *Venenum Bufonis* (蟾酥), and *Realgar* (雄黄), used as an antiphlogistic for treating acute tonsilitis, sore throat, and boils

金不换膏 [jīn bù huàn gāo]
***Jinbuhuan* Plaster; Priceless Plaster:** plaster prepared from *Radix et Rhizoma Rhei* (大黄), *Myrrha* (没药), *Sanguis Draconis* (血竭), *Scolopendra* (蜈蚣), *Herba Ephedrae* (麻黄), *Radix Aconiti*

Kusnezoffii (草乌), etc., used externally to expel wind and cold, promote blood flow and relieve pain, for treating muscle and joint pains due to cold, also for treating sprains and other injuries

伤湿止痛膏 [shāng shī zhǐ tòng gāo]
Shangshi Zhitong **Plaster; Rheumatic-pain-relieving Plaster:** plaster prepared from *Radix Aconiti* (川乌), *Olibanum* (乳香), *Myrrha* (没药), *Cortex Cinnamomi* (肉桂), *Flos Caryophylli* (丁香), *Mentholum* (薄荷脑), *Semen Strychni* (马钱子), etc., used externally for treating rheumatic pains, sprains and other injuries

七厘散 [qī lí sǎn]
Qili **Powder; Anti-bruise Powder:** powder prepared from *Sanguis Draconis* (血竭), *Flos Carthami* (红花), *Olibanum* (乳香), *Myrrha* (没药), *Catechu* (儿茶), *Borneolum* (冰片), *Moschus* (麝香), etc., used to promote blood flow and relieve pain in cases of traumatic wounds with local ecchymosis

冰硼散 [bīng péng sǎn]
Bingpeng **Powder; Borneolum-Borax Powder:** powder prepared from *Borneolum* (冰片), *Borax* (硼砂), *Cinnabaris* (朱砂) and *Natrii Sulfas Exsiccatus* (玄明粉), used externally for treating sore throat, painful swelling of the gums, and ulcers in the mouth or on the tongue

如意金黄散 [rú yì jīn huáng sǎn]
Ruyi Jinhuang **Powder; Golden Powder for Alleviation:** powder prepared from *Rhizoma Curcumae Longae* (姜黄), *Radix et Rhizoma Rhei* (大黄), *Cortex Phellodendri* (黄柏), *Rhizoma Atractylodis* (苍术), *Cortex Magnoliae Officinalis* (厚朴), *Rhizoma Arisaematis* (天南星), *Radix Angelicae Dahuricae* (白芷), etc., used externally to promote subsidence of swelling and alleviate pain for treating abscesses, erysipelas and traumatic wounds

养血生发胶囊 [yǎng xuè shēng fà jiāo náng]
Yangxue Shengfa **Capsules; Blood-nourishing Hair-growing Capsules:** capsules prepared from *Radix Polygoni Multiflori* (何首乌), *Radix Angelicae Sinensis* (当归), *Radix Rehmanniae Preparata* (熟地黄), *Rhizoma Gastrodiae* (天麻), *Rhizoma Chuanxiong* (川芎), *Fructux Chaenomelis* (木瓜), etc., used to promote the growth of hair in cases of alopecia areata, seborrheic alopecia, and alopecia after childbirth or after a serious disease

石斛夜光丸 [shí hú yè guāng wán]
Shihu Yeguang **Pills; Dendrobium Eyesight-improving Pills:** pills prepared from *Herba Dendrobi* (石斛), *Radix Ginseng* (人参), *Herba Cistanches* (肉苁蓉), *Fructus Lycii* (枸杞子), *Semen Cuscutae* (菟丝子), *Radix Rehmanniae* (地黄), *Fructus Schisandrae* (五味子), *Radix Asparagi* (天冬), *Radix Ophiopogonis* (麦冬), *Rhizoma Chuanxiong* (川芎), *Rhizoma Coptidis* (黄连), *Radix Achyanthis Bidentatae* (牛膝), *Flos Chrysanthemi* (菊花), *Fructus Tribuli* (蒺藜), *Semen Celosiae* (青葙子), *Semen Cassiae* (决明子), *Cornu Bubali* (水牛角), *Cornu Saigae Tataricae* (羚羊角),

etc., used to replenish kidney yin, quench liver fire and improve eyesight for treating cataracts

耳聋左慈丸 [ěr lóng zuǒ cí wán]
Erlong Zuoci **Pills; Zuoci's Deafness Pills:** pills prepared from *Magnetitum* (磁石), *Radix Rehmanniae Preparata* (熟地黄), *Fructus Corni* (山茱萸), *Cortex Moutan* (牡丹皮), *Rhizoma Discoreae* (山药), *Poria* (茯苓), *Rhizoma Alismatis* (泽泻), and *Radix Bupleuri Marginati* (竹叶柴胡), used to replenish the kidney and subdue hyperactivity of the liver for treating tinnitus and impairment of hearing

针灸学 Acupuncture and Moxibustion

经络
Meridians/Channels and Collaterals

经络学说 [jīng luò xué shuō]
theory of meridians/channels and collaterals: basic component of traditional Chinese medical theory that there exists, within the human body, a system of conduits through which *qi* and blood flow, and by which the internal organs are connected with one another as well as with the superficial organs and tissues, and in this way the body is made an organic whole

经络 [jīng luò]
meridian/channel and collateral: system of conduits through which *qi* and blood flow and by which the internal organs are connected with one another as well as with superficial organs and tissues, making the body an organic whole

经脉 [jīng mài]
meridians; channels: cardinal conduits of *qi* and blood coursing vertically, composed of twelve regular meridians/channels and eight extra meridians/channels

络脉 [luò mài]
collateral vessel: (1) branch of a meridian/channel; (2) collective term for all branches of the meridians/channels consisting of the fifteen collateral vessels (十五络脉 [shí wǔ luò mài]), divergent collateral vessels (别络 [bié luò]), tertiary collateral vessels (孙络 [sūn luò]) and superficial collateral vessels (浮络 [fú luò]), a network linking all the various aspects of the body

经隧 [jīng suì]
meridian passage; channel passage: pathway of meridians/channels under the body surface

十二经 [shí èr jīng]
twelve meridians; twelve channels: collective term for lung meridian/channel of hand greater yin (LU), large intestine meridian/channel of hand yang brightness (LI), stomach meridian/channel of foot yang brightness (ST), spleen meridian/channel of foot greater yin (SP), heart meridian/channel of hand lesser yin (HT), small intestine meridian/channel of hand greater yang (SI), bladder meridian/channel of foot greater yang (BL), kidney meridian/channel of foot lesser yin (KI), pericardium meridian/channel of hand reverting yin (PC), triple energizer meridian/channel of hand lesser yang (TE), gallbladder meridian/channel of foot lesser yang (GB), and liver meridian/channel of foot reverting yin (LR), the main passages of *qi* and blood, also known as regular meridians/channels (正经 [zhèng jīng])

十二经脉 [shí èr jīng mài]
twelve meridians/channels: same as 十二经 [shí èr jīng]

正经 [zhèng jīng]
regular meridians/channels: another

name for the twelve meridians/channels (十二经 [shí èr jīng])

手三阴经 [shǒu sān yīn jīng]
three yin meridians/channels of the hand: collective term for the meridians/channels running through the anterior side of the upper limbs from the chest to the hands, namely, lung meridian/channel, heart meridian/channel, and pericardium meridian/channel

手三阳经 [shǒu sān yáng jīng]
three yang meridians/channels of the hand: collective term for the meridians/channels running through the posterior side of the upper limbs from the hands to the head, namely, large intestine meridian/channel, small intestine meridian/channel, and triple energizer meridian/channel

足三阳经 [zú sān yáng jīng]
three yang meridians/channels of the foot: collective term for the meridians/channels running from the head through the trunk downward to the feet, namely, stomach meridian/channel, bladder meridian/channel, and gallbladder meridian/channel

足三阴经 [zú sān yīn jīng]
three yin meridians/channels of the foot: collective term for the meridians/channels running through the inner side of the lower limbs from the feet to the abdomen and chest, namely, spleen meridian/channel, kidney meridian/channel, and liver meridian/channel

六经 [liù jīng]
six meridians/channels: collective term for greater yang meridian/channel, yang brightness meridian/channel, lesser yang meridian/channel, greater yin meridian/channel, lesser yin meridian/channel, and reverting yin meridian/channel, which, in conformity with the rules of classification of the twelve meridians/channels, may be subdivided into the six meridians/channels of the hand and the six meridians/channels of the foot

阳经 [yáng jīng]
yang meridians/channels: collective term for the three yang meridians/channels of the hand and the foot, plus governor vessel, yang link vessel, and yang heel vessel

阴经 [yīn jīng]
yin meridians/channels: collective term for the three yin meridians/channels of the hand and the foot, plus conception vessel, thoroughfare vessel, yin link vessel, and yin heel vessel

三阴 [sān yīn]
(I) three yin: collective term for the three yin meridians/channels of both the hand and the foot, six in all; **(II) third yin:** greater yin meridian/channel

二阴 [èr yīn]
second yin: lesser yin meridian/channel

一阴 [yī yīn]
first yin: reverting yin meridian/channel

三阳 [sān yáng]
(I) three yang: collective term for the three yang meridians/channels of both the hand and the foot, six in all; **(II) third yang:** greater yang meridian/channel

二阳 [èr yáng]

second yang: yang brightness meridian/channel

一阳 [yī yáng]

first yang: lesser yang meridian/channel

六阳脉 [liù yáng mài]

(I) six yang meridians/channels: collective term for the six yang meridians/channels of the hands and the feet, three on each side; **(II) six yang pulses:** presence of surging pulse at inch, bar and cubit of both hands in a normal person

六阴脉 [liù yīn mài]

six yin meridians/channels: collective term for the six yin meridians/channels of the hands and the feet, three on each side

外经 [wài jīng]

external meridian; external channel: part of a meridian/channel distributed in the outer part of the body, in contrast with that of the meridian/channel connecting with the visceral organ

十四经 [shí sì jīng]

fourteen meridians/channels: twelve meridians/channels plus governor and conception vessels

手太阴肺经 [shǒu tài yīn fèi jīng]

lung meridian/channel of hand greater yin; lung meridian/channel (LU): one of the twelve meridians/channels, which originates internally in the middle energizer, descends to connect with the large intestine, then ascends to the lung and throat, courses laterally and exits superficially at *Zhongfu* (LU 1), descends along the lateral side of the arm and forearm, and terminates at *Shaoshang* (LU 11), with 11 points on either side (Fig. 1)

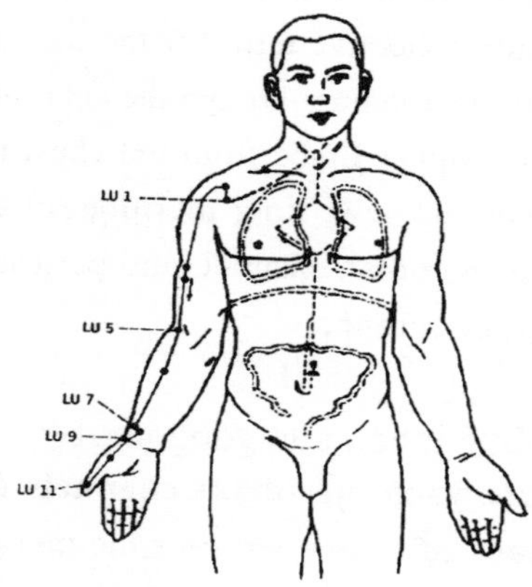

Fig. 1 Lung Meridian

手阳明大肠经 [shǒu yáng míng dà cháng jīng]

large intestine meridian/channel of hand yang brightness; large intestine meridian/channel (LI): one of the twelve meridians/channels, which originates at *Shangyang* (LI 1) and ascends the dorsal surface of the hand and forearm, the lateral side of the arm, the dorsal side of the shoulder to *Jugu* (LI 16) where the meridian/channel enters internally and travels posteriorly to *Dazhui* (GV 14), and then courses anteriorly to the supraclavicular fossa, where it descends past the diaphragm to connect with the large intestine. The superficial supraclavicular branch ascends the anterior lateral neck and the mandible, connects internally with the lower teeth, encircles the lips and terminates at the opposite *Yingxiang* (LI 20), with 20 points on either side. (Fig. 2)

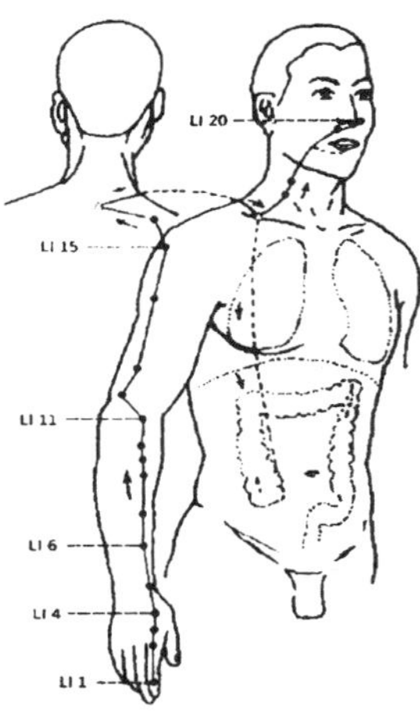

Fig. 2 Large Intestine Meridian

足阳明胃经 [zú yáng míng wèi jīng] **stomach meridian/channel of foot yang brightness; stomach meridian/channel (ST):** one of the twelve meridians/channels, which originates internally at the lateral edge of the nose, ascends to the medial canthus of the eye, then reaches the first superficial point *Chenqi* (ST 1) at the inferior border of the orbit, descends to the upper gum, courses around the mouth, and travels up to *Touwei* (ST 8) at the hairline of the temple, where it runs into the internal and terminates at *Shenting* (GV 24). The facial branch descends from *Daying* (ST 5) where it turns to run internally and descends past the diaphragm to connect with the stomach and spleen. The supraclavicular fossa branch descends along the midclavicular line to *Qichong* (ST 30) in the inguinal region, then anteriorly along the lateral margin of the femur to the patella, and terminates at *Lidui* (ST 45) on the lateral side of the tip of the second toe. The gastric branch descends internally past the umbilicus and terminates at *Qichong* (ST 30). The tibial branch leaves *Zusanli* (ST 36) and descends along the fibula, and terminates at the lateral side of the tip of the middle toe. The dorsal foot branch leaves *Chongyang* (ST 42) and descends to terminate at *Yinbai* (SP 1) on the medial side of the great toe. There are 45 points on either side. (Fig. 3)

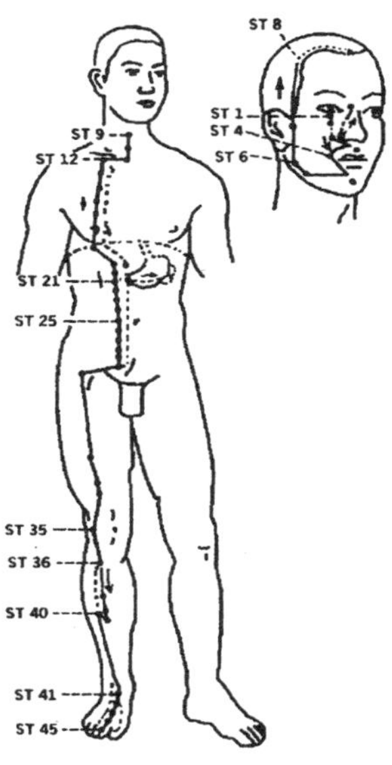

Fig. 3 Stomach Meridian

足太阴脾经 [zú tài yīn pí jīng] **spleen meridian/channel of foot greater yin; spleen meridian/channel (SP):** one of the twelve meridians/channels, which runs from *Yinbai* (SP 1) at the medial side of the great toe, ascends along the medial side of the foot and tibia, and anteromedial side of the thigh to the lower abdomen, then enters the abdomen and connects with the spleen and stomach, ascends again along the abdomen at a distance of 4.0 *cun* lateral to the conception vessel, and terminates superficially at *Dabao* (SP 21) in the sixth intercostal space on the midaxillary line. The meridian/channel continues internally past the supraclavicular fossa, and terminates at the base of the tongue. The gastric branch leaves the stomach and ascends internally past the diaphragm, and connects with the heart. There are 21 points on either side. (Fig. 4)

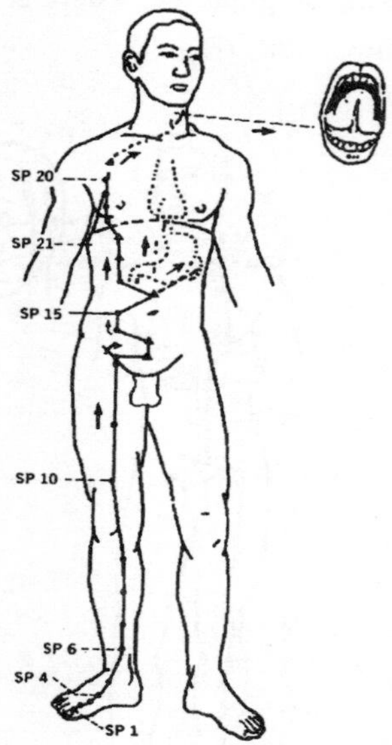

Fig. 4 Spleen Meridian

手少阴心经 [shǒu shào yīn xīn jīng]

heart meridian/channel of hand lesser yin; heart meridian/channel (HT): one of the twelve meridians/channels, which originates in the heart, descends internally past the diaphragm, and connects with the small intestine. The cardiac branch ascends internally paralateral to the esophagus, and terminates at the eye. The main branch leaves the heart, traverses the lung and emerges superficially in the midaxilla at *Jiquan* (HT 1), descends along the ulnar side of the forearm medially, and terminates at *Shaochong* (HT 9) on the radial side of the tip of the small finger, with 9 points on either side. (Fig. 5)

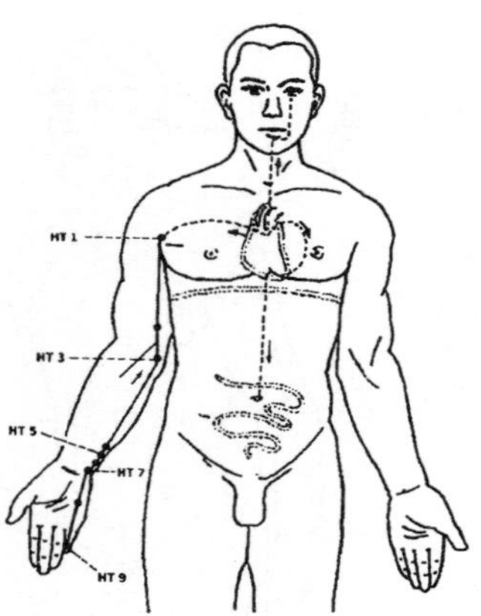

Fig. 5 Heart Meridian

手太阳小肠经 [shǒu tài yáng xiǎo cháng jīng]

small intestine meridian/channel of hand greater yang; small intestine meridian/channel (SI): one of the twelve meridians/channels, which originates at *Shaoze* (SI 1) at the ulnar side of the little finger, ascends the ulnar side of the forearm, and up the arm, over the scapula to *Dazhui* (GV 14) between the spinous processes of the 7th cervical and 1st thoracic vertebrae, then descends internally to the heart following the esophagus past the diaphragm to connect with the small intestine. The supraclavicular fossa branch ascends superficially along the lateral side of the neck past the cheek to the lateral corner of the eye, and terminates at *Tinggong* (SI 19). The buccal branch leaves the main meridian at the cheek, and ascends to the medial canthus of the eye. There are 19 points on either side. (Fig. 6)

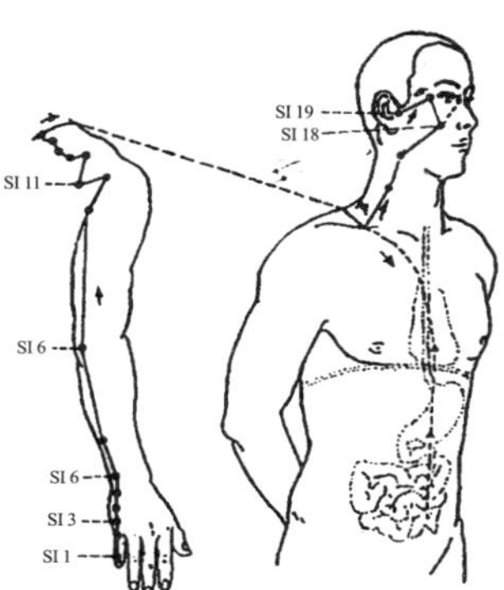

Fig. 6 Small Intestine Meridian

足太阳膀胱经 [zú tài yáng páng guāng jīng]

bladder meridian/channel of foot greater yang; bladder meridian/channel (BL): one of the twelve meridians/channels, which runs from *Jingming* (BL 1) at the medial canthus of the eye, ascends the forehead to the vertex and then enters the brain and exits at the nape of the neck where it divides into two parallel branches: the first branch descends the back at a distance of 1.5 *cun* from the spine, and during its course it connects with kidney and urinary bladder, and continues along the posterior side of the thigh to the popliteal fold; the second branch descends the back at a distance of 3 *cun* from the spine, continues along the latero-posterior side of the thigh to the popliteal fold where it meets the first branch. The meridian/channel continues to descend along the posterior side of the calf to the lateral malleolus, and terminates at *Zhiyin* (BL 67) on the lateral side of the tip of the little toe. There are 67 points on either side. (Fig. 7)

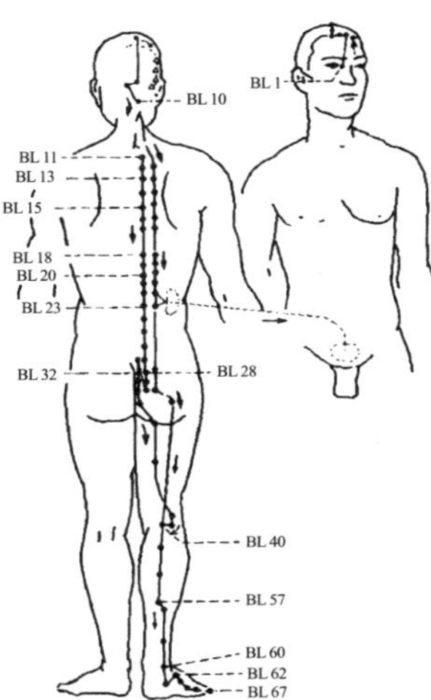

Fig. 7 Bladder Meridian

足少阴肾经 [zú shào yīn shèn jīng]

kidney meridian/channel of foot lesser yin; kidney meridian/channel (KI): one of the twelve meridians/channels, which begins on the plantar tip of the little toe, travels to *Yongquan* (KI 1) in the center of the sole of the foot, continues along the inner side of the lower limb to the symphysis pubis, runs internally to the kidney and urinary bladder, and back to the symphysis pubis, ascends along the

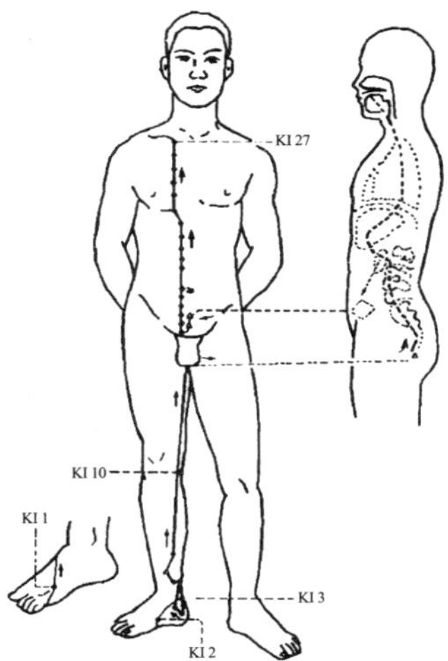

Fig. 8 Kidney Meridian

abdomen and chest up to *Shufu* (KI 27) in the depression between the first rib and the lower border of the clavicle, with 27 points on either side (Fig. 8)

手厥阴心包经 [shǒu jué yīn xīn bāo jīng]

pericardium meridian/channel of hand reverting yin; pericardium meridian/channel (PC): one of the twelve meridians/channels, which originates in the center of the thorax, connects with the pericardium, and descends to the lower abdomen, linking all three energizers. The thoracic branch exits superficially at *Tianchi* (PC 1) near the nipple, and descends along the midline of the anterior side of the arm to *Zhongchong* (PC 9) at the midpoint of the tip of the middle finger, with 9 points on either side. (Fig. 9)

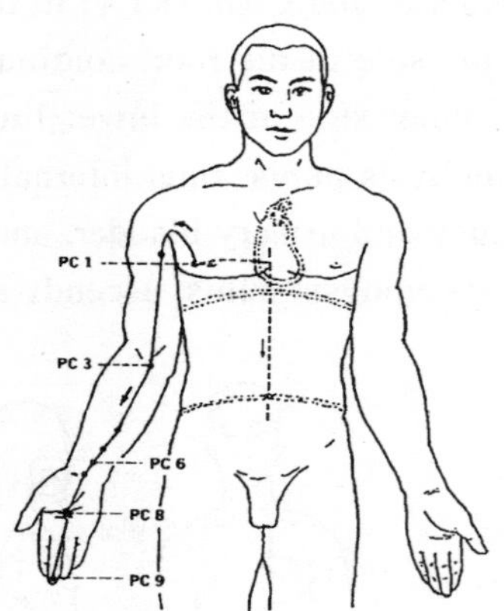

Fig. 9 Pericardium Meridian

手少阳三焦经 [shǒu shào yáng sān jiāo jīng]

triple energizer meridian/channel of hand lesser yang; triple energizer meridian/channel (TE): one of the twelve meridians/channels, which originates at *Guanchong* (TE 1) at the ulnar side of the ring finger, travels along the midline of the posterior side of the arm and through the regions of the shoulder, neck, ear and eye, and terminates at *Sizhukong* (TE 23) at the lateral canthus, with 23 points on either side. A branch goes from the supraclavicular fossa to the pericardium and down through the thorax and abdomen, linking the upper, middle and lower energizers. (Fig. 10)

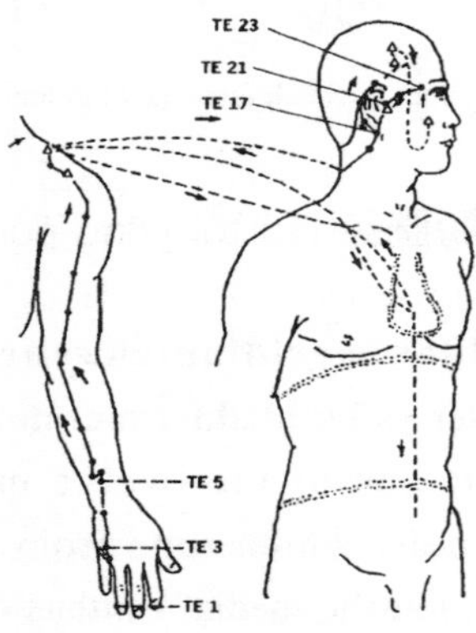

Fig. 10 Triple Energizer Meridian

足少阳胆经 [zú shào yáng dǎn jīng]

gallbladder meridian/channel of foot lesser yang; gallbladder meridian/channel (GB): one of the twelve meridians/channels, which orignates at *Tongziliao* (GB 1) at the lateral canthus of the eye, runs through the regions of the temple, ear, neck, shoulder, flank, and the outer side of the lower limb, and terminates at *Zuqiaoyin* (GB 44) on the lateral side of the tip of the 4th toe, with 44 points on either side. The post-auricular branch travels into the ear and down to the supraclavicular fossa, where it joins the mother meridian/channel, continues to run down into the chest, past the diaphragm, connecting with the gallbladder and liver, and further down to the lower abdomen into the inguinal canal. The dorsal foot branch leaves the mother meridian/channel at *Zulinqi* (GB 41), descends between the first and second metatarsals, and terminates at the base of the big toe nail. (Fig. 11)

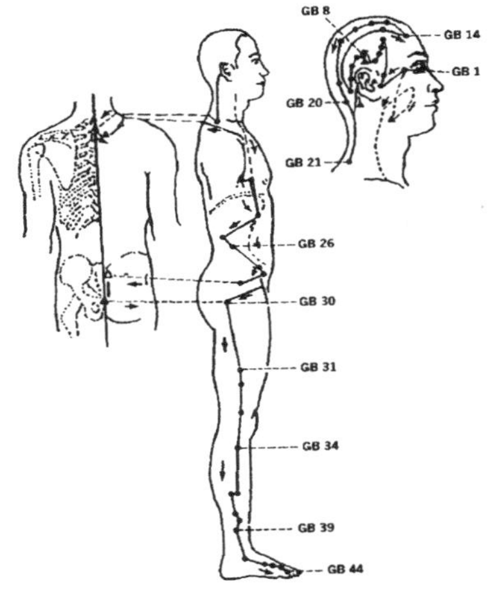

Fig. 11 Gallbladder Meridian

足厥阴肝经 [zú jué yīn gān jīng]

liver meridian/channel of foot reverting yin; liver meridian/channel (LR): one of the twelve meridians/channels, which originates at *Dadun* (LR 1) on the big toe just behind the nail, runs through the inner side of the lower limb, external genitalia and abdomen, to *Qimen* (LR 14), a point approximately 2 *cun* below the nipple, with

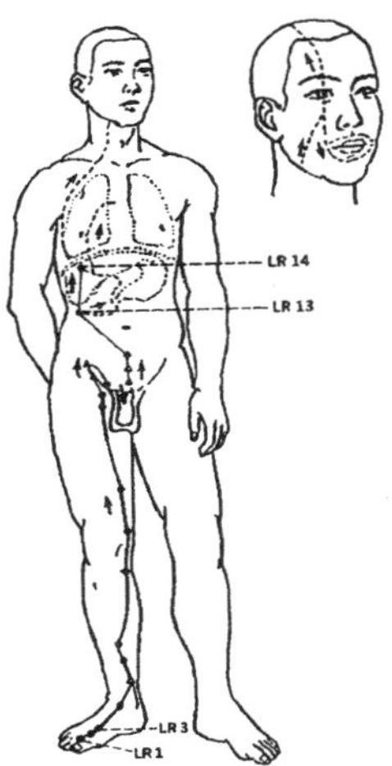

Fig. 12 Liver Meridian

14 points on either side. From *Qimen* (LR 14) the meridian/channel enters the abdomen, and travels para-laterally along the stomach to the gallbladder. From the liver, the meridian/channel ascends past the diaphragm along the trachea, larynx, and sinus cavity, connecting with the eye, and then ascends further to the vertex, where it meets the governor vessel. (Fig. 12)

奇经八脉 [qí jīng bā mài]

eight extra meridians/channels: collective term for governor vessel, conception vessel, thoroughfare vessel, belt vessel, yin heel vessel, yang heel vessel, yin link vessel, and yang link vessel

督脉 [dū mài]

governor vessel (GV): one of the eight extra meridians/channels, which begins at *Changqiang* (GV 1), a point at the back of the anus, sending one branch forward to *Huiyin* (CV 1), while the main portion of the meridian/channel ascending the midline of the back to the top of the head and then descending the midline of the face down to *Yinjiao* (GV 28), a point between the upper lip and the upper gum in the labia frenum, with 28 points (Fig. 13)

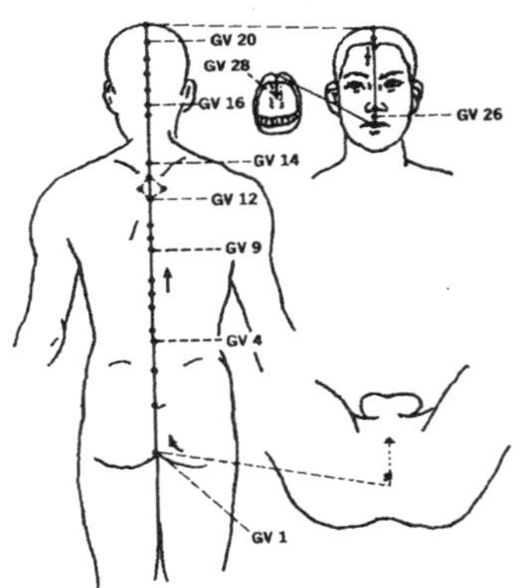

Fig. 13 Governor Vessel

任脉 [rèn mài]

conception vessel (CV): one of the eight extra meridians/channels, which originates at *Huiyin* (CV1), a point in the center of the perineum, ascends the midline of the abdominal wall and chest to *Chengjiang* (CV 24), midpoint of the mentolabial sulcus, with 24 points. One internal branch of the meridian/channel ascends from *Chengjiang* (CV 24), encircles the mouth and reaches the eyes, while the other internal branch travels from the pelvic cavity, ascending the spine, to the throat. (Fig. 14)

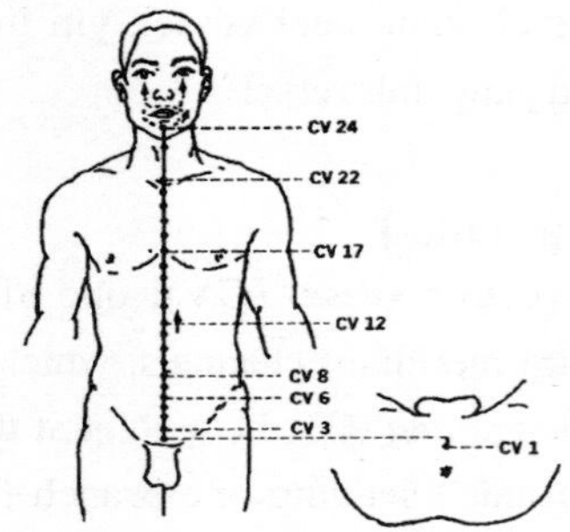

Fig. 14 Conception Vessel

冲脉 [chōng mài]

thoroughfare vessel (TV): one of the eight extra meridians/channels, which originates at the uterus or *Guanyuan* (CV4), merges with the kidney meridian/channel, and then runs upward along both sides of the abdomen to the chest

带脉 [dài mài]

belt vessel (BV): one of the eight extra meridians/channels, which originates from the lower part of the hypochondria, and encircles the waist

阴跷脉 [yīn qiāo mài]

yin heel vessel (YinHV): one of the eight extra meridians/channels, which originates at the inner side of the heel, runs upward along the inner side of the lower limb, through the front private parts, abdomen, chest, neck, and either side of the nose, and terminates at the eye

阳跷脉 [yáng qiāo mài]

yang heel vessel (YangHV): one of the eight extra meridians/channels, which originates at the outer side of the heel, runs upward along the outer ankle and then the outer side of the lower limb, through the abdomen, chest, shoulder and cheek, and terminates at the back of the neck

阴维脉 [yīn wéi mài]

yin link vessel (YinLV): one of the eight extra meridians/channels, which originates at the upper part of the inner ankle, runs upward along the inner side of the lower limb, through the abdomen, chest and throat, and terminates at the back of the neck

阳维脉 [yáng wéi mài]

yang link vessel (YangLV): one of the eight extra meridians/channels, which originates at the lower part of the outer ankle, runs upward along the outer side of the lower limb, through the side of the trunk, shoulder, and neck, and terminates at the top of the head

十二经筋 [shí èr jīng jīn]

twelve meridian/channel sinews: sinew systems distributed to the twelve meridians/channels, also called meridian/channel sinews (经筋 [jīng jīn]) for short

经筋 [jīng jīn]

(I) meridian/channel sinew: sinew

system attributed to a particular meridian/channel; **(II) meridian/channel sinews:** abbreviation for twelve meridian/channel sinews (十二经筋 [shí èr jīng jīn])

十二经别 [shí èr jīng bié]
twelve meridian/channel divergences: divergent passages of the regular meridians/channels running deep in the body to facilitate communication between the interior and exterior, and to play a supplementary role in conducting the flow of *qi* of the regular meridians/channels, also called meridian/channel divergences (经别 [jīng bié]) for short

经别 [jīng bié]
(I) meridian/channel divergence: divergent passage of a regular meridian/channel running deep in the body; **(II) meridian/channel divergences:** abbreviation for twelve meridian/channel divergences (十二经别 [shí èr jīng bié])

十二皮部 [shí èr pí bù]
twelve cutaneous regions: regions of the skin reflecting the functioning conditions of the twelve regular meridians/channels, respectively

十五络脉 [shí wǔ luò mài]
fifteen collateral vessels: collective term for the main collateral vessels of the fourteen meridians/channels and the great collateral vessel of the spleen, responsible for communication between the exterior and interior of the body.

脾之大络 [pí zhī dà luò]
great collateral vessel of the spleen: collateral vessel that issues from *Dabao* (SP 21), and spreads over the thoracic and hypochondriac regions

别络 [bié luò]
divergent collateral vessel: larger branch of a collateral vessel

孙络 [sūn luò]
tertiary collateral vessel: (1) subdivided branch of a collateral vessel; (2) capillary

浮络 [fú luò]
superficial collateral vessel: collateral vessel lying just beneath the skin

鱼络 [yú luò]
thenar collateral vessel: collateral vessel in the thenar eminence, the congestion of which shows disorder of the large intestinal meridian.

胞络 [bāo luò]
uterine collateral vessel: collateral vessel distributed on the uterus

胞脉 [bāo mài]
uterine vessel: vessel that connects with the uterus, chiefly referring to the conception vessel or thoroughfare vessel, governing menstruation, conception and pregnancy

阴络 [yīn luò]
yin collateral: (1) collateral or branch of yin meridian/channel of the hand or foot; (2) collateral running downward or deep in the body

阳络 [yáng luò]
yang collateral: (1) collateral or branch of yang meridian/channel of the hand or foot;

(2) collateral or branch running upward or superficially

经络辨证 [jīng luò biàn zhèng]
meridian/channel syndrome differentiation; meridian/channel pattern identification: syndrome differentiation (pattern identification) on the basis of meridian/channel theory

经络证候 [jīng luò zhèng hòu]
meridian/channel syndrome: syndrome indicating that a certain meridian/channel is being attacked by single or multiple pathogenic factors

所生病 [suǒ shēng bìng]
viscus-induced disease: (1) disease caused by disorder of the viscus itself but not that of its related meridian/channel, e.g., cough with dyspnea is a disease caused by disorder of the lung; (2) symptoms induced by a viscus disease at the site where the corresponding meridian/channel passes, e.g., lung disease may have such symptoms as pain in the interio-anterior aspect of the arm and heat sensation in the palms of the hands where the greater yin (*taiyin*) meridian/channel of the hand reaches

是动病 [shì dòng bìng]
meridian/channel induced disease: (1) disease caused by a disordered meridian/channel, e.g., toothache caused by disorder of the hand *yangming* (yang brightness) meridian/channel; (2) viscus disease induced by the disordered connecting meridian/channel, e.g., cough and dyspnea due to disordered hand *taiyin* (greater yin) meridian/channel but not the lung itself

俞穴 Acupoints

经穴
Meridian/Channel Points

俞穴 [shù xué]
acupuncture point; acupoint: a place on the surface of the body where *qi* and blood of the meridians/channels and collateral vessels gather or pass, also known as 腧穴 [shù xué]

腧穴 [shù xué]
acupoint: same as 俞穴 [shù xué]

经穴 [jīng xué]
meridian/channel point: acupuncture-moxibustion point of a regular meridian/channel

手太阴肺经穴 [shǒu tài yīn fèi jīng xué]
points of the lung meridian/channel: acupuncture-moxibustion points distributed on the lung meridian/channel (LI)

中府 [zhōng fǔ]
***Zhongfu* (LU 1):** point on the superior lateral part of the anterior thoracic wall, at the level of the 1st intercostal space, 6 *cun* lateral to the anterior midline (Fig. 16)

云门 [yún mén]
***Yunmen* (LU 2):** point in the depression of the infraclavicular fossa, 6 *cun* lateral to the anterior midline (Fig. 16)

天府 [tiān fǔ]
***Tianfu* (LU 3):** point on the medial side of the upper arm, 3 *cun* below the anterior

end of the axillary fold (Fig. 15)

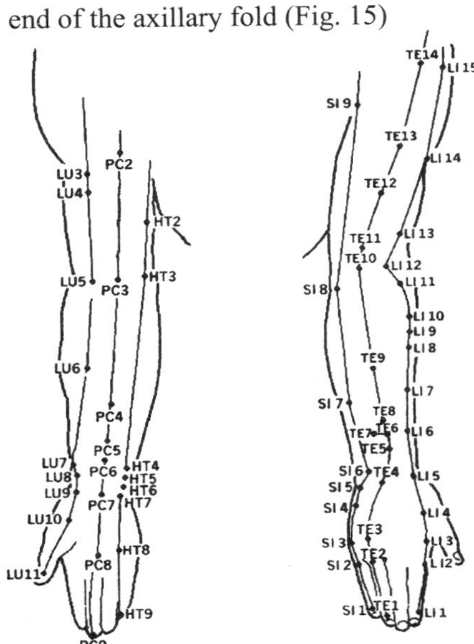

Fig. 15 Regular points on the upper limb

侠白 [xiá bái]

***Xiabai* (LU 4):** point on the medial side of the upper arm, 4 *cun* below the anterior end of the axillary fold (Fig. 15)

尺泽 [chǐ zé]

***Chize* (LU 5):** point in the cubital crease, in the depression of the radial side of the tendon of the biceps muscle of the arm (Fig. 15)

孔最 [kǒng zuì]

***Kongzui* (LU 6):** point on the radial side of the palmar surface of the forearm, 7 *cun* above the cubital crease (Fig. 15)

列缺 [liè quē]

***Lieque* (LU 7):** point on the radial side of the forearm, proximal to the styloid process of the radius, 1.5 *cun* above the crease of the wrist (Fig. 15)

经渠 [jīng qú]

***Jingqu* (LU 8):** point on the radial side of the palmar surface of the forearm, 1 *cun* above the crease of the wrist (Fig. 15)

太渊 [tài yuān]

***Taiyuan* (LU 9):** point at the radial end of the crease of the wrist, where the pulsation of the radial artery is palpable (Fig. 15)

鱼际 [yú jì]

***Yuji* (LU 10):** point on the radial side of the midpoint of the 1st metacarpal bone, and on the junction of the red and white skin (Fig. 15)

少商 [shào shāng]

***Shaoshang* (LU 11):** point on the radial side of the distal segment of the thumb, 0.1 *cun* from the corner of the fingernail (Fig. 15)

手阳明大肠经穴 [shǒu yáng míng dà cháng jīng xué]

points of the large intestine meridian/channel: acupuncture-moxibustion points distributed on the large intestine meridian/channel (LI)

商阳 [shāng yáng]

***Shangyang* (LI 1):** point on the radial side of the distal segment of the index finger, 0.1 *cun* proximal to the corner of the nail (Fig. 15)

二间 [èr jiān]

***Erjian* (LI 2):** point in the depression on the radial side, distal to the 2nd metacarpophalangeal joint (Fig. 15)

三间 [sān jiān]

***Sanjian* (LI 3):** point in the depression on the radial side, proximal to the 2nd metacarpophalangeal joint (Fig. 15)

合谷 [hé gǔ]

***Hegu* (LI 4):** point on the dorsum of the hand, between the 1st and 2nd metacarpal bones, and on the radial side of the midpoint of the 2nd metacarpal bone (Fig. 15)

阳溪 [yáng xī]

***Yangxi* (LI 5):** point at the radial end of the crease of the wrist, in the depression between the tendons of the short extensor and long extensor muscles of the thumb when tilted upward (Fig. 15)

偏历 [piān lì]

***Pianli* (LI 6):** point on the radial side of the dorsal surface of the forearm, 3 *cun* above the crease of the wrist (Fig. 15)

温溜 [wēn liū]

***Wenliu* (LI 7):** point on the radial side of the dorsal surface of the forearm, 5 *cun* above the crease of the wrist (Fig. 15)

下廉 [xià lián]

***Xialian* (LI 8):** point on the radial side of the dorsal surface of the forearm, 4 *cun* below the cubital crease (Fig. 15)

上廉 [shàng lián]

***Shanglian* (LI 9):** point on the radial side of the dorsal surface of the forearm, 3 *cun* below the cubital crease (Fig. 15)

手三里 [shǒu sān lǐ]

***Shousanli* (LI 10):** point on the radial side of the dorsal surface of the forearm, 2 *cun* below the cubital crease (Fig. 15)

曲池 [qū chí]

***Quchi* (LI 11):** point at the lateral end of the cubital crease with the elbow flexed (Fig. 15)

肘髎 [zhǒu liáo]

***Zhouliao* (LI 12):** point on the lateral side of the upper arm, 1 *cun* above *Quchi* (LI 11) with the elbow flexed, on the border of the humerus (Fig. 15)

手五里 [shǒu wǔ lǐ]

***Shouwuli* (LI 13):** point on the lateral side of the upper arm, 3 *cun* above *Quchi* (LI 11) (Fig. 15)

臂臑 [bì nào]

***Binao* (LI 14):** point on the lateral side of the arm, 7 *cun* above *Quchi* (LI 11) (Fig. 15)

肩髃 [jiān yú]

***Jianyu* (LI 15):** point on the shoulder, in the depression anterior and inferior to the acromion when the arm is abducted (Fig. 15)

巨骨 [jù gǔ]

***Jugu* (LI 16):** point on the shoulder, in the depression between the acromial extremity of the clavicle and scapular spine (Fig. 16)

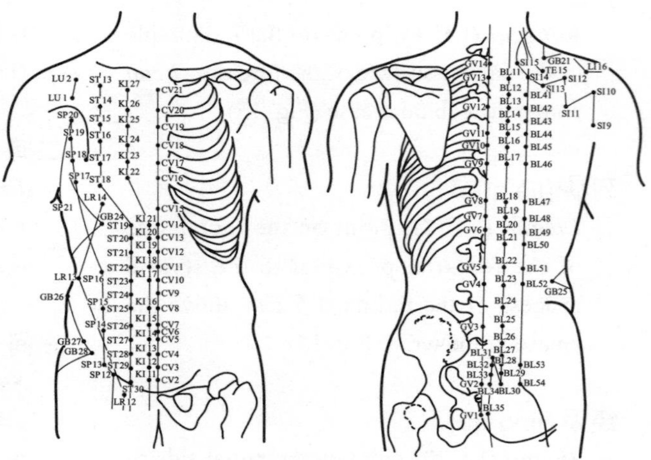

Fig. 16 Regular points on the trunk

天鼎 [tiān dǐng]

***Tianding* (LI 17):** point on the lateral side of the neck, at the posterior border of the sternocleidomastoid muscle beside the laryngeal protuberance (Fig. 17a and b)

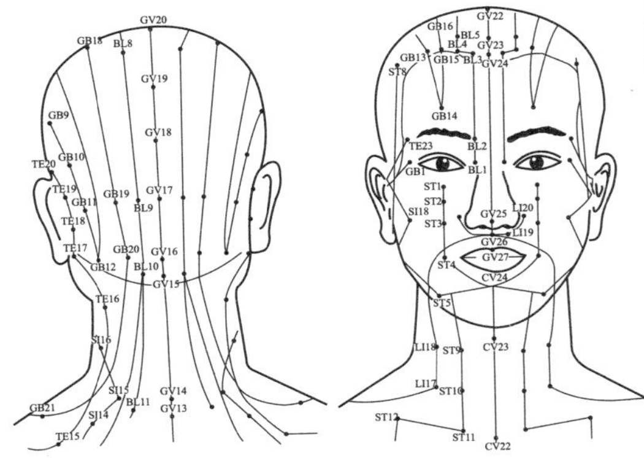

Fig. 17a Regular points on the head

扶突 [fú tū]

***Futu* (LI 18):** point on the lateral side of the neck, beside the laryngeal protuberance, between the anterior and posterior borders of the sternocleidomastoid muscle (Fig. 17a and b)

口禾髎 [kǒu hé liáo]

***Kouheliao* (LI 19):** point on the upper lip, directly below the lateral border of the nostril, on the level of *Shuigou* (GV 26) (Fig. 17a and b)

禾髎 [hé liáo]

***Heliao* (LI 19):** same as 口禾髎 [kǒu hé liáo]

迎香 [yíng xiāng]

***Yingxiang* (LI 20):** point in the nasolabial groove, beside the midpoint of the lateral border of the nasal ala (Fig. 17a and b)

足阳明胃经穴 [zú yáng míng wèi jīng xué]

points of the stomach meridian/channel: acupuncture-moxibustion points distributed on the stomach meridian/channel (ST)

承泣 [chéng qì]

***Chengqi* (ST 1):** point on the face, directly below the pupil, between the eyeball and the infraorbital ridge (Fig. 17a and b)

四白 [sì bái]

***Sibai* (ST 2):** point on the face, directly below the pupil, in the depression of the infraorbital foramen (Fig. 17a and b)

巨髎 [jù liáo]

***Juliao* (ST 3):** point on the face, directly below the pupil, on the level of the lower border of the nasal ala (Fig. 17a and b)

地仓 [dì cāng]

***Dicang* (ST 4):** point on the face, directly below the pupil, beside the mouth angle (Fig. 17a and b)

大迎 [dà yíng]

***Daying* (ST 5):** point anterior to the mandibular angle, on the anterior border of the masseter muscle, where the pulsation of the facial artery is palpable (Fig. 17a and b)

颊车 [jiá chē]

***Jiache* (ST 6):** point on the cheek, one finger breadth anterior and superior to the mandibular angle (Fig. 17a and b)

下关 [xià guān]

***Xiaguan* (ST 7):** point on the face, anterior to the ear, in the depression between the zygomatic arch and mandibular notch (Fig. 17a and b)

头维 [tóu wéi]

***Touwei* (ST 8):** point on the lateral side of the head, 0.5 *cun* above the anterior hairline at the corner of the forehead (Fig. 17a and b)

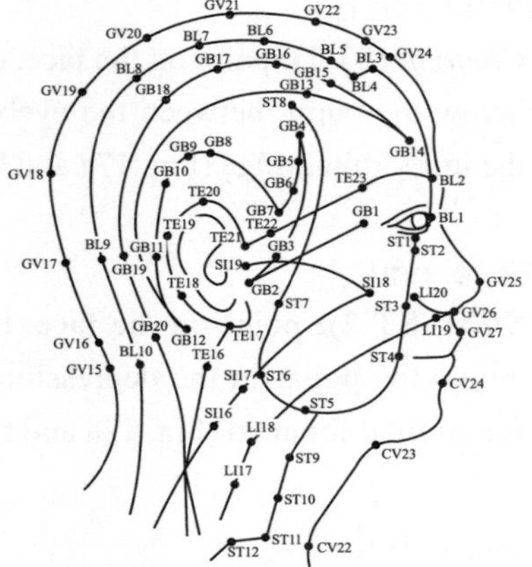

Fig. 17b Regular points on the head

人迎 [rén yíng]

***Renying* (ST 9):** point on the neck, beside the laryngeal protuberance, and on the anterior border of the sternocleidomastoid muscle where the pulsation of the common carotid artery is palpable (Fig. 17a and b)

水突 [shuǐ tū]

***Shuitu* (ST 10):** point on the neck and on the anterior border of the sternocleidomastoid muscle, at the midpoint of the line connecting *Renying* (ST 9) and *Qishe* (ST 11) (Fig. 17a and b)

气舍 [qì shè]

***Qishe* (ST 11):** point on the neck and on the upper border of the medial end of the clavicle, between the sternal and clavicular heads of the sternocleidomastoid muscle (Fig. 17a and b)

缺盆 [quē pén]

***Quepen* (ST 12):** point at the center of the supraclavicular fossa, 4 *cun* lateral to the anterior midline (Fig. 17a and b)

气户 [qì hù]

***Qihu* (ST 13):** point on the chest, below the midpoint of the lower border of the clavicle, 4 *cun* lateral to the anterior midline (Fig. 16)

库房 [kù fáng]

***Kufang* (ST 14):** point on the chest, in the 1st intercostal space, 4 *cun* lateral to the anterior midline (Fig. 16)

屋翳 [wū yì]

***Wuyi* (ST 15):** point on the chest, in the 2nd intercostal space, 4 *cun* lateral to the anterior midline (Fig. 16)

膺窗 [yīng chuāng]

***Yingchuang* (ST 16):** point on the chest, in the 3rd intercostal space, 4 *cun* lateral to the anterior midline (Fig. 16)

乳中 [rǔ zhōng]

***Ruzhong* (ST 17):** point at the center of the nipple (Fig. 16)

乳根 [rǔ gēn]

***Rugen* (ST 18):** point on the chest, in the 5th intercostal space, 4 *cun* lateral to the anterior midline (Fig. 16)

不容 [bù róng]

***Burong* (ST 19):** point on the upper abdomen, 6 *cun* above the center of the umbilicus and 2 *cun* lateral to the anterior midline (Fig. 16)

承满 [chéng mǎn]

***Chengman* (ST 20):** point on the upper abdomen, 5 *cun* above the center of the umbilicus and 2 *cun* lateral to the anterior midline (Fig. 16)

梁门 [liáng mén]

***Liangmen* (ST 21):** point on the upper abdomen, 4 *cun* above the center of the umbilicus and 2 *cun* lateral to the anterior midline (Fig. 16)

关门 [guān mén]

***Guanmen* (ST 22):** point on the upper abdomen, 3 *cun* above the center of the umbilicus and 2 *cun* lateral to the anterior midline (Fig. 16)

太乙 [tài yǐ]

***Taiyi* (ST 23):** point on the upper abdomen, 2 *cun* above the center of the umbilicus and 2 *cun* lateral to the anterior midline (Fig. 16)

滑肉门 [huá ròu mén]

***Huaroumen* (ST 24):** point on the upper abdomen, 1 *cun* above the center of the umbilicus and 2 *cun* lateral to the anterior midline (Fig. 16)

天枢 [tiān shū]

***Tianshu* (ST 25):** point on the middle abdomen, 2 *cun* lateral to the center of the umbilicus (Fig. 16)

外陵 [wài líng]

***Wailing* (ST 26):** point on the lower abdomen, 1 *cun* below the center of the umbilicus and 2 *cun* lateral to the anterior midline (Fig. 16)

大巨 [dà jù]

***Daju* (ST 27):** point on the lower abdomen, 2 *cun* below the center of the umbilicus and 2 *cun* lateral to the anterior midline (Fig. 16)

水道 [shuǐ dào]

***Shuidao* (ST 28):** point on the lower abdomen, 3 *cun* below the center of the umbilicus and 2 *cun* lateral to the anterior midline (Fig. 16)

归来 [guī lái]

***Guilai* (ST 29):** point on the lower abdomen, 4 *cun* below the center of the umbilicus and 2 *cun* lateral to the anterior midline (Fig. 16)

气冲 [qì chōng]

***Qichong* (ST 30):** point slightly above the inguinal groove, 5 *cun* below the center of the umbilicus and 2 *cun* lateral to the anterior midline (Fig. 16)

髀关 [bì guān]

***Biguan* (ST 31):** point on the anterior side of the thigh and on the line connecting the anteriosuperior iliac spine and the superiolateral corner of the patella, in the depression lateral to the sartorius muscle (Fig. 18)

伏兔 [fú tù]

***Futu* (ST 32):** point on the anterior side of the thigh, 6 *cun* above the superiolateral corner of the patella (Fig. 18)

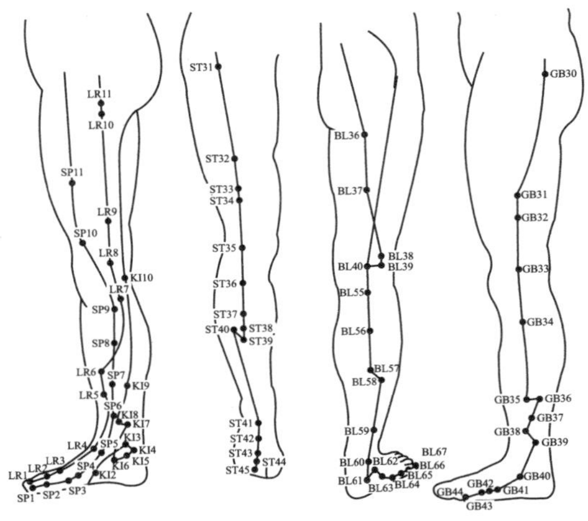

Fig. 18 Regular points on the lower limb

阴市 [yīn shì]
***Yinshi* (ST 33):** point on the anterior side of the thigh, 3 *cun* above the superiolateral corner of the patella (Fig. 18)

梁丘 [liáng qīu]
***Liangqiu* (ST 34):** point on the anterior side of the thigh, 2 *cun* above the superiolateral corner of the patella (Fig. 18)

犊鼻 [dú bí]
***Dubi* (ST 35):** point on the knee, in the depression lateral to the patella and its ligament when the knee is flexed (Fig. 18)

足三里 [zú sān lǐ]
***Zusanli* (ST 36):** point on the anteriolateral side of the leg, 3 *cun* below *Dubi* (ST 35), one finger breadth from the anterior crest of the tibia (Fig. 18)

上巨虚 [shàng jù xū]
***Shangjuxu* (ST 37):** point on the anteriolateral side of the leg, 6 *cun* below *Dubi* (ST 35), one finger breadth from the anterior crest of the tibia (Fig. 18)

条口 [tiáo kǒu]
***Tiaokou* (ST 38):** point on the anteriolateral side of the leg, 8 *cun* below *Dubi* (ST 35), one finger breadth from the anterior crest of the tibia (Fig. 18)

下巨虚 [xià jù xū]
***Xiajuxu* (ST 39):** point on the anteriolateral side of the leg, 9 *cun* below *Dubi* (ST 35), one finger breadth from the anterior crest of the tibia (Fig. 18)

丰隆 [fēng lóng]
***Fenglong* (ST 40):** point on the anteriolateral side of the leg, 8 *cun* above the tip of the external malleolus, lateral to *Tiaokou* (ST 38), and two finger breadths from the anterior crest of the tibia (Fig. 18)

解溪 [jiě xī]
***Jiexi* (ST 41):** point in the central depression of the crease between the instep of the foot and the leg (Fig. 18)

冲阳 [chōng yáng]
***Chongyang* (ST 42):** point on the dome of the instep of the foot, where the pulsation of the dorsal artery of the foot is palpable (Fig. 18)

陷谷 [xiàn gǔ]
***Xiangu* (ST 43):** point on the instep of the foot, in the depression distal to the commissure of the 2nd and 3rd metatarsal bone (Fig. 18)

内庭 [nèi tíng]
***Neiting* (ST 44):** point on the instep of the foot, at the junction of the red and white skin proximal to the margin of the web between the 2nd and 3rd toes (Fig. 18)

厉兑 [lì duì]
***Lidui* (ST 45):** point on the lateral side of the distal segment of the 2nd toe, 0.1 *cun* proximal to the corner of the nail (Fig. 18)

足太阴脾经穴 [zú tài yīn pí jīng xué]
points of the spleen meridian/channel: acupuncture-moxibustion points distributed on the spleen meridian/channel (SP)

隐白 [yǐn bái]

***Yinbai* (SP 1):** point on the medial side of the distal segment of the big toe, 0.1 *cun* proximal to the corner of the nail (Fig. 18)

大都 [dà dū]

***Dadu* (SP 2):** point on the medial border of the foot, in the depression just distal to the metatarsophalangeal joint (Fig. 18)

太白 [tài bái]

***Taibai* (SP 3):** point on the medial border of the foot, in the depression proximal and inferior to the metatarsophalangeal joint (Fig. 18)

公孙 [gōng sūn]

***Gongsun* (SP 4):** point on the medial border of the foot, anterior and inferior to the proximal end of the 1st metatarsal bone (Fig. 18)

商丘 [shāng qiū]

***Shangqiu* (SP 5):** point on the medial side of the ankle in the depression anterior and inferior to the medial malleolus (Fig. 18)

三阴交 [sān yīn jiāo]

***Sanyinjiao* (SP 6):** point on the medial side of the leg, 3 *cun* above the tip of the medial malleolus, just posterior to the tibia (Fig. 18)

漏谷 [lòu gǔ]

***Lougu* (SP 7):** point on the medial side of the leg, 6 *cun* above the tip of the medial malleolus, just posterior to the tibia (Fig. 18)

地机 [dì jī]

***Diji* (SP 8):** point on the medial side of the leg, 3 *cun* below *Yinlingquan* (SP 9) (Fig. 18)

阴陵泉 [yīn líng quán]

***Yinlingquan* (SP 9):** point on the medial side of the leg, in the depression posterior and inferior to the medial condyle of the tibia (Fig. 18)

血海 [xuè hǎi]

***Xuehai* (SP 10):** point with the knee flexed, on the medial side of the thigh, 2 *cun* above the superior medial corner of the patella, on the prominence of the medial head of the quadriceps muscle (Fig. 18)

箕门 [jī mén]

***Jimen* (SP 11):** point on the medial side of the thigh, on the line connecting *Xuehai* (SP 10) and *Chongmen* (SP 12), and 6 *cun* above *Xuehai* (SP 10) (Fig. 18)

冲门 [chōng mén]

***Chongmen* (SP 12):** point at the lateral end of the inguinal groove, 3.5 *cun* lateral to the midpoint of the upper border of the symphysis pubis, lateral to the pulsating external iliac artery (Fig. 16)

府舍 [fǔ shè]

***Fushe* (SP 13):** point on the lower abdomen, 4 *cun* below the center of the umbilicus, 0.7 *cun* above *Chongmen* (SP 12), and 4 *cun* lateral to the anterior midline (Fig. 16)

腹结 [fù jié]

***Fujie* (SP 14):** point on the lower abdomen, 1.3 *cun* below *Daheng* (SP 15), and 4 *cun* lateral to the anterior midline (Fig. 16)

大横 [dà héng]

***Daheng* (SP 15):** point on the middle abdomen, 4 *cun* lateral to the center of the umbilicus (Fig. 16)

腹哀 [fù āi]

***Fu'ai* (SP 16):** point on the upper abdomen, 3 *cun* above the center of the umbilicus, and 4 *cun* lateral to the anterior midline (Fig. 16)

食窦 [shí dòu]

***Shidou* (SP 17):** point on the lateral side of the chest and in the 5th intercostal space, 6 *cun* lateral to the anterior midline (Fig. 16)

天溪 [tiān xī]

***Tianxi* (SP 18):** point on the lateral side of the chest and in the 4th intercostal space, 6 *cun* lateral to the anterior midline (Fig. 16)

胸乡 [xiōng xiāng]

***Xiongxiang* (SP 19):** point on the lateral side of the chest and in the 3rd intercostal space, 6 *cun* lateral to the anterior midline (Fig. 16)

周荣 [zhōu róng]

***Zhourong* (SP 20):** point on the lateral side of the chest and in the 2nd intercostal space, 6 *cun* lateral to the anterior midline (Fig. 16)

大包 [dà bāo]

***Dabao* (SP 21):** point on the lateral side of the chest and on the middle axillary line, in the 6th intercostal space (Fig. 16)

手少阴心经穴 [shǒu shào yīn xīn jīng xué]

points of the heart meridian/channel: acupuncture-moxibustion points distributed on the heart meridian/channel (HT)

极泉 [jí quán]

***Jiquan* (HT 1):** point at the apex of the axillary fossa, where the pulsation of the axillary artery is palpable (Fig. 5)

青灵 [qīng líng]

***Qingling* (HT 2):** point on the medial side of the arm, 3 *cun* above the cubital crease, in the groove medial to the biceps muscle (Fig. 15)

少海 [shào hǎi]

***Shaohai* (HT 3):** point at the midpoint of the line connecting the medial end of the cubital crease and the medial epicondyle of the humerus when the elbow is flexed (Fig. 15)

灵道 [líng dào]

***Lingdao* (HT 4):** point on the palmar side of the forearm and on the radial side of the tendon of the ulnar flexor muscle of the wrist, 1.5 *cun* proximal to the crease of the wrist (Fig. 15)

通里 [tōng lǐ]

***Tongli* (HT 5):** point on the palmar side of the forearm and on the radial side of the tendon of the ulnar flexor muscle of the wrist, 1 *cun* proximal to the crease of the wrist (Fig. 15)

阴郄 [yīn xì]

***Yinxi* (HT 6):** point on the palmar side of

the forearm and on the radial side of the tendon of the ulnar flexor muscle of the wrist, 0.5 *cun* proximal to the crease of the wrist (Fig. 15)

神门 [shén mén]

***Shenmen* (HT 7):** point on the wrist, at the ulnar end of the crease of the wrist, in the depression of the radial side of the tendon of the ulnar flexor muscle of the wrist (Fig. 15)

少府 [shào fǔ]

***Shaofu* (HT 8):** point on the palm, between the 4th and 5th metacarpal bones, at the part of the palm touching the tip of the little finger when a fist is made (Fig. 15)

少冲 [shào chōng]

***Shaochong* (HT 9):** point on the radial side of the distal segment of the little finger, 0.1 *cun* proximal to the corner of the nail (Fig. 15)

手太阳小肠经穴 [shǒu tài yáng xiǎo cháng jīng xué]

points of the small intestine meridian/channel: acupuncture-moxibustion points distributed on the small intestine meridian/channel (SI)

少泽 [shào zé]

***Shaoze* (SI 1):** point on the ulnar side of the distal segment of the little finger, 0.1 *cun* proximal to the corner of the nail (Fig. 15)

前谷 [qián gǔ]

***Qiangu* (SI 2):** point at the junction of the red and white skin along the ulnar border of the hand, at the ulnar end of the crease of the 5th metacarpophalangeal joint when a loose fist is made (Fig. 15)

后溪 [hòu xī]

***Houxi* (SI 3):** point at the junction of the red and white skin along the ulnar border of the hand, at the ulnar end of the distal palmar crease, proximal to the 5th metacarpophalangeal joint when a loose fist is made (Fig. 15)

腕骨 [wàn gǔ]

***Wangu* (SI 4):** point on the ulnar border of the hand, in the depression between the proximal end of the 5th metacarpal bone and hamate bone, and at the junction of the red and white skin (Fig. 15)

阳谷 [yáng gǔ]

***Yanggu* (SI 5):** point on the ulnar border of the wrist, in the depression between the styloid process of the ulna and triangular bone (Fig. 15)

养老 [yǎng lǎo]

***Yanglao* (SI 6):** point on the ulnar side of the posterior surface of the forearm, in the depression proximal to and on the radial side of the head of the ulna (Fig. 15)

支正 [zhī zhèng]

***Zhizheng* (SI 7):** point on the ulnar side of the posterior surface of the forearm, 5 *cun* proximal to the dorsal crease of the wrist (Fig. 15)

小海 [xiǎo hǎi]

***Xiaohai* (SI 8):** point on the medial side of the elbow, in the depression between the olecranon of the ulna and the medial epicondyle of the humerus (Fig. 15)

肩贞 [jiān zhēn]

***Jianzhen* (SI 9):** point posterior and inferior to the shoulder joint, 1 *cun* above the posterior end of the axillary fold with the arm adducted (Fig. 15 and 16)

臑俞 [nào shù]

***Naoshu* (SI 10):** point on the shoulder, above the posterior end of the axillary fold, in the depression below the lower border of the scapular spine (Fig. 16)

天宗 [tiān zōng]

***Tianzong* (SI 11):** point on the scapula, in the depression of the center of the subscapular fossa, and on the level of the 4th thoracic vertebra (Fig. 16)

秉风 [bǐng fēng]

***Bingfeng* (SI 12):** point on the scapula, at the center of the suprascapular fossa, in the depression found when the arm is raised (Fig. 16)

曲垣 [qū yuán]

***Quyuan* (SI 13):** point on the scapula, at the medial end of the suprascapular fossa, at the midpoint of the line connecting *Naoshu* (SI 10) and the spinous process of the 2nd thoracic vertebra (Fig. 16)

肩外俞 [jiān wài shù]

***Jianwaishu* (SI 14):** point on the back, below the spinous process of the 1st thoracic vertebra, 3 *cun* lateral to the posterior midline (Fig. 16)

肩中俞 [jiān zhōng shù]

***Jianzhongshu* (SI 15):** point on the back, below the spinous process of the 7th cervical vertebra, 2 *cun* lateral to the posterior midline (Fig. 16)

天窗 [tiān chuāng]

***Tianchuang* (SI 16):** point on the lateral side of the neck, posterior to the sternocleidomastoid muscle and *Futu* (LI 18), on the level of the laryngeal protuberance (Fig. 17b)

天容 [tiān róng]

***Tianrong* (SI 17):** point on the lateral side of the neck, posterior to the mandibular angle, in the depression of the anterior border of the sternocleidomastoid muscle (Fig. 17b)

颧髎 [quán liáo]

***Quanliao* (SI 18):** point on the face, directly below the outer canthus, in the depression below the zygomatic bone (Fig. 17a and b)

听宫 [tīng gōng]

***Tinggong* (SI 19):** point on the face, anterior to the tragus and posterior to the mandibular condyloid process, in the depression found when the mouth is open (Fig. 17b)

足太阳膀胱经穴 [zú tài yáng páng guāng jīng xué]

points of the bladder meridian/channel: acupuncture-moxibustion points distributed on the bladder meridian/channel (BL)

睛明 [jīng míng]

***Jingming* (BL 1):** point on the face, in the depression slightly above the inner canthus (Fig. 17a and b)

攒竹 [cuán zhú]
***Cuanzhu* (BL 2):** point on the face, in the depression of the medial end of the eyebrow, at the supraorbital notch (Fig. 17a and b)

眉冲 [méi chōng]
***Meichong* (BL 3):** point on the head, directly above *Cuanzhu* (BL2), 0.5 *cun* above the anterior hairline (Fig. 17a and b)

曲差 [qū chā] [qū chāi]
***Qucha (Quchai)* (BL 4):** point on the head, 0.5 *cun* above the anterior hairline and 1.5 *cun* lateral to *Shenting* (GV 24) (Fig. 17a and b)

五处 [wǔ chù]
***Wuchu* (BL 5):** point on the head, 1 *cun* directly above the midpoint of the anterior hairline and 1.5 *cun* lateral to the midline (Fig. 17a and b)

承光 [chéng guāng]
***Chengguang* (BL 6):** point on the head, 2.5 *cun* directly above the midpoint of the anterior hairline and 1.5 *cun* lateral to the midline (Fig. 17a)

通天 [tōng tiān]
***Tongtian* (BL 7):** point on the head, 4 *cun* directly above the midpoint of the anterior hairline and 1.5 *cun* lateral to the midline (Fig. 17b)

络却 [luò què]
***Luoque* (BL 8):** point on the head, 5.5 *cun* directly above the midpoint of the anterior hairline and 1.5 *cun* lateral to the midline (Fig. 17a and b)

玉枕 [yù zhěn]
***Yuzhen* (BL 9):** point on the occiput, 2.5 *cun* directly above the midpoint of the posterior hairline and 1.3 *cun* lateral to the midline, in the depression on the level of the upper border of the external occipital protuberance (Fig. 17a and b)

天柱 [tiān zhù]
***Tianzhu* (BL 10):** point on the nape, in the depression of the lateral border of the trapezius muscle and 1.3 *cun* lateral to the midpoint of the posterior hairline (Fig. 17a and b)

大杼 [dà zhù]
***Dazhu* (BL 11):** point on the back, below the spinous process of the 1st thoracic vertebra, 1.5 *cun* lateral to the posterior midline (Fig. 17a and 16)

风门 [fēng mén]
***Fengmen* (BL 12):** point on the back, below the spinous process of the 2nd thoracic vertebra, 1.5 *cun* lateral to the posterior midline (Fig. 16)

肺俞 [fèi shù]
***Feishu* (BL 13):** point on the back, below the spinous process of the 3rd thoracic vertebra, 1.5 *cun* lateral to the posterior midline (Fig. 16)

厥阴俞 [jué yīn shù]
***Jueyinshu* (BL 14):** point on the back, below the spinous process of the 4th thoracic vertebra, 1.5 *cun* lateral to the posterior midline (Fig. 16)

心俞 [xīn shù]
***Xinshu* (BL 15):** point on the back, below

the spinous process of the 5th thoracic vertebra, 1.5 *cun* lateral to the posterior midline (Fig. 16)

督俞 [dū shù]

Dushu **(BL 16):** point on the back, below the spinous process of the 6th thoracic vertebra, 1.5 *cun* lateral to the posterior midline (Fig. 16)

膈俞 [gé shù]

Geshu **(BL 17):** point on the back, below the spinous process of the 7th thoracic vertebra, 1.5 *cun* lateral to the posterior midline (Fig. 16)

肝俞 [gān shù]

Ganshu **(BL 18):** point on the back, below the spinous process of the 9th thoracic vertebra, 1.5 *cun* lateral to the posterior midline (Fig. 16)

胆俞 [dǎn shù]

Danshu **(BL 19):** point on the back, below the spinous process of the 10th thoracic vertebra, 1.5 *cun* lateral to the posterior midline (Fig. 16)

脾俞 [pí shù]

Pishu **(BL 20):** point on the back, below the spinous process of the 11th thoracic vertebra, 1.5 *cun* lateral to the posterior midline (Fig. 16)

胃俞 [wèi shù]

Weishu **(BL 21):** point on the back, below the spinous process of the 12th thoracic vertebra, 1.5 *cun* lateral to the posterior midline (Fig. 16)

三焦俞 [sān jiāo shù]

Sanjiaoshu **(BL 22):** point on the lower back, below the spinous process of the 1st lumbar vertebra, 1.5 *cun* lateral to the posterior midline (Fig. 16)

肾俞 [shèn shù]

Shenshu **(BL 23):** point on the lower back, below the spinous process of the 2nd lumbar vertebra, 1.5 *cun* lateral to the posterior midline (Fig. 16)

气海俞 [qì hǎi shù]

Qihaishu **(BL 24):** point on the lower back, below the spinous process of the 3rd lumbar vertebra, 1.5 *cun* lateral to the posterior midline (Fig. 16)

大肠俞 [dà cháng shù]

Dachangshu **(BL 25):** point on the lower back, below the spinous process of the 4th lumbar vertebra, 1.5 *cun* lateral to the posterior midline (Fig. 16)

关元俞 [guān yuán shù]

Guanyuanshu **(BL 26):** point on the lower back, below the spinous process of the 5th lumbar vertebra, 1.5 *cun* lateral to the posterior midline (Fig. 16)

小肠俞 [xiǎo cháng shù]

Xiaochangshu **(BL 27):** point on the sacrum and on the level of the 1st posterior sacral foramen, 1.5 *cun* lateral to the median sacral crest (Fig. 16)

膀胱俞 [páng guāng shù]

Pangguangshu **(BL 28):** point on the sacrum and on the level of the 2nd posterior sacral foramen, 1.5 *cun* lateral to the median sacral crest (Fig. 16)

中膂俞 [zhōng lǚ shù]
***Zhonglushu* (BL 29):** point on the sacrum and on the level of the 3rd posterior sacral foramen, 1.5 *cun* lateral to the median sacral crest (Fig. 16)

白环俞 [bái huán shù]
***Baihuanshu* (BL 30):** point on the sacrum and on the level of the 4th posterior sacral foramen, 1.5 *cun* lateral to the median sacral crest (Fig. 16)

上髎 [shàng liáo]
***Shangliao* (BL 31):** point on the sacrum, at the midpoint between the posteriosuperior iliac spine and the posterior midline, just at the 1st posterior sacral foramen (Fig. 16)

次髎 [cì liáo]
***Ciliao* (BL 32):** point on the sacrum, medial and inferior to the posteriosuperior iliac spine, just at the 2nd posterior sacral foramen (Fig. 16)

中髎 [zhōng liáo]
***Zhongliao* (BL 33):** point on the sacrum, medial and inferior to *Ciliao* (GL 32), just at the 3rd posterior sacral foramen (Fig. 16)

下髎 [xià liáo]
***Xialiao* (BL 34):** point on the sacrum, medial and inferior to *Zhongliao* (BL 33), just at the 4th posterior sacral foramen (Fig. 16)

会阳 [huì yáng]
***Huiyang* (BL 35):** point on the sacrum, 0.5 *cun* lateral to the tip of the coccyx (Fig. 16)

承扶 [chéng fú]
***Chengfu* (BL 36):** point on the posterior side of the thigh, at the midpoint of the inferior gluteal crease (Fig. 18)

殷门 [yīn mén]
***Yinmen* (BL 37):** point on the posterior side of the thigh and on the line connecting *Chengfu* (BL 36) and *Weizhong* (BL 40), 6 *cun* below *Chengfu* (BL 36) (Fig. 18)

浮郄 [fú xì]
***Fuxi* (BL 38):** point at the lateral end of the popliteral crease, 1 *cun* above *Weiyang* (BL 39), medial to the tendon of the biceps muscle of the thigh (Fig. 18)

委阳 [wěi yáng]
***Weiyang* (BL 39):** point at the lateral end of the popliteal crease, medial to the tendon of the biceps muscle of the thigh (Fig. 18)

委中 [wěi zhōng]
***Weizhong* (BL 40):** point at the midpoint of the popliteal crease, between the tendon of the biceps muscle of the thigh and the semitendinous muscle (Fig. 18)

附分 [fù fēn]
***Fufen* (BL 41):** point on the back, below the spinous process of the 2nd thoracic vertebra, 3 *cun* lateral to the posterior midline (Fig. 16)

魄户 [pò hù]
***Pohu* (BL 42):** point on the back, below the spinous process of the 3rd thoracic vertebra, 3 *cun* lateral to the posterior midline (Fig. 16)

膏肓 [gāo huāng]
***Gaohuang* (BL 43):** point on the back, below the spinous process of the 4th thoracic vertebra, 3 *cun* lateral to the posterior midline (Fig. 16)

神堂 [shén táng]
***Shentang* (BL 44):** point on the back, below the spinous process of the 5th thoracic vertebra, 3 *cun* lateral to the posterior midline (Fig. 16)

譩譆 [yī xī]
***Yixi* (BL 45):** point on the back, below the spinous process of the 6th thoracic vertebra, 3 *cun* lateral to the posterior midline (Fig. 16)

膈关 [gé guān]
***Geguan* (BL 46):** point on the back, below the spinous process of the 7th thoracic vertebra, 3 *cun* lateral to the posterior midline (Fig. 16)

魂门 [hún mén]
***Hunmen* (BL 47):** point on the back, below the spinous process of the 9th thoracic vertebra, 3 *cun* lateral to the posterior midline (Fig. 16)

阳纲 [yáng gāng]
***Yanggang* (BL 48):** point on the back, below the spinous process of the 10th thoracic vertebra, 3 *cun* lateral to the posterior midline (Fig. 16)

意舍 [yì shè]
***Yishe* (BL 49):** point on the back, below the spinous process of the 11th thoracic vertebra, 3 *cun* lateral to the posterior midline (Fig. 16)

胃仓 [wèi cāng]
***Weicang* (BL 50):** point on the back, below the spinous process of the 12th thoracic vertebra, 3 *cun* lateral to the posterior midline (Fig. 16)

肓门 [huāng mén]
***Huangmen* (BL 51):** point on the lower back, below the spinous process of the 1st lumbar vertebra, 3 *cun* lateral to the posterior midline (Fig. 16)

志室 [zhì shì]
***Zhishi* (BL 52):** point on the lower back, below the spinous process of the 2nd lumbar vertebra, 3 *cun* lateral to the posterior midline (Fig. 16)

胞肓 [bāo huāng]
***Baohuang* (BL 53):** point on the buttock and on the level of the 2nd posterior sacral foramen, 3 *cun* lateral to the median sacral crest (Fig. 16)

秩边 [zhì biān]
***Zhibian* (BL 54):** point on the buttock and on the level of the 4th posterior sacral foramen, 3 *cun* lateral to the median sacral crest (Fig. 16)

合阳 [hé yáng]
***Heyang* (BL 55):** point on the posterior side of the leg and on the line connecting *Weizhong* (BL 40) and *Chengshan* (BL 57), 2 *cun* below *Weizhong* (BL 40) (Fig. 18)

承筋 [chéng jīn]
***Chengjin* (BL 56):** point on the posterior side of the leg and on the line connecting *Weizhong* (BL 40) and *Chengshan* (BL

57), at the center of the gastrocnemius muscle belly, 5 *cun* below *Weizhong* (BL 40) (Fig. 18)

承山 [chéng shān]
***Chengshan* (BL 57):** point on the posterior midline of the leg, between *Weizhong* (BL 40) and *Kunlun* (BL 60), in a pointed depression formed below the gastrocnemius muscle belly when the leg is stretched or the heel is lifted (Fig. 18)

飞阳 [fēi yáng]
***Feiyang* (BL 58):** point on the posterior side of the leg, 7 *cun* directly above *Kunlun* (BL 60) and 1 *cun* lateral and inferior to *Chengshan* (BL 57) (Fig. 18)

跗阳 [fū yáng]
***Fuyang* (BL 59):** point on the posterior side of the leg, posterior to the lateral malleolus, 3 *cun* directly above *Kunlun* (BL 60) (Fig. 18)

昆仑 [kūn lún]
***Kunlun* (BL 60):** point posterior to the external malleolus, in the depression between the tip of the external malleolus and Achilles tendon (Fig. 18)

仆参 [pú cān]
***Pucan* (BL 61):** point on the lateral side of the foot, posterior and inferior to the external malleolus, directly below *Kunlun* (BL 60), lateral to the calcaneum, at the junction of the red and white skin (Fig. 18)

申脉 [shēn mài]
***Shenmai* (BL 62):** point on the lateral side of the foot, in the depression directly below the external malleolus (Fig. 18)

金门 [jīn mén]
***Jinmen* (BL 63):** point on the lateral side of the foot, directly below the anterior border of the external malleolus, on the lower border of the cuboid bone (Fig. 18)

京骨 [jīng gǔ]
***Jinggu* (BL 64):** point on the lateral side of the foot, below the tuberosity of the 5th metatarsal bone, at the junction of the red and white skin (Fig. 18)

束骨 [shù gǔ]
***Shugu* (BL 65):** point on the lateral side of the foot, posterior to the 5th metatarsophalangeal joint, at the junction of the red and white skin (Fig. 18)

足通谷 [zú tōng gǔ]
***Zutonggu* (BL 66):** point on the lateral side of the foot, anterior to the 5th metatarsophalangeal joint, at the junction of the red and white skin (Fig. 18)

至阴 [zhì yīn]
***Zhiyin* (BL 67):** point on the lateral side of the distal segment of the little toe, 0.1 *cun* from the corner of the toenail (Fig. 18)

足少阴肾经穴 [zú shào yīn shèn jīng xué]
points of the kidney meridian/channel: acupuncture-moxibustion points distributed on the kidney meridian/channel (KI)

涌泉 [yǒng quán]
***Yongquan* (KI 1):** point on the sole, in the depression at the junction of the anterior third and posterior two-thirds of the line connecting the base of the 2nd and 3rd toes and the heel (Fig. 8)

然谷 [rán gǔ]

***Rangu* (KI 2):** point on the medial border of the foot, below the tuberosity of the navicular bone, and at the junction of the red and white skin (Fig. 18)

太溪 [tài xī]

***Taixi* (KI 3):** point on the medial side of the foot, posterior to the medial malleolus, in the depression between the tip of the medial malleolus and the Achilles tendon (Fig. 18)

大钟 [dà zhōng]

***Dazhong* (KI 4):** point on the medial side of the foot, posterior and inferior to the medial malleolus, in the depression medial and anterior to the attachment of the Achilles tendon (Fig. 18)

水泉 [shuǐ quán]

***Shuiquan* (KI 5):** point on the medial side of the foot, posterior and inferior to the medial malleolus, 1 *cun* directly below *Taixi* (KI 3), in the depression of the medial side of the tuberosity of the calcaneum (Fig. 18)

照海 [zhào hǎi]

***Zhaohai* (KI 6):** point on the medial side of the foot, in the depression below the tip of the medial malleolus (Fig. 18)

复溜 [fù liū]

***Fuliu* (KI 7):** point on the medial side of the leg, 2 *cun* directly above *Taixi* (KI 3), anterior to the Achilles tendon (Fig. 18)

交信 [jiāo xìn]

***Jiaoxin* (KI 8):** point on the medial side of the leg, 2 *cun* above *Taixi* (KI 3) and 0.5 *cun* anterior to *Fuliu* (KI 7), posterior to the medial border of the tibia (Fig. 18)

筑宾 [zhù bīn]

***Zhubin* (KI 9):** point on the medial side of the leg and on the line connecting *Taixi* (KI 3) and *Yingu* (KI 10), 5 *cun* above *Taixi* (KI 3), medial and inferior to the gastrocnemius muscle belly (Fig. 18)

阴谷 [yīn gǔ]

***Yingu* (KI 10):** point on the medial side of the popliteal fossa, between the tendons of the semitendinous and semimembranous muscles when the knee is flexed (Fig. 18)

横骨 [héng gǔ]

***Henggu* (KI 11):** point on the lower abdomen, 5 *cun* below the center of the umbilicus and 0.5 *cun* lateral to the anterior midline (Fig. 16)

大赫 [dà hè]

***Dahe* (KI 12):** point on the lower abdomen, 4 *cun* below the center of the umbilicus and 0.5 *cun* lateral to the anterior midline (Fig. 16)

气穴 [qì xué]

***Qixue* (KI 13):** point on the lower abdomen, 3 *cun* below the center of the umbilicus and 0.5 *cun* lateral to the anterior midline (Fig. 16)

四满 [sì mǎn]

***Siman* (KI 14):** point on the lower abdomen, 2 *cun* below the center of the umbilicus and 0.5 *cun* lateral to the anterior midline (Fig. 16)

中注 [zhōng zhù]

***Zhongzhu* (KI 15):** point on the lower

abdomen, 1 *cun* below the center of the umbilicus and 0.5 *cun* lateral to the anterior midline (Fig. 16)

肓俞 [huāng shù]

***Huangshu* (KI 16):** point on the middle abdomen, 0.5 *cun* lateral to the center of the umbilicus (Fig. 16)

商曲 [shāng qū]

***Shangqu* (KI 17):** point on the upper abdomen, 2 *cun* above the center of the umbilicus, and 0.5 *cun* lateral to the anterior midline (Fig. 16)

石关 [shí guān]

***Shiguan* (KI 18):** point on the upper abdomen, 3 *cun* above the center of the umbilicus, and 0.5 *cun* lateral to the anterior midline (Fig. 16)

阴都 [yīn dū]

***Yindu* (KI 19):** point on the upper abdomen, 4 *cun* above the center of the umbilicus and 0.5 *cun* lateral to the anterior midline (Fig. 16)

腹通谷 [fù tōng gǔ]

***Futonggu* (KI 20):** point on the upper abdomen, 5 *cun* above the center of the umbilicus and 0.5 *cun* lateral to the anterior midline (Fig. 16)

幽门 [yōu mén]

***Youmen* (KI 21):** point on the upper abdomen, 6 *cun* above the center of the umbilicus and 0.5 *cun* lateral to the anterior midline (Fig. 16)

步廊 [bù láng]

***Bulang* (KI 22):** point on the chest, in the 5th intercostal space, 2 *cun* lateral to the anterior midline (Fig. 16)

神封 [shén fēng]

***Shenfeng* (KI 23):** point on the chest, in the 4th intercostal space, 2 *cun* lateral to the anterior midline (Fig. 16)

灵墟 [líng xū]

***Lingxu* (KI 24):** point on the chest, in the 3rd intercostal space, 2 *cun* lateral to the anterior midline (Fig. 16)

神藏 [shén cáng]

***Shencang* (KI 25):** point on the chest, in the 2nd intercostal space, 2 *cun* lateral to the anterior midline (Fig. 16)

彧中 [yù zhōng]

***Yuzhong* (KI 26):** point on the chest, in the 1st intercostal space, 2 *cun* lateral to the anterior midline (Fig. 16)

俞府 [shù fǔ]

***Shufu* (KI 27):** point on the chest, below the lower border of the clavicle, 2 *cun* lateral to the anterior midline (Fig. 16)

手厥阴心包经穴 [shǒu jué yīn xīn bāo jīng xué]

points of the pericardium meridian/channel: acupuncture-moxibustion points distributed on the pericardium meridian/channel (PC)

天池 [tiān chí]

***Tianchi* (PC 1):** point on the chest, in the 4th intercostal space, 1 *cun* lateral to the nipple and 5 *cun* lateral to the anterior midline (Fig. 9)

天泉 [tiān quán]

***Tianquan* (PC 2):** point on the medial side of the arm, 2 *cun* below the anterior end of the axillary fold, between the long and short heads of the biceps muscle of the arm (Fig. 15)

曲泽 [qū zé]

***Quze* (PC 3):** point at the midpoint of the cubital crease, on the ulnar side of the tendon of the biceps muscle of the arm (Fig. 15)

郄门 [xì mén]

***Ximen* (PC 4):** point on the palmar side of the forearm and on the line connecting *Quze* (PC 3) and *Daling* (PC 7), 5 *cun* above the crease of the wrist (Fig. 15)

间使 [jiān shǐ]

***Jianshi* (PC 5):** point on the palmar side of the forearm and on the line connecting *Quze* (PC 3) and *Daling* (PC 7), 3 *cun* above the crease of the wrist, between the tendons of the long palmar muscle and radial flexor muscle of the wrist (Fig. 15)

内关 [nèi guān]

***Neiguan* (PC 6):** point on the palmar side of the forearm and on the line connecting *Quze* (PC 3) and *Daling* (PC 7), 2 *cun* above the crease of the wrist, between the tendons of the long palmar muscle and radial flexor muscle of the wrist (Fig. 15)

大陵 [dà líng]

***Daling* (PC 7):** point at the midpoint of the crease of the wrist, between the tendons of the long palmar muscle and radial flexor muscle of the wrist (Fig. 15)

劳宫 [láo gōng]

***Laogong* (PC 8):** point at the center of the palm, between the 2nd and 3rd metacarpal bones, but closer to the latter, and in the part touching the tip of the middle finger when a fist is made (Fig. 15)

中冲 [zhōng chōng]

***Zhongchong* (PC 9):** point at the center of the tip of the middle finger (Fig. 15)

手少阳三焦经穴 [shǒu shào yáng sān jiāo jīng xué]

points of the triple energizer meridian/channel: acupuncture-moxibustion points distributed on the triple energizer meridian/channel (TE)

关冲 [guān chōng]

***Guanchong* (TE 1):** point on the ulnar side of the distal segment of the ring finger, 0.1 *cun* from the corner of the nail (Fig. 15)

液门 [yè mén]

***Yemen* (TE 2):** point on the dorsum of the hand, between the ring and small fingers, at the junction of the red and white skin, proximal to the margin of the web (Fig. 15)

中渚 [zhōng zhǔ]

***Zhongzhu* (TE 3):** point on the dorsum of the hand, proximal to the 4th metacarpophalangeal joint, in the depression between the 4th and 5th metacarpal bones (Fig. 15)

阳池 [yáng chí]

***Yangchi* (TE 4):** point at the midpoint of the dorsal crease of the wrist, in the depression on the ulnar side of the tendon of the extensor muscle of the fingers (Fig. 15)

外关 [wài guān]

***Waiguan* (TE 5):** point on the dorsal side of the forearm and on the line connecting *Yangchi* (TE 4) and the tip of the olecranon, 2 *cun* proximal to the dorsal crease of the wrist, between the radius and ulna (Fig. 15)

支沟 [zhī gōu]

***Zhigou* (TE 6):** point on the dorsal side of the forearm and on the line connecting *Yangchi* (TE 4) and the tip of the olecranon, 3 *cun* proximal to the dorsal crease of the wrist, between the radius and ulna (Fig. 15)

会宗 [huì zōng]

***Huizong* (TE 7):** point on the dorsal side of the forearm, 3 *cun* proximal to the dorsal crease of the wrist, on the ulnar side of *Zhigou* (TE 6) and on the radial border of the ulna (Fig. 15)

三阳络 [sān yáng luò]

***Sanyangluo* (TE 8):** point on the dorsal side of the forearm, 4 *cun* proximal to the dorsal crease of the wrist, between the radius and ulna (Fig. 15)

四渎 [sì dú]

***Sidu* (TE 9):** point on the dorsal side of the forearm and on the line connecting *Yangchi* (TE 4) and the tip of the olecranon, 5 *cun* distal to the tip of the olecranon, between the radius and ulna (Fig. 15)

天井 [tiān jǐng]

***Tianjing* (TE 10):** point on the lateral side of the upper arm, in the depression 1 *cun* proximal to the tip of the olecranon when the elbow is flexed (Fig. 15)

清冷渊 [qīng lěng yuān]

***Qinglengyuan* (TE 11):** point on the lateral side of the upper arm, 2 *cun* above the tip of the olecranon when the elbow is flexed and 1 *cun* above *Tianjing* (TE 10) (Fig. 15)

消泺 [xiāo luò]

***Xiaoluo* (TE 12):** point on the lateral side of the upper arm, at the midpoint of the line connecting *Qinglengyuan* (TE 11) and *Naohui* (TE 13) (Fig. 15)

臑会 [nào huì]

***Naohui* (TE 13):** point on the lateral side of the upper arm and on the line connecting the tip of the olecranon and *Jianliao* (TE 14), 3 *cun* below *Jianliao* (TE 14), and on the posterioinferior border of the deltoid muscle (Fig. 15)

肩髎 [jiān liáo]

***Jianliao* (TE 14):** point on the shoulder, posterior to *Jianyu* (LI 15), in the depression inferior and posterior to the acromion when the arm is abducted (Fig. 15)

天髎 [tiān liáo]

***Tianliao* (TE 15):** point on the scapula, at the midpoint between *Jianjing* (GB 21) and *Quyuan* (SI 13), at the superior angle of the scapula (Fig. 17a)

天牖 [tiān yǒu]

***Tianyou* (TE 16):** point on the lateral side of the neck, directly below the posterior border of the mastoid process, on the level of the mandibular angle, and on the posterior border of the sternocleidomastoid muscle (Fig. 17a and b)

翳风 [yì fēng]
***Yifeng* (TE 17):** point posterior to the ear lobe, in the depression between the mastoid process and mandibular angle (Fig. 17a and b)

瘛脉 [chì mài]
***Chimai* (TE 18):** point on the head, at the center of the mastoid process, and at the junction of the middle third and lower third of the line connecting *Jiaosun* (TE 20) and *Yifeng* (TE 17) along the curve of the ear helix (Fig. 17a and b)

颅息 [lú xī]
***Luxi* (TE 19):** point on the head, at the junction of the upper third and middle third of the line connecting *Jiaosun* (TE 20) and *Yifeng* (TE 17) along the curve of the ear helix (Fig. 17a and b)

角孙 [jiǎo sūn]
***Jiaosun* (TE 20):** point on the head, above the ear apex and within the hairline (Fig. 17a and b)

耳门 [ěr mén]
***Ermen* (TE 21):** point on the face, anterior to the supratragic notch, in the depression behind the posterior border of the condyloid process of the mandible (Fig. 17b)

耳和髎 [ěr hé liáo]
***Erheliao* (TE 22):** point on the lateral side of the head, on the posterior margin of the temples, anterior to the anterior border of the root of the ear auricle and posterior to the superficial temporal artery (Fig. 17b)

和髎 [hé liáo]
***Heliao* (TE 22):** same as *Erheliao* (耳和髎[ěr hé liáo])

丝竹空 [sī zhú kōng]
***Sizhukong* (TE 23):** point on the face, in the depression of the lateral end of the eyebrow (Fig. 17a and b)

足少阳胆经穴 [zú shào yáng dǎn jīng xué]
points of the gallbladder meridian/ channel: acupuncture-moxibustion points distributed on the gallbladder meridian/ channel (GB)

瞳子髎 [tóng zǐ liáo]
***Tongziliao* (GB 1):** point on the face, lateral to the outer canthus, on the lateral border of the orbit (Fig. 17a and b)

听会 [tīng huì]
***Tinghui* (GB 2):** point on the face, anterior to the intertragic notch, in the depression posterior to the condyloid process of the mandible when the mouth is open (Fig. 17b)

上关 [shàng guān]
***Shangguan* (GB 3):** point anterior to the ear, directly above *Xiaguan* (ST 7), in the depression above the upper border of the zygomatic arch (Fig. 17b)

颔厌 [hàn yàn]
***Hanyan* (GB 4):** point on the head, in the hair above the temple, at the junction of the upper fourth and lower three fourths of

the curved line connecting *Touwei* (ST 8) and *Qubin* (GB 7) (Fig. 17b)

悬颅 [xuán lú]
***Xuanlu* (GB 5):** point on the head, in the hair above the temple, at the midpoint of the curved line connecting *Touwei* (ST 8) and *Qubin* (GB 7) (Fig. 17b)

悬厘 [xuán lí]
***Xuanli* (GB 6):** point on the head, in the hair above the temples, at the junction of the upper three fourths and lower fourth of the curved line connecting *Touwei* (ST 8) and *Qubin* (GB 7) (Fig. 17b)

曲鬓 [qū bìn]
***Qubin* (GB 7):** point on the head, at the crossing point of the vertical posterior border of the temples and horizontal line through the ear apex (Fig. 17b)

率谷 [shuài gǔ]
***Shuaigu* (GB 8):** point on the head, directly above the ear apex, 1.5 *cun* above the hairline, directly above *Jiaosun* (TE 20) (Fig. 17b)

天冲 [tiān chōng]
***Tianchong* (GB 9):** point on the head, directly above the posterior border of the ear root, 2 *cun* above the hairline and 0.5 *cun* posterior to *Shuaigu* (GB 8) (Fig. 17a and b)

浮白 [fú bái]
***Fubai* (GB 10):** point on the head, posterior and superior to the mastoid process, at the junction of the middle third and upper third of the curved line connecting *Tianchong* (GB 9) and *Wangu* (GB 12) (Fig. 17a and b)

头窍阴 [tóu qiào yīn]
***Touqiaoyin* (GB 11):** point on the head, posterior and superior to the mastoid process, at the junction of the middle third and lower third of the curved line connecting *Tianchong* (GB 9) and *Wangu* (GB 12) (Fig. 17a and b)

完骨 [wán gǔ]
***Wangu* (GB 12):** point on the head, in the depression posterior and inferior to the mastoid process (Fig. 17b)

本神 [běn shén]
***Benshen* (GB 13):** point on the head, 0.5 *cun* above the anterior hairline, 3 *cun* lateral to *Shenting* (GV 24), at the junction of the medial two thirds and lateral third of the line connecting *Shenting* (GV 24) and *Touwei* (ST 8) (Fig. 17a and b)

阳白 [yáng bái]
***Yangbai* (GB 14):** point on the forehead, directly above the pupil, 1 *cun* above the eyebrow (Fig. 17a and b)

头临泣 [tóu lín qì]
***Toulinqi* (GB 15):** point on the head, directly above the pupil and 0.5 *cun* above the anterior hairline, at the midpoint of the line connecting *Shenting* (GV 24) and *Touwei* (ST 8) (Fig. 17a and b)

目窗 [mù chuāng]
***Muchuang* (GB 16):** point on the head, 1.5 *cun* above the anterior hairline and 2.25 cun lateral to the midline of the head (Fig. 17a and b)

正营 [zhèng yíng]
***Zhengying* (GB 17):** point on the head, 2.5

cun above the anterior hairline and 2.25 *cun* lateral to the midline of the head (Fig. 17b)

承灵 [chéng líng]
***Chengling* (GB 18):** point on the head, 4 *cun* above the anterior hairline and 2.25 *cun* lateral to the midline of the head (Fig. 17a and b)

脑空 [nǎo kōng]
***Naokong* (GB 19):** point on the head and on the level of the upper border of the external occipital protuberance or *Naohu* (GV 17) , 2.25 *cun* lateral to the midline of the head (Fig. 17a and b)

风池 [fēng chí]
***Fengchi* (GB 20):** point on the nape, below the occipital bone, on the level of *Fengfu* (GV 16), in the depression between the upper ends of the sternocleidomastoid and trapezius muscles (Fig. 17a and b)

肩井 [jiān jǐng]
***Jianjing* (GB 21):** point on the shoulder, directly above the nipple, at the midpoint of the line connecting *Dazhui* (GV 14) and the acromion (Fig. 17a and 24)

渊液 [yuān yè]
***Yuanye* (GB 22):** point on the lateral side of the chest, on the midaxillary line when the arm is raised, 3 *cun* below the axilla, in the 4th intercostal space

辄筋 [zhé jīn]
***Zhejin* (GB 23):** point on the lateral side of the chest, 1 *cun* anterior to *Yuanye* (GB 22), on the level of the nipple, and in the 4th intercostal space

日月 [rì yuè]
***Riyue* (GB 24):** point on the upper abdomen, directly below the nipple, in the 7th intercostal space, 4 *cun* lateral to the anterior midline (Fig. 16)

京门 [jīng mén]
***Jingmen* (GB 25):** point on the lateral side of the waist, 1.8 *cun* posterior to *Zhangmen* (LR 13), below the free end of the 12th rib (Fig. 16)

带脉 [dài mài]
***Daimai* (GB 26):** point on the lateral side of the abdomen, 1.8 *cun* below *Zhangmen* (LR 13), at the crossing point of a vertical line through the free end of the 11th rib and a horizontal line through the umbilicus (Fig. 16)

五枢 [wǔ shū]
***Wushu* (GB 27):** point on the lateral side of the abdomen, anterior to the anteriosuperior iliac spine, 3 *cun* below the level of the umbilicus (Fig. 16)

维道 [wéi dào]
***Weidao* (GB 28):** point on the lateral side of the abdomen, anterior and inferior to the anteriosuperior iliac spine, 0.5 *cun* anterior and inferior to *Wushu* (GB 27) (Fig. 16)

居髎 [jū liáo]
***Juliao* (GB 29):** point on the hip, at the midpoint of the line connecting the anteriosuperior iliac spine and the prominence of the great trochanter

环跳 [huán tiào]
***Huantiao* (GB 30):** point on the lateral side of the thigh, at the junction of the

middle third and lateral third of the line connecting the prominence of the great trochanter and the sacral hiatus when the patient is in a lateral recumbent position with the thigh flexed (Fig. 18)

风市 [fēng shì]
***Fengshi* (GB 31):** point on the lateral midline of the thigh, 7 *cun* above the popliteal crease, or at the place touching the tip of the middle finger when the patient stands erect with the arms hanging down freely (Fig. 18)

中渎 [zhōng dú]
***Zhongdu* (GB 32):** point on the lateral side of the thigh, 2 *cun* below *Fengshi* (GB 31), or 5 *cun* above the popliteal crease, between the lateral vastus muscle and biceps muscle of the thigh (Fig. 18)

膝阳关 [xī yáng guān]
***Xiyangguan* (GB 33):** point on the lateral side of the knee, 3 *cun* above *Yanglingquan* (GB 34) , in the depression above the external epicondyle of the femur (Fig. 18)

阳陵泉 [yáng líng quán]
***Yanglingquan* (GB 34):** point on the lateral side of the leg, in the depression anterior and inferior to the head of the fibula (Fig. 18)

阳交 [yáng jiāo]
***Yangjiao* (GB 35):** point on the lateral side of the leg, 7 *cun* above the tip of the external malleolus, on the posterior border of the fibula (Fig. 18)

外丘 [wài qiū]
***Waiqiu* (GB 36):** point on the lateral side of the leg, 7 *cun* above the tip of the external malleolus, on the anterior border of the fibula and on the level of *Yangjiao* (GB 35) (Fig. 18)

光明 [guāng míng]
***Guangming* (GB 37):** point on the lateral side of the leg, 5 *cun* above the tip of the external malleolus, on the anterior border of the fibula (Fig. 18)

阳辅 [yáng fǔ]
***Yangfu* (GB 38):** point on the lateral side of the leg, 4 *cun* above the tip of the external malleolus, slightly anterior to the anterior border of the fibula (Fig. 18)

悬钟 [xuán zhōng]
***Xuanzhong* (GB 39):** point on the lateral side of the leg, 3 *cun* above the tip of the external malleolus, on the anterior border of the fibula (Fig. 18)

丘墟 [qiū xū]
***Qiuxu* (GB 40):** point anterior and inferior to the external malleolus, in the depression lateral to the tendon of the long extensor muscle of the toes (Fig. 18)

足临泣 [zú lín qì]
***Zulinqi* (GB 41):** point on the lateral side of the instep of the foot, posterior to the 4th metatarsophalangeal joint, in the depression lateral to the tendon of the extensor muscle of the little toe (Fig. 18)

地五会 [dì wǔ huì]
***Diwuhui* (GB 42):** point on the lateral side of the instep of the foot, posterior to the 4th metatarsophalangeal joint, between the 4th and 5th metatarsal bones, medial to the

tendon of the extensor muscle of the little toe (Fig. 18)

侠溪 [xiá xī]

***Xiaxi* (GB 43):** point on the lateral side of the instep of the foot, between the 4th and 5th toes, at the junction of the red and white skin, proximal to the margin of the web (Fig. 18)

足窍阴 [zú qiào yīn]

***Zuqiaoyin* (GB 44):** point on the lateral side of the distal segment of the 4th toe, 0.1 *cun* from the corner of the toenail (Fig. 18)

足厥阴肝经穴 [zú jué yīn gān jīng xué]

points of the liver meridian/channel: acupuncture-moxibustion points distributed on the liver meridian/channel (LR)

大敦 [dà dūn]

***Dadun* (LR 1):** point on the lateral side of the distal segment of the big toe, 0.1 *cun* proximal to the corner of the nail (Fig. 18)

行间 [xíng jiān]

***Xingjian* (LR 2):** point on the instep of the foot, between the 1st and 2nd toes, at the junction of the red and white skin proximal to the margin of the web (Fig. 18)

太冲 [tài chōng]

***Taichong* (LR 3):** point on the instep of the foot, in the depression of the posterior end of the 1st interosseous metatarsal space (Fig. 18)

中封 [zhōng fēng]

***Zhongfeng* (LR 4):** point on the instep of the foot, anterior to the medial malleolus, on the line connecting *Shangqiu* (SP 5) and *Jiexi* (ST 41), in the depression medial to the tendon of the anterior tibial muscle (Fig. 18)

蠡沟 [lí gōu]

***Ligou* (LR 5):** point on the medial side of the leg, 5 *cun* above the tip of the medial malleolus, on the midline of the medial surface of the tibia (Fig. 18)

中都 [zhōng dū]

***Zhongdu* (LR 6):** point on the medial side of the leg, 7 *cun* above the tip of the medial malleolus, on the midline of the medial surface of the tibia (Fig. 18)

膝关 [xī guān]

***Xiguan* (LR 7):** point on the medial side of the leg, posterior and inferior to the medial epicondyle of the tibia, 1 *cun* posterior to *Yinlingquan* (SP 9), at the upper end of the medial head of the gastrocnemius muscle (Fig. 18)

曲泉 [qū quán]

***Ququan* (LR 8):** point on the medial side of the knee, at the medial end of the popliteal crease when the knee is flexed, posterior to the medial epicondyle of the tibia, in the depression of the anterior border of the insertion of the semimemebranous and semitendinous muscles (Fig. 18)

阴包 [yīn bāo]

***Yinbao* (LR 9):** point on the medial side of the thigh, 4 *cun* above the medial epicondyle of the femur, between the medial vastus muscle and sartorius muscle (Fig. 18)

足五里 [zú wǔ lǐ]
Zuwuli (LR 10): point on the medial side of the thigh, 3 *cun* directly below *Qichong* (ST 30), at the proximal end of the thigh, below the pubic tubercle and on the lateral border of the long abductor muscle of the thigh (Fig. 18)

阴廉 [yīn lián]
Yinlian (LR 11): point on the medial side of the thigh, 2 *cun* directly below *Qichong* (ST 30), at the proximal end of the thigh, below the pubic tubercle and on the lateral border of the long abductor muscle of the thigh (Fig. 18)

急脉 [jí mài]
Jimai (LR 12): point lateral to the pubic tubercle, lateral and inferior to *Qichong* (ST 30), in the inguinal groove where the pulsation of the femoral artery is palpable, 2.5 *cun* lateral to the anterior midline (Fig. 16)

章门 [zhāng mén]
Zhangmen (LR 13): point on the lateral side of the abdomen, below the free end of the 11th rib (Fig. 16)

期门 [qī mén]
Qimen (LR 14): point on the chest, directly below the nipple, in the 6th intercostal space, 4 *cun* lateral to the anterior midline (Fig. 16)

督脉穴 [dū mài xué]
points of the governor vessel: acupuncture-moxibustion points distributed on the governor vessel (GV)

长强 [cháng qiáng]
Changqiang (GV 1): point below the tip of the coccyx, at the midpoint of the line connecting the tip of the coccyx and anus (Fig. 16)

腰俞 [yāo shù]
Yaoshu (GV 2): point on the sacrum and on the posterior midline, just at the sacral hiatus (Fig. 16)

腰阳关 [yāo yáng guān]
Yaoyangguan (GV 3): point on the lower back and on the posterior midline, in the depression below the spinous process of the 4th lumbar vertebra (Fig. 16)

命门 [mìng mén]
Mingmen (GV 4): point on the lower back and on the posterior midline, in the depression below the spinous process of the 2nd lumbar vertebra (Fig. 16)

悬枢 [xuán shū]
Xuanshu (GV 5): point on the lower back and on the posterior midline, in the depression below the spinous process of the 1st lumbar vertebra (Fig. 16)

脊中 [jǐ zhōng]
Jizhong (GV 6): point on the back and on the posterior midline, in the depression below the spinous process of the 11th thoracic vertebra (Fig. 16)

中枢 [zhōng shū]
Zhongshu (GV 7): point on the back and on the posterior midline, in the depression below the spinous process of the 10th thoracic vertebra (Fig. 16)

筋缩 [jīn suō]

***Jinsuo* (GV 8):** point on the back and on the posterior midline, in the depression below the spinous process of the 9th thoracic vertebra (Fig. 16)

至阳 [zhì yáng]

***Zhiyang* (GV 9):** point on the back and on the posterior midline, in the depression below the spinous process of the 7th thoracic vertebra (Fig. 16)

灵台 [líng tái]

***Lingtai* (GV 10):** point on the back and on the posterior midline, in the depression below the spinous process of the 6th thoracic vertebra (Fig. 16)

神道 [shén dào]

***Shendao* (GV 11):** point on the back and on the posterior midline, in the depression below the spinous process of the 5th thoracic vertebra (Fig. 16)

身柱 [shēn zhù]

***Shenzhu* (GV 12):** point on the back and on the posterior midline, in the depression below the spinous process of the 3rd thoracic vertebra (Fig. 16)

陶道 [táo dào]

***Taodao* (GV 13):** point on the back and on the posterior midline, in the depression below the spinous process of the 1st thoracic vertebra (Fig. 17a and 16)

大椎 [dà zhuī]

***Dazhui* (GV 14):** point on the posterior midline, in the depression below the 7th cervical vertebra (Fig. 17a and 16)

哑门 [yǎ mén]

***Yamen* (GV 15):** point on the nape, 0.5 *cun* directly above the midpoint of the posterior hairline, below the 1st cervical vertebra (Fig. 17a and b)

风府 [fēng fǔ]

***Fengfu* (GV 16):** point on the nape, 1 *cun* directly above the midpoint of the posterior hairline, directly below the external occipital protuberance, in the depression between the trapezius muscle of both sides (Fig. 17a and b)

脑户 [nǎo hù]

***Naohu* (GV 17):** point on the head, 2.5 *cun* directly above the midpoint of the posterior hairline, in the depression on the upper border of the external occipital protuberance (Fig. 17a and b)

强间 [qiáng jiān]

***Qiangjian* (GV 18):** point on the head, 4 *cun* directly above the midpoint of the posterior hairline and 1.5 *cun* above *Naohu* (GV 17) (Fig. 17a and b)

后顶 [hòu dǐng]

***Houding* (GV 19):** point on the head, 5.5 *cun* directly above the midpoint of the posterior hairline and 3 *cun* above *Naohu* (GV 17) (Fig. 17a and b)

百会 [bǎi huì]

***Baihui* (GV 20):** point on the head, 5 *cun* directly above the midpoint of the anterior hairline, at the midpoint of the line connecting the apexes of both ears (Fig. 17a and b)

前顶 [qián dǐng]
***Qianding* (GV 21):** point on the head, 3.5 *cun* directly above the midpoint of the anterior hairline and 1.5 *cun* anterior to *Baihui* (GV 20) (Fig. 17a and b)

囟会 [xìn huì]
***Xinhui* (GV 22):** point on the head, 2 *cun* directly above the midpoint of the anterior hairline and 3 *cun* anterior to *Baihui* (GV 20) (Fig. 17a and b)

上星 [shàng xīng]
***Shangxing* (GV 23):** point on the head, 1 *cun* directly above the midpoint of the anterior hairline (Fig. 17a and b)

神庭 [shén tíng]
***Shenting* (GV 24):** point on the head, 0.5 *cun* directly above the midpoint of the anterior hairline (Fig. 17a and b)

素髎 [sù liáo]
***Suliao* (GV 25):** point at the center of the apex of the nose (Fig. 17a and b)

水沟 [shuǐ gōu]
***Shuigou* (GV 26):** point at the junction of the upper third and middle third of the philtrum (Fig. 17a and b)

兑端 [duì duān]
***Duiduan* (GV 27):** point on the labial tubercle of the upper lip, on the vermilion border between the philtrum and upper lip (Fig. 17a and b)

龈交 [yín jiāo]
***Yinjiao* (GV 28):** point inside the upper lip, at the junction of the labial frenum and upper gum (Fig. 17a and b)

任脉穴 [rèn mài xué]
points of the conception vessel: acupuncture-moxibustion points distributed on the conception vessel (CV)

会阴 [huì yīn]
***Huiyin* (CV 1):** point on the perineum, at the midpoint between the posterior border of the scrotum and anus in male, and between the posterior commissure of the large labia and anus in female (Fig. 20)

曲骨 [qū gǔ]
***Qugu* (CV 2):** point on the lower abdomen and on the anterior midline, at the midpoint of the upper border of the pubic symphysis (Fig. 16)

中极 [zhōng jí]
***Zhongji* (CV 3):** point on the lower abdomen and on the anterior midline, 4 *cun* below the center of the umbilicus (Fig. 16)

关元 [guān yuán]
***Guanyuan* (CV 4):** point on the lower abdomen and on the anterior midline, 3 *cun* below the center of the umbilicus (Fig. 16)

石门 [shí mén]
***Shimen* (CV 5):** point on the lower abdomen and on the anterior midline, 2 *cun* below the center of the umbilicus (Fig. 16)

气海 [qì hǎi]
***Qihai* (CV 6):** point on the lower abdomen and on the anterior midline, 1.5 *cun* below the center of the umbilicus (Fig. 16)

阴交 [yīn jiāo]

***Yinjiao* (CV 7):** point on the lower abdomen and on the anterior midline, 1 *cun* below the center of the umbilicus (Fig. 16)

神阙 [shén què]

***Shenque* (CV 8):** point on the middle abdomen and at the center of the umbilicus (Fig. 16)

水分 [shuǐ fēn]

***Shuifen* (CV 9):** point on the upper abdomen and on the anterior midline, 1 *cun* above the center of the umbilicus (Fig. 16)

下脘 [xià wǎn]

***Xiawan* (CV 10):** point on the upper abdomen and on the anterior midline, 2 *cun* above the center of the umbilicus (Fig. 16)

建里 [jiàn lǐ]

***Jianli* (CV 11):** point on the upper abdomen and on the anterior midline, 3 *cun* above the center of the umbilicus (Fig. 16)

中脘 [zhōng wǎn]

***Zhongwan* (CV 12):** point on the upper abdomen and on the anterior midline, 4 *cun* above the center of the umbilicus (Fig. 16)

上脘 [shàng wǎn]

***Shangwan* (CV 13):** point on the upper abdomen and on the anterior midline, 5 *cun* above the center of the umbilicus (Fig. 16)

巨阙 [jù què]

***Juque* (CV 14):** point on the upper abdomen and on the anterior midline, 6 *cun* above the center of the umbilicus (Fig. 16)

鸠尾 [jiū wěi]

***Jiuwei* (CV 15):** point on the upper abdomen and on the anterior midline, 1 *cun* below the xiphosternal synchondrosis (Fig. 16)

中庭 [zhōng tíng]

***Zhongting* (CV 16):** point on the chest and on the anterior midline, on the level of the 5th intercostal space, on the xiphosternal synchondrosis (Fig. 16)

膻中 [dàn zhōng]

***Danzhong* (CV 17):** point on the chest and on the anterior midline, on the level of the 4th intercostal space, at the midpoint of the line connecting both nipples (Fig. 16)

玉堂 [yù táng]

***Yutang* (CV 18):** point on the chest and on the anterior midline, on the level of the 3rd intercostal space (Fig. 16)

紫宫 [zǐ gōng]

***Zigong* (CV 19):** point on the chest and on the anterior midline, on the level of the 2nd intercostal space (Fig. 16)

华盖 [huágài]

***Huagai* (CV 20):** point on the chest and on the anterior midline, on the level of the 1st intercostal space (Fig. 16)

璇玑 [xuán jī]

***Xuanji* (CV 21):** point on the chest and on

the anterior midline, 1 *cun* below *Tiantu* (CV 22) (Fig. 16)

天突 [tiān tū]
***Tiantu* (CV 22):** point on the neck and on the anterior midline, at the center of the suprasternal fossa (Fig. 16)

廉泉 [lián quán]
***Lianquan* (CV 23):** point on the neck and on the anterior midline, in the depression of the upper border of the hyoid bone (Fig. 16)

承浆 [chéng jiāng]
***Chengjiang* (CV 24):** point on the face, in the depression at the midpoint of the mentolabial sulcus (Fig. 16)

特定穴 [tè dìng xué]
specific points: points on the meridians/channels with specific therapeutic effects, hence, specific names. They embrace the five transport points, source points, connecting points, alarm points, back transport points, eight influential points, cleft points, crossing points, eight confluence points, and lower sea points.

五输穴 [wǔ shū xué]
five transport points: five points on the twelve meridians/channels distributing distal to the elbow and knees, varying in their condition of the flow of *qi* and blood. They consist of well points, spring points, stream points, river points and sea points.

井穴 [jǐng xué]
well points: transport points located at the ends of the fingers or toes. Each of the twelve meridians/channels has a well point. They are *Shaoshang* (LU 11), *Shangyang* (LI 1), *Zhongchong* (PC 9), *Guanchong* (TE 1), *Shaochong* (HT 9), *Shaoze* (SI 1), *Yinbai* (SP 1), *Lidui* (ST 45), *Dadun* (LR 1), *Zuqiaoyin* (GB 44), *Yongquan* (KI 1), and *Zhiyin* (BL 67). They are mainly used for emergency revival.

荥穴 [yíng xué]
spring points: transport points located at the distal ends of the limbs mainly in the metacarpal and metatarsal regions. Each of the twelve regular meridians/channels has a spring point, namely, *Yuji* (LU 10), *Erjian* (LI 2), *Laogong* (PC 8), *Yeman* (TE 2), *Shaofu* (HT 8), *Qiangu* (SI 2), *Dadu* (SP 2), *Neiting* (ST 44), *Xingjian* (LR 2), *Xiaxi* (GB 43), *Rangu* (KI 2), and *Tonggu* (BL 66). They are mainly used for treating febrile diseases.

输穴 [shū xué]
(I) acupoints: acupuncture points in general, also known as 俞穴 [shù xué] and 腧穴 [shù xué]; **(II) stream points:** transport points located on the hands or feet. Each of the twelve regular meridians/channels has a stream point, namely, *Taiyuan* (LU 9), *Sanjian* (LI 3), *Daling* (PC 7), *Zhongzhu* (TE 3), *Shenmen* (HT 7), *Houxi* (SI 3), *Taibai* (SP 3), *Xiangu* (ST 43), *Taichong* (LR 3), *Zulinqi* (GB 41), *Taixi* (KI 3), and *Shugu* (BL 65). They are mainly used for treating arthralgia.

经穴 [jīng xué]
(I) meridian/channel points: points on the fourteen meridians/channels, 361 in all; **(II) river points:** transport points mostly located on the legs and forearms. Each

of the twelve regular meridians/channels has a river point, namely, *Jingqu* (LU 8), *Yangxi* (LI 5), *Jianshi* (PC 5), *Zhigou* (TE 6), *Lingdao* (HT 4), *Yanggu* (SI 5), *Shangqiu* (SP 5), *Jiexi* (ST 41), *Zhongfeng* (LR 4), *Yangfu* (GB 38), *Fuliu* (KI 7), and *Kunlun* (BL 60). They are mainly used for treating cough, asthma, and disorders of the throat.

合穴 [hé xué]

sea points: transport points mostly located at the elbow or the knee. Each of the twelve regular meridians/channels has a sea point, namely, *Chize* (LU 5), *Quchi* (LI 11), *Quze* (PC 3), *Tianjing* (TE 10), *Shaohai* (HT 3), *Xiaohai* (SI 8), *Yinlingquan* (SP 9), *Zusanli* (ST 36), *Ququan* (LR 8), *Yanglingquan* (GB 34), *Yingu* (KI 10), and *Weizhong* (BL 40). They are mainly used for treating diseases of the *fu* organs, such as the stomach and intestines.

原穴 [yuán xué]

source points: points where the original *qi* of *zang-fu* organs passes or stays. Each of the twelve regular meridians/channels has a source point, namely, *Taiyuan* (LU 9), *Jinggu* (BL 64), *Hegu* (LI 4), *Taixi* (KI 3), *Chongyang* (ST 42), *Daling* (PC 7), *Taibai* (SP 3), *Yangchi* (TE 4), *Shenmen* (HT 7), *Qiuxu* (GB 40), *Wangu* (SI 4), and *Taichong* (LR 3).

络穴 [luò xué]

connecting points: points for the fourteen meridians/channels to connect the respective yin and yang meridians/channels interior-exteriorly. The spleen meridian/channel has two connecting points, hence fifteen in all. They are *Pianli* (LI 6), *Dazhong* (KI 4), *Lieque* (LU 7), *Feiyang* (BL 58), *Gongsun* (SP 4), *Waiguan* (TE 5), *Fenglong* (ST 40), *Neiguan* (PC 6), *Zhizheng* (SI 7), *Ligou* (LR 5), *Tongli* (HT 5), *Guangming* (GB 37), *Dabao* (SP 21), *Changqiang* (GV 1), and *Jiuwei* (CV 15).

郄穴 [xì xué]

cleft point: point where the meridian/channel *qi* accumulates deeply. Each of the twelve regular meridians/channels, together with the yin heel, yang heel, yin link, and yang link vessels has a cleft point, hence sixteen in all. They are *Kongzui* (LU 6), *Huizong* (TE 7), *Ximen* (PC 4), *Yanglao* (SI 6), *Yinxi* (HT 6), *Liangqiu* (ST 34), *Wenliu* (LI 7), *Waiqiu* (GB 36), *Jinmen* (UB 63), *Fuyang* (UB 59), *Diji* (SP 8), *Jiaoxin* (KI 8), *Zhongdu* (LR 6), *Yangjiao* (GB 35), *Shuiquan* (K I5), and *Zhubin* (K I9). The cleft point is mainly used to treat acute disorders and pains in the area related to its respective meridian/channel, and diseases of the corresponding internal organ.

募穴 [mù xué]

alarm point: point located on the chest or abdomen, where the *qi* of the respective internal organ is concentrated, and so pathological reactions such as tenderness will be found if the internal organ is diseased. *Zhongfu* (LU 1), *Zhongwan* (CV 12), *Danzhong* (CV 17), *Shimen* (CV 5), *Juque* (CV 14), *Jingmen* (GB 25), *Qimen* (LR 4), *Tianshu* (ST 25), *Riyue* (GB 24), *Guanyuan* (CV 4), *Zhangmen* (LR 13), and *Zhongji* (CV 3) are all the alarm points.

背俞穴 [bèi shù xué]
back transport points: specific points located along the bladder meridian/channel on the back whither the *qi* of the *zang-fu* organs flows, and pain upon pressure is often found when the corresponding *zang-fu* organ is diseased. The points and their corresponding organs are: *Feishu* (BL 13) – lung; *Jueyinshu* (BL 14) – pericardium; *Xinshu* (BL 15) – heart; *Ganshu* (BL 18) – liver; *Danshu* (BL 19) – gallbladder; *Pishu* (BL 20) – spleen; *Sanjiaoshu* (BL 22) – triple energizer; *Shenshu* (BL 23) – kidney; *Dachangshu* (BL 25) – large intestine; *Xiaochangshu* (BL 27) – small intestine; *Pangguanshu* (BL 28) – urinary bladder.

八会穴 [bā huì xué]
eight influential points: eight important points which are closely related to the *zang*, *fu*, *qi*, blood, bones, marrow, tendons and blood vessels respectively, namely, *Zhangmen* (LR 13) to the *zang*-organs, *Zhongwan* (CV 12) to the *fu*-organs, *Danzhong* (CV 17) to *qi*, *Geshu* (BL 17) to blood, *Dazhu* (BL 11) to the bones, *Xuanzhong* (GB 39) to the marrow, *Yanglingquan* (GB 34) to the tendons, and *Taiyuan* (LU 9) to the vessels

交会穴 [jiāo huì xué]
crossing point: a point where two or more meridians/channels intersect

八脉交会穴 [bā mài jiāo huì xué]
eight confluence points: points where the regular meridians/channels communicate with the eight extra meridians/channels, namely, *Gongsun* (SP4), *Neiguan* (PC 6), *Houxi* (SI 3), *Shenmai* (BL 62), *Waiguan* (TE 5), *Zulinqi* (GB 41), *Lieque* (LU 7), and *Zhaohai* (KI 6)

下合穴 [xià hé xué]
lower confluent points; lower sea points: specific points on the three yang meridians/channels of the foot where the *qi* of the six *fu*-organs flows into the meridian/channel, namely, *Zusanli* (ST 36) for the stomach, *Shangjuxu* (ST 37) for the large intestine, *Xiajuxu* (ST 39) for the small intestine, *Yanglingquan* (GB 34) for the gallbladder, *Weizhong* (BL 40) for the urinary bladder, and *Weiyang* (BL 39) for the triple energizer. Since three of them, i.e., ST 36, GB 34 and BL 40 are the same as the sea points, they are also called lower sea points.

经外穴 Extra Points

经外穴 [jīng wài xué]
extra points: acupuncture-moxibustion points not distributed on the meridians

头颈部穴 [tóu jǐng bù xué]
points of the head and neck (HN): extra points located on the head and neck

四神聪 [sì shén cōng]
***Sishencong* (EX-HN 1):** four points on the head, 1 *cun* anterior, posterior and lateral to *Baihui* (GV 20) (Fig. 19)

当阳 [dāng yáng]
***Dangyang* (EX-HN 2):** point at the forehead, directly above the pupil, 1 *cun* above the anterior hairline (Fig. 19)

印堂 [yìn táng]

***Yintang* (EX-HN 3):** point on the forehead, at the midpoint between the eyebrows (Fig. 19)

鱼腰 [yú yāo]

***Yuyao* (EX-HN 4):** point on the forehead, directly above the pupil, in the eyebrow (Fig. 19)

太阳 [tài yáng]

***Taiyang* (EX-HN 5):** point at the temporal part of the head, between the lateral end of the eyebrow and the outer canthus, in the depression one finger breadth behind (Fig. 19)

耳尖 [ěr jiān]

***Erjian* (EX-HN 6):** point at the apex of the auricle when the ear is folded forward (Fig. 19)

球后 [qiú hòu]

***Qiuhou* (EX-HN 7):** point on the face, at the junction of the lateral fourth and medial three fourths of the infraorbital margin (Fig. 19)

上迎香 [shàng yíng xiāng]

***Shangyingxiang* (EX-HN 8):** point on the face, at the junction of the alar cartilage of the nose and the nasal concha, near the upper end of the nasolabial groove (Fig. 19)

内迎香 [nèi yíng xiāng]

***Neiyingxiang* (EX-HN 9):** point in the nostril, at the junction between the alar cartilage of the nose and the nasal concha (Fig. 19)

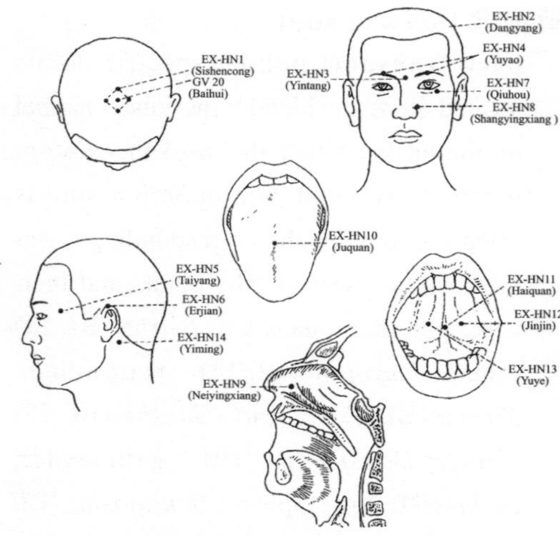

Fig. 19 Extra points on the head and neck

聚泉 [jù quán]

***Juquan* (EX-HN 10):** point in the mouth, at the midpoint of the dorsal midline of the tongue (Fig. 19)

海泉 [hǎi quán]

***Haiquan* (EX-HN 11):** point in the mouth, at the midpoint of the frenulum of the tongue (Fig. 19)

金津 [jīn jīn]

***Jinjin* (EX-HN 12):** point in the mouth, on the vein on the left side of the frenulum of the tongue (Fig. 19)

玉液 [yù yè]

***Yuye* (EX-HN 13):** point in the mouth, on the vein on the right side of the frenulum of the tongue (Fig. 19)

翳明 [yì míng]

***Yiming* (EX-HN 14):** point on the nape, 1 *cun* posterior to *Yifen* (TE 17) (Fig. 19)

颈白劳 [jǐng bái láo]

***Jingbailao* (EX-HN 15):** point on the nape, 2 *cun* above *Dazhui* (GV 14) and 1 *cun* lateral to the posterior midline (Fig. 19)

胸腹部穴 [xiōng fù bù xué]

points on the chest and abdomen (CA): extra points located on the chest and abdomen

子宫 [zǐ gōng]

***Zigong* (EX-CA 1):** point on the lower abdomen, 4 *cun* below the center of the umbilicus and 3 *cun* lateral to *Zhongji* (CV 3) (Fig. 20)

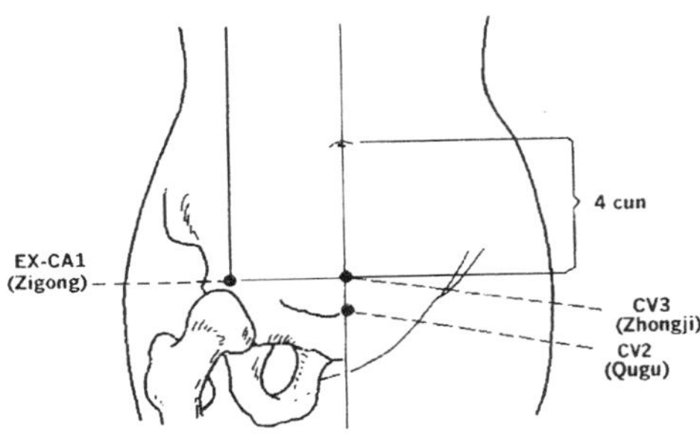

Fig. 20 Extra points on the abdomen

背部穴 [bèi bù xué]

points on the back (B): extra points located on the back

定喘 [dìng chuǎn]

***Dingchuan* (EX-B 1):** point on the back, below the spinous process of the 7th cervical vertebra, 0.5 *cun* lateral to the posterior midline (Fig. 21)

夹脊 [jiá jǐ]

***Jiaji* (EX-B 2):** 17 points on each side of the back, below the spinous processes from the 1st thoracic to the 5th lumbar vertebrae, 0.5 *cun* lateral to the posterior midline (Fig. 21)

胃脘下俞 [wèi wǎn xià shù]

***Weiwanxiashu* (EX-B 3):** point on the back, below the spinous process of the 8th thoracic vertebra, 1.5 *cun* lateral to the posterior midline (Fig. 21)

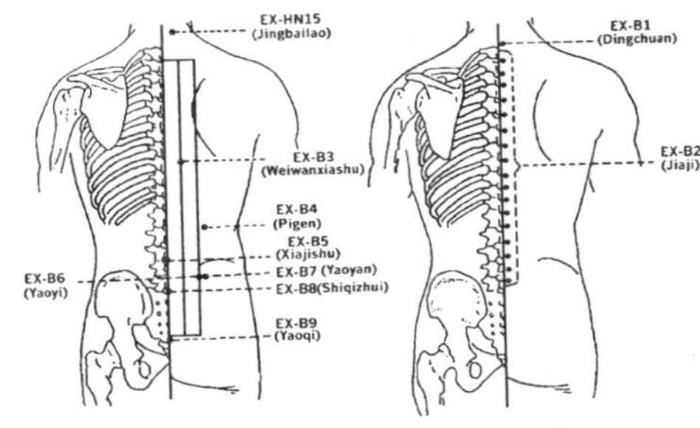

Fig. 21 Extra points on the back

痞根 [pǐ gēn]

***Pigen* (EX-B 4):** point on the lower back, below the spinous process of the 1st lumbar vertebra, 3.5 *cun* lateral to the posterior midline (Fig. 21)

下极俞 [xià jí shù]

***Xiajishu* (EX-B 5):** point on the midline of the lower back, below the spinous process of the 3rd lumbar vertebra (Fig. 21)

腰宜 [yāo yí]

***Yaoyi* (EX-B 6):** point on the lower back, below the spinous process of the 4th lumbar vertebra, 3 *cun* lateral to the posterior midline (Fig. 21)

腰眼 [yāo yǎn]

***Yaoyan* (EX-B 7):** point on the lower back, below the spinous process of the 4th lumbar vertebra, in the depression 3.5 *cun* lateral to the posterior midline (Fig. 21)

十七椎 [shí qī zhuī]

***Shiqizhui* (EX-B 8):** point on the lower back and on the posterior midline, below the spinous process of the 5th lumbar vertebra (Fig. 21)

腰奇 [yāo qí]

***Yaoqi* (EX-B 9):** point on the lower back, 2 cun directly above the tip of the coccyx, in the depression between the sacral horns (Fig. 21)

上肢穴 [shàng zhī xué]

points of the upper extremities (UE): extra points located on the upper extremities

肘尖 [zhǒu jiān]

***Zhoujian* (EX-UE 1):** point on the posterior side of the elbow, at the tip of the olecranon when the elbow is flexed (Fig. 22)

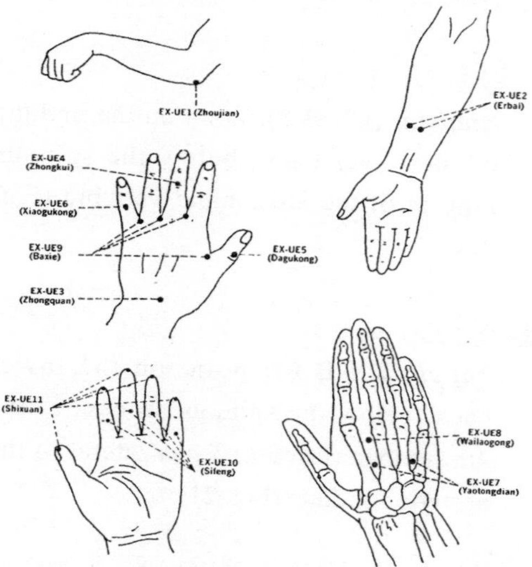

Fig. 22 Extra points on the upper extremity

二白 [èr bái]

***Erbai* (EX-UE 2):** two points on the palmar side of each forearm, 4 *cun* proximal to the crease of the wrist, on each side of the tendon of the radial flexor muscle of the wrist (Fig. 22)

中泉 [zhōng quán]

***Zhongquan* (EX-UE 3):** point on the dorsal crease of the wrist, in the depression on the radial side of the tendon of the common extensor muscle of the fingers (Fig. 22)

中魁 [zhōng kuí]

***Zhongkui* (EX-UE 4):** point on the dorsal side of the middle finger, at the center of the proximal interphalangeal joint (Fig. 22)

大骨空 [dà gǔ kōng]

***Dagukong* (EX-UE 5):** point on the dorsal side of the thumb, at the center of the interphalangeal joint (Fig. 22)

小骨空 [xiǎo gǔ kōng]

***Xiaogukong* (EX-UE 6):** point on the dorsal side of the little finger, at the center of the proximal interphalangeal joint (Fig. 22)

腰痛点 [yāo tòng diǎn]

***Yaotongdian* (EX-UE 7):** two points on the dorsum of each hand, between the 2nd and 3rd, and between the 4th and 5th metacarpal bones, and at the midpoint between the dorsal crease of the wrist and the metacarpo-phalangeal joint (Fig. 22)

外劳宫 [wài láo gōng]

***Wailaogong* (EX-UE 8):** point on the dorsum of the hand, between the 2nd and 3rd metacarpal bones, and 0.5 *cun* proximal to the metacarpo-phalangeal joint (Fig. 22)

八邪 [bā xié]

***Baxie* (EX-UE 9):** four points on the dorsum of each hand, at the junction of the red and white skin proximal to the margin of the four webs between the fingers (Fig. 22)

四缝 [sì fèng]

Sifeng **(EX-UE 10):** four points on each hand, on the palmar side of the 2nd to 5th fingers and at the center of the proximal interphalangeal joints (Fig. 22)

十宣 [shí xuān]

Shixuan **(EX-UE 11):** ten points on both hands, at the tips of the 10 fingers, 0.1 *cun* from the free margin of the nails (Fig. 22)

下肢穴 [xià zhī xué]

points of the lower extremities (LE): extra points located on the lower extremities

髋骨 [kuān gǔ]

Kuangu **(EX-LE 1):** two points on each thigh, in the lower part of the anterior surface of the thigh, 1.5 *cun* lateral and medial to *Liangqiu* (ST34) (Fig. 23)

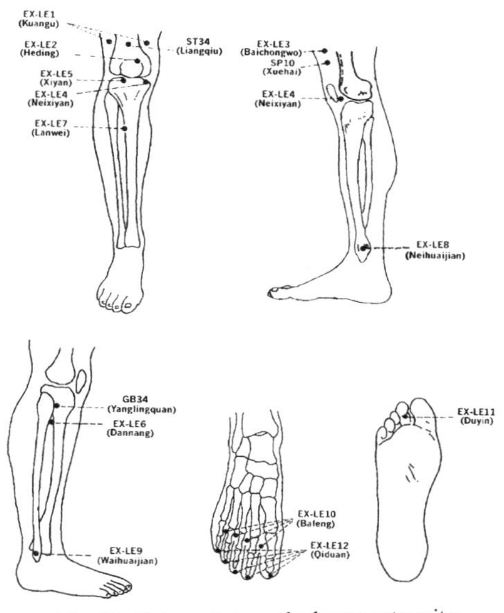

Fig. 23 Extra points on the lower extremity

鹤顶 [hè dǐng]

Heding **(EX-LE 2):** point above the knee, in the depression of the midpoint of the upper border of the patella (Fig. 23)

百虫窝 [bǎi chóng wō]

Baichongwo **(EX-LE 3):** point 3 *cun* above the medial superior corner of the patella of the thigh with the knee flexed, i.e., 1 *cun* above *Xuehai* (SP 10) (Fig. 23)

内膝眼 [nèi xī yǎn]

Neixiyan **(EX-LE 4):** point in the depression medial to the patellar ligament when the knee is flexed (Fig. 23)

膝眼 [xī yǎn]

Xiyan **(EX-LE 5):** point in the depression on the lateral side of the patellar ligament when the knee is flexed (Fig. 23)

胆囊 [dǎn náng]

Dannang **(EX-LE 6):** point at the upper part of the lateral surface of the leg, 2 *cun* directly below the depression anterior and inferior to the head of the fibula or 2 *cun* below *Yanglingquan* (GB 34) (Fig. 23)

阑尾 [lán wěi]

Lanwei **(EX-LE 7):** point at the upper part of the anterior surface of the leg, 5 *cun* below *Dubi* (ST 35), one finger breadth lateral to the anterior crest of the tibia (Fig. 23)

内踝尖 [nèi huái jiān]

Neihuajian **(EX-LE 8):** point on the medial side of the foot, at the tip of the medial malleolus (Fig. 23)

外踝尖 [wài huái jiān]

Waihuaijian **(EX-LE 9):** point on the lateral side of the foot, at the tip of the lateral malleolus (Fig. 23)

八风 [bā fēng]

Bafeng **(EX-LE 10):** eight points on the

insteps of both feet, at the junction of the red and white skin proximal to the margin of the webs between each two neighboring toes (Fig. 23)

独阴 [dú yīn]
***Duyin* (EX-LE 11):** point on the plantar side of the 2nd toe, at the center of the distal interphalangeal joint (Fig. 23)

气端 [qì duān]
***Qiduan* (EX-LE 12):** ten points at the tips of the 10 toes of both feet, 0.1 *cun* from the free margin of each toenail (Fig. 23)

阿是穴 [ā shì xué]
***Ashi* point; "Yes-no" point:** a category of points that have no fixed location and are found by eliciting tenderness at the diseased site

针法 Acupuncture

针灸学 [zhēn jiǔ xué]
(science of) acupuncture and moxibustion: a branch of traditional Chinese medicine that studies the meridians/channels, acupoints, and stimulation of the acupoints by needling or igniting moxa, as well as the stimulation techniques in disease treatment and prevention (through regulation of *qi*, blood and *zang-fu* functions)

针灸师 [zhēn jiǔ shī]
acupuncturist: one who practices acupuncture and moxibustion

针灸疗法 [zhēn jiǔ liáo fǎ]
acupuncture and moxibustion therapy: collective term for treatment of illness by means of acupuncture and moxibustion

针刺疗法 [zhēn cì liáo fǎ]
acupuncture therapy: traditional Chinese therapy in which the functions of the body are regulated for curing disease by way of stimulating certain sites of the body (acupoints) with specially designed needles

针法 [zhēn fǎ]
(I) acupuncture: abbreviation for acupuncture therapy (针刺疗法 [zhēn cì liáo fǎ]); **(II) needling (technique):** technique of acupuncture therapy

刺法 [cì fǎ]
puncturing (technique): synonym for needling (针法 [zhēn fǎ])

刺灸法 [cì jiǔ fǎ]
puncturing and moxibustion: collective term for the techniques of acupuncture and moxibustion

针灸 [zhēn jiǔ]
acupuncture-moxibustion: collective term for acupuncture and moxibustion

寸 [cùn]
***cun*:** abbreviation for body *cun* (同身寸 [tóng shēn cùn])

同身寸 [tóng shēn cùn]
body *cun*; body inch: unit of length for measurement in locating acupoints, abbreviated as *cun* (寸[cùn]). A certain part of the patient's body is divided into certain divisions of equal length, each of which is taken as one proportional unit for measurement.

中指同身寸 [zhōng zhǐ tóng shēn cùn]
middle finger body-*cun*; middle finger body-inch: the length between the two

medial ends of twisted folds of the patient's middle finger when bent, which is taken as one *cun*, a unit of measurement (Fig. 24)

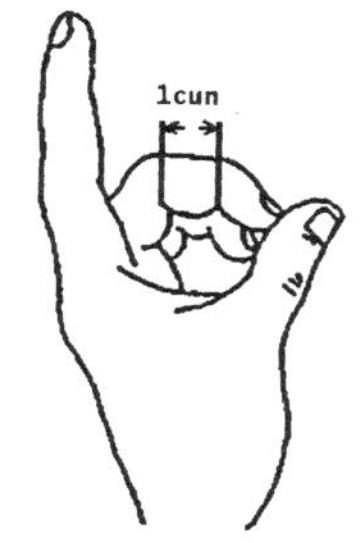

Fig. 24 Middle finger cun

拇指同身寸 [mǔ zhǐ tóng shēn cùn]

thumb body-*cun*; thumb body-inch: the width of the phalangeal joint of the patient's thumb, which is taken as one *cun*, a unit of measurement (Fig. 25)

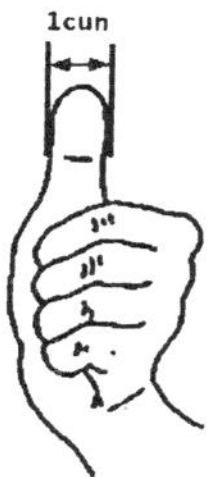

Fig. 25 Thumb cun

横指同身寸 [héng zhǐ tóng shēn cùn]

finger-breadth body-*cun*; finger-breadth body-inch: the maximal width of the four fingers (namely, the index finger, middle finger, ring finger and little finger) held together with the hand open, which is taken as 3 *cun*, a unit of measurement (Fig. 26)

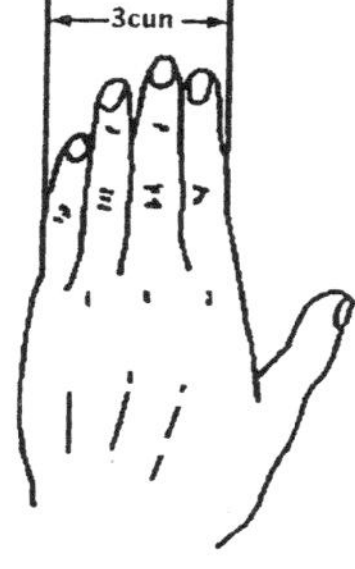

Fig. 26 Palm measurement

一夫法 [yī fū fǎ]

palm measurement: another name for measurement by finger-breadth body-*cun* (横指同身寸 [héng zhǐ tóng shēn cùn])

骨度分寸定穴法 [gǔ dù fēn cùn dìng xué fǎ]

location of point by bone measurement: the length of equally divided portions of a certain long bone or of the distance between two anatomical landmarks taken as one *cun*, a unit of measurement for locating points (Fig. 27), sometimes simply called bone measurement (骨度法 [gǔ dù fǎ])

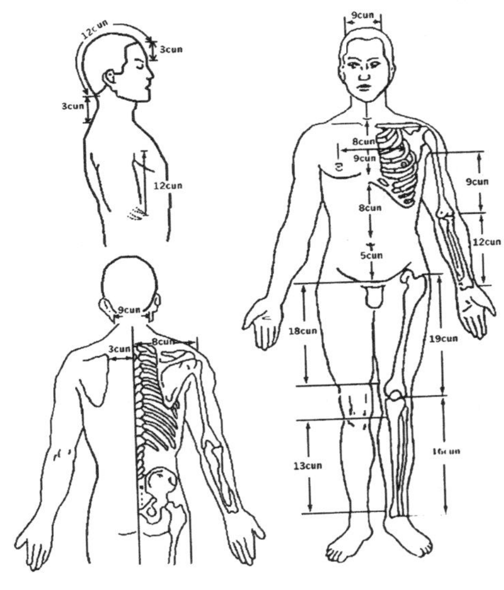

Fig. 27 Bone-length measurement

骨度法 [gǔ dù fǎ]

bone measurement: abbreviation for location of points by bone measurement (骨度分寸定穴法 [gǔ dù fēn cùn dìng xué fǎ])

选穴法 [xuǎn xué fǎ]

selection of points: determination of appropriate points for acupuncture treatment, also known as 取穴法 [qǔ xué fǎ]

取穴法 [qǔ xué fǎ]
selection of points: same as 选穴法 [xuǎn xué fǎ]

局部选穴法 [jú bù xuǎn xué fǎ]
selection of local points: selecting points in the local area of the disease site for treatment

邻近选穴法 [lín jìn xuǎn xué fǎ]
selection of adjacent points: selecting points in the adjacent or nearby area of the disease site for treatment

远道选穴法 [yuǎn dào xuǎn xué fǎ]
selection of distant points: selecting points in the area far from the disease site for treatment

循经选穴法 [xún jīng xuǎn xué fǎ]
selection of points along the affected meridian/channel: selecting points, either local or distant, along the meridian/channel affected by the disease for treatment

异经选穴法 [yì jīng xuǎn xué fǎ]
selection of points on other meridian(s)/channel(s): selecting points on the meridian(s)/channel(s) other than the directly affected one, e.g., selecting *Gongsun* (SP 4) to treat gastralgia, which affects the stomach meridian/channel; selecting *Sanyinjiao* (SP 6) other than a point on the conception vessel to treat metrorrhagia due to conception vessel disorder, also called 他经选穴法 [tā jīng xuǎn xué fǎ]

他经选穴法 [tā jīng xuǎn xué fǎ]
selection of points on other meridians/channels: same as异经选穴法 [yì jīng xuǎn xué fǎ]

对症选穴法 [duì zhèng xuǎn xué fǎ]
point selection according to symptoms: selecting points according to the patient's symptoms for treatment. Some points are traditionally noted for their effectiveness in treating specific symptoms, e.g., *Dazhui* (GV 14) for allaying fever, *Shenmen* (HT 7) for treating insomnia, and *Lieque* (LU 7) for relieving cough.

表里选穴法 [biǎo lǐ xuǎn xué fǎ]
selection of points on the exterior-interiorly related meridians/channels: selecting points on the meridian/channel directly related to the diseased organ as well as points on its exterior-interiorly related meridian/channel, e.g., selecting points of lung meridian/channel of hand greater yin and large intestine meridian/channel of hand yang brightness to treat lung diseases

对应选穴法 [duì yìng xuǎn xué fǎ]
selection of points opposite to the affected area: selecting points in the area opposite to that affected, e.g., selecting points on the ventral part of the body for treating diseases of the dorsal part, selecting points on the lower part of the body for treating diseases of the upper part, selecting points on the left side of the body for treating diseases of the right side, etc.

辨证选穴法 [biàn zhèng xuǎn xué fǎ]
point selection according to syndrome differentiation; point selection according to pattern identification: selecting points according to the syndrome/pattern identified in the diagnosis for treatment, e.g., in the treatment of prolapse of the anus, selecting *Baihui* (GV 20), *Zusanli* (ST 36) and *Changqiang* (GV 1) if the

syndrome/pattern is middle *qi* sinking, while selecting *Dachangshu* (BL 25) and *Tianshu* (ST 25) if the syndrome/pattern is large intestinal accumulation of heat

交叉选穴法 [jiāo chā xuǎn xué fǎ]
contralateral point selection: selecting points lying on the side of the body opposite to that of the disease site for treatment

交会选穴法 [jiāo huì xuǎn xué fǎ]
crossing point selection: selecting the relevant crossing point for treatment, e.g., selecting *Sanyinjiao* (SP 6) to treat diseases of the liver, spleen or kidney meridian/channel

配穴法 [pèi xué fǎ]
point combination: combined use of points in acupuncture for achieving desired therapeutic effect

上下配穴法 [shàng xià pèi xué fǎ]
upper-lower point combination: method of point combination in which points on an upper limb are paired with points on a lower limb or points on the head and face paired with points on the limbs

左右配穴法 [zuǒ yòu pèi xué fǎ]
right-left point combination: method of point combination in which bilateral points of a given meridian/channel are selected

前后配穴法 [qián hòu pèi xué fǎ]
anterior-posterior point combination: method of point combination in which points on the anterior aspect of the trunk are paired with corresponding points on the posterior aspect, also called ventro-dorsal point combination (腹背配穴法 [fù bèi pèi xué fǎ])

腹背配穴法 [fù bèi pèi xué fǎ]
ventro-dorsal point combination: same as anterior-posterior point combination (前后配穴法 [qián hòu pèi xué fǎ])

阴阳配穴法 [yīn yáng pèi xué fǎ]
yin-yang point combination: method of point combination in which points of a yin meridian/channel are paired with points of the corresponding yang meridian/channel

本经配穴法 [běn jīng pèi xué fǎ]
point combination of the same meridian/channel: method of point combination in which only the points of the involved meridian/channel are selected

表里配穴法 [biǎo lǐ pèi xué fǎ]
exterior-interior point combination: method of point combination based on the exterior-interior relationship of the meridians/channels, also called exterior-interior meridian/channel point combination (表里经配穴法 [biǎo lǐ jīng pèi xué fǎ])

表里经配穴法 [biǎo lǐ jīng pèi xué fǎ]
exterior-interior meridian/channel point combination: same as exterior-interior point combination (表里配穴法 [biǎo lǐ pèi xué fǎ])

原络配穴法 [yuán luò pèi xué fǎ]
source-connecting point combination: method of point combination in which the source point of the corresponding meridian/channel is paired with the connecting point of the exterior-interiorly related meridian/channel

同名经配穴法 [tóng míng jīng pèi xué fǎ]

combination of points from the meridians/channels with the same name: method of point combination in which points are selected from meridians/channels bearing the same name of the hand and foot, e.g., from the yang brightness meridians/channels of the hand and foot, namely, from the large intestine meridian/channel and stomach meridian/channel

子母配穴法 [zǐ mǔ pèi xué fǎ]

mother-son point combination: method of point combination in which the points are selected according to the therapeutic principle of reinforcing the "mother" in cases of deficiency or reducing the "son" in cases of excess

交会经配穴法 [jiāo huì jīng pèi xué fǎ]

crossing meridian/channel point combination: method of point combination in which the points are selected on the meridians/channels that cross the diseased meridian/channel

内外配穴法 [nèi wài pèi xué fǎ]

medial-lateral point combination: method of point combination in which points on the medial side are paired with those on the lateral side, usually taken as the major method for regulating yin-yang disharmony

远近配穴法 [yuǎn jìn pèi xué fǎ]

distant-local point combination: method of point combination in which local points are paired with points distant from the diseased area

主应配穴法 [zhǔ yìng pèi xué fǎ]

primary-secondary point combination: method of point combination in which points distant from the diseased area are taken as the primary ones while those close to the diseased area are taken as the secondary ones

五输配穴法 [wǔ shū pèi xué fǎ]

five-transport-points combination: method of point combination in which the chief points are selected from the five transport points according to their indications

俞募配穴法 [shù mù pèi xué fǎ]

transport-alarm point combination: method of point combination in which points are selected from the transport points and alarm points of the diseased visceral organ, e.g., selecting *Weishu* (BL 21) and *Zhongwan* (CV 12) to treat stomach diseases

俞原配穴法 [shù yuán pèi xué fǎ]

transport-source point combination: method of point combination in which points are selected from the back transport points and the source point of the corresponding meridian/channel

募合配穴法 [mù hé pèi xué fǎ]

alarm-sea point combination: method of point combination in which points are selected from the related alarm points and lower sea points

郄会配穴法 [xī huì pèi xué fǎ]

cleft-influential point combination: method of point combination in which points are selected from the cleft points and eight influential points

通经接气配穴法 [tōng jīng jiē qì pèi xué fǎ]

meridian/channel-*qi*-connecting point combination: method of point combination in which points of the relevant meridian/channel are sequentially selected after the presence of needling sensation to conduct it to the diseased site

针尖 [zhēn jiān]

tip of the needle: pointed end of the needle (Fig. 28)

针体 [zhēn tǐ]

body of the needle: part of the needle between the tip and the handle (Fig. 28)

针根 [zhēn gēn]

needle root: junction between the handle and the body of the needle (Fig. 28)

针柄 [zhēn bǐng]

handle of the needle: part of the needle held with the fingers when in use (Fig. 28)

毫针 [háo zhēn]

filiform needle: most commonly used acupuncture needle at present, with length ranging from 15 to 125mm, and caliber ranging from gauge 26 to gauge 32 (Fig. 28)

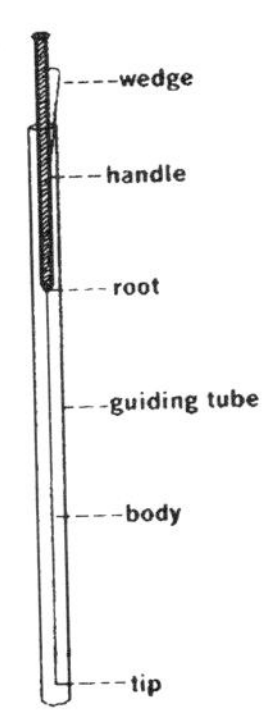

Fig. 28 Filiform acupuncture needle

三棱针 [sān léng zhēn]

three-edged needle: special kind of acupuncture needle with a triangular head and sharp point used for quick puncture and bloodletting

三棱针疗法 [sān léng zhēn liáo fǎ]

three-edged needle therapy: therapeutic method in which a three-edged needle is applied to patients using the techniques of pricking, open picking, scattered needling, and collateral puncture

点刺 [diǎn cì]

quick pricking: needling technique of fast piercing followed by immediate removal of the needle, usually with a three-edged one

散刺 [sǎn cì]

scattered needling: needling technique in which a three-edged needle is used to prick around the local lesion, also known as leopard-spot needling (豹文刺[bào wén cì])

刺络 [cì luò]

collateral puncture: needling technique in which a venule is pricked with a three-edged needle, for letting out a small amount of blood

挑刺法 [tiǎo cì fǎ]

pricking method: therapeutic method using a three-edged needle, involving picking out a small piece of fibrous substance and squeezing out a small amount of fluid

皮肤针 [pí fū zhēn]

dermal needle: needling instrument, including plum-blossom needle and seven-star needle, in which a bundle of five and seven short needles, respectively, are attached to a handle, used for tapping and pricking certain points or areas of the body

皮肤针疗法 [pí fū zhēn liáo fǎ]
dermal needle therapy: therapeutic method whereby points are tapped with a dermal needle

梅花针 [méi huā zhēn]
plum-blossom needle: dermal needling instrument with a bundle of five short fine needles fixed vertically at the end of a handle, the tips of which are clustered in the pattern of plum blossom petals

七星针 [qī xīng zhēn]
seven-star needle: dermal needling instrument with a bundle of seven short needles attached vertically to the end of a handle

罗汉针 [luó hàn zhēn]
arhat needle: hammer-shaped dermal needling instrument with eighteen needles attached to the head

皮内针 [pí nèi zhēn]
intradermal needle: small needle embedded in the skin for continuous stimulation

皮内针疗法 [pī nèi zhēn liáo fǎ]
intradermal needle therapy: therapeutic method whereby a disease is treated by embedding in the skin a small needle or needles at certain point(s), also called needle-embedding therapy (埋针疗法 [mái zhēn fǎ])

埋针疗法 [mái zhēn liáo fǎ]
needle-embedding therapy: another name for intradermal needle therapy (皮内针疗法 [pí nèi zhēn liáo fǎ])

揿针 [qìn zhēn]
thumbtack needle: small needle which is usually embedded in the auricle, also called thumbtack intradermal needle (图钉型皮内针 [tú dīng xíng pí nèi zhēn])

图钉型皮内针 [tú dīng xíng pí nèi zhēn]
thumbtack intradermal needle: small needle with a head like a thumbtack for subcutaneous embedding, also known as thumbtack needle (揿针 [qìn zhēn])

麦粒型皮内针 [mài lì xíng pí nèi zhēn]
wheatgrain intradermal needle: small needle with the head resembling a grain of wheat, which may be embedded subcutaneously at any part of the body, also known as granular intradermal needle (颗粒型皮内针[kē lì xíng pí nèi zhēn])

颗粒型皮内针 [kē lì xíng pí nèi zhēn]
granular intradermal needle: same as wheatgrain intradermal needle (麦粒型皮内针 [mài lì xíng pí nèi zhēn])

火针 [huǒ zhēn]
fire needle: needle heated red-hot, also known as burnt needle (燔针 [fán zhēn] or 烧针 [shāo zhēn])

火针疗法 [huǒ zhēn liáo fǎ]
fire needling therapy: acupuncture method which involves heating the needles red hot, inserting them into the diseased part immediately and withdrawing them at once, often used for treating scrofula and rheumatism

燔针 [fán zhēn]
burnt needle: another name for fire needle (火针[huǒ zhēn])

烧针 [shāo zhēn]
burnt needle: another name for fire needle (火针 [huǒ zhēn])

小针刀 [xiǎo zhēn dāo]
acupotome: therapeutic instrument bearing a needle and a tiny surgical knife in combination, also called needle knife

小针刀疗法 [xiǎo zhēn dāo liáo fǎ]
acupotomy: therapeutic treatment with a needle knife (an acupotome) , mostly indicated for treating soft tissue injuries

蜂针疗法 [fēng zhēn liáo fǎ]
bee sting therapy: special acupuncture treatment in which a particular point is allowed to be stung by a bee, for a therapeutic purpose

砭石 [biān shí]
healing stone; stone needle: needle made of stone, used as a primitive tool for acupuncture and surgical incision in ancient times

九针 [jiǔ zhēn]
nine classical needles: collective term for nine kinds of needles used in ancient times, namely, shear needle or arrow-headed needle (镵针 [chán zhēn]), round-pointed needle (圆针 [yuán zhēn]), spoon-like needle (鍉针 [chí zhēn]), lance needle or sharp three-edged needle (锋针 [fēng zhēn]), stiletto needle or sword needle (铍针 [pī zhēn] or 剑针 [jiàn zhēn]), round sharp needle (圆利针 [yuán lì zhēn]), filiform needle (毫针 [háo zhēn]), long needle (长针 [cháng zhēn]) and large needle (大针 [dà zhēn]) (Fig. 29)

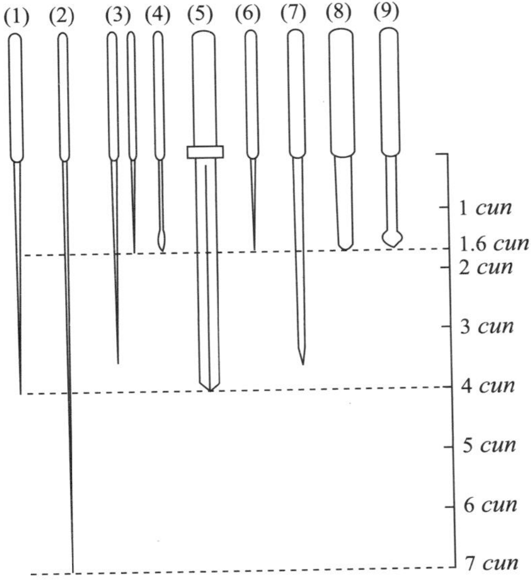

Fig. 29 Nine classical needles: (1) large needle, (2) long needle, (3) filiform needle, (4) round sharp needle, (5) stiletto needle (sword needles), (6) round-sharp needle, (7) spoon-like needle, (8) round-pointed needle, (9) shear needle (arrow-headed needle)

镵针 [chán zhēn]
shear needle: one of the nine classical needles, characterized by a big head and sharp tip, used for reducing yang *qi*, also called arrow-headed needle (箭头针[jiàn tóu zhēn])

箭头针 [jiàn tóu zhēn]
arrow-headed needle: same as shear needle (镵针 [chán zhēn])

圆针 [yuán zhēn]
round-pointed needle: one of the nine classical needles, characterized by an oval tip, used for massage as in the treatment of rheumatic conditions

鍉针 [chí zhēn]
spoon-like needle: one of the nine

classical needles, characterized by a thick shaft and a round and slightly pointed tip, used to press the meridian vessels for directing the flow of *qi* and blood

锋针 [fēng zhēn]
lance needle: one of the nine classical needles, characterized by triple sharp edges in one needle, also called triple-edged needle (三棱针 [sān léng zhēn])

铍针 [pī zhēn]
stiletto needle: one of the nine classical needles, characterized by the shape of a double-edged sword, for draining pus, also called sword needle 剑针[jiàn zhēn]

剑针 [jiàn zhēn]
sword needle: same as stiletto needle (铍针 [pī zhēn])

圆利针 [yuán lì zhēn]
round-sharp needle: one of the nine classical needles, 1.6 *cun* long with a somewhat large and round-sharp end, used for treating abscesses and rheumatic conditions

长针 [cháng zhēn]
long needle: one of the nine classical needles, 7 *cun* in length, used for deep puncturing

大针 [dà zhēn]
large needle: one of the nine classical needles, a large-gauge needle with a length of 4 *cun* and a somewhat round tip, primarily used for treating swelling due to retention of water

金针 [jīn zhēn]
metal needle: needle made of metal

银针 [yín zhēn]
silver needle: needle made of silver

合金针 [hé jīn zhēn]
alloy needle: needle made of alloy

不锈钢针 [bù xiù gāng zhēn]
stainless steel needle: needle made of stainless steel

一次性针 [yī cì xìng zhēn]
disposable needle: needle intended for single use only

滚刺［针］筒 [gǔn cì (zhēn) tǒng]
needle roller: a metallic roller embedded with short needles designed for dermal needling

滚刺疗法 [gǔn cì liáo fǎ]
roller needle therapy: therapeutic treatment using a needle roller

针灸铜人 [zhēn jiǔ tóng rén]
bronze model of meridians/channels and acupoints: model in bronze marked with meridians/channels and acupuncture points, used for teaching purposes, originating in the 11th century A.D.

进针 [jìn zhēn]
needle insertion: penetration of a needle into the body through the skin, usually with the tip of the needle reaching a certain depth

进针法 [jìn zhēn fǎ]
needle insertion method: technique of inserting a needle through the skin (Fig. 30)

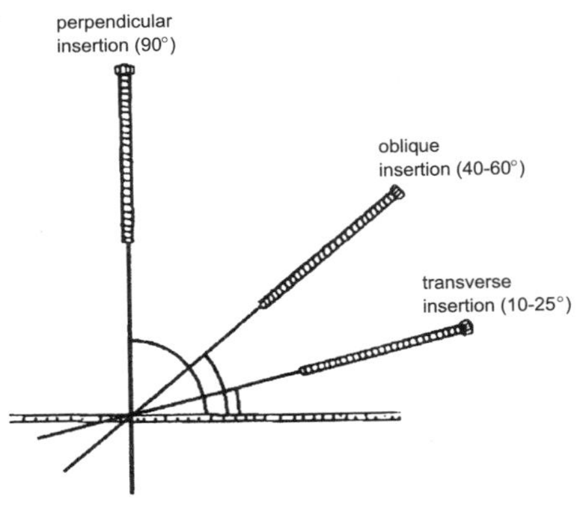

Fig. 30 Methods of needle insertion

刺手 [cì shǒu]
needling hand: pratitioner's hand that holds and inserts the needle

押手 [yā shǒu]
pressing hand: practitioner's hand that presses the puncturing site to facilitate the needle insertion, usually with one or two fingers

单手进针法 [dān shǒu jìn zhēn fǎ]
single-handed needle insertion: needle insertion technique performed with one hand alone

双手进针法 [dān shǒu jìn zhēn fǎ]
double-handed needle insertion: needle insertion technique performed with two hands in cooperation, with one as the needling hand and the other the pressing hand

指切进针法 [zhǐ qiē jìn zhēn fǎ]
fingernail-pressing needle insertion: needle insertion technique for short filiform needles performed with the help of finger-tip pressure,

夹持进针法 [jiā chí jìn zhēn fǎ]
hand-holding needle insertion: double-handed needle insertion technique whereby the thumb and index finger of the pressing hand hold a sterilized cotton ball with which the shaft of the needle is wrapped

舒张进针法 [shū zhāng jìn zhēn fǎ]
skin-spreading needle insertion: double-handed needle insertion technique whereby the skin is stretched with the pressing hand to facilitate needle insertion

提捏进针法 [tí niē jìn zhēn fǎ]
pinching needle insertion: double-handed needle insertion technique whereby the needle is inserted with one hand while the other hand pinches and lifts the surrounding flesh

插入法 [chā rù fǎ]
thrusting insertion: method of needle insertion whereby the needle is directly thrust through the skin without being twisted after the tip of the needle is brought into contact with the skin

飞入法 [fēi rù fǎ]
needle-flying insertion: method of needle insertion whereby the practitioner holds and twirls the handle of the needle with the thumb and index finger, and inserts the needle while the thumb is moving backward and the other fingers are extending along with the index finger, resembling the wing movement of a flying bird

弹入法 [tán rù fǎ]
flicking-in insertion: method of needle

insertion whereby the practitioner inserts the needle rapidly by flicking the handle of the needle with a finger and the thumb of the needling hand

随咳进针法 [suí ké jìn zhēn fǎ]
needle insertion during coughing: method of needle insertion whereby the practitioner asks the patient to cough while the needle is being inserted

管针进针法 [guǎn zhēn jìn zhēn fǎ]
needle insertion with tube: needle insertion technique whereby a fine tube is used as a guide for insertion

直刺 [zhí cì]
perpendicular insertion: needle insertion at a 90 degree angle to the local skin surface (Fig. 30)

斜刺 [xié cì]
oblique insertion: needle insertion at an angle of roughly 45 degrees to the local skin surface (Fig. 30)

横刺 [héng cì]
transverse insertion: needle insertion at an angle of roughly 15 degrees to the local skin surface (Fig. 30), also known as horizontal insertion (平刺 [píng cì])

平刺 [píng cì]
horizontal insertion: same as transverse insertion (横刺 [héng cì])

透刺 [tòu cì]
penetration needling: puncture of two or more adjoining points with one needle insertion

直透 [zhí tòu]
perpendicular penetration: puncture of two adjoining points on the anterior and posterior aspects or interior and exterior aspects of a limb with one needle insertion

横透 [héng tòu]
transverse penetration: puncture of two neighboring points on the same aspect with one needle insertion

深刺 [shēn cì]
deep insertion: inserting a needle deeply into the tissue

浅刺 [qiǎn cì]
shallow insertion: inserting a needle to the level where the tip of the needle is only a short distance away from the skin surface or just beneath the skin

催气法 [cuī qì fǎ]
***qi*-hastening method:** method of hastening the arrival of needling sensation with needle manipulations

行针 [xíng zhēn]
needle manipulation: manipulating a needle after insertion to produce the desired effect, also known as 运针 [yùn zhēn]

运针 [yùn zhēn]
needle manipulation: same as 行针 [xíng zhēn]

捻转法 [niǎn zhuǎn fǎ]
twirling method: needle manipulation technique whereby the inserted needle is rotated rapidly after insertion to a proper depth, as an auxiliary method to promote needling sensation

提插法 [tí chā fǎ]
lifting-thrusting method: a needle manipulation technique whereby the inserted needle is pulled up and pushed down after insertion to a proper depth, as an auxiliary method to promote needling sensation

刮柄法 [guā bǐng fǎ]
handle-scrapng method: needle manipulation technique whereby the handle of the needle is scraped with a finger nail after insertion to the proper depth, as an auxiliary method to promote needling sensation

弹柄法 [tán bǐng fǎ]
handle-flicking method: needle manipulation technique whereby the handle of the needle is flicked after insertion to the proper depth, as an auxiliary method to promote needling sensation

搓柄法 [cuō bǐng fǎ]
handle-twisting method: needle manipulation technique whereby the handle of the needle is twisted after insertion to the proper depth, as an auxiliary method to promote needling sensation

摇柄法 [yáo bǐng fǎ]
handle-waggling method: needle manipulation technique whereby the handle of the needle is moved from side to side in a rapid manner after insertion to the proper depth, as an auxiliary method to promote needling sensation

震颤法 [zhèn chàn fǎ]
trembling method: needle manipulation technique whereby the handle of the needle is lifted, thrust and twisted, alternately and at a high frequency with small amplitude, as an auxiliary method to promote needling sensation

努法 [nǔ fǎ]
shaft-flicking method: needle manipulation technique whereby the shaft of the needle is flicked with the middle finger while being held with the thumb and index finger at the handle after insertion to the proper depth, as an auxiliary method to promote needling sensation , also known as 弩法 [nǔ fǎ]

弩法 [nǔ fǎ]
shaft-flicking method: same as 努法 [nǔ fǎ]

捣法 [dǎo fǎ]
repeated lifting-thrust method: needle manipulation technique whereby the needle is lifted and thrust repeatedly with a considerable amplitude after insertion to the proper depth, as an auxiliary method to promote needling sensation

循法 [xún fǎ]
massage along the meridian/channel: manipulation for promoting needling sensation, in which the practitioner applies massage along the meridian/channel after inserting a needle, also known as 循按法 [xún àn fǎ]

循按法 [xún àn fǎ]
massage along the meridian/channel: same as 循法 [xún fǎ]

导气 [dǎo qì]
inducing *qi*: manipulating the needle to

promote the arrival of needling sensation and conduct its transmission pathway

候气 [hòu qì]
awaiting *qi*: waiting for the arrival of needling sensation after a needle insertion

行针候气 [xíng zhēn hòu qì]
manipulating the needle to await *qi*: maneuvering the handle of a needle after insertion by the practitioner, using various techniques, such as twirling and flicking, while the patient is awaiting the arrival of needling sensation

留针候气 [liú zhēn hòu qì]
retaining the needle to await *qi*: after inserting the needle to the proper depth, keeping it unmoved to wait for the arrival of needling sensation

得气 [dé qì]
obtaining *qi*; arrival of *qi*: state of acupunture application in which the patient senses soreness, heaviness, numbness, and a feeling of distension at or around the acupuncture site, while in the meantime the practitioner feels tightness in needle manipulation, indicative of a successful acupuncture application, also known as 气至 [qì zhì]

气至 [qì zhì]
arrival of *qi*: same as 得气 [dé qì]

针感 [zhēn gǎn]
needling sensation: unique physical sensation felt by the patient in response to needling, which may be described as soreness, heaviness, numbness or distension, or the mixed sensation of two or more of those feelings

守气 [shǒu qì]
keeping *qi*: keeping the needling sensation at the needling point after its arrival

补泻法 [bǔ xiè fǎ]
method of reinforcement and reduction: method of bringing back normal functions by way of reinforcement and reduction. Reinforcement means activating and restoring a decreased function to normal, while reduction means expelling pathogenic factors and thereby restoring hyperactivity to normal.

提插补泻 [tí chā bǔ xiè]
lifting-thrusting reinforcement and reduction: form of needle manipulation in which reinforcement or reduction is attained by lifting and thrusting with different degrees of force

提插补泻法 [tí chā bǔ xiè fǎ]
lifting-thrusting reinforcement-reduction method: acupuncture method in which the needle is thrust in forcefully and lifted gently for reinforcement effect, or thrust in gently and lifted rapidly for reduction effect

紧按慢提 [jǐn àn màn tí]
swift thrusting and slow lifting: acupuncture method whereby the needle is thrust swiftly and forcefully but lifted slowly and gently, usually used to achieve a reinforcement effect

重插轻提 [zhòng chā qīng tí]
forceful thrusting and light lifting: synonymous with swift thrusting and slow lifting (紧按慢提[jǐn àn màn tí])

紧提慢按 [jǐn tí màn àn]
swift lifting and slow thrusting: acupuncture method whereby the needle is lifted swiftly and forcefully but thrust slowly and gently, used to achieve a reduction effect

重提轻插 [zhòng tí qīng chā]
forceful lifting and light thrusting: synonymous with swift lifting and slow thrusting (紧提慢按 [jǐn tí màn àn])

捻转补泻 [niǎn zhuǎn bǔ xiè]
twirling reinforcement and reduction: form of needle manipulation in which reinforcementor reduction effect is achieved by controlling the degree of twirling and the strength with which the needle is twirled

捻转补泻法 [niǎn zhuǎn bǔ xiè fǎ]
twirling reinforcing-reducing method: acupuncture method in which the needle is twirled exceeding 360 degrees with forceful manipulation for reduction effect, or less than 180 degrees with gentle manipulation for reinforcement effect

呼吸补泻 [hū xī bǔ xiè]
respiratory reinforcement and reduction: form of needle manipulation in which reinforcement or reduction effect is achieved by timing the insertion and withdrawal of the needle according to the phases of the patient's respiration.

呼吸补泻法 [hū xī bǔ xiè fǎ]
respiratory reinforcing-reducing method: acupuncture method whereby the needle is inserted when the patient exhales and withdrawn when the patient has inhaled to the fullest capacity for reinforcement effect, or insertion is made during the patient's inspiration and withdrawal at the end of expiration for reduction effect

迎随补泻 [yíng suí bǔ xiè]
directional reinforcement and reduction: form of needle manipulation in which reinforcement or reduction is achieved by the direction of needle insertion

迎随补泻法 [yíng suí bǔ xiè fǎ]
directional reinforcing-reducing method: acupuncture method whereby the needle is pointed obliquely along the meridian/channel during insertion for reinforcement effect, or against the direction of the meridian/channel for reduction effect

开阖补泻 [kāi hé bǔ xiè]
open-closed reinforcement and reduction: form of needle manipulation in which reinforcement or reduction effect is achieved by closing or opening the acupuncture hole respectively, after withdrawing the needle

开阖补泻法 [kāi hé bǔ xiè fǎ]]
open-closed reinforcement-reduction method: acupuncture method whereby the needle hole is closed with light finger pressure to prevent the *qi* from escaping, for reinforcement effect, or the needle hole is left open to let the pathogenic factors out for reduction effect

疾徐补泻 [jǐ xú bǔ xiè]
quick-slow reinforcement and reduction: form of needle manipulation in which reinforcement or reduction is achieved by insertion and withdrawal of the needle at different speeds

疾徐补泻法 [jí xú bǔ xiè fǎ]
quick-slow reinforcing-reducing method: acupunture method whereby needling is performed with slow insertion and rapid withdrawal for reinforcement effect, or swift insertion and slow withdrawal for reduction effect

平补平泻 [píng bǔ píng xiè]
neutral reinforcement and reduction: form of needle manipulation indicated in cases of combined excess and deficiency or a diseased state with no distinct excess or deficiency

平补平泻法 [píng bǔ píng xiè fǎ]
neutral reinforcing-reducing method: acupuncture method whereby the needle is lifted, thrust and twirled evenly with a proper amplitude and favorable angle

大补大泻法 [dà bǔ dà xiè fǎ]
heavy reinforcing-reducing method: acupuncture method whereby the needle is manipulated to induce a strong stimulus for either reinforcement or reduction

子母补泻法 [zǐ mǔ bǔ xiè fǎ]
mother-son reinforcing and reducing method: acupuncture method which follows the principle of reinforcing the "mother" organ in cases of deficiency and purging the "child" organ in cases of excess

盘旋法 [pán xuán fǎ]
circular needling method: acupuncture method in which the needle is tilted after insertion through the skin and a circular movement of the handle of the needle is made, clockwise for reinforcement and anticlockwise for reduction, often abbreviated as盘法 [pán fǎ]

盘法 [pán fǎ]
circular needling method: same as盘旋法 [pán xuán fǎ]

白虎摇头法 [bái hǔ yáo tóu fǎ]
"white tiger shaking its head": acupuncture method whereby the needle is twirled to the left while being inserted, and twirled to the right while being lifted, and then shaken gently to promote blood circulation

青龙摆尾法 [qīng lóng bǎi wěi fǎ]
"blue dragon wagging its tail": acupuncture method whereby the inserted needle is directed toward the diseased site and its handle is gently moved from side to side in order to guide the flow of *qi*, also known as 苍龙摆尾法 [cāng lóng bǎi wěi fǎ]

苍龙摆尾法 [cāng lóng bǎi wěi fǎ]
"blue dragon wagging its tail": same as 青龙摆尾法 [qīng lóng bǎi wěi fǎ]

烧山火 [shāo shān huǒ]
"burning the mountain": form of needle manipulation to achieve reinforcement with a local or generalized feeling of intense heat

透天凉 [tòu tiān liáng]
"cooling the sky": form of needle manipulation to achieve reduction with a local or generalized feeling of cooling

循经感传 [xún jīng gǎn chuán]
transmission of sensation along the meridian/channel: transmission of

needling sensation, a complex feeling of soreness, numbness, distension and heaviness, along the meridian/channel

行气法 [xíng qì fǎ]
***qi*-conducting method:** method of conducting the *qi* or acupuncture feeling to a certain site, usually the diseased site

指压行气法 [zhǐ yā xíng qì fǎ]
finger-pressure conduction of *qi*: method of inducing the acupuncture feeling to travel proximally or distally along the meridian/channel by applying pressure with the finger to the meridian/channel proximal or distal to the acupoint, respectively

针向行气法 [zhēn xiàng xíng qì fǎ]
needle-direction conduction of *qi*: method of inducing the transmission of acupuncture feeling by varying the direction of insertion, i.e., inserting the needle in the same direction as that of the desired *qi* transmission

子午流注 [zǐ wǔ liú zhù]
midnight-midday ebb flow: ancient medical theory that the state of *qi* and blood in the meridians/channels and receptivity of different points vary with time and thus that the most effective needling time can be calculated in terms of the Heavenly Stems and Earthly Branches

子午流注针法 [zǐ wǔ liú zhù zhēn fǎ]
midnight-midday ebb flow acupuncture: acupuncture performed according to the midnight-midday flow calculation

纳甲法 [nà jiǎ fǎ]
day-prescription of points: selection of points based upon their "opening days" of a month calculated from the Heavenly Stems as well as the correspondence with the viscera and meridians/channels, also known as 纳干法 [nà gān fǎ]

纳干法 [nà gān fǎ]
day-prescription of points: same as 纳甲法 [nà jiǎ fǎ]

纳子法 [nà zǐ fǎ]
hour-prescription of points: selection of the points based upon their "opening hours" of a day calculated from the earthly branches as well as the correspondence with the viscera and meridians/channels, also known as 纳支法 [nà zhī fǎ]

纳支法 [nà zhī fǎ]
hour-prescription of points: same as 纳子法 [nà zǐ fǎ]

五刺 [wǔ cì]
five needling methods: collective term for five ancient needling techniques, i.e., half needling (半刺 [bàn cì]), leopard-spot needling (豹文刺 [bào wén cì]), joint needling (关刺 [guān cì]), joined valley needling (合谷刺 [hé gǔ cì]), and transport point needling (输刺 [shū cì])

半刺 [bàn cì]
half needling: one of the five needling methods, characterized by shallow insertion and swift withdrawal of the needle

豹文刺 [bào wén cì]
leopard-spot needling: one of the five needling methods, characterized by pricking with a triple-edged needle around

the point, for treating blood stasis in the vessels

关刺 [guān cì]
joint needling: one of the five needling methods, characterized by puncturing the sinew close to the joint, for treating sinew impediment

合谷刺 [hé gǔ cì]
joined valley needling: one of the five needling methods, characterized by puncturing the affected region directly with the needle going obliquely in different directions and the pathways taking a shape like a chicken claw, for treating numbness and muscle pains

输刺 [shū cì]
transport needling: (1) one of the five needling methods, characterized by deep perpendicular puncture to the bone, for treating bone impediment; (2) one of the nine needling methods, characterized by puncturing the transport points on the back as well as the five transport points on the limbs

九刺 [jiǔ cì]
nine needling methods: collective term for nine ancient techniques of needling, i.e., transport needling (输刺 [shū cì]), distant needling (远道刺 [yuǎn dào cì]), meridian/channel needling (经刺 [jīng cì]), collateral needling (络刺 [luò cì]), intermuscular needling (分刺 [fēn cì]), drainage needling (大泻刺 [dà xiè cì]), red-hot needling (焠刺 [cuì cì]), contralateral meridian/channel needling (巨刺 [jù cì]), and superficial needling (毛刺 [máo cì])

远道刺 [yuǎn dào cì]
distant needling: ancient needling method in which the needling points are selected on the lower extremities while the diseased site is on the upper body

经刺 [jīng cì]
meridian/channel needling: ancient needling method whereby puncture is executed at the site of the meridian/channel where stagnation exists

络刺 [luò cì]
collateral needling: ancient needling method whereby the relevant small vessels are pricked for bloodletting

分刺 [fēn cì]
intermuscular needling: ancient needling method whereby the needle goes directly into the interstice between muscles

大泻刺 [dà xiè cì]
drainage needling: ancient needling method referring to incision and drainage of pus and blood with a stiletto needle

焠刺 [cuì cì]
red-hot needling: ancient needling method involving swift pricking with a red-hot needle in the treatment of cold arthralgia, scrofula, etc.

巨刺 [jù cì]
contralateral meridian/channel needling: ancient needling method whereby puncture is executed on the point of the meridian/channel contralateral to the diseased side

毛刺 [máo cì]
superficial needling: ancient needling

method referring to shallow needling of the skin with a short filiform needle for treating skin impediment disease

缪刺 [miù cì]
contralateral collateral needling: ancient needling method whereby needling is executed on the point of the collateral contralateral to the diseased side

十二刺 [shí èr cì]
twelve needling methods: collective term for twelve ancient techniques of needling, i.e., paired needling (偶刺 [ǒu cì]), successive trigger needling (报刺 [bào cì]), relaxing needling (恢刺 [huī cì]), triple needling (齐刺 [qí cì]), shallow surround needling (扬刺 [yáng cì]), direct needling (直针刺 [zhí zhēn cì]), transport needling (输刺 [shū cì]), short thrust needling (短刺 [duǎn cì]), superficial needling (浮刺 [fú cì]), yin needling (阴刺 [yīn cì]), proximate needling (傍针刺 [bàng zhēn cì]), and repeated shallow needling (赞刺 [zàn cì])

偶刺 [ǒu cì]
paired needling: ancient needling method characterized by puncturing with a pair of needles, one anterior to and the other posterior to the diseased site, i.e., one on the chest and the other on the back, for treating heart impediment

报刺 [bào cì]
successive trigger needling: ancient needling method characterized by searching for tender points over the diseased area and needling in succession, for treating diseases with wandering pain

恢刺 [huī cì]
relaxing needling: ancient needling method characterized by inserting the needle on one side and then puncturing the contracted muscle in different directions to induce relaxation, for treating muscular contracture

齐刺 [qí cì]
triple needling: ancient needling method characterized by simultaneous needling of three points in the diseased area, i.e., one point in the center and two by its side, used for treating small-area deep-located cold impediment

扬刺 [yáng cì]
shallow surround needling: ancient needling method characterized by simultaneous needling of five points in the diseased area, i.e., one point in the center, and four other points anterior, posterior, right and left of the center, used for treating large-area shallow-located cold impediment

直针刺 [zhí zhēn cì]
direct needling: ancient needling method characterized by inserting the needle directly beneath the lifted skin

短刺 [duǎn cì]
short thrust needling: ancient needling method characterized by inserting the needle to the bone while gently shaking the handle, followed by short and swift lift and thrust, used for treating bone impediment

浮刺 [fú cì]
superficial needling: ancient needling

method characterized by shallow oblique puncturing, used for treating muscular spasm

阴刺 [yīn cì]
yin needling: ancient needling method characterized by puncturing the selected points of bilateral foot lesser yin meridian/channel (kidney meridian/channel), for treating cold reversal

傍针刺 [bàng zhēn cì]
proximate needling: ancient needling method characterized by perpendicular needling one point followed by oblique needling of another point in close proximity

赞刺 [zàn cì]
repeated shallow needling: ancient needling method characterized by multiple shallow needle insertions to induce bleeding

留针 [liú zhēn]
needle retention: retaining the needle in the point for a time to maintain and prolong the puncture effect

静留针法 [jìng liú zhēn fǎ]
actionless needle retention: no needle manipulation during retention of the needle after the arrival of *qi* (needling sensation)

动留针法 [dòng liú zhēn fǎ]
active needle retention: repeated needle manipulation during retention of the needle after the arrival of *qi* (needling sensation)

出针 [chū zhēn]
needle withdrawal: removing the needle from the point in which it has been inserted, also known as 起针 [qǐ zhēn]

起针 [qǐ zhēn]
needle withdrawal: same as 出针 [chū zhēn]

出针法 [chū zhēn fǎ]
needle withdrawal method: method of taking the needle away from the point in which it has been inserted, also called 起针法 [qǐ zhēn fǎ]

起针法 [qǐ zhēn fǎ]
needle withdrawal method: same as 出针法 [chū zhēn fǎ]

引针 [yǐn zhēn]
withdrawal of the needle: synonymous with 出针 [chū zhēn]

轻捻出针法 [qīng niǎn chū zhēn fǎ]
withdrawal of the needle with gentle twirling: method of withdrawing the needle while gently twirling its handle with the thumb and index finger or with the thumb, index finger and middle finger

平稳出针法 [píng wěn chū zhēn fǎ]
steady withdrawal of the needle: method of steadily withdrawing the needle along the exact course of its insertion but in the opposite direction

迅速出针法 [xùn sù chū zhēn fǎ]
quick withdrawal of the needle: method of quickly withdrawing the needle from its puncturing position with the thumb and

index finger, also called 快速起针法 [kuài sù qǐ zhēn fǎ]

快速起针法 [kuài sù qǐ zhēn fǎ]
quick withdrawal of the needle: same as 迅速出针法 [xùn sù chū zhēn fǎ]

退法 [tuì fǎ]
needle-retreating method: method of needle withdrawal in which the needle is lifted to the superficial portion, allowed to rest for a short while until resistance disappears, and then pulled out

晕针 [yùn zhēn]
fainting during acupuncture: an acupuncture complication, manifested by dizziness, dim eyesight, pale complexion, nausea, palpitations, cold sweat and drop of blood pressure

滞针 [zhì zhēn]
sticking of the needle: an abnormal condition occurring in acupuncture in which the needle is grasped so tightly that it is impossible to be twirled, lifted, thrust, or even withdrawn after it is inserted

弯针 [wān zhēn]
bending of the needle: an abnormal condition occurring during acupuncture after insertion of the needle, often due to change of the patient's posture

折针 [shé zhēn]
breaking of the needle: an acupuncture accident mostly due to using needles of poor quality, too forceful manipulation that causes powerful muscle contraction, or sudden change of the patient's posture, also called 断针 [duàn zhēn]

断针 [duàn zhēn]
breaking of the needle: same as 折针 [shé zhēn]

禁针穴 [jìn zhēn xué]
needling-prohibited point: point to which needling must not be applied

灸法及其他由针刺演变之疗法
Moxibustion and Other Techniques Derived from Acupuncture

灸疗法 [jiǔ liáo fǎ]
moxibustion: therapeutic procedure involving ignited material (usually moxa) to apply heat to certain points or areas of the body surface for curing disease through regulation of the function of meridians/channels and *zang-fu* organs, also called 灸法 [jiǔ fǎ] or simply 灸 [jiǔ]

灸法 [jiǔ fǎ]
moxibustion: same as 灸疗法 [jiǔ liáo fǎ]

灸 [jiǔ]
moxibustion: abbreviation for 灸法 [jiǔ fǎ] or 灸疗法 [jiǔ liáo fǎ]

艾 [ài]
moxa (*Artemisia vulgaris*): plant from which moxa floss is prepared

艾绒 [ài róng]
moxa floss: cottony material for moxibustion made from moxa leaves

艾炷 [ài zhù]
moxa cone: cone-shaped mass made of moxa floss

壮 [zhuàng]
cone: time taken for burning a moxa cone as a unit of measuring the amount of moxibustion

艾条 [ài tiáo]
moxa stick: round long stick made of moxa, also called moxa roll (艾卷 [ài juǎn])

艾卷 [ài juǎn]
moxa roll: same as moxa stick (艾条 [ài tiáo])

温灸器 [wēn jiǔ qì]
moxa burner: device for moxibustion, usually a square or round box designed to hold ignited moxa floss

艾条灸 [ài tiáo jiǔ]
moxa-stick moxibustion; moxibustion with moxa stick: moxibustion by using an ignited moxa stick (Fig. 31), also called moxa-roll moxibustion (艾卷灸 [ài juǎn jiǔ])

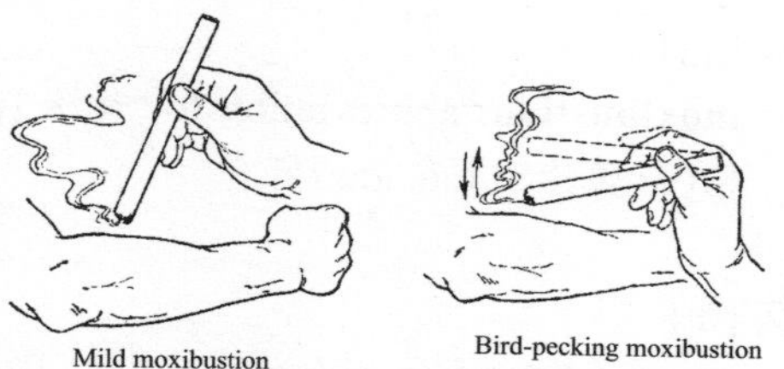

Fig. 31 Moxa-stick moxibustion

艾卷灸 [ài juǎn jiǔ]
moxa-roll moxibustion; moxibustion with an ignited moxa roll: same as moxa-stick moxibustion (艾条灸 [ài tiáo jiǔ])

悬起灸 [xuán qǐ jiǔ]
suspended moxibustion: type of moxa-stick moxibustion, in which the ignited moxa stick is held above the skin, including mild moxibustion, pecking moxibustion, and revolving moxibustion, also called 悬灸 [xuán jiǔ]

悬灸 [xuán jiǔ]
suspended moxibustion: same as 悬起灸 [xuán qǐ jiǔ]

温和灸 [wēn hé jiǔ]
mild moxibustion; gentle moxibustion: type of moxa-stick moxibustion, performed by holding an ignited moxa stick approximately an inch away from the patient's skin surface, on top of the selected spot, keeping the spot warm or making it reddened but not burned (Fig. 30)

雀啄灸 [què zhuó jiǔ]
bird-pecking moxibustion; pecking moxibustion: type of moxa-stick moxibustion, performed by holding an ignited moxa stick near the patient's skin surface, and moving it up and down on top of the selected spot so as to give more than mild heat to the spot (Fig. 30)

回旋灸 [huí xuán jiǔ]
circling moxibustion; revolving moxibustion: type of moxa-stick moxibustion, performed by keeping an ignited moxa stick at a fixed distance away from the patient's skin surface, while moving it in a circular direction centered on the selected spot

艾炷灸 [ài zhù jiǔ]
moxa-cone moxibustion: moxibustion with an ignited moxa cone, which may be applied directly or indirectly

大炷灸 [dà zhù jiǔ]
large cone moxibustion: moxibustion with a large moxa cone, the base of which is no less than 1 cm in diameter

小炷灸 [xiǎo zhù jiǔ]
small cone moxibustion: moxibustion with a small moxa cone, the base of which is approximately 0.3 cm in diameter

麦粒灸 [mài lì jiǔ]
wheat-grain-sized cone moxibustion: moxibustion with a small moxa cone with the shape and size of a wheat grain

直接灸 [zhí jiē jiǔ]
direct moxibustion: moxibustion by applying an ignited moxa cone directly to the skin surface, also called 明灸 [míng jiǔ] or direct contact moxibustion (着肤灸 [zháo fū jiǔ])

明灸 [míng jiǔ]
direct moxibustion: same as直接灸 [zhí jiē jiǔ]

着肤灸 [zháo fū jiǔ]
direct contact moxibustion: another name for direct moxibustion (直接灸 [zhí jiē jiǔ])

瘢痕灸 [bān hén jiǔ]
scarring moxibustion: type of direct moxibustion performed by applying an ignited moxa cone till the skin of the applied spot is burned, blisters and then pustulates, leaving a scar, also known as pustulating moxibustion (化脓灸 [huà nóng jiǔ])

化脓灸 [huà nóng jiǔ]
pustulating moxibustion: another name for scarring moxibustion (瘢痕灸 [bān hén jiǔ])

无瘢痕灸 [wú bān hén jiǔ]
non-scarring moxibustion: type of direct moxibustion performed by applying an ignited moxa cone till the skin of the applied spot turns red but not burned, leaving no scar, also known as non-pustulating moxibustion (非化脓灸 [fēi huà nóng jiǔ])

非化脓灸 [fēi huà nóng jiǔ]
non-pustulating moxibustion: another name for non-scarring moxibustion (无瘢痕灸 [wú bān hén jiǔ])

间接灸 [jiàn jiē jiǔ]
indirect moxibustion: moxibustion using an ignited moxa cone, performed by placing something (e.g., a slice of ginger, garlic, some salt, or a cake of crushed medicinal) between the moxa cone and the skin, also known as interposed moxibustion (隔物灸 [gé wù jiǔ] or 间隔灸 [jiàn gé jiǔ])

隔物灸 [gé wù jiǔ]
interposed moxibustion: another name for indirect moxibustion (间接灸 [jiān jiē jiǔ])

间隔灸 [jiàn gé jiǔ]
interposed moxibustion: same as 隔物灸 [gé wù jiǔ]

隔姜灸 [gé jiāng jiǔ]
ginger-interposed moxibustion: indirect moxibustion mediated by ginger, performed by placing beneath the moxa cone and on

the applied spot a piece of fresh ginger approximately 3mm thick with pores made on it, used for treating vomiting, abdominal pain and diarrhea due to endogenous cold

隔蒜灸 [gé suàn jiǔ]
garlic-interposed moxibustion: indirect moxibustion mediated by garlic, performed by placing beneath the moxa cone and on the applied spot a piece of fresh garlic approximately 3 mm thick with some pores made on it, used for treating sores and boils

隔盐灸 [gé yán jiǔ]
salt-interposed moxibustion: indirect moxibustion mediated by salt, performed by filling the umbilical depression to the brim with salt and then putting a large ignited moxa cone on the salt, used for treating prostration, abdominal pain due to cold, acute vomiting and diarrhea

附子饼灸 [fù zǐ bǐng jiǔ]
aconite-interposed moxibustion: indirect moxibustion mediated by aconite, performed by placing beneath the moxa cone and on the applied spot a cake of *Radix Aconiti Lateralis* mixed with wine, used for treating impotence, or chronic diarrhea

温针灸 [wēn zhēn jiǔ]
warming needle moxibustion: a practice used for treating rheumatic pains, performed by placing a segment of ignited moxa stick on the handle of the needle after insertion of the needle

实按灸 [shí àn jiǔ]
pressing moxibustion: moxibustion performed by placing several layers of cloth or paper on the selected spot and then pressing the ignited end of a moxa stick on the cloth or paper

雷火神针 [léi huǒ shén zhēn]
thunder-fire miraculous moxibustion: type of pressing moxibustion performed by using a special kind of medicinal moxa roll containing mugwort, frankincense, wolfsbane, realgar, and other medicinal herbs

温灸器灸 [wēn jiǔ qì jiǔ]
moxa-burner moxibustion: moxibustion using a moxa burner

天灸 [tiān jiǔ]
natural moxibustion: practice equivalent to moxibustion, performed by applying irritant medicinal on the selected spots of the skin to induce vesiculation or local congestion, also known as medicinal moxibustion (药物灸 [yào wù jiǔ]) or vesiculating moxibustion (发泡灸 [fā pào jiǔ])

药物灸 [yào wù jiǔ]
medicinal moxibustion: same as natural moxibustion (天灸[tiān jiǔ])

发泡灸 [fā pào jiǔ]
vesiculating moxibustion: same as natural moxibustion (天灸 [tiān jiǔ])

蒜泥灸 [suàn ní jiǔ]
ground garlic moxibustion: type of vesiculating moxibustion performed by applying ground garlic to the selected spots of the skin

斑蝥灸 [bān máo jiǔ]

cantharis moxibustion: type of vesiculating moxibustion performed by applying powdered cantharis to the selected spots of the skin

白芥子灸 [bái jiè zǐ jiǔ]

white mustard moxibustion: type of vesiculating moxibustion performed by applying powdered white mustard seed to the selected spots of the skin

电灸器 [diàn jiǔ qì]

electric moxibustion device: device for moxibustion with the heat generated by electricity

电灸 [diàn jiǔ]

electric moxibustion: moxibustion with the heat generated by electricity, also called 电热灸 [diàn rè jiǔ]

电热灸 [diàn rè jiǔ]

electric moxibustion: same as 电灸[diàn jiǔ]

红外线灸 [hóng wài xiàn jiǔ]

infrared moxibustion: moxibustion with the heat generated by infrared radiation

晕灸 [yùn jiǔ]

fainting during moxibustion: feeling of faintness during moxibustion as an adverse reaction to the treatment

灸禁 [jiǔ jìn]

moxibustion contraindication: conditions that make moxibustion therapy inadvisable, e.g., high fever with rapid floating pulse, also called 灸忌 [jiǔ jì]

灸忌 [jiǔ jì]

moxibustion contraindication: same as 灸禁 [jiǔ jìn]

禁灸穴 [jìn jiǔ xué]

moxibustion-prohibited point: point to which moxibustion must not be applied

拔罐 [bá guàn]

cupping: suction by using a vacuumized (usually by fire) cup or jar

拔罐疗法 [bá guàn liáo fǎ]

cupping therapy: therapeutic method involving the application of suction of certain body area by placing a cup or jar onto the surface, followed by vacuumization

竹罐 [zhú guàn]

bamboo cup: cup made of bamboo as a cupping device (Fig. 32)

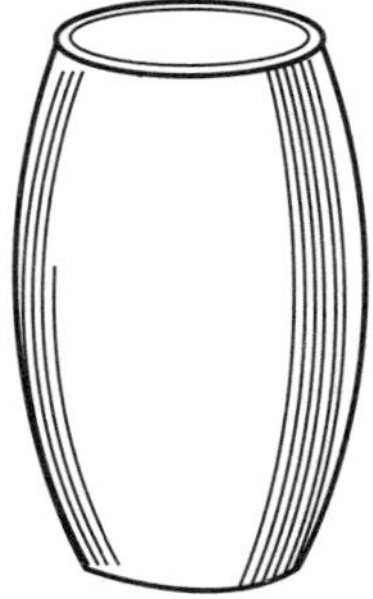

Fig. 32 Bamboo cup

陶罐 [táo guàn]

pottery cup: cup made of pottery as a cupping device

玻璃罐 [bō lí guàn]

glass cup: cup made of glass as a cupping device (Fig. 33)

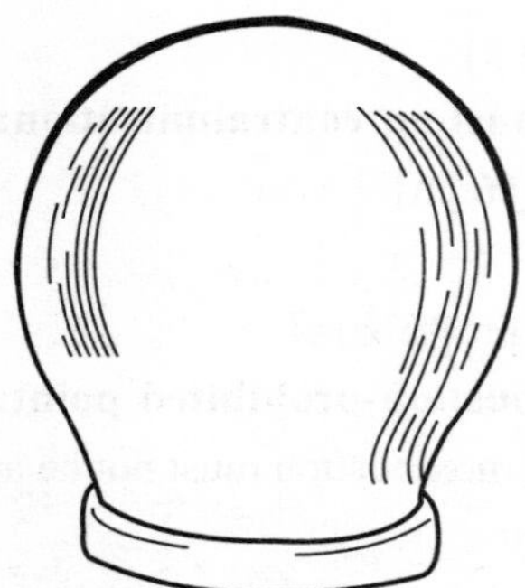
Fig. 33 Glass cup

抽气罐 [chōu qì guàn]
suction cup: cup or jar with a rubber valve through which the air inside can be sucked out

火罐法 [huǒ guàn fǎ]
fire cupping: cupping therapy with the cup or jar vacuumized by fire

闪火法 [shǎn huǒ fǎ]
flash-fire cupping: cupping procedure which involves flashing the fire of a small ignited alcohol-cotton ball once around the cup/jar interior, and pressing the cup/jar onto the applied area immediately after removing the ignited cotton (Fig. 34)

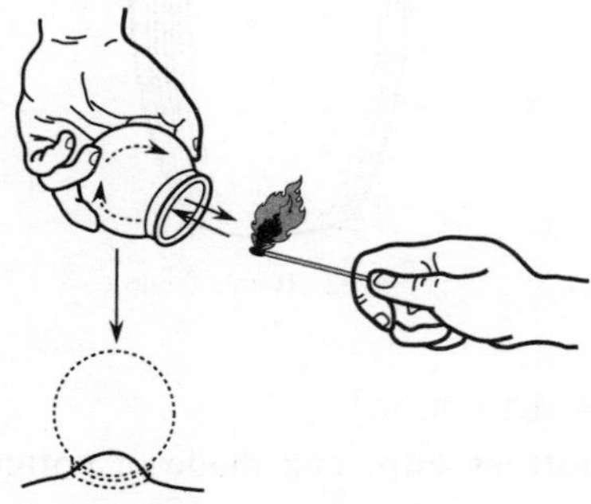
Fig. 34 Flash-fire cupping

投火法 [tóu huǒ fǎ]
fire-insertion cupping: cupping procedure which involves inserting a small ignited alcohol-cotton ball or crunched piece of paper into a cup/jar and pressing the cup/jar transversely onto the applied area of the lateral side of the body

架火法 [jià huǒ fǎ]
fire-rack cupping: cupping procedure which involves placing at the applied area a piece of incombustible substance with a small alcohol-cotton ball on it, and covering with a cup/jar immediately after igniting the cotton ball (Fig. 35)

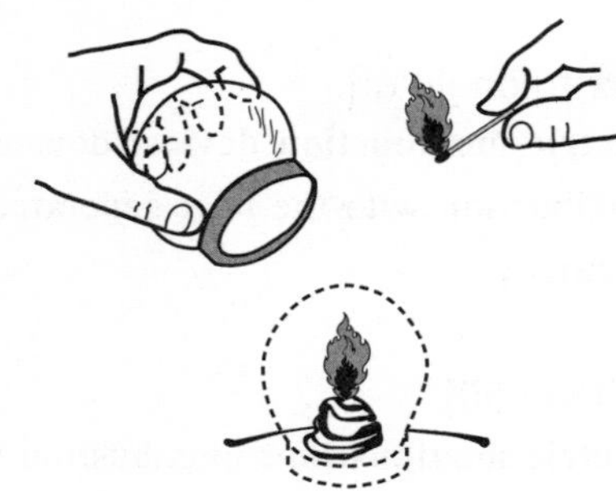
Fig. 35 Fire-racking cupping

贴棉法 [tiē mián fǎ]
cotton-burning cupping: cupping procedure which involves affixing a thin layer of alcohol-cotton pad on the wall of the cup/jar, and pressing the cup/jar onto the applied area after igniting the cotton

滴酒法 [dī jiǔ fǎ]
alcohol fire cupping: cupping procedure which involves spreading 1-3 drops of alcohol solution on the bottom of the cup/jar and pressing the cup/jar onto the applied area after igniting the alcohol

抽气罐法 [chōu qì guàn fǎ]
suction cupping: cupping therapy by using suction cups/jars

煮罐法 [zhǔ guàn fǎ]
cup-boiling method: cupping procedure

which involves putting a bamboo cup/jar onto the applied area, after being boiled in water or a herbal decoction for a short period of time, usually 1-2 minutes

留罐 [liú guàn]
retained cupping: common method of cupping in which the cup/jar is kept suctioned on the spot for a period of time, usually10-15 minutes, to maximize the therapeutic effect, also called 坐罐 [zuò guàn]

坐罐 [zuò guàn]
retained cupping: same as 留罐 [liú guàn]

推罐 [tuī guàn]
glide cupping: cupping method in which the cup/jar is moved to and fro on the skin surface lubricated with vaseline in advance, also known as slide cupping (走罐 [zǒu guàn]) (Fig. 36)

走罐 [zǒu guàn]
slide cupping: synonymous with glide cupping (推罐 [tuī guàn]) (Fig. 36)

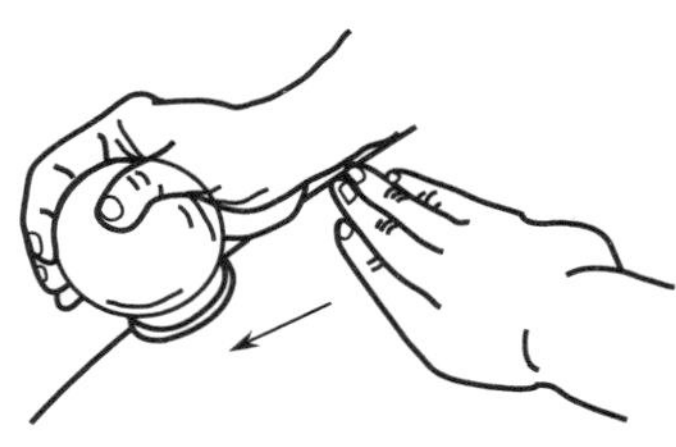

Fig. 36 Glide cupping (slide cupping)

留针拔罐 [liú zhēn bá guàn]
cupping with needle retention: combined method of acupuncture and cupping in which cupping is applied to the acupuncture site with the needle retained after the arrival of *qi*

刺血拔罐 [cì xuè bá guàn]
bloodletting pricking and cupping: combined method of pricking and cupping in which cupping is applied to the site pricked with a three-edged needle for bloodletting, also known as collateral pricking and cupping (刺络拔罐 [cì luò bá guàn])

刺络拔罐 [cì luò bá guàn]
collateral pricking and cupping: same as bloodletting pricking and cupping (刺血拔罐 [cì xuè bá guàn])

药罐 [yào guàn]
medicated cupping: type of cupping therapy in which the cup or jar is dipped into boiling medicinal solution before use

起罐 [qǐ guàn]
cup removal: removing the cup or jar at the end of cupping therapy

刮痧板 [guā shā bǎn]
scraping bar: bar made of hard material such as ox horn, stone or jade, used in scraping therapy

刮痧疗法 [guā shā liáo fǎ]
scraping therapy: therapeutic method whereby the skin of a certain area is repeatedly scraped with a bar until local congestion occurs

撮痧疗法 [cuō shā liáo fǎ]
pinching therapy: therapy whereby a disease is treated by pinching a certain area of the body surface such as the area around an acupoint to induce local congestion, also called 抓痧疗法 [zhuā shā liáo fǎ]

抓痧疗法 [zhuā shā liáo fǎ]
pinching therapy: same as 撮痧疗法 [cuō shā liáo fǎ]

电针 [diàn zhēn]
electro-acupuncture; galvano-acupuncture: acupuncture with electric stimulation after the needle is inserted and normal sensation is felt

电针仪 [diàn zhēn yí]
electric stimulator: instrument that provides electric stimulation for electro-acupuncture

电针疗法 [diàn zhēn liáo fǎ]
electro-acupuncture therapy: treatment of disease with electro-acupuncture

激光针 [jī guāng zhēn]
laser acupuncture: variant of acupuncture in which needling is replaced by laser irradiation

微波针灸 [wēi bō zhēn jiǔ]
microwave acumoxibustion: variant of acupuncture which incorporates microwave radiation technique with needling so that both acupuncture and moxibustion effects are produced

微波针灸疗法 [wēi bō zhēn jiǔ liáo fǎ]
microwave acupuncture therapy: treatment of disease with incorperaton of microwave radiation with acupuncture

穴位注射 [xué wèi zhù shè]
acupoint injection: method whereby liquid medicine is injected into the selected point so as to obtain a combined therapeutic effect of both needling stimulation and pharmaceutical reaction

水针 [shuǐ zhēn]
hydro-acupuncture: same as acupoint injection (穴位注射 [xué wèi zhù shè])

穴位封闭 [xué wèi fēng bì]
acupoint block: block anesthesia accomplished by injecting anaesthetics into selected points for treating pains of various kinds

针刺麻醉 [zhēn cì má zuì]
acupuncture anesthesia: method of inducing anaesthetic effect by way of needling, often applied in a surgical operation during which the patient remains conscious

电针麻醉 [diàn zhēn má zuì]
electro-acupuncture anesthesia: method of inducing anesthesia by way of electro-acupuncture

针麻诱导 [zhēn má yòu dǎo]
induction of acupuncture anesthesia: process of manual or electric stimulation to raise the pain threshold of the patient, usually performed before a surgical operation

头针 [tóu zhēn]
scalp acupuncture: acupuncture at the specific lines located on the scalp, also called 头皮针 [tóu pí zhēn]

头皮针 [tóu pí zhēn]
scalp acupuncture: same as 头针 [tóu zhēn]

头针疗法 [tóu zhēn liáo fǎ]
scalp acupuncture therapy: method of acupuncture in which points along specific lines on the scalp are needled for therapeutic purpose，also called 头皮针疗法 [tóu pí zhēn liáo fǎ]

头皮针疗法 [tóu pí zhēn liáo fǎ]
scalp acupuncture therapy: same as 头针疗法 [tóu zhēn liáo fǎ]

头穴线 [tóu xué xiàn]
scalp acupuncture lines: virtual lines used in scalp acupuncture, labeled with the alphabetic code MS (derived from "micro-system" and "scalp point") for positioning along the middle of the head

额中线 [é zhōng xiàn]
middle line of the forehead (MS 1): the line 1 *cun* from *Shenting* (GV 24) straight down along the meridian/channel of GV

额旁1线 [é páng yī xiàn]
lateral line 1 of the forehead (MS 2): the line 1 *cun* from *Meichong* (BL 3) straight down along the bladder meridian/channel

额旁2线 [é páng èr xiàn]
lateral line 2 of the forehead (MS 3): the line 1 *cun* from *Toulingqi* (GB 15) straight down along the gallbladder meridian/channel

额旁3线 [é páng sān xiàn]
lateral line 3 of the forehead (MS 4): the line 1 *cun* from and 0.75 cun medial to *Touwei* (ST 8), straight down

顶中线 [dǐng zhōng xiàn]
middle line of the vertex (MS 5): the line from *Baihui* (GV 20) to *Qianding* (GV 21)

顶颞前斜线 [dǐng niè qián xié xiàn]
anterior oblique line of the vertex-temporal (MS 6): the line from *Qianshencong*, 1 *cun* anterior to *Baihui* (GV 20) obliquely to *Xuanli* (GB 6)

顶颞后斜线 [dǐng niè hòu xié xiàn]
posterior oblique line of the vertex-temporal (MS 7): the line from *Baihui* (GV 20) obliquely to *Qubin* (GB 7)

顶旁1线 [dǐng páng yī xiàn]
lateral line 1 of the vertex (MS 8): the line 1.5 *cun* lateral to the middle line of the vertex, 1.5 *cun* from *Chengguang* (BL 6) backward along the bladder meridian/channel

顶旁2线 [dǐng páng èr xiàn]
lateral line 2 of the vertex (MS 9): the line 2.25 *cun* lateral to the middle line of the vertex, 1.5 *cun* from *Zhengying* (GB 17) backward along the gallbladder meridian/channel

颞前线 [niè qián xiàn]
anterior temporal line (MS 10): the line from GB 4 to GB 5

颞后线 [niè hòu xiàn]
posterior temporal line (MS 11): the line from *Shuaigu* (GB 8) to *Qubin* (GB 7)

枕上正中线 [zhěn shàng zhèng zhōng xiàn]
upper-middle line of the occiput (MS 12): the line from *Qiangjian* (GV 18) to *Naohu* (GV 17)

枕上旁线 [zhěn shàng páng xiàn]

upper-lateral line of the occiput (MS 13): the line 0.5 *cun* lateral and parallel to the upper-middle line of the occiput

枕下旁线 [zhěn xià páng xiàn]

lower-lateral line of the occiput (MS 14): the line 2 *cun* from *Yuzhen* (BL 9), straight down

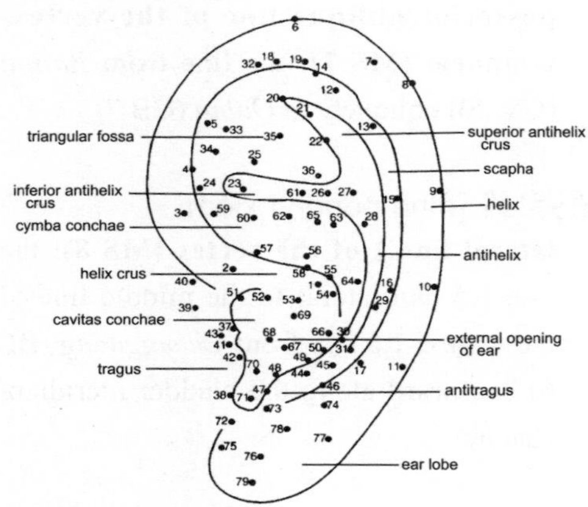

Fig. 37 Points on the anterior aspect of the auricle

耳针 [ěr zhēn]

ear acupuncture: needling of the points located on the ear

耳针疗法 [ěr zhēn liáo fǎ]

ear acupuncture therapy: variety of acupuncture therapy in which specific points on the ear are needled for treating a large variety of diseases, such as asthma, gastric troubles, neurasthenia, skin diseases, hypertension, and enuresis as well as achieving anesthesia

耳轮 [ěr lún]

helix: the prominent rim of the auricle

耳轮结节 [ěr lún jié jié]

helix tubercle: small tubercle at the posterosuperior aspect of the helix

耳轮脚 [ěr lún jiǎo]

helix crus: transverse part of the helix that runs backward to the ear cavity

耳轮尾 [ěr lún wěi]

helix cauda: inferior part of the helix which the earlobe adjoins

对耳轮 [duì ěr lún]

antihelix: elevated Y-shaped ridge opposite the helix, including the trunk, superior and inferior crura

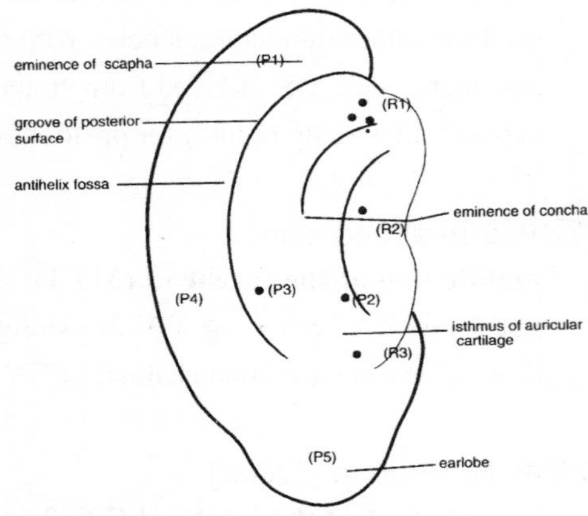

Fig. 38 Points on the posterior aspect of the auricle

对耳轮体 [duì ěr lún tǐ]

trunk of the antihelix: main vertical part of the antihelix

对耳轮上脚 [duì ěr lún shàng jiǎo]

superior crus of the antihelix: upper (upward) branch of the antihelix

对耳轮下脚 [duì ěr lún xià jiǎo]

inferior crus of the antihelix: lower (forward) branch of the antihelix

三角窝 [sān jiǎo wō]

triangular fossa: triangular depression between the two crura of the antihelix

耳舟 [ěr zhōu]
scapha: curved depression between the helix and antihelix

耳屏 [ěr píng]
tragus: cartilaginous projection anterior to external opening of the ear

对耳屏 [duì ěr píng]
antitragus: projection opposite the tragus

屏上切迹 [píng shàng qiē jì]
supratragic notch: depression between the helix crux and the upper border of the tragus

屏间切迹 [píng jiān qiē jì]
intertragic notch: depression between the tragus and antitragus

轮屏切迹 [lún píng qiē jì]
helix notch: depression between the antitragus and antihelix

耳垂 [ěr chuí]
earlobe: lower part of the auricle where there is no cartilage

耳甲 [ěr jiǎ]
concha auricularis; concha: hollow of the auricle of the external ear, bounded anteriorly by the tragus and posteriorly by the antihelix

耳甲艇 [ěr jiǎ tǐng]
cymba conchae: upper part of the concha of the auricle, superior to the helix crus

耳甲腔 [ěr jiǎ qiāng]
cavity of the concha; cavitas conchae: part of the concha of the auricle inferior to the helix crus

外耳门 [wài ěr mén]
external opening of the ear: orifice of the external auditory meatus

上耳根 [shàng ěr gēn]
superior auricular root: area where the upper border of the auricle is attached to the scalp

下耳根 [xià ěr gēn]
inferior auricular root: area where the earlobe is attached to the face

耳穴 [ěr xué]
ear acupoints: points used in ear acupuncture (see the table below and Fig. 37 and 38)

Chinese	Pinyin	English	Location
耳中	ěr zhōng	ear center	at the helix crus (1)
直肠	zhí cháng	rectum	at the helix anterosuperior to the helix crus (2)
尿道	niào dào	urethra	at the helix above the rectum area (3)
外生殖器	wài shēng zhí qì	external genitals	at the helix anterior to the inferior crus of the antihelix (4)
肛门	gāng mén	anus	at the helix anterior to the triangular fossa (5)
耳尖	ěr jiān	ear apex	at the tip of the auricle when the ear is folded toward the tragus (6)

结节	jié jié	node	at the helix tubercle (7)
轮 1	lún yī	helix 1	at the helix below the helix tubercle (8)
轮 2	lún èr	helix 2	at the helix below helix 1 (9)
轮 3	lún sān	helix 3	at the helix below helix 2 (10)
轮 4	lún sì	helix 4	at the helix below helix 3 (11)
指	zhǐ	finger	at the top of the scapha (12)
腕	wàn	wrist	just below the finger area (13)
风溪	fēng xī	wind stream	at the junction of the finger and wrist areas, anterior to the helix tubercle (14)
肘	zhǒu	elbow	below the wrist area (15)
肩	jiān	shoulder	below the elbow area (16)
锁骨	suǒ gǔ	clavicle	below the shoulder area (17)
跟	gēn	heel	at the front part of the top of the superior crus of the antihelix (18)
趾	zhǐ	toe	at the back part of the top of the superior crus of the antihelix, just below the ear apex (19)
踝	huái	ankle	below the heel and toe areas (20)
膝	xī	knee	at the middle 1/3 of the superior crus of antihelix (21)
髋	kuān	hip	at the lower 1/3 of the superior crus of the antihelix (22)
坐骨神经	zuò gǔ shén jīng	sciatic nerve	at the front 2/3 of the inferior crus of the antihelix (23)
交感	jiāo gǎn	sympathesis	at the junction between the inferior crus of the antihelix and the inner border of the helix (24)
臀	tún	gluteus	at the back 1/3 of the inferior crus of the antihelix (25)
腹	fù	abdomen	at the upper 2/5 of the anterior part of the trunk of the antihelix (26)
腰骶椎	yāo dǐ zhuī	lumbosacral vertebrae	just behind the abdomen area (27)
胸	xiōng	chest	at the middle 2/5 of the front part of the antihelix (28)
胸椎	xiōng zhuī	thoracic vertebrae	just behind the chest area (29)
颈	jǐng	neck	at the lower 1/5 of the front part of the antihelix (30)
颈椎	jǐng zhuī	cervical vertebrae	just behind the neck area (31)

角窝上	jiǎo wō shàng	superior triangular fossa	in the upper part of the front 1/3 of the triangular fossa (32)
内生殖器	nèi shēng zhí qì	internal genitals	in the lower part of the front 1/3 of the triangular fossa (33)
角窝中	jiǎo wō zhōng	middle triangular fossa	at the middle 1/3 of the triangular fossa (34)
神门	shén mén	*shenmen*	in the upper part of the back 1/3 of the triangular fossa (35)
盆腔	pén qiāng	pelvis	in the lower part of the back 1/3 of the triangular fossa (36)
上屏	shàng píng	upper tragus	at the upper 1/2 of the outer side of the tragus (37)
下屏	xià píng	lower tragus	at the lower 1/2 of the outer side of the tragus (38)
外耳	wài ěr	external ear	in front of the supratragic notch, close to the helix (39)
屏尖	píng jiān	apex of the tragus	at the upper end of the free border of the tragus (40)
外鼻	wài bí	external nose	at the middle of the outer side of the tragus (41)
肾上腺	shèn shàng xiàn	adrenal gland	at the lower end of the free border of the tragus (42)
咽喉	yān hóu	throat	at the upper 1/2 of the inner side of the tragus (43)
内鼻	nèi bí	internal nose	at the lower 1/2 of the inner side of the tragus
屏间前	píng jiān qián	anterior intertragal notch	in the lowest part of the tragus, in front of the intertragal notch
额	é	forehead	in the front part of the outer side of the antitragus (44)
屏间后	píng jiān hòu	posterior intertragal notch	in the anteroinferior part of the antitragus, behind the intertragal notch
颞	niè	temple	in the middle part of the outer side of the antitragus (45)
枕	zhěn	occiput	in the back part of the outer side of the antitragus (46)
皮质下	pí zhì xià	subcortex	in the inner side of the antitragus (47)
对屏尖	duì píng jiān	apex of the antitragus	at the apex of the free border of the antitragus (48)
缘中	yuán zhōng	central rim	on the free border of the antitragus, at the mid-point between the apex of the antitragus and the helix notch (49)

脑干	nǎo gàn	brain stem	at the helix notch (50)
口	kǒu	mouth	at the front 1/3 below the helix crus (51)
食道	shí dào	esophagus	at the middle 1/3 below the helix crus (52)
贲门	bēn mén	cardia	at the back 1/3 below the helix crus (53)
胃	wèi	stomach	at the place where the helix crus ends (54)
十二指肠	shī èr zhǐ cháng	duodenum	at the back 1/3 of the superior helix crux (55)
小肠	xiǎo cháng	small intestine	at the middle 1/3 of the superior helix crus (56)
大肠	dà cháng	large intestine	at the front 1/3 of the superior helix crus (57)
阑尾	lán wěi	appendix	between the small and large intestine areas (58)
艇角	tǐng jiǎo	angle of the superior concha	at the front part below the inferior crus of the antihelix (59)
膀胱	páng guāng	bladder	at the middle part below the inferior crus of the antihelix (60)
肾	shèn	kidney	at the back part below the inferior crus of the antihelix (61)
输尿管	shū niào guǎn	ureter	between the kidney and bladder areas (62)
胰胆	yí dǎn	pancreas and gallbladder	at the posterosuperior part of the cymba conchae (63)
肝	gān	liver	at the posteroinferior part of the cymba conchae (64)
艇中	tǐng zhōng	center of the superior concha	between the small intestine and kidney areas (65)
脾	pí	spleen	at the posterosuperior part of the cavitas conchae (66)
心	xīn	heart	in the center of the cavitas conchae (67)
气管	qì guǎn	trachea	between the heart area and the external opening of the ear (68)
肺	fèi	lung	around the heart and trachea areas (69)
三焦	sān jiāo	triple energizer	posteroinferior to the external opening of the ear, between the lung and endocrine areas (70)
内分泌	nèi fēn mì	endocrine	inside the intertragic notch, at the anteroinferior part of the cavitas conchae (71)
牙	yá	tooth	in the anterosuperior part of the front side of the earlobe (72)
舌	shé	tongue	in the mediosuperior part of the front side of the earlobe (73)

颌	hé	jaw	in the posterosuperior part of the front side of the earlobe (74)
垂前	chuí qián	anterior ear lobe	in the anteromedial part of the front side of the earlobe (75)
眼	yǎn	eye	in the central part of the front side of the earlobe (76)
内耳	nèi ěr	internal ear	in the posteromedial part of the front side of the earlobe (77)
面颊	miàn jiá	cheek	at the junction between the internal ear and eye areas (78)
扁桃体	biǎn táo tǐ	tonsil	in the lower part of the front side of the earlobe (79)
耳背心	ěr bèi xīn	heart of the posterior surface	in the upper part of the posterior surface of the auricle (P1)
耳背肺	ěr bèi fèi	lung of the posterior surface	in the middle and inner part of the posterior surface of the auricle (P2)
耳背脾	ěr bèi pí	spleen of the posterior surface	at the center of the posterior surface of the auricle (P3)
耳背肝	ěr bèi gān	liver of the posterior surface	in the middle and outer part of the posterior surface of the auricle (P4)
耳背肾	ěr bèi shèn	kidney of the posterior surface	in the lower part of the posterior surface of the auricle (P5)
耳背沟	ěr bèi gōu	groove of the posterior surface	in the groove of the inferior crus of the antihelix
上耳根	shàng ěr gēn	upper ear root	at the upper border of the auricular root (R1)
耳迷根	ěr mí gēn	root of the ear vagus	at the junction of the retroauricle and the mastoid, at the level of the helix crus (R2)
下耳根	xià ěr gēn	lower ear root	at the lower border of the auricular root (R3)

Note: The figures in parentheses refer to the points or areas shown in Fig. 37 and 38.

耳穴探测仪 [ěr xué tàn cè yí]

auricular point detector: apparatus to test electric conductivity, for locating needling points in ear acupuncture

鼻针 [bí zhēn]

nose acupuncture: needling the points located on the nose

鼻针疗法 [bí zhēn liáo fǎ]

nose acupuncture therapy:variety of acupuncture therapy in which specific points on the nose are needled for treating a range of symptoms similar to those listed under ear acupuncture

面针 [miàn zhēn]

facial acupuncture: needling the points located on the face

面针疗法 [miàn zhēn liáo fǎ]

facial acupuncture therapy: variety of acupuncture therapy in which specific points on the face are needled for treating various disorders including those elsewhere in the body

手针 [shǒu zhēn]

hand acupuncture: needling the points located on the hand

手针疗法 [shǒu zhēn liáo fǎ]

hand acupuncture therapy: variety of acupuncture in which specific points on the hand are needled for therapeutic purposes

足针 [zú zhēn]

foot acupuncture: needling the points located on the foot

足针疗法 [zú zhēn liáo fǎ]

foot acupuncture therapy: variety of acupuncture in which specific points on the foot are needled for treating various disorders including those elsewhere in the body

穴位埋线疗法 [xué wèi mái xiàn liáo fǎ]

acupoint catgut-embedding therapy: form of acutherapy in which catgut is imbedded in the acupoint for prolonged stimulation

穿刺针埋线法 [chuān cì zhēn mái xiàn fǎ]

catgut-embedding with lumbar puncture needle: method of embedding catgut in an acupoint by means of a lumbar puncture needle

切开埋线法 [qiē kāi mái xiàn fǎ]

catgut-embedding by incision: method of embedding catgut in anacupoint by means of a local incision

三角针埋线法 [sān jiǎo zhēn mái xiàn fǎ]

catgut-embedding with triangular needle: method of embedding catgut in an acupoint by means of a suture needle

割治疗法 [gē zhì liáo fǎ]

incision therapy: form of acutherapy in which a certain point is incised and a small amount of subcutaneous tissue is removed at the point

磁珠疗法 [cí zhū liáo fǎ]

magnetic bead therapy: form of acutherapy in which magnetized steel beads are taped to selected points as substitutes for needles and retained in place for prolonged stimulation, for treating chronic diseases, also called acupoint magnetic therapy (穴位磁疗法 [xué wèi cí liáo fǎ] or 磁穴疗法 [cí xué liáo fǎ])

穴位磁疗法 [xué wèi cí liáo fǎ]

acupoint magnetic therapy: same as magnetic bead therapy (磁珠疗法 [cí zhū liáo fǎ])

磁穴疗法 [cí xué liáo fǎ]

acupoint magnetic therapy: same as magnetic bead therapy (磁珠疗法 [cí zhū liáo fǎ])

紫外线穴位照射疗法 [zǐ wài xiàn xué wèi zhào shè liáo fǎ]

acupoint ultraviolet irradiation therapy: form of acutherapy in which selected acupoints are irradiated with artificial ultraviolet rays

指压疗法 [zhǐ yā liáo fǎ]

finger-pressure therapy: procedure performed by pressing and rubbing a selected point with the finger(s), indicated in treating syncope, hysteria, epilepsy, toothache, etc.

指压麻醉 [zhǐ yā má zuì]

finger-pressure anesthesia: method of inducing anesthesia by pressing selected point(s) with the finger(s), usually used during tooth extraction

金针拨障法 [jīn zhēn bō zhàng fǎ]

needle couching; needle cataractopiesis: procedure of extracting cataracts by way of acupuncture, in which a special needle is inserted into the eye through an incision followed by removal of the cataract from the pupil, for restoring eyesight

其他疗法与保健 Other Therapies and Health Preservation

推拿按摩 *Tuina* and Massage

按摩 [àn mó]
(I) massage: application of various manipulations to certain points or areas of the patient's body in coordination with movement of the patient's limbs so as to achieve the goals of prevention and treatment of disease, also called 推拿 [tuī ná]; **(II) pressing and rubbing:** two of the eight methods of bone-setting

推拿 [tuī ná]
(I) *tuina*: traditional Chinese medical massage, also called massage (按摩 [àn mó]); **(II) pushing and kneading:** two of the eight methods of bone-setting

推拿疗法 [tuī ná liáo fǎ]
***tuina* therapy:** treatment of disease by *tuina* [massage]

按摩疗法 [àn mó liáo fǎ]
massotherapy: treatment of disease by massage

按跷 [àn qiāo]
"limb-pressing": ancient term for massage

按摩师 [àn mó shī]
massage practitioner; masseur; masseuse: one who practices massage

按摩手法 [àn mó shǒu fǎ]
massage manipulation: different ways of massaging including utilization of different parts of the body of the massager such as the hand or elbow, as well as application of different maneuvers onto certain points or areas of a massagee's body in a skilled manner

按法 [àn fǎ]
pressing: massage manipulation performed by pressing the point or affected area of the patient with the thumb, palm of the hand, or knuckle of the practitioner

按压法 [àn yā fǎ]
sustained pressing: massage manipulation performed by pressing the point or affected area of the patient forcefully with sustained pressure, usually by using the forearm or elbow of the practitioner

掐法 [qiā fǎ]
fingernail pressing: massage manipulation performed by pressing a selected point on the patient's body with a finger-nail of the practitioner to produce a strong stimulation, usually used for treating syncope and convulsions

揉法 [róu fǎ]
kneading: massage technique applicable to all parts of the body, performed by pressing and moving to and fro or circularly on a point or affected area of the patient with the flat of the thumb, tips of the index, middle and ring fingers, thenar eminence, or the root of the palm of the hand of the practitioner

捻法 [niǎn fǎ]
twisting: massage manipulation performed by holding a digital joint or the skin of the patient with the thumb and index finger of the practitioner and twisting it as if twisting a thread, used for relieving rigidity of the joints and ensuring smooth flow of *qi* and blood

刮法 [guā fǎ]
scraping: massage manipulation performed by scraping the area between the eyebrows, nape, or costal regions of the patient with the outer side of the thumb, edge of a spoon or rim of a coin downward or outward to cause local congestion

刮痧 [guā shā]
scraping to congestion: a popular massage manipulation for treating contraction of excess heat, performed by scraping the patient's neck, chest or back to cause local congestion (cf.刮法 [guā fǎ])

拧法 [nǐng fǎ]
pinching and lifting: massage manipulation performed by pinching and lifting a portion of the skin with the second segments of the flexed index and middle fingers like a vice to cause local congestion until the skin turns red and purple

点法 [diǎn fǎ]
point pressing: massage manipulation performed by pressing with light, moderate or intense force as required on a point with the tip of the middle finger while the index and ring fingers are slightly flexed, also called pounding (捣法 [dǎo fǎ] or 捣击法[dǎo jī fǎ]), point hitting (点击法 [diǎn jī fǎ]), and finger puncture (指针法 [zhǐ zhēn fǎ])

捣法 [dǎo fǎ]
pounding: synonym for point pressing (点法 [diǎn fǎ])

捣击法 [dǎo jī fǎ]
pounding: synonym for point pressing (点法 [diǎn fǎ])

点击法 [diǎn jī fǎ]
point-hitting: synonym for point pressing (点法 [diǎn fǎ])

指针法 [zhǐ zhēn fǎ]
finger puncture: synonym for point pressing (点法 [diǎn fǎ])

笃击法 [dǔ jī fǎ]
hitting with the knuckle: massage manipulation performed by hitting a selected point on the patient's body, chiefly the head and upper limbs, with the knuckle of the practitioner's middle finger

抠法 [kōu fǎ]
digging: massage manipulation performed by digging into a depressed part, such as armpit, groin or cubital fossa of the patient with the thumb, middle or index finger of the practitioner and plucking a selected tendon and vessel with force, for treating numbness of a limb

滚法 [gǔn fǎ]
rolling: massage manipulation performed by moving a hollow fist formed with the thumb bent over the fingers by turning it on the selected skin area of the patient back and forth continuously, with moderate force and small amplitude

挠法 [náo fǎ]
scratching: massage manipulation performed by making the index, middle and ring fingers of one hand into a hook, pressing the fingertips of the "hook"onto the top of the patient's back and sliding it down to the lower back

挪法 [núo fǎ]
shifting: massage manipulation performed by rubbing the body surface of the patient slowly but forcibly with the ulnar side of the palm of the hand up and down and to and fro, applied chiefly to the abdomen

摸法 [mō fǎ]
palpating: (1) technique performed by palpating a selected area of the patient's body surface with the hand or fingers of the practitioner, chiefly for diagnosis; (2) one of the eight manipulations of bone-setting, used for examining a traumatic injury and adjacent soft tissues

擦法 [cā fǎ]
rubbing: massage manipulation performed by rubbing with the flat of the fingers, thenar or palms of the hands to and fro on the skin continuously, applied to the patient's forehead, limbs or back

捏法 [niē fǎ]
pinching: massage manipulation performed by holding, lifting and releasing the tissue of the patient by using the thumb and the middle segment of the crooked index finger of the practitioner, often applied to the muscles along the spine on the back

摩法 [mó fǎ]
circular rubbing: massage manipulation performed by rubbing the affected area with the finger tips or the palm of the hand of the practitioner in a circular motion with moderate force and frequency

抹法 [mǒ fǎ]
wiping (with the palm or thumb): massage manipulation performed by rubbing the patient's skin with the palmar side of the practitioner's thumbs or the palms of the hands up and down, right and left, with moderate force to promote the flow of *qi* and blood

推法 [tuī fǎ]
pushing: massage manipulation performed by pushing and squeezing the patient's muscles with the practitioner's fingers, palms of the hands or elbow forward, apart or spirally with force

一指禅推法 [yī zhǐ chán tuī fǎ]
single-finger meditation pushing: massage manipulation performed by pushing the patient's tissue with the tip, flat or outer side of the thumb of the practitioner, on which the practitioner's *qi* is concentrated by meditation, also called single-finger meditation manipulation (一指禅功 [yī zhǐ chán gōng]) (Fig. 39)

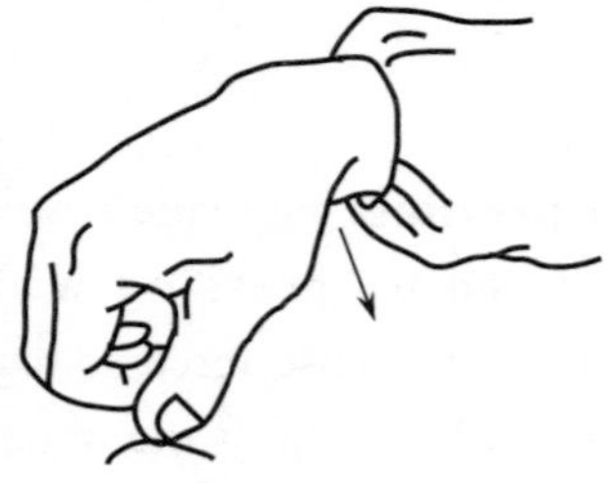

Fig. 39 Single-finger meditation

一指禅功 [yī zhǐ chán gōng]
single-finger meditation manipulation:

synonym for single-finger meditation pushing (一指禅推法 [yī zhǐ chán tuī fǎ])

拳击法 [quán jī fǎ]
rapping: manipulation performed by rapping with the back of the practitioner's fist, chiefly applied to the patient's back

拿法 [ná fǎ]
grasping: massage manipulation performed by lifting and squeezing or lifting and rapidly releasing the patient's affected muscles with three or five fingers of one or both of the practitioner's hands

抓法 [zhuā fǎ]
grasping with the whole hand: massage manipulation performed by grasping the local tissue with the whole palm of the hand and fingers of the practitioner after positioning the center of the palm over a selected area of the patient's body

拿捏法 [ná niē fǎ]
grasping and pinching: massage manipulation performed by combined use of grasping and pinching

捺法 [nà fǎ]
pressing-grasping: massage manipulation performed by pressing a selected area of the patient's body surface with the palm of the hand, grasping the local tissue and the relevant muscle, releasing them, and then repeating the sequence

梳法 [shū fǎ]
combing: massage manipulation performed by combing a selected area of the patient's body surface, usually the abdomen, briskly with the fingertips of the two hands, alternately

拂法 [fú fǎ]
whisking: massage manipulation characterized by a quick and light brushing movement

掸拂法 [dǎn fú fǎ]
brushing and whisking: massage manipulation performed by brushing the patient's spine with the palm(s) of the hand(s), but finishing with a whisk at the end of a brush

运法 [yùn fǎ]
circular kneading: massage manipulation performed by kneading in a circular motion slowly and repeatedly with the thumb and juxtaposed fingers, or the base of the palm of the hand, to promote circulation of *qi* and blood

扯法 [chě fǎ]
pulling: massage manipulation performed by grasping the skin with the thumb and the middle segment of the index finger and giving it a pull before releasing it so as to cause local congestion, also called 揪法 [jiū fǎ]

揪法 [jiū fǎ]
dragging: synonym for pulling (扯法 [chě fǎ])

拍法 [pāi fǎ]
patting: massage manipulation performed by patting gently with one or both palms of the hands on a selected area of the patient's body, often applied at the beginning and end of massotherapy for relaxation

托提法 [tuō tí fǎ]
supporting and lifting: massage manipulation performed by putting the hands under the patient's armpits and lifting him or her up

挤法 [jǐ fǎ]
squeezing: massage manipulation performed by squeezing a selected area of the patient's skin with the thumb and index and middle fingers till the local tissues turn red and purple

搓法 [cuō fǎ]
twisting rubbing: massage manipulation performed by holding the limb or the chest of the patient with both palms of the hands, one on the front and the other from behind, and rubbing in opposite directions (Fig. 40)

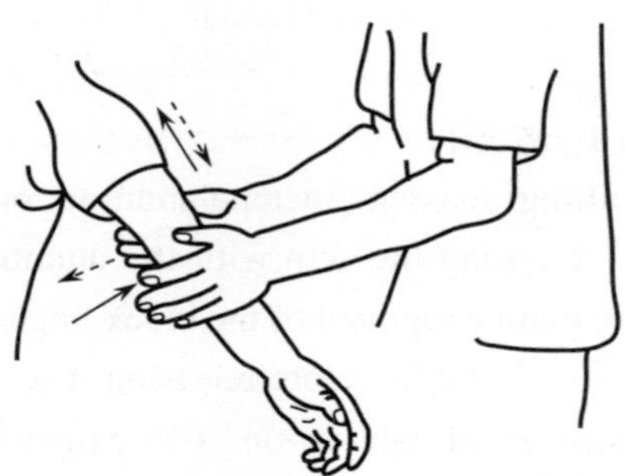

Fig. 40 Twisting manipulation

撮法 [cuō fǎ]
taking up with fingers: massage manipulation performed by grasping a selected area of the skin on the patient's body with three fingers gently, then releasing it and moving on for another grasp

振法 [zhèn fǎ]
vibrating: massage manipulation performed by placing the palm of the hand on a selected area of the patient's body to make rapid local vibrations, also called 颤法 [chàn fǎ]

颤法 [chàn fǎ]
vibrating: synonym for 振法 [zhèn fǎ]

扼法 [è fǎ]
holding tight: massage manipulation performed by placing the palms of the hands on a selected area of the patient's body surface or placing the thumbs and finger tips around the area with the palms lifted untouched, and then grasping and holding the local tissues and the relevant muscle with force for a moment, chiefly applied to the back

叩［扣］法 [kòu fǎ]
tapping: massage manipulation performed by tapping with the tips of the thumb and fingers held together, chiefly applied to the top of the head, also called 啄击法 [zhuó jī fǎ]

啄击法 [zhuó jī fǎ]
pecking: synonym for tapping (扣法 [kòu fǎ])

击法 [jī fǎ]
striking: massage manipulation performed by striking the affected limb of the patient with the palm of the hand or fist of the practitioner, or an aid such as a specially made rod

弹击法 [tán jī fǎ]
flicking: massage manipulation performed by hitting a selected point on the patient's body with the back of a fingertip of the practitioner by flicking it against the latter's thumb

弹筋 [tán jīn]
tendon-plucking: massage manipul-ationperformed by repeatedly pulling up and immediately releasing a tendon or muscle

捶法 [chuí fǎ]
hammering: massage manipulation performed by hitting the patient's back with the ulnar side of the practitioner's hollow fist

棒击法 [bàng jī fǎ]
rodstroking: massage manipulation performed by beating the patient's head or lower back gently with a rod made of mulberry twigs bound together and wrapped in tough paper or cloth

扳法 [bān fǎ]
pulling: massage manipulation performed by pulling, stretching and rotating the joints of the limbs or the waist to relieve rigidity, separate adhesion and restore dislocated bones

扳腿推拿手法 [bān tuǐ tuī ná shǒu fǎ]
leg pulling: massage manipulation utilizing pulling for treating lumbar hyperextension

拨法 [bō fǎ]
poking: massage maniplation performed by poking or plucking a selected tendon of the patient with the fingers of the practitioner forcibly for relieving pain and separating adhesion

摇法 [yáo fǎ]
rotating: massage manipulation performed by turning the patient's head and neck, shoulder, wrist, hip joint, knee joint, or ankle, to and fro for relieving rigidity

伸法 [shēn fǎ]
stretching: massage manipulation performed by extending the disordered joints of the neck and limbs, including pulling and stretching (引伸法 [yǐn shēn fǎ]) and lifting and stretching (提伸法 [tí shēn fǎ])

引伸法 [yǐn shēn fǎ]
pulling and stretching: massage manipulation utilizing both stretching and pulling

提伸法 [tí shēn fǎ]
lifting and stretching: massage maniplation utilizing both stretching and lifting

屈法 [qū fǎ]
flexing: massage manipulation performed by bending the neck, lumbus, elbow, wrist, ankle, fingers, or toes of the patient for relieving rigidity

拨络法 [bō luò fǎ]
collateral-poking: massage manipulation performed by poking a relevant collateral meridian/channel and the affected musculature of the patient with the practitioner's fingers

踩法 [cǎi fǎ]
treading: massage performed by stepping on the affected area, such as the lumbar area, with one or both feet of the practitioner, also called stamping (跷法 [qiāo fǎ]) or treading-stamping (踩跷法 [cǎi qiāo fǎ])

跷法 [qiāo fǎ]
stamping: synonym for treading (踩法 [cǎi fǎ])

踩跷法 [cǎi qiāo fǎ]
treading-stamping: synonym for treading (踩法 [cǎi fǎ])

踏跳法 [tà tiào fǎ]
rhythmic stepping: massage performed by stepping rhythmically on the patient's body along the selected meridians/channels, on the selected acupoints, or directly on the affected area

拉腿手法 [lā tuǐ shǒu fǎ]
leg-pulling manipulation: massage manipulation performed by pulling the leg, for treating lumbago

扭痧 [niǔ shā]
twisting for congestion: massage manipulation by grasping, pulling and turning a selected area of the patient's skin with force to cause local congestion, for treating sunstroke and other related ailments, also called pulling for congestion (扯痧 [chě shā]) or dragging for congestion (揪痧 [jiū shā])

扯痧 [chě shā]
pulling for congestion: synonym for twisting for congestion (扭痧 [niǔ shā])

揪痧 [jiū shā]
dragging for congestion: synonym for twisting for congestion (扭痧 [niǔ shā])

推扳手法 [tuī bān shǒu fǎ]
pushing-pulling: massage manipulation performed by pressing tightly on a selected muscle of the patient with the thumb and fingers while pushing forward or pulling backward the muscle, for relaxing muscular spasm

三板推拿疗法 [sān bǎn tuī ná liáo fǎ]
tri-tabular *tuina*-therapy; tri-tabular massotherapy: massotherapy utilizing three types of boards, i.e., finger pushing board, leg board and oblique board, for treating disorders of the spine and lower limbs

小儿推拿疗法 [xiǎo ér tuī ná liáo fǎ]
infantile *tuina*-therapy; infantile massotherapy: massotherapy performed on a selected area of an infant patient's body, for treating disease or inducing passive movement of the limbs

捏脊 [niē jǐ]
pinching along the spine: massage manipulation performed by pinching and kneading the skin and muscles along the spine, for treating digestive disorders and malnutrition in children, also called pinching (捏积 [niē jī])

捏积 [niē jī]
pinching: synonym for pinching along the spine (捏脊 [niē jǐ])

自我按摩 [zì wǒ àn mó]
automassage: massaging oneself

栉头 [zhì tóu]
combing the head: automassage performed by combing the head with the fingertips from the anterior to the posterior hairline to promote the flow of *qi* and blood

击头 [jī tóu]
tapping the head: automassage performed by tapping the head with the tips of the slightly bent fingers, for refreshing and improving the flow of *qi* and blood

抹前额 [mǒ qián é]
wiping the forehead (with fingers): automassage performed by wiping the forehead with the flat of the index, middle and ring fingers of the right and left hand alternately till the forehead feels hot, or repeatedly rubbing the forehead from the middle to the frontal eminences with the radial side of the index fingers while the thumbs are pressing the temples and the fingers are slightly bent

存泥丸 [cún ní wán]
rubbing the forehead to the top: automassage performed by rubbing the head from the forehead to the top with the right and left palms of the hands alternately for refreshment of the mind

拧眉心 [nǐng méi xīn]
pinching the glabella: automassage performed by pinching the tissues of the central area between the eyebrows with the tip of the thumb and index finger till red and purple spots appear, for treating headache, hypertension and insomnia

按太阳 [àn tài yáng]
pressing the temples: automassage performed by pressing the temples with the tips of the thumbs or the middle fingers, for relieving headache, common cold and facial paralysis

摩面 [mó miàn]
rubbing the face: automassage performed by rubbing the face with the palms of the hands till the whole face grows warm, to promote facial blood circulation

熨目 [yùn mù]
compressing the eyes (with the hot palms): automassage performed by rubbing the palms of the hands till a hot sensation appears and then pressing them on the closed eyes, repeatedly for 30 minutes, for improving eyesight

揉攒竹 [róu cuán zhú]
kneading *Cuanzhu* (BL 2): automassage performed by pressing at the inner ends of the eyebrows with the tips of the thumbs till local soreness and distension are experienced

揉四白 [róu sì bái]
kneading *Sibai* (ST 2): automassage performed by kneading the points below the eyes with the tips of the middle fingers till local soreness and distension are experienced, for improving vision and preventing near-sightedness

按目四眦 [àn mù sì zì]
pressing the four canthi: automassage performed by pressing and rubbing the inner and outer canthi of the eyes with the knuckles of the thumbs bent over the fists till local soreness and distension are felt, for improving vision and preventing near-sightedness

刮眼眶 [guā yǎn kuàng]
scraping the orbital rims: automassage performed by scraping with the radial side of the index fingers or the knuckles of the

thumbs from the inner to the outer canthi along the upper and lower rims of the orbit alternately, for improving vision and preventing near-sightedness

旋耳 [xuán ěr]

revolving the ears: automassage performed by pulling and twisting the ears with the fingers, for improving acuity of hearing

按压耳穴 [àn yā ěr xué]

pressing the auricular points: automassage performed by pressing selected points on the ear as a form of auriculo-acupuncture, for treating various diseases

按捺耳窍 [àn nà ěr qiào]

pressing the ear orifice: automassage performed by pressing the ears with the palms of the hands or stopping the opening of the external auditory canals with the tips of the middle fingers on and off, for improving hearing

按捏鼻梁 [àn niē bí liáng]

pressing and pinching the nose bridge: automassage performed by pressing and pinching the bridge of the nose, for preventing common cold

按迎香 [àn yíng xiāng]

pressing *Yingxiang* (LI 20): automassage performedby pressing bilateral *Yingxiang* (LI20) (the point beside the wing of the nose) with the tips of the middle fingers till soreness and distension are experienced, for treating common cold or rhinitis

揉颊车 [róu jiá chē]

kneading *Jiache* (ST 6): automassage performed by kneading *Jiache* (ST6), one finger breath anterior and superior to the mandibular angles, with the tips of the middle fingers till soreness and distension are experienced, for relieving toothache

叩 [扣] 齿 [kòu chǐ]

tapping the teeth: automassage performed by tapping the upper and lower teeth on each other

搅舌 [jiǎo shé]

stirring the tongue: automassage performed by moving the tongue right and left and up and down to massage the teeth and promote salivation

鸣天鼓 [míng tiān gǔ]

"sounding the celestial drum": automassage performed by pressing the ears with the palms of the hands and beating the occiput with the fingers

摩颈项 [mó jǐng xiàng]

rubbing the neck: automassage performed by rubbing the neck with the right and left palms of the hands alternately till a hot sensation is experienced, for preventing and treating stiff neck

按揉颈项 [àn róu jǐng xiàng]

pressing and kneading the neck: automassage performed by pressing and kneading the large muscles on the back of the neck till local soreness and distension are experienced

拿颈项 [ná jǐng xiàng]

grasping the neck: automassage performed by grasping and rubbing the tendons of the large muscles on both sides of the neck with the thumbs, index and middle fingers moving downward with increasing force until soreness and pain result

按揉风池 [àn róu fēng chí]
pressing and kneading *Fengchi* (GB 20): automassage performed by pressing and kneading with the thumbs while the palms of the hands are placed over the ears till local soreness, distension and pain are experienced, for treating common cold, headache, stiff neck and hypertension

摩击上肢 [mó jī shàng zhī]
rubbing and stroking the arm: automassage performed by rubbing and stroking the arm with the hands (left hand for the right arm and vice versa) to promote circulation of *qi* and blood, for treating numbness and soreness of the arm

拿合谷 [ná hé gǔ]
grasping *Hegu* (LI 4): automassage performed by grasping the tissues of the region between the first and second metacarpal bones of one hand with the thumb and index finger of the other to cause local soreness and pain, for relieving headache and toothache, and treating lockjaw and wry mouth

洗手 [xǐ shǒu]
wringing the hands: automassage performed by rubbing and wringing the hands all over till they grow warm to promote circulation of *qi* and blood, for treating stiffness, numbness and frostbite of the hands

摩腹 [mó fù]
rubbing the abdomen: automassage performed by rubbing the abdomen with both hands in a clockwise direction, for promoting digestion

摩脐 [mó qí]
rubbing the navel: automassage performed by rubbing the navel with the thenar eminence or base of the palm of the hand slowly but forcibly till one feels comfortable, used for treating gastralgia, belching, and abdominal distension and pain

捶腰背 [chuí yāo bèi]
hammering the lower back: automassage performed by hitting the lower back with the back of the fists or with a wooden rod, for relieving lower back pain

揉腰眼 [róu yāo yǎn]
kneading the sides of the small of the back: automassage performed by kneading the sides of the small of the back with the knuckles of the bent thumbs, for strengthening the kidney and relieving lumbar aching and menstrual disorders

击下肢 [jī xià zhī]
striking the lower limb: automassage performed by striking the lower limb with the root of the palms of the hands to promote the flow of *qi* and blood

按摩足三里 [àn mó zú sān lǐ]
massaging *Zusanli* (ST 36): automassage performed by pressing and rubbing *Zusanli* (ST 36) with the tips of the thumbs while sitting, till soreness and distension are experienced, to reinforce *qi* and blood, for treating abdominal pain, indigestion, diarrhea, constipation, fatigue, and insomnia

擦涌泉 [cā yǒng quán]
rubbing *Yongquan* (KI 1): automassage performed by rubbing *Yongquan* (located in the center of the soles of the feet) with the hands, e.g., placing the left foot on the right leg while sitting and holding it with the left hand, rubbing the center of the sole with the palm thenar of the right hand till the point grows warm, and vice versa, for treating dizziness, blurring of vision, insomnia, and hypertension

复合手法 [fù hé shǒu fǎ]
compound manipulation: massage manipulation utilizing a combination of two or more manipulations, such as grasping-pinching and kneading-vibrating

一指禅推拿 [yī zhǐ chán tuī ná]
single-finger meditation *tuina*; single-finger meditation massage: massotherapy performed by massaging a selected point or area with a single finger on which the practitioner's *qi* is concentrated via meditation

滚法推拿 [gǔn fǎ tuī ná]
rolling *tuina*; rolling massage: massotherapy characterized by rolling manipulations, also combined with kneading, pressing, grasping, holding and twisting, and twisting rubbing

内功推拿 [nèi gōng tuī ná]
internal exercise *tuina*; internal exercise massage: massotherapy characterized by vigorous but comfortable palm pushing manipulations

指压推拿 [zhǐ yā tuī ná]
finger-pressing *tuina*; finger-pressing massage: massotherapy characterized by digital point pressing manipulations

点穴疗法 [diǎn xué liáo fǎ]
digital point pressure therapy: therapy characterized by stimulating the selected points with various manipulations such as fingernail pressing, tapping, rapping, etc.

耳穴推拿疗法 [ěr xué tuī ná liáo fǎ]
ear-point *tuina* therapy; ear-point massotherapy: massotherapy performed by pressing and rubbing a vaccaria seed fixed onto a tender point on the auricle with adhesive plaster

保健球按摩 [bǎo jiàn qiú àn mó]
health-ball massage: massage performed by holding two balls of similar size, such as walnuts or balls made of stone or steel, in one hand and rolling them within the hand with the thumb and fingers, a method not only beneficial to the health of the hands, but also to the health in general, especially for the aged

药摩 [yào mó]
medicinal massage: massage mediated by selected medicine chiefly in the form of balm or ointment, also called ointment massage (膏摩 [gāo mó]) in ancient times, for which hundreds of formulas have been prescribed as the effective ingredients of the ointment

膏摩 [gāo mó]
ointment massage: massage performed with ointment as the medium

推拿的补泻手法 [tuī ná de bǔ xiè shǒu fǎ]

reinforcement and reduction manipulations in *tuina* therapy; reinforcement and reduction manipulations in massotherapy: a collective term for massage manipulations effective for either reinforcing the deficient or reducing the excessive, achieved chiefly by altering the force, speed and direction of the massage

轻重徐疾补泻法 [qīng zhòng xú jí bǔ xiè fǎ]

reinforcement-reduction by varying the force and speed: massage guided by the principle that force and speed of a massage decide the outcome – gentle and slow massage gives a reinforcement effect, while quick and forcible massage induces reduction

迎随顺逆补泻法 [yíng suí shùn nì bǔ xiè fǎ]

reinforcement-reduction by massaging along or against the meridian/channel: massage guided by the principle that the direction of a massage in relation to that of a meridian/channel decides the outcome – massage in the direction of the course of the meridian/channel gives a reinforcement effect, while massage in the direction opposed to that of the meridian/channel induces reduction

择向补泻法 [zé xiàng bǔ xiè fǎ]

reinforcement-reduction by choosing direction: massage guided by the principle that direction in a general sense decides the outcome – afferent, upward, inward, or clockwise manipulations give a reinforcement effect, while efferent, downward, outward and counterclockwise manipulations induce reduction; and for men, turning from the right to the left is reinforcement and from the left to the right is reduction, while for women, just the contrary

徒手整复 [tú shǒu zhěng fù]

manual restoration: bare-handed restoration of the normal position of a body part

气功 *Qigong*

气功 [qì gōng]

***qigong*:** systematic exercises encompassing taking proper postures, adjusting breathing, and concentrating to achieve the union of the essence, *qi* and mind as a whole, for physical training, health preservation and prevention and treatment of diseases

导引 [dǎo yǐn]

***daoyin*; conducting (exercise):** ancient Chinese physical exercise associated with respiratory movement and self-massage performed by conducting the mind and *qi*, for health preservation and disease prevention and treatment

静功 [jìng gōng]

static *qigong*: *qigong* exercise practiced without any movement of the body and limbs, also called internal exercise (内功 [nèi gōng])

内功 [nèi gōng]

internal exercise: synonym for static *qigong* (静功 [jìng gōng])

动功 [dòng gōng]
dynamic *qigong*: *qigong* exercise practiced with movement of the body and limbs, also called external exercise (外功 [wài gōng])

外功 [wài gōng]
external exercise: synonym for dynamic *qigong* (动功[dòng gōng])

硬气功 [yìng qì gōng]
hard *qigong*: *qigong* aiming for hardening muscles and joints and mobilizing the forces of the body for a concentrated blow, also called martial-art *qigong* (武术气功 [wǔ shù qì gōng])

武术气功 [wǔ shù qì gōng]
martial-art *qigong*: *qigong* as a kind of martial art, cultivated for self-defense, or as a form of physical training, also called hard *qigong* (硬气功[yìng qì gōng])

软气功 [ruǎn qì gōng]
soft *qigong*: *qigong* aiming to train enduring force through posturization, breathing and mental concentration, for preserving general health, and preventing and treating diseases

医用气功 [yī yòng qì gōng]
medical *qigong*: *qigong* exercises aiming to achieve therapeutic effects, especially for treating functional and chronic diseases

气功疗法 [qì gōng liáo fǎ]
***qigong* therapy:** therapeutic treatment by practicing *qigong*

儒家气功 [rú jiā qì gōng]
Confucian *qigong*: *qigong* developed by the Confucian school, focused on the cultivation of quietude in mind and body, and their coordination

道家气功 [dào jiā qì gōng]
Taoist *qigong*: *qigong* initiated and developed by Tao's priests, based on the principles of self-physiological alchemy and the microcosm of the universe, aiming to discover an elixir of life and the "fountain of perpetual youth"

佛家气功 [fó jiā qì gōng]
Buddhist *qigong*: *qigong* developed by Buddhists, based on the wisdom of liberation from reincarnation and self-observation, as a tool to search for the perfection of purity of mind, and the ultimate union between the individual and the universe

动静相兼功 [dòng jìng xiāng jiān gōng]
static-dynamic *qigong*: *qigong* involving both static and dynamic exercises

动中有静 [dòng zhōng yǒu jìng]
quiescence within motion: quietness coexisting with motion, particularly referring or as a guideline to the practice of a dynamic *qigong* exercise, which appears to be motive, but requires quietness of mind or high concentration

静中有动 [jìng zhōng yǒu dòng]
motion within quiescence: motion coexisting with quietness, particularly referring or as a guideline to the practice of a static *qigong* exercise, which appears to be static, but actually requires ability or elements of motion in order to make the movements go smoothly

内景 [nèi jǐng]
inner scene: the image of the activities of *zang-fu* organs, *qi* and blood formed in the mind

松 [sōng]
relaxation: principle of *qigong* exercise, referring to relaxation of both the body and mind

入静 [rù jìng]
entering quiescence; falling into static state: restful state of the mind attained, via directional exercise of mental activity during the awakened state, in which the mind is aware of changes in physiological functions inside the body while maximally eliminating both internal and external interferences

内视 [nèi shì]
inward vision: seeing inward at a certain part of the body to induce corresponding changes by means of the mind

调身 [tiáo shēn]
posture management: making the body suitable and convenient for *qigong* exercise to guarantee a smooth flow of internal *qi*, also called posturization (姿式 [zī shì])

身法 [shēn fǎ]
posture management: same as 调身 [tiáo shēn]

姿式 [zī shì]
posturization: synonym for posture management (调身 [tiáo shēn])

调身要领 [tiáo shēn yào lǐng]
essentials of posture management: fundamental elements of adjusting the posture, viz., loosening the clothing, keeping the head upright, shrinking the chest, straightening the back, drooping the shoulders, relaxing the waist and abdomen, contracting the buttocks, etc.

宽解衣带 [kuān jiě yī dài]
loosening clothes: wearing loose clothes or loosening the clothes so that one can move freely (during *qigong* practice), a prerequisite for posture management

头如顶物 [tóu rú dǐng wù]
keeping the head upright as if carrying something on the top: holding the head properly (for *qigong* practice), one of the fundamental elements of posture management

头正 [tóu zhèng]
head upright: the way to hold the head, i.e., keeping the head upright as if the head were hung up at the vertex

颈松 [jǐng sōng]
neck relaxed: keeping the neck relaxed so that the cervical vertebrae can be well spread out

沉肩 [chén jiān]
drooping the shoulders: keeping the shoulders relaxed to prevent shrugging which causes muscular tension

坠肘 [zhuì zhǒu]
dropping the elbows: having the elbows hanging down naturally while the shoulders are drooping, also called down-hanging elbows (垂肘 [chuí zhǒu])

垂肘 [chuí zhǒu]
down-hanging elbows: same as dropping the elbows (坠肘 [zhuì zhǒu])

伸腰沉胯 [shēn yāo chén kuà]
stretching the waist and keeping the hips sunk: one of the fundamental elements of posture management

含胸拔背 [hán xiōng bá bèi]
shrinking the chest and straightening the back: one of the fundamental elements of posture management

舒腰松腹 [shū yāo sōng fù]
keeping the waist and abdomen relaxed: one of the fundamental elements of posture management

收臀松膝 [shōu tún sōng xī]
contracting the buttocks and relaxing the knees: one of the fundamental elements of posture management

五趾抓地 [wǔ zhǐ zhuā dì]
clutching the ground with the toes: standing firmly, one of the fundamental elements of posture management

两目垂帘内视 [liǎng mù chuí lián nèi shì]
curtain-falling and inward vision: drooping the eyelids to create inward vision

塞兑反听 [sè duì fǎn tīng]
blocking the ears and inward listening: rejecting the sounds from outside and listening to the breathing sounds within the body

舌抵上腭 [shé dǐ shàng è]
sticking the tongue against the palate: licking the palate with the tongue just behind the upper gums in order to communicate with the conception and governor vessels, also called tongue propping the palate (舌柱上腭 [shé zhù shàng è]), tongue propping (柱舌 [zhù shé]) or building the magpie bridge (搭鹊桥 [dā què qiáo])

舌柱上腭 [shé zhù shàng è]
tongue propping the palate: same as sticking the tongue against the palate (舌抵上腭 [shé dǐ shàng è])

柱舌 [zhù shé]
tongue propping: abbreviation for tongue propping the palate (舌柱上腭 [shé zhù shàng è])

搭鹊桥 [dā què qiáo]
building the magpie bridge: another expression for sticking the tongue against the palate (舌抵上腭 [shé dǐ shàng è])

鹊桥 [què qiáo]
magpie bridge: name referring to two body portions in *qigong* exercise – the upper one is situated at the part between the glabella and the nostrils, and the lower one between the coccyx and the anus

胎食 [tāi shí]
fetal feeding; saliva-swallowing: swallowing of refluxed saliva in *qigong* exercise

坐式 [zuò shì]
sitting posture: variety of basic postures for *qigong* exercises, including plain

sitting, leaning sitting and cross-legged sitting

平坐 [píng zuò]
plain sitting: sitting on a bench or in a chair with the shoulders relaxed, the palms of the hands resting on the thighs, and the feet on the ground and set apart about the width of the shoulders

靠坐 [kào zuò]
leaning sitting: sitting with the back leaning against a cushion to make an angle of 120-140 degrees between the trunk and the thighs

盘坐 [pán zuò]
cross-legged sitting: sitting on a large bench or cushion spread on the ground with the legs crossed and the hands crossed on each other before the abdomen

单盘坐 [dān pán zuò]
single cross-legged sitting: sitting with one leg folded under the other, and the hands crossed on each other on or in front of the lower abdomen

双盘坐 [shuāng pán zuò]
double cross-legged sitting: sitting with the feet folded to face each other on the medial aspects of the thighs with both soles facing upwards, and the hands placed in front of the lower abdomen

卧式 [wò shì]
lying posture: basic postures for *qigong* exercises, including supine, recumbent, and reclining postures

仰卧式 [yǎng wò shì]
supine posture: lying on the back, with the legs stretched naturally and the hands stretched along the sides or crossed on each other over the abdomen

侧卧式 [cè wò shì]
lateral recumbent posture: lying on one side, with the body slightly bent like a bow, the upper hand placed on the hip and the lower hand on the pillow, with the thumbs and fingers spread naturally

三接式 [sān jiē shì]
three-contact posture: lying on one side with the upper leg flexed and its sole placed on the knee of the other leg, and the lower arm flexed with the palm of the hand placed on the elbow of the upper arm

半卧式 [bàn wò shì]
semi-recumbent posture: reclining on a couch or bed with the upper part of the body and the head raised with pillows or cushions

站式 [zhàn shì]
standing posture: variety of basic postures for *qigong* exercises, including natural stance, horseman's stance, ball-holding and downward-pressing postures

自然站式 [zì rán zhàn shì]
natural standing posture: standing naturally with the feet set apart about the width of the shoulders and the hands hanging naturally at the sides

骑马式 [qí mǎ shì]
horseman's stance: half squatting with the legs set apart, the heels turned outward, and the fists placed in front of the abdomen or at the sides

三圆式 [sān yuán shì]
three-circle posture: standing with the feet set apart about the width of the shoulders and the toes turned inward to form a circle, with the knees slightly bent and the arms raised before the chest in a circle as if embracing a tree trunk and the fingers spread as if holding a basketball, also called ball-holding posture (抱球式 [bào qiú shì])

抱球式 [bào qiú shì]
ball-holding posture: another name for three-circle posture (三圆式 [sān yuán shì])

下按式 [xià àn shì]
downward-pressing posture: standing in the three-circle posture but with the arms hanging naturally at the sides, with the palms of the hands facing downward and the fingers pointing to the front, as if pressing a floating ball into water

走式 [zǒu shì]
walking posture: collective term for a variety of basic postures for *qigong* exercises, including *taiji* walking, eight-diagram walking, etc.

矮步 [ǎi bù]
half-squatting walking: walking in a half-squatting position with the upper part of the body and head held upright and eyes looking forward, smiling and performing various exercise at the same time

弓步 [gōng bù]
bow step: step in which one leg is kept straight while the other is bent and holds the body's weight

太极步 [tài jí bù]
***taiji* walking:** walking with the legs slightly bent and hands pressed at the sides or placed upon one another before the abdomen, and the weight of the body shifting from side to side alternately

八卦步 [bā guà bù]
eight-diagram walking: walking with the tips of the toes turned slightly inward and clutching the ground with the toes when stepping forward with the heels slightly elevated, the knees slightly bent, and the eyes looking forward while smiling

上丹田 [shàng dān tián]
upper *dantian*; upper elixir field: location on which the mind is concentrated during *qigong* exercise, considered to be the seat of mentality, beneath the area between the eyebrows approximately 3 *cun* deeper than the point *Yintang* (Ex-HN 3), also called mud ball (泥丸 [ní wán])

泥丸 [ní wán]
mud ball: (1) another name for upper *dantian* (上丹田 [shàng dān tián]); (2) another name for *Baihui* (GV 20)

中丹田 [zhōng dān tián]
middle *dantian*; middle elixir field: location on which the mind is concentrated during *qigong* exercise, considered to be the seat of *qi* and a place where *qi* is trained and emitted to the outside of the body, underneath the area between the nipples in the chest approximately 3 *cun* deeper than the point *Danzhong* (CV 17)

下丹田 [xià dān tián]
lower *dantian*; lower elixir field: location on which the mind is concentrated during *qigong* exercise, approximately 3 *cun* below the umbilicus with point *Qihai* (CV 6) as its center, where essence is transformed into *qi*, and *qi* is trained and emitted to the outside of the body

丹田 [dān tián]
***dantian*; elixir field:** the place where *qi* is stored and the mind is focused in *qigong* exercises, compared by the Taoists in ancient China to the furnace in alchemy where elixir is tempered, hence the name

调息 [tiáo xī]
management of breath: training of breathing to bring the functions of *qi* into full play, also called management of *qi* (调气 [tiáo qì]), and known as breathing in and out (吐纳 [tǔ nà]) in ancient times

调气 [tiáo qì]
management of *qi*: same as management of breath (调息 [tiáo xī])

吐纳 [tǔ nà]
breathing in and out: synonym for management of breath (调息 [tiáo xī])

自然呼吸 [zì rán hū xī]
natural breathing: breathing while no special attention is paid to the breath at all, embracing thoracic breathing, abdominal breathing and mixed breathing

顺腹式呼吸 [shùn fù shì hū xī]
orthodromic abdominal breathing: breathing marked by dilating the abdomen while inhaling and contracting it while exhaling

逆腹式呼吸 [nì fù shì hū xī]
antidromic abdominal breathing: breathing marked by contracting the abdomen while inhaling and dilating it while exhaling

潜呼吸 [qián hū xī]
latent breathing: abdominal breathing performed almost unnoticeably, with gentle rising and falling of the lower abdomen

脐呼吸 [qí hū xī]
navel breathing: finest abdominal breathing with the abdomen remaining almost motionless, while the practitioner imagines that he or she is breathing through the umbilicus just as a fetus does in the womb, and hence also called fetal breathing (胎息 [tāi xī])

胎息 [tāi xī]
fetal breathing: synonymous with navel breathing (脐呼吸 [qí hū xī])

鼻吸鼻呼 [bí xī bí hū]
nasal breathing: inhaling and exhaling through the nose, a form of breathing usually adopted during static *qigong* practice

吐字呼吸 [tǔ zì hū xī]
word-articulating breathing: form of breathing in which particular words are articulated while exhaling

提肛呼吸 [tí gāng hū xī]
anus-lifting breathing: breathing with the anus contracted while inhaling, and relaxed

while exhaling, used in the treatment of visceral prolapse and hemorrhoids

数吸 [shǔ xī]
breath counting: combining mental concentration with breathing by counting the number of respirations

听息 [tīng xī]
breath listening: combining mental concentration with breathing by listening to one's own respiration

意呼吸 [yì hū xī]
imaginary breathing: breathing coupled with certain thoughts and ideas that exchange of *qi* can be performed through the skin or pores to communicate with the universe

停息 [tíng xī]
breathing with pause: breathing in which the breath is temporarily held at the end of inhalation or exhalation

随息 [suí xī]
following one's own breathing: process in *qigong* exercises involving mentally following and being aware of one's own breathing for the concentration of the mind

调心 [tiáo xīn]
management of the mind: method of attaining mental concentration and guarding against distraction in *qigong* exercises, also called training of the mind (练神 [liàn shén]), preservation of the mind (存神 [cún shén]), and preservation of the breath (存息 [cún xī]) in ancient times

练神 [liàn shén]
training of the mind: same as management of the mind (调心 [tiáo xīn])

存神 [cún shén]
preservation of the mind: same as management of the mind (调心[tiáo xīn])

存息 [cún xī]
preservation of the breath: same as management of the mind (调心 [tiáo xīn])

坐忘 [zuò wàng]
sitting in forgetfulness: one of the Confucian techniques of self-cultivation, marked by sitting while forgetting the existence of the body, mind, and all subjects and objects

精、气、神 [jīng、qì、shén]
essence, *qi*, and mind: three elements as both the bases and the purposes of *qigong* exercises

炼丹 [liàn dān]
(I) alchemy: ancient quasi-chemical art through which practitioners sought a panacea for disease and the secret of eternal youth; **(II) physiological alchemy:** traditional Taoist static *qigong* exercise for training essence, *qi*, and mentality, also known as inner elixir exercise (内丹功 [nèi dān gōng])

内丹 [nèi dān]
inner elixir: imaginary substance in the body, which was believed to have the power to make one live forever

内丹功 [nèi dān gōng]
inner elixir exercise: static exercise in *qigong* practice for producing inner elixir, i.e., self-physiological cultivation

内丹术 [nèi dān shù]
inner elixir art: same as inner elixir exercise (内丹功[nèi dān gōng])

炼己 [liàn jǐ]
cultivating oneself: the process of concentrating one's mind and getting rid of mental distraction during a *qigong* exercise

炼精 [liàn jīng]
cultivating essence: the process of reinforcing the inborn essence during a *qigong* exercise

炼气 [liàn qì]
cultivating *qi*: training the breathing and strengthening the vitality during a *qigong* excercise

炼神 [liàn shén]
cultivating the mind: training the mental faculties during a *qigong* exercise

炼精化气 [liàn jīng huà qì]
cultivating essence to become *qi*: transforming essence into energy by conducting *qi* through the small complete cycle of circulation during a *qigong* excercise

炼气化神 [liàn qì huà shén]
cultivating *qi* to become mentality: transforming energy into mental faculties by conducting *qi* through large complete cycle of circulation during a *qigong* excercise

练功 [liàn gōng]
practicing *qigong*: doing *qigong* exercises with appropriate postures, breathing, and mental concentration

意守 [yì shǒu]
concentration of the mind: focusing one's concentration on one specific object

排除杂念 [pái chú zá niàn]
getting rid of mental distractions: concentrating one's mind on one single object to replace all other thoughts and ideas

意守自身 [yì shǒu zì shēn]
concentration on oneself: concentration of the mind on a certain part of the body, or a particular organ, meridian/channel or point

意守丹田 [yì shǒu dān tián]
concentration on *dantian*: concentration of the mind on *dantian*, or the elixir field where *qi* is stored

意守体外 [yì shǒu tǐ wài]
concentration on something outside the body: concentration of the mind on an object, sign, sound or some past experience recalled

面壁 [miàn bì]
facing a wall: standing motionless as if facing a wall in order to get rid of all external disturbances and internal worries, also called looking at a wall (壁观 [bì guān])

壁观 [bì guān]
looking at a wall: same as facing a wall (面壁 [miàn bì])

存想 [cún xiǎng]
**preservation of thought; imaginary

concentration: concentration on an imaginary object to get rid of distractions and induce a desired feeling

内气 [nèi qì]
inner *qi*: *qi* within the body that circulates through the meridians/channels and induces a *qi* sensation in the process of *qigong* exercise, also called 真气 [zhēn qì]

真气 [zhēn qì]
genuine *qi*: dynamic force of life activities of the human body, same as inner *qi* (内气 [nèi qì])

外气 [wài qì]
out-going *qi*: *qi* that is emitted from a *qigong* master's body into a certain part of the patient for therapeutic purposes

周天 [zhōu tiān]
heavenly circuit; cosmic cycle: complete cycle of *qi* circulation within the body

小周天 [xiǎo zhōu tiān]
small heavenly circuit; microcosmic cycle: part of the complete cycle of *qi* circulation in the body, referring to *qi* circulation within the conception and governor vessels

大周天 [dà zhōu tiān]
large heavenly circuit; macrocosmic cycle: major part of the complete cycle of *qi* circulation, referring to *qi* circulation within the regular and extra meridians/channels (except the conception and governor vessels)

离体周天 [lí tǐ zhōu tiān]
extracorporeal heavenly circuit; extracorporeal cosmic cycle: the part of the *qi* circulation cycle outside the body, either going out of the body through the coccyx and coming back into the body through *Baihui* (GV 20) or going out through the feet and coming back through the head

禅定 [chán dìng]
meditating fixation: one of the representative exercises of Buddhist *qigong*, marked by meditation and fixation, or stoppage of thinking

放松功 [fàng sōng gōng]
relaxation exercise: basic exercise in static *qigong* for rehabilitation by lessening tension of both the body and mind

内养功 [nèi yǎng gōng]
inner nourishing exercise: *qigong* characterized by combining silent reading of words or phrases with training of breathing, taking a lying or sitting posture with abdominal breathing, for invigorating the functional activities of the digestive and respiratory systems

强壮功 [qiáng zhuàng gōng]
roborant exercise: *qigong* exercise by means of breathing and mind concentration on *dantian* to reinforce intrinsic *qi* and build up health

头面功 [tóu miàn gōng]
head-face exercise: exercise including bathing the face, combing the hair, kneading the temples and *Fenchi* (GB 20), and tapping the back of the head to regulate the meridians/channels of the head and face, promote the flow of *qi* and

blood, invigorate the brain, and refresh the mind

眼功 [yǎn gōng]
eye exercise: exercise by focusing on the movements of the eye to regulate the flow of *qi* and blood through the liver meridian/channel, and improve acuity of vision

鼻齿功 [bí chǐ gōng]
nose-teeth exercise: exercise for clearing the nasal passage and consolidating the teeth

耳功 [ěr gōng]
ear exercise: exercise including pressing and "bathing" the ears, and rubbing the helix to improve hearing

颈项功 [jǐng xiàng gōng]
neck exercise: exercise for preventing and curing neck troubles

肩臂功 [jiān bì gōng]
shoulder-arm exercise: exercise for promoting the flow of *qi* and blood along the three yang and three yin meridians/channels of the hands

胸胁功 [xiōng xié gōng]
chest-hypochondrium exercise: exercise for preventing and treating diseases in the chest and hypochondriac regions

腹部功 [fù bù gōng]
abdomen exercise: common *qigong* exercise of rubbing the abdomen and *dantian*, for preventing and treating digestive disorders

腰部功 [yāo bù gōng]
waist exercise: exercise characterized by rubbing the waist to strengthen the lumbar muscles and replenish the kidney

下肢功 [xià zhī gōng]
lower limb exercise: exercise consisting of kneading the kneecaps and rubbing *Yongquan* (KI 1) to activate the flow of *qi* and blood and to relax and strengthen the muscles and tendons of the lower limbs

理心功 [lǐ xīn gōng]
heart-regulation exercise: exercise to regulate *qi* and blood of the heart meridian/channel for preventing and treating heart troubles

理脾功 [lǐ pí gōng]
spleen-regulation exercise: exercise to regulate *qi* and blood of the spleen meridian/channel for promoting digestion

理肺功 [lǐ fèi gōng]
lung-regulation exercise: exercise to regulate *qi* and blood of the lung meridian/channel

周天功 [zhōu tiān gōng]
heavenly circuit exercise: *qigong* exercise in which *qi* is activated to travel in the small and large heavenly circuits for strengthening the mind and body, preserving health and prolonging life

小周天功 [xiǎo zhōu tiān gōng]
small heavenly circuit exercise: *qigong* exercise in which *qi* is activated to travel in the small heavenly circuit, i.e., the circuit composed of the conception and governor vessels

大周天功 [dà zhōu tiān gōng]
large heavenly circuit exercise: *qigong* exercise in which *qi* is activated to travel in the large heavenly circuit, i.e., the circuit composed of the regular and extra meridians/channels (except the conception and governor vessels)

周天自转功 [zhōu tiān zì zhuàn gōng]
automatic *qi* circulation exercise: exercise to conduct circulation of *qi*, with the navel as the center, by mental activities and breathing in coordination with saying words silently

疏肝明目功 [shū gān míng mù gōng]
liver-soothing and vision-improving exercise: exercise which has the function of improving the eyesight, relaxing the neck and back muscles, relieving muscular strain of the eye, and promoting recovery from fatigue

铁裆功 [tiě dāng gōng]
iron-crotch exercise: an important exercise for training the physical strength and nimbleness of the lower part of the body in ancient times, now chiefly used for preserving health and reinforcing sexual competence of the male

虎步功 [hǔ bù gōng]
tiger-striding exercise: *qigong* exercise for strengthening the waist and legs externally and the liver and kidney internally

叫化功 [jiào huā gōng]
beggar's exercise: *qigong* exercise for poor people to ward off hunger and cold in ancient times and now to increase the resistance of the stomach and intestines to cold

五禽戏 [wǔ qín xì]
five fauna-mimic frolics: movements in imitation of those of five types of wildlife – tiger, bear, monkey, deer, and bird, believed to have been initiated by Hua Tou (华佗 [huà tuó])

八段锦 [bā duàn jǐn]
eight-section brocade: physical exercise in eight forms, widely practiced by people of all ages in both ancient and modern times

站桩功 [zhàn zhuāng gōng]
stake-standing exercise: *qigong* exercises characterized by taking a standing posture

自然站桩功 [zì rán zhàn zhuāng gōng]
natural stake-standing exercise: standing exercise in which one stands upright with the knees slightly bent, the eyes looking straight ahead, and both hands placed in front of the lower abdomen

三圆站桩功 [sān yuán zhàn zhuāng gōng]
triple-round stake-standing exercise: standing exercise in which one stands naturally, moves the hands up over the shoulders with the elbows and the palms facing each other as if holding a ball or up to the level of the chest with the elbows bent and palms facing the body as if embracing the trunk of a big tree

下按式站桩功 [xià àn shì zhàn zhuāng gōng]
hand-pressing postural stake-standing

exercise: standing exercise in which one takes the natural stake-standing position with the knees bent, raises the hands to the level of the waist with the palms of the hands facing the ground, the fingers spread and pointing ahead, and the forearms kept horizontal as if pressing something downward

七星功 [qī xīng gōng]
seven-star exercise: simple, graceful and useful exercise with seven postures, beneficial to all parts of the body

易筋功 [yì jīn gōng]
sinew-transforming exercise: dynamic exercise for training *qi* derived from the *Sinew Transforming Classic* credited to Dharma in the sixth century

九九阳功 [jiǔ jiǔ yáng gōng]
double-nine yang exercise: dynamic exercise for training *qi*

运气 [yùn qì]
moving *qi*: moving *qi* to a certain part of the body by mental concentration

练气 [liàn qì]
training *qi*: basic step of emitting *qi*

却谷食气 [què gǔ shí qì]
feeding on *qi* instead of food: principle of a certain school of health preservation that the practitioner can be nourished by *qi* through *qigong* exercises instead of taking food

辟谷功 [bì gǔ gōng]
food-restricting exercise; fasting exercise: *qigong* exercise performed for the purpose of decreasing the practitioner's food-taking

减肥功 [jiǎn féi gōng]
slimming exercise: *qigong* exercise performed for the purpose of reducing body weight

震桩式 [zhèn zhuāng shì]
pile-driving standing posture: standing with the knees slightly bent, the heels turned outward, and the hands held apart in front as if holding a ball, a basic posture commonly used for training *qi*

导气 [dǎo qì]
conducting *qi*: guiding *qi* flow to a portion or a point of the hand, to be emitted as out-going *qi*

合掌震桩导气 [hé zhǎng zhèn zhuāng dǎo qì]
conducting *qi* with pile-driving standing and palms put together: form of conducting *qi* from *dantian* to the palms of the hands through the governor vessel and then back to *dantian* through the three yin meridians/channels of the hands

一指禅导气 [yī zhǐ chán dǎo qì]
conducting *qi* with single-finger meditation: conducting *qi* performed by taking a stake-standing posture with the left hand held at shoulder level and the right hand on the right side of the abdomen with the tips of the forefingers pointing to each other

对掌推拉导气 [duì zhǎng tuī lā dǎo qì]
palm-to-palm pushing-pulling conduction of *qi*: conducting *qi* performed by taking

a standing posture and putting the palms of the hands together in the front, and then rubbing the palms of the hands against each other, with *qi* emitted from *Laogong* (PC 8) of one palm to the other

三点拉线导气 [sān diǎn lā xiàn dǎo qì]
three-point aligning conduction of *qi*: conducting *qi* performed by placing an ignited incense stick on a table in the front, taking a standing posture and holding the right arm to the front with the palm of the right hand open naturally and its *Laogong* (PC 8) facing the burning tip of the incense stick, in the meantime placing the left hand with a single finger stretched out behind the tip of the incense stick and aligning the tip of the stretched finger, the tip of the incense stick and point *Laogong* along the same line

三点求圆导气 [sān diǎn qiú yuán dǎo qì]
three-point circle-drawing conduction of *qi*: conducting *qi* by placing an ignited incense stick on a table in the front, taking a standing posture and making the ignited end of an incense stick and *Laogong* (PC 8) of the two palms of the hands an equalateral triangle and an imaginary circle

腾跃爆发导气 [téng yuè bào fā dǎo qì]
prancing to conduct *qi* in a burst: conducting *qi* by taking a standing posture with the knees slightly bent, making both hands into fists and holding them in front of the chest, and then prancing and spreading the fingers suddenly to emit *qi* from *Laogong* (PC 8) in a burst

发气 [fā qì]
emission of *qi*: sending *qi* out, also called emission of trained *qi* (发功 [fā gōng]) and emission of outgoing *qi* (发放外气 [fā fàng wài qì]), or distributing *qi* (布气 [bù qì]) in ancient times

发功 [fā gōng]
emission of trained *qi*: same as emission of *qi* (发气 [fā qì])

发放外气 [fā fàng wài qì]
emission of outgoing *qi*: same as emission of *qi* (发气 [fā qì])

布气 [bù qì]
distributing *qi*: ancient term for emission of *qi* (发气 [fā qì])

发气手势 [fā qì shǒu shì]
***qi*-emitting hand gesture:** hand gesture for emitting outgoing *qi*

一指禅式 [yī zhǐ chán shì]
single-finger meditation gesture: hand gesture for emitting *qi* with a single finger via meditation

平掌式 [píng zhǎng shì]
flat-palm gesture: hand gesture for emitting *qi* with an open palm of the hand

探爪式 [tàn zhuǎ shì]
spreading-claw gesture: hand gesture for emitting *qi* with the thumb and fingers slightly bent, shaped like a claw

剑决式 [jiàn jué shì]
sword-thrusting gesture: hand gesture for emitting *qi* with the index and middle fingers pointing forward

中指独立式 [zhōng zhǐ dú lì shì]
middle-finger-propping gesture: hand gesture for emitting *qi* with only the middle finger pointing forward

龙衔式 [lóng xián shì]
dragon-mouth gesture: hand gesture for emitting *qi* with the thumb and fingers shaped like the mouth of a dragon

气感 [qì gǎn]
sensation of *qi*: sensation of both genuine *qi* and evil *qi*

真气气感 [zhēn qì qì gǎn]
sensation of genuine *qi*: sensation of the direction, density, nature and volume of genuine *qi*, by which the condition of body resistance can be judged

秽气气感 [huì qì qì gǎn]
sensation of filthy *qi*: sensation experienced by the *qigong* master while treating a patient, by which the nature and severity of the patient's condition can be judged

收功 [shōu gōng]
closing form: (1) end or winding up of *qigong* exercise; (2) closing form of emission of *qi*, including that for the patient who receives *qigong* treatment and that for the *qigong* master who provides *qigong* treatment

气功偏差 [qì gōng piān chā]
deviation of *qigong*: adverse reaction in the course of *qigong* exercise, physical or mental, such as headache, dizziness, palpitations, shortness of breath, hand tremors, cold sweats, mental disorders and even schizophrenia

出偏 [chū piān]
deviation: abbreviation for deviation of *qigong* (气功偏差 [qì gōng piān chā])

走火入魔 [zǒu huǒ rù mó]
evil reactions: a popular term for deviation of *qigong* (气功偏差 [qì gōng piān chā])

保健 Health Preservation

保健功 [bǎo jiàn gōng]
health-preserving exercise: exercise for preventing a certain disease or diseases in general and promoting health

静坐 [jìng zuò]
silent sitting: sitting silently with the eyes closed, the legs crossed, the tongue resting against the palate, and the mind concentrated on *dantian*, for cultivating genuine *qi*

耳功 [ěr gōng]
ear exercise: exercise performed by flicking the occiput to cause a mild stimulation with the index fingers while pressing the bilateral tragi with the palmar prominences to close the external auditory canals, for regulating the brain function

叩齿 [kòu chǐ]
clicking the teeth: tapping the upper and lower teeth on each other to make short hard sounds to firm the teeth and improve digestion

舌功 [shé gōng]
tongue exercise: exercise performed by

stirring the tongue in the mouth to produce saliva

赤龙搅海 [chì lóng jiǎo hǎi]
"red dragon stirring the sea": elegant expression for tongue exercise (舌功 [shé gōng])

漱津 [shù jīn]
gargling with saliva: gargling with the saliva produced by stirring of the tongue, swallowing it, and then sending it mentally to the lower *dantian*

擦鼻 [cā bí]
rubbing the nose: rubbing the sides of the nose with the backs of the thumbs up and down around the point *Yingxiang* (LI20), for preventing colds and rhinitis

目功 [mù gōng]
eye exercise: excerise performed by gently rubbing the bilateral eyelids with the digital joints of the slightly bent thumbs and then rubbing the eyebrows, followed by rotating the eyeballs and looking into the distance, for improving vision

擦面 [cā miàn]
rubbing the face: rubbing the face with both palms of the hands from the top of the forehead down to the chin, and then from the chin up to the forehead, for improving one's facial features

项功 [xiàng gōng]
nape exercise: exercise performed by placing the palms of the hands on the occiput with fingers crossed, repeatedly bending and lifting the head with force, for training the neck muscles and improving the local blood circulation

揉肩 [róu jiān]
kneading the shoulders: kneading the right shoulder with the left hand in a rotary motion and kneading the left shoulder with the right hand similarly, for improving the function of the shoulders

夹脊 [jiā jǐ]
pressing the spine: swinging the right and left arms to and fro alternately with the elbows bent 90 degrees and the hands making fists, for training the shoulders and pectoral muscles and preventing disorders of the spine

搓腰 [cuō yāo]
rubbing the waist: rubbing the waist with the palms of the hands up and down, and right and left, around the points *Mingmen* (GV 4) and *Shenshu* (BL 23)

搓内肾 [cuō nèi shèn]
rubbing the inner kidney: traditional term for rubbing the waist (搓腰 [cuō yāo])

擦丹田 [cā dān tián]
rubbing *dantian*: rubbing the lower abdomen first with one hand and then the other in a circular motion around *dantian*, for invigorating the spleen and tonifying the kidney

揉膝 [róu xī]
kneading the knees: kneading both knees with the hands simultaneously, for soothing the tendons and strengthening the bones

擦涌泉 [cā yǒng quán]
rubbing *Yongquan* (KI 1): rubbing

the sole of the left foot with the index and middle fingers of the right hand, surrounding the point *Yongquan* (KI 1), and then the sole of the right foot with the index and middle fingers of the left hand, for preventing hypertension

养生十常 [yǎng shēng shí cháng]
ten health-preserving routines: doing the following ten things routinely for health preservation: (1) tapping the teeth, (2) swallowing the saliva, (3) rubbing the face, (4) massaging the soles of the feet, (5) making the ears pop, (6) rubbing the nose, (7) moving the eyeballs, (8) massaging the abdomen in a circular way, (9) stretching the limbs, and (10) contracting the anus

睡眠十忌 [shuì mián shí jì]
ten items of avoidance for sleep: (1) avoiding lying on the back while sleeping, (2) avoiding anxiety, (3) avoiding anger, (4) avoiding overeating before going to bed, (5) avoiding talking too much before going to sleep, (6) avoiding sleeping facing the light, (7) avoiding sleeping with the mouth open, (8) avoiding sleeping with the head covered, (9) avoiding sleeping in a draught, and (10) avoiding sleeping with the head against a stove

饮食有节 [yǐn shí yǒu jié]
temperance in eating and drinking

药膳 [yào shàn]
medicated diet: food cooked with medicinal materials for therapeutic purpose

药粥 [yào zhōu]
medicated porridge: porridge cooked with medicinal materials, such as lotus seeds, Chinese dates, etc.

药酒 [yào jiǔ]
medicated wine: wine containing medicinal substances to be taken regularly for therapeutic purpose, such as acanthopanax-bark wine for rheumatism

药茶 [yào chá]
medicated tea: herbal medicines mixed and prepared to be infused with boiling water and taken as tea or together with tea

常用引文 Commonly Used Citations

真气存内，邪不可干。
[zhēn qì cún nèi, xié bù kě gān]
If the body's resisting forces prevail, attack of pathogens will not avail.

恬淡虚无，真气从之；精神内守，病从安来。
[tiǎn dàn xū wú, zhēn qì cóng zhī; jīng shén nèi shǒu, bìng cóng ān lái]
Uncluttered mind preserves vitality, good spirit alienates fatality.

虚邪贼风，避之有时。
[xū xié zéi fēng, bì zhī yǒu shí]
Evil winds and draughts must be avoided wisely.

治未病。

[zhì wèi bìng]
Treat diseases before they get a hold.

春夏养阳，秋冬养阴。
[chūn xià yǎng yáng, qiū dōng yǎng yīn]
Cultivate yang in spring and summer, and nourish yin in autmn and winter.

勿药为中医。
[wù yào wéi zhōng yī]
No medication is better than wrong medication.

若要安，三里常不干。
[ruò yào ān, sān lǐ cháng bù gān]
If you want to stay healthy, always keep *Sanli* moist: Moxibustion frequently applied to *Zusanli* (ST 36) makes one healthy.

背要常暖，胸要常护。
[bèi yào cháng nuǎn, xiōng yào cháng hù]
Keep your back warm and your chest well covered all the time.

足要常搓，腹要常摩。
[zú yào cháng cuō, fù yào cháng mó]
Rub the soles of your feet and massage your abdomen frequently.

修性以保神，安心以全身。
[xiū xìng yǐ bǎo shén, ān xīn yǐ quán shēn]
Good character preserves one's soul, good temperament preserves one's life.

以动养形，以形养神。
[yǐ dòng yǎng xíng, yǐ xíng yǎng shén]
Exercise builds up the physique and the physique buoys up the spirit.

户枢不蠹，流水不腐，人之形体，其亦由是。
[hù shū bù dù, liú shuǐ bù fǔ, rén zhī xíng tǐ, qí yì yóu shì]
A rolling stone gathers no moss, neither does the human body.

人欲劳于形，百病不能成。
[rén yù láo yú xíng, bǎi bìng bù néng chéng]
Proper physical labor keeps diseases away.

贪吃贪睡，添病减岁。
[tān chī tān shuì, tiān bìng jiǎn suì]
Overeating and oversleeping lead to disease and earlier death.

食饱不可睡，睡则诸疾生。
[shí bǎo bù kě shuì, shuì zé zhū jí shēng]
One should not go to sleep immediately after having a heavy meal, otherwise disease will follow quickly.

饭后百步走，活到九十九。
[fàn hòu bǎi bù zǒu, huó dào jiǔ shí jiǔ]
A hundred steps after each meal make one live up to ninety-nine.

先睡心，后睡眼。
[xiān shuì xīn, hòu shuì yǎn]
For a good sleep, ease your mind first and then close your eyes.

少思以养神，少欲以养精。
[shǎo sī yǐ yǎng shén, shǎo yù yǐ yǎng jīng]
Free of cares, your mind will be restful; free of inordinate desires, your body will be full of vigor.

多思则神殆，多念则智散。
[duō sī zé shén dài, duō niàn zé zhì sǎn]
Worries make one's spirit low, and cares make one's mind distracted.

多欲则智昏，多事则劳形。
[duō yù zé zhì hūn, duō shì zé láo xíng]
Lust retards the mind, and overwork exhausts the body.

心胸宽，人快活；心胸窄，忧愁多。
[xīn xiōng kuān, rén kuài huó; xīn xiōng zhǎi, yōu chóu duō]
A broad mind makes one happy while a narrow mind makes one worry.

笑口常开，青春常在。
[xiào kǒu cháng kāi, qīng chūn cháng zài]
If mirth stays with you, youth will cling to you.

笑一笑，少一少；恼一恼，老一老。
[xiào yī xiào, shào yī shào; nǎo yī nǎo, lǎo yī lǎo]
Mirth makes one younger while fretting makes one older.

歌咏所以养性情，舞蹈所以养血脉。
[gē yǒng suǒ yǐ yǎng xìng qíng, wǔ dǎo suǒ yǐ yǎng xuè mài]
Singing can remould one's temperament, and dancing can promote one's blood flow.

诗书悦心，山林逸兴，可以延年。
[shī shū yuè xīn, shān lín yì xìng, kě yǐ yán nián]
Poetry pleases one's heart and scenery one's eye, both does life benefit by.

精神到处文章老，学问深处意气平。
[jīng shén dào chù wén zhāng lǎo, xué wèn shēn chù yì qì píng]
The best essay is written by the most concentrated mind, and a peaceful mood comes from the most learned head.

下棋可忘忧，慢跑可长寿。
[xià qí kě wàng yōu, màn pǎo kě cháng shòu]
Chess playing can relieve one's cares, and jogging can make one live longer.

七情之病，看花解闷，听曲消愁，胜于服药。
[qī qíng zhī bìng, kàn huā jiě mèn, tīng qǔ xiāo chóu, shèng yú fú yào]
A flower show or a musical performance is a better cure for emotional disturbances than a medicine.

欲不可纵，纵欲成灾；乐不可极，乐极生灾。
[yù bù kě zòng, zòng yù chéng zāi; lè bù kě jí, lè jí shēng zāi]
Sexual desire should not be indulged in, neither should enjoyment be sought to excess, otherwise disaster will follow.

起居有常，养其神也，不妄作劳，养其精也。
[qǐ jū yǒu cháng, yǎng qí shén yě, bù wàng zuò láo, yǎng qí jīng yě]
Regularity in daily life helps preserve vitality, temperance in sexual life helps preserve essence.

衣着寒暖适体，勿侈华艳。
[yī zhuó hán nuǎn shì tǐ, wù chǐ huá yàn]
Being dressed warmly and comfortably

is better than being dressed in luxurious and gaudy clothes.

晨起三百步，睡前一盆汤。
[chén qǐ sān bǎi bù, shuì qián yī pén tāng]
Walk three hundred steps after rising in the morning and bathe your feet in warm water before retiring at night.

立如松，坐如钟，卧如弓。
[lì rú sōng, zuò rú zhōng, wò rú gōng]
Stand upright like a pine, sit firm like a bell, and sleep on the side like a bow.

冬不欲极温，夏不欲极凉。
[dōng bù yù jí wēn, xià bù yù jí liáng]
Don't crave excessive warmth in winter, or excessive coldness in summer.

饮食自倍，脾胃乃伤。
[yǐn shí zì bèi, pí wèi nǎi shāng]
Eating to excess injures the spleen and stomach.

烹调有方。
[pēng tiáo yǒu fāng]
Food should be cooked in the right way.

五谷为养，五果为助，五畜为益，五菜为充。
[wǔ gǔ wéi yǎng, wǔ guǒ wéi zhù, wǔ chù wéi yì, wǔ cài wéi chōng]
Cereals supply main nutrients while fruits are auxiliary, meats salutary and veggies complementary.

菜饭宜清淡，少盐少疾患。
[cài fàn yì qīng dàn, shǎo yán shǎo jí huàn]
Light food and not so salty, such a diet keeps one healthy.

乳贵有时，食贵有节。
[rǔ guì yǒu shí, shí guì yǒu jié]
Proper breast feeding is achieved by controlling feeding time, and proper food intake by food amount.

先饥而食，先渴而饮；食欲数而少，不欲顿而多。
[xiān jī ér shí, xiān kě ér yǐn; shí yù shuò ér shǎo, bù yù dùn ér duō]
Eat before becoming hungry and drink before becoming thirsty, frequent feeding with less food at a time is better than too much food taken at a single meal.

病从口入。
[bìng cóng kǒu rù]
Disease usually breaks in through the mouth.

药补不如食补。
[yào bǔ bù rú shí bǔ]
Taking healthy food is better than taking tonics.

酒通血脉，消愁遣兴，少饮壮神，过多损命。
[jiǔ tōng xuè mài, xiāo chóu qiǎn xìng, shǎo yǐn zhuàng shén, guò duō sǔn mìng]
Wine can promote blood flow, quench one's sorrow and heighten one's sense of merriment. It may keep up one's spirits if drunk in moderation, but endanger one's life if drunk to excess.

气大伤人，酒多伤身。
[qì dà shāng rén, jiǔ duō shāng shēn]

Both raving anger and overdrinking are harmful to health.

宁可三日无粮，不可一日无茶。

[nìng kě sān rì wú liáng, bù kě yī rì wú chá]

One would rather go three days without food than a single day without tea.

莫吃空心茶，休饮卯时酒，更兼戌后饭，禁之当谨守。

[mò chī kōng xīn chá, xiū yǐn mǎo shí jiǔ, gēng jiān xū hòu fàn, jìn zhī dāng jǐn shǒu]

Don't drink too much tea with empty stomach, don't drink too much wine in the early morning, and don't eat too much food in the late evening; these three don'ts should be abided by carefully.

饥不暴食，渴不狂饮。

[jī bù bào shí, kě bù kuáng yǐn]

Don't eat to excess when hungry or drink to excess when thirsty.

胃不和，卧不安。

[wèi bù hé, wò bùān]

Indigestion disturbs sleep.

临床各科
Clinical Medicine

温病 Warm Diseases

天受 [tiān shòu]

(I) air- or water-borne; (II) air- or water-borne infection: infection mediated by air or water, such as inhalation of pathogen-contaminated air or contact with pathogen-contaminated aqueous source

传染 [chuán rǎn]

contagion: transmission of a disease by contact

时行 [shí xíng]

(I) epidemic: affecting a large number of individuals in the same place at the same time; **(II) epidemicity:** the state of being epidemic, also called 天行 [tiān xíng]

天行 [tiān xíng]

synonymous with 时行[shí xíng]

时行戾气 [shí xíng lì qì]

seasonal pestilential *qi*; epidemic pathogen: pathogen that causes an outbreak of epidemic infectious disease

时毒 [shí dú]

(I) seasonal toxin: pathogen that causes an infectious seasonal disease; **(II) seasonal toxicosis:** an acute infectious disease marked by high fever together with local redness, and swelling and pain in the face, also known as erysipelas facialis (大头瘟 [dà tóu wēn])

温邪 [wēn xié]

warm pathogen: collective term for various pathogens that cause acute febrile diseases

温毒 [wēn dú]

warm toxin: (1) warm pathogen combined with heat toxin, usually causing acute inflammatory diseases in winter and spring, marked by high fever with swelling of the head, face or throat, or with skin eruption; (2) any acute inflammatory disease attributed to contraction of warm toxin, e.g., measles, scarlet fever, mumps. erysipelas, and typhus

时病 [shí bìng]

seasonal diseases: diseases closely related to the climatic influence of a certain season, also called 时令病 [shí lìng bìng]

时令病 [shí lìng bìng]

seasonal diseases: same as时病 [shí bìng]

时疫 [shí yì]

seasonal epidemic: epidemic of an acute infectious disease in a certain season, particularly referring to pestilence in summer, also known as prevalent seasonal epidemic (天行时疫 [tiān xíng shí yì])

天行时疫 [tiān xíng shí yì]

prevalent seasonal epidemic: synonymous with seasonal epidemic (时疫 [shí yì])

阴病 [yīn bìng]

yin disease: (1) general designation for diseases with deficiency syndromes/patterns and/or of cold nature; (2) disease of yin meridian

阳病 [yáng bìng]
yang disease: (1) general designation for diseases with excess syndromes/patterns and/or heat syndromes/patterns; (2) disease of yang meridian

卒病 [cù bìng]
abrupt illness: sudden onset of disease

暴病 [bào bìng]
sudden illness: sudden attack of a serious disease

新病 [xīn bìng]
recent illness: disease occurring recently, usually referring to the onset of a new disease in addition to a chronic illness

新感 [xīn gǎn]
recent contraction: onset of a disease soon after contraction of a pathogen

伤寒 [shāng hán]
cold damage: (1) general term for various externally contracted febrile diseases; (2)morbid condition caused by cold, manifested as chills and fever, absence of sweating, headache, and floating and tense pulse

热病 [rè bìng]
febrile disease: (1) disease due to exogenous pathogenic factors with fever as its main manifestation; (2) one of the cold damage diseases; (3) febrile disease caused by summerheat

温病 [wēn bìng]
warm disease: (1) general term for acute externally contracted febrile diseases caused by warm pathogens, clinically manifested chiefly as fever; (2) acute febrile disease occurring in spring

伏气 [fú qì]
latent *qi*: (1) latent pathogen, another name for 伏邪 [fú xié]; (2) abbreviation for latent-*qi* warm disease (伏气温病 [fú qì wēn bìng])

伏气温病 [fú qì wēn bìng]
latent-*qi* warm disease: epidemic febrile disease caused by latent warm pathogen, marked by syndrome of internal heat with fever, and thirst and fidgetiness at the onset

温［瘟］疫 [wēn yì]
pestilence: general term for virulent infectious epidemic diseases

顺传 [shùn chuán]
sequential transmission: ordinary proceeding of a febrile disease from the exterior to the interior

逆传 [nì chuán]
adverse transmission: extraordinary proceeding of a febrile disease, for instance, directly from the superficies to the pericardium

感冒 [gǎn mào]
common cold; colds: affliction of the lung-superficies by pathogenic wind, mainly manifested as fever, chills, headache, general aching, congested nose, sneezing, itching throat and coughing

时行感冒 [shí xíng gǎn mào]
influenza: invasion of the lung-superficies by a seasonal epidemic pathogen causing

acute fever, sore throat, headache and general aching

风寒感冒 [fēng hán gǎn mào]
wind-cold common cold: disease caused by wind and cold, manifested as aversion to cold with mild fever, absence of sweating, headache, stuffed and running nose, sneezing, general aching, and floating and tense pulse

风热感冒 [fēng rè gǎn mào]
wind-heat common cold: disease caused by wind and heat, manifested as fever with mild aversion to cold, headache, sore throat, cough and expectoration of yellowish sputum, thirst, and rapid pulse

气虚感冒 [qì xū gǎn mào]
***qi*-deficiency common cold:** common cold in one with a constitution of *qi* deficiency

阳虚感冒 [yáng xū gǎn mào]
yang-deficiency common cold: common cold in one with a constitution of yang deficiency

血虚感冒 [xuè xū gǎn mào]
blood-deficiency common cold: common cold in one with a constitution of blood deficiency

阴虚感冒 [yīn xū gǎn mào]
yin-deficiency common cold: common cold in one with a constitution of yin deficiency

风温 [fēng wēn]
(I) wind-warmth (disease): acute externally contracted febrile disease caused by pathogenic wind-heat, marked by exterior heat syndrome at the onset; **(II) wind-warmth (syndrome/pattern):** wind syndrome/pattern in cases of acute febrile disease, usually occurring after diaphoresis, marked by high fever, spontaneous sweating, heaviness of the body and sleepiness

风温病 [fēng wēn bìng]
wind-warmth disease: full name of wind-warmth (风温 [fēng wēn]) as a disease

春温 [chūn wēn]
spring warmth: acute febrile disease caused by latent warm-heat pathogen, marked by presence of interior heat at the onset

春温病 [chūn wēn bìng]
spring warmth disease: full name of spring warmth (春温 [chūn wēn]) as a disease

冒暑 [mào shǔ]
summerheat affliction: ailment of the nose and throat with catarrh, sneezing and coughing in summer

暑秽 [shǔ huì]
summerheat filth: heat stroke occurring in summer, marked by sudden syncope

暑秽病 [shǔ huì bìng]
summerheat filth disease: full name of summerheat filth (暑秽 [shǔ huì])

暑湿流注 [shǔ shī liú zhù]
multiple abscesses of summerheat-dampness: multiple abscesses deep in muscles occurring in summer and autumn, ascribed to the invasion of summerheat-dampness

暑病 [shǔ bìng]
summerheat disease: collective term for acute diseases caused by summerheat

阳暑 [yáng shǔ]
yang summerheat: affliction by heat in summer, usually referring to heatstroke

阴暑 [yīn shǔ]
yin summerheat: affliction by cold in summer, e.g., affliction due to exposure to cold draught or excessive cold drinks

伤暑 [shāng shǔ]
summerheat damage: general term for various conditions caused by summerheat, especially for mild cases of heatstroke and sunstroke

感暑 [gǎn shǔ]
summerheat affection: same as summerheat damage (伤暑 [shāng shǔ])

中暑 [zhòng shǔ]
summerheat stroke; heatstroke: acute disease caused by summerheat, marked by sudden loss of consciousness or high fever with restlessness, trismus, and even convulsions

暑厥 [shǔ jué]
summerheat syncope: severe case of sunstroke marked by loss of consciousness and cold limbs

暑厥证 [shǔ jué zhèng]
summerheat syncope syndrome/pattern: full name of summerheat syncope (暑厥 [shǔ jué]) as a syndrome/pattern

暑痉 [shǔ jìng]
summerheat convulsion: convulsions in children caused by pathogenic summerheat-warmth, a type of summerheat-wind (暑风 [shǔ fēng])

暑痫 [shǔ xián]
summerheat epilepsy: severe heatstroke in summer with sudden loss of consciousness and convulsions

暑温 [shǔ wēn]
summerheat-warmth: acute externally contracted febrile disease caused by summerheat pathogen, marked by heat syndrome/pattern of the stomach meridian/channel at the onset

暑温病 [shǔ wēn bìng]
summerheat-warmth disease: full name of summerheat-warmth (暑温 [shǔ wēn]) as a disease

暑瘵 [shǔ zhài]
summerheat phthisis: sudden onset of cough and hemoptysis caused by summerheat, resembling phthisis

暑风 [shǔ fēng]
summerheat-wind: disease marked by sudden onset of opisthotonos and convulsions caused by summerheat

暑风证 [shǔ fēng zhèng]
summerheat-wind syndrome/pattern: syndrome/pattern marked by sudden onset of opisthotonos and convulsions caused by summerheat

暑入阳明 [shǔ rù yáng míng]
summerheat entering *yangming* (yang brightness): syndrome/pattern occurring

in the initial stage of summerheat-warmth disease, manifested by high fever, profuse sweating, thirst, fidgetiness, dry yellow tongue coating, and surging rapid pulse

暑入阳明证 [shǔ rù yáng míng zhèng]
syndrome/pattern of summerheat entering *yangming* (yang brightness): full name of summerheat entering *yangming* (暑入阳明 [shǔ rù yáng míng]) as a syndrome / pattern

湿病 [shī bìng]
dampness disease: any disease caused by dampness, usually with such symptoms as distending pain and swelling of joints, heavy sensation of the body, watery diarrhea, and edema

湿阻 [shī zǔ]
dampness impediment: externally contracted disease characterized by impairment of the lung and defense system by pathogenic dampness, with such manifestations as aching and heavy sensation of the head and body, anorexia, and epigastric stuffiness, also known as dampness damage (伤湿 [shāng shī]) or dampness affliction (冒湿 [mào shī])

冒湿 [mào shī]
dampness affliction: synonym for dampness impediment (湿阻 [shī zǔ])

伤湿 [shāng shī]
dampness damage: synonym for dampness impediment (湿阻 [shī zǔ])

湿温 [shī wēn]
dampness-warmth: infectious febrile disease caused by dampness-heat, prevalent in summer and autumn, marked by prolonged fever, general aches and pains with heaviness, stuffiness in the chest and distension in the abdomen, and greasy coating of the tongue, usually referring to typhoid and paratyphoid fever

湿温病 [shī wēn bìng]
dampness-warmth disease: full name of dampness-warmth (湿温 [shī wēn])

伏暑 [fú shǔ]
latent summerheat: acute febrile disease caused by latent summerheat or summerheat-dampness pathogen, occurring in autumn or winter

伏暑病 [fú shǔ bìng]
latent summerheat disease: full name of latent summerheat (伏暑 [fú shǔ]) as a disease

秋燥 [qiū zào]
autumn dryness: externally contracted febrile disease caused by dryness-heat in autumn, marked by fever with dry throat, dry cough, dry skin, and other symptoms of dryness

秋燥病 [qiū zào bìng]
autumn dryness disease: full name of autumn dryness (秋燥 [qiū zào]) as a disease

凉燥 [liáng zào]
cool dryness: seasonal disease caused by coolness and dryness in autumn, marked by aversion to cold, headache, fever, absence of sweating, dryness of the nasal cavity and mouth, dry cough, and thin whitish tongue coating

凉燥病 [liáng zào bing]
cool dryness disease: full name of cool dryness (凉燥 [liáng zào]) as a disease

温燥 [wēn zào]
warm dryness: seasonal disease caused by warmth and dryness in autumn, marked by fever, headache, absence of sweating, dry cough, dryness of the throat, thirst, reddened tongue tip and margin, and rapid floating pulse

温燥病 [wēn zào bìng]
warm dryness disease: full name of warm dryness (温燥[wēn zào]) as a disease

冬温 [dōng wēn]
winter warmth: febrile disease in winter

外感 [wài gǎn]
external contraction: disease or morbid condition caused by exogenous pathogenic factors

潮热 [cháo rè]
tidal fever: fever recurring daily, in most cases in the afternoon, like the regular rise and fall of the tide

阴虚潮热 [yīn xū cháo rè]
yin-deficiency tidal fever: tidal fever due to consumption of essence, as seen in cases of tuberculosis

午后潮热 [wǔ hòu cháo rè]
afternoon tidal fever: fever recurring daily, more marked in the afternoon

日晡潮热 [rī bū cháo rè]
late afternoon tidal fever: tidal fever in the afternoon, usually 3-5 p.m., especially that caused by accumulation of pathogenic heat in the intestines, also called late afternoon fever (日晡发热 [rī bū fā rè]) (cf. 阳明腑证 [yáng míng fǔ zhèng])

日晡发热 [rī bū fā rè]
late afternoon fever: synonym for late afternoon tidal fever (日晡潮热 [rī bū cháo rè])

上火 [shàng huǒ]
up-rising of fire: morbid condition caused by excessive internal heat, manifested by constipation, inflammation of the nasal and oral cavities, conjunctival congestion, etc.

结胸 [jié xiōng]
chest bind; thoracic accumulation: accumulation of pathogenic factors (such as heat or cold in combination with retained fluid or phlegm or stagnant blood) in the chest, often manifested by tenderness and fullness sensation in the costal region with fever and sweating, or by pain and tenderness from the epigastrium to the lower abdomen with constipation and thirst

大结胸 [dà jié xiōng]
major chest bind; major thoracic accumulation: massive accumulation of phlegm-heat in the chest, a serious disease characterized by fullness, pain and tenderness of the chest and abdomen

小结胸 [xiǎo jié xiōng]
minor chest bind; minor thoracic accumulation: mild case of accumulation of phlegm-heat in the chest, marked by epigastric distension, stuffiness and tenderness

寒结胸 [hán jié xiōng]
cold chest bind; thoracic accumulation of cold: accumulation of pathogenic cold in the chest, marked by thoracic fullness and tenderness, constipation, absence of fever and thirst, whitish slippery coating of the tongue, and deep and slow pulse

血结胸 [xuè jié xiōng]
blood chest bind; thoracic accumulation of blood: accumulation of stagnant blood in the chest, marked by thoracic distension, pain and tenderness

大头瘟 [dà tóu wēn]
epidemic swollen-head infection; erysipelas facialis: acute infection of the face marked by high fever and local redness, swelling, hotness and pain

虾蟆瘟 [há ma wēn]
epidemic toad-like infection: another name for erysipelas facialis (大头瘟[dà tóu wēn])

烂喉痧 [làn hóu shā]
scarlatina: acute infectious disease caused by toxic warmth-heat and marked by swelling and erosion of the throat with an erythematous rash, also called 疫喉痧 [yì hóu shā] or simply 疫痧 [yì shā], 烂喉丹痧 [làn hóu dān shā] or simply 丹痧 [dān shā] or 喉痧 [hóu shā]

疫喉痧 [yì hóu shā]
scarlet fever: another name for scarlatina (烂喉痧 [làn hóu shā])

疫痧 [yì shā]
scarlet fever: same as scarlatina (烂喉痧 [làn hóu shā])

烂喉丹痧 [làn hóu dān shā]
scarlatina angionosa: scarlet fever with painful pharyngitis, another name for scarlatina (烂喉痧 [làn hóu shā])

丹痧 [dān shā]
scarlatina: another name for 烂喉痧 [làn hóu shā]

喉痧 [hóu shā]
scarlatina: another name for 烂喉痧 [làn hóu shā]

瘴气 [zhàng qì]
miasma: noxious effluvium alleged to cause malaria

瘴疟 [zhàng nüè]
miasmic malaria: severe malaria with loss of consciousness or jaundice

疟疾 [nüè ji]
malaria: externally contracted disease caused by malarial parasites, marked by paroxysms of shivering chills, high fever and sweating, also called 疟病 [nüè bìng], and abbreviated as 疟 [nüè]

疟病 [nüè bìng]
malaria: same as 疟疾 [nüè ji]

疟 [nüè]
malaria: abbreviation for 疟疾 [nüè ji]

正疟 [zhèng nüè]
ordinary malaria: malaria with regular attacks of chills, fever and sweating

温疟 [wēn nüè]
warm malaria: malaria with higher fever and fewer chills than in an ordinary attack

暑疟 [shǔ nüè]
summerheat malaria: malaria with manifestations of summerheat with dampness

湿疟 [shī nüè]
dampness malaria: malaria marked by internal dampness-heat, manifested by submerged fever, continuous light sweating, nausea and vomiting

寒疟 [hán nüè]
cold malaria: malaria with more chills and less fever than in an ordinary attack

热瘴 [rè zhàng]
heat miasmic malaria: miasmic malaria with marked heat symptoms

寒瘴 [hán zhàng]
cold miasmic malaria: miasmic malaria with trembling chills, also called 冷瘴 [lěng zhàng]

冷瘴 [lěng zhàng]
cold miasmic malaria: same as 寒瘴 [hán zhàng]

瘴毒 [zhàng dú]
miasmic toxin: pathogenic factor that causes miasmic malaria

瘴疟 [zhàng nüè]
miasmic malaria: malignant malaria

劳疟 [láo nüè]
consumptive malaria: chronic malaria with general debility and frequent recurrence following physical exertion

疟母 [nüè mǔ]
malarial mass: splenomegaly in chronic malaria, also called malarial lump (疟痞 [nüè pǐ]) or malarial accumulation (疟积 [nüè jī])

疟痞 [nüè pǐ]
malarial lump: synonymous with malarial mass (疟母 [nüè mǔ])

疟积 [nüè jī]
malarial accumulation: synonymous with malarial mass (疟母 [nüè mǔ])

牝疟 [pìn nüè]
yin malaria: chronic malaria in a debilitated patient, with severe shivering chills but low-grade fever

久疟 [jiǔ nüè]
chronic malaria: malaria that has been persisting for a long time with frequent recurrence

痢疾 [lì ji]
dysentery: disease characterized by abdominal pain, tenesmus, and diarrhea with stools containing blood and mucus

湿热痢 [shī rè lì]
dampness-heat dysentery: dysentery with frequent bloody mucoid stools, tenesmus, and burning sensation in the anus

寒湿痢 [hán shī lì]
cold-dampness dysentery: dysentery characterized by passage of whitish, thin mucoid stools, absence of fever and thirst, distending distress of the epigastrium and dull pain in the abdomen, tenesmus, poor appetite, pale tongue with whitish coating, and slow pulse

时疫痢 [shí yì lì]
epidemic dysentery: dysentery that becomes epidemic, also known as 疫痢 [yì lì]

疫痢 [yì lì]
epidemic dysentery: same as 时疫痢 [shí yì lì]

疫毒痢 [yì dú lì]
epidemic toxic dysentery: severe case of dysentery with acute onset of high fever, vomiting and frequent passage of bloody-mucoid stools, severe tenesmus, and even impaired consciousness

噤口痢 [jìn kǒu lì]
food-denial dysentery: severe case of dysentery with utter loss of appetite and vomiting upon eating and drinking

休息痢 [xiū xī lì]
intermittent dysentery: chronic dysentery with frequent relapse

迁延痢 [qiān yán lì]
protracted dysentery: dysentery lasting for a long time

久痢 [jiǔ lì]
chronic dysentery: dysentery lasting for a long time or continually recurring

虚寒痢 [xū hán lì]
deficiency-cold dysentery: chronic dysentery due to deficiency cold of the spleen and kidney, characterized by passage of thin mucous stools accompanied by dull pain in the lower abdomen, poor appetite, lassitude, coolness of the limbs, weakness of the loins and aversion to cold

赤痢 [chì lì]
red dysentery: dysentery marked by passage of bloody stools

白痢 [bái lì]
white dysentery: dysentery marked by passage of whitish mucous purulent stools

赤白痢 [chì bái lì]
red-white dysentery: dysentery with frequent passage of stools containing blood and mucus

霍乱 [huò luàn]
(I) cholera: acute infectious disease caused by *Vibrio cholerae* (as defined in modern medicine); **(II) choleraic turmoil:** disease characterized by sudden and drastic vomiting and diarrhea, including acute gastro-enteritis, food poisoning and cholera (as defined before 1820)

霍乱病 [huò luàn bìng]
cholera: acute infectious disease caused by *Vibrio cholerae*

干霍乱 [gān huò luàn]
dry choleraic turmoil: acute disease marked by severe abdominal pain associated with an urgent but ineffectual desire to vomit and defecate, also called colicky intestinal turmoil (绞肠痧 [jiǎo cháng shā] or 搅肠痧 [jiǎo cháng shā])

绞肠痧 [jiǎo cháng shā]
colicky intestinal turmoil: another name for dry choleraic turmoil (干霍乱 [gān huò luàn])

搅肠痧 [jiǎo cháng shā]
colicky intestinal turmoil: same as 绞肠痧 [jiǎo cháng shā]

寒霍乱 [hán huò luàn]
cold choleraic turmoil: choleraic turmoil due to attack by pathogenic cold, also called cold-*qi* choleraic turmoil (寒气霍乱 [hán qì huò luàn])

寒气霍乱 [hán qì huò luàn]
cold-*qi* choleraic turmoil: synonymous with cold choleraic turmoil (寒霍乱 [hán huò luàn])

热霍乱 [rè huò luàn]
heat choleraic turmoil: choleraic turmoil with high fever and other heat symptoms

霍乱转筋 [huò luàn zhuàn jīn]
cramp in choleraic turmoil: cramp in the muscles of the calf of the leg following drastic vomiting and diarrhea

转筋霍乱 [zhuàn jīn huò luàn]
choleraic turmoil with cramps: sudden and drastic vomiting and diarrhea accompanied by cramps in the calf muscles of the leg

胃家实 [wèi jiā shí]
excessiveness in the stomach and intestines: accumulation of pathogenic heat in the stomach and intestines, which often results in fluid damage and brings on such symptoms as high fever, persistent thirst, profuse sweating, full and gigantic pulse, constipation or discharge of hard fecal masses, and abdominal pain

发黄 [fā huáng]
yellow discoloration: a yellowish pigmentation of the skin and sclera

黄疸 [huáng dǎn]
jaundice: diseased state characterized by yellow discoloration of the skin and sclera

阳黄 [yáng huáng]
yang jaundice: jaundice characterized by bright yellow discoloration of the skin and sclera, usually acute at the onset and accompanied by dampness-heat symptoms

阴黄 [yīn huáng]
yin jaundice: jaundice characterized by dim yellow discoloration of the skin and sclera, usually chronic in progress, and accompanied by cold-dampness or deficiency-cold symptoms

急黄 [jí huáng]
fulminant jaundice: critical case of jaundice with sudden onset, rapid deterioration and poor prognosis, accompanied by high fever, impairment of consciousness, abdominal distension, ascites, and hematemesis

内科 Internal Medicine

内科杂病 [nèi kē zá bìng]
miscellaneous internal diseases: various internal disease excluding cold-damage and warm diseases, and abbreviated as 杂病 [zá bìng]

杂病 [zá bìng]
miscellaneous diseases: abbreviation for miscellaneous internal diseases (内科杂病 [nèi kē zá bìng])

宿疾 [sù jí]
old disease; long illness: disease that has a long history and is not cured

固［痼］疾 [gù jí]
obstinate disease: chronic disease difficult to cure

隐疾 [yǐn jí]
occult disease: euphemism for venereal disease or impotence

失音 [shī yīn]
aphonia: loss of voice

失音病 [shī yīn bìng]
aphonia (disease): diseased state characterized by loss of voice

咳嗽 [ké sou]
cough: Strictly speaking, the two Chinese characters have different meanings. 咳 [ké] means the expelling of air from the lungs suddenly with an explosive noise but no expectoration, while 嗽 [sòu] refers to the expectoration of sputum without explosive noise. Generally, the two Chinese characters are used together to denote "cough", regardless of noise or expectoration.

心经咳嗽 [xīn jīng ké sou]
heart meridian/channel cough: cough accompanied by precordial pain, and sore throat or choking sensation in the throat, indicating the involvement of the heart meridian/channel, also abbreviated as heart cough (心咳 [xīn ké])

心咳 [xīn ké]
heart cough: abbreviation for heart meridian/channel cough (心经咳嗽 [xīn jīng ké sou])

肝经咳嗽 [gān jīng ké sou]
liver meridian/channel cough: cough due to liver fire invading the lung, usually accompanied by hypochondriac and lower abdominal pain or alternate attacks of chills and fever, irascibility and dizziness, also abbreviated as liver cough (肝咳 [gān ké])

肝咳 [gān ké]
liver cough: abbreviation for liver meridian/channel cough (肝经咳嗽 [gān jīng ké sou])

脾经咳嗽 [pí jīng ké sou]
spleen meridian/channel cough: cough related to disorders of the spleen, usually accompanied by right hypochondriac pain radiating to the shoulder and back, and aggravated upon exertion, also abbreviated as spleen cough (脾咳 [pí ké])

脾咳 [pí ké]
spleen cough: abbreviation for spleen meridian/channel cough (脾经咳嗽 [pí jīng ké sòu]

肺经咳嗽 [fèi jīng ké sou]
lung meridian/channel cough: cough ascribed to disorders of the lung, either excessive or deficient in nature, usually marked by loud cough or bloody sputum, also abbreviated as lung cough (肺咳 [fèi ké])

肺咳 [fèi ké]
lung cough: abbreviation for lung meridian/channel cough (肺经咳嗽 [fèi jīng ké sou])

肾经咳嗽 [shèn jīng ké sou]
kidney meridian/channel cough: cough accompanied by lumbago or back pain, usually due to kidney deficiency, also abbreviated as kidney cough (肾咳 [shèn ké])

肾咳 [shèn ké]
kidney cough: abbreviation for kidney meridian/channel cough (肾经咳嗽[shèn jīng ké sou])

胃咳 [wèi ké]
stomach cough: cough accompanied by vomiting

小肠咳 [xiǎo cháng ké]
small intestinal cough: cough accompanied by breaking wind

大肠咳 [dà cháng ké]
large intestinal cough: cough accompanied by fecal incontinence

胆咳 [dǎn ké]
gallbladder cough: cough accompanied by vomiting of bile

膀胱咳 [páng guāng ké]
bladder cough: cough accompanied by incontinence of urine

三焦咳 [sān jiāo ké]
triple energizer cough: cough accompanied by abdominal distension and anorexia

干咳 [gān ké]
dry cough: cough with no or scanty expectoration, also called 干咳嗽 [gān ké sou]

干咳嗽 [gān ké sou]
cough with no expectoration: cough indicating consumption of fluid in the lung, also abbreviated as dry cough (干咳 [gān ké])

外感咳嗽 [wài gǎn ké sou]
externally contracted cough: cough due to external contraction, characterized by acute onset often accompanied by chills and fever

风寒咳嗽 [fēng hán ké sou]
wind-cold cough: cough caused by wind-cold, marked by association with frothy expectoration, stuffed-up nose, chills or aversion to cold, general aching and no sweating

风热咳嗽 [fēng rè ké sou]
wind-heat cough: cough caused by windheat, marked by association with sticky expectoration, fever, thirst, and sore throat

风燥咳嗽 [fēng zào ké sou]
wind-dryness cough: cough caused by wind-dryness, marked by dry cough with itching of the throat and other symptoms of dryness

内伤咳嗽 [nèi shāng ké sou]
internal damage cough: cough due to internal damage, characterized by a chronic course, often accompanied by dyspnea or shortness of breath

痰湿咳嗽 [tán shī ké sou]
phlegm-dampness cough: cough due to accumulation of phlegm-dampness in the lung, marked by association with copious expectoration, relieved when phlegm is discharged, also known as phlegm cough (痰咳 [tán ké])

痰咳 [tán ké]
phlegm cough: synonym for phlegm-dampness cough (痰湿咳嗽 [tán shī ké sou])

肺虚咳嗽 [fèi xū ké sou]
lung-deficiency cough: cough due to deficiency in the lung (mostly yin deficiency), marked by dry cough or blood-stained sputum, accompanied by emaciation, fidgetiness, insomnia, night sweats, malar flush and afternoon fever

气虚咳嗽 [qì xū ké sou]
***qi*-deficiency cough:** cough due to deficiency of lung *qi*, marked by chronic cough with feeble sound, profuse thin expectoration, lassitude, spontaneous sweating, and vulnerability to colds

五更咳 [wǔ gēng ké]
fifth-watch cough: cough occurring or exaggerated daily before dawn, usually due to spleen insufficiency with profuse production of phlegm in the early morning

劳咳 [láo ké]
consumptive cough: (1) chronic persistent cough that causes comsumption; (2) cough occurring in phthisis or due to consumption by overfatigue or sexual intemperance, also called 劳嗽 [láo sòu]

劳嗽 [láo sòu]
consumptive cough: another name for 劳咳 [láo ké]

短气 [duǎn qì]
shortness of breath: rapid labored breathing

少气 [shǎo qì]
shortage of *qi*: weak or faint breathing

上气 [shàng qì]
(I) abnormal rising of *qi*; dyspnea: state characterized by reversed upward flow of *qi* in the lung, usually seen in the case of an external contraction when the airway is obstructed by phlegm; **(II) the upper *qi*:** *qi* in the upper part of the body, including heart *qi* and lung *qi*

咳逆上气 [ké nì shàng qì]
cough with reversed ascent of *qi*: cough with counterflow of *qi* in the air passage, usually abbreviated as cough with dyspnea (咳逆 [ké nì])

咳逆 [ké nì]
cough with dyspnea: abbreviation for 咳逆上气 [ké nì shàng qì]

喘 [chuǎn]
dyspnea: difficult and labored breathing

喘证 [chuǎn zhèng]
dyspnea (syndrome): morbid state characterized by difficult and labored breathing

喘病 [chuǎn bìng]
dyspnea (disease): synonym for dyspnea (syndrome) (喘证 [chuǎn zhèng])

实喘 [shí chuǎn]
dyspnea of excess type: dyspnea caused by excessive pathogenic factors marked by rapid, forceful and coarse breathing with acute onset and short duration

虚喘 [xū chuǎn]
dyspnea of deficiency type: dyspnea due to insufficient function of the lung and kidney, marked by shortness of breath and dyspnea upon exertion

哮 [xiào]
wheezing: difficult and labored breathing with a whistling sound

哮病 [xiào bìng]
wheezing disease: morbid state characterized by difficult and labored breathing with a whistling sound

哮喘 [xiào chuǎn]
asthma: general term for dyspnea with wheezing

寒哮 [hán xiào]
cold wheezing: asthma due to invasion of pathogenic cold, marked by dyspnea with wheezing, cough with thin mucous expectoration, stuffiness in the chest, whitish and slippery tongue coating, and floating and tense pulse, also called 冷哮 [lěng xiào]

冷哮 [lěng xiào]
cold wheezing: same as 寒哮 [hán xiào]

热哮 [rè xiào]
heat wheezing: asthma due to retention of heat-phlegm which causes obstruction of the respiratory tract, marked by dyspnea, wheezing, thick and yellowish sputum, distress in the chest, flushed face, dry mouth with desire to drink, reddened tongue with yellow and greasy coating, and slippery and rapid pulse

痰喘 [tán chuǎn]
phlegm dyspnea: dyspnea caused by excessive phlegm in the lung, marked by tachypnea with phlegmatic sound, cough, and stuffiness in the chest

寒痰 [hán tán]
cold phlegm: phlegm syndrome characterized by expectoration of thin and foamy sputum, usually due to cold

水饮 [shuǐ yǐn]
fluid retention; retained fluid: clear and watery pathoglocial product that comes from the internal organs as a result of disordered fluid metabolism, also abbreviated as 饮 [yǐn]

饮 [yǐn]
fluid retention: abbreviation for 水饮 [shuǐ yǐn]

饮证 [yǐn zhèng]

fluid retention syndrome: collective term for various diseases resulting from fluid retention in the body, generally including phlegm-fluid retention (痰饮 [tán yǐn]), pleural fluid retention (悬饮 [xuán yǐn]), subcutaneous fluid retention (溢饮 [yì yǐn]), and thoracic fluid retention (支饮 [zhī yǐn])

痰饮 [tán yǐn]

phlegm-fluid retention: (1) general term for retention of phlegm and fluid in any part of the body; (2) particular designation for retention of fluid in the gastrointestinal tract, e.g., gastric retention in pyloric stenosis

悬饮 [xuán yǐn]

pleural fluid retention: excessive fluid retained in the side of the thorax with stretching pain during respiration

溢饮 [yì yǐn]

subcutaneous fluid retention: excessive fluid in the body flooding the body surface and muscles

支饮 [zhī yǐn]

thoracic fluid retention: retention of excessive fluid in the lung and chest

伏饮 [fú yǐn]

latent fluid retention: disease characterized by phlegm-fluid latent in the body with episodes brought on by external contractions and manifested by frequent recurrence of backache, feeling of fullness and distension in the chest and hypochondrium, cough, vomiting, chills and fever

热痰 [rè tán]

heat phlegm: (1) morbid condition caused by combined pathogens of phlegm and heat, and characterized by cough and dyspnea with thick yellow sputum difficult to expectorate; (2) phlegm lingering in the heart meridian, joined and aggravated by heat, giving rise to mania, and palpitations, also known as fire phlegm 火痰 [huǒ tán]

火痰 [huǒ tán]

fire phlegm: synonym for heat phlegm (热痰 [rè tán])

顽痰 [wán tán]

obstinate phlegm: chronic case of phlegm retention difficult to cure, e.g., bronchial asthma with persistent recurrence, mania, and epilepsy

肺痈 [fèi yōng]

lung abscess: abscess occurring in the lung, marked by fever, cough, chest pain, and expectoration of foul turbid or bloody purulent sputum

肺胀 [fèi zhàng]

lung distension: disease of the lung characterized by persistent distension of the lung, resulting from chronic cough or asthma, manifested by a sensation of pressure in the chest, profuse expectoration, shortness of breath upon mild exertion, and cyanosis or even edema of the limbs, seen in cases of pulmonary emphysema and pulmonary heart disease

肺萎 [痿] [fèi wěi]

lung atrophy: disease of the lung due to chronic cough, marked by atrophy of the lung with shortness of breath and expectoration

虚劳（病）[xū láo (bìng)]
consumptive disease: disease characterized by consumption, either infectious or non-infectious, the latter also known as 虚损 [xū sǔn], and the former 劳［痨］瘵 [láo zhài]

虚损 [xū sǔn]
consumption: deficiency and impairment of yin, yang, *qi* or blood in *zang-fu* organs, usually due to non-infectious factors such as emotional intemperance, overexertion, improper diet, and sexual overindulgence

劳［痨］瘵 [láo zhài]
phthisis: term for chronic infectious consumptive diseases such as pulmonary tuberculosis

痨病 [láo bìng]
phthisis (disease): old name for pulmonary tuberculosis

骨蒸 [gǔ zhēng]
bone steaming: subjective feeling of fever deep in the body, which appears to emanate from the bones, a term for hectic fever with night sweats, as seen in cases of consumptive diseases

五劳 [wǔ láo]
(I) five kinds of overstrain: collective term for over-protracted looking, lying, sitting, standing or walking; **(II) five kinds of consumptive diseases:** collective term for consumption of the lung, liver, heart, spleen, and kidney

肺痨 [fèi láo]
lung phthisis: wasting of the lung, an old name for pulmonary tuberculosis

肺劳 [fèi láo]
(1) lung consumption: consumptive disease of the lung due to overstrain, manifested by cough, shortness of breath, back pain, lassitude and emaciation; **(2) lung phthisis:** also known as 肺痨 [fèi láo]

肝劳 [gān láo]
liver consumption: disease due to impairment of the liver by emotional upset, manifested by blurred vision, pain in the chest and hypochondrium, flaccid muscles and tendons, and difficulty in movement

心劳 [xīn láo]
heart consumption: consumptive disease of the heart marked by exhaustion of the heart blood due to overstrain, manifested by fidgetiness, insomnia, palpitations, and liability to panic

脾劳 [pí láo]
spleen consumption: consumptive disease of the spleen due to improper diet or mental stress, marked by muscular wasting, manifested by weakness of limbs, anorexia, abdominal distension, and loose stools

肾劳 [shèn láo]
kidney consumption: consumptive disease of the kidney due to excessive sexual activities, manifested by lumbago, spermatorrhea or menoxenia, night sweats, hectic fever, and weakness of the legs

虚烦 [xū fán]
vexation of deficiency type: vexation due to deficiency of yin, which brings on endogenous heat

虚热 [xū rè]

fever of deficiency type: fever due to deficiency of yin, yang, *qi* or blood

内伤发热 [nèi shāng fā rè]

internal damage fever: fever due to disorder of internal organs caused by emotional stress, improper diet, overwork, sexual intemperance, etc.

阴虚发热 [yīn xū fā rè]

yin-deficiency fever: fever due to yin deficiency, marked by appearance of fever in the afternoon or at night, sensation of heat in the chest, palms of the hands and soles of the feet, accompanied by night sweats, dry mouth, reddened tongue, and thready rapid pulse

阳虚发热 [yáng xū fā rè]

yang-deficiency fever: fever due to yang deficiency, marked by appearance of fever in the morning, accompanied by spontaneous sweating, intolerance of wind, lassitude, anorexia, and feeble pulse

血虚发热 [xuè xū fā rè]

blood-deficiency fever: fever due to blood deficiency, marked by low fever with dizziness, lassitude, palpitations, pallor, pale tongue, and thin weak pulse

劳蒸 [láo zhēng]

consumptive steaming (fever): hectic fever due to consumption

干血痨 [gān xuè láo]

dry blood consumption: consumptive disease seen mostly in women, often accompanied by menopenia or amenorrhea

心悸 [xīn jì]

palpitations: diseased state marked by a subjective feeling of unduly rapid or violent heart beat

惊悸 [jīng jì]

fright palpitations: palpitations ascribed to being frightened

怔忡 [zhēng chōng]

fearful throbbing: severe case of palpitations

胸痛 [xiōng tòng]

chest pain: pain in the middle or lateral part of the chest, usually ascribed to disorders of the heart, lung or liver

胸痹 [xiōng bì]

chest impediment: disease marked by paroxysmal attacks of pectoral pain, sometimes accompanied by a feeling of suffocation

心痛 [xīn tòng]

heart pain: general term for pain in the precordial and epigastric regions

真心痛 [zhēn xīn tòng]

real heart pain: disease characterized by sudden occurrence of severe pain in the precordial region accompanied by sweating, cyanotic lips and cold limbs, so named to distinguish it from gastralgia which was also called heart pain in ancient times

厥心痛 [jué xīn tòng]

heart pain with cold limbs: (1) extreme pain in the precordial region leading to collapse with cold limbs; (2) heart pain caused by cold that blocks the *qi* flow, manifested as cold limbs

冷心痛 [lěng xīn tòng]
cold heart pain: severe pain in the region over the heart, accompanied by cold limbs and cold sweats

卒心痛 [cù xìn tòng]
sudden heart pain: sudden attack of precordial pain due to invasion of the heart meridian/channel by pathogenic cold, heat or wind, which causes stagnation of *qi* and blood within the meridian/channel

肝郁胁痛 [gān yù xié tòng]
liver-depressive hypochondriac pain: hypochondriac pain due to liver stagnation, mostly caused by emotional upset, accompanied by stuffy feeling in the chest, poor appetite, and wiry pulse, also known as liver *qi* hypochondriac pain (肝气胁痛 [gān qì xié tòng])

肝气胁痛 [gān qì xié tòng]
liver *qi* hypochondriac pain: synonym for liver-depressive hypochondriac pain (肝郁胁痛 [gān yù xié tòng])

汗证 [hàn zhèng]
sweating syndrome: state characterized by abnormal sweating due to yin-yang disharmony or infirmity of the subcutaneous interstices and pores, also known as sweating disease (汗病 [hàn bìng])

汗病 [hàn bìng]
sweating disease: synonym for sweating syndrome (汗证 [hàn zhèng])

自汗 [zì hàn]
spontaneous sweating: abnormal sweating in the daytime aggravated by mild exertion and unconnected with environmental factors

盗汗 [dào hàn]
night sweats: sweating during sleep, which stops upon awakening

脱汗 [tuō hàn]
sweating in shock: profuse sweating accompanied by listlessness, cold limbs, and hardly perceivable pulse, usually occurring in a critical case

战汗 [zhàn hàn]
shiver sweating: sweating occurring in cases of acute febrile diseases, characterized by sudden occurrence of shivering chills and then generalized sweating, indicating a sharp struggle of healthy *qi* against the pathogen

黄汗 [huáng hàn]
yellow sweat: disease marked by yellow-colored sweat accompanied by bitterness and stickiness in the mouth, dry mouth with no desire to drink, and yellow and greasy tongue coating, ascribed to the interior accumulation of dampness-heat

气虚自汗 [qì xū zì hàn]
spontaneous sweating in *qi* deficiency: spontaneous sweating resulting from deficiency of defense *qi*, usually accompanied by fatigue, weakness, and aversion to wind

阳虚自汗 [yáng xū zì hàn]
spontaneous sweating in yang deficiency:

abnormal state characterized by spontaneous sweating accompanied by intolerance of cold

阴虚盗汗 [yīn xū dào hàn]
night sweating in yin deficiency: night sweating due to deficiency of yin with exuberant yang which stimulates the discharge of sweat during sleep, when defense *qi* goes inward

眩晕 [xuàn yùn]
(I) dizziness: disordered state characterized by a sensation of unsteadiness with a feeling of movement within the head; **(II) vertigo:** more serious state of dizziness characterized by a sensation that either the environment or one's own body is revolving

风寒眩晕 [fēng hán xuàn yùn]
wind-cold dizziness; wind-cold vertigo: dizziness or vertigo due to exogenous affection by wind-cold, usually accompanied by headache, joint pain or general aching, and aversion to wind and cold

风热眩晕 [fēng rè xuàn yùn]
wind-heat dizziness; wind-heat vertigo: dizziness or vertigo due to upward drive of pathogenic wind-heat, often accompanied by distress in the chest and vomiting, and even fainting

肝阳眩晕 [gān yáng xuàn yùn]
liver yang dizziness; liver yang vertigo: intermittent dizziness or vertigo due to uprising of liver yang, often accompanied by headache, insomnia, irritability, and wiry pulse

肝火眩晕 [gān huǒ xuàn yùn]
liver fire dizziness; liver fire vertigo: dizziness or vertigo due to liver fire induced by an emotional upset, usually accompanied by headache, blood-shot eyes, irritability, bitter taste in the mouth, reddened tongue with yellowish coating, and wiry and rapid pulse

风痰眩晕 [fēng tán xuàn yùn]
wind-phlegm dizziness; wind-phlegm vertigo: dizziness or vertigo due to wind-phlegm, usually accompanied by headache, blurred vision, tightness of the chest, palpitations, vomiting, and expectoration of sticky sputum

肾虚眩晕 [shèn xū xuàn yùn]
kidney insufficiency dizziness; kidney insufficiency vertigo: dizziness or vertigo due to insufficient kidney essence for nourishing the brain, usually accompanied by tinnitus, listlessness, forgetfulness and weakness of the loins and legs

血虚眩晕 [xuè xū xuàn yùn]
blood deficiency dizziness; blood deficiency vertigo: dizziness or vertigo due to blood deficiency, marked by aggravation upon exertion, pallor, insomnia, pale tongue, and thready pulse

气虚眩晕 [qì xū xuàn yùn]
***qi* deficiency dizziness; *qi* deficiency vertigo:** dizziness or vertigo due to *qi* deficiency, marked by aggravation upon exertion, listlessness, poor appetite, pale tongue, and weak pulse

感暑眩晕 [gǎn shǔ xuàn yùn]
summerheat dizziness; summerheat vertigo: dizziness or vertigo due to affection by summerheat, also known as

heatstroke dizziness or heatstroke vertigo (中暑眩晕 [zhòng shǔ xuàn yùn])

中暑眩晕 [zhòng shǔ xuàn yùn]
heatstroke dizziness; heatstroke vertigo: synonym for summerheat dizziness or summerheat vertigo (感暑眩晕 [gǎn shǔ xuàn yùn])

头痛 [tóu tòng]
headache: diseased state marked by pain in the head either due to external contraction or internal injury

真头痛 [zhēn tóu tòng]
real headache; true headache: critical case of headache marked by sudden attack of pain in the head accompanied by counterflow of cold from the extremities upward to the elbows and knees

头风 [tóu fēng]
head wind; recurrent headache: chronic headache with repeated recurrence

偏头风 [piān tóu fēng]
hemilateral head wind; migraine: chronic recurrent headache occurring on one side of the head, also called hemilateral headache (偏头痛 [piān tóu tòng])

偏头痛 [piān tóu tòng]
hemilateral headache; migraine: same as hemilateral head wind (偏头风 [piān tóu fēng])

雷头风 [léi tóu fēng]
thunder head wind: diseased state characterized by pain with loud noise in the head

外感头痛 [wài gǎn tóu tòng]
externally contracted headache: collective term for various types of headache ascribed to exogenous contractions

风寒头痛 [fēng hán tóu tòng]
wind-cold headache: headache due to attack of external wind-cold, marked by pain in the head extending to the nape and back, aversion to cold and wind, soreness and pain in the joints, watery nasal discharge, thin and whitish tongue coating and floating tense pulse

风热头痛 [fēng rè tóu tòng]
wind-heat headache: headache due to attack of external wind-heat, usually accompanied by fever, thirst, constipation, and floating and rapid pulse

风湿头痛 [fēng shī tóu tòng]
wind-dampness headache: headache due to attack of external wind-dampness, marked by pain in the head as if it were tightly bound, accompanied by heaviness of the limbs, stuffiness in the chest, anorexia, white greasy tongue coating, and soft pulse

痰浊头痛 [tán zhuó tóu tòng]
phlegm-turbidity headache: headache resulting from turbid phlegm, marked by pain and distension of the head accompanied by stuffiness in the chest, nausea, expectoration, white greasy tongue coating, and slippery pulse

内伤头痛 [nèi shāng tóu tòng]
internal damage headache: headache marked by slow onset and intermittent recurrence, accompanied by deficiency

syndromes of *qi*, blood, or *zang-fu* organs, or with manifestations indicating the presence of endogenous pathogenic factors

肝阳头痛 [gān yáng tóu tòng]
liver-yang headache: headache ascribed to exuberant liver yang, usually accompanied by dizziness, irritability, irascibility, dream-disturbed sleep and wiry pulse

风痰头痛 [fēng tán tóu tòng]
wind-phlegm headache: headache ascribed to wind-phlegm, usually accompanied by dizziness, heaviness of the body, distress in the chest, and expectoration of sticky sputum

气虚头痛 [qì xū tóu tòng]
***qi*-deficiency headache:** headache ascribed to *qi* deficiency, usually aggravated during exertion, accompanied by anorexia and lassitude

瘀血头痛 [yū xuè tóu tòng]
blood-stasis headache: chronic headache, stabbing in character and fixed in location, often occurring after traumatic injury

血虚头痛 [xuè xū tóu tòng]
blood-deficiency headache: headache ascribed to blood deficiency, marked by dull pain of the head, usually accompanied by dizziness, pallor, and palpitations

百合病 [bǎi hé bìng]
"lily disease": ancient term for neurosis with mental strain, listlessness, sleeplessness, anorexia, sham heat and sham cold, bitterness in the mouth, yellow urine, rapid pulse, etc. It is so called because it can be effectively treated by administering *Bulbus Lilii*.

癫狂 [diān kuáng]
depressive-manic psychosis: term referring to depression and mania in combination

癫病 [diān bìng]
depressive psychosis: mental disorder characterized by severe depression, often abbreviated as depression in the strict sense (癫 [diān])

癫 [diān]
depression: used in the strict sense, a synonym for depressive psychosis

狂病 [kuáng bìng]
manic psychosis: psychotic disorder characterized by mental and physical hyperactivity, disorganization of behavior, and elevation of mood, often abbreviated as mania (狂 [kuáng])

狂 [kuáng]
mania: abbreviation for manic psychosis (狂病 [kuáng bìng])

痫病 [xián bìng]
epilepsy (disease): disease or syndrome characterized by paroxysmal transient loss of consciousness with generalized tonic-clonic seizures, up-staring of the eyes and stertorous breathing, often preceded by an aura, also called epilepsy (syndrome) (痫证 [xián zhèng]) or epilepsy (癫痫 [diān xián]) and "bleating convulsions" (羊痫风 [yáng xián fēng])

痫证 [xián zhèng]
epilepsy (syndrome): same as 痫病 [xián bìng]

癫痫 [diān xián]
epilepsy: synonym for 痫病 [xián bìng]

羊痫风 [yáng xián fēng]
"bleating convulsions": popular name for epilepsy (癫痫 [diān xián])

阳痫 [yáng xián]
yang epilepsy: epilepsy associated with a yang syndrome characterized by convulsive attacks with transient loss of consciousness

阴痫 [yīn xián]
yin epilepsy: epilepsy associated with a yin syndrome characterized by transient clouding of consciousness without convulsions

惊痫 [jīng xián]
fright epilepsy: (1) epilepsy induced by fright; (2) infantile convulsions

脏躁 [zàng zào]
hysteria: morbid condition characterized by violent emotional paroxysms, anxiety, and disturbances of sensory and motor functions

梅核气 [méi hé qì]
"plum-stone *qi*"; globus hystericus: disturbing subjective sensation of a lump in the throat commonly experienced in cases of hysteria

奔豚 [bēn tún]
"running piglet": ancient name for the morbid condition characterized by a feeling of masses of gas ascending within the abdomen like running piglets

奔豚气 [bēn tún qì]
"running piglet *qi*": (1) synonym for running piglet (奔豚 [bēn tún]); (2) another name for hernia (疝气 [shàn qì])

嗜睡 [shì shuì]
somnolence: excessive sleepiness

失眠 [shī mián]
insomnia: prolonged inability to obtain normal sleep, also known as 不得卧 [bù dé wò]

不得卧 [bù dé wò]
inability to sleep: synonym for insomnia (失眠 [shī mián])

肝火不得卧 [gān huǒ bù dé wò]
liver fire insomnia: insomnia with dream-disturbed sleep and irritability due to exuberant liver fire

心血虚不得卧 [xīn xuè xū bù dé wò]
heart blood deficiency insomnia: insomnia with abnormal wakefulness and forgetfulness due to deficiency of heart blood

心气虚不得卧 [xīn qì xū bù dé wò]
heart *qi* deficiency insomnia: insomnia with fidgetiness, lassitude, and spontaneous sweating due to deficiency of heart *qi*

健忘 [jiàn wàng]
amnesia: loss of memory, also known as forgetfulness (善忘 [shàn wàng])

善忘 [shàn wàng]
forgetfulness: synonym for amnesia (健忘 [jiàn wàng])

痴呆 [chī dāi]
dementia: deteriorated mentality characterized by marked decline of the intellectual function and emotional apathy

卒中 [cù zhòng]
stroke: (1) same as wind stroke (中风 [zhòng fēng]); (2) sudden loss of consciousness

中风 [zhòng fēng]
wind stroke; apoplexy: disease characterized by sudden appearance of hemiplegia, deviated eye and mouth, and impeded speech, also called stroke disease (中风病 [zhòng fēng bìng])

中风病 [zhòng fēng bìng]
wind stroke disease: synonym for wind stroke (中风 [zhòng fēng])

中风闭证 [zhòng fēng bì zhèng]
blockage pattern of wind stroke: wind-stroke characterized by blockage of the orifices, manifested by loss of consciousness, trismus, and spastic tonus of the limbs, pertaining to an excess condition which can be further classified into yin blockage and yang blockage

中风阴闭 [zhòng fēng yīn bì]
yin blockage of wind stroke: blocking of the orifices by dampness-phlegm in cases of wind stroke, manifested by pallor, lying in quiescence, cool limbs, excessive secretion in the mouth, and white greasy tongue coating

中风阳闭 [zhòng fēng yáng bì]
yang blockage of wind stroke: blocking of the orifices by phlegm-heat in cases of wind stroke, manifested by fever, flushing of the face, coarse breathing, foul breath, restlessness, and yellow greasy tongue coating

中风脱证 [zhòng fēng tuō zhèng]
collapse pattern of wind stroke: wind stroke characterized by prostration of yang *qi* during the attack, manifested by loss of consciousness, closed eyes with opened mouth, flaccid paralysis of the limbs, profuse cold sweat, incontinence of urine and feces, and faint breathing

真中风 [zhēn zhòng fēng]
real wind stroke; true wind stroke: apoplexy caused by exogenous pathogenic wind marked by sudden loss of consciousness, wry mouth, hemiplegia and aphasia, often abbreviated as real stroke or true stroke (真中 [zhēn zhòng])

真中 [zhēn zhòng]
real stroke; true stroke: abbreviation for real wind stroke or true wind stroke (真中风 [zhēn zhòng fēng])

类中风 [lèi zhòng fēng]
apoplectic wind stroke: apoplexy caused by endogenous pathogenic wind, usually ascribed to internal stirring of liver wind or transformation of dampness-phlegm into heat and wind, also abbreviated as apoplectic stroke (类中 [lèi zhòng])

类中 [lèi zhòng]
apoplectic stroke: abbreviation for apoplectic wind stroke (类中风 [lèi zhòng fēng])

中脏 [zhòng zàng]
***zang*(-organ) stroke; visceral stroke:**

most serious form of apoplexy with sudden loss of consciousness, aphasia, and paralysis of the lips with salivation

中腑 [zhòng fǔ]
***fu*(-organ) stroke; bowel stroke:** serious form of apoplexy with fainting, hemiplegia, distortion of the face and dysphasia

中经 [zhòng jīng]
meridian stroke; channel stroke: mild form of apoplexy with paralysis of the face and limbs, and dysphasia, but no impairment of consciousness

中络 [zhòng luò]
collateral stroke: mildest form of apoplexy with slight distortion of the face and numbness of the limbs

口噤 [kǒu jìn]
trismus: lockjaw with difficulty in opening the mouth

失语 [shī yǔ]
aphasia: loss of the ability of expression by speech

偏枯 [piān kū]
hemiplegia: paralysis of one side of the body

半身不遂 [bàn shēn bù suí]
hemiplegia: same as 偏枯 [piān kū]

㖞僻不遂 [wāi pì bù suí]
hemiplegia with wry mouth: paralysis of one side of the body with retraction of the angle of the mouth, which often occurs after a stroke

口僻 [kǒu pì]
deviation of the mouth: retraction of the angle of the mouth in the case of unilateral facial paralysis, also known as wry mouth (口㖞 [kǒu wāi])

口㖞 [kǒu wāi]
wry mouth: synonym for deviation of the mouth (口僻 [kǒu pì])

麻木 [má mù]
numbness: reduced sensibility to touch. Strictly speaking, 麻 [má] and 木 [mù] have different meanings, the former referring to a tingling sensation, while the latter to loss of the ability to feel and move; but the term composed of the two characters in combination often means loss of sensation or numbness.

中风昏迷 [zhòng fēng hūn mí]
apoplectic coma: coma occurring in cases of wind stroke

中风后遗症 [zhòng fēng hòu yí zhèng]
sequelae of wind stroke: functional disturbances following an attack of apoplexy, such as hemiplegia, dysphasia and dementia

厥 [jué]
(I) syncope: temporary loss of consciousness; **(II) reversed cold extremities:** pronounced cold of the limbs originating from the extremeties

厥证 [jué zhèng]
syncope: morbid state characterized by temporary loss of consciousness with cold limbs resulting from disordered flow of *qi* and blood

大厥 [dà jué]
major syncope: severe sudden loss of consciousness as if the patient were suddenly deceased

薄厥 [pò jué]
sudden syncope: ancient term for sudden fainting in a fit of rage

脏厥 [zàng jué]
visceral syncope: syncope due to yang debilitation of the visceral organs

食厥 [shí jué]
crapulent syncope: syncope due to eating and drinking too much at one sitting

气厥 [qì jué]
***qi* syncope:** syncope induced by emotional upset or spiritual stimulation, marked by sudden fainting, loss of consciousness, cold limbs, and trismus

血厥 [xuè jué]
blood syncope: syncope following a fit of rage that causes an upward reverse flow of *qi* and blood, marked by flushed face and stringy forceful pulse

痰厥 [tán jué]
phlegm syncope: syncope occurring after a fit of serious coughing in one with chronic cough, asthma and expectoration, marked by gurgling sounds in the throat, white greasy tongue coating and deep slippery pulse

昏厥 [hūn jué]
fainting: sudden loss of consciousness

手足厥冷 [shǒu zú jué lěng]
reversed cold of hands and feet: pronounced cold of the limbs starting from the extremities, usually up to the knees and elbows or beyond, with sudden loss of consciousness, occurring in syncope or shock, also called 手足逆冷 [shǒu zú nì lěng] and abbreviated as 四逆 [sì nì]

手足逆冷 [shǒu zú nì lěng]
reversed cold of hands and feet: same as 手足厥冷 [shǒu zú jué lěng]

四逆 [sì nì]
reversed cold of extremities: abbreviation for 手足逆冷 [shǒu zú nì lěng]

蛔厥 [huí jué]
ascariasis syncope: syncope due to acute abdominal pain caused by ascarides, as seen in cases of biliary ascariasis

热厥 [rè jué]
heat syncope: collapse due to excessive pathogenic heat in the interior of the body, a symptom of syncope or shock in cases of acute febrile diseases

寒厥 [hán jué]
cold syncope: collapse due to yang debilitation with excessive cold in the body

痉病 [jìng bìng]
convulsive disease: diseased state characterized by rigidity of the nape, convulsion of the limbs and opisthotonos

热甚发痉 [rè shèn fā jìng]
febrile convulsions: convulsions induced by high fever

抽搐 [chōu chù]
convulsions: a violent involuntary contraction or series of contractions

痿 [wěi]
atrophy-flaccidity: flaccid paralysis with muscular atrophy

痿病 [wěi bìng]
atrophy-flaccidity disease: diseased condition characterized by flaccid paralysis with muscular atrophy of a limb

痿证 [wěi zhèng]
atrophy-flaccidity syndrome: syndrome characterized by flaccid paralysis with muscular atrophy of a limb

痿躄 [wěi bì]
atrophic crippling: crippling with muscular atrophy of a lower limb

脚弱 [jiǎo ruò]
leg weakness: lack of strength with muscular atrophy of a lower limb

脚气 [jiǎo qì]
leg *qi*: (1) leg flaccidity; (2) beriberi

脚气冲心 [jiǎo qì chōng xīn]
beriberi involving the heart: serious case of beriberi with heart failure, manifested by palpitations and shortness of breath

筋痿 [jīn wěi]
sinew atrophy-flaccidity: one of the atrophy-flaccidity syndromes ascribed to exuberant liver heat which wilts the sinews with contracture of the limbs, also called liver atrophy-flaccidity (肝痿 [gān wěi])

肝痿 [gān wěi]
liver atrophy-flaccidity: another name for sinew atrophy-flaccidity (筋痿 [jīn wěi])

脉痿 [mài wěi]
vessel atrophy-flaccidity: one of the atrophy-flaccidity syndromes ascribed to up-flaming of heart fire with emptiness of blood vessels in the lower part that makes the legs extremely flaccid and the patient unable to stand, also called heart atrophy-flaccidity (心痿 [xīn wěi])

心痿 [xīn wěi]
heart atrophy-flaccidity: another name for vessel atrophy-flaccidity (脉痿 [mài wěi])

肉痿 [ròu wěi]
flesh atrophy-flaccidity: one of the atrophy-flaccidity syndromes ascribed to heat or dampness in the spleen that causes damage to the flesh and leads to numbness or even immobility of the limbs, also called spleen atrophy-flaccidity (脾痿 [pí wěi])

脾痿 [pí wěi]
spleen atrophy-flaccidity: another name for flesh atrophy-flaccidity (肉痿 [ròu wěi])

骨痿 [gǔ wěi]
bone atrophy-flaccidity: one of the atrophy-flaccidity syndromes ascribed to impairment of the kidney with consumption of essence, manifested by limpness of the loins and flaccidity of the legs with the patient's inability to walk, also called kidney atrophy-flaccidity (肾痿 [shèn wěi])

肾痿 [shèn wěi]
kidney atrophy-flaccidity: another name for bone atrophy-flaccidity (骨痿 [gǔ wěi])

颤震［振］ [chàn zhèn]
tremor: diseased state characterized by involuntary shaking or trembling of the head or hands, also called trembling (振掉 [zhèn diào])

振掉 [zhèn diào]
trembling: synonym for tremor (颤震 [chàn zhèn])

痹（病） [bì (bìng)]
(I) impediment disease: group of diseases characterized by invasion of the pathogenic factors that cause stagnation of *qi* and blood, and blockage of the collateral meridians; **(II) arthralgia:** impediment disease in the narrow sense involving the joints of the limbs, marked by joint pain with difficulty in movement

历节风 [lì jié fēng]
joint-running wind; multiple arthralgia: disease characterized by redness and swelling of multiple joints with acute pain and limitation of motion

三痹 [sān bì]
three kinds of impediment; three kinds of arthralgia: collective term for arthralgia caused by wind, by cold and by dampness

热痹 [rè bì]
heat impediment; heat arthralgia: arthritis due to heat, marked by pain, heat, and redness and swelling of the joints, usually accompanied by fever

风痹 [fēng bì]
wind impediment; wind arthralgia: impediment disease ascribed to invasion by wind, marked by migratory joint pains, also called migratory impediment or migratory arthralgia (行痹 [xíng bì])

行痹 [xíng bì]
migratory impediment; migratory arthralgia: another name for wind impediment or wind arthralgia (风痹 [fēng bì])

寒痹 [hán bì]
cold impediment; cold arthralgia: impediment disease with severe joint pain exaggerated by cold, also known as bone impediment (骨痹 [gǔ bì]) or agonizing impediment or agonizing arthralgia (痛痹 [tòng bì])

痛痹 [tòng bì]
agonizing impediment; agonizing arthralgia: synonym for cold impediment or cold arthralgia (寒痹 [hán bì])

湿痹 [shī bì]
dampness impediment; dampness arthralgia: impediment disease with arthralgia ascribed to invasion by dampness, marked by swelling with heavy sensation in the joints with fixed or localized pain, also known as muscle impediment (肌痹 [jī bì]) or fixed impediment or fixed arthralgia (着痹 [zhuó bì])

着痹 [zhuó bì]
fixed impediment; fixed arthralgia: another name for dampness impediment or

dampness arthralgia (湿痹 [shī bì])

尪痹 [wāng bì]
lameness impediment; ankylosing arthralgia: disease characterized by arthralgia with joint deformities

骨痹 [gǔ bì]
bone impediment: disease characterized by invasion of pathogenic wind-cold-dampness to the bones that produces severe joint pain with cold sensation and difficulty in moving, synonymous with cold impediment or cold arthralgia (寒痹 [hán bì]), also agonizing impediment or agonizing arthralgia (痛痹 [tòng bì])

肌痹 [jī bì]
muscle impediment: (1) disease characterized by invasion of the joints and superficial muscles by cold-dampness, synonymous with dampness impediment or dampness arthralgia (湿痹 [shī bì]) and fixed impediment or fixed arthralgia (着痹 [zhuó bì]); (2) impediment disease mainly involving the muscles, marked by weakness and atrophy of the limbs

脉痹 [mài bì]
vessel impediment: impediment disease mainly involving the vessels, marked by sluggish blood flow

筋痹 [jīn bì]
sinew impediment: impediment disease mainly involving the sinews, marked by joint pain and accompanied by hypertonicity of the sinews

皮痹 [pí bì]
skin impediment: impediment disease mainly involving the skin, marked by urticaria and rubella with a sensation of insects crawling on the skin

心痹 [xīn bì]
heart impediment: impediment disease mainly involving the heart and developing from vessel impediment, manifested by palpitations, precordial pain and stuffy sensation in the chest

肝痹 [gān bì]
liver impediment: impediment disease mainly involving the liver and developing from longstanding sinew impediment, manifested by fright during sleep in the night, thirst with increased fluid intake, frequent urination, hypochondriac pain, and abdominal distension

脾痹 [pí bì]
spleen impediment: impediment disease mainly involving the spleen and developing from muscle impediment, manifested by slothfulness of the limbs, dull pain in the abdomen, no desire for food or drink, sallow complexion, and loose stools

肺痹 [fèi bì]
lung impediment: impediment disease mainly involving the lung and developing from persistent skin impediment, manifested by severe pain in the chest and back, dyspnea with quick breathing, and in some cases vomiting

肾痹 [shèn bì]
kidney impediment: impediment disease mainly involving the kidney and developing from persistent bone

impediment, manifested by inability to straighten the lumbus and back, lumbago, hypertonicity of the lower limbs, and seminal emission

肠痹 [cháng bì]
intestinal impediment: impediment disease mainly involving the large and small intestines, manifested by excessive intake of fluid with inhibited urination, or diarrhea with fluid stools containing undigested food

血痹 [xuè bì]
blood impediment: impediment disease occurring in patients with *qi*-blood deficiency after sleeping in drafts or sweating from exertion, marked by numbness and pain in the limbs

肝胃气痛 [gān wèi qì tòng]
liver-*qi* stomachache: pain in the stomach ascribed to a perverted flow of liver *qi*, usually related to emotional disturbance

胃脘痛（病）[wèi wǎn tòng (bìng)]
epigastric pain (disease): diseased state characterized by pain in the epigastric region

痞 [pǐ]
stuffiness: diseased state characterized by a tightly full sensation due to impairment of *qi* movement or retention of *qi*, often in the middle energizer, but sometimes in the chest

实痞 [shí pǐ]
stuffiness of excess type: stuffiness caused by accumulation of pathogenic factors

虚痞 [xū pǐ]
stuffiness of deficiency type: stuffiness without accumulation of pathogenic factors

气痞 [qì pǐ]
***qi* stuffiness:** stuffiness caused by accumulation of stagnant *qi*

痰痞 [tán pǐ]
phlegm stuffiness: stuffiness caused by accumulation of phlegm and stagnant *qi*

胃痞 [wèi pǐ]
stomach stuffiness: stuffiness in the stomach region, also called epigastric stuffiness (心下痞 [xīn xià pǐ])

心下痞 [xīn xià pǐ]
epigastric stuffiness: synonym for stomach stuffiness (胃痞 [wèi pǐ])

呕吐 [ǒu tù]
vomiting: forcible expulsion of the stomach contents through the mouth. Making sounds of vomiting while casting up the matter from the stomach is called 呕 [ǒu], and vomiting without sound is 吐 [tù].

热呕 [rè ǒu]
heat vomiting: vomiting immediately after food intake due to accumulated heat in the stomach or attack on the stomach by pathogenic heat

寒呕 [hán ǒu]
cold vomiting: vomiting due to invasion of the stomach by cold or deficiency-cold, characterized by vomiting upon exposure to cold or long after eating, cyanotic complexion and cool limbs

泛酸 [fàn suān]
acid regurgitation: flow of the acid gastric contents in the opposite direction – from the stomach to the mouth

吐酸 [tù suān]
acid vomiting: vomiting of the acid gastric contents in the reverse flow – from the stomach to the mouth

吞酸 [tūn suān]
acid swallowing: swallowing of the acid gastric contents flowing backward – from the stomach to the mouth

嘈杂 [cáo zá]
gastric upset: disturbing feeling in the stomach, often accompanied by acid regurgitation

呃逆 [è nì]
hiccup; hiccough: upward counterflow of stomach *qi* with an involuntary movement of the diaphragm, causing a short and sharp sound

哕 [yuě]
hiccup: ancient term for 呃逆 [è nì]

反胃 [fǎn wèi]
stomach reflux; regurgitation: flowing back of the stomach contents into the mouth a long time after eating

胃反 [wèi fǎn]
stomach reflux: same as 反胃 [fǎn wèi]

噎嗝 [yē gé]
dysphagia: difficulty in swallowing caused by narrowing or obstruction of the esophagus, also called 膈噎 [gé yē] or aphagopraxia (鬲咽 [gé yān])

膈噎 [gé yē]
dysphagia: same as 噎嗝 [yē gé]

鬲咽 [gé yān]
aphagopraxia: another name for dysphagia (噎嗝 [yē gé])

上膈 [shàng gé]
upper obstruction: obstruction in the upper portion, characterized by vomiting instantly after intake of food

下膈 [xià gé]
lower obstruction: obstruction in the lower portion, characterized by vomiting in the evening of undigested food taken during the day

伤食 [shāng shí]
food damage; dyspepsia: damage to the spleen and stomach caused by improper diet or overeating

伤食证 [shāng shí zhèng]
food damage syndrome; dyspepsia syndrome: syndrome characterized by indigestion ascribed to improper diet or overeating

食滞 [shí zhì]
food stagnation: diseased state characterized by retention of undigested food in the stomach and intestines, also known as food retention (停食 [tíng shí] or 宿食 [sù shí])

停食 [tíng shí]
food retention: synonym for food stagnation (食滞 [shí zhì])

宿食 [sù shí]

food retention: synonym for food stagnation (食滞 [shí zhì])

嗜偏食 [shì piān shí]

food partiality: diseased state marked by special liking for some unusual food such as raw rice in cases of parasitosis

关格 [guān gé]

blockage and repulsion: (1) anuria and vomiting occurring simultaneously; (2) simultaneous retention of urine and stool; (3) unique strong pulse indicating disunion of yin and yang

关格病 [guān gé bìng]

blockage-repulsion disease: diseased state characterized by anuria and incessant vomiting

吐矢 [tù shǐ]

vomiting fecal matter: symptom seen in cases of intestinal obstruction

便秘 [biàn mì]

constipation: infrequent or difficult evacuation of feces

脾约 [pí yuē]

splenic constipation: infrequent passage of dry hardened feces as a consequence of dysfunction of the spleen

实秘 [shí mì]

constipation of excess type: collective term referring to various types of constipation ascribed to such pathogenic factors as heat, cold, stagnant *qi* and phlegm

虚秘 [xū mì]

constipation of deficiency type: collective term for various types of constipation related to deficiency conditions, such as deficiency of *qi*, yang or yin, usually seen in aged or debilitated subjects or postpartum cases

热秘 [rè mì]

heat constipation: constipation accompanied by fever, flushed face, thirst, abdominal distension, and yellow and dry tongue coating

气秘 [qì mì]

***qi* constipation:** (1) constipation due to stagnation of *qi*, accompanied by frequent eructation, stuffiness in the chest, impaired appetite, and even abdominal pain; (2) constipation due to deficiency of *qi*, marked by difficulty in defecation while the feces are neither dry nor hard, usually accompanied by other symptoms of *qi* deficiency

痰秘 [tán mì]

phlegm constipation: constipation accompanied by stuffy sensation in the chest, dyspnea, and sweating from the head, ascribed to accumulation of phlegm and dampness-heat in the intestines

冷秘 [lěng mì]

cold constipation: constipation ascribed to the binding of yin cold in the intestines, also known as yin bind (阴结 [yīn jié]) or cold bind (寒结 [hán jié]), manifested by difficulty in passing stool with abdominal colic, distension, tenderness and cold limbs

寒结 [hán jié]

cold bind: synonym for cold constipation

(冷秘 [lěng mì])

阴结 [yīn jié]
yin bind: synonym for cold constipation (冷秘 [lěng mì])

泄泻（病）[xiè xiè (bìng)]
diarrhea (disease): diseased condition characterized by abnormal frequency and liquidity of fecal discharge

暴泻（病）[bào xiè (bìng)]
fulminant diarrhea (disease): diseased condition characterized by sudden onset of diarrhea with profuse discharge

久泄 [泻] [jiǔ xiè]
chronic diarrhea: diarrhea lasting for a long time or continually recurring

五更泄 [泻] [wǔ gēng xiè]
fifth-watch diarrhea: diarrhea daily before dawn, usually due to deficiency of the vital gate fire (kidney yang) to warm the spleen

下利 [xià lì]
diarrhea: ancient designation for diarrhea including dysentery

下利清谷 [xià lì qīng gǔ]
diarrhea with undigested food: frequent discharge of fluid stools containing undigested food

滑泄 [huá xiè]
(I) efflux diarrhea: chronic diarrhea with fecal incontinence; **(II) spermatorrhea:** same as 滑精 [huá jīng]

飧泄 [泻] [sūn xiè]
lienteric diarrhea: diarrhea due to spleen insufficiency induced by stagnation of liver *qi*, marked by watery stool containing undigested food, borborygmi and abdominal pain

脾虚泄泻 [pí xū xiè xiè]
spleen deficiency diarrhea: recurrent diarrhea with stools containing undigested food, aggravated by eating fatty food, and marked by sallow complexion, lassitude, pale tongue with whitish coating, and weak pulse

肾虚泄泻 [shèn xū xiè xiè]
kidney deficiency diarrhea: chronic diarrhea occurring before dawn daily, accompanied by abdominal pain and borborygmi, aversion to cold, and cold limbs

伤食泄泻 [shāng shí xiè xiè]
indigestion diarrhea: diarrhea occurring as a result of impairment of the stomach and spleen by immoderate eating and drinking, usually accompanied by belching with fetid odor, abdominal distension and pain, and thick greasy tongue coating

热泻 [rè xiè]
heat diarrhea: diarrhea due to accumulated heat in the large intestine, marked by passage of foul-smelling, yellow stool accompanied by abdominal pain, and burning sensation at the anus

湿热泄泻 [shī rè xiè xiè]
dampness-heat diarrhea: diarrhea due to accumulation of pathogenic dampness-heat in the intestines, usually accompanied by burning sensation at the anus, scanty

deep-colored urine, and yellowish greasy tongue coating

寒泻 [hán xiè]
cold diarrhea: diarrhea due to accumulation of pathogenic cold in the interior, marked by passage of watery stools with undigested food, dull abdominal pain, slippery whitish tongue coating, and deep and slow pulse

虚寒泄泻 [xū hán xiè xiè]
deficiency-cold diarrhea: chronic diarrhea accompanied by abdominal pain and borborygmi, aversion to cold, cold limbs, pale tongue with white coating, and deep and thready pulse

腹痛 [fù tòng]
abdominal pain: pain in the abdomen below the epigastrium and above the pubic hair

气滞腹痛 [qì zhì fù tòng]
***qi*-stagnant abdominal pain:** abdominal pain unfixed in location, usually aggravated by emotional changes, and accompanied by distension, eructation, and wiry pulse

血瘀腹痛 [xuè yū fù tòng]
blood-stasis abdominal pain: persistent abdominal pain fixed in location, accompanied by tenderness, purplish tongue and choppy pulse

寒冷腹痛 [hán lěng fù tòng]
cold abdominal pain: lingering abdominal pain due to the presence of pathogenic cold, which may be aggravated by exposure to cold and alleviated by warmth, also known as cold-*qi* abdominal pain (寒气腹痛 [hán qì fù tòng])

寒气腹痛 [hán qì fù tòng]
cold-*qi* abdominal pain: synonym for cold abdominal pain (寒冷腹痛 [hán lěng fù tòng])

虚寒腹痛 [xū hán fù tòng]
deficiency-cold abdominal pain: diseased state ascribed to deficiency-cold of the spleen and stomach, characterized by lingering abdominal pain on and off, aggravated by hunger and exposure to cold, and alleviated by warmth and pressing, often accompanied by lassitude, aversion to cold, loose bowels, pale tongue with whitish coating, and deep thready pulse

食积腹痛 [shí jī fù tòng]
food-retention abdominal pain: abdominal pain due to accumulation of undigested food in the stomach and intestines

虫积腹痛 [chóng jī fù tòng]
parasitic abdominal pain: abdominal pain due to intestinal parasitosis

胃缓 [wèi huǎn]
relaxed stomach: gastroptosis

肠痈 [cháng yōng]
intestinal abscess: (1) acute appendicitis; (2) periappendicular abscess

胁痛（病）[xié tòng (bìng)]
lateropectoral pain; hypochondriac pain: diseased state characterized by unilateral or bilateral pain in the

lateropectoral or hypochondriac region. It more definitely refers to hypochondriac pain according to its old names 胁下痛 [xié xià tòng] or 季胁痛 [jì xié tòng].

胁下痛 [xié xià tòng]
hypochondriac pain: pain in the lower part of the lateropectoral region

季胁痛 [jì xié tòng]
hypochondriac pain: pain over the region of the last few ribs

胆胀（病）[dǎn zhàng (bìng)]
gallbladder distension: diseased state due to stagnation of gallbladder *qi*, manifested by right hypochondriac distension and pain

臌胀（病）[gǔ zhàng (bìng)]
abdominal distension: diseased state characterized by distension of the abdomen with the accumulation of gas or fluid in it

单腹胀 [dān fù zhàng]
simple abdominal distension: abdominal distension without edema of the limbs

气臌（病）[qì gǔ (bìng)]
tympanites: abdominal distension with accumulation of gas in the abdomen

水臌（病）[shuǐ gǔ (bìng)]
ascites: abdominal distension with accumulation of fluid in the abdomen

血臌（病）[xuè gǔ (bìng)]
ascites with engorgement: abdominal distension with fluid accumulation, varicose veins, and vascular spiders

萎黄 [wěi huáng]
sallowness: yellowish and withered complexion often seen in such chronic cases as anemia

萎黄病 [wěi huáng bìng]
sallow disease: diseased state characterized by yellowish and withered complexion associated with general weakness, lassitude, and loose stools, often seen in such chronic cases as anemia

黄胖 [huáng pàng]
yellowish puffiness: yellowish puffy complexion often seen in cases of ankylostomiasis, malnutrition, and other chronic diseases

黄胖病 [huáng pàng bìng]
yellowish puffy disease: chronic diseased state characterized by yellowish and puffy complexion, often seen in cases of ankylostomiasis, malnutrition and other chronic diseases

虫积（证）[chóng jī (zhèng)]
worm accumulation (syndrome): painful movable mass in the abdomen ascribed to the aggregation of parasitic worms in the intestines

狐惑 [hú huò]
throat-anus-genital syndrome: ancient term for a disease marked by erosion of the mouth, throat and genitalia, red eyes and black canthi, resembling Behçet's syndrome

痞块 [pǐ kuài]
stuffy lump: lump in the abdomen with a sensation of stuffiness and fullness, usually

caused by undigested food, stagnant blood, and retained phlegm

癥瘕积聚 [zhēng jiǎ jī jù]
accumulation-aggregation masses: collective term for various kinds of masses formed in the abdomen

癥瘕 [zhēng jiǎ]
abdominal mass: collective term for 癥 [zhēng] and 瘕 [jiǎ], the masses formed in the abdomen, the former of which is a product of aggregation of static blood, the latter a product of accumulation of stagnant *qi*. 癥 has a definite shape and causes fixed pain, while 瘕 has no fixed shape and is easily movable, or appears and disappears from time to time, and causes a migratory pain, if present.

积聚 [jī jù]
accumulation-aggregation: term referring to mass formation in the abdomen with distension or pain due to *qi* stagnation, blood stasis, or phlegm retention

积证 [jī zhèng]
accumulation syndrome: syndrome characterized by mass formation in the abdomen, immovable with definite shape and fixed local pain, ascribed to accumulation of pathogenic factors, particularly stagnant blood and turbid phlegm

聚证 [jù zhèng]
aggregation syndrome: syndrome characterized by mass formation in the abdomen, with no definite shape and easily movable, accompanied by distending pain, usually ascribed to gathering of stagnant *qi*

水肿 [shuǐ zhǒng]
edema: (1) an abnormal excess accumulation of fluid in the body, usually ascribed to dysfunction of the lung, spleen, kidney or bladder; (2) any of the morbid states in which abnormally excess body fluid is accumulated

水肿病 [shuǐ zhǒng bìng]
edematous disease: same as edema (水肿 [shuǐ zhǒng])

水气 [shuǐ qì]
water *qi*: (1) ancient term for edema (水肿 [shuǐ zhǒng]); (2) another name for retained fluid (水饮 [shuǐ yǐn])

水胀 [shuǐ zhàng]
water distension: edema due to insufficiency of yang *qi* that leads to accumulation of water-dampness, marked initially by abdominal distension, and then swelling of the extremities

虚肿 [xū zhǒng]
edema of deficiency type: edema occurring in deficiency conditions of the spleen, of the liver and kidney, or of the lung

阳水 [yáng shuǐ]
yang edema: edema due to attack of wind or immersion of water-dampness involving the lung and the spleen, usually with an acute onset and a short course accompanied by heat and excess symptoms

风水 [fēng shuǐ]

wind edema: edema especially of the face and head, ascribed to attack on the lung by pathogenic wind, manifested by sudden onset of edema accompanied by aching joints, fever, chills, and floating pulse

皮水 [pí shuǐ]

skin edema: generalized pitting edema accompanied by floating pulse

里水 [lǐ shuǐ]

interior edema: generalized edema accompanied by oliguria and sunken pulse

正水 [zhèng shuǐ]

typical edema; regular edema: edema accompanied by dyspnea and slow sunken pulse

石水 [shí shuǐ]

stony edema: edema marked by stony hardness of the swollen lower abdomen

阴水 [yīn shuǐ]

yin edema: edema due to dysfunction of the spleen and the kidney, usually with a gradual onset and a long course, associated with cold and deficiency symptoms

五水 [wǔ shuǐ]

five kinds of edema: collective term for edemas due to dysfunction of the heart, liver, spleen, lung and kidney

心水 [xīn shuǐ]

heart edema: edema due to dysfunction of the heart, marked by anasarca, orthopnea and difficulty in lying flat

肝水 [gān shuǐ]

liver edema: edema due to dysfunction of the liver, marked by enlarged abdomen and hypochondriac pain

脾水 [pí shuǐ]

spleen edema: edema due to dysfunction of the spleen, marked by abdominal distension, heaviness of the limbs, lassitude, and oliguria

肺水 [fèi shuǐ]

lung edema: edema due to dysfunction of the lung, marked by general anasarca, oliguria, and loose stools

肾水 [shèn shuǐ]

kidney edema: edema due to dysfunction of the kidney, marked by swelling and distension of the abdomen, accompanied by lumbago, oliguria, and cold feet

郁病 [yù bìng]

depression; depressive disease: diseased state characterized by a depressed mood with feelings of despair or uneasiness, caused by emotional factors with stagnant *qi*

血证 [xuè zhèng]

(I) hemorrhagic syndrome: general term for various hemorrhages; **(II) blood troubles:** a group of disorders involving the blood, including bleeding, blood stasis, and blood heat

失血 [shī xuè]

loss of blood; hemorrhage: general term for various kinds of profuse bleeding, also known as 夺血 [duó xuè]

夺血 [duó xuè]

(I) loss of blood: same as 失血 [shī xuè]; **(II)**

dehydration of blood: decrease of the blood volume resulting from massive sweating

鼻衄 [bí nǜ]

nosebleed; epistaxis: hemorrhage from the nose unconnected with trauma or vicarious menstruation

齿衄 [chǐ nǜ]

gum bleeding: bleeding from the gums unconnected with trauma

咳血 [ké xuè]

hemoptysis with coughing: expectoration of blood or blood-stained sputum together with coughing

咯血 [kǎ xuè]

hemoptysis without coughing: spontaneous expectoration of blood without coughing

吐血 [tù xuè]

hematemesis: vomiting of blood

尿血 [niào xuè]

hematuria: discharge of bloody urine or urine with blood streaks, but with no pain during urination

血尿 [xuè niào]

bloody urine: urine containing blood

便血 [biàn xuè]

hematochezia: bleeding from the rectum, including bloody stools and passage of pure blood through the anus

近血 [jìn xuè]

proximal bleeding: bleeding into the alimentary tract near the anus, with the discharged blood being fresh red, usually referring to anal or rectal bleeding

远血 [yuǎn xuè]

distal bleeding: bleeding into the alimentary tract far from the anus, with the discharged blood being dark or black, generally referring to bleeding from the upper digestive tract

蓄血 [xù xuè]

blood accumulation: disease caused by stagnant blood accumulated in a meridian/channel or organ, e.g., in the uterus (manifested by distension and pain in the lower abdomen, chills and fever, delirium or other mental disorders at night), or in the middle energizer (manifested by pain, tenderness and resistance to touch over the epigastrium)

紫斑 [zǐ bān]

purpura: (1) any of a group of conditions characterized by ecchymoses or small hemorrhages in the skin and mucous membrane; (2) purplish discoloration resulting from extravasation of blood in the skin and mucous membrane

血脱 [xuè tuō]

blood collapse: diseased state characterized by pale and withered complexion, dizziness, blurred vision or accompanied by bleeding, usually ascribed to consumption of genuine yin and emptiness of the blood chamber

津脱 [jīn tuō]

fluid collapse: collapse with profuse sweating

液脱 [yè tuō]

liquid collapse: diseased state characterized

by extreme consumption of body fluids, usually manifested by emaciation, parched lips, wizened skin, sunken eyes, and dry tongue

消渴（病） [xiāo kě (bìng)]
wasting thirst; diabetes: general term for diseases characterized by excessive thirst, polyuria, and polyphagia with emaciation, but chiefly referring to diabetes mellitus

三消 [sān xiāo]
three types of wasting-thirst; three types of diabetes: collective term for diabetes marked by three "polys", namely polydipsia, polyphagia and polyuria

上消 [shàng xiāo]
upper wasting-thirst: a case of wasting-thirst (diabetes) , in which the upper energizer is mainly involved, characterized by polydipsia, also called lung wasting-thirst (肺消 [fèi xiāo])

肺消 [fèi xiāo]
lung wasting-thirst: synonym for upper wasting-thirst (上消 [shàng xiāo])

中消 [zhōng xiāo]
middle wasting-thirst: a case of wasting-thirst (diabetes), in which the middle energizer is mainly involved, characterized by polyphagia, emaciation, and constipation, also called stomach wasting-thirst (胃消 [wèi xiāo]) or spleen wasting-thirst (脾消 [pí xiāo])

胃消 [wèi xiāo]
stomach wasting-thirst: synonym for middle wasting-thirst (中消 [zhōng xiāo])

脾消 [pí xiāo]
spleen wasting-thirst: synonym for middle wasting-thirst (中消 [zhōng xiāo])

下消 [xià xiāo]
lower wasting-thirst: a case of wasting-thirst (diabetes), in which the lower energizer is mainly involved, characterized by polyuria with thick suspension in the urine, also called kidney wasting-thirst (肾消 [shèn xiāo])

肾消 [shèn xiāo]
kidney wasting-thirst: synonym for lower wasting-thirst (下消 [xià xiāo])

尿浊 [niào zhuó]
turbid urine (disease): discharge of turbid urine without difficulty or pain in urination, a condition different from stranguria with turbid discharge (淋浊 [lìn zhuó]) or chylous stranguria (膏淋 [gāo lìn])

淋（证） [lìn (zhèng)]
stranguria: general term for a class of diseases characterized by frequent, painful and dripping urination

淋浊 [lìn zhuó]
stranguria with turbid discharge: frequent painful discharge of turbid urine and sometimes pus-like fluid, ascribed to the down-pouring of dampness-heat and phlegm-turbidity to the bladder

淋病 [lìn bìng]
gonorrhea: sexually transmitted infection marked by inflammation of the urethral orifice and frequent painful dripping of turbid urine

五淋 [wǔ lìn]

five kinds of stranguria: (1) urolithic stranguria, *qi* stranguria, chylous stranguria, strain stranguria, and heat stranguria; (2) *qi* stranguria, blood stranguria, chylous stranguria, urolithic stranguria, and strain stranguria

石淋 [shí lìn]

urolithic stranguria: painful and difficult urination due to the passage of urinary calculi

砂（石）淋 [shā (shí) lìn]

urolithic stranguria: same as 石淋 [shí lìn]

气淋 [qì lìn]

***qi* stranguria:** stranguria due to *qi* disorders, either stagnation or deficiency

劳淋 [láo lìn]

overstrain stranguria: stranguria ascribed to overstrain, marked by dripping of urine with dull pain, usually seen in chronic cases

膏淋 [gāo lìn]

chylous stranguria: stranguria characterized by painful discharge of turbid, milky urine like rice-water

血淋 [xuè lìn]

blood stranguria: stranguria characterized by painful discharge of bloody urine

热淋 [rè lìn]

heat stranguria: stranguria ascribed to heat, marked by discharge of reddened urine with acute onset, and accompanied by burning pain and fever

白淫 [bái yín]

white ooze: an ancient term referring to the presence of seminal fluid in urine in males or persistent vaginal discharge in females

癃闭 [lóng bì]

ischuria: reduction in the flow of urine (癃 [lóng]) or anuria (闭 [bì]), seen in cases of urinary bladder and urethra diseases with retention of urine, or in cases of renal failure with extreme suppression of urine secretion

遗精 [yí jīng]

seminal emission: involuntary emission of semen

梦遗 [mèng yí]

nocturnal emission: involuntary emission of semen during sleep, usually accompanied by an erotic dream

滑精（病） [huá jīng (bìng)]

spermatorrhea: (diseased state characterized by) involuntary and frequent discharge of semen without copulation

早泄（病） [zǎo xiè (bìng)]

premature ejaculation: (diseased state characterized by) ejaculation of semen immediately after or even prior to penetration

阳痿（病） [yáng wěi (bìng)]

impotence: (abnormal state of a male characterized by) inability to initiate or maintain an erection in sexual intercourse

血精 [xuè jīng]

hemospermia: presence of blood in the semen

不育 [bù yù]
sterility: inability to produce offspring

精冷 [jīng lěng]
cold semen: diseased state characterized by thin seminal fluid with inadequate spermatozoa due to decline of life gate fire, which often leads to sterility, also called 精寒 [jīng hán]

精寒 [jīng hán]
cold semen: same as 精冷 [jīng lěng]

精少 [jīng shǎo]
scant semen: (1) defective ejaculation; (2) oligospermia

阴阳易 [yīn yáng yì]
yin-yang transmission: disease contracted by a healthy person after sexual intercourse with one who has not yet recovered from an external contraction

遗尿（病） [yí niào (bìng)]
enuresis: (diseased state characterized by) involuntary discharge of urine

腰痛 [yāo tòng]
lumbago: pain in the lumbar region caused by disordered *qi* and blood flow in the related collateral vessels in cases of exogenous afflictions, traumatic injuries or kidney insufficiency

外感腰痛 [wài gǎn yāo tòng]
externally contracted lumbago: pain in the lumbar region ascribed to an affection by external factors, such as living in a damp place, exposure to wind after sweating, or rain-drenching

寒湿腰痛 [hán shī yāo tòng]
cold-dampness lumbago: lumbago ascribed to attack of cold-dampness, manifested by severe pain in the lumbar region together with a cold and heavy sensation, aggravated upon lying down and on rainy days

湿热腰痛 [shī rè yāo tòng]
dampness-heat lumbago: lumbar pain while stretching, ascribed to attack of dampness-heat, usually accompanied by local hotness, dry mouth with no desire to drink, and reddened tongue with yellow greasy coating

风寒腰痛 [fēng hán yāo tòng]
wind-cold lumbago: lumbago ascribed to attack of wind-cold, manifested as the presence of pain together with a cold sensation, ameliorated by warmth and aggravated by coldness

风热腰痛 [fēng rè yāo tòng]
wind-heat lumbago: pain and heat sensation in the lumbar region, usually accompanied by sore throat, mild sweating and rapid floating pulse

风湿腰痛 [fēng shī yāo tòng]
wind-dampness lumbago: lumbar pain ascribed to attack of wind-dampness, usually occurring after exposure to wind while sleeping in a damp place, marked by contracture, heaviness and pain of the lower back with limited motility, or accompanied by fever and aversion to wind

内伤腰痛 [nèi shāng yāo tòng]
internal damage lumbago: lumbago

ascribed to internal damage, such as chronic overstrain, general debility in the aged, overindulgence in sex, and emotional depression

肾虚腰痛 [shèn xū yāo tòng]
kidney-insufficiency lumbago: lumbar pain ascribed to deficiency of kidney *qi* and essence, usually aggravated upon exertion and ameliorated upon lying down, and accompanied by weakness of the loins and legs

血虚腰痛 [xuè xū yāo tòng]
blood-deficiency lumbago: pain in the lumbar region ascribed to blood deficiency, usually occurring in women with metrorrhagia

气滞腰痛 [qì zhì yāo tòng]
***qi*-stagnation lumbago:** lumbar pain ascribed to *qi* stagnation, stabbing in character but not fixed in location, often accompanied by distension of the abdomen and hypochondriac regions

血瘀腰痛 [xuè yū yāo tòng]
blood-stasis lumbago: lumbago ascribed to blood stasis, marked by pain with fixed location, ameliorated in the daytime and aggravated in the night time

沥血腰痛 [lì xuè yāo tòng]
blood-stasis lumbago: same as 血瘀腰痛 [xuè yū yāo tòng]

腰软 [yāo ruǎn]
lumbar weakness: lack of strength in the lower back, due to either invasion of wind-dampness or kidney insufficiency

疝 [shàn]
(I) hernia: protrusion of a part of an organ or tissue from the body cavity through an abnormal opening, also called 疝气 [shàn qì] or 小肠气 [xiǎo cháng qì]; **(II) genital disease:** collective term for diseases of the male and female genitalia; **(III) lower abdominal colic:** severe colicky pain in the lower abdomen usually accompanied by constipation and ischuria

疝气 [shàn qì]
hernia: synonym for 疝 [shàn] (I)

小肠气 [xiǎo cháng qì]
hernia: another name for 疝 [shàn] (I)

妇产科 Gynecology and Obstetrics

胞 [bāo]

(I) uterus: same as 胞宫 [bāo gōng]; **(II) placenta:** abbreviation for 胞衣 [bāo yī]; **(III) bladder:** abbreviation for 尿胞 [niào bāo]; **(IV) eyelid:** same as 胞睑 [bāo jiǎn]

玉门 [yù mén]

virginal orifice: external opening of the vagina in a virgin

龙门 [lóng mén]

nulliparous vaginal orifice: external opening of the vagina in a nulliparous married woman

胞门 [bāo mén]

parous vaginal orifice: external opening of the vagina in a para

产门 [chǎn mén]

parturient vaginal orifice: external opening of the vagina of a parturient

子门 [zǐ mén]

cervical orifice: external opening of the cervix of the uterus into the vagina

人胞 [rén bāo]

placenta: organ lining the uterus, which is formed during pregnancy to support the growth of the fetus by delivering nutrients through the umbilical cord, and expelled after birth

胞衣 [bāo yī]

afterbirth: placenta and membranes delivered from the uterus after the birth of a child, also called 胎衣 [tāi yī]

胎衣 [tāi yī]

afterbirth: another name for 胞衣 [bāo yī]

血室 [xuè shì]

blood chamber: (1) another name for the uterus (胞宫 [bāo gōng]); (2) another name for the thoroughfare vessel (冲脉 [chōng mài]); (3) another name for the liver (肝 [gān])

阴户 [yīn hù]

(I) vulva: region of the external female genital organs including the labia majora, labia minora, mons pubis, clitoris, and vestibule of vagina; **(II) (external) vaginal orifice**

阴道 [yīn dào]

vagina: the genital canal in the female, leading from the uterus to the vulva, also called 子肠 [zǐ cháng]

子肠 [zǐ cháng]

vagina: another name for 阴道 [yīn dào]

胞宫 [bāo gōng]

uterus: female organ in which menstruation is formed and the developing fetus is nourished, also called 子宫 [zǐ gōng], 子脏 [zǐ zàng], 女子胞 [nǚ zǐ bāo], 胞脏 [bāo zàng], and 血脏 [xuè zàng]

子宫 [zǐ gōng]

uterus: same as 胞宫 [bāo gōng]

子脏 [zǐ zàng]
uterus: same as 胞宫 [bāo gōng]

女子胞 [nǚ zǐ bāo]
uterus: same as 胞宫 [bāo gōng]

胞脏 [bāo zàng]
uterus: same as 胞宫 [bāo gōng]

血脏 [xuè zàng]
uterus: same as 胞宫 [bāo gōng]

经带胎产 [jīng dài tāi chǎn]
menstrual disorders, leukorrheal diseases, gravid troubles, and parturition problems: the four general categories of gynecological and obstetrical diseases

月经 [yuè jīng]
menstruation: cyclic discharge from the genital tract of women, usually at approximately one-month intervals, also called menstrual discharge (经水 [jīng shuǐ]), monthly discharge (月水 [yuè shuǐ]), "monthly matter" (月事 [yuè shì]), or "monthly message" (月信 [yuè xìn])

经血 [jīng xuè]
menstrual blood: blood discharged through the vagina during menstruation

经水 [jīng shuǐ]
menstrual discharge: another term for menstruation, also called monthly discharge (月水 [yuè shuǐ])

月水 [yuè shuǐ]
monthly discharge: another term for menstruation, same as menstrual discharge (经水 [jīng shuǐ])

月事 [yuè shì]
"monthly matter": another term for menstruation

月信 [yuè xìn]
"monthly message": another term for menstruation

并月 [bìng yuè]
bimonthly menstruation: menstruation occurring once every two months

居经 [jū jīng]
tri-monthly menstruation: menstruation occurring once every three months, also called seasonal menstruation (季经 [jì jīng])

季经 [jì jīng]
seasonal menstruation: menstruation occurring once each season, same as tri-monthly menstruation (居经 [jū jīng])

避年 [bì nián]
annual menstruation: menstruation occurring once a year

暗经 [àn jīng]
latent menstruation: life-long absence of menstrual discharge, but with the potential for pregnancy

天癸 [tiān guǐ]
(I) *tiangui*; sex-stimulating substance: substance that promotes human growth, development and reproduction; **(II) menstruation**

天癸竭 [tiān guǐ jié]
(I) exhaustion of *tiangui*; *tiangui* exhaustion; exhaustion of the sex-stimulating essence; (II) ceasing of menstruation; menopause

月经病 [yuè jīng bìng]
menstrual disease; emmeniopathy: collective term for disorders of menstruation, including abnormal cycles, intervals and amount of discharge as well as accompanying symptoms

月经不调 [yuè jīng bù tiáo]
menstrual irregularities: general term for irregular menstruation and other menstrual complaints, such as abnormal duration, amount, color and quality of menstrual discharge, also called 月水不调 [yuè shuǐ bù tiáo] or 经水不调 [jīng shuǐ bù tiáo]

月水不调 [yuè shuǐ bù tiáo]
menstrual irregularities: same as 月经不调 [yuè jīng bù tiáo]

经水不调 [jīng shuǐ bù tiáo]
menstrual irregularities: same as 月经不调 [yuè jīng bù tiáo]

月经先期 [yuè jīng xiān qī]
early periods; polymenorrhea: periods that come one week or more ahead of due time, also known as 经行先期 [jīng xíng xiān qī], 经水先期 [jīng shuǐ xiān qī] or 经早 [jīng zǎo]

经水先期 [jīng shuǐ xiān qī]
early periods: same as 月经先期 [yuè jīng xiān qī]

经行先期 [jīng xíng xiān qī]
early periods; shortened menstrual cycles: same as 月经先期 [yuè jīng xiān qī]

经早 [jīng zǎo]
early periods: synonym for 月经先期 [yuè jīng xiān qī]

血热经行先期 [xuè rè jīng xíng xiān qī]
blood-heat early periods; early periods due to blood heat: periods coming before due time, with massive discharge deep red in color, accompanied by irritability, reddened tongue with yellow coating, and slippery, rapid and forceful pulse

气虚经行先期 [qì xū jīng xíng xiān qī]
***qi*-deficient early periods; early periods due to *qi* deficiency:** periods coming before due time, with the release of thin and pinkish discharge, accompanied by lassitude, pallor, pale tongue, and weak pulse

月经后期 [yuè jīng hòu qī]
late periods; oligomenorrhea: periods that come one week or more after due time, also called 经行后期 [jīng xíng hòu qī], 经水后期 [jīng shuǐ hòu qī], lengthened menstrual cycles (经期错后 [jīng qī cuò hòu]), or 经迟 [jīng chí]

经行后期 [jīng xíng hòu qī]
late periods: same as 月经后期 [yuè jīng hòu qī]

经水后期 [jīng shuǐ hòu qī]
late periods: same as 月经后期 [yuè jīng hòu qī]

经期错后 [jīng qī cuò hòu]
lengthened menstrual cycles: same as 月经后期 [yuè jīng hòu qī]

经迟 [jīng chí]
late periods: abbreviation for 月经后期 [yuè jīng hòu qī]

血寒经行后期 [xuè hán jīng xíng hòu qī]
blood-cold late periods; late periods due to blood cold: periods coming after due time with the release of scanty discharge of dark colored blood, accompanied by aversion to cold, cold limbs, and lower abdominal pain which is alleviated by warmth

血虚经行后期 [xuè xū jīng xíng hòu qī]
blood-deficient late periods; late periods due to blood deficiency: periods coming after due time with the release of scanty discharge of light-colored blood, accompanied by sallow complexion, dizziness, pale tongue, and weak thready pulse

气滞经行后期 [qì zhì jīng xíng hòu qī]
***qi*-stagnant late periods; late periods due to *qi* stagnation:** periods coming after due time with the release of scanty discharge of normal-colored blood, accompanied by mammary distension, discomfort in the chest, hypochondriac pain, and distending pain in the lower abdomen

月经先后无定期 [yuè jīng xiān hòu wú dìng qī]
irregular periods; irregular menstrual cycles: periods that come with irregular cycles, more than one week earlier or later, also called 经乱 [jīng luàn]

经乱 [jīng luàn]
irregular periods: abbreviation for 月经先后无定期 [yuè jīng xiān hòu wú dìng qī]

月经过少 [yuè jīng guò shǎo]
scant menorrhea; hypomenorrhea: menstrual discharge of less than the normal amount occurring at regular intervals, with the period of flow being less than the usual duration, also known as scant inhibited menorrhea (月经涩少 [yuè jīng sè shǎo] or 经水涩少 [jīng shuǐ sè shǎo])

月经涩少 [yuè jīng sè shǎo]
scant inhibited menorrhea: same as scant menorrhea or hypomenorrhea (月经过少 [yuè jīng guò shǎo])

经水涩少 [jīng shuǐ sè shǎo]
scant inhibited menorrhea: same as scant menorrhea (月经过少 [yuè jīng guò shǎo])

血虚月经过少 [xuè xū yuè jīng guò shǎo]
blood deficiency hypomenorrhea: scant menstruation due to blood deficiency marked by menstrual discharge of abnormally small amount, pinkish in color, accompanied by sallow complexion, dizziness, palpitations, pale tongue, and thready weak pulse

肾虚月经过少 [shèn xū yuè jīng guò shǎo]
kidney insufficiency hypomenorrhea: scant menstruation due to kidney insufficiency marked by menstrual discharge of abnormally small amount, bright red in color, accompanied by aching of loins and knees, dizziness, tinnitus, and deep pulse

血滞月经过少 [xuè zhì yuè jīng guò shǎo]
blood stagnation hypomenorrhea:

scant menstration due to blood stagnation marked by menstrual discharge of abnormally small amount, purple-red in color or containing blood clots, accompanied by distending pain in the lower abdomen

停经 [tíng jīng]
ceasing of menstruation: general term for stoppage of the menses, referring to abnormal stoppage in a diseased state or normal stoppage during pregnancy and lactation, or even the ending of a period with no more menstrual discharge

闭经 [bì jīng]
amenorrhea: failure of menstruation to occur at puberty or abnormal stoppage of the menses for more than three months after menarche, also called 经闭 [jīng bì]

经闭 [jīng bì]
amenorrhea: same as 闭经 [bì jīng]

火邪经闭 [huǒ xié jīng bì]
fire amenorrhea: amenorrhea ascribed to endogenous heat and fire, usually accompanied by cough and shoulder pain if the lung is involved, by restlessness at night if the heart is involved, by hypochondriac pain if the liver is involved, and by constipation if the spleen is involved

虫积经闭 [chóng jī jīng bì]
helminthic amenorrhea: amenorrhea caused by intestinal worms that consume yin and blood

血瘀经闭 [xuè yū jīng bì]
blood stasis amenorrhea: amenorrhea caused by stagnation of *qi* or accumulation of cold, either of which leads to blood stasis in the thoroughfare and conception vessels, usually accompanied by lower abdominal pain and tenderness

血亏经闭 [xuè kuī jīng bì]
blood deficiency amenorrhea: amenorrhea caused by deficiency of yin and blood due to chronic loss of blood, multiple deliveries, or intemperate sexual life, usually accompanied by anorexia, emaciation, pallor, or sallow complexion

血枯经闭 [xuè kū jīng bì]
blood exhaustion amenorrhea: severe case of anemorrhea due to blood deficiency

心虚经闭 [xīn xū jīng bì]
heart insufficiency amenorrhea: amenorrhea caused by depression or anxiety that involves the heart in the function of governing the blood

脾虚经闭 [pí xū jīng bì]
spleen insufficiency amenorrhea: amenorrhea usually accompanied by anorexia, stuffiness in the abdomen, and loose bowels

肾虚经闭 [shèn xū jīng bì]
kidney insufficiency amenorrhea: amenorrhea caused by congenital defect, marrying too early, intemperate sexual life, or multiple deliveries, usually marked by tinnitus, dizziness, aching in the loins, and weakness of the legs

经期延长 [jīng qī yán cháng]
prolonged menstruation; menostaxis: excessively prolonged menstruation at regular cycles

经间期出血 [jīng jiān qī chū xuè]
intermenstrual bleeding: periodic uterine bleeding occurring between two menstrual periods at the ovulatory time

痛经 [tòng jīng]
painful menstruation; dysmenorrhea: lower abdominal pain with referring pain in the lower back occurring around or during the menstrual period, also called abdominal pain during menstruation (经行腹痛 [jīng xíng fù tòng])

经行腹痛 [jīng xíng fù tòng]
abdominal pain during menstruation: synonymous with painful menstruation or dysmenorrhea (痛经 [tòng jīng])

气滞痛经 [qì zhì tòng jīng]
***qi* stagnation dysmenorrhea:** dysmenorrhea caused by emotional depression, and marked by distending pain in the lower abdomen accompanied by distension and discomfort in the chest and breasts before or during menstruation

血瘀痛经 [xuè yū tòng jīng]
blood stasis dysmenorrhea: dysmenorrhea characterized by stabbing pain in the lower abdomen with tenderness, occurring before or during menstruation with little menstrual discharge. The pain is usually alleviated after discharge of blood clots.

寒凝痛经 [hán níng tòng jīng]
cold congealing dysmenorrhea: dysmenorrhea marked by sluggish menstrual flow with cold feeling and pain in the lower abdomen, which can be alleviated by warmth

湿热痛经 [shī rè tòng jīng]
dampness-heat dysmenorrhea: dysmenorrhea accompanied by leukorrhagia with yellowish discharge

气血虚弱痛经 [qì xuè xū ruò tòng jīng]
***qi*-blood deficiency dysmenorrhea:** dysmenorrhea marked by reduced amount of thin and pink-colored menstrual flow associated with persistent dull pain in the lower abdomen which usually occurs during the late period of menstruation and can be alleviated by pressing

肾虚痛经 [shèn xū tòng jīng]
kidney insuffciency dysmenorrhea: dysmenorrhea caused by congenital defect, marrying too early, intemperate sexual life or multiple deliveries, and usually accompanied by dizziness, aching in the loins, and weakness of the legs

倒经 [dǎo jīng]
vicarious menstruation: menstrual flow from some part other than the vagina, especially from nose, also called inverted menstruation (逆经 [nì jīng])

逆经 [nì jīng]
inverted menstruation: synonym for vicarious menstruation (倒经 [dǎo jīng])

月经过多 [yuè jīng guò duō]
profuse menstruation; menorrhagia; hypermenorrhea: excessive uterine bleeding occurring at regular intervals, also called 经水过多 [jīng shuǐ guò duō] or 月水过多 [yuè shuǐ guò duō]

经水过多 [jīng shuǐ guò duō]
hypermenorrhea: same as 月经过多 [yuè

jīng guò duō]

月水过多 [yuè shuǐ guò duō]
hypermenorrhea: same as 月经过多 [yuè jīng guò duō]

崩漏 [bēng lòu]
flooding and spotting; metrorrhagia and metrostaxis: excessive uterine bleeding with a sudden onset occurring not in the regular menstruation period (崩 [bēng]), or incessant dripping of blood (漏 [lòu])

血崩 [xuè bēng]
flooding; metrorrhagia: sudden massive uterine bleeding, also called uterine flooding (崩中 [bēng zhōng]) or sudden flooding (暴崩 [bào bēng])

崩中 [bēng zhōng]
uterine flooding: synonym for flooding or metrorrhagia (血崩 [xuè bēng])

暴崩 [bào bēng]
sudden flooding: synonym for flooding or metrorrhagia (血崩 [xuè bēng])

漏下 [lòu xià]
spotting; metrostaxis: slight but persistent escape of blood from the uterus

崩证 [bēng zhèng]
flooding syndrome; metrorrhagic syndrome: syndrome marked by sudden profuse uterine bleeding

经崩 [jīng bēng]
menstrual flooding; menorrhagia: profuse uterine bleeding in a prolonged menstrual period of more than two weeks

经漏 [jīng lòu]
menstrual dripping: incessant escape of small amounts of blood from the uterus in a prolonged menstrual period of more than two weeks

血热崩漏 [xuè rè bēng lòu]
blood heat metrorrhagia and metrostaxis: excessive uterine bleeding, deep red in color, usually occurring in women with constitution of exuberant yang or after an emotional upset, accompanied by flushed face, dry mouth, insomnia, deep red tongue, and full and rapid pulse

血瘀崩漏 [xuè yū bēng lòu]
blood stasis metrorrhagia and metrostaxis: excessive uterine bleeding containing blood clots, accompanied by lower abdominal pain with tenderness, dark red tongue, and choppy pulse

气虚崩漏 [qì xū bēng lòu]
***qi* deficiency metrorrhagia and metrostaxis:** excessive uterine bleeding or incessant dripping of thin and pinkish blood, accompanied by lassitude, anorexia, loose stools, and weak pulse

肾虚崩漏 [shèn xū bēng lòu]
kidney insufficiency metrorrhagia and metrostaxis: excessive uterine bleeding accompanied by weakness of loins and knees, usually caused by intemperance in sexual life, multiple deliveries, or marrying too early

气陷血崩 [qì xiàn xuè bēng]
***qi* sinking metrorrhagia:** excessive uterine bleeding due to spleen insufficiency with sunken *qi*, marked by thin and pinkish

discharge accompanied by lassitude and shortness of breath, and aggravated upon exertion

气郁血崩 [qì yù xuè bēng]
***qi* stagnation metrorrhagia:** excessive uterine bleeding after a fit of rage, marked by sudden onset of profuse discharge of purplish-red blood with clots, accompanied by irritability, and discomfort in the hypochondriac region

经行发热 [jīng xíng fā rè]
menstrual fever; fever during menstruation: fever occurring during or around each menstrual period, also known as 经来发热 [jīng lái fā rè]

经来发热 [jīng lái fā rè]
menstrual fever: same as 经行发热 [jīng xíng fā rè]

经期水肿 [jīng qī shuǐ zhǒng]
menstrual edema; edema during menstruation: edema of the face and limbs occurring during or prior to each menstrual period either due to yang deficiency of the spleen and kidney or due to *qi* stagnation with dampness retention, also known as 经行浮肿 [jīng xíng fú zhǒng]

经行浮肿 [jīng xíng fú zhǒng]
menstrual edema: same as 经期水肿 [jīng qī shuǐ zhǒng]

经行头痛 [jīng xíng tóu tòng]
menstrual headache; headache during menstruation: headache occurring during or around each menstrual period

经行眩晕 [jīng xíng xuàn yùn]
menstrual dizziness; dizziness during menstruation: dizziness occurring during or around each menstrual period

经行身痛 [jīng xíng shēn tòng]
menstrual body pain; general aching during menstruation: generalized aching over the body occurring during or prior to each menstrual period, usually accompanied by fever and aversion to cold

经行吐衄 [jīng xíng tù nǜ]
menstrual hematemesis and epistaxis; hematemesis and epistaxis during menstruation: vicarious or supplementary menstruation manifested by hematemesis and epistaxis

经行衄血 [jīng xíng nǜ xuè]
menstrual epistaxis; epistaxis during menstruation: vicarious or supplementary menstruation manifested by epistaxis

经行吐血 [jīng xíng tù xuè]
menstrual hematemesis; hematemesis during menstruation: vicarious or supplementary menstruation manifested by hematemesis

经行便血 [jīng xíng biàn xuè]
ano-urethral bleeding during menstruation: discharge of blood through the anus and urethra during each menstrual period, also called crossed menstruation (错经 [cuò jīng] or 差经 [chà jīng])

错经 [cuò jīng]；差经 [chà jīng]
crossed menstruation: synonym for ano-urethral bleeding during menstruation (经行便血 [jīng xíng biàn xuè])

经行泄泻 [jīng xíng xiè xiè]
menstrual diarrhea; diarrhea during menstruation: diarrhea occurring during each menstruation, and stopping spontaneously when the period is over, also called 经来泄泻 [jīng lái xiè xiè]

经来泄泻 [jīng lái xiè xiè]
menstrual diarrhea: same as 经行泄泻 [jīng xíng xiè xiè]

经行乳房胀痛 [jīng xíng rǔ fáng zhàng tòng]
distending pain in the breasts during menstruation: distension or sensation of fullness and pain in the breasts during or prior to each menstrual period

经行情志异常 [jīng xíng qíng zhì yì cháng]
moodiness during menstruation; menstrual mental disorder; premenstrual syndrome: depression, gloominess, irritability and other changes of mood occurring prior to or during each menstrual period, and returning to normal after the period

经行口糜 [jīng xíng kǒu mí]
menstrual oral ulcer; oral ulcer during menstruation: ulceration in the mouth or on the tongue occurring prior to or during each menstrual period

经行隐疹 [jīng xíng yǐn zhěn]
menstrual urticaria; urticaria during menstruation: raised red patches of skin with intense itching occurring prior to or during each menstrual period, also called hives during menstruation (经行风疹块 [jīng xíng fēng zhěn kuài]) or 经行瘖瘤 [jīng xíng pēi léi]

经行风疹块 [jīng xíng fēng zhěn kuài]
hives during menstruation: same as menstrual urticaria or urticaria during menstruation (经行隐疹 [jīng xíng yǐn zhěn]

经行瘖瘤 [jīng xíng pēi léi]
hives during menstruation: same as menstrual urticaria or urticaria during menstruation (经行隐疹 [jīng xíng yǐn zhěn]

断经前后诸证 [duàn jīng qián hòu zhū zhèng]
menopausal syndromes: syndromes related to menopause, such as hot flushes, excessive sweating, lassitude, irritability, dizziness, tinnitus, palpitations, insomnia, amnesia, backache, heat sensation in the palms of the hands and soles of the feet

绝经前后诸病 [jué jīng qián hòu zhū bìng]
menopausal diseases: same as menopausal syndromes (断经前后诸证 [duàn jīng qián hòu zhū zhèng])

经断复来 [jīng duàn fù lái]
postmenopausal hemorrhage: uterine bleeding occurring two years or more after menopause

带下 [dài xià]
(I) vaginal discharge; leukorrhea: normal vaginal discharge in physiological conditions or abnormal discharge in morbid conditions; **(II) gynecological disease:** collective term used in ancient times for various kinds of gynecological diseases, for all of them occur below the belt around the waist or the belt vessel.

The Chinese character 带 refers to the belt or the belt vessel and 下 means below.

白带 [bái dài]
white vaginal discharge; leukorrhea: whitish discharge from the vagina

黄带 [huáng dài]
yellowish leukorrhea: yellowish viscid discharge from the vagina, usually indicating the presence of pathogenic dampness

赤白带 [chì bái dài]
reddish leukorrhea: profuse leukorrhea mixed with reddish discharge, usually indicating the presence of dampness-heat

带下病 [dài xià bìng]
leukorrheal diseases: group of morbid states characterized by excessive leukorrhea with abnormal color, quality and smell, accompanied by general or local symptoms

脾虚带下 [pí xū dài xià]
spleen insufficiency leukorrhagia: leukorrhagia due to deficiency of spleen yang, marked by incessant profuse leukorrhea, thin and whitish or pale yellow with no unpleasant smell, accompanied by lassitude, anorexia, loose bowels, edema of the legs, pale tongue with white greasy coating, and relaxed pulse

肾虚带下 [shèn xū dài xià]
kidney insufficiency leukorrhagia: leukorrhagia due to deficiency of kidney yang, marked by continuous profuse watery leukorrhea, accompanied by dizziness, tinnitus, lumbar pain, aversion to cold, cold limbs, cold sensation in the lower abdomen, frequent micturition, darkish complexion, and deep, thready and slow pulse

湿热带下 [shī rè dài xià]
dampness-heat leukorrhagia: leukorrhagia caused by down-pouring of dampness-heat, marked by profuse, sticky yellow leukorrhea with an unpleasant odor, usually accompanied by bitterness in the mouth, dry throat, lower abdominal pain, reddened tongue with yellow greasy coating, and soggy rapid pulse

湿毒带下 [shī dú dài xià]
toxic dampness leukorrhagia: leukorrhagia caused by invasion of toxic dampness, marked by excessive purulent and bloody leukorrhea with an offensive odor, accompanied by lower abdominal pain, lumbar aching, bitterness in the mouth, dry throat, reddened tongue with yellow greasy coating, and slippery rapid pulse

交接出血 [jiāo jiē chū xuè]
copulative bleeding: vaginal bleeding during sexual intercourse

阴挺 [yīn tǐng]
prolapse of the uterus: downward displacement of the uterus, sometimes with the entire uterus outside the vaginal orifice

妊娠 [rèn shēn]
pregnancy: condition of having a developing embryo or fetus in the body from conception to delivery

重身 [chóng shēn]
gravidity: synonym for pregnancy (妊娠 [rèn shēn])

不孕 [bù yùn]
infertility: lack of capacity to produce offspring

全不产 [quán bù chǎn]
primary infertility: ancient name for infertility occurring in those who have never conceived

断绪 [duàn xù]
secondary infertility: ancient name for infertility occurring in those who have previously conceived

肾虚不孕 [shèn xū bù yùn]
kidney insufficiency infertility: infertility ascribed to deficiency of kidney *qi*, yin or yang

宫冷不孕 [gōng lěng bù yùn]
uterus coldness infertility: infertility ascribed to deficiency-cold of the kidney which fails to warm the uterus, usually marked by coldness in the lower abdomen, aversion to cold, cold limbs, retarded menstruation, and even frigidity, also called 胞寒不孕 [bāo hán bù yùn]

胞寒不孕 [bāo hán bù yùn]
uterus coldness infertility: same as 宫冷不孕 [gōng lěng bù yùn]

血虚不孕 [xuè xū bù yùn]
blood deficiency infertility: infertility caused by insufficiency of the spleen and stomach or chronic loss of blood, marked by general weakness, lassitude, and sallow complexion

血滞不孕 [xuè zhì bù yùn]
blood stagnation infertility: infertility due to impeded blood flow, often accompanied by lower abdominal pain and late periods

肝郁不孕 [gān yù bù yùn]
liver depression infertility: infertility due to depression of the liver, often accompanied by irregularity of the menstrual cycle, distension and pain in the breasts before the periods, hypochondriac discomfort, depression and irritability

嫉妒不孕 [jí dù bù yùn]
infertility due to jealousy: infertility in women with depression of the liver caused by emotional factors such as jealousy

痰湿不孕 [tán shī bù yùn]
phlegm-dampness infertility: infertility caused by accumulation of phlegm-dampness, marked by late periods or even amenorrhea, profuse leukorrhea, dizziness, palpitations and discomfort in the chest, also called dampness phlegm infertility (湿痰不孕 [shī tán bù yùn])

湿痰不孕 [shī tán bù yùn]
dampness-phlegm infertility: same as phlegm-dampness infertility (痰湿不孕 [tán shī bù yùn])

血瘀不孕 [xuè yū bù yùn]
blood stasis infertility: infertility caused by blood stasis, usually marked by retarded menstruation, presence of blood clots in the menstrual discharge, and pain in the lower abdomen with tenderness

肥胖不孕 [féi pàng bù yùn]
obesity infertility: infertility occurring in obese women who eat too much fat, which turns to phlegm-dampness and then blocks

the conception vessel, often accompanied by palpitations, shortness of breath, and leukorrhagia

脂塞不孕 [zhī sè bù yùn]
fat infertility: infertility due to excessive fat, which blocks the uterine vessel

胎元 [tāi yuán]
fetal origin: (1) embryo within the mother's womb; (2) the mother's original *qi* that nourishes the fetus; (3) placenta

脐带 [qí dài]
umbilical cord: structure by which the fetus is attached to the placenta

激经 [jī jīng]
stimulated menses; menstruation during pregnancy: regular menstruation during early pregnancy, which stops spontaneously when the fetus is fully grown, also known as 盛胎 [shèng tāi] or 垢胎 [gòu tāi]

盛胎 [shèng tāi]
menstruation during pregnancy: another name for 激经 [jī jīng]

垢胎 [gòu tāi]
menstruation during pregnancy: another name for 激经 [jī jīng]

妊娠病 [rèn shēn bìng]
diseases of pregnancy: diseases that occur during the period of pregnancy and are related to pregnancy

妊娠恶阻 [rèn shēn è zǔ]
morning sickness: nausea and vomiting during early pregnancy, also abbreviated as 恶阻 [è zǔ]

恶阻 [è zǔ]
morning sickness: same as 妊娠恶阻 [rèn shēn è zǔ]

妊娠呕吐 [rèn shēn ǒu tù]
vomiting of pregnancy; hyperemesis gravidarum: synonym for morning sickness (妊娠恶阻 [rèn shēn è zǔ])

妊娠腹痛 [rèn shēn fù tòng]
abdominal pain in pregnancy: lower abdominal pain occurring in pregnancy, usually due to the fetal impediment to the flow of *qi* and blood, also called uterine obstruction (胞阻 [bāo zǔ])

胞阻 [bāo zǔ]
uterine obstruction: synonym for abdominal pain in pregnancy (妊娠腹痛 [rèn shēn fù tòng])

妊娠眩晕 [rèn shēn xuàn yùn]
vertigo in pregnancy: vertigo or even fainting occurring in pregnancy, also called gravidic vertigo (子晕 [zǐ yùn])

子晕 [zǐ yùn]
gravidic vertigo: synonym for vertigo in pregnancy (妊娠眩晕 [rèn shēn xuàn yùn])

妊娠痫证 [rèn shēn xián zhèng]
eclampsia (in pregnancy): sudden onset of convulsions and loss of consciousness occurring during pregnancy, also known as 子痫 [zǐ xián] or 子冒 [zǐ mào]

子痫 [zǐ xián]
eclampsia: same as 妊娠痫证 [rèn shēn xián zhèng]

子冒 [zǐ mào]
eclampsia: same as 妊娠痫证 [rèn shēn xián zhèng]

妊娠小便淋痛 [rèn shēn xiǎo biàn lìn tòng]
stranguria in pregnancy: difficult and painful discharge of urine during pregnancy, also known as gravidic stranguria (子淋 [zǐ lìn])

子淋 [zǐ lìn]
gravidic stranguria: synonym for stranguria during pregnancy (妊娠小便淋痛 [rèn shēn xiǎo biàn lìn tòng])

胎气上逆 [tāi qì shàng nì]
upward reversal of fetal *qi*: feeling of oppression in the abdomen and thorax, even with dyspnea during pregnancy, also known as gravid oppression (子悬 [zǐ xuán])

子悬 [zǐ xuán]
gravid oppression: synonym for upward reversal of fetal *qi* (胎气上逆 [tāi qì shàng nì])

子死腹中 [zǐ sǐ fù zhōng]
dead fetus in the uterus: death of a fetus in the uterus, also called 胎死腹中 [tāi sǐ fù zhōng]

胎死腹中 [tāi sǐ fù zhōng]
dead fetus in the uterus: same as 子死腹中 [zǐ sǐ fù zhōng]

死胎 [sǐ tāi]
dead fetus: abbreviation for dead fetus in the uterus (子死腹中 [zǐ sǐ fù zhōng] or 胎死腹中 [tāi sǐ fù zhōng])

胎死不下 [tāi sǐ bù xià]
missed labor: retention of a dead fetus in the uterus beyond the normal period of pregnancy, also called 死胎不下 [sǐ tāi bù xià]

死胎不下 [sǐ tāi bù xià]
missed labor: same as 胎死不下 [tāi sǐ bù xià]

鬼胎 [guǐ tāi]
pseudopregnancy: (1) abnormal mass in the uterine; (2) pseudocyesis, some physical symptoms of pregnancy appearing without conception, such as cessation of menses, enlargement of the abdomen, and apparent fetal movement; (3) hydatidiform mole (cf. 葡萄胎 [pú táo tāi])

葡萄胎 [pú táo tāi]
hydatidiform mole: abnormal pregnancy resulting in a mass of cysts resembling a bunch of grapes

胎水肿满 [tāi shuǐ zhǒng mǎn]
excess amniotic fluid: such fluid causing abnormally enlarged abdomen, sensation of fullness and dyspnea, also known as hydramnios (子满 [zǐ mǎn])

子满 [zǐ mǎn]
hydramnios: synonym for excess amniotic fluid (胎水肿满 [tāi shuǐ zhǒng mǎn])

妊娠心烦 [rèn shēn xīn fán]
vexation during pregnancy: state of being annoyed or worried during pregnancy, also called gravidic vexation (子烦 [zǐ fán])

子烦 [zǐ fán]
gravidic vexation: vexation occurring

during pregnancy, same as 妊娠心烦 [rèn shēn xīn fán]

妊娠咳嗽 [rèn shēn ké sòu]
cough during pregnancy: persistent cough during pregnancy, also called gravidic cough (子嗽 [zǐ sòu])

子嗽 [zǐ sòu]
gravidic cough: synonym for cough during pregnancy (妊娠咳嗽 [rèn shēn ké sòu])

妊娠失音 [rèn shēn shī yīn]
aphonia of pregnancy: hoarseness or loss of voice due to pregnancy, also called gravid aphonia (子喑 [zǐ yīn])

子喑 [zǐ yīn]
gravid aphonia: synonym for aphonia of pregnancy (妊娠失音 [rèn shēn shī yīn])

妊娠肿胀 [rèn shēn zhǒng zhàng]
edema of pregnancy: edema of the face and limbs occurring in the late stage of pregnancy, also called gravid edema (子肿 [zǐ zhǒng])

子肿 [zǐ zhǒng]
gravid edema: synonym for edema of pregnancy (妊娠肿胀 [rèn shēn zhǒng zhàng])

胎寒 [tāi hán]
(I) cold syndrome of the gravida: disorder in pregnant women due to immoderate eating of raw and cold food, or exposure to wind during pregnancy, manifested by excessive movements of the fetus, increased borborygmi, diarrhea, distending pain in the chest and abdomen and spasms of the limbs; **(II) fetal cold:** digestive disorders in the newborn attributed to contraction of cold from the mother during pregnancy

胎热 [tāi rè]
(I) heat syndrome of the gravida: loss of vision of a pregnant woman in labor, attributed to eating too much hot and spicy and/or barbecued food; **(II) fetal heat:** heat syndrome of the newborn marked by bloodshot eyes with crusting at the margins of the eyelids, attributed to the mother's contraction of heat during pregnancy

胎动不安 [tāi dòng bù ān]
threatened miscarriage: continuous moving of the fetus with lumbar pain and lower abdominal pain which may be accompanied by small amount of vaginal bleeding

分娩 [fēn miǎn]
delivery; childbirth; parturition: the act of giving birth to offspring, including the expulsion of the fetus, placenta and membranis from the uterus through the vagina

临产 [lín chǎn]
labor: the process of giving birth to offspring

试胎 [shì tāi]
testing labor: abdominal pain that goes on for a short time and then stops during the eighth or ninth month of pregnancy, also called 试月 [shì yuè]

试月 [shì yuè]
testing labor: same as 试胎 [shì tāi]

弄胎 [nòng tāi]
agitated fetus; false labor: intermittent abdominal pain that occurs toward the end of the term without backache

试水 [shì shuǐ]
early leakage of amniotic fluid: condition characterized by leakage of amniotic fluid which is not followed by childbirth

堕胎 [duò tāi]
(I) abortion: spontaneous expulsion of a fetus during the first twelve weeks of pregnancy; **(II) induced abortion:** abortion brought on intentionally

小产 [xiǎo chǎn]
miscarriage: spontaneous expulsion of a fetus after the twelfth week and before the twenty-eighth week of pregnancy

伤产 [shāng chǎn]
injury-induced labor: premature delivery induced by traumatic injury

胎漏 [tāi lòu]
vaginal bleeding during pregnancy: a sign of threatened miscarriage

胎元不固 [tāi yuán bù gù]
insecurity of fetus: provision of inadequate support for the fetus, which leads to liability to abortion

临产病 [lín chǎn bìng]
parturient diseases: diseases related to labor, occurring in the birth process and within four hours after delivery

难产 [nán chǎn]
difficult labor; dystocia: slow and difficult delivery, also called 产难 [chǎn nán]

产难 [chǎn nán]
difficult labor; dystocia: same as 难产 [nán chǎn]

胞衣先破 [bāo yī xiān pò]
premature rupture of fetal membrane: rupture of the fetal membrane at the end of the term of pregnancy but not followed by childbirth

沥浆产 [lì jiāng chǎn]
premature amniotic rupture: rupture of the fetal membrane before the proper time during the delivery, also known as 沥浆生 [lì jiāng shēng] and 沥胞生 [lì bāo shēng]

沥浆生 [lì jiāng shēng]
premature amniotic rupture: same as 沥浆产 [lì jiāng chǎn])

沥胞生 [lì bāo shēng]
premature amniotic rupture: same as 沥浆产 [lì jiāng chǎn]

滑胎 [huá tāi]
habitual abortion: spontaneous abortion in three or more consecutive pregnancies

气虚滑胎 [qì xū huá tāi]
***qi* deficiency habitual abortion:** habitual abortion due to deficiency of *qi*

血虚滑胎 [xuè xū huá tāi]
blood deficiency habitual abortion: habitual abortion due to deficiency of blood

血热滑胎 [xuè rè huá tāi]
blood heat habitual abortion: habitual abortion due to heat in blood

肾虚滑胎 [shèn xū huá tāi]
kidney insufficiency habitual abortion: habitual abortion due to deficiency of kidney *qi*

交骨不开 [jiāo gǔ bù kāi]
fixation of pubic cartilage: condition which impedes the passage of the fetus during parturition

胞衣不下 [bāo yī bù xià]
detention of afterbirth: retarded delivery of afterbirth, also called 息胞 [xī bāo]

息胞 [xī bāo]
detention of afterbirth: same as 胞衣不下 [bāo yī bù xià]

恶露 [è lù]
lochia: vaginal discharge in the puerperium

恶露不下 [è lù bù xià]
retention of lochia: retarded discharge of lochia

恶露不绝 [è lù bù jué]
lochiorrhea: prolonged discharge of lochia, which usually lasts over 3 weeks after childbirth, also called incessant discharge of lochia (恶露不止 [è lù bù zhǐ])

恶露不止 [è lù bù zhǐ]
incessant discharge of lochia: synonym for lochiorrhea (恶露不绝 [è lù bù jué])

产后恶露不绝 [chǎn hòu è lù bù jué]
(postpartum) lochiorrhea: same as 恶露不绝 [è lù bù jué]

产后病 [chǎn hòu bìng]
postpartum diseases: diseases occurring after childbirth in the puerperal period, related to labor and puerperium

产后三病 [chǎn hòu sān bìng]
three postpartum diseases: collective term for convulsions, depression-drowsiness, and dyschezia following delivery

产后三急 [chǎn hòu sān jí]
three postpartum emergencies: collective term for continuous vomiting, profuse sweating and diarrhea following delivery

产后三脱 [chǎn hòu sān tuō]
three kinds of postpartum collapses: collective term for collapse of blood, *qi* and mental power following delivery

产后三冲 [chǎn hòu sān chōng]
three postpartum crises: collective term for heart crisis, lung crisis, and stomach crisis, the three critical conditions caused by putrid blood derived from lochioschesis following childbirth

败血冲心 [bài xuè chōng xīn]
putrid-blood-induced heart crisis: critically diseased state following childbirth characterized by impaired consciousness and mania, ascribed to invasion of the heart by putrid blood derived from lochioschesis

败血冲肺 [bài xuè chōng fèi]
putrid-blood-induced lung crisis: critically diseased state following childbirth characterized by stuffiness in the chest, shortness of breath and epistaxis, ascribed to invasion of the lung by putrid blood derived from lochioschesis

败血冲胃 [bài xuè chōng wèi]
putrid-blood-induced stomach crisis: critically diseased state after childbirth characterized by nausea, vomiting, and abdominal distension and pain, ascribed to invasion of the stomach by putrid blood derived from lochioschesis

产后血晕 [chǎn hòu xuè yùn]
postpartum fainting: fainting occurring following childbirth due to excessive loss of blood

产后血崩 [chǎn hòu xuè bēng]
postpartum metrorrhagia: sudden profuse uterine bleeding following childbirth

产后郁冒 [chǎn hòu yù mào]
(I) postpartum depression and dizziness: condition usually ascribed to excessive blood loss, profuse sweating, or affection by external pathogens in the puerperal period; **(II) postpartum fainting:** synonym for 产后血晕 [chǎn hòu xuè yùn]

产后身痛 [chǎn hòu shēn tòng]
postpartum general aching: general aching involving the trunk, limbs and joints during the puerperal period

产后小便不通 [chǎn hòu xiǎo biàn bù tōng]
postpartum retention of urine: retention of urine following childbirth, usually accompanied by distension and pain in the lower abdomen

产后小便失禁 [chǎn hòu xiǎo biàn shī jìn]
postpartum incontinence of urine: incontinence of urine following childbirth

产后大便难 [chǎn hòu dà biàn nán]
postpartum dyschezia: difficult evacuation of feces from the rectum following childbirth

产后发热 [chǎn hòu fā rè]
postpartum fever: fever following childbirth due to various causes, particularly puerperal infection

产后头痛 [chǎn hòu tóu tòng]
postpartum headache: headache following childbirth, often due to excessive blood loss and sometimes due to blood stasis

产后怔忡 [chǎn hòu zhèng chōng]
postpartum palpitations: palpitations following childbirth, usually due to excessive blood loss

产后自汗 [chǎn hòu zì hàn]
spontaneous sweating after childbirth: abnormal condition of sweating occurring after childbirth usually due to weak constitution and consumption of *qi* and blood during labor

产后盗汗 [chǎn hòu dào hàn]
night sweating after childbirth: abnormal condition of sweating after childbirth usually due to consumption of blood and yin during labor

产后病温 [chǎn hòu bìng wēn]
postpartum warm disease; puerperal epidemic febrile disease: general term for various epidemic febrile diseases occurring following delivery

产后尿血 [chǎn hòu niào xuè]
postpartum hematuria: hematuria following childbirth, usually due to affection

by heat in a state of deficiency of *qi* and blood

产后腰痛 [chǎn hòu yāo tòng]
postpartum lumbago: dull pain in the lower back following childbirth, usually due to injury to kidney *qi* and stagnation of blood in the belt vessel

产后腹痛 [chǎn hòu fù tòng]
postpartum abdominal pain: pain in the lower abdomen following childbirth, accompanied by dizziness, lassitude, palpitations and shortness of breath if it is due to deficiency of blood with impaired blood supply to the uterine vessels, and accompanied by mass formation and tenderness in the lower abdomen and purplish tongue if it is due to stagnation of blood and cold in uterine vessels

产后胁痛 [chǎn hòu xié tòng]
postpartum hypochondriac pain: pain in the hypochondriac regions following childbirth, usually due to stagnation of *qi* and blood or impairment of the liver meridian/channel by excessive blood loss

产后腹胀 [chǎn hòu fù zhàng]
postpartum abdominal distension: abdominal distension due to stagnant blood which impairs the flow of *qi* with involvement of the spleen and stomach, or due to improper diet

产后水肿 [chǎn hòu shuǐ zhǒng]
postpartum edema: edema occurring following childbirth, usually seen in one with spleen and kidney yang deficiency which is worsened by labor

产后痹证 [chǎn hòu bì zhèng]
postpartum arthralgia: arthralgia following childbirth, usually due to the invasion of pathogenic wind-cold-dampness in a deficiency condition of *qi* and blood

产后痉证 [chǎn hòu jìng zhèng]
postpartum convulsions: sudden onset of rigidity, convulsions, trismus and opisthotonos in the puerperal period, also called 产后痉病 [chǎn hòu jìng bìng] or 产后病痉 [chǎn hòu bìng jìng]

产后痉病 [chǎn hòu jīng bìng]
postpartum convulsive disease: synonym for postpartum convulsions (产后痉证 [chǎn hòu jìng zhèng])

产后病痉 [chǎn hòu bìng jìng]
postpartum convulsions: same as 产后痉病 [chǎn hòu jìng bìng]

蓐劳 [rù láo]
puerperal phthisis: general weakness following childbirth accompanied by cough, dyspnea, stuffiness in the chest, chills, and fever

蓐风 [rù fēng]
puerperal tetanus: disease marked by opisthotonos and trismus following childbirth

缺乳 [quē rǔ]
oligogalactia; hypogalactia: deficient milk secretion

产后缺乳 [chǎn hòu quē rǔ]
postpartum oligogalactia; postpartum

hypogalactia: deficient milk secretion following childbirth

乳汁不行 [rǔ zhī bù xíng]
agalactia: no milk secretion following childbirth, also called 乳汁不通 [rǔ zhī bù tōng]

乳汁不通 [rǔ zhī bù tōng]
agalactia: same as 乳汁不行 [rǔ zhī bù xíng]

乳汁自出 [rǔ zhī zì chū]
galactorrhea: spontaneous flow of milk irrespective of nursing, also called 乳溢 [rǔ yì]

产后乳汁自出 [chǎn hòu rǔ zhī zì chū]
postpartum galactorrhea: spontaneous flow of milk following childbirth, irrespective of nursing

乳溢 [rǔ yì]
galactorrhea: same as 乳汁自出 [rǔ zhī zì chū]

儿科 Pediatrics

龆龀 [tiáo chèn]
seven- or eight-year-old child

稚子 [zhì zǐ]
ten-year-old child

纯阳之体 [chún yáng zhī tǐ]
pure yang constitution: constitution of infants or children characterized by fullness of vitality while healthy and exuberance of yang (e.g., liability to high fever and impairment of fluid) while ill

稚阴稚阳 [zhì yīn zhì yáng]
immature yin-yang: yin and yang that have not yet fully developed in young children

易虚易实 [yì xū yì shí]
liability to change from excess to deficiency and vice versa: a distinctive characteristic of children's diseases in the transformation between excess and deficiency syndromes/patterns

易寒易热 [yì hán yì rè]
liability to change from heat to cold and vice versa: distinctive characteristic of children's diseases in the transformation between cold and heat natures

初生不啼 [chū shēng bù tí]
failure to cry in the newborn; asphyxia neonatorum: perinatal asphyxia in the newborn

初生不乳 [chū shēng bù rǔ]
failure to suck in the newborn: condition marked by inability of the newborn to suck milk, often due to inadequacy of genuine *qi*, deficiency cold of the spleen and stomach, or accumulation of filthy heat

惊风 [jīng fēng]
infantile convulsions: series of muscular contractions associated with opisthotonus and loss of consciousness, occurring in infants and young children

惊风病 [jīng fēng bìng]
infantile convulsive disease: full name of infantile convulsions (惊风 [jīng fēng]) as a disease

惊风八候 [jīng fēng bā hòu]
eight signs of infantile convulsions: collective term for the signs of infantile convulsions – including clonic contraction of the hands, twitching of the fingers, forward bending of the back, hyperextension of the body, turning of the head, stretching of the arms, up-staring of the eyes, and immobility of the eyeballs

急惊风 [jí jīng fēng]
acute infantile convulsions: infantile convulsions of acute onset accompanied by high fever and loss of consciousness, mostly due to exogenous contraction, sometimes caused by fright

慢惊风 [màn jīng fēng]
chronic infantile convulsions: repeated infantile convulsions of gradual onset associated with loss of consciousness or

paralysis, indicative of poor prognosis

慢脾风 [màn pí fēng]
chronic convulsions due to spleen disorder: chronic infantile convulsions usually occurring after protracted vomiting and diarrhea with spleen *qi* deficiency

慢惊夹痰 [màn jīng jiā tán]
chronic convulsions with phlegm: chronic convulsions complicated by heat-phlegm symptoms, manifested as afternoon fever, thirst, epigastric distension, shortness of breath, expectoration, insomnia, and periodic convulsions

慢惊自汗 [màn jīng zì hàn]
chronic convulsions with incessant sweating: a critical case of chronic convulsions with impending shock

惊厥 [jīng jué]
(I) syncope from terror; (II) convulsions

瘛疭 [chì zòng]
clonic convulsions: convulsions marked by alternating contraction and relaxation of the muscles (瘛 [chì] means contraction, and 疭 [zòng], relaxation.)

婴儿瘛疭 [yīng ér chì zòng]
infantile clonic convulsions: clonic convulsions occurring in infants

天钓 [tiān diào]
upward-staring convulsions: infantile convulsions usually due to accumulation of heat in the heart and lung, marked by convulsions with tossed head and upward staring eyes, high fever, cyanosis, and salivation

内钓 [nèi diào]
visceral convulsions: infantile convulsions mainly manifested as visceral contraction and abdominal colic

脐风 [qí fēng]
neonatal tetanus: severe form of infectious tetanus occurring in the newborn during the first few days after birth, mostly due to unhygienic practice in dressing the umbilical stump

脐风三证 [qí féng sān zhèng]
three signs of neonatal tetanus: collective term for pursed mouth, lockjaw, and locked abdomen

撮口 [cuō kǒu]
pursed mouth: sign of neonatal tetanus marked by spasms of the buccal muscles which make the lips form a small tight round shape involuntarily, with difficulty in opening the mouth

噤风 [jìn fēng]
lockjaw: sign of neonatal tetanus marked by spasms of the muscles of mastication resulting in inability to cry or suck milk

锁肚 [suǒ dù]
locked abdomen: sign of neonatal tetanus marked by protruding of the swollen umbilicus and distension of the abdomen with stoppage of bowel movements

惊风抽搐 [jīng fēng chōu chù]
infantile convulsive seizure: series of involuntary contractions of muscles in a case of infantile convulsions

惊风腹痛 [jīng fēng fù tòng]
infantile convulsions with abdominal pain: morbid condition characterized by convulsions complicated by abdominal pain, often caused by accumulated undigested food impairing the stomach, stagnant heat producing phlegm and contraction of external wind

惊风烦渴 [jīng fēng fán kě]
infantile convulsions with vexing thirst: vexing thirst due to consumption of body fluids following a seizure of infantile convulsions

硬肿症 [yìng zhǒng zhèng]
sclerederma neonatorum: hardening and thickening of the skin in the newborn

胎赤 [tāi chì]
fetal redness; erythroderma neonatorum: abnormal redness of the skin in a newborn, often due to affection of toxic heat at the fetal stage

胎禀 [tāi bǐng]
fetal endowment: quality of the newborn inherited from its parents

胎弱 [tāi ruò]
fetal weakness: congenitally weak constitution, also known as 胎怯 [tāi qiè]

胎怯 [tāi qiè]
fetal feebleness: synonym for fetal weakness (胎弱 [tāi ruò])

胎寒 [tāi hán]
(I) fetal cold: cold syndrome of the newborn, marked by abdominal pain with cold huddling extremities, shivering, incessant crying or lockjaw; **(II) cold syndrome of gravida:** cf. 胎寒 [tāi hán] on p.568

胎热 [tāi rè]
(I) fetal heat: febrile disease of the newborn attributed to the mother's improper diet and medication during pregnancy; **(II) heat syndrome of gravida:** cf. 胎热 [tāi rè] on p.568

胎毒 [tāi dú]
(I) fetal toxicosis: boils, blisters, eczema, etc. of newborns, considered in ancient times to result from infection of endogenous toxicity of the pregnant mother before birth; **(II) fetal toxin:** cf. 胎毒 [tāi dú] on p. 69

胎黄 [tāi huáng]
neonatal jaundice; icterus neonatorum: jaundice in a newborn, also called 胎疸 [tāi dǎn]

胎疸 [tāi dǎn]
neonatal jaundice: same as 胎黄 [tāi huáng]

胎黄病 [tāi huáng bìng]
neonatal jaundice (disease); icterus neonatorum: full name of neonatal jaundice (胎黄 [tāi huáng]) as a disease

囟填 [xìn tián]
bulging fontanel: outward swelling of the fontanel in an infant, often seen in cases of infectious disease with excessive internal heat or indigestion with retention of undigested food, and also as a prodromal sign of infantile convulsions if accompanied by high fever and vomiting

囟陷 [xìn xiàn]
sunken fontanel: depressed fontanel in an infant, often due to consumption of yin fluid in cases of acute febrile disease or diarrhea, and sometimes due to congenital defect

解颅 [jiě lú]
ununited skull; hydrocephalus: abnormal accumulation of excess fluid within the skull marked by enlargement of the head and persistent non-closure of the skull sutures

解颅病 [jiě lú bìng]
ununited skull (disease); hydrocephalus (disease): disease characterized by accumulation of excess fluid within the skull

百晬内嗽 [bǎi zuì nèi sòu]
neonatal cough: coughing by a newborn within one hundred days after its birth, often due to common cold or respiratory infection (晬 [zuì] means a whole day, and 百晬内 [bǎi zuì nèi], within one hundred days.)

小儿哮喘 [xiǎo ér xiào chuǎn]
infantile asthma: infantile disease characterized by paroxysmal labored breathing accompanied by wheezing

夜啼 [yè tí]
night crying: morbid night crying in babies, in most cases due to cold in the spleen or heat in the heart, and sometimes due to being frightened

热夜啼 [rè yè tí]
night crying due to heat: night crying in babies caused by heart heat, marked by flushed face, fever, and irritability

寒夜啼 [hán yè tí]
night crying due to cold: night crying in babies caused by spleen cold, marked by pallor, hands and abdomen cold to the touch, and coiled posture suggesting abdominal pain

客忤 [kè wǔ]
fright seizure: seizure of fright that causes vomiting, diarrhea, abdominal pain, and even convulsions

客忤夜啼 [kè wǔ yè tí]
night crying due to fright: night crying in babies caused by fright

伤乳 [shāng rǔ]
milk damage; infantile dyspepsia: dyspepsia caused by improper breast feeding

溢乳 [yì rǔ]
milk regurgitation: such ailment resulting from overfeeding or improper way of nursing, also called vomiting of milk (呕乳 [ǒu rǔ])

呕乳 [ǒu rǔ]
vomiting of milk: synonym for milk regurgitation (溢乳 [yì rǔ])

五迟 [wǔ chí]
five kinds of retardation: collective term for retarded development in infants covering standing, walking, hair-growth, tooth eruption and speaking

立迟 [lì chí]
retardation of standing: inability to stand

in children till 2 ～ 3 years of age

行迟 [xíng chí]

retardation of walking: chronic inability to walk in children

发迟 [fà chí]

retardation of hair-growth: retarded growth of hair in children

齿迟 [chǐ chí]

retardation of tooth-eruption: retarded eruption of teeth in children

语迟 [yǔ chí]

retardation of speaking: inability to speak in children till 4 ～ 5 years of age

五硬 [wǔ yìng]

five types of stiffness: collective term for stiffness of the hand, foot, waist, flesh and neck in children

五软 [wǔ ruǎn]

five types of flaccidity: collective term for flaccidity of the neck, nape, extremities, muscles, and mastication as striking features of delayed growth and mental retardation in infants

鸡胸 [jī xiōng]

chicken breast; pigeon chest: deformity of the chest in which the sternum is prominent, usually due to rickets, also called tortoise chest (龟胸 [guī xiōng])

龟胸 [guī xiōng]

tortoise chest: synonym for pigeon chest (鸡胸 [jī xiōng])

龟背 [guī bèi]

kyphosis; humpback: the back shaped like a tortoise-shell, a condition of deformity in children due to underdevelopment and malnutrition, as seen in cases of rickets

脐疮 [qí chuāng]

umbilical sore; omphalelcosis: ulceration of the umbilicus

脐湿 [qí shī]

umbilical dampness; omphalorrhea: effusion of body fluid at the umbilicus

脐血 [qí xuè]

umbilical bleeding; omphalorrhagia: hemorrhage or oozing of blood from the umbilicus

脐疝 [qí shàn]

umbilical hernia: abdominal hernia in which part of the intestine protrudes at the umbilicus and is covered with skin, also called umbilical protrusion (脐突 [qí tū])

脐突 [qí tū]

umbilical protrusion: another name for umbilical hernia (脐疝 [qí shàn])

差颓［癞］[cī tuí]

unilateral swollen testicle: swelling of the testicle on one side (差[cī] means asymmetrical, 颓 [tuí] or 癞[tuí], a disease marked by testicular swelling.)

流涎 [liú xián]

drooling: flowing of saliva from the mouth

小儿多涎 [xiǎo ér duō xián]

infantile slobbering: excessive discharge of thick saliva due to heat in the spleen or excessive discharge of thin saliva due to deficiency-cold of the spleen and stomach

滞颐 [zhì yí]
dribbling with wet cheeks: another expression for infantile slobbering (小儿多涎 [xiǎo ér duō xián])

龂齿 [xiè chǐ]
teeth grinding: grinding of teeth during sleep, often due to exuberant fire in the heart and stomach or due to deficiency of *qi* and blood

马牙 [mǎ yá]
gingival eruption: sporadic eruption of small round yellowish nodules on the gums in the newborn, causing difficulty in sucking milk

螳螂子 [táng láng zǐ]
corpus adiposum bucca: encapsulated mass of fat (looking like a mantis egg, and hence the Chinese name) in the cheek of an infant, causing difficulty in sucking, also called buccal fat pad (颊脂垫 [jiá zhī diàn])

颊脂垫 [jiá zhī diàn]
buccal fat pad: another name for corpus adiposum bucca (螳螂子 [táng láng zǐ])

木舌 [mù shé]
wooden tongue: swollen, hardened tongue, as stiff as a piece of wood, seen in newborns suffering from glossitis

地图舌 [dì tú shé]
geographic tongue: irregular shedding of the tongue coating indicating deficiency of stomach *qi* and yin

连舌 [lián shé]
adhered tongue; ankyloglossia: restricted movement of the tongue that causes difficulty in sucking, also called tongue-tie (结舌 [jié shé])

结舌 [jié shé]
tongue-tie: synonym for adhered tongue or ankyloglossia (连舌 [lián shé])

鹅口疮 [é kǒu chuāng]
thrush: disease of infants and young children of poor health, characterized by the presence of white patches of soft material on the buccal mucosa and tongue, looking like the mouth of a goose, also known as snow-white mouth (雪口 [xuě kǒu])

雪口 [xuě kǒu]
snow-white mouth: another name for thrush (鹅口疮 [é kǒu chuāng])

口疮 [kǒu chuāng]
aphtha: small oral ulcer

口糜 [kǒu mí]
ulcerative stomatitis: stomatitis by the appearance of shallow ulcers on the cheeks, tongue, gums and palate

燕口疮 [yàn kǒu chuāng]
angular stomatitis; perlèche: superficial inflammation of the angles of the mouth with fissuring, usually attributed to accumulation of heat in the lung and stomach, also called 燕口[yàn kǒu] or 口吻疮 [kǒu wěn chuāng]

燕口 [yàn kǒu]
angular stomatitis: abbreviation for 燕口疮 [yàn kǒu chuāng]

口吻疮 [kǒu wěn chuāng]
angular stomatitis: same as 燕口疮 [yàn kǒu chuāng]

口疳 [kǒu gān]
oral sore: aphthous ulcer, usually occurring in malnourished children

疳 [gān]
(infantile) malnutrition: chronic nutritional disorder in infants due to improper feeding, digestive impairment or intestinal parasitosis with symptoms of wasting, pallid or sallow complexion, potbelly, and chronic diarrhea

疳证 [gān zhèng]
(infantile) malnutrition syndrome: syndrome characterized by malnutrition in infants

疳病 [gān bìng]
(infantile) malnutrition disease: synonymous with (infantile) malnutrition (疳 [gān])

疳气 [gān qì]
(infantile) malnutrition *qi*; mild (infantile) malnutrition: infantile malnutrition at the early stage with mild symptoms, characterized by leanness, lusterless complexion, and anorexia

疳气证 [gān qì zhèng]
(infantile) malnutrition *qi* syndrome: syndrome characterized by early-stage malnutrition in infants

疳积 [gān jī]
(infantile) malnutrition with accumulation: infantile malnutrition at the intermediate stage, characterized by marked leanness, sallow complexion, distended abdomen, and listlessness

疳积证 [gān jī zhèng]
(infantile) malnutrition-accumulation syndrome: syndrome of malnutrition in infants at the intermediate stage with marked leanness and distended abdomen

干疳 [gān gān]
dryness (infantile) malnutrition: infantile malnutrition at the extreme stage with drying up of *qi* and blood, marked by a dry and shriveled body worn to a shadow

干疳证 [gān gān zhèng]
dryness (infantile) malnutrition syndrome: syndrome of malnutrition in infants at the extreme stage, with a dry and shriveled body worn to a shadow

丁奚疳 [dīng xī gān]
T-shaped (infantile) malnutrition: severe case of infantile malnutrition, leaving the patient with an emaciated T-shaped figure

五疳 [wǔ gān]
five (infantile) malnutrition syndromes: collective term for malnutrition involving the spleen, liver, heart, lung, and kidney, in accordance with an ancient classification of infantile malnutrition

脾疳 [pí gān]
spleen (infantile) malnutrition; (infantile) malnutrition involving the spleen: basic syndrome of infantile malnutrition due to accumulation of dampness-heat in the spleen, marked by sallow complexion, fever, distended abdomen, emaciation, anorexia, compulsive eating of dirt and mud, and

loose bowels, also called feeding (infantile) malnutrition (食疳 [sì gān])

食疳 [sì gān]
feeding (infantile) malnutrition: another name for spleen (infantile) malnutrition or (infantile) malnutrition involving the spleen (脾疳 [pí gān])

肺疳 [fèi gān]
lung (infantile) malnutrition; (infantile) malnutrition involving the lung: one of the five malnutrition syndromes named in ancient times, characterized by damage to the lung meridian/channel by accumulated heat, manifested by oral and nasal sores and dyspnea, also called *qi* (infantile) malnutrition (气疳 [qì gān])

气疳 [qì gān]
***qi* (infantile) malnutrition:** another name for lung (infantile) malnutrition or (infantile) malnutrition involving the lung (肺疳 [fèi gān])

心疳 [xīn gān]
heart (infantile) malnutrition; (infantile) malnutrition involving the heart: one of the five malnutrition syndromes according to an ancient classification, caused by improper feeding with sweet stuff that produces heat affecting the heart, manifested as flushed face, fever with sweats, frightened restlessness, grinding of the teeth, oral sores, anorexia, and leanness, also called fright (infantile) malnutrition (惊疳 [jīng gān])

惊疳 [jīng gān]
fright (infantile) malnutrition: another name for heart (infantile) malnutrition (心疳 [xīn gān])

肝疳 [gān gān]
liver (infantile) malnutrition; (infantile) malnutrition involving the liver: one of the five malnutrition syndromes according to an ancient classification, caused by improper feeding with damage to the liver by heat, manifested by cyanotic complexion, night-blindness, emaciation with a distended abdomen, also called sinew (infantile) malnutrition (筋疳 [jīn gān])

筋疳 [jīn gān]
sinew (infantile) malnutrition: another name for liver (infantile) malnutrition (肝疳 [gān gān])

肾疳 [shèn gān]
kidney (infantile) malnutrition; (infantile) malnutrition involving the kidney: one of the five malnutrition syndromes according to an ancient classification, which is ascribed to congenital defect with weak constitution and excessive eating of sweet stuff that produces heat to consume kidney yin, manifested as heat in the upper portion and cold in the lower portion, vomiting and diarrhea, rectal prolapse, genital sores, and night crying, also known as bone (infantile) malnutrition (骨疳 [gǔ gān])

骨疳 [gǔ gān]
bone (infantile) malnutrition: another name for kidney (infantile) malnutrition (肾疳 [shèn gān])

眼疳 [yǎn gān]
eye (infantile) malnutrition; (infantile)

malnutrition involving the eyes: attack of liver fire to the eyes in a malnourished child, manifested by inflammation of the eyes first, and then corneal opacity associated with emaciation

蛔疳 [huí gān]
ascariasis (infantile) malnutrition; (infantile) malnutrition due to ascariasis: infantile malnutrition due to ascaris infestation

虫积 [chóng jī]
worm accumulation; intestinal parasitosis: infestation of parasitic worms in the intestines, marked by sallow complexion, emaciation, potbelly, and fits of umbilical pain

哺乳疳 [bǔ rǔ gān]
lactational malnutrition: malnutrition of an infant due to improper breast-feeding

乳积 [rǔ jī]
milk retention; infantile dyspepsia: indigestion or dyspepsia due to improper milk feeding

食积 [shí jī]
food retention; dyspepsia; indigestion: diseased state characterized by accumulation of undigested food in the stomach and intestines, manifested by abdominal distension and pain, vomiting, diarrhea, and impaired appetite

厌食 [yàn shí]
anorexia: diseased state in children characterized by loss of appetite for food

苦夏 [kǔ xià]
summer affliction: children's suffering marked by anorexia and loss of weight in summer

疰夏 [zhù xià]
summer non-acclimation: children's disease usually occurring in summer, with symptoms of dyspepsia, dizziness, lassitude and frequent yawning, or with persistent fever

疰夏病 [zhù xià bìng]
summer non-acclimation disease: the full name of summer non-acclimation (疰夏 [zhù xià]) as a disease

夏季热 [xià jì rè]
summer fever: disease of young children, characterized by prolonged fever in summer owing to lack of adaptability to hot weather

夏季热病 [xià jì rè bìng]
summer fever disease: full name of summer fever (夏季热 [xià jì rè]) as a disease

小儿暑温 [xiǎo ér shǔ wēn]
epidemic summer fever in children: epidemic disease in children caused by warm toxins in summer and characterized by high fever, convulsions and coma with sudden onset, usually referring to encephalitis B

小儿诸热 [xiǎo ér zhū rè]
fevers in children: collective term for various kinds of fever in children

夜热 [yè rè]
fever at night: fever usually due to improper feeding or exogenous affection which impairs

the function of the spleen and lung

惊热 [jīng rè]
fever due to fright: fever in children induced by fright

客热 [kè rè]
irregular recurrent fever: fever which comes and goes from time to time as if being visited by guests once in a while

血热 [xuè rè]
(I) blood fever: fever in children, which recurs daily at noon and subsides in the evening; **(II) fever at blood aspect:** fever accompanied by bleeding symptoms

癖热 [pǐ rè]
fever with hypochondriac mass: irregular fever accompanied by abdominal distension, vomiting, and formation of hypochondriac mass

骨蒸热 [gǔ zhēng rè]
bone-steaming fever; consumptive fever: hectic fever in children, accompanied by emaciation, night sweating or mass formation in the abdomen, usually due to improper feeding without timely treatment or remnant heat after a severe disease which consumes the vital essence and body fluid

食积寒热 [shí jī hán rè]
food retention with chills and fever: indigestion with retention of undigested food accompanied by chills and fever

小儿虚热 [xiǎo ér xū rè]
asthenic fever in children: low or tidal fever caused by excessive diaphoresis or purgation or after a serious disease

变蒸 [biàn zhēng]
growth fever: fever of a child due to the growth and development

痧 [shā]
(I) rash; exanthem: (1) skin eruption, generally referring to fine, sand-like papules; (2) disease in which skin eruptions or rashes are a prominent manifestation; **(II) filthy attack:** sudden attack of impaired consciousness or vomiting and diarrhea in children in summer, attributed to invasion of a filthy factor which can often be driven out by scraping the skin

小儿发痧 [xiǎo ér fā shā]
filthy attack in children: popular name for sudden attack of acute vomiting and diarrhea or heat stroke in children

闷痧 [mèn shā]
drowsy filthy attack: filthy attack with mental confusion

寒痧 [hán shā]
cold filthy attack: filthy attack in children marked by tidal fever, cool fingertips, and aversion to cold

热痧 [rè shā]
heat filthy attack: filthy attack in children marked by fever with restlessness, flushed face, and dire thirst

风疹 [fēng zhěn]
rubella: infectious eruptive disease caused by a wind-heat pathogen, manifested by low fever, cough, enlargement of the

postauricular and suboccipital lymph nodes, and generalized pink skin rash, also called wind rash (风痧 [fēng shā])

风痧 [fēng shā]
wind rash: same as rubella (风疹 [fēng zhěn])

麻疹 [má zhěn]
measles: highly contagious disease caused by a specific seasonal pathogen, clinically marked by fever and generalized maculopapular rash preceded by coryza, characteristic spots on the buccal mucosa, and palpebral conjunctivitis, also called 痧子 [shā zǐ]

痧子 [shā zǐ]
measles: another term for 麻疹 [má zhěn]

麻毒内攻 [má dú nèi gōng]
inward invasion of measles: severe case of measles with inadequate eruption to expel the toxins

麻毒入营 [má dú rù yíng]
measles toxin entering the nutrient aspect: measles with the toxin penetrating into the nutrient aspect, manifested by high fever, delirium, convulsions, or loss of consciousness

麻毒闭肺 [má dú bì fèi]
measles toxin blocking the lung: measles complicated by pneumonia, also known as measles toxin penetrating into the lung (麻毒陷肺 [má dú xiàn fèi])

麻毒陷肺 [má dú xiàn fèi]
measles toxin penetrating into the lung: measles complicated by pneumonia, same as measles toxin blocking the lung (麻毒闭肺[má dú bì fèi])

麻毒攻目 [má dú gōng mù]
measles toxin attacking the eyes: measles complicated by keratoconjunctivitis

麻疹顺证 [má zhěn shùn zhèng]
favorable syndrome/pattern of measles: case of measles with favorable prognosis

麻疹逆证 [má zhěn nì zhèng]
unfavorable syndrome/pattern of measles: case of measles with complications and poor prognosis

麻疹闭证 [má zhěn bì zhèng]
block syndrome/pattern of measles: measles without adequate eruption to expel toxins

麻疹险证 [má zhěn xiǎn zhèng]
critical case of measles: life-threatening case of measles

奶麻 [nǎi má]
roseola infantum; exathema subitum: acute eruptive disease in infants, characterized by sudden subsidence of a high fever of 3-4 days duration with simultaneous appearance of a macular rash

痘 [dòu]
pox: pea-like skin sores, as seen on the skin of smallpox and chickenpox patients

水痘 [shuǐ dòu]
chickenpox; varicella: acute contagious disease caused by an epidemic pathogen, marked by fever and formation of vesicles followed by incrustation, also called 水疱

[shuǐ pào], 水花 [shuǐ huā], or 水疮 [shuǐ chuāng]

水疱 [shuǐ pào]
chickenpox: another name for 水痘 [shuǐ dòu]

水花 [shuǐ huā]
chickenpox: another name for 水痘 [shuǐ dòu]

水疮 [shuǐ chuāng]
chickenpox: another name for 水痘 [shuǐ dòu]

天花 [tiān huā]
smallpox: acute contagious febrile disease characterized by skin eruption with pustules, sloughing, and scar formation, also known as variola (痘疮 [dòu chuāng])

痘疮 [dòu chuāng]
variola: another name for smallpox (天花 [tiān huā])

疫喉 [yì hóu]
epidemic throat diseases: general term for epidemic diseases involving the throat, such as diphtheria and scarlatina

白喉 [bái hóu]
diphtheria: acute contagious febrile disease marked by the formation of a false membrane in the throat, also called 白缠喉 [bái chán hóu]

白缠喉 [bái chán hóu]
diphtheria: another name for 白喉 [bái hóu]

丹痧 [dān shā]
scarlatina; scarlet fever: infection characterized by inflammation of the throat with erythematous rash, also called throat infection with erythema (喉痧 [hóu shā]), epidemic erythema (疫痧 [yì shā]), or erosion of the throat with erythema (烂喉丹痧 [làn hóu dān shā])

疫痧 [yì shā]
epidemic erythema: another name for scarlatina (丹痧 [dān shā])

烂喉丹痧 [làn hóu dān shā]
erosion of the throat with erythema: another name for scarlatina (丹痧 [dān shā])

喉痧 [hóu shā]
throat infection with erythema: another name for scarlatina (丹痧 [dān shā])

杨莓舌 [yáng méi shé]
strawberry tongue: crimson, prickly tongue with peeled coating, resembling a strawberry, a sign of scarlatina at the stage when the toxin enters the nutrient aspect

痄腮 [zhà sāi]
mumps; epidemic parotitis: epidemic disease caused by wind-heat toxin and characterized by painful swelling of one or both parotid glands, also called swollen cheek (腮肿 [sāi zhǒng])

腮肿 [sāi zhǒng]
swollen cheek: another name for mumps (痄腮 [zhà sāi])

肺风痰喘 [fèi fēng tán chuǎn]
lung wind with phlegmatic dyspnea: dyspnea in children due to obstruction of

qi by phlegm in the case of a wind-cold affection of the lung meridian/channel

肺炎喘嗽 [fèi yán chuǎn sòu]
lung inflammation with dyspnea and cough: external contraction with obstruction of the lung collaterals by the pathogen, manifested mainly by fever, cough, dyspnea, and flaring nares

马脾风 [mǎ pí fēng]
horse-spleen wind; acute asthmatic attack in children: emergency case of acute asthma in children, also called sudden dyspnea. (暴喘 [bào chuǎn]) (This critical condition is attributed to attack of wind-heat on the heart and spleen. Horse-spleen wind is a folk rendering of heart-spleen wind. One reason for the replacement of *heart* by *horse* is that both pertain to fire according to the five-element/phase theory.)

暴喘 [bào chuǎn]
sudden dyspnea: same as horse-spleen wind (马脾风 [mǎ pí fēng])

百日咳 [bǎi rì ké]
pertussis; whooping cough: acute contagious infection of the respiratory system with characteristic paroxysmal cough, consisting of a deep inspiration, followed by a series of quick, short coughs which end with a long shrill, whooping inspiration, also known as egret's cough (鹭鸶咳 [lù sī ké]), 顿咳 [dùn ké], and epidemic cough (疫咳 [yì ké])

顿咳 [dùn ké]
whooping cough: same as pertussis (百日咳 [bǎi rì ké])

鹭鸶咳 [lù sī ké]
egret's cough: another name for pertussis (百日咳 [bǎi rì ké])

疫咳 [yì ké]
epidemic cough: another name for pertussis (百日咳 [bǎi rì ké])

食积盗汗 [shí jī dào hàn]
food-retention night sweating: sweating during sleep due to accumulation of undigested food

胃虚汗 [wèi xū hàn]
stomach-insufficiency sweating: abnormal spontaneous sweating due to decreased function of the stomach, distributed from the head to the umbilicus, and accompanied by pallor and lassitude

气鬲 [qì gé]
***qi* dysphagia:** dysphagia due to *qi* disorder

小儿呕吐 [xiǎo ér ǒu tù]
infantile vomiting: vomiting in infants usually due to excess nursing

寒吐 [hán tù]
cold vomiting: vomiting in infants due to deficiency-cold in the stomach

热吐 [rè tù]
heat vomiting: vomiting in infants due to heat in the stomach, also called stomach heat vomiting (胃热呕吐 [wèi rè ǒu tù])

胃热呕吐 [wèi rè ǒu tù]
stomach heat vomiting: same as heat vomiting (热吐 [rè tù])

伤食吐 [shāng shí tù]
food damage vomiting: vomiting in infants due to improper feeding

伤乳吐 [shāng rǔ tù]
milk damage vomiting: vomiting of milk in infants due to overfeeding, also known as milk vomiting (呕乳 [ǒu rǔ]) and milk regurgitation (溢乳 [yì rǔ])

呕乳 [ǒu rǔ]
milk vomiting: simplified expression for milk damage vomiting (伤乳吐 [shāng rǔ tù])

溢乳 [yì rǔ]
milk regurgitation: synonymous with milk vomiting (呕乳 [ǒu rǔ])

积吐 [jī tù]
food-retention vomiting: vomiting due to retention of undigested food

虫吐 [chóng tù]
ascariasis vomiting: vomiting due to intestinal ascariasis, occurring when the ascarides enter the stomach

惊吐 [jīng tù]
fright vomiting: vomiting due to being frightened, usually accompanied by fever in the morning and evening, with disturbed sleep and restlessness, also called vomiting with fright (夹惊吐 [jiā jīng tù])

夹惊吐 [jiā jīng tù]
vomiting with fright: same as fright vomiting 惊吐 [jīng tù]

小儿卒利 [xiǎo ér cù lì]
sudden infantile diarrhea: sudden occurrence of diarrhea in infants, also called 小儿暴泻 [xiǎo ér bào xiè]

小儿暴泻 [xiǎo ér bào xiè]
sudden infantile diarrhea: same as 小儿卒利 [xiǎo ér cù lì]

小儿泄泻 [xiǎo ér xiè xiè]
infantile diarrhea: diseased state in infants characterized by abnormally frequent passage of thin, watery stools

小儿寒湿泻 [xiǎo ér hán shī xiè]
infantile cold-dampness diarrhea: infantile diarrhea caused by cold-dampness which impairs the spleen, marked by frequent discharge of watery stools with abdominal pain, cold limbs, pallor, and no desire to drink

小儿湿热泻 [xiǎo ér shī rè xiè]
infantile dampness-heat diarrhea: infantile diarrhea caused by dampness-heat which invades the stomach and intestines, usually occurring in summer, marked by frequent discharge of watery stools with abdominal pain, fever and thirst

小儿热泻 [xiǎo ér rè xiè]
infantile heat diarrhea: infantile diarrhea caused by invasion of the large intestine by summer-heat, marked by frequent discharge of blood-tinged or foamy stools, accompanied by spells of borborygmi, abdominal pain and restlessness

小儿火泻 [xiǎo ér huǒ xiè]
infantile fire diarrhea: infantile diarrhea caused by accumulation of intense heat in the large intestine, marked by spouting discharge of large amounts of watery stools, accompanied by a burning

sensation at the anus, abdominal pain, fever and flushed face

脐寒泻 [qí hán xiè]
umbilical cold diarrhea: infantile diarrhea due to wind-cold invasion of the cut end of the umbilicus which has not been properly protected, marked by discharge of thin stools accompanied by abdominal pain and borborygmi, also called visceral cold diarrhea (脏寒泻 [zàng hán xiè])

脏寒泻 [zàng hán xiè]
visceral cold diarrhea: same as umbilical cold diarrhea (脐寒泻 [qí hán xiè)

脾虚泻 [pí xū xiè]
spleen-insufficiency diarrhea: chronic infantile diarrhea marked by discharge of loose stools containing undigested food soon after meals, accompanied by emaciation, sallow complexion and listlessness

中寒泻 [zhòng hán xiè]
cold-stroke diarrhea: infantile diarrhea caused by direct attack of cold to the spleen and stomach, marked by loose stools, anorexia, abdominal pain, cold limbs, and pallor

伤食泻 [shāng shí xiè]
indigestion diarrhea: infantile diarrhea due to indigestion either as a result of improper feeding or due to decreased function of the stomach, marked by loose stools containing undigested food with sour fetid odor, also called 食泻 [shí xiè] or 食泄 [shí xiè]

食泻 [泄] [shí xiè]
indigestion diarrhea: same as 伤食泻 [shāng shí xiè]

飧水泻 [sūn shuǐ xiè]
watery lienteric diarrhea: infantile diarrhea characterized by discharge of watery stools containing undigested food

肾虚泻 [shèn xū xiè]
kidney insufficiency diarrhea: infantile diarrhea due to deficiency of kidney yang as a result of congenital defect or after a protracted disease, marked by discharge of liquid stools daily before dawn

小儿腹痛 [xiǎo ér fù tòng]
abdominal pain in children

盘肠气痛 [pán cháng qì tòng]
intestinal *qi* colic: abdominal pain often occurring in a child with a weak spleen after exposure to cold

气积腹痛 [qì jī fù tòng]
***qi*-accumulation abdominal pain:** abdominal pain due to accumulation of stagnant *qi*, marked by dull pain accompanied by abdominal distension and belching

虫积腹痛 [chóng jī fù tòng]
parasitic abdominal pain: abdominal pain due to intestinal ascariasis

食积腹痛 [shí jī fù tòng]
food-retention abdominal pain: abdominal pain due to retention of undigested food

小儿腹胀 [xiǎo ér fù zhàng]
abdominal distension in children

虚胀 [xū zhàng]
abdominal distension of deficiency type: abdominal distension due to *qi* deficiency or blood deficiency

实胀 [shí zhàng]
abdominal distension of excess type: abdominal distension due to food retention, dampness stagnation, dampness-heat accumulation, or blood stasis

伤食腹胀 [shāng shí fù zhàng]
abdominal distension with indigestion: abdominal distension due to overeating

小儿瘿气 [xiǎo ér yǐng qì]
endemic goiter in children

小儿消渴 [xiǎo ér xiāo kě]
diabetes in children

消上 [xiāo shàng]
upper diabetes: diabetes in children marked by polydipsia

消肌 [xiāo jī]
muscle-wasting diabetes: diabetes in children marked by polyphagia and emaciation

消浊 [xiāo zhuó]
turbid diabetes: diabetes marked by discharge of turbid urine

癫痫 [diān xián]
epilepsy: paroxysmal transient disturbance of the mind manifested as episodic loss of consciousness with generalized tonic-clonic seizures, also called 颠疾 [diān jí] or 痫证 [xián zhèng]

颠疾 [diān jí]
epilepsy (in older children): epilepsy occurring in children over ten years of age

痫证 [xián zhèng]
epilepsy (in younger children): epilepsy occurring in children under ten years of age

阴痫 [yīn xián]
(I) yin epilepsy: epilepsy accompanied by such yin symptoms as cold limbs, pallor and feeble voice; **(II) yin convulsions:** same as chronic infantile convulsions (慢惊风 [màn jīng fēng])

阳痫 [yáng xián]
(I) yang epilepsy: epilepsy accompanied by such yang symptoms as fever, sweating, flushed face, trismus or incessant crying; **(II) yang convulsions:** same as acute infantile convulsions (急惊风 [jí jīng fēng])

暴痫 [bào xián]
fulminant epilepsy: sudden occurrence of epilepsy without any predisposing factor

食痫 [shí xián]
food-induced epilepsy: epileptic seizure induced by overfeeding, marked by convulsions accompanied by vomiting and diarrhea

风痫 [fēng xián]
wind epilepsy: (1) epilepsy with aphasia after seizure; (2) convulsive seizure induced by affection of exogenous wind

惊痫 [jīng xián]
fright epilepsy: epileptic seizure induced by fright

痰痫 [tán xián]
phlegm epilepsy: epileptic seizure caused by phlegm-heat, marked by salivation, phlegmatic sounds in the throat, and mental confusion with the eyes staring straight ahead

寒痫 [hán xián]
cold epilepsy: epileptic seizure predisposed by cold

热痫 [rè xián]
heat epilepsy: epileptic seizure induced by internally accumulated heat

虫痫 [chóng xián]
parasitic epilepsy: epilepsy caused by parasitosis, e.g., cysticercosis

胎痫 [tāi xián]
neonatal epilepsy: epilepsy in a newborn due to injury to it at its fetal stage

瘀血痫 [yū xuè xián]
blood-static epilepsy: epilepsy in children caused by trauma or birth injury

小儿麻痹 [xiǎo ér má bì]
infantile paralysis; poliomyelitis: acute infectious disease characterized by fever, sore throat, and paralysis of the limbs, subsequently with permanent disability and deformity

小儿浮肿 [xiǎo ér fú zhǒng]
edema in children: edema occurring in children mostly 2-7 years old, also called 小儿水肿 [xiǎo ér shuǐ zhǒng]

小儿水肿 [xiǎo ér shuǐ zhǒng]
edema in children: same as 小儿浮肿 [xiǎo ér fú zhǒng]

小儿水气肿 [xiǎo ér shuǐ qì zhǒng]
anasarca in children: generalized edema occurring in children

小儿遗尿 [xiǎo ér yí niào]
enuresis in children; bed-wetting: urinating while asleep, ascribed to inadequacy of genuine *qi* and immaturity of the internal organs in children

遗尿 [yí niào]
enuresis; bed-wetting: urinary incontinence during sleep, mostly occurring in children

兔唇 [tù chún]
harelip: congenital cleft or defect of the upper lip

腭裂 [é liè]
cleft palate: congenital fissure of the palate

侏儒 [zhū rú]
dwarfism: unusual shortness of stature

外科 External Medicine

外证 [wài zhèng]

external disease: collective term for diseases with lesions visible or palpable from without, mostly referring to skin diseases and some surgical conditions

疹 [zhěn]

rash: temporary eruption on the skin, mostly referring to papule

斑 [bān]

macula: general term for any spot or area distinguishable by color from its surroundings

疱疹 [pào zhěn]

vesicle: small circumscribed elevation of the outer layer of the skin enclosing a watery liquid

痂 [jiá]

crust: outer layer of solid matter formed by the drying of a body exudate or secretion

丘疹 [qiū zhěn]

papule: small conical elevation of the skin

脓疱 [nóng pào]

pustule: small circumscribed elevation of the skin containing pus

肿疡 [zhǒng yáng]

swelling (sore): any swelling in an external disease that has not ruptured

溃疡 [kuì yáng]

ulcer: any lesion in an external disease with a local defect of the surface produced by the sloughing of the necrotic tissue

结核 [jié hé]

subcutaneous node: general term for any round mass formed under the skin

疮疡 [chuāng yáng]

sore and ulcer: any pyogenic infection on the body surface

疮 [chuāng]

(I) sore: localized sore spot on the body with the tissues ruptured or abraded and with infection; **(II) wound:** physical injury to the body consisting of laceration or breaking of the skin

疡 [yáng]

(I) ulcer; (II) injury; (III) surgical conditions: general term for surgical conditions on the body surface

肿毒 [zhǒng dú]

toxic swelling: swelling in a pyogenic inflammation

漏 [lòu]

fistula: abnormal passage leading from an abscess or a hollow organ to the body surface

疖 [jiē]

furuncle; boil: localized swelling and inflammation of the skin, having a hard central core, and forming pus

暑疖 [shǔ jiē]
summerheat boil: boil secondary to miliaria or small furuncle, occurring in summer

蝼蛄疖 [lóu gū jiē]
mole cricket boil: multiple abscesses of the scalp, referring to folliculitis abscedens et suffodiens

发际疮 [fà jì chuāng]
hairline boil: boil occurring at the nape close to the hairline

疖病 [jiē bìng]
furunculosis: the condition of tending to develop multiple furuncles

坐板疮 [zuò bǎn chuāng]
seat sore: boil on the buttock

疔 [dīng]
deep-rooted boil: boil with its central core deeply rooted

蛇眼疔 [shé yǎn dīng]
snake-eye whitlow; snake-eye felon: paronychia with inflammation of both sides of a fingernail, resembling the eyes of a snake

蛇头疔 [shé tóu dīng]
snake-head whitlow; snake-head felon: digital pyogenic inflammation of a swollen fingertip, resembling the head of a snake

蛇肚疔 [shé dù dīng]
snake-body whitlow; snake-body felon: digital pyogenic inflammation with swelling of the middle segment of a finger, resembling the body of a snake

托盘疔 [tuō pán dīng]
tray-like palmar infection; palmar pustule: acute pyogenic inflammation of the central part of the palm, making the hand unable to close, with pustule formed in the palm looking like a pearl placed on a tray, also called palmar infection (掌心毒 [zhǎng xīn dú] or 手心毒 [shǒu xīn dú])

掌心毒 [zhǎng xīn dú]
palmar infection; palmar pustule: synonymous with 托盘疔 [tuō pán dīng]

手心毒 [shǒu xīn dú]
palmar infection; palmar pustule: synonymous with 托盘疔 [tuō pán dīng]

足底疔 [zú dǐ dīng]
plantar pustule: acute pyogenic inflammation of the sole of the foot with pustule formation

红丝疔 [hóng sī dīng]
(I) red-streaked boil: boil complicated by acute inflammation of the adjacent lymph vessel or vessels forming a painful red streak or streaks under the skin; **(II) acute lymphangitis:** acute inflammation of the lymph vessel

疫疔 [yì dīng]
pestilent boil; cutaneous anthrax: infectious zoonotic disease transmitted to humans by contact with infected animals, manifested as a small, painless, pruritic papular lesion that enlarges, ulcerates, and becomes crusted with a dense black eschar

烂疔 [làn dīng]
ulcerated gangrene; gas gangrene: acute

severe infection, often occurring in a dirty, lacerated wound, in which the lesion is filled with thin purulent fluid and gas, followed by sloughing of a large amount of necrotic tissue

颜面疔疮 [yán miàn dīng chuāng]
deep-rooted facial boil: deep-rooted furuncle or carbuncle occurring on the face, which may easily progress to pyosepticemia, a critical condition

痈 [yōng]
(I) abscess: pyogenic infection with localized collection of pus buried in tissues or organs; **(II) carbuncle:** necrotizing infection of skin and subcutaneous tissue, composed of a cluster of boils with multiple drainage sinuses

内痈 [nèi yōng]
internal abscess: abscess formed in an internal organ

外痈 [wài yōng]
external abscess: abscess occurring on the body surface

颈痈 [jǐng yōng]
cervical abscess: pyogenic infection with abscess formation at the lateral aspect of the neck

腋痈 [yè yōng]
axillary abscess: pyogenic infection with abscess formation in the axillary region

胯腹痈 [kuà fù yōng]
inguinal abscess: acute pyogenic inflammation in the inguinal region with enlarged painful lymph node and difficulty in walking

委中毒 [wěi zhōng dú]
popliteal sore: acute pyogenic inflammation in the popliteal region with localized stiffness and pain, which causes difficulty in bending and extending the leg

脐痈 [qí yōng]
(I) omphalitis: inflammation of the umbilicus; **(II) umbilical abscess:** acute pyogenic inflammation in the umbilical region with pus collection, usually easy to heal after rupture

脐疮 [qí chuāng]
umbilical sore: acute inflammation in the umbilical region

脐漏 [qí lòu]
umbilical fistula: abnormal passage communicating with the gut or with the urachus at the umbilicus

锁喉痈 [suǒ hóu yōng]
throat-blocking abscess: (1) pyogenic infection of the neck, which causes obstruction of the throat and difficulty in swallowing; (2) abscess at the laryngeal protuberance; also called throat-blocking infection (锁喉毒 [suǒ hóu dú])

锁喉毒 [suǒ hóu dú]
throat-blocking infection: same as throat-blocking abscess (锁喉痈 [suǒ hóu yōng])

丹毒 [dān dú]
erysipelas: acute infection of the skin marked by intense local redness, also called 火丹 [huǒ dān]

火丹 [huǒ dān]
erysipelas: same as 丹毒 [dān dú]

抱头火丹 [bào tóu huǒ dān]
head erysipelas; facial erysipelas: erysipelas that affects the head or face

流火 [liú huǒ]
"flowing fire"; shank erysipelas: erysipelas that effects the leg

赤游丹 [chì yóu dān]
wandering erysipelas: erysipelas in infants characterized by changing the location of the lesion either from the trunk to the extremities or vice versa

无名肿毒 [wú míng zhǒng dú]
innominate toxic swelling: local inflammation that may appear on any part of the body surface, often hard, red and painful

发 [fā]
(I) cellulitis: acute, diffuse and suppurative inflammation of deep subcutaneous tissue; **(II) phlegmon:** diffuse purulent inflammation and infiltration of connective tissue. (In both cases, the lesion is widespread, and hence the name 发 [fā] is given to it, meaning diffuse or diffusion.)

发背 [fā bèi]
dorsal carbuncle: carbuncle occurring on the back

搭手 [dā shǒu]
lumbodorsal carbuncle: carbuncle occurring on the back in a location which the sufferer can reach with a hand

手发背 [shǒu fā bèi]
phlegmon of the dorsum of the hand: acute pyogenic infection of the dorsum of the hand, characterized by diffuse swelling and inflammation, forming a suppurative or gangrenous lesion that may extend into deep subcutaneous tissues and muscles

足发背 [zú fā bèi]
phlegmon of the dorsum of the foot: acute pyogenic infection of the dorsum of the foot with diffuse swelling and inflammation

臀痈 [tún yōng]
gluteal abscess: suppurative inflammation of subcutaneous tissue of the buttock with abscess formation

疽 [jū]
phlegmon; cellulitis: purulent inflammation and infiltration of connective tissue

有头疽 [yǒu tóu jū]
headed phlegmon; carbuncle: necrotizing infection of the skin and subcutaneous tissue with multiple openings for the discharge of pus and sloughing of dead tissue

瘭疽 [biāo jū]
whitlow; felon: an extremely painful suppurative inflammation of a finger or toe near the end or around the nail

发颐 [fā yí]
suppurative parotitis: inflammation of the parotid gland, associated with suppuration

肩胛疽 [jiān jiǎ jū]
scapular cellulitis: cellulitis occurring in the scapular region

股疽 [gǔ jū]
thigh cellulitis: suppurative inflammation

of deep subcutaneous tissue of the thigh

股阴疽 [gǔ yīn jū]
thigh yin cellulitis: cellulitis on the medial aspect of the thigh

股阳疽 [gǔ yáng jū]
thigh yang cellulitis: cellulitis on the lateral aspect of the thigh

流注 [liú zhù]
metastatic abscess: secondary abscess, usually multiple, deeply located, and distant from the primary lesion

髂窝流注 [qià wō liú zhù]
metastatic abscess of the iliac fossa: metastatic abscess occurring in the iliac fossa

无头疽 [wú tóu jū]
deep abscess: pyogenic inflammation located deeply with no color change of the skin surface, usually difficult to rupture and heal

附骨疽 [fù gǔ jū]
bone-attached abscess; suppurative osteomyelitis: suppurative inflammatory bone disease, marked by local death and separation of tissues, occurring on the lateral side of the thigh

咬骨疽 [yǎo gǔ jū]
medial suppurative osteomyelitis: suppurative inflammatory bone disease, marked by local death and separation of tissues, occurring on the medial side of the thigh

环跳疽 [huán tiào jū]
cellulitis at *Huantiao* (GB 30); suppurative coxitis: suppurative inflammation at the hip joint where acupoint *Huantiao* (GB 30) is located

臁疮 [lián chuāng]
shank sore: chronic ulcer on the shank

脱疽 [tuō jū]
digital gangrene: gangrene of the extremities, especially referring to thromboangiitis, also called gangrene of the extremities (脱骨疽 [tuō gǔ jū])

脱骨疽 [tuō gǔ jū]
gangrene of the extremities: synonymous with digital gangrene (脱疽 [tuō jū])

走黄 [zǒu huáng]
pyosepticemia: generalized septicemia in which secondary foci of suppuration occur and multiple abscesses are formed. (走黄 [zǒu huáng] is a popular term derived from the ancient term 癀走 [huáng zǒu], in which 癀 [huáng] means heat toxin, and the whole term means wide spreading of the heat toxin pathogen in the body.)

疔疮走黄 [dīng chuāng zǒu huáng]
deep-rooted boil with pyosepticemia: deep-rooted boil complicated by pyemia or septicemia, cf. 走黄 [zǒu huáng]

内陷 [nèi xiàn]
inward invasion: penetration (of pyogenic toxin) into blood and the internal organs

干陷 [gān xiàn]
non-festering inward invasion: inward invasion marked by impaired consciousness and collapse but scanty suppuration of the pyogenic lesion

火陷 [huǒ xiàn]
inward invasion of fire: inward invasion with penetration of fire toxin into the nutrient aspect, manifested by high fever, thirst, restlessness and delirium associated with the dark-colored and dehydrated inflamed lesion

疮毒内陷 [chuāng dú nèi xiàn]
inward invasion of sore toxin: penetration of pyogenic toxin into the blood and internal organs, resulting in generalized pyogenic infection

瘰疬 [luǒ lì]
scrofula: chronic inflammation or tuberculosis of the cervical lymph node

流痰 [liú tán]
"flowing phlegm": tuberculosis of bone or joint, also known as bone phthisis (骨痨 [gǔ láo]) and phthisis sore (疮痨 [chuāng láo]). (Pus formed in the lesion is as thin as phlegm and often flows to other places, hence 流痰 [liú tán] is the name given to it. 流 [liú] means flow and 痰 [tán], phlegm.)

骨痨 [gǔ láo]
bone phthisis: tuberculosis of bone or joint, same as "flowing phlegm" (流痰 [liú tán])

疮痨 [chuāng láo]
phthisis sore: tuberculosis of bone or joint, same as "flowing phlegm" (流痰 [liú tán])

乳头破碎 [rǔ tóu pò suì]
cracked nipple: ailment of the nipple characterized by painful fissuring, bleeding and exudation, also called nipple wind (乳头风 [rǔ tóu fēng])

乳头风 [rǔ tóu fēng]
nipple wind: synonymous with cracked nipple (乳头破碎 [rǔ tóu pò suì])

乳痈 [rǔ yōng]
acute mastitis: acute pyogenic inflammation of the breast

内吹乳痈 [nèi chuī rǔ yōng]
"internal blowing" mastitis; pregnancy mastitis: mastitis occurring during pregnancy, also called 内吹 [nèi chuī] which means internal blowing (so called because such mastitis was originally considered to be the consequence of wind blowing on the breast from inside due to movement of the fetus)

内吹 [nèi chuī]
"internal blowing": abbreviation for "internal blowing" mastitis (内吹乳痈 [nèi chuī rǔ yōng])

外吹乳痈 [wài chuī rǔ yōng]
"external blowing" mastitis; puerperal mastitis: mastitis occurring after delivery, also called 外吹 [wài chuī] which means external blowing (so called because such mastitis was originally considered to be attributed to wind blowing on the breast due to the breathing of the infant)

外吹 [wài chuī]
"external blowing": abbreviation for "external blowing" mastitis (外吹乳痈 [wài chuī rǔ yōng])

乳发 [rǔ fā]
phlegmonous mastitis: inflammation of

the breast leading to necrosis and abscess formation

乳疽 [rǔ jū]
intramammary abscess: acute mastitis characterized by early formation of abscess and rupture

乳痨 [rǔ láo]
mammary phthisis: tuberculosis of the breast, also called mammary phlegm (乳痰 [rǔ tán])

乳痰 [rǔ tán]
mammary phlegm: another name for mammary phthisis (乳痨 [rǔ láo]), so called because of the discharged thin pus resembling phlegm

乳漏 [rǔ lòu]
mammary fistula: abnormal passage between the mammary duct and the cutaneous surface of the breast or the areola of the nipple

乳癖 [rǔ pǐ]
mammary hyperplasia: presence of nodular masses in the breast, painful, movable and not firm, often related to the menstrual cycle and emotional change

乳中结核 [rǔ zhōng jié hé]
nodule in the breast: benign tumor of the breast, usually referring to fibro-adenoma of the mammary gland, often abbreviated as breast nodule (乳核 [rǔ hé])

乳核 [rǔ hé]
breast nodule: abbreviation for nodule in the breast (乳中结核 [rǔ zhōng jié hé])

乳疬 [rǔ lì]
(I) gynecomastia: excessive development of the breast in males; **(II) mastauxy in children:** enlargement of the breast in children

乳衄 [rǔ nǜ]
thelorrhagia: bleeding from the nipple

瘿 [yǐng]
goiter: enlargement of the thyroid gland, causing a swelling on the front part of the neck

气瘿 [qì yǐng]
***qi* goiter:** goiter due to emotional depression or geographical factors, mainly referring to simple goiter or endemic goiter

肉瘿 [ròu yǐng]
fleshy goiter: goiter soft or beefy, often accompanied by irritability, palpitations, discomfort in the chest, or menstrual disorder, mostly referring to the thyroid enlargement in Graves' disease or adenoma of the thyroid gland

石瘿 [shí yǐng]
stony goiter: enlarged thyroid, nodulated and as hard as stone, mostly referring to carcinoma of the thyroid

筋瘿 [jīn yǐng]
goiter with varicose veins: goiter with prominent varicose veins

瘿痈 [yǐng yōng]
thyroiditis: acute inflammation of the thyroid gland, with mass formation, swelling, heat and pain

瘤 [liú]

tumor: neoplasm which persists and has no physiological use, often caused by stagnant blood, retained phlegm, and lingering turbid *qi*

气瘤 [qì liú]

***qi* tumor:** term for multiple pedunculated soft tumors arising superficially under the skin, becoming flat on pressing and bulging again when the pressure is removed as if they were filled with air (*qi*), mostly referring to neurofibroma

血瘤 [xuè liú]

blood tumor; hemangioma: vascular tumor composed of dilated blood vessels in the skin or subcutaneously, including capillary hemangioma and cavernous hemangioma

肉瘤 [ròu liú]

fat tumor; lipoma: tumor of subcutaneous fatty tissue

筋瘤 [jīn liú]

sinew tumor; varix: dilated and tortuous vein, usually in the leg

骨瘤 [gǔ liú]

bone tumor; osteoma: benign tumor composed of bone tissue

脂瘤 [zhī liú]

sebaceous cyst: cyst derived from the sebaceous gland, filled with lipid-rich debris, also called 粉瘤 [fěn liú]

粉瘤 [fěn liú]

sebaceous cyst: same as 脂瘤 [zhī liú]

岩 [yán]

cancer; carcinoma: malignant tumor palpable on the body surface, hard and unsmooth like a rock, a homograph of 岩 [yán], which means rock

舌菌 [shé jūn]

tongue cancer: carcinoma of the tongue, also called 舌岩 [shé yán]

舌岩 [shé yán]

carcinoma of the tongue: same as tongue cancer (舌菌 [shé jūn])

茧唇 [jiǎn chún]

lip cancer: carcinoma of the lip

失荣 [shī róng]

cervical malignancy with cachexia: advanced case of malignant tumor of the cervical lymph node, either primary or metastatic, accompanied by cachexia

乳岩 [rǔ yán]

mammary cancer: malignant tumor occurring in the breast

肾岩 [shèn yán]

penial cancer: carcinoma of the penis, also known as carcinoma of the penis (肾癌 [shèn ái])

肾癌 [shènái]

carcinoma of the penis: same as penial cancer (肾岩 [shèn yán])

肾岩翻花 [shèn yán fān huā]

carcinoma of the penis with ulceration

痔 [zhì]

hemorrhoid; pile: varicose dilatation of a

vein of the superior or inferior hemorrhoidal plexus

内痔 [nèi zhì]
internal hemorrhoid: varicose dilatation of a vein of the superior hemorrhoidal plexus, situated above the pectinate line

外痔 [wài zhì]
external hemorrhoid: varicose dilatation of a vein of the inferior hemorrhoidal plexus, situated distal to the pectinate line

内外痔 [nèi wài zhì]
mixed hemorrhoid: varicose dilatation of a vein connecting the superior and inferior hemorrhoidal plexuses, forming an external and an internal hemorrhoid in continuity

血箭痔 [xuè jiàn zhì]
blood-spurting hemorrhoid: internal hemorrhoid with massive bleeding

脱肛 [tuō gāng]
prolapse of the rectum: protrusion of the rectal mucous membrane through the anus

肛漏 [gāng lòu]
anal fistula: fistula opening on the cutaneous surface near the anus, which may communicate with the rectum, also called 肛瘘 [gāng lòu]

肛瘘 [gāng lòu]
anal fistula: same as 肛漏 [gāng lòu]

肛裂 [gāng liè]
anal fissure: painful linear ulcer at the margin of the anus

肛痈 [gāng yōng]
anorectal abscess: abscess arising in the anorectum

息肉痔 [xī ròu zhì]
rectal polyp: polyp of the rectum

肠痔 [cháng zhì]
perianal abscess: superficial abscess occurring beneath the perianal skin

交肠 [jiāo cháng]
rectovesical fistula: fistula between the rectum and urinary bladder

子痈 [zǐ yōng]
testicular abscess: inflammatory infection of the testis and epididymis marked by local pain and swelling, referring to epididymitis and orchitis

囊痈 [náng yōng]
scrotal abscess: acute pyogenic inflammation of the scrotum

子痰 [zǐ tán]
tuberculosis of epididymis: tuberculosis involving the epididymis which gradually increase in size, suppurates, and ruptures to discharge thin purulent fluid resembling phlegm

水疝 [shuǐ shàn]
hydrocele: accumulation of fluid in the testicle

精浊 [jīng zhuó]
seminal turbidity: inflammatory disease of male genital organs marked by frequent discharge of turbid secretion from the urethra, referring to prostitis, gonorrhea or seminal vesiculitis

精癃 [jīng lóng]
prostatic hypertrophy: hypertrophy of the prostate that causes difficulty in urination or retention of urine

睾丸萎缩 [gāo wán wěi suō]
testicular atrophy: atropy of the testis

睾丸肿痛 [gāo wán zhǒng tòng]
painful and swollen testis: pain and swelling of the testis

偏坠 [piān zhuì]
hemilateral sagging: unilateral swelling of the testis which is often accompanied by a bearing-down pain

热疮 [rè chuāng]
heat sore; herpes febrilis: herpes simplex usually occurring as a concomitant of fever

蛇串疮 [shé chuàn chuāng]
herpes zoster: acute eruptive disease characterized by severe pain along the girdled distribution of clustered vesicles, also called zoster (缠腰火丹 [chán yāo huǒ dān] or 缠腰蛇丹 [chán yāo shé dān]) and shingles (火带疮 [huǒ dài chuāng])

缠腰火丹 [chán yāo huǒ dān]
zoster: another name for herpes zoster (蛇串疮[shé chuàn chuāng])

缠腰蛇丹 [chán yāo shé dān]
zoster: another name for herpes zoster (蛇串疮[shé chuàn chuāng])

火带疮 [huǒ dài chuāng]
shingles: another name for herpes zoster (蛇串疮[shé chuàn chuāng])

蛇丹 [shé dān]
zoster: another name for herpes zoster (蛇串疮[shé chuàn chuāng])

疣 [yóu]
wart; verruca: horny projection on the skin

瘊子 [hóu zi]
wart: popular name for verruca (疣 [yóu])

疣目 [yóu mù]
wart eye; verruca vulgaris: lobulated hyperplastic epidermal lesion with a horny surface, usually occurring on the back of the hand, fingers or scalp

扁瘊 [biǎn hóu]
flat wart; verruca plana: small, smooth, slightly raised wart, occurring on the face, back of the hands, or wrists

跖疣 [zhí yóu]
plantar wart; verruca plantaris: wart on the sole of the foot

鼠乳 [shǔ rǔ]
"mouse nipple"; molluscum contagiosum: small papular, umbilicated skin lesion transmitted by contact, containing white cheese-like substance, and usually occurring on the trunk or face

丝状疣 [sī zhuàng yóu]
verruca filiformis: wart with soft, thin, threadlike projections on its surface, also called filiform wart (线瘊 [xiàn hóu])

线瘊 [xiàn hóu]
filiform wart: another name for verruca filiformis (丝状疣 [sī zhuàng yóu]

趼子 [jiǎn zi]
callus: popular name for 胼胝 [piàn zhī]

胼胝 [pián zhī]
(I) callus: hard thickened area on the skin;
(II) callosity: state of being callous

鸡眼 [jī yǎn]
clavus; corn: small area of hard thickened skin on the foot, especially the toe, sometimes painful, also called 肉刺 [ròu cì]

肉刺 [ròu cì]
clavus; corn: same as 鸡眼 [jī yǎn]

皴揭 [cūn jiē]
chap: crack in or sore roughening of the skin, also called rhagas (皲裂 [jūn liè])

皲裂 [jūn liè]
rhagas: synonymous with chap (皴揭 [cūn jiē])

皲裂疮 [jūn liè chuāng]
rhagades: linear cracks or fissures in the skin, especially such lesions around the mouth or other regions subjected to frequent movement

痱（子） [fèi (zi)]
miliaria; prickly heat: inflammatory disorder of the skin characterized by redness, eruption, and itching due to blockage of sweat ducts

粉刺 [fěn cì]
acne: inflammatory disease of the follicles and sebaceous glands, occurring on the face, chest and back, also known as 酒刺 [jiǔ cì]

酒刺 [jiǔ cì]
acne: sama as 粉刺 [fěn cì]

雀斑 [què bān]
freckle: small brown spot in the skin

血缕 [xuè lǚ]
vascular spider; spider nevus: red area on the skin formed of dilated capillaries or arterioles radiating from a central point like the legs of a spider

酒皶鼻 [jiǔ zhā bí]
brandy nose; rosacea: chronic hyperemic disease of the skin, usually involving the middle part of the face, particularly the nose, also known as red nose 赤鼻[chì bí]

赤鼻 [chì bí]
red nose: another name for rosacea (酒皶鼻 [jiǔ zhā bí])

瓜藤缠 [guā téng chán]
erythema nodosum: panniculitis which most often affects young women and is characterized by the development of crops of transient, inflammatory nodules that are usually tender, multiple, and bilateral, most commonly located on the shin as if the latter were wound by melon vines (瓜藤[guā téng])

猫眼疮 [māo yǎn chuāng]
erythema multiforme: acute self-limited inflammatory skin disease characterized by the sudden onset of an erythematous, macular, bullous, papular, nodose, or vesicular eruption resembling the cat's eye

红蝴蝶疮 [hóng hú dié chuāng]
lupus erythematosus: a systemic or non-

systemic disease marked by butterfly rash

皮痹 [pí bì]
skin numbness: disease marked by numbness of the skin accompanied by an abnormal sensation resembling that made by insects creeping in or on the skin

白癜风 [bái diàn fēng]
vitiligo: skin disease manifested by smooth white spots on various parts of the body, also called 白驳风 [bái bó fēng]

白驳风 [bái bó fēng]
vitiligo: same as 白癜风 [bái diàn fēng]

白屑风 [bái xiè fēng]
seborrhea sicca: scaly seborrheic dermatitis

牛皮癣 [niú pí xuǎn]
neurodermatitis: chronic disorder of the skin characterized by patches of itching lichenoid eruption resembling cattlehide, and hence the Chinese term which literally means oxhide lichen, also known as stubborn lichen (顽癣 [wán xuǎn]) because of its chronicity

摄领疮 [shè lǐng chuāng]
cervical neurodermatitis: neurodermatitis occurring on the nape and neck

顽癣 [wán xuǎn]
stubborn lichen: another name for neurodermatitis (牛皮癣 [niú pí xuǎn])

风热疮 [fēng rè chuāng]
wind-heat sore; pityriasis rosea: acute or subacute, self-limited exanthematous disease, the onset of which is marked by the presence of a solitary rose-colored herald plaque, most often seen on the trunk, followed by the development of papular or macular lesions which have vesicular borders subsequently that tend to peel and produce a scaly collarette, also known as wind itch (风痒 [fēng yǎng])

风痒 [fēng yǎng]
wind itch: another name for wind-heat sore or pityriasis rosea (风热疮 [fēng rè chuāng])

白疕 [bái bì]
psoriasis: chronic skin disease marked by round, circumscribed, erythematous, dry, scaling patches, covered by silvery white, lamellar scales, resembling the bark of a pine tree, and hence the Chinese term which literally means white crust, also called pine-bark lichen (松皮癣 [sōng pí xuǎn])

松皮癣 [sōng pí xuǎn]
pine-bark lichen: another name for psoriasis (白疕 [bái bì])

面游风 [miàn yóu fēng]
seborrhea; seborrheic dermatitis: chronic inflammation of the skin marked by excessive secretion of sebum

发落 [fà luò]
alopecia: disease causing the hair to fall

发蛀脱发 [fà zhù tuō fà]
alopecia seborrheica: alopecia associated with seborrheic dermatitis

斑秃 [bān tū]
alopecia areata: patchy loss of hair, occurring in sharply defined areas

油风 [yóu fēng]
alopecia: disease marked by sudden patchy loss of hair, which usually occurs in sharply defined areas, referring to alopecia areata (斑秃 [bān tū]), but may involve the whole scalp and the beard

疥疮 [jiè chuāng]
scabies: contagious skin disease caused by mite, also called 疥癞 [jiè lài]

疥癞 [jiè lài]
scabies: same as 疥疮 [jiè chuāng]

风团 [fēng tuán]
wheal: suddenly formed itching elevation of the skin surface

风瘙痒 [fēng sào yǎng]
wind pruritus: generalized itching of the skin with sudden onset

隐［瘾］疹 [yǐn zhěn]
urticaria; hives: allergic disorder of the skin, marked by red or pale wheals, on and off, and usually by intense itching, also known as 风瘾疹 [fēng yǐn zhěn]

风瘾疹 [fēng yǐn zhěn]
urticaria: same as 隐疹 [yǐn zhěn]

虫咬皮炎 [chóng yǎo pí yán]
insect dermatitis: dermatitis caused by insect bite or the toxin-containing irritant hairs of certain insects

接触性皮炎 [jiē chù xìng pí yán]
contact dermatitis: dermatitis caused by substances coming in contact with the skin

漆疮 [qī chuāng]
lacquer dermatitis: contact dermatitis produced by lacquer

膏药风 [gāo yào fēng]
plaster dermatitis: contact dermatitis caused by the application of adhesive plaster

药毒 [yào dú]
(I) dermatitis medicamentosa; drug eruption: adverse cutaneous reaction produced by ingestion or local application of a drug; **(II) medicinal toxicity:** the toxic quality of a drug

湿疮 [shī chuāng]
eczema: inflammatory skin disease characterized by symmetrical distribution, itching, vesiculation, watery discharge, and the development of scales and crusts, also called 湿疹 [shī zhěn]

湿疹 [shī zhěn]
eczema: same as 湿疮 [shī chuāng]

旋耳疮 [xuán ěr chuāng]
auricular eczema: eczema occurring in the auricular region

四弯风 [sì wān fēng]
cubito-popliteal eczema: eczema occurring in the cubital and popliteal fossae

肾囊风 [shèn náng fēng]
scrotal eczema: eczema of the scrotum

脐疮 [qí chuāng]
umbilical eczema: eczema occurring in the umbilical region

浸淫疮 [jìn yín chuāng]
exudative eczema: eczema in the acute

stage characterized by erythema associated with serous exudate

婴儿湿疮 [yīng ér shī chuāng]
infantile eczema: eczema common in infants, which usually occurs on the cheeks and then may extend to other areas, also called milk lichen (奶癣 [nǎi xuǎn])

奶癣 [nǎi xuǎn]
milk lichen: another name for infantile eczema (婴儿湿疮 [yīng ér shī chuāng])

湿癣 [shī xuǎn]
damp lichen: dermatitis marked by itching and exudation, mostly referring to acute eczema

脚湿气 [jiǎo shī qì]
tinea pedis: tinea involving the feet, also known as 脚气疮 [jiǎo qì chuāng]

脚气疮 [jiǎo qì chuāng]
tinea pedis: same as 脚湿气 [jiǎo shī qì]

黄水疮 [huáng shuǐ chuāng]
yellow-water sore; impetigo: contagious pyoderma which is usually seen in children and is characterized by discrete fragile vesicles that become pustular, and rupture to discharge a thin yellow seropurulent fluid

癣 [xuǎn]
ringworm; tinea: superficial fungal infection caused by a dermatophyte and involving the skin, hair and nails

白秃疮 [bái tū chuāng]
white bald scalp sore; tinea alba; white ringworm: ringworm of the scalp, manifested by multiple whitish or gray scaly lesions, and abbreviated as bald scalp sore (秃疮 [tū chuāng]) or white bald (白秃 [bái tū])

秃疮 [tū chuāng]
bald scalp sore: abbreviation for white bald scalp sore (白秃疮 [bái tū chuāng]), referring to white ringworm

白秃 [bái tū]
white bald: abbreviation for white bald scalp sore (白秃疮 [bái tū chuāng])

肥疮 [féi chuāng]
fat sore; tinea favosa; favus: ringworm characterized by formation of yellow cup-shaped crusts

圆癣 [yuán xuǎn]
round ringworm; tinea circinata: tinea involving glabrous skin areas other than hands and feet, characterized by one or more well-demarcated erythematous, scaly macules with raised borders, producing annular outlines, also called tinea corparis (风癣 [fēng xuǎn])

风癣 [fēng xuǎn]
tinea corporis: synonymous with round ringworm or tinea circinata (圆癣 [yuán xuǎn])

股癣 [gǔ xuǎn]
tinea cruris: tinea in the groin or perineal area

鹅掌风 [é zhǎng fēng]
tinea manuum: ringworm affecting the interdigital spaces and palmar surfaces of the hands

鹅爪风 [é zhuǎ fēng]
tinea unguium: ringworm affecting the nails and causing them opaque, white, thickened and brittle

马桶癣 [mǎ tǒng xuǎn]
chamber-pot dermatitis: contact dermatitis of buttocks

干癣 [gān xuǎn]
dry ringworm: chronic skin disease characterized by clearly circumscribed thickening of the skin, fissuring, itching and scaling, mostly referring to (1) chronic eczema, (2) neurodermatitis

紫白癜风 [zǐ bái diàn fēng]
tinea versicolor: skin disorder characterized by multiple macular patches, of all sizes and shapes, varying from white in pigmented skin to tan or brown in pale skin

腋臭 [yè chòu]
armpit odor; hircismus: strong odor of the axillae caused by apocrine sweat, also called foxy odor (狐臭 [hú chòu])

狐臭 [hú chòu]
foxy odor: synonymous with armpit odor (腋臭 [yè chòu])

麻风 [má fēng]
leprosy: chronic infectious disease characterized by the formation of nodules on the surface of the body and especially on the face, accompanied by loss of sensation of the infected area, also called 大风 [dà fēng], 疠风 [lì fēng], 癞病 [lài bìng]

大风 [dà fēng]
leprosy: same as 麻风 [má fēng]

疠风 [lì fēng]
leprosy: same as 麻风 [má fēng]

癞病 [lài bìng]
leprosy: same as 麻风 [má fēng]

烧伤 [shāo shāng]
burn: injury to tissue caused by contact with fire, also called 火伤 [huǒ shāng]

火伤 [huǒ shāng]
burn: same as 烧伤 [shāo shāng]

金疮 [jīn chuāng]
incised wound: wound made by a knife or other cutting tools, also called 金创 [jīn chuàng]

金创 [jīn chuàng]
incised wound: same as 金疮 [jīn chuāng]

破伤风 [pò shāng fēng]
tetanus: acute, often fatal disease caused by toxic wind pathogen introduced through a wound, manifested by lockjaw, glottal spasm, generalized muscle spasm, opisthotonos and respiratory spasm, also called 金疮痉 [jīn chuāng jìng]

金疮痉 [jīn chuāng jìng]
tetanus: another name for 破伤风 [pò shāng fēng]

冻疮 [dòng chuāng]
chilblain; frostbite: inflammatory swelling or sore caused by exposure to cold, also called 冻风 [dòng fēng]

冻风 [dòng fēng]
chilblain; frostbite: same as 冻疮 [dòng chuāng]

褥疮 [rù chuāng]
bedsore; decubitus ulcer: ulceration caused by prolonged pressure, usually occurring in a patient allowed to lie in bed for a long period of time, circumscribed to the areas that hold the pressue, also called 席疮 [xí chuāng]

席疮 [xí chuāng]
bedsore: ancient term for 褥疮 [rù chuāng]

青蛇毒 [qīng shé dú]
blue snake toxin sore; superficial thrombophlebitis: inflammation of a superficial vein at the calf associated with thrombus formation, resembling a blue snake lying on the leg

股肿 [gǔ zhǒng]
thigh swelling; deep thrombophlebitis: thrombus formation and inflammation of a deep-located vein of the thigh

毒蛇咬伤 [dú shé yǎo shāng]
venomous snake bite: wound and intoxication made by a venomous snake's bite

毒虫咬伤 [dú chóng yǎo shāng]
insect bite: wound and intoxication made by a poisonous insect's bite

眼科 Ophthalmology

眼科（学）[yǎn kē (xué)]
ophthalmology: branch of medicine that studies the eye and its diseases

五轮 [wǔ lún]
five orbiculi: collective term for eyelid, canthus, white of the eye, black of the eye and pupil. A theory of ophthalmology holds that each *zang* organ is physio-pathologically associated with a different orbiculus (cf. 肉轮 [ròu lún], 血轮 [xuè lún], 气轮 [qì lún], 风轮 [fēng lún]，水轮 [shuǐ lún])

肉轮 [ròu lún]
flesh orbiculus: eyelid, one of the five orbiculi which is believed to be strongly associated with the spleen

血轮 [xuè lún]
blood orbiculus: canthus, one of the five orbiculi which is believed to be strongly associated with the heart

气轮 [qì lún]
***qi* orbiculus:** white of the eye, one of the five orbiculi which is believed to be strongly associated with the lung

风轮 [fēng lún]
wind orbiculus: black of the eye, one of the five orbiculi which is believed to bestrongly associated with the liver

水轮 [shuǐ lún]
water orbiculus: pupil, one of the five orbiculi which is believed to be strongly associated with the kidney

八廓 [bā kuò]
eight regions of the eye: ancient hypothesis of dividing the eye into eight regions, each of which is thought to be strongly associated with a particular internal organ pathologically. This hypothesis has been abandoned due to controversies over location of the regions and determination of their relationship with the internal organs.

眼睑 [yǎn jiǎn]
palpebra; eyelid: either of the two movable folds of the eye that can be closed over the eyeball, also called 胞睑 [bāo jiǎn], 目胞 [mù bāo] or 目裹 [mù guǒ]

胞睑 [bāo jiǎn]
palpebra; eyelid: same as 眼睑 [yǎn jiǎn]

目胞 [mù bāo]
palpebra; eyelid: same as 眼睑 [yǎn jiǎn]

目裹 [mù guǒ]
palpebra; eyelid: same as 眼睑 [yǎn jiǎn]

目眦 [mù zì]
canthus: corner of the eye formed by the meeting of the upper and lower eyelids

眦 [zì]
abbreviation for 目眦 [mù zì]

目锐眦 [mù ruì zì]
lateral canthus: lateral corner of the eye,

also called 锐眦 [ruì zì] or outer canthus (目外眦 [mù wài zì] or 外眦 [wài zì])

锐眦 [ruì zì]
lateral canthus: same as 目锐眦 [mù ruì zì]

目外眦 [mù wài zì]
outer canthus: same as lateral canthus (目锐眦 [mù ruì zì])

外眦 [wài zì]
outer canthus: same as lateral canthus (目锐眦 [mù ruì zì]), also called small canthus (小眦 [xiǎo zì])

目内眦 [mù nèi zì]
inner canthus; medial canthus: medial corner of the eye, also called 内眦 [neì zì] or big canthus (大眦 [dà zì])

内眦 [nèi zì]
inner canthus; medial canthus: same as 目内眦 [mù nèi zì]

大眦 [dà zì]
big canthus: another name for inner canthus or medial canthus (内眦 [nèi zì])

小眦 [xiǎo zì]
small canthus: another name for outer canthus (外眦 [wài zì])

目眶 [mù kuàng]
eye socket; orbit: bony cavity that encloses and protects the eye

目眶骨 [mù kuàng gǔ]
orbit bone: bone forming the eye socket

目纲 [mù gāng]
tarsi of the eyelid: plates forming the framework of the eyelid

目上纲 [mù shàng gāng]
upper palpebral musculature: muscles controlling the upper eyelid, chiefly referring to the superior tarsal muscle, also called 目上网 [mù shàng wǎng]

目上网 [mù shàng wǎng]
upper palpebral musculature: same as 目上纲 [mù shàng gāng]

目下纲 [mù xià gāng]
lower palpebral musculature: muscles controlling the lower eyelid, chiefly referring to the inferior tarsal muscle

目下网 [mù xià wǎng]
lower palpebral musculature: same as 目下纲[mù xià gāng]

睑弦 [jiǎn xián]
palpebral margin: edge of the free margin of eyelid, from which the eyelashes arise, also called margin of the eyelid (目弦 [mù xián])

目弦 [mù xián]
margin of the eyelid: same as palpebral margin (睑弦 [jiǎn xián])

上睑 [shàng jiǎn]
upper eyelid: the superior of the paired movable folds that protect the anterior surface of the eyeball, also called 目上胞 [mù shàng bāo]

目上胞 [mù shàng bāo]
upper eyelid: same as 上睑 [shàng jiǎn]

目上弦 [mù shàng xián]
upper eyelid margin: margin of the upper eyelid

下睑 [xià jiǎn]
lower eyelid: the inferior of the paired movable folds that protect the anterior surface of the eyeball, also called 目下胞 [mù xià bāo]

目下胞 [mù xià bāo]
lower eyelid: same as 下睑 [xià jiǎn]

目下弦 [mù xià xián]
lower eyelid margin: margin of the lower eyelid

睑内 [jiǎn nèi]
palpebral conjunctiva: membrane that lines the inner side of the eyelid

白睛 [bái jīng]
white of the eye: the white part of the eyeball, also called white kernel (白仁 [bái rén]) or 白珠 [bái zhū]

白仁 [bái rén]
white kernel: another name for the white of the eye (白睛 [bái jīng])

白珠 [bái zhū]
white of the eye: same as 白睛 [bái jīng]

泪泉 [lèi quán]
lacrimal gland: gland that secretes tears

泪窍 [lèi qiào]
lacrimal punctum: opening of the lacrimal duct at the inner canthus of the eye, also called 泪堂 [lèi táng] or 泪点 [lèi diǎn]

泪堂 [lèi táng]
lacrimal punctum: same as 泪窍 [lèi qiào]

泪点 [lèi diǎn]
lacrimal point: same as lacrimal punctum (泪窍 [lèi qiào])

黑睛 [hēi jīng]
dark of the eye: the central anterior part of the eye, referring to the cornea

瞳神 [tóng shén]
(I) pupil: opening at the center of the iris of the eye; **(II) pupil and intra-ocular tissues**

瞳子 [tóng zǐ]
pupil: same as 瞳神 [tóng shén]

瞳人 [tóng rén]
pupil: same as 瞳神 [tóng shén]

瞳仁 [tóng rén]
pupil: same as 瞳神 [tóng shén]

金井 [jīn jǐng]
pupil: another name for 瞳神 [tóng shén] (金井 [jīn jǐng] literally means metallic well. It is so called because the pupil resembles a well with aqueous humor at the bottom, and metal generates water according to the five-element/phase theory.)

睛帘 [jīng lián]
iris: muscular membrane suspended in front of the lens of the eye, also called 虹彩 [hóng cǎi]

虹彩 [hóng cǎi]
iris: another name for 睛帘 [jīng lián]

黄仁 [huáng rén]
yellow kernel: traditional name for iris

神水 [shén shuǐ]
(I) aqueous humor: fluid produced in the eye, occupying the space between the crystalline lens and cornea; **(II) tears:** watery secretion of the lacrimal glands which serves to moisten the conjunctiva

精珠 [jīng zhū]
lens: transparent lens-shaped body in the eye, also called crystalline lens (晶珠 [jīng zhū]) or yellowish lens (黄精 [huángjīng])

晶珠 [jīng zhū]
crystalline lens: another name for lens of the eye (精珠 [jīng zhū])

黄精 [huáng jīng]
yellowish lens: another name for lens of the eye (精珠 [jīng zhū])

神膏 [shén gāo]
vitreous: clear colorless transparent jelly that fills the eyeball

视衣 [shì yī]
coats of the eyeball; chorioretina: choroid and retina of the eye

目珠 [mù zhū]
eyeball: round part of the eye within the eyelids and socket, also called 眼珠 [yǎn zhū]

眼珠 [yǎn zhū]
eyeball: same as 目珠 [mù zhū]

眼带 [yǎn dài]
extra-ocular muscles: muscles that move the eyeball

目系 [mù xì]
ocular connector: cord connecting the eye with the brain, including the ocular nerves and blood vessels associated with the eye, also called 眼系 [yǎn xì] or 目本 [mù běn]

眼系 [yǎn xì]
ocular connector: same as 目系 [mù xì]

目本 [mù běn]
ocular connector: same as 目系 [mù xì]

羞明 [xiū míng]
photophobia: abnormal fear of light, also called 畏明 [wèi míng] or 羞明畏日 [xiū míng wèi rì]

畏明 [wèi míng]
photophobia: same as 羞明 [xiū míng]

羞明畏日 [xiū míng wèi rì]
photophobia: same as 羞明 [xiū míng]

目痛 [mù tòng]
eye pain: pain of the eye, one of the common symptoms indicating an eye disease

目眵 [mù chī]
eye gum: secretion of the eye, thin or mucilaginous or even pus-like, often occurring in external ocular diseases, abbreviated as gum (眵 [chī])

眵 [chī]
gum (in the eyes): abbreviation for eye gum 目眵 [mù chī]

眵泪 [chī lèi]
eye gum and tears: secretion of the eye mixed with tears

眵泪胶粘 [chī lèi jiāo nián]
sticky eye gum and tears: mucopurulent secretion of the eye mixed with tears

迎风流泪 [yíng fēng liú lèi]
lacrimination induced by wind: abnormal or excessive secretion of tears induced by exposure to wind

迎风冷泪 [yíng fēng lěng lèi]
cold tear shedding induced by wind: abnormal or excessive secretion of cold tears, often due to deficiency of *qi*-blood or of the liver and kidney

迎风热泪 [yíng fēng rè lèi]
warm tear shedding induced by wind: abnormal or excessive secretion of warm tears, often seen in inflammatory external ophthalmopathies

不时泪溢 [bù shí lèi yì]
watering of the eyes from time to time; epiphora: watering of the eyes due to excessive secretion of tears or to obstruction of lacrimal passages

白睛红赤 [bái jīng hóng chì]
redness of the white of the eye; hyperemia of the bulbar conjunctiva: increased blood flow in the bulbar conjunctiva, also called turbid redness of the white of the eye (白睛混赤 [bái jīng hún chì])

白睛混赤 [bái jīng hún chì]
turbid redness of the white of the eye: same as redness of the white of the eye or hyperemia of the bulbar conjunctiva (白睛红赤 [bái jīng hóng chì])

白睛暴赤 [bái jīng bào chì]
sudden redness of the bulbar conjunctiva: sudden onset of hyperemia of the bulbar conjunctiva

白睛浮壅 [bái jīng fú yōng]
chemosis: swelling of the conjunctival tissue around the cornea

白睛赤肿 [bái jīng chì zhǒng]
redness and swelling of the bulbar conjunctiva: hyperemia with swelling of the bulbar conjunctiva

白睛涩痛 [bái jīng sè tòng]
irritation and pain of the bulbar conjunctiva: irritation and pain of the conjunctival tissue around the cornea

抱轮红赤 [bào lún hóng chì]
ciliary hyperemia: redness of the bulbar conjunctiva surrounding the ciliary body, also called 白睛抱红 [bái jīng bào hóng] or 赤带抱轮 [chì dài bào lún]

白睛抱红 [bái jīng bào hóng]
ciliary hyperemia: same as 抱轮红赤 [bào lún hóng chì]

赤带抱轮 [chì dài bào lún]
ciliary hyperemia: same as 抱轮红赤 [bào lún hóng chì]

赤脉传睛 [chì mài chuán jīng]
red vessels passing the eye; angular conjunctivitis: conjunctivitis with reddening at the canthus and spreading

to the white of the eye, and sometimes stretching to the dark of the eye, also called red vessels crossing the eye (赤脉贯睛 [chì mài guàn jīng]) or red vessels invading the eye (赤脉侵睛 [chì mài qīn jīng])

赤脉贯睛 [chì mài guàn jīng]
red vessels crossing the eye; angular conjunctivitis: same as 赤脉传睛 [chì mài chuán jīng]

赤脉侵睛 [chì mài qīn jīng]
red vessels invading the eye; angular conjunctivitis: same as 赤脉传睛 [chì mài chuán jīng]

结膜红赤 [jié mó hóng chì]
conjunctival hyperemia: redness of the palpebral conjunctiva

障 [zhàng]
vision obstruction; ophthalmopathy: general term for any disease of the eye causing visual disturbance

外障 [wài zhàng]
external ophthalmopathy: any of the external ocular diseases

内障 [nèi zhàng]
internal ophthalmopathy: any of the internal ocular diseases

目盲 [mù máng]
blindness: lack or loss of the ability to see, also called 盲 [máng]

盲 [máng]
blindness: same as 目盲 [mù máng]

赤膜 [chì mó]
red membrane; pannus: red membranous vascular tissue causing a superficial opacity of the cornea, also called 红膜 [hóng mó]

红膜 [hóng mó]
red membrane; pannus: same as 赤膜 [chì mó]

翳 [yì]
nebula: cloudy opacity of the cornea which may impair the vision to different degrees depending upon the location of the opaque area

新翳 [xīn yì]
fresh nebula: newly developed opacity of the cornea with the formation of a coarse surface and indistinct margins, tending to further development

宿翳 [sù yì]
chronic corneal opacity: opacity of the cornea with a smooth surface and clear-cut margins, usually due to scar formation

星翳 [xīng yì]
dotted nebula:opacity due to small opaque dots on the cornea

蛛丝飘浮 [zhū sī piāo fú]
floaters; muscae volitantes: threads or spots before the eyes due to fine filaments in the vitreous body

针眼 [zhēn yǎn]
stye; hordeolum: small furuncle occurring on the eyelid, also known as 偷针 [tōu zhēn], 土疡 [tǔ yáng] or 土疳 [tǔ gān]

偷针 [tōu zhēn]
stye; hordeolum: another name for stye (针眼 [zhēn yǎn])

土疡 [tǔ yáng]
stye; hordeolum: another name for stye (针眼 [zhēn yǎn])

土疳 [tǔ gān]
stye; hordeolum: another name for stye (针眼 [zhēn yǎn])

胞生痰核 [bāo shēng tán hé]
phlegm node on the eyelid; chalazion: small lump formed on the eyelid, without redness or pain, also called 胞睑肿核 [bāo jiǎn zhǒng hé] or 睥生痰核 [pì shēng tán hé]

胞睑肿核 [bāo jiǎn zhǒng hé]
chalazion: another name for 胞生痰核 [bāo shēng tán hé]

睥生痰核 [pì shēng tán hé]
chalazion: another name for 胞生痰核 [bāo shēng tán hé]

椒疮 [jiāo chuāng]
trachoma: eye disease marked by innumerable granulations, red and hard, shaped like Chinese prickly ash (and hence the Chinese name "prickly-ash sore") accumulating on the conjunctival surface

倒睫 [dào jié]
trichiasis: ingrowing of eyelashes, also called 睫毛倒入 [jié máo dào rù]

睫毛倒入 [jié máo dào rù]
trichiasis: same as 倒睫 [dào jié]

倒睫拳毛 [dào jié quán máo]
trichiasis and entropion: inversion of the margin of the eyelid with ingrowing eyelashes, one of the sequelae of trachoma

睥翻粘睑 [pì fān zhān jiǎn]
cicatrical ectropion of the eyelid: eversion of the margin of an eyelid caused by scar tissue

睥肉粘轮 [pì ròu zhān lún]
symblepharon: adhesion between the tarsal conjunctiva and bulbar conjunctiva, also called 睑粘睛珠 [jiǎn zhān jīng zhū]

睑粘睛珠 [jiǎn zhān jīng zhū]
symblepharon: same as 睥肉粘轮 [pì ròu zhān lún]

粟疮 [sù chuāng]
millet sore; follicular conjunctivitis: eye disease marked by formation on the conjunctival surface of numerous follicles with the shape and size of millet seeds

睑弦赤烂 [jiǎn xián chì làn]
erosion of the palpebral margin; marginal blepharitis: inflammation and ulceration of the margin of the eyelid, also called 眼缘赤烂 [yǎn yuán chì làn] or 风弦赤烂 [fēng xián chì làn]

眼缘赤烂 [yǎn yuán chì làn]
erosion of the palpebral margin; marginal blepharitis: same as 睑弦赤烂 [jiǎn xián chì làn]

风弦赤烂 [fēng xián chì làn]
erosion of the palpebral margin; marginal blepharitis: same as 睑弦赤烂 [jiǎn xián chì làn]

睑弦糜烂 [jiǎn xián mí làn]
ulceration of the palpebral margin; ulcerative marginal blepharitis: inflammation of the margin of the eyelid with ulcer formation

眦帷赤烂 [zì wéi chì làn]
erosion of the canthal eyelid; blepharitis angularis: inflammation of the eyelid affecting the inner canthus

风赤疮痍 [fēng chì chuāng yí]
wind red sore of the eyelid; eczematous dermatitis of the eyelid: disease of the eyelid characterized by redness of the palpebral skin with the formation of vesicles or even local erosion, also called 风赤疮疾 [fēng chì chuāng jí]

风赤疮疾 [fēng chì chuāng jí]
wind red sore of the eyelid; eczematous dermatitis of the eyelid: another name for 风赤疮痍 [fēng chì chuāng yí]

胞肿 [bāo zhǒng]
swollen eyelid: swelling of the eyelid either inflammatory or non-inflammatory

胞肿如桃 [bāo zhǒng rú táo]
peach-like eyelid swelling; inflammatory swelling of the eyelid: severe swelling of the eyelid with redness resembling a ripe peach

胞虚如球 [bāo xū rú qiú]
ball-like eyelid swelling; non-inflammatory edema of the eyelid: severe swelling of the eyelid, but without change of local skin color, also called 睥虚如球 [pì xū rú qiú]

睥虚如球 [pì xū rú qiú]
ball-like eyelid swelling; non-inflammatory edema of the eyelid: same as 胞虚如球 [bāo xū rú qiú]

上胞下垂 [shàng bāo xià chuí]
blepharoptosis: drooping of the upper eyelid, also called 睑皮垂缓 [jiǎn pí chuí huǎn]

睑皮垂缓 [jiǎn pí chuí huǎn]
blepharoptosis: same as 上胞下垂 [shàng bāo xià chuí]

睑废 [jiǎn fèi]
invalid eyelid: serious blepharoptosis

胞轮振跳 [bāo lún zhèn tiào]
tic of the eyelid: involuntary twitching of the eyelid, also called 睥轮振跳 [pì lún zhèn tiào]

睥轮振跳 [pì lún zhèn tiào]
tic of the eyelid: same as 胞轮振跳 [bāo lún zhèn tiào]

目连劄 [mù lián zhá]
frequent nictitation: involuntary frequent winking, often abbreviated as nictitation (目劄 [mù zhá])

目劄 [mù zhá]
nictitation: abbreviation for frequent nictitation (目连劄 [mù lián zhá])

睑内结石 [jiǎn nèi jié shí]
calculus of the conjunctiva: single or multiple granules formed in the palpebral conjunctiva, fine, firm, hard and yellowish in color

流泪证 [liú lèi zhèng]
dacryorrhea syndrome: general term

for various conditions characterized by overabundant flow of tears, also called dacryorrhea disease (流泪病症 [liú lèi bìng zhèng])

流泪病症 [liú lèi bìng zhèng]
dacryorrhea disease: same as 流泪证 [liú lèi zhèng]

热泪 [rè lèi]
heat dacryorrhea: dacryorrhea occurring in inflammatory eye diseases as a symptom

冷泪 [lěng lèi]
cold dacryorrhea: dacryorrhea without redness, pain or opacity of the eyes

漏睛 [lòu jīng]
dacryopyorrhea; chronic dacryocystitis: chronic inflammation of the lacrimal sac with frequent outflow of fluid or pus from the inner canthus, known also as canthus pyorrhea (眦漏 [zì lòu]), orifice pyorrhea (窍漏 [qiào lòu]), or dacryopyorrheal eye (漏睛眼 [lòu jīng yǎn])

眦漏 [zì lòu]
canthus pyorrhea: synonym for dacryopyorrhea (漏睛 [lòu jīng])

窍漏 [qiào lòu]
orifice pyorrhea: another name for dacryopyorrheal (漏睛 [lòu jīng])

漏睛眼 [lòu jīng yǎn]
dacryopyorrheal eye: same as dacryopyorrhea (漏睛 [lòu jīng])

漏睛脓出 [lòu jīng nóng chū]
dacryopyorrhea: frequent discharge of tears mixed with pus, also known as inner-canthus dacryopyorrhea (大眦脓漏 [dà zì nóng lòu])

大眦脓漏 [dà zì nóng lòu]
inner-canthus dacryopyorrhea: synonym for dacryopyorrhea (漏睛脓出 [lòu jīng nóng chū])

漏睛疮 [lòu jīng chuāng]
dacryocyst sore; acute dacryocystitis: acute inflammation of the lacrimal sac with purulent discharge

胬肉攀睛 [nǔ ròu pān jīng]
pterygium: partial coverage of the cornea by a triangular fleshy mass formed at the canthus, even disturbing the vision, also called 胬肉扳睛 [nǔ ròu bān jīng] or 胬肉侵睛 [nǔ ròu qīn jīng]

胬肉扳睛 [nǔ ròu bān jīng]
pterygium: same as 胬肉攀睛 [nǔ ròu pān jīng]

胬肉侵睛 [nǔ ròu qīn jīng]
pterygium: same as 胬肉攀睛 [nǔ ròu pān jīng]

流金凌木 [liú jīn líng mù]
pseudopterygium: condition in which a conjunctival scar is attached to the cornea, resembling a ptyergyum except that the attachment is not as firm as in the latter case. (The term may be literally translated as "a flow of metal invading wood", in which metal refers to the bulbar conjunctiva and wood the cornea.)

风火眼 [fēng huǒ yǎn]
wind-fire eye; acute conjunctivitis: acute attack of wind-fire to the eye, marked

by an acute onset of redness and pain of the eye accompanied by photophobia and lacrimation, also known as wind-fire painful eye (风火眼痛 [fēng huǒ yǎn tòng]) or wind-heat eye (风热眼 [fēng rè yǎn]), usually abbreviated as inflamed eye (火眼 [huǒ yǎn])

风火眼痛 [fēng huǒ yǎn tòng]
wind-fire painful eye; acute conjunctivitis: same as 风火眼 [fēng huǒ yǎn]

风热眼 [fēng rè yǎn]
wind-heat eye; acute conjunctivitis: same as 风火眼 [fēng huǒ yǎn]

火眼 [huǒ yǎn]
inflammed eye; conjunctivitis: same as wind-fire eye (风火眼 [fēng huǒ yǎn]), also called red eye (赤眼 [chì yǎn])

赤眼 [chì yǎn]
red eye: same as inflammed eye (火眼 [huǒ yǎn])

暴发火眼 [bào fā huǒ yǎn]
fulminant conjunctivitis: acute contagious inflammation of the conjunctiva occurring suddenly and with great severity

暴风客热 [bào fēng kè rè]
sudden attack of wind-heat on the eye; sudden attack of bulbar conjunctivitis: acute inflammatory eye disease involving the bulbar conjunctiva (white of the eye) with sudden onset, due to external contraction of wind-heat, also called cold-damaged eye (伤寒眼 [shāng hán yǎn])

伤寒眼 [shāng hán yǎn]
cold-damaged eye: popular name for sudden attack of wind-heat on the eye or sudden attack of bulbar conjunctivitis (暴风客热 [bào fēng kè rè]) (伤寒 [shāng hán] or "cold damage" actually refers to exogenous contraction of febrile diseases.)

天行赤眼 [tiān xíng chì yǎn]
epidemic red eye; epidemic conjunctivitis: highly infectious eye disease characterized by sudden onset of inflammation of the bulbar conjunctiva (white of the eye), usually bilateral, and quickly contagious, also called 天行赤目 [tiān xíng chì mù] or epidemic fulminant red eye (天行暴赤 [tiān xíng bào chì])

天行赤目 [tiān xíng chì mù]
epidemic red eye; epidemic conjunctivitis: same as 天行赤眼 [tiān xíng chì yǎn]

天行暴赤 [tiān xíng bào chì]
epidemic fulminant red eye: same as 天行赤眼 [tiān xíng chì yǎn]

暴赤生翳 [bào chì shēng yì]
fulminant red eye with nebula formation; acute kerato-conjunctivitis: acute inflammation of the conjunctiva and cornea

天行赤眼暴翳 [tiān xíng chì yǎn bào yì]
epidemic red eye with fulminant nebula; epidemic kerato-conjunctivitis: highly infectious disease that may form an epidemic, characterized by simultaneous inflammation of the cornea and conjunctiva, also called 天行赤目暴翳 [tiān xíng chì mù bào yì]

天行赤目暴翳 [tiān xíng chì mù bào yì]
epidemic red eye with fulminant nebula;

epidemic kerato-conjunctivitis: same as 天行赤眼暴翳 [tiān xíng chì yǎn bào yì]

金疳 [jīn gān]
metal ulcer (of the eye); phlyctenular conjunctivitis: variety of conjunctivitis marked by presence of small vesicles or ulcerated nodules, also called 金疡 [jīn yáng]. (金疳 [jīn gān] and 金疡 [jīn yáng] literally mean "metal ulcer", so called because the lung pertains to metal according to the five-element/phase theory, and phlyctenular conjunctivitis or vesicular or ulcerative lesion is believed to be induced by exuberant lung fire.)

金疡 [jīn yáng]
metal ulcer (of the eye); phlyctenular conjunctivitis: same as 金疳 [jīn gān]

火疳 [huǒ gān]
fire ulcer (of the eye); episcleritis: eye disease caused by excessive fire which invades the inner surface of the white of the eye, resulting in bulging of localized dark violet patches, also called 火疡 [huǒ yáng]

火疡 [huǒ yáng]
fire ulcer (of the eye); episcleritis: same as 火疳 [huǒ gān]

白膜侵睛 [bái mó qīn jīng]
white membrane invading the eye; phlyctenular kerato-conjunctivitis: a form of kerato-conjunctivitis marked by formation of a small whitish circumscribed lesion at the corneal limbus

白膜蔽睛 [bái mó bì jīng]
white membrane covering the eye; pannus: membranous tissue causing a superficial opacity of the cornea, usually occurring in trachoma

白睛青蓝 [bái jīng qīng lán]
blueing the white of the eye: bluish discoloration of the bulbar conjunctiva surrounding the cornea after recurrent inflammation of the sclera with violet bulging, generally referring to deep scleritis or scleral staphyloma, also called 白珠俱青 [bái zhū jù qīng]

白珠俱青 [bái zhū jù qīng]
blueing the white of the eye: same as 白睛青蓝 [bái jīng qīng lán]

白睛溢血 [bái jīng yì xuè]
subconjunctival ecchymosis: extravasation beneath the conjunctiva

白涩症 [bái sè zhèng]
white xerotic syndrome: eye disease characterized by an uncomfortable feeling of dryness and roughness without apparent redness or swelling, generally referring to chronic conjunctivitis or superficial punctate keratitis, also called white xerotic disease (白涩病 [bái sè bìng])

白涩病 [bái sè bìng]
white xerotic disease: synonym for white xerotic syndrome (白涩症 [bái sè zhèng])

赤丝虬脉 [chì sī qiú mài]
hyperemia of subconjunctival capillaries: excess of blood in the capillaries beneath the bulbar conjunctiva resembling imaginary scenes of dragon's flying, also called 白睛虬脉 [bái jīng qiú mài]

白睛虬脉 [bái jīng qiú mài]
hyperemia of subconjunctival capillaries: same as 赤丝虬脉 [chì sī qiú mài]

黄油障 [huáng yóu zhàng]
pinguecula: yellowish triangular patch of proliferation on the bulbar conjunctiva close to the inner canthus, also called 黄油证 [huáng yóu zhèng]

黄油证 [huáng yóu zhèng]
pinguecula: same as 黄油障 [huáng yóu zhàng]

聚星障 [jù xīng zhàng]
star-cluster nebula; superficial punctate keratitis: eye disease characterized by sudden appearance of multiple minute opacities on the cornea, generally referring to virus keratitis

花翳白陷 [huā yì bái xiàn]
petaloid nebula with sunken center; ulcerative keratitis: keratitis with ulceration of the corneal surface forming scars with flower pattern, also called scaly nebula with sunken center (白陷鱼鳞 [bái xiàn yú lín])

白陷鱼鳞 [bái xiàn yú lín]
scaly nebula with sunken center; ulcerative keratitis: same as 花翳白陷 [huā yì bái xiàn]

凝脂翳 [níng zhī yì]
fat-congealed nebula; purulent keratitis: severe keratitis with purulent disintegration of the cornea

黄液上冲 [huáng yè shàng chōng]
upsurging of the yellow fluid; hypopyon: accumulation of pus between the cornea and iris (i.e., the anterior chamber), also called upsurging of the yellow pus (黄脓上冲 [huáng nóng shàng chōng]) or upsurging of the yellow membrane (黄膜上冲 [huáng mó shàng chōng])

黄脓上冲 [huáng nóng shàng chōng]
upsurging of the yellow pus; hypopyon: same as 黄液上冲 [huáng yè shàng chōng]

黄膜上冲 [huáng mó shàng chōng]
upsurging of the yellow membrane; hypopyon: same as 黄液上冲 [huáng yè shàng chōng]

蟹睛病 [xiè jīng bìng]
crab's eye disease; corneal perforation with irridoptosis: severe eye disease marked by perforation of the cornea with prolapse of the iris, making the affected eye look like a crab's eye, also called crab's eye (蟹目 [xiè mù] or 蟹珠 [xiè zhū])

蟹目 [xiè mù]
crab's eye; corneal perforation with irridoptosis: same as 蟹睛病 [xiè jīng bìng]

蟹珠 [xiè zhū]
crab's eye; corneal perforation with irridoptosis: same as 蟹睛病 [xiè jīng bìng]

混睛障 [hún jīng zhàng]
murky eye nebula; interstitial keratitis: eye disease with visual disturbance marked by deep deposits in the substance of the cornea, making the cornea grayish and opaque, also called 混睛外障 [hún jīng wài zhàng], murky nebula (混障症 [hún zhàng zhèng]) or *qi* nebula (气翳[qì yì])

混睛外障 [hún jīng wài zhàng]
murky eye nebula: same as 混睛障 [hún jīng zhàng]

混障症 [hún zhàng zhèng]
murky nebula: synonym for interstitial keratitits (混睛障 [hún jīng zhàng])

气翳 [qì yì]
***qi* nebula:** synonym for interstitial keratitits (混睛障 [hún jīng zhàng])

风轮赤豆 [fēng lún chì dòu]
wind-orbiculus red bean; fascicular keratitis: corneal lesion of the granular vesicle surrounded by small blood vessels, resulting in a cluster shaped like a red bean, which leaves a scar after recurrent attacks, causing disturbance of vision, mostly referring to fascicular keratitis

赤膜下垂 [chì mó xià chuí]
drooping pannus; trachomatous pannus: membranous vascular tissue extending downward into the cornea, most frequently occurring in trachoma, also known as drooping nebula (垂帘翳 [chuí lián yì])

垂帘翳 [chuí lián yì]
drooping nebula: same as drooping pannus or trachomatous pannus (赤膜下垂 [chì mó xià chuí])

血翳包睛 [xuè yì bāo jīng]
keratic pannus: superficial vascularization covering the entire cornea, also called rosy clouds shining on the cornea (红霞映日 [hóng xiá yìng rì])

红霞映日 [hóng xiá yìng rì]
rosy clouds shining on the cornea: euphemism for keratic pannus (血翳包睛 [xuè yì bāo jīng])

瞳神紧小 [tóng shén jǐn xiǎo]
miosis: contraction of the pupil, often caused by iridocyclitis or panuveitis, also called 瞳神细小 [tóng shén xì xiǎo] or 瞳神缩小 [tóng shén suō xiǎo]

瞳神细小 [tóng shén xì xiǎo]
miosis: same as 瞳神紧小 [tóng shén jǐn xiǎo]

瞳神缩小 [tóng shén suō xiǎo]
miosis: same as 瞳神紧小 [tóng shén jǐn xiǎo]

瞳神散大 [tóng shén sǎn dà]
mydriasis: dilation of the pupil

瞳神干缺 [tóng shén gān quē]
pupillary metamorphosis: loss of normal round shape of the pupil, usually seen in chronic iridocyclitis, also called 瞳人干缺 [tóng rén gān quē] or 瞳神缺陷 [tóng shén quē xiàn]

瞳人干缺 [tóng rén gān quē]
pupillary metamorphosis: same as 瞳神干缺[tóng shén gān quē]

瞳神缺陷 [tóng shén quē xiàn]
pupillary metamorphosis: same as 瞳神干缺 [tóng shén gān quē]

绿风内障 [lǜ fēng nèi zhàng]
greenish glaucoma: acute eye disease characterized by hardening of the eyeball, impaired vision, and dilation of the pupil with a greenish discoloration, also called 绿风 [lǜ fēng]

绿风 [lǜ fēng]
greenish glaucoma: abbreviation for 绿风内障 [lǜ fēng nèi zhàng]

青风内障 [qīng fēng nèi zhàng]
bluish glaucoma: mild case of simple glaucoma, also called 青风 [qīng fēng]

青风 [qīng fēng]
bluish glaucoma: abbreviation for 青风内障 [qīng fēng nèi zhàng]

黄风内障 [huáng fēng nèi zhàng]
yellowish glaucoma: advanced stage of glaucoma with the pupil discolored to yellowish, also called 黄风 [huáng fēng]

黄风 [huáng fēng]
yellowish glaucoma: abbreviation for 黄风内障 [huáng fēng nèi zhàng]

圆翳内障 [yuán yì nèi zhàng]
cataract: chronic eye disease marked by opacity in the lens, impairing vision or causing blindness, also called 圆翳 [yuán yì]

圆翳 [yuán yì]
cataract: abbreviation for 圆翳内障 [yuán yì nèi zhàng]

惊震内障 [jīng zhèn nèi zhàng]
traumatic cataract: cataract resulting from eye injury

胎患内障 [tāi huàn nèi zhàng]
congenital cataract: any of various kinds of ocular opacity present at birth, usually bilateral

云雾移睛 [yún wù yí jīng]
fog floating before the eye; vitreous opacity: cloudy or star-shaped opacity in the vitreous humor, also called flying fly shadow (蝇影飞越 [yíng yǐng fēi yuè]) or fly-wing-like shadow (蝇翅黑花 [yíng chì hēi huā])

蝇影飞越 [yíng yǐng fēi yuè]
flying fly shadow: another name for vitreous opacity (云雾移睛 [yún wù yí jīng])

蝇翅黑花 [yíng chì hēi huā]
fly-wing-like shadow: another name for vitreous opacity (云雾移睛 [yún wù yí jīng])

暴盲 [bào máng]
sudden blindness: sudden loss of vision without abnormalities in the appearance of the eye

视瞻昏渺 [shì zhān hūn miǎo]
blurring of vision: impaired vision without abnormality of the external eye, also called 瞻视昏渺 [zhān shì hūn miǎo]

瞻视昏渺 [zhān shì hūn miǎo]
blurring of vision: same as 视瞻昏渺 [shì zhān hūn miǎo]

青盲 [qīng máng]
bluish blindness: general term for a group of eye diseases characterized by increasing impairment of vision to total blindness with no abnormal appearance of the external eye, usually referring to optic atrophy

高风内障 [gāo fēng nèi zhàng]
pigmentary retinopathy: hereditary pro-

gressive degenerative disease characterized by night blindness, constriction of the visual field, and eventual blindness, also called 高风雀目 [gāo fēng què mù]

高风雀目 [gāo fēng què mù]
pigmentary retinopathy: same as 高风内障 [gāo fēng nèi zhàng]

异物入目 [yì wù rù mù]
foreign body entering the eye: condition in which a small foreign body is attached to or embedded on the surface of the eyeball

撞击伤目 [zhuàng jī shāng mù]
ocular contusion: eye injury due to a knock or strike with no ruptured wound

真睛破损 [zhēn jīng pò sǔn]
ruptured wound of the eyeball: penetrating injury to the eyeball or other eye injuries with a ruptured wound, also called traumatic injury to the eyeball (物损真睛 [wù sǔn zhēn jīng])

物损真睛 [wù sǔn zhēn jīng]
traumatic injury to the eyeball: synonym for ruptured wound of the eye ball (真睛破损 [zhēn jīng pò sǔn])

电光伤目 [diàn guāng shāng mù]
electric ophthalmia; flash ophthalmia: inflammation of the eye caused by electric light or flash

疳积上目 [gān jī shàng mù]
(malnutritional) keratomalacia: softening and ulceration of the cornea of the eye due to malnutrition, also called 疳眼 [gān yǎn]

疳眼 [gān yǎn]
keratomalacia: same as 疳积上目 [gān jī shàng mù]

近视 [jìn shì]
myopia: condition in which one is only able to see clearly things that are close to the eyes, also called nearsightedness (能近怯远症 [néng jìn qiè yuǎn zhèng])

能近怯远症 [néng jìn qiè yuǎn zhèng]
nearsightedness: another expression for myopia (近视 [jìn shì])

远视 [yuǎn shì]
hyperopia: condition in which vision is better for distant than for near objects, also called farsightedness (能远怯近症 [néng yuǎn qiè jìn zhèng])

能远怯近症 [néng yuǎn qiè jìn zhèng]
farsightedness: another expression for hyperopia (远视 [yuǎn shì])

视物易色 [shì wù yì sè]
chromatopsia: disturbance of vision in which colored objects appear unnaturally colored or colorless objects appear colored

视直为曲 [shì zhí wéi qū]
metamorphopsia: disturbance of vision in which objects are seen distorted in shape

雀盲 [què máng]
sparrow's blindness; night blindness; nyctalopia: loss of vision at night or in a dim light, also called sparrow's vision (雀目 [què mù]) or sparrow's cataract (雀目内障 [què mù nèi zhàng])

雀目 [què mù]
sparrow's vision: another name for night blindness (雀盲 [què máng])

雀目内障 [què mù nèi zhàng]
sparrow's cataract: same as sparrow's vision (雀盲[què máng])

目偏视 [mù piān shì]
squint; strabismus: condition in which the eyes do not align with each other properly, leading to failure of directing both eyes towards the same object at the same time, also called 偏斜瞻视 [piān xié zhān shì]

偏斜瞻视 [piān xié zhān shì]
strabismus: another name for 目偏视 [mù piān shì]

风牵偏视 [fēng qiān piān shì]
wind-induced squint; paralytic strabismus: squint caused by attack of wind on the collateral meridian/channel

突起睛高 [tū qǐ jīng gāo]
sudden protrusion of the eyeball: eye disease characterized by acute onset of painful protrusion and distension of the eyeball, often referring to purulent ophthalmia, also known as 睛高突起 [jīng gāo tū qǐ] or distension of the eyeball (睛胀 [jīng zhàng])

睛高突起 [jīng gāo tū qǐ]
sudden protrusion of the eyeball: same as 突起睛高[tū qǐ jīnggāo]

睛胀 [jīng zhàng]
distension of the eyeball: synonym for 突起睛高 [tū qǐ jīng gāo]

目痒 [mù yǎng]
eye itching: condition characterized by intense itching of the eye, often referring to catarrhal conjunctivitis

瞽症 [gǔ zhèng]
blindness in ophathalmosteresis: blindness with loss of both eyes

眇目 [miǎo mù]
monocular blindness: blindness of a single eye

耳鼻喉科 Otorhinolaryngology

耳科（学）[ěr kē xué]
otology: branch of medicine that deals with the ear and its diseases

完骨 [wán gǔ]
mastoid bone: mastoid part of temporal bone

耳疔 [ěr dīng]
ear boil: boil of the external auditory meatus, also called ear furuncle (耳疖 [ěr jiē])

黑疔 [hēi dīng]
black boil: (1) blackish boil of the external auditory meatus; (2) blackish gingival boil

耳疖 [ěr jiē]
ear furuncle: synonym for 耳疔 [ěr dīng]

耳疮 [ěr chuāng]
ear sore: diffuse inflammation of the external auditory meatus

旋耳疮 [xuán ěr chuāng]
peri-auricular sore; eczema of the external ear: redness, itching, exudation and oozing vesicular lesions surrounding the ear, also known as eclipsed lunar sore (月蚀疮 [yuè shí chuāng])

月蚀疮 [yuè shí chuāng]
eclipsed lunar sore; eczema of the external ear: another name for periauricular eczema (旋耳疮 [xuán ěr chuāng])

耳壳流痰 [ěr qiào liú tán]
auricular pseudocyst: cystic collection of fluid on the auricle, soft with no hotness or tenderness, nor change in skin color, referring to exudative perichondritis of the auricle

耳胀 [ěr zhàng]
ear distension: feeling of distension with pain in the ear, a symptom often occurring in acute non-suppurative otitis media

耳闭 [ěr bì]
ear block: feeling of blocking in the ear developed after a long course of ear distension, often occurring in chronic non-suppurative otitis media

脓耳 [nóng ěr]
otopyorrhea; suppurative otitis media: disease of the ear characterized by perforation of the tympanitic membrane and discharge of pus

脓耳变证 [nóng ěr biàn zhèng]
deteriorated otopyorrhea; complications of suppurative otitis media: secondary conditions or diseases that develop in the course of suppurative otitis media, including postauricular infection (耳根毒 [ěr gēn dú]), postauricular abscess (耳根痈 [ěr gēn yōng]), otopyorrhea with facial paralysis (脓耳口眼㖞斜 [nóng ěr kǒu yǎn wāi xié]) and otogenic intracranial infection (黄耳伤寒 [huáng ěr shāng hán])

耳根毒 [ěr gēn dú]
postauricular infection: disease marked by pain and tenderness at the mastoid region, local swelling and even rupture with discharge of pus

耳根痈 [ěr gēn yōng]
postauricular abscess: postauricular infection with formation of abscess, also called postauricular subperiosteal abscess (耳后附骨痈 [ěr hòu fù gǔ yōng])

耳后附骨痈 [ě hòu fù gǔ yōng]
postauricular subperiosteal abscess: synonym for postauricular abscess (耳根痈 [ěr gēn yōng])

脓耳口眼㖞斜 [nóng ěr kòu yǎn wāi xié]
otopyorrhea with facial paralysis: suppurative otitis media complicated by wry eye and mouth

黄耳伤寒 [huáng ěr shāng hán]
otogenic intracranial infection: suppurative otitis media complicated by mental derangements or convulsions

耳鸣 [ěr míng]
tinnitus: ringing in the ear

风热耳鸣 [fēng rè ěr míng]
wind-heat tinnitus: ringing in the ear occurring in a wind-heat affliction, characterized by hearing a low-pitched sound, usually unilateral

肝火耳鸣 [gān huǒ ěr míng]
liver-fire tinnitus: ringing in the ear occurring in a liver-fire affliction, characterized by hearing a rumbling sound, usually unilateral, and sudden onset accompanied by hypochondriac distension, irritability, and wiry rapid pulse

痰火耳鸣 [tán huǒ ěr míng]
phlegm-fire tinnitus: ringing in the ear occurring in a phlegm-fire affliction, characterized by hearing a soft sound, accompanied by local pain and distension, or even discharge of pus from the ear, usually unilateral

脏腑虚损耳鸣 [zàng fǔ xū sǔn ěr míng]
***zang-fu* insufficiency tinnitus:** ringing in the ear due to insufficiency of *zang-fu* organs, characterized by hearing a high-pitched sound, usually bilateral, accompanied by deficiency syndrome of the corresponding organ

肾虚耳鸣 [shèn xū ěr míng]
kidney-insufficiency tinnitus: ringing in the ear due to insufficiency of the kidney, characterized by hearing a high-pitched sound, usually bilateral, accompanied by dizziness, aching lumbus and weak legs

重听 [chóng tīng] [zhòng tīng]
hardness of hearing: decreased sense of hearing or distorted hearing

耳聋 [ěr lóng]
deafness: lack or loss, complete or partial, of the sense of hearing

暴聋 [bào lóng]
sudden deafness: deafness occurring suddenly, also called 卒聋 [cù lóng]

卒聋 [cù lóng]
sudden deafness: same as 暴聋 [bào lóng]

渐聋 [jiàn lóng]
progressive deafness: deafness happening or developing gradually over a period of time

干聋 [gān lóng]
dry deafness: deafness due to impacted earwax

耵聍 [dīng níng]
cerumen; earwax: yellow waxy secretion in the external ear

耵耳 [dīng ěr]
impacted cerumen: condition in which accumulated cerumen forms a solid mass that adheres to the wall of external auditory meatus

耳眩晕 [ěr xuàn yùn]
aural vertigo: vertigo due to otopathy

脓耳眩晕 [nóng ěr xuàn yùn]
otopyorrheal vertigo: vertigo due to suppurative otitis media

耳瘘 [ěr lòu]
ear fistula: fistula in front of or behind the ear with exudation

耳菌 [ěr jūn]
ear polyp: polyp of the external auditory meatus, also called 耳蕈 [ěr xùn]

耳蕈 [ěr xùn]
ear polyp: same as 耳菌 [ěr jūn]

耳挺 [ěr tǐng]
ear protuberance: long-stemmed papilloma of the external auditory meatus

耳痔 [ěr zhì]
ear pile; nodular vegetation of the ear: nodular papilloma of the external auditory meatus

耳疳 [ěr gān]
ulcerated ear: chronic suppurative otitis media with fetid purulent discharge

聤耳 [tíng ěr]
otopyorrhea; suppurative otitis media: disease characterized by purulent discharge from the ear

耳后发 [ěr hòu fā]
postauricular phlegmon: acute suppurative or gangrenous mastoiditis

耳聋口哑 [ěr lóng kǒu yǎ]
deaf-mutism: absence of both the sense of hearing and the ability to speak

鼻科（学） [bí kē (xué)]
rhinology: branch of medicine that deals with the nose and its diseases

明堂 [míng táng]
(I) "bright hall": ancient term for the nose, especially the apex of the nose. (It is so called because the face is the place where yang meridians/channels gather, and the nose is situated in the center of the face and hence is considered to be the meeting place of bright yang.) **(II) point marks:** marks indicating acupuncture points on a model

畜门 [xiù mén]
"opening of smelling": ancient term for the nostril. (In ancient times, the Chinese character 畜 was the same as 臭 or 嗅, which means smelling.)

鼻尖 [bí jiān]
nose tip: tip of the nose

鼻准 [bí zhǔn]
apex of the nose; apex nasi: the most distal portion of the nose

山根 [shān gēn]
root of the nose; radix nasi: the upper portion of the nose, which is attached to the frontal bone

频 [é]
(I) radix nasi: root of the nose; **(II) nose stem**: the dorsal middle part of the nose as a whole

鼻柱 [bí zhù]
nose stem: dorsal middle part of the nose, also called bridge of the nose (鼻梁 [bí liáng])

鼻梁 [bí liáng]
bridge of the nose: popular name for the nose stem (鼻柱 [bí zhù])

鼻翼 [bí yì]
ala nasi: nostril wing

鼻前孔 [bí qián kǒng]
anterior naris; nostril: either of the two openings in the nose

鼻前庭 [bí qián tíng]
nasal vestibule: cavity of the nose

鼻病 [bí bìng]
nasal disease: collective term for diseases of the nose

鼻塞 [bí sāi]
nasal congestion; stuffy nose: inability to breathe smoothly through the nose, also called 鼻窍不利 [bí qiào bù lì]

鼻窍不利 [bí qiào bù lì]
nasal congestion; stuffy nose: same as nasal congestion (鼻塞 [bí sāi])

鼻燥 [bí zào]
(I) dry nose: dryness of the nasal cavity; **(II) rhinitis sicca:** atrophic rhinitis without secretion

鼻涕 [bí tì]
nasal discharge: discharge from the nose

不闻香臭 [bù wén xiāng chòu]
anosmia: loss or impairment of the sense of smell

鼻疔 [bí dīng]
nasal boil: boil occurring at the nasal vestibule, or at the tip or the wing of the nose

鼻疮 [bí chuāng]
nasal sore; nasal vestibulitis: disease marked by recurrent inflammation of the nasal vestibule with ulceration, crusting, itching and pain, also called 鼻疳疮 [bí gān chuāng] or 鼻疳 [bí gān]

鼻疳疮 [bí gān chuāng]
nasal sore; nasal vestibulitis: same as 鼻疮 [bí chuāng]

鼻疳 [bí gān]
nasal sore; nasal vestibulitis: abbreviation for 鼻疳疮 [bí gān chuāng]

伤风鼻塞 [shāng fēng bí sāi]
nasal obstruction in common cold; acute

rhinitis: disease marked by acute nasal congestion due to common cold

鼻窒 [bí zhì]

stuffy nose; chronic rhinitis: chronic nasal disease marked by recurrent nasal obstruction, sometimes accompanied by impairment of the sense of smell

鼻槁［藁］[bí gǎo]

atrophic rhinitis: disease of the nose characterized by dry mucous membrane with atrophy, enlarged nasal passages and a foul smell, progressing to ozena

鼻臭证 [bí chòu zhèng]

ozena: chronic atrophic rhinitis with a strong offensive smell

鼻鼽 [bí qiú]

running nose; allergic rhinits: disease characterized by sudden and recurrent attacks of nasal itching, sneezing, thin discharge and stuffy nose, also known as running nose with sneezing (鼽嚏 [qiú tì])

鼽嚏 [qiú tì]

running nose with sneezing: synonym for 鼻鼽 [bí qiú]

鼻渊 [bí yuān]

rhinorrhea with turbid discharge; sinusitis: a nasal disease characterized by persistent excessive flow of turbid nasal discharge, often seen in case of the inflammation of a paranasal sinus, also called 脑漏 [nǎo lòu], 脑渗 [nǎo shèn] , 脑崩 [nǎo bēng] and 控脑砂 [kòng nǎo shā]

脑漏 [nǎo lòu]

rhinorrhea with turbid discharge; sinusitis: another name for 鼻渊 [bí yuān]

脑渗 [nǎo shèn]

rhinorrhea with turbid discharge; sinusitis: another name for 鼻渊 [bí yuān]

脑崩 [nǎo bēng]

rhinorrhea with turbid discharge; sinusitis: another name for 鼻渊 [bí yuān]

控脑砂 [kòng nǎo shā]

rhinorrhea with turbid discharge; sinusitis: another name for 鼻渊 [bí yuān]

鼻息肉 [bí xī ròu]

nasal polyp: a growth protruding from the nasal mucous membrane, also called 鼻痔 [bí zhì] or 鼻菌 [bí jūn]

鼻痔 [bí zhì]

nasal polyp: another name for 鼻息肉 [bí xī ròu]

鼻菌 [bí jūn]

nasal polyp: another name for 鼻息肉 [bí xī ròu]

鼻赘 [bí zhuì]

(I) nasal polyp: same as 鼻息肉 [bí xī ròu];
(II) rhinophyma: rosacea at hypertrophic stage involving the lower half of the nose

鼻息肉病 [bí xī ròu bìng]

nasal polyposis: the development of multiple polyps on the nasal mucosa

鼻衄 [bí nǜ]

nosebleed; epistaxis: bleeding from the nose

鼻沥血 [bí lì xuè]
nosebleed: same as 鼻衄 [bí nù]

鼻洪 [bí hóng]
profuse nasal bleeding: profuse bleeding from the nose

脑衄 [nǎo nù]
severe epistaxis: severe case of bleeding from the nose

鼻梁骨折 [bí liáng gǔ zhé]
fracture of the nose bridge: breaking of the nasal bone

咽喉科学 [yān hóu kē xué]
pharyngolaryngology: branch of medicine that studies the throat, pharynx, larynx and nasopharynx, and their diseases

喉核 [hóu hé]
tonsil: either of a pair of prominent masses that lie one on each side of the throat between the anterior and posterior pillars of the fauces

喉关 [hóu guān]
faucial isthmus: passage between the cavity of the mouth and the pharynx

喉嗌 [hóu yì]
pharynx: passage between the cavity of mouth and the esophagus

颃颡 [háng sǎng]
nasopharynx: part of the pharynx above the soft palate

喉底 [hóu dǐ]
retropharynx: posterior part of the pharynx

悬雍垂 [xuán yōng chuí]
uvula: fleshy lobe in the middle of the posterior border of the soft palate, also called 小舌 ([xiǎo shé]), 蒂丁 [dì dīng] or 蒂中 [dì zhōng]

小舌 [xiǎo shé]
"little tongue": popular name for the palatine uvula

蒂丁 [dì dīng]
uvula: same as 悬雍垂 [xuán yōng chuí]

蒂中 [dì zhōng]
uvula: same as 蒂丁 [dì dīng]

乳蛾 [rǔ é]
tonsillitis: redness and swelling of painful tonsils, resembling a moth, often covered with a yellowish-white secretion like milk, hence the Chinese name 乳蛾 [rǔ é] which literally means "milky moth", also known as "throat moth" (喉蛾 [hóu é])

喉蛾 [hóu é]
throat moth: another name for tonsillitis (乳蛾[rǔ é])

单蛾 [dān é]
unilateral tonsillitis: inflammation of the tonsil of only one side

双蛾 [shuāng é]
bilateral tonsillitis: inflammation of the tonsils of both sides

风热乳蛾 [fēng rè rǔ é]
wind-heat tonsillitis: acute tonsillitis caused by attack of wind-heat

虚火乳蛾 [xū huǒ rǔ é]
deficiency-fire tonsillitis: chronic tonsillitis caused by fire of deficiency type

石蛾 [shí é]
"stony moth"; hypertrophy of the tonsil: hard hypertrophied tonsils in children with no inflammation

咽喉肿痛 [yān hóu zhǒng tòng]
sore throat: painful swelling of the throat

喉痹 [hóu bì]
throat impediment; pharyngitis: redness, swelling and pain of the throat with difficulty in swallowing, also called pharynx impediment (咽痹 [yān bì])

咽痹 [yān bì]
pharynx impediment; pharyngitis: same as throat impediment (喉痹 [hóu bì])

风热喉痹 [fēng rè hóu bì]
wind-heat pharyngitis: acute pharyngitis caused by wind-heat

风寒喉痹 [fēng hán hóu bì]
wind-cold pharyngitis: acute pharyngitis caused by wind-cold, occasionally occurring in a debilitated person

虚火喉痹 [xū huǒ hóu bì]
deficiency-fire pharyngitis: chronic pharyngitis caused by fire of deficiency type

帘珠喉痹 [lián zhū hóu bì]
granular pharyngitis: chronic pharyngitis with granules on the posterior wall of the pharynx

喉痈 [hóu yōng]
throat abscess: abscess of the throat, including retropharyngeal abscess and peritonsillar abscess

猛疽 [měng jū]
ominous throat abscess: abscess of the laryngopharynx that causes obstruction of breathing and is often fatal if not properly treated in time

喉关痈 [hóu guān yōng]
(I) faucial abscess: abscess of the fauces; **(II) peritonsillar abscess:** abscess in the peritonsillar tissue, resulting from suppuration of the tonsil

咽后痈 [yān hòu yōng]
retropharyngeal abscess: suppurative inflammation in the posterior wall of the pharynx, also called 里喉痈 [lǐ hóu yōng]

里喉痈 [lǐ hóu yōng]
retropharyngeal abscess: same as 咽后痈[yān hòu yōng]

颌下痈 [hé xià yōng]
submandibular abscess: suppurative inflammation beneath the mandible

喉癣 [hóu xuǎn]
tinea-like erosion of the throat: ulceration of the laryngopharyngeal mucosa resembling tinea, often referring to laryngeal tuberculosis, also called throat tinea with moth-eaten holes (天白蚁 [tiān bái yǐ])

天白蚁 [tiān bái yǐ]
throat tinea with moth-eaten holes: advanced case of laryngeal tuberculosis

喉喑［瘖］[hóu yīn]
hoarseness or aphonia: harsh quality of voice or loss of voice

急喉喑［瘖］[jí hóu yīn]
acute hoarseness or aphonia: acute onset of harshness or loss of voice

暴喑［瘖］[bào yīn]
sudden hoarseness or aphonia: sudden harshness or loss of voice, also called 卒喑 [cù yīn]

卒喑［瘖］[cù yīn]
sudden hoarseness or aphonia: same as 暴喑 [bào yīn]

慢喉喑［瘖］[màn hóu yīn]
chronic hoarseness or aphonia: chronic harshness of voice or loss of voice

悬雍肿 [xuán yōng zhǒng]
swollen uvula; uvulitis: inflammation of the uvula

悬痈 [xuán yōng]
(I) uvular abscess: abscess of the uvula; **(II) perineal abscess:** pyogenic infection of the perineum with abscess formation

悬旗小舌 [xuán qí xiǎo shé]
uvular hematoma: hematoma on the uvula, also called uvular wind (悬旗风 [xuán qí fēng])

悬旗风 [xuán qí fēng]
uvular wind: another name for uvular hematoma (悬旗小舌 [xuán qí xiǎo shé])

喉风 [hóu fēng]
throat wind; acute throat trouble: general term for serious conditions of swelling and pain of the throat with difficulty in breathing and swallowing

急喉风 [jí hóu fēng]
acute throat wind; acute throat infection: acute laryngitis with difficulty in breathing and speaking

紧喉风 [jǐn hóu fēng]
constrictive throat wind; constrictive throat infection: acute laryngitis mainly manifested by sensation of suffocation, and difficulty in breathing and swallowing

缠喉风 [chán hóu fēng]
entwining throat wind; entwining throat infection: severe throat infection with redness entwining the fauces in the interior and swelling surrounding the neck in the exterior

锁喉风 [suǒ hóu fēng]
obstructive throat wind; acute laryngemphraxis: acute throat infection with obstruction or closure of the larynx

喉痹 [hóu bì]
throat impediment; pharyngitis: inflammation of the pharynx with marked painful swelling that causes difficulty in breathing and swallowing

急喉痹 [jí hóu bì]
acute throat impediment; acute pharyngitis: acute inflammation of the pharynx, also called 卒喉痹 [cù hóu bì]

卒喉痹 [cù hóu bì]
sudden onset of throat impediment: same as acute pharyngitis (急喉痹 [jí hóu bì])

飞扬喉 [fēi yáng hóu]
diffuse palatitis: wide-spread inflammation of the palate involving the throat

喉疳 [hóu gān]
throat necrosis: ulcerative necrosis of the throat

梅核气 [méi hé qì]
plum-stone *qi*; globus hystericus: disease characterized by the subjective sensation of being choked with a lump in the throat which can be neither swallowed nor ejected

骨鲠 [gǔ gěng]
bone stuck in the throat: condition in which a fishbone or bone of another kind becomes lodged in the throat or esophagus

喉瘤 [hóu liú]
tumor of the throat: new growth in the throat, unilateral or bilateral

喉岩 [hóu yán]
throat cancer; carcinoma of the throat: malignant tumor of the throat as hard as a rock, also called 喉菌 [hóu jūn]

喉菌 [hóu jūn]
throat cancer; carcinoma of the throat: malignant tumor of the throat in the shape of a mushroom, another name for 喉岩 [hóu yán]

口齿科 Stomatology and Dentistry

口齿科（学）[kǒu chǐ kē (xué)]
stomatology and dentistry: the branch of medicine that studies the teeth, oral cavity and associated structures, as well as their diseases

智齿 [zhì chǐ]
wisdom tooth: the third molar that is the last tooth to erupt, also called third molar tooth (真牙[zhēn yá])

真牙 [zhēn yá]
third molar tooth: same as wisdom tooth (智齿 [zhì chǐ])

齿更 [chǐ gēng]
dental transition: eruption of permanent teeth to replace deciduous teeth

齿落 [chǐ luò]
dedentition: shedding or loss of teeth

齿龂 [chǐ xiè]
teeth grinding: grinding of teeth during sleep, also called 龂齿 [xiè chǐ]

龂齿 [xiè chǐ]
grinding of teeth: same as 齿龂 [chǐ xiè]

牙痛 [yá tòng]
toothache: pain in a tooth or teeth

风热牙痛 [fēng rè yá tòng]
wind-heat toothache: paroxysmal attacks of toothache, ameliorated by cold and aggravated by heat, accompanied by redness and swelling of the gums, also known as wind-fire toothache (风火牙痛 [fēng huǒ yá tòng])

风火牙痛 [fēng huǒ yá tòng]
wind-fire toothache: same as wind-heat toothache (风热牙痛 [fēng rè yá tòng])

风寒牙痛 [fēng hán yá tòng]
wind-cold toothache: paroxysmal attacks of toothache aggravated by cold

胃火牙痛 [wèi huǒ yá tòng]
stomach-fire toothache: intense toothache with marked gingival redness, swelling, and discharge of pus or oozing of blood

虚火牙痛 [xū huǒ yá tòng]
deficiency-fire toothache: slight, dull toothache with mild gingival redness and swelling or even atrophy

齿龋 [chǐ qǔ]
dental caries: localized destruction of the tooth leading to cavity formation, also called dental decay (齿蠹 [chǐ dù])

齿蠹 [chǐ dù]
dental decay: same as dental caries (齿龋 [chǐ qǔ])

龋齿 [qǔ chǐ]
carious tooth: a tooth with caries

龋齿牙痛 [qǔ chǐ yá tòng]
carious toothache: toothache due to dental caries

龋脱 [qǔ tuō]
carious odontoptosis: loss of teeth due to caries

牙痈 [yá yōng]
gingival abscess: localized, painful, inflammatory lesion of the gums with pyorrhea

牙龄[咬]痈 [yá yǎo yōng]
distal gingival abscess: gingival abscess occurring at the most distal end, accompanied by difficulty in opening the mouth, usually referring to wisdom tooth pericoronitits

牙宣 [yá xuān]
exposure of dental root; gingival recession: exposure of the root surfaces of teeth due to the drawing back of gingivae from the necks of the teeth, also known as 齿龈宣露 [chǐ yín xuān lù], 齿挺 [chǐ tǐ ng] or 食床 [shí chuáng]

齿龈宣露 [chǐ yín xuān lù]
gingival recession: another name for 牙宣 [yá xuān]

齿挺 [chǐ tǐng]
exposure of dental root: another name for 牙宣 [yá xuān]

食床 [shí chuáng]
gingival recession: an ancient name for 牙宣 [yá xuān]

牙疳 [yá gān]
ulcerative gingivitis: disease marked by painful inflammation of the gums with necrosis and fetid discharge

风热牙疳 [fēng rè yá gān]
wind-heat ulcerative gingivitis: acute ulcerative gingivitis

走马牙疳 [zǒu mǎ yá gān]
noma; cancrum oris: ulcerative gingivitis with development as rapid as a horse running, spreading to large-area destruction of buccal mucosa and tissue of the face, often abbreviated as 走马疳 [zǒu mǎ gān]

走马疳 [zǒu mǎ gān]
noma: same as 走马牙疳 [zǒu mǎ yá gān]

口疮 [kǒu chuāng]
aphtha: small superficial ulcer on the buccal mucosa, also called 口疳 [kǒu gān]

口疳 [kǒu gān]
aphtha: same as 口疮 [kǒu chuāng]

口糜 [kǒu mí]
oral erosion: condition marked by multiple spots of erosion on the buccal mucosa

唇风 [chún fēng]
exfoliative cheilitis: persistent exfoliation of the lip caused by inflammation of the mucous membrane

骨槽风 [gǔ cáo fēng]
maxillary osteomyelitis: infectious inflammatory disease of the jaw bone with local death and separation of tissue

重舌 [chóng shé]
double tongue; sublingual swelling: hypertrophy of bilateral sublingual glands,

making a shape of a double tongue

莲花舌 [lián huā shé]
lotus tongue: hypertrophy of the sublingual glands, making a shape of a lotus flower

绊舌 [bàn shé]
ankyloglossia: restricted movement of the tongue, often resulting from a short lingual frenum

舌痈 [shé yōng]
tongue abscess: suppurative inflammation of the tongue

舌疔 [shé dīng]
tongue pustule: localized painful swelling and inflammation of the tongue, having a hard core, and forming pus

舌疮 [shé chuāng]
tongue sore: sore occurring on the tongue with local cracking, swelling and discharge of blood, accompanied by foul breath and constipation

唇疮 [chún chuāng]
lip sore: sore occurring on the lip, itching or painful, sometimes with purulent discharge

唇疔 [chún dīng]
lip pustule: furuncle on the lip or at the corner of the mouth, small but deep-rooted with pustule formation

唇疽 [chún jū]
lip abscess: infectious inflammation of the lip leading to abscess formation

痰包 [tán bāo]
phlegm cyst: retention cyst of the floor of the mouth, also called sublingual cyst (舌下痰包 [shé xià tán bāo])

舌下痰包 [shé xià tán bāo]
sublingual cyst: same as phlegm cyst (痰包 [tán bāo])

鹅口疮 [é kǒu chuāng]
thrush: disease usually of infants, marked by milky-white adhesion in the mouth and throat with pus formation

齿龈肿痛 [chǐ yín zhǒng tòng]
painful swollen gum: inflammation of the gum with pain and swelling

齿龈结瓣 [chǐ yín jié bàn]
petaloid gum: inflammation of the gum with the appearance of petals

雀舌 [què shé]
lingual hyperplasia: lingual vegetation that makes the entire tongue look like a sparrow's, with pain at the beginning and then erosion

唇菌 [chún jūn]
lip cancer: mushroom-like cancer occurring on the lip

舌菌 [shé jūn]
tongue cancer: mushroom-like cancer occurring on the tongue

骨伤科 Traumato-orthopedics

骨伤科（学）[gǔ shāng kē (xué)]
traumato-orthopedics: branch of medicine that encompasses orthopedics and traumatology

正骨（科）[zhèng gǔ (kē)]
orthopedics: branch of medicine that studies preservation and restoration of the function of the skeletal system, its articulation and associated structures

伤科 [shāng kē]
traumatology: branch of medicine that studies wounds and disability from injuries and their treatment

疡 [yáng]
trauma: injury to living tissue caused by an extrinsic agent

疡医 [yáng yī]
traumato-orthopedist: ancient name for a specialist in traumato-orthopedics

折疡 [zhé yáng]
trauma and fracture: ancient name for various traumatic conditions

金创 [jīn chuāng]
incised wound: wound made by a metallic cutting device, also called 金疡 [jīn yáng]

金疡 [jīn yáng]
incised wound: same as 金创 [jīn chuāng]

踠跌 [wǎn diē]
fracture from a fall: fracture of a limb caused by a fall

折骨绝筋 [zhé gǔ jué jīn]
fracture with broken tendon: breaking of the bone that produces rupture of the tendons but without open wound in the skin

折骨列肤 [zhé gǔ liè fū]
fracture with split skin; open fracture: breaking of the bone producing an open wound in the skin

断端移位 [duàn duān yí wèi]
displacement of fractured ends: movement of the fractured ends from the usual or correct place

骨折 [gǔ zhé]
fracture: breaking of a bone. The terms for various types of fracture commonly used in contemporary traumatology of Chinese medicine are the same as those used in Western medicine and are listed in the following table.

锁骨骨折	suǒ gǔ gǔ zhé	clavicle fracture
肩胛骨骨折	jiān jiǎ gǔ gǔ zhé	scapula fracture
肱骨外科颈骨折	gōng gǔ wài kē jǐng gǔ zhé	humerus surgical neck fracture
肱骨干骨折	gōng gǔ gàn gǔ zhé	humerus shaft fracture

肱骨髁上骨折	gōng gǔ kē shàng gǔ zhé	humerus supracondylar fracture
肱骨髁间骨折	gōng gǔ kē jiān gǔ zhé	humerus intercondylar fracture
肱骨外髁骨折	gōng gǔ wài kē gǔ zhé	humerus external condyle fracture
肱骨内上髁骨折	gōng gǔ nèi shàng kē gǔ zhé	humerus internal epicondyle fracture
尺骨鹰嘴骨折	chǐ gǔ yīng zuǐ gǔ zhé	ulna coronoid process fracture
桡骨头骨折	ráo gǔ tóu gǔ zhé	radius head fracture
尺骨干骨折	chǐ gǔ gàn gǔ zhé	ulna shaft fracture
尺骨上 1/3 骨折合并桡骨头脱位	chǐ gǔ shàng 1/3 gǔ zhé hé bìng ráo gǔ tóu tuō wèi	ulna (upper third) fracture with radius proximal end dislocation
桡骨下 1/3 骨折合并下桡尺骨关节脱位	ráo gǔ xià 1/3 gǔ zhé hé bìng xià ráo chǐ gǔ guān jié tuō wèi	radius (lower third) fracture with distal radio-ulnar dislocation
桡骨下端骨折	ráo gǔ xià duān gǔ zhé	radius lower end fracture
腕舟骨骨折	wàn zhōu gǔ gǔ zhé	hand scaphoid fracture
掌骨骨折	zhǎng gǔ gǔ zhé	metacarpal fracture
指骨骨折	zhǐ gǔ gǔ zhé	phalanx fracture
股骨颈骨折	gǔ gǔ jǐng gǔ zhé	femur/femoral neck fracture
股骨粗隆间骨折	gǔ gǔ cū lóng jiān gǔ zhé	femur/femoral intertrochanteric fracture
股骨干骨折	gǔ gǔ gàn gǔ zhé	femur/femoral shaft fracture
股骨髁上骨折	gǔ gǔ kē shàng gǔ zhé	femur/femoral epicondyles fracture
股骨髁部骨折	gǔ gǔ kē bù gǔ zhé	femur/femoral condyles fracture
髌骨骨折	bìn gǔ gǔ zhé	patella fracture
胫骨髁骨折	jìng gǔ kē gǔ zhé	tibia condyles fracture
胫腓骨干双骨折	jìng féi gǔ gàn shuāng gǔ zhé	tibia and fibula shaft fracture
腓骨干骨折	féi gǔ gàn gǔ zhé	tibia shaft fracture
踝骨骨折	huái gǔ gǔ zhé	ankle bone fracture
距骨骨折	jù gǔ gǔ zhé	astragalus fracture
跟骨骨折	gēn gǔ gǔ zhé	calcaneous fracture; heel bone fracture
足舟骨骨折	zú zhōu gǔ gǔ zhé	foot navicular fracture; foot scaphoid fracture
跖骨骨折	zhí gǔ gǔ zhé	metatarsal bone fracture
趾骨骨折	zhǐ gǔ gǔ zhé	toe fracture
胫骨干骨折	jìng gǔ gàn gǔ zhé	tibia shaft fracture
脊柱骨折	jǐ zhù gǔ zhé	spine fracture
寰枢椎骨折	huán shū zhuī gǔ zhé	atlantoaxial fracture
颈椎单纯骨折	jǐng zhuī dān chún gǔ zhé	cervical vertebral simple fracture

胸腰椎骨折	xiōng yāo zhuī gǔ zhé	thoraco-lumbar vertebral fracture
外伤性截瘫	wài shāng xìng jié tān	traumatic paraplegia
骨盆骨折	gǔ pén gǔ zhé	pelvic fracture
肋骨骨折	lèi gǔ gǔ zhé	rib fracture
裂缝骨折	liè fèng gǔ zhé	fissured fracture
青枝骨折	qīng zhī gǔ zhé	greenstick fracture
骨骺分离	gǔ hóu fēn lí	epiphysiolysis

脱位 [tuō wèi]

dislocation; luxation: displacement of a bone, also called 脱臼 [tuō jiù], 脱骱 [tuō jiè], 脱髎 [tuō liáo]. The terms for various types of dislocation commonly used in contemporary Chinese traumatology are the same as those used in Western medicine and are listed in the following table.

脱臼 [tuō jiù]

dislocation: another name for 脱位 [tuō wèi]

脱骱 [tuō jiè]

dislocation: an ancient term for 脱位 [tuō wèi]

脱髎 [tuō liáo]

dislocation: an ancient term for 脱位 [tuō wèi]

下颌关节脱位	xià hé guān jié tuō wèi	mandible dislocation
胸锁关节脱位	xiōng suǒ guān jié tuō wèi	sternoclavicular dislocation
肩关节脱位	jiān guān jié tuō wèi	shoulder dislocation
肩锁关节脱位	jiān suǒ guān jié tuō wèi	acromioclavicular dislocation
肘关节脱位	zhǒu guān jié tuō wèi	elbow dislocation
桡骨头半脱位	ráo gǔ tóu bàn tuō wèi	radius head subluxation
月骨前脱位	yuè gǔ qián tuō wèi	lunate anterior dislocation
拇指腕掌关节脱位	mǔ zhǐ wàn zhǎng guān jié tuō wèi	thumb carpometacarpal dislocation
拇指掌指关节脱位	mǔ zhǐ zhǎng zhǐ guān jié tuō wèi	thumb metacarpophalangeal dislocation
掌指关节脱位	zhǎng zhǐ guān jié tuō wèi	metacarpophalangeal dislocation
指间关节脱位	zhǐ jiān guān jié tuō wèi	interphalangeal dislocation
髋关节脱位	kuān guān jié tuō wèi	hip dislocation
髌骨脱位	bìn gǔ tuō wèi	patella dislocation
膝关节脱位	xī guān jié tuō wèi	knee dislocation
踝关节脱位	huái guān jié tuō wèi	ankle dislocation
距骨脱位	jù gǔ tuō wèi	astragalus/talus dislocation

跖跗关节脱位	zhí fū guān jié tuō wèi	tarsometatarsal dislocation
跖趾关节脱位	zhí zhǐ guān jié tuō wèi	metatarsophalangeal dislocation
足趾间关节脱位	zú zhǐ jiān guān jié tuō wèi	foot interphalangeal dislocation

正骨手法 [zhèng gǔ shǒu fǎ]
bone-setting manipulation: manual correction of a fracture or dislocation

正骨八法 [zhèng gǔ bā fǎ]
eight bone-setting manipulations: commonly used manipulations in bone-setting, comprising palpating, rejoining, hold-carrying, lifting, pressing, circular rubbing, pushing, and grasping

断骨接整 [duàn gǔ jiē zhěng]
reduction of fracture: reunion of a fracture in its normal position

平整复元 [píng zhěng fù yuán]
correction and reduction: restoration to the original normal position of a fractured bone in bone-setting, often called reduction (整复 [zhěng fù]) for short

整复 [zhěng fù]
reduction: correction of a fracture, abbreviation for correction and reduction (平整复元[píng zhěng fù yuán])

手摸心会 [shǒu mō xīn huì]
comprehending (perceiving) by touching: comprehending or perceiving the condition of a fracture such as the location of the fractured ends by careful palpation

拔伸牵引 [bá shēn qiān yǐn]
pulling, stretching and traction: basic procedure for fracture reduction in which the limb is pulled and stretched along its long axis, and tracted in a proper direction

旋转屈伸 [xuán zhuǎn qū shēn]
rotating, bending and stretching: manipulative procedure for reducing a fracture near a uniaxial joint with an angulation deformity, i.e., restoring the normal physiological axis first by rotating the distal part, and then correcting the dislocated bone by bending and stretching

提按端挤 [tí àn duān jǐ]
lifting, pressing, holding, and squeezing: collective term for the manipulative procedures for reducing a dislocation after the overlapping, rotation and angulation deformities have been corrected, lifting and pressing for reduction of upper-lower dislocation, and holding and squeezing for right-left dislocation

摇摆触碰 [yáo bǎi chù pèng]
rocking and tapping: manipulative procedure for further reduction of a transverse, serrated fracture, rocking to make a close contact of the broken ends, and tapping after splintage to make the proper embedment

夹挤分骨 [jiā jǐ fēn gǔ]
separate bones by squeezing: manipulative procedure for reducing a fracture of two long bones in parallel, such as ulnar and radial dual fracture

端法 [duān fǎ]
hold-carrying: manipulation of massotherapy and bone setting performed by carrying the diseased extremity of the patient upwards and downwards with its distal end held in one or both hands of the practitioner

提法 [tí fǎ]
lifting: manipulation of bone fracture reduction performed by lifting the broken bone upwards and outwards with the hand or a cord so as to obtain a complete reduction directly or indirectly

拉法 [lā fǎ]
traction: drawing or exerting a pulling force, a basic reduction manipulation for treating overlapping and displacement of fractured bones, also called 牵拉法 [qiān lā fǎ]

牵拉法 [qiān lā fǎ]
traction: same as 拉法 [lā fǎ]

接法 [jiē fǎ]
rejoining; (bone-)setting: method of restoring the original normal position of the broken ends or fragments of a fractured bone

接骨续筋 [jiē gǔ xù jīn]
reunion of the bone, muscle and ligament: rejoining of the fractured bone and restoration of the soft tissues

折顶 [zhé dǐng]
turning to the opposite: manipulative procedure for reducing a transverse or serrated fracture when traction force is inadequate for complete correction of the overlapping or displacement, i.e., increasing the angulation by pressing to make the broken ends touch each other, and then placing them into the correct position by turning the angulation in the opposite direction

回旋 [huí xuán]
reverse rotation: manipulative procedure for reducing an oblique or spiral fracture with dorsal displacement by holding the proximal and distal parts and rotating them in the direction opposite to the displacement

足蹬 [zú dēng]
pressing down with the foot: manipulative procedure for reducing forward dislocation of the shoulder, elbow or hip joint by pressing down the dislocated region of the patient with the foot while pulling the patient's distal part of the related extremity with the hands

膝顶 [xī dǐng]
pushing with the knee; knee-pushing (reduction): manipulative procedure for reducing dislocation of the shoulder or elbow performed by pushing the dislocated region of the patient with a knee while pulling the patient's arm with the hands

杠杆支撑 [gàng gǎn zhī chēng]
propping with a lever: procedure for reducing a long-standing dislocation difficult to reduce merely by the hands in which a propping lever is used as an aid

端提捺正 [duān tí nà zhèng]
holding, lifting, and restoring to the

right location: collective term for manipulations for reduction of dislocation

捺正 [nà zhèng]
manual correction: therapeutic method of restoring the dislocated ends of a fracture or luxation with the hands

续筋接骨 [xù jīn jiē gǔ]
reunion of fractured bone and tendon: rejoining a fractured bone and restoring the normal function of injured muscles and tendons

拔伸复位 [bá shēn fù wèi]
pulling-stretching reduction: reduction by exerting a pulling force along the long axis of a bone

拔伸捏正 [bá shēn niē zhèng]
pulling-kneading reduction: bone-setting manipulation performed by pulling the fractured bone and kneading the displaced ends simultaneously for restoration

挺腿拔伸 [tǐng tuǐ bá shēn]
leg-straightening traction: bone-setting manipulation performed by first straightening the leg and then applying traction

顺骨捋筋 [shùn gǔ lǚ jīn]
tendon-stroking along the bone: bone-setting manipulation performed by stroking the tendons and muscles along the long axis of the bone

欲合先离 [yù hé xiān lí]
separation before reunion: bone-setting manipulation performed by separating the overlapping fracture ends before restoring them to normal position

离而复合 [lí ér fù hé]
reunion after separation: reduction manipulation performed by restoring the fractured ends to the normal position after separation

纳入原位 [nà rù yuán wèi]
manual restoration: restoration of a dislocated bone to its normal position with the hands

外固定 [wài gù dìng]
external fixation: immobilization of the parts of a fractured bone by the use of attachments from outside

夹板固定 [jiā bǎn gù dìng]
splintage: application of splints for fixation

夹板固定疗法 [jiā bǎn gù dìng liáo fǎ]
splintage therapy: fracture fixation treatment by the use of splints and pads

托板 [tuō bǎn]
supporting board: rectangular wooden board used to support the diseased part in bone-setting

后侧夹板 [hòu cè jiā bǎn]
posterior splint: splint fixed at the posterior aspect of an extremity

鼎式夹板固定 [dǐng shì jiā bǎn gù dìng]
tripod-shaped splint fixation: fixation beyond the joint with a tripod-shaped splint

棉枕固定 [mián zhěn gù dìng]
fixation with cotton pads: stabilization of

a fractured bone by means of cotton pads

固定垫 [gù dìng diàn]
fixation pad: pad made of paper or cotton to be placed in between the skin and the splint for fixing fractured ends after reduction, also called pressure pad (压力垫 [yā lì diàn] or 压垫 [yā diàn])

压力垫 [yā lì diàn]
pressure pad: synonym for fixation pad (固定垫 [gù dìng diàn])

压垫 [yā diàn]
pressure pad: same as 压力垫 [yā lì diàn]

平垫 [píng diàn]
flat pad: square or rectangular pad, 4-8 cm long and 1.5-4 cm thick, suitable for being placed on the flat part of a limb and often used for the fixation of a shaft fracture

高低垫 [gāo dī diàn]
high-low pad: pad thick on one side, used for fixation of a clavicle fracture

葫芦垫 [hú lú diàn]
calabash pad: pad of even thickness with wider ends, in the shape of a calabash or a dumbbell, useful for a radius head fracture or dislocation

横垫 [héng diàn]
transverse pad: strip of padding 6-7cm long and 1.5-2 cm wide and approximately 0.3 cm thick, useful for treating lower-end fracture of the radius

抱骨垫 [bào gǔ diàn]
bone-holding pad: semilunar-shaped pad used for fixation of a fractured bone in cases of ulna coronoid process fracture or patella fracture

分骨垫 [fēn gǔ diàn]
bone-separating pad: pressure pad used to separate the double fracture of two parallel bones

合骨垫 [hé gǔ diàn]
bone-combining pad: pad thicker around the sides, suitable for fixation of lower ulna-radial joint separation

大头垫 [dà tóu diàn]
megacaput pad: fixation pad with cotton wrapped on one end of the splint, forming a mushroom shape, used for fixation of fractured surgical neck of the humerus

一垫固定法 [yī diàn gù dìng fǎ]
fixation with one pad: fixation method by using a single pad at the site of a fracture

二垫固定法 [èr diàn gù dìng fǎ]
fixation with two pads: fixation method for fracture with lateral displacement by using two pads, each on the displacement side of the two broken ends in order to prevent recurrence

三垫固定法 [sān diàn gù dìng fǎ]
fixation with three pads: fixation method for a fracture with angulation deformity by placing one pad at the prominence of the angle and the other two on the counter side close to the two broken ends

抱膝器 [bào xī qì]
peripatellapexor: an appliance for patellapexy

扎带 [zhā dài]
bandage: strip of cloth or ribbon for binding a splint

内固定 [nèi gù dìng]
internal fixation: immobilization of the parts of a fractured bone by the use of attachments from inside

复位 [fù wèi]
reduction: correction of a fracture or dislocation

坐式复位 [zuò shì fù wèi]
sitting reduction: reduction of a dislocated shoulder joint by traction with the patient in a sitting position

慢性复位 [màn xìng fù wèi]
gradual reduction: manipulation for gradual restoration of a fractured bone by traction

入臼 [rù jiù]
joint reduction: restoration of a joint to its normal position by manipulation

熨药 [yùn yào]
hot-compress medicinal: medicinal used for hot compress

手法牵引 [shǒu fǎ qiān yǐn]
manual traction: pulling with the hands

牵推法 [qiān tuī fǎ]
pulling-pushing manipulation: manual reduction of temporomandibular joint by pulling downward and then pushing upward

攀索叠砖 [pān suǒ dié zhuān]
holding a rope and standing on a pile of bricks: ancient method of traction for a lumbar or thoracic injury (fracture or dislocation) whereby the patient is asked to stand on a pile of bricks (usually three under each foot), holding a rope hanging from above, while the practitioner takes away the bricks one by one for gradual increase of traction

牵引疗法 [qiān yǐn liáo fǎ]
traction therapy: treatment of bone disorders by means of pulling. In contemporary Chinese medicine, most of the terms for various traction therapies are the same as those in Western medicine, and the rest are self-explanatory from the Western medical perspectives. The commonly used ones are listed in the following table.

皮肤牵引	pí fū qiān yǐn	skin traction
骨牵引	gǔ qiān yǐn	bone traction
颅骨牵引	lú gǔ qiān yǐn	skull traction
尺骨鹰嘴牵引	chǐ gǔ yīng zuǐ qiān yǐn	traction through ulnar olecranon
股骨下端牵引	gǔ gǔ xià duān qiān yǐn	traction through femoral distal end
胫骨结节牵引	jìng gǔ jié jié qiān yǐn	traction through tibial tubercle
跟骨牵引	gēn gǔ qiān yǐn	transcalcaneal traction
肋骨牵引	lèi gǔ qiān yǐn	rib traction

布托牵引	bù tuō qiān yǐn	cloth-wrapping traction
颌枕带牵引	hé zhěn dài qiān yǐn	madibulo-occipital bandage traction
骨盆悬吊牵引	gǔ pén xuán diào qiān yǐn	pelvic sling traction
骨盆牵引带牵引	gǔ pén qiān yǐn dài qiān yǐn	pelvic bandage traction

筋断 [jīn duàn]

musculotendinous rupture: complete or partial disruption of muscle and tendon

筋缩 [jīn suō]

(I) muscle contracture: permanent shortening of a muscle with deformity and dysfunction; **(II) *Jinsuo* (GV 8):** an acupoint on the back and on the posterior midline

筋痿 [jīn wěi]

(I) muscle flaccidity: weakness and softness of a muscle; **(II) impotence**: lack of copulative power in the male because of failure to have or maintain an erection

筋粗 [jīn cū]

musculotendinous thickening: thickening of a tendon and muscle after injury, due to blood stasis, or due to regeneration, degeneration or spasm of the tissue

筋结 [jīn jié]

musculotendinous nodulation: occurrence of a cystic mass of a muscle or tendon due to stagnation of *qi* and blood following a soft tissue injury

筋柔 [jīn róu]

musculotendinous softening: relaxation and weakness of a joint following a soft tissue injury

筋伤 [jīn shāng]

soft tissue injury: injury of soft tissues, including muscle, muscle tendon, tendon sheath, ligament, joint capsule, synovial bursa, intervertebral disc, peripheral nerve, and blood vessel. The terms for various soft tissue injuries used in contemporary traumatology of Chinese medicine are essentially the same as those used in Western medicine and are listed in the following table.

Soft tissue injuries of the shoulder		
肩部扭挫伤	jiān bù niǔ cuò shāng	shoulder sprain and contusion
肩凝症	jiān níng zhèng	frozen shoulder
肩袖损伤	jiān xiù sǔn shāng	rotator cuff injury
肱二头肌长头肌腱炎	gōng èr tóu jī cháng tóu jī jiàn yán	brachial biceps long head tendonitis
肱二头肌短头肌腱捩伤	gōng èr tóu jī duǎn tóu jī jiàn liè shāng	brachial biceps short head tendon sprain
肱二头肌腱断裂	gōng èr tóu jī jiàn duàn liè	rupture of brachial biceps tendon
肩关节周围炎	jiān guān jié zhōu wéi yán	periarthritis of shoulder
肩峰下滑液囊炎	jiān fēng xià huá yè náng yán	subacromial bursitis

Soft tissue injuries of the elbow		
肘关节扭挫伤	zhǒu guān jié niǔ cuò shāng	elbow sprain and contusion
肱骨外上髁炎	gōng gǔ wài shàng kē yán	external humeral epicondylitis
肱骨内上髁炎	gōng gǔ nèi shàng kē yán	internal humeral epicondylitis
旋前圆肌综合征	xuán qián yuán jī zōng hé zhēng	pronator syndrome
旋后肌综合征	xuán hòu jī zōng hé zhēng	supinator syndrome
肘关节骨化性肌炎	zhǒu guān jié gǔ huà xìng jī yán	ossifying myositis of elbow
尺骨鹰嘴滑膜囊炎	chǐ gǔ yīng zuǐ huá mó náng yán	bursitis of olecranon
Soft tissue injuries of the wrist and hand		
腕关节扭伤	wàn guān jié niǔ shāng	wrist sprain
桡侧伸腕肌腱周围炎	ráo cè shēn wàn jī jiàn zhōu wéi yán	radial extensor perimyotenositis of wrist
腕管综合征	wàn guǎn zōng hé zhēng	carpal tunnel syndrome
指伸、指屈肌腱断裂	zhǐ shēn、zhǐ qū jī jiàn duàn liè	tendinous rupture of digital flexor or extensor muscle
腱鞘囊肿	jiàn qiào náng zhǒng	thecal cyst
桡骨茎突狭窄性腱鞘炎	ráo gǔ jìng tū xiá zhǎi xìng jiàn qiào yán	tenosynovitis stenosans (of processus styloideus radii)
指屈肌腱鞘炎	zhǐ qū jī jiàn qiào yán	tenosynovititis of digital flexor muscle
Soft tissue injuries of the hip and thigh		
股四头肌损伤	gǔ sì tóu jī sǔn shāng	injury of quadriceps femoris
股内收肌群损伤	gǔ nèi shōu jī qún sǔn shāng	injury of femoral adductors
髋关节一过性滑膜炎	kuān guān jié yī guò xìng huá mó yán	transient bursitis of hip joint
弹响髋	tán xiǎng kuān	snapping hip
股骨大转子滑膜囊炎	gǔ gǔ dà zhuàn zǐ huá mó náng yán	trochanteric bursitis of femur
Soft tissue injuries of the knee and shin		
膝关节内、外侧副韧带损伤	xī guān jié nèi、wài cè fù rèn dài sǔn shāng	injury of medial/lateral collateral ligament of knee joint
膝交叉韧带损伤	xī jiāo chā rèn dài sǔn shāng	cruciate ligament injury of knee
半月板损伤	bàn yuè bǎn sǔn shāng	meniscus injury
膝关节创伤性滑膜炎	xī guān jié chuāng shāng xìng huá mó yán	traumatic synovitis of knee
髌腱断裂	bìn jiàn duàn liè	rupture of patellar tendon

髌前、髌下滑膜囊炎	bìn qián、bìn xià huá mó náng yán	prepatellar or infrapatellar bursitis
髌骨软化症	bìn gǔ ruǎn huà zhèng	chondromalacia patellae
髌下脂肪垫肥厚	bìn xià zhī fáng diàn féi hòu	hypertrophy of subpatellar fat pad
腘窝囊肿	guó wō náng zhǒng	popliteal cyst
腓肠肌损伤	féi cháng jī sǔn shāng	injury of gastrocnemius muscle
Soft tissue injuries of the ankle and foot		
距小腿关节内、外侧韧带损伤	jù xiǎo tuǐ guān jié nèi、wài cè rèn dài sǔn shāng	injury of medial or lateral ligament of talocrural joint
跗跖关节扭伤	fū zhí guān jié niǔ shāng	tarsometatarsal sprain
跟腱断裂	gēn jiàn duàn liè	rupture of Achilles tendon
跟腱滑膜囊炎	gēn jiàn huá mó náng yán	Achilles bursitis
跟腱炎	gēn jiàn yán	Achilles tendinitis
踝管综合征	huái guǎn zōng hé zhēng	tarsal tunnel syndrome
腓骨长、短肌腱滑脱	féi gǔ cháng、duǎn jī jiàn huá tuō	olisthy of long or short peroneal tendon
跟痛症	gēn tòng zhèng	heel pain; calcaneodynia
跖痛症	zhí tòng zhèng	metatarsal pain
跗跖滑膜囊炎	mǔ zhí huá mó náng yán	hallucal bursitis
Soft tissue injuries of the chin and neck		
颞颌关节紊乱症	niè hé guān jié wěn luàn zhèng	disorder of temporomandibular joint
颈部急性扭挫伤	jǐng bù jí xìng niǔ cuò shāng	acute sprain and contusion of neck
落枕	lào zhěn	stiff neck
颈椎病	jǐng zhuī bìng	cervical spondylosis
肌性斜颈	jī xìng xié jǐng	myogenic torticollis
颈椎关节突关节错缝	jǐng zhuī guān jié tū guān jié cuò fèng	fissured fracture of cervical vertebral process
Soft tissue injuries of the chest and back		
胸部扭挫伤	xiōng bù niǔ cuò shāng	thoracic sprain and contusion
项背急性扭挫伤	xiàng bèi jí xìng niǔ cuò shāng	acute nuchal sprain and contusion
胸廓出口综合征	xiōng kuò chū kǒu zōng hé zhēng	thoracic outlet syndrome
胸椎小关节错缝	xiōng zhuī xiǎo guān jié cuò fèng	minor joint dislocation of thoracic vertebrae
Soft tissue injuries of the lumbosaccral region		
急性腰扭伤	jí xìng yāo niǔ shāng	acute lumbar sprain

慢性腰肌劳损	màn xìng yāo jī láo sǔn	chronic lumbar muscle strain
第三腰椎横突综合征	dì sān yāo zhuī héng tū zōng hé zhēng	transverse process syndrome of the third lumbar vertebra
腰椎间盘突出症	yāo zhuī jiān pán tū chū zhèng	prolapse of lumbar intervertebral disc
腰椎椎管狭窄症	yāo zhuī zhuī guǎn xiá zhǎi zhèng	lumbar spinal canal stenosis
骶髂关节损伤	dǐ qià guān jié sǔn shāng	sacro-iliac injury
腰椎退行性滑脱	yāo zhuī tuì xíng xìng huá tuō	lumbar retrograde spondylolisthesis
腰臀部筋膜炎	yāo tún bù jīn mó yán	lumbogluteal fasciitis
臀肌挛缩症	tún jī luán suō zhèng	contraction of gluteal muscles
梨状肌综合征	lí zhuàng jī zōng hé zhēng	periform muscle syndrome
坐骨结节滑膜囊炎	zuò gǔ jié jié huá mó náng yán	bursitis of ischial tuberosity
骶尾部挫伤	dǐ wěi bù cuò shāng	sacrococcygeal contusion
Peripheral nerve injuries		
正中神经损伤	zhèng zhōng shén jīng sǔn shāng	median nerve injury
尺神经损伤	chǐ shén jīng sǔn shāng	ulnar nerve injury
桡神经损伤	ráo shén jīng sǔn shāng	radial nerve injury
臂丛神经损伤	bì cóng shén jīng sǔn shāng	brachial plexus nerve injury
坐骨神经损伤	zuò gǔ shén jīng sǔn shāng	sciatic nerve injury
腓神经损伤	féi shén jīng sǔn shāng	peroneal nerve injury
腓总神经损伤	féi zǒng shén jīng sǔn shāng	common peroneal nerve injury
胫神经损伤	jìng shén jīng sǔn shāng	tibial nerve injury

撕裂伤 [sī liè shāng]
laceration; lacerated wound: torn and ragged wound

断裂伤 [duàn liè shāng]
rupture; ruptured wound: wound with disruption of the tissues

骨错缝 [gǔ cuò fèng]
fissured fracture: crack extending from the surface into, but not through a long bone

扭伤 [niǔ shāng]
sprain: sudden or violent twist or wrench of a joint causing stretching or tearing of ligaments

挫伤 [cuò shāng]
contusion: injury of the subcutaneous or deeper tissues without a break in the skin

碾挫伤 [niǎn cuò shāng]
crushing-contusion: crushed and contused wound

牵拉肩 [qiān lā jiān]
dragged shoulder: sprain of the short head tendon of the brachial biceps

弹响指 [tán xiǎng zhǐ]
snapping finger: another name for tenovaginitis of flexor digitorum. It is so called as the finger is liable to have a momentary spasmodic arrest of flexion or extension followed by a snapping into place.

理筋手法 [lǐ jīn shǒu fǎ]
tendon-regulating manipulation; therapeutic manipulation for tendon injury: collective term for various manipulations for treating injured tendons and other soft tissues, including pressing, rubbing, kneading, pinching, pushing, grasping, lifting, plucking and shaking

理筋 [lǐ jīn]
tendon regulation: manipulation performed by pressing and pushing the injured tendon along its course with the fingers slowly and repeatedly, to regulate and soothe the tendon and promote the flow of *qi* and blood

分筋 [fēn jīn]
tendon separation: manipulation performed by pressing deeply with the tip of the thumb the area close to the nodulation or tender point of the tendon and slowly kneading and plucking for separating adhesion or relieving spasm

筋正 [jīn zhèng]
tendon restoration: restoration of the tendon or soft tissue to its normal position

筋合 [jīn hé]
tendon reunion: reuniting of the tendon and muscle after an injury

搓法 [cuō fǎ]
twisting manipulation; foulage: twisting an injured limb with both palms in opposite directions

揉法 [róu fǎ]
kneading manipulation: pressing and moving to and fro or circularly on an affected area with the flat of the thumb, the tips of the index, middle and ring fingers, the thenar or root of a palm of the hand

指揉法 [zhǐ róu fǎ]
finger-kneading manipulation: kneading with the index and middle fingers or with the index, middle and ring fingers (Fig. 41)

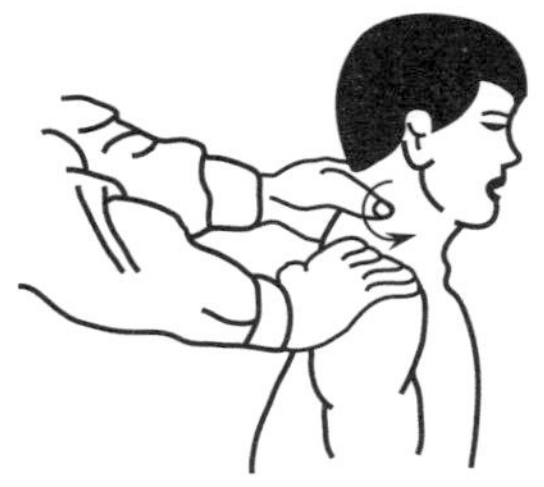

Fig. 41 Finger-kneading manipulation

掌揉法 [zhǎng róu fǎ]
palm-kneading manipulation: kneading with the palm of the hand circularly (Fig. 42)

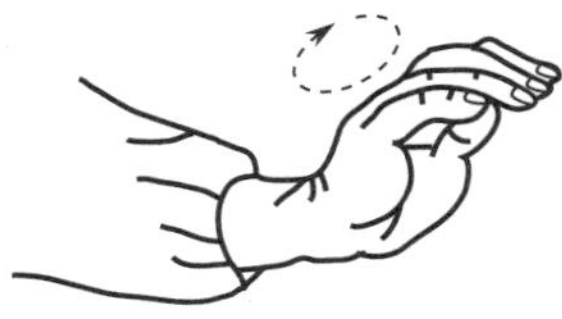

Fig. 42 Palm-kneading manipulation

拳揉法 [quán róu fǎ]
fist-kneading manipulation: kneading with the ulnar aspect of a fist circularly (Fig. 43)

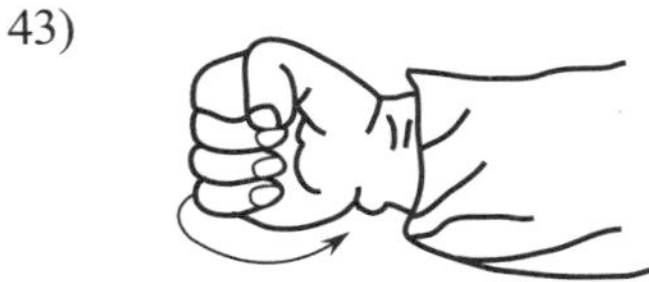

Fig. 43 Fist-kneading manipulation

肘揉法 [zhǒu róu fǎ]

elbow-kneading manipulation: kneading with the olecranon of an elbow on the affected area for massaging deep muscles (Fig. 44)

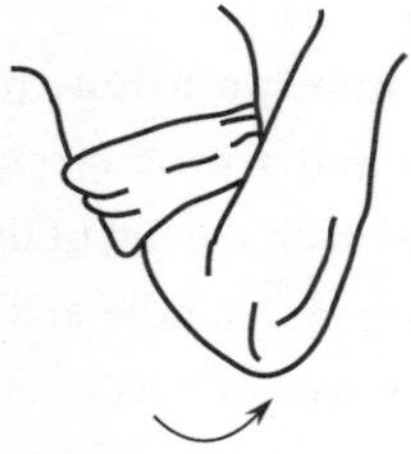

Fig. 44 Elbow-kneading manipulation

抱踝手法 [bào huái shǒu fǎ]

peri-ankle manipulation: kneading the ankle

撙令平正 [zǔn lìng píng zhèng]

kneading restoration: restoration of a local injury to its normal condition by way of kneading

撙捺皮相 [zǔn nà pí xiàng]

evaluation via kneading-pressing: evaluating a fractured bone via kneading and pressing of the fractured ends

撙捺相近 [zǔn nà xiāng jìn]

kneading-pressing (the fractured ends) close: manipulation in bone-setting performed by kneading and pressing the fractured ends and bringing them close to each other

推法 [tuī fǎ]

pushing manipulation: pushing and squeezing muscles with the fingers, palms of the hands, or elbow forward, apart, or spirally with force

一指禅推法 [yī zhǐ chán tuī fǎ]

***qi*-concentrated single-finger pushing manipulation:** pushing tissues with the tip, flat or outer side of the thumb,on which the operator's *qi* is concentrated by meditation, also called 一指禅推拿疗法 [yī zhǐ chán tuī ná liáo fǎ] (Fig. 45)

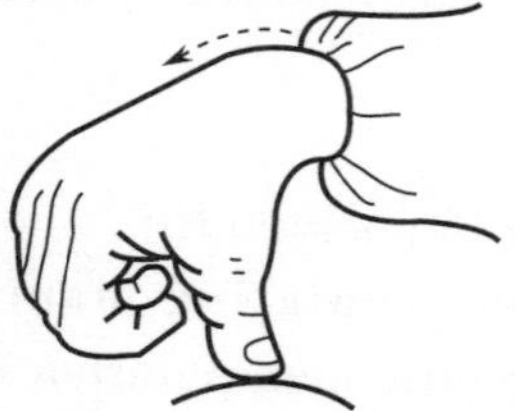

Fig. 45 *Qi*-concentrated single-finger pushing

一指禅推拿疗法 [yī zhǐ chán tuī ná liáo fǎ]

***qi*-concentrated single-finger pushing therapy:** same as 一指禅推法 [yī zhǐ chán tuī fǎ]

指推法 [zhǐ tuī fǎ]

finger-pushing manipulation: pushing with the ventral side of the thumb while the other fingers are slightly bent, usually along the course of a meridian/channel or muscle fibers

掌推法 [zhǎng tuī fǎ]

palm-pushing manipulation: pushing with the root of a palm of the hand alone or with the root of one palm of the hand overlapped by that of the other (Fig. 46)

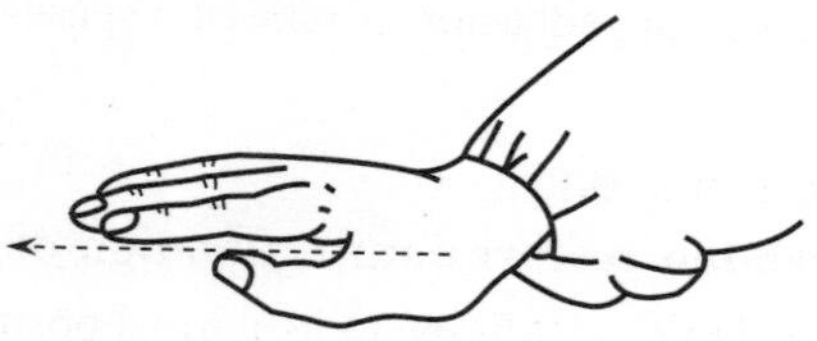

Fig. 46 Palm-pushing manipulation

肘推法 [zhǒu tuī fǎ]

elbow pushing manipulation: pushing with the olecranon of the elbow, usually giving stronger force (Fig. 47)

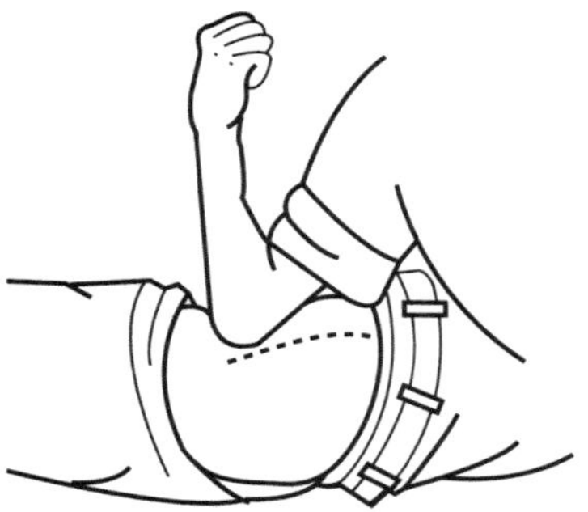

Fig. 47 Elbow-pushing manipulation

滚法 [gǔn fǎ]

rolling manipulation: manipulation performed by turning the back of a hollow fist over the skin back and forth continuously with moderate force and small amplitude

拍击法 [pāi jī fǎ]

patting-striking manipulation: combined manipulation of patting and striking

击法 [jī fǎ]

striking manipulation: manipulation performed by striking the affected area of the body with the palm of the hand, fist, or a specially made rod

拳击法 [quán jī fǎ]

fist-striking manipulation: striking the selected area of the body surface with the ulnar side of one or both fists (Fig. 48)

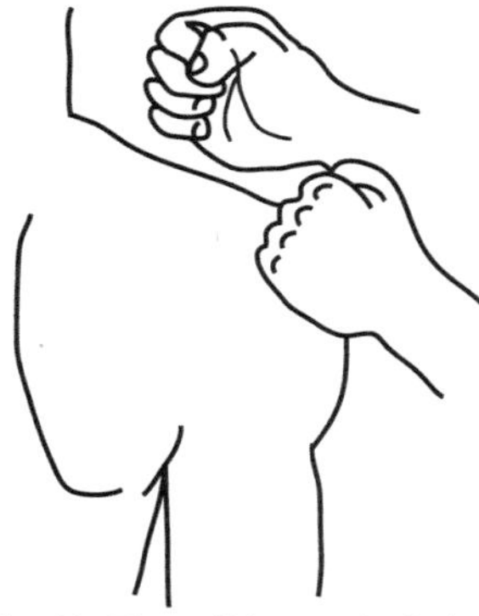

Fig. 48 Fist-striking manipulation

掌击法 [zhǎng jī fǎ]

palm-striking manipulation: striking the selected area of the body surface with the root of a palm of the hand (Fig. 49)

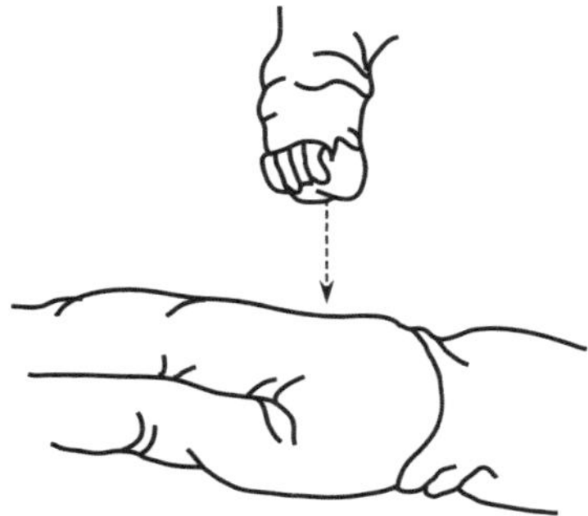

Fig. 49 Palm-striking manipulation

指节拍法 [zhǐ jié pāi fǎ]

knuckle-patting manipulation: patting a certain part of the body with the dorsal side of the finger joints with the fingers lightly bent (Fig. 50)

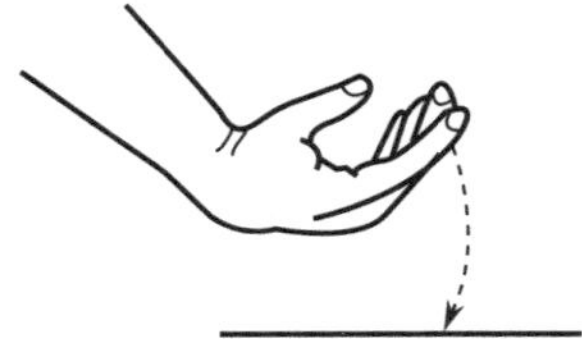

Fig. 50 Knuckle-patting manipulation

劈法 [pī fǎ]

vertical palm-striking manipulation: striking a selected area of the body surface by using the ulnar side of the palms of the hands with the fingers extended as if tending to split the treated area (Fig. 51)

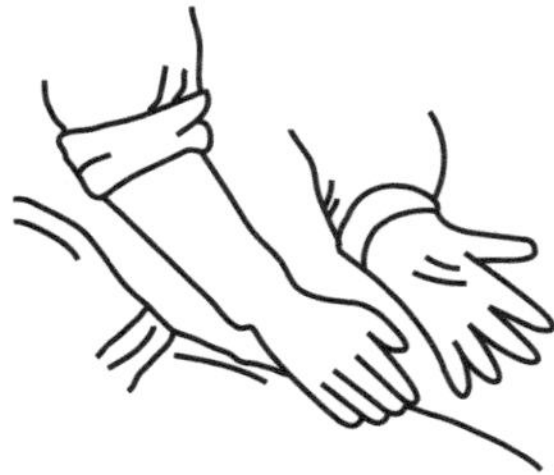

Fig. 51 Vertical palm-striking manipulation

啄法 [zhuó fǎ]

pecking manipulation: patting the selected area of the body surface with the finger tips when the fingers are slightly bent, resembling a bird's pecking (Fig. 52)

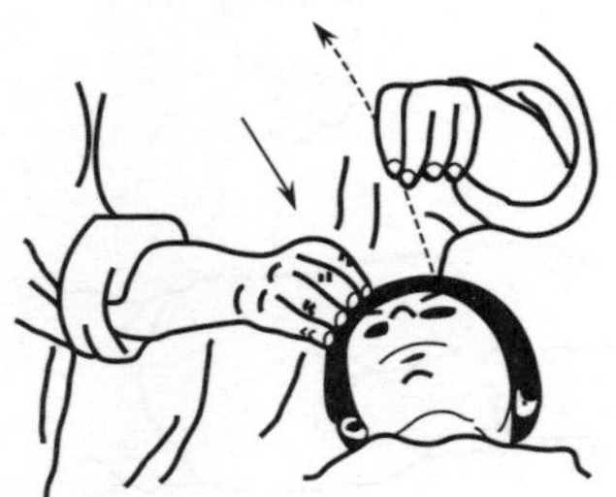

Fig. 52 Pecking manipulation

棒击法 [bàng jī fǎ]

rod-striking manipulation: striking the selected area of the body surface with a mulberry branch

摩法 [mó fǎ]

circular rubbing manipulation: rubbing the affected part with the ventral aspect of the finger tips or the palm in a circular motion with moderate force and frequency

掌摩法 [zhǎng mó fǎ]

palmar circular rubbing manipulation: circular rubbing performed on the surface of the affected area by using the palm of a hand (Fig. 53)

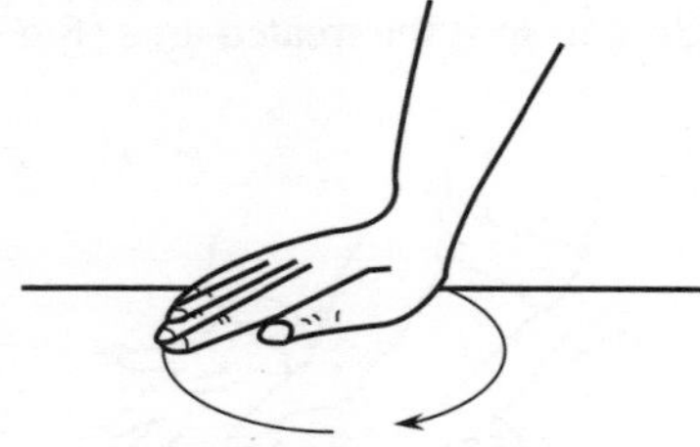

Fig. 53 Palmar circular rubbing manipulation

指摩法 [zhǐ mó fǎ]

digital circular rubbing manipulation: rotary rubbing performed on the surface of the affected area by using the ventral aspect of the thumb, index finger and middle finger in combination (Fig. 54)

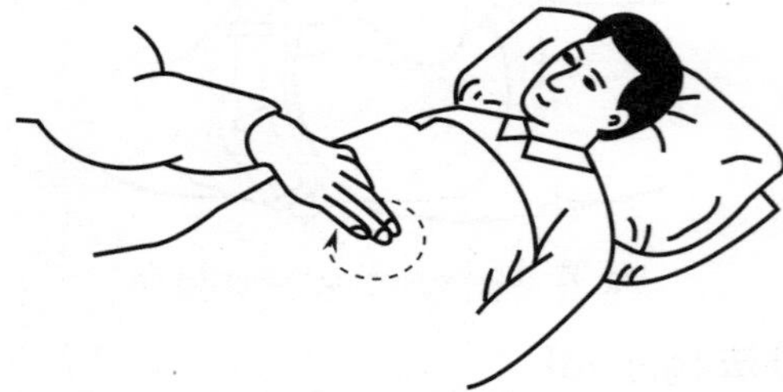

Fig. 54 Digital circular rubbing manipulation

擦法 [cā fǎ]

rubbing manipulation: rubbing with the flat of the finger, the thenar, or the palm of the hand to and fro over the selected area of the body surface continuously and with a high frequency

掌擦法 [zhǎng cā fǎ]

palm-rubbing manipulation: rubbing the selected area of the body surface with the whole palm of the hand (Fig. 55)

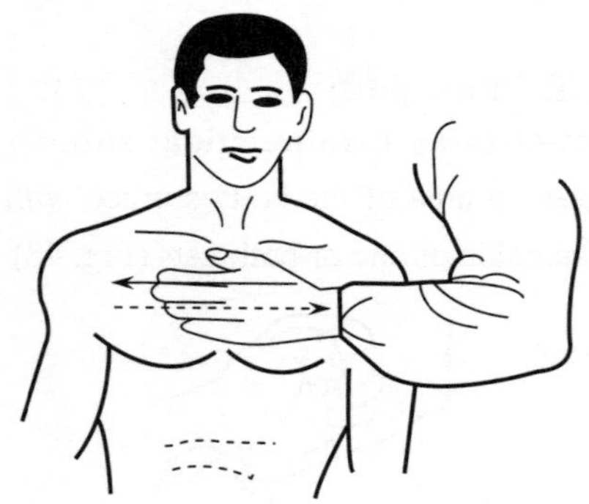

Fig. 55 Palm-rubbing manipulation

鱼际擦法 [yú jì cā fǎ]

eminence-rubbing manipulation: rubbing the selected area of the body surface with the thenar eminence (Fig. 56)

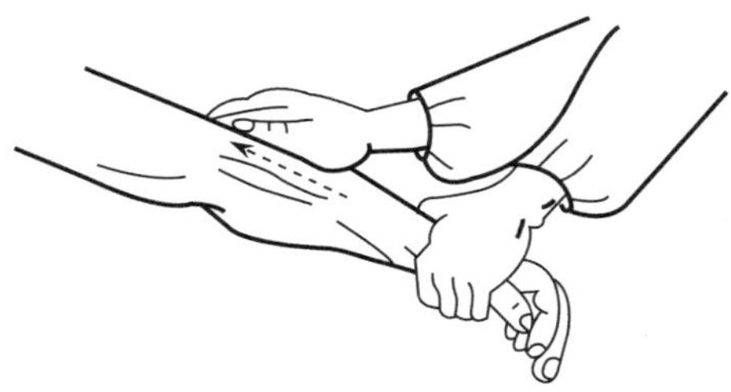

Fig. 56 Eminence-rubbing manipulation

侧擦法 [cè cā fǎ]

side-rubbing manipulation: rubbing the selected area of the body surface with the ulnar side of the palm of the hand (Fig. 57)

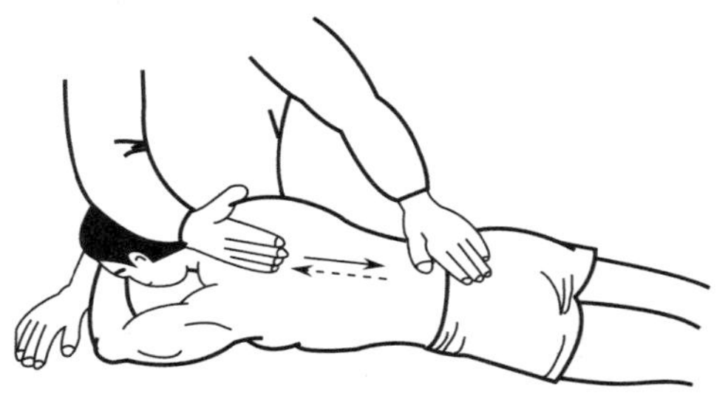

Fig. 57 Side-rubbing manipulation

抖法 [dǒu fǎ]

shaking manipulation: holding down and pulling outwards the distal end of the affected extremity, which is then shaken up and down within the limit of movement (Fig. 58)

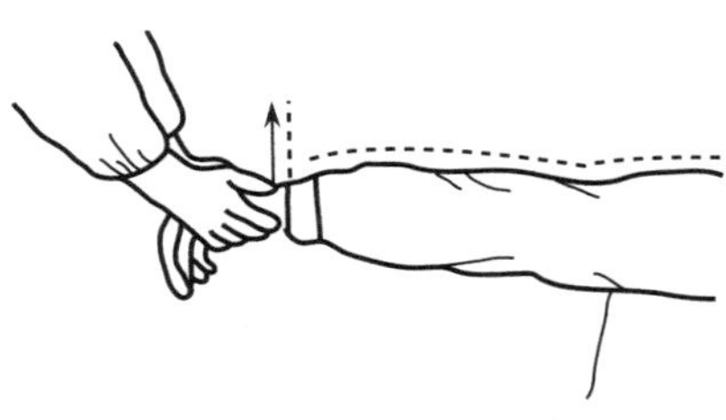

Fig. 58 Shaking manipulation

弹法 [tán fǎ]

flicking manipulation: hitting the affected area with the back of the index or middle fingertip by flicking it against the thumb (Fig. 59)

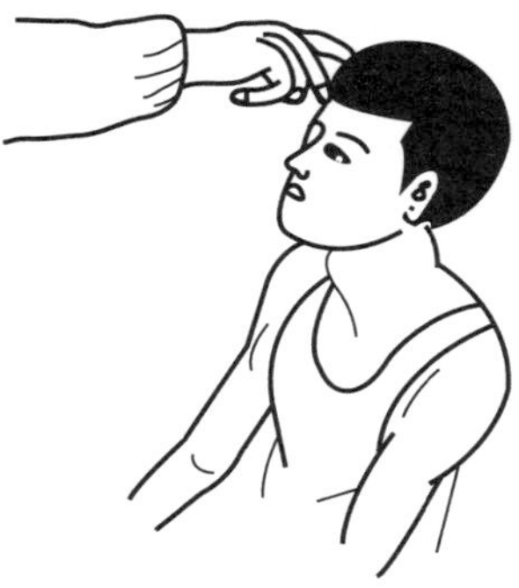

Fig. 59 Flicking manipulation

弹筋法 [tán jīn fǎ]

tendon-plucking manipulation: repeating the actions of pulling up the tendon or muscle and immediately releasing it

按法 [àn fǎ]

pressing manipulation: pushing steadily in a direction vertical to the body surface

指按法 [zhǐ àn fǎ]

finger-pressing manipulation: pressing with the ventral part of the thumb or with the ventral part of the index, middle and ring fingers in combination

掌按法 [zhǎng àn fǎ]

palm-pressing manipulation: pressing the selected area with the radial eminence, ventral surface or root part of the palm of the hand. An overlapping hand may be added if forceful pressing is necessary.

肘按法 [zhǒu àn fǎ]

elbow-pressing manipulation: pressing with the olecranon of the elbow

拿法 [ná fǎ]

grasping manipulation: manual treatment for soft-tissue injury by lifting and squeezing or lifting and rapidly releasing the affected muscles with the thumb, index and middle fingers or with the thumb and the other four fingers of one or both of the practitioner's hands

捏法 [niē fǎ]

pinching manipulation: holding and lifting the superficial tissues by using the thumb with the index and middle fingers or the thumb with the other four fingers, and squeezing and pushing forward

合指捏法 [hé zhǐ niē fǎ]

finger-combining pinching manipulation: referring to pinching with the thumb, the index and middle fingers or pinching with the thumb and the other four fingers

双手捏法 [shuāng shǒu niē fǎ]

bimanual pinching manipulation: pinching with the fingers of both hands or the roots of the palms of both hands

屈指捏法 [qū zhǐ niē fǎ]

bent-finger pinching manipulation: pinching a muscle firmly with the thumb and index finger bent like a pair of pliers, followed by kneading the treated area

踩跷法 [cǎi qiào fǎ]

treading manipulation: manipulation seldom used at present, performed by treading the affected area for reduction, e.g., treading on the back for the reduction of protruded intervertebral disc

摇法 [yáo fǎ]

rotating manipulation: turning the patient's head and neck, or shoulder, wrist, hip joint, knee joint, and ankle to and fro to relieve rigidity

扳法 [bān fǎ]

pulling manipulation: extending, bending or rotating the spine or a limb by pulling with two hands of the practitioner in an opposite direction and beyond a limited range instantaneously

扳颈椎法 [bān jǐng zhuī fǎ]

cervical pulling manipulation: reduction of a dislocated cervical vertebra by pulling

颈椎单人旋转复位法 [jǐng zhuī dān rén xuán zhuǎn fù wèi fǎ]

single-handed rotating reduction of cervical vertebra: reduction manipulation often used for treating dislocation of an upper cervical vertebra

颈椎角度复位法 [jǐng zhuī jiǎo dù fù wèi fǎ]

angular reduction of cervical vertebra: reduction manipulation often used for treating dislocation of a middle cervical vertebra

颈椎侧旋复位法 [jǐng zhuī cè xuán fù wèi fǎ]

laterally-rotating reduction of cervical vertebra: reduction manipulation often used for treating dislocation of a lower cervical vertebra

扳胸椎法 [bān xiōng zhuī fǎ]

thoracic pulling manipulation: pulling to reduce a dislocated thoracic vertebra

掌推扳胸椎法 [zhǎng tuī bān xiōng zhuī fǎ]

palm-pushing thoracic pulling manipulation: manipulation for reduction of a displaced thoracic vertebra, performed by placing the palm root of one hand on the spinous process of the affected vertebra while the patient is lying prone, pushing forward and upward with the aid of the other hand at the end of deep expiration by the patient, with a nimble action which causes a click

膝顶扳胸椎法 [xī dǐng bān xiōng zhuī fǎ]
knee-pushing thoracic pulling manipulation: manipulation for reduction of a displaced thoracic vertebra while the patent is sitting on a low stool, performed by pushing upward and forward with the practitioner's right knee and simultaneously pressing the upper chest backward and downward with the practitioner's hands at the end of inspiration by the patient, with a nimble action which causes a click

扳腰椎法 [bān yāo zhuī fǎ]
lumbar pulling manipulation: pulling to reduce a dislocated lumbar vertebra

斜扳腰椎法 [xié bān yāo zhuī fǎ]
oblique lumbar pulling manipulation: manipulation to reduce a dislocated lumbar vertebra while the patient is lying on his (her) side, performed by placing one hand on the anterior aspect of the patient's shoulder and the other hand on the patient's buttock, then pulling the shoulder while pushing the buttock simultaneouly with a nimble forceful action which causes a click

腰椎旋转复位法 [yāo zhuī xuán zhuǎn fù wèi fǎ]
lumbar rotating reduction manipulation: rotating the lumbar spine for reducing a dislocated lumbar vertebra

后伸扳腰法 [hòu shēn bān yāo fǎ]
lumbar extending-counterpulling manipulation: manipulation to reduce a dislocated lumbar vertebra while the patient is lying prone, performed by pressing the patient's lumbar or sacro-iliac region with one hand and lifting the legs with the other hand to cause lumbar extension

拔伸法 [bá shēn fǎ]
pulling-stretching manipulation: combined manipulation of pulling and stretching

屈伸法 [qū shēn fǎ]
flexing-stretching manipulation: combined manipulation of flexing and stretching

背法 [bēi fǎ]
back-carrying manipulation: manipulation for reducing a protruded lumbar intervertebral disc, performed by lifting the patient onto the practitioner's back while the two stand back to back

练功 [liàn gōng]
functional training: physical exertion for the improvement of body functions

肩臂功 [jiān bì gōng]
shoulder-arm exercise; acromiobrachial functional training: functional training of the shoulder and arm

腿功 [tuǐ gōng]
leg training: method of training the lower limb during convalescence after bone-setting

双手攀足式 [shuāng shǒu pān zú shì]
grasping the feet with both hands: lumbar training by grasping the feet with both own hands

双手托天式 [shuāng shǒu tuō tiān shì]
pushing upwards with both hands: training the functional activity of the upper limbs by pushing the hands upward as if lifting a weight

拧拳反掌式 [nǐng quán fǎn zhǎng shì]
clenching a fist, turning over and opening the hand: an exercise for training the carpal joint

振挺 [zhèn tǐng]
patting stick: a wooden stick, 2-3 cm in diameter, used as a patting device for dispersing swelling and dissipating ecchymosis in traumatology

通利关节 [tōng lì guān jié]
easing the joint: restoring natural mobility to a joint

骨病 [gǔ bìng]
osteopathy: bone disease. The terms for various bone diseases used in contemporary Chinese medicine are the same as those used in Western medicine and are listed in the following table.

Suppurative bone inflammation		
急性化脓性骨髓炎	jí xìng huà nóng xìng gǔ suǐ yán	acute suppurative osteomyelitis
慢性化脓性骨髓炎	màn xìng huà nóng xìng gǔ suǐ yán	chronic suppurative osteomyelitis
化脓性关节炎	huà nóng xìng guān jié yán	suppurative arthritis
硬化性骨髓炎	yìng huà xìng gǔ suǐ yán	sclerosing osteomyelitis
Bone tuberculosis		
脊柱结核	jǐ zhù jié hé	tuberculosis of spine
髋关节结核	kuān guān jié jié hé	tuberculosis of hip joint
膝关节结核	xī guān jié jié hé	tuberculosis of knee joint
骶髂关节结核	dǐ qià guān jié jié hé	tuberculosis of sacro-iliac joint
骨干结核	gǔ gàn jié hé	diaphysial tuberculosis
Osteoarthiritis		
骨性关节炎	gǔ xìng guān jié yán	osteoarthritis
类风湿性关节炎	lèi fēng shī xìng guān jié yán	rheumatoid arthritis
强直性脊柱炎	jiāng zhí xìng jǐ zhù yán	ankylosing spondylitis
髋关节骨性关节炎	kuān guān jié gǔ xìng guān jié yán	osteoarthritis of hip
膝关节骨性关节炎	xī guān jié gǔ xìng guān jié yán	osteoarthritis of knee
牛皮癣性关节炎	niú pí xuǎn xìng guān jié yán	psoriatic arthritis
痛风性关节炎	tòng fēng xìng guān jié yán	gouty arthritis
神经性关节炎	shén jīng xìng guān jié yán	neuropathic arthritis
Atrophy-flaccidity of bone		
骨质疏松症	gǔ zhì shū sōng zhèng	osteoporosis

佝偻病	gōu lóu bìng	rickets
骨软化症	gǔ ruǎn huà zhèng	osteomalacia
Sequelae of poliomyelitis		
臀肌瘫痪	tún jī tān huàn	paralysis of gluteal muscles
股四头肌瘫痪	gǔ sì tóu jī tān huàn	paralysis of quadriceps femoris
小腿肌瘫痪	xiǎo tuǐ jī tān huàn	paralysis of crural muscles
Osteonecrosis		
股骨头缺血性坏死	gǔ gǔ tóu quē xuè xìng huài sǐ	ischemic necrosis of caput femoris
胫骨结节骨骺炎	jìng gǔ jié jié gǔ hóu yán	epiphysitis of tibial tuberosity
脊椎骨骺骨软骨炎	jǐ zhuī gǔ hóu gǔ ruǎn gǔ yán	osteochondritis of epiphysis of the spine
距骨缺血性坏死	jù gǔ quē xuè xìng huài sǐ	ischemic necrosis of the talus
Congenital osteoarticular deformities		
先天性斜颈	xiān tiān xìng xié jǐng	congenital torticollis
颈肋	jǐng lèi	cervicle rib
脊柱侧凸症	jǐ zhù cè tū zhèng	scoliosis
脊柱裂	jǐ zhù liè	rachischisis; spina bifida
先天性高肩胛症	xiān tiān xìng gāo jiān jiǎ zhèng	congenital elevation of scapula
先天性桡骨缺如	xiān tiān xìng ráo gǔ quē rú	congenital absence of radius
先天性髋关节脱位	xiān tiān xìng kuān guān jié tuō wèi	congenital hip luxation
膝内翻	xī nèi fān	genu varum
膝外翻	xī wài fān	genu valgum
踇外翻	mǔ wài fān	hallux valgus
先天性胫骨假关节	xiān tiān xìng jìng gǔ jiǎ guān jié	congenital tibia pseudoarthrosis
先天性马蹄内翻足	xiān tiān xìng mǎ tí nèi fān zú	congenital equinovarus
Developmental bone disturbances		
成骨不全	chéng gǔ bù quán	osteogenesis imperfecta
软骨发育不全	ruǎn gǔ fā yù bù quán	achondroplasia
石骨症	shí gǔ zhèng	marble bone; osteopetrosis
Bone tumors		
骨瘤	gǔ liú	osteoma
软骨瘤	ruǎn gǔ liú	chondroma
骨软骨瘤	gǔ ruǎn gǔ liú	osteochondroma

骨样骨瘤	gǔ yàng gǔ liú	osteoid osteoma
骨巨细胞瘤	gǔ jù xì bāo liú	giant cell tumor of bone
骨血管瘤	gǔ xuè guǎn liú	hemangioma of bone
骨肉瘤	gǔ ròu liú	osteosarcoma
软骨肉瘤	ruǎn gǔ ròu liú	chondrosarcoma
纤维肉瘤	xiān wéi ròu liú	fibrosarcoma
骨髓瘤	gǔ suǐ liú	myeloma
骨转移瘤	gǔ zhuǎn yí liú	metastatic tumor of bone
Endemic and professional osteo-articular diseases		
大骨节病	dà gǔ jié bìng	Kaschin-Beck disease
氟骨病	fú gǔ bìng	skeletal fluorosis
振动病	zhèn dòng bìng	vibration disease
Syphilis of bones and joints		
骨梅毒	gǔ méi dú	bone syphilis
关节梅毒	guān jié méi dú	joint syphilis

内翻 [nèi fān]

inversion: the condition of being turned inward (as of the foot)

外翻 [wài fān]

eversion: the condition of being turned outward (as of the foot)

附骨疽 [fù gǔ jū]

bone-attached abscess: suppurative osteomyelitis including osteomyelitits and bone tuberculosis

骨痨 [gǔ láo]

bone phthisis: osteoarticular tuberculosis

医学史
Medical History

名医 Distinguished Physicians

岐伯 [qí bó]

Qi Bo: physician in the reign of Huangdi (the Yellow Emperor) (trad. 2698-2589 B.C.). He was requested by Huangdi to taste various kinds of herbs and to study medicine and pharmacy. His dialogues with Huangdi on broad aspects of medical issues were recorded and compiled as the major content of the first comprehensive medical work in China – *Huangdi Nei Jing* (黄帝内经), or *Yellow Emperor's Internal Classic*, or *Yellow Emperor's Canon of Medicine*.

雷公 [léi gōng]

Lei Gong: (1) physician in the reign of Huangdi (the Yellow Emperor). Discussions between Huangdi and Lei Gong on medicine including pharmacy, acupuncture and moxibustion were recorded and compiled in the *Canon of Medicine*; (2) the style name of 雷敩 [léi xiào], a pharmacist in the period of the Northern and Southern Dynasties (420-589) who wrote the *Lei Gong Pao Zhi Lun* (雷公炮炙论), or *Lei's Treatise on Medicinal Processing*

医和 [yī hé]

Yi He: physician in the Spring and Autumn Period (c. 600 B.C.), who put forward the theory that abnormality in the six climatic conditions, namely, cloudiness, sunniness, windiness, raininess, gloominess, and brightness, would lead to illnesses of different natures

扁鹊 [biǎn què]

Bian Que: another name for Qin Yueren (秦越人) (c. 500B.C.), the earliest Chinese physician versed in diagnosis and treatment, especially in pulse taking and acupuncture. To him is ascribed the authorship of such medical works as *Bian Que Nei Jing* (扁鹊内经), or *The Internal Classic of Bian Que*, and *Bian Que Wai Jing* (扁鹊外经), or *The External Classic of Bian Que*, both of which have been lost.

秦越人 [qín yuè rén]

Qin Yueren: the original name of Bian Que (扁鹊 [biǎn què])

淳于意 [chún yú yì]

Chunyu Yi: physician (c. 205-? B.C.) styled Cang Gong (仓公 [cāng gōng]), the Reverend Master of the Granary, for having been put in charge of the public granary of the State of Qi. He is said to have attached great importance to pulse taking and record keeping of complete clinical data.

仓公 [cāng gōng]

Cang Gong: style name of Chunyu Yi (淳于意)

张机 [zhāng jī]

Zhang Ji: one of the most influential physicians in the history of Chinese medicine (150?-219?), also called Zhang Zhongjing (张仲景). He was the first to propose the theory of syndrome differentiation (pattern identification)

in accordance with the six meridians/channels, identify the eight principal syndromes/patterns and establish the corresponding principles of treatment. To him is ascribed the authorship of several books on various medical topics, the most important of which now extant are the *Shang Han Za Bing Lun* (伤寒杂病论), or *Treatise on Cold Damage and Miscellaneous Diseases*, and the *Jin Gui Yao Lue Fang Lun* (金匮要略方论), or *Synopsis of Prescriptions of the Golden Chamber.*

张仲景 [zhāng zhòng jǐng]
Zhang Zhongjing: another name for Zhang Ji (张机)

华佗 [huà tuó]
Hua Tuo: surgeon and at the same time master of all other branches of medicine, also known as Hua Fu (华旉) or Hua Yuan-hua (华元化) (?-203). He was said to have performed many major surgical operations including abdominal section with herbal anesthesia and to be the inventor of therapeutic gymnastics called Wu Qin Xi (五禽戏), or the *Frolics of Five Animals*. The book *Zhong Zang Jing* (中藏经), or *Treasured Classic* was once ascribed to him but it was in fact compiled by an unknown author during the Six Dynasties period (220-589).

华旉 [huà fū]
Hua Fu: another name for Hua Tuo (华佗)

王熙 [wáng xī]
Wang Xi: commissioner of the Imperial Academy of Medicine, also called Wang Shuhe (王叔和) (c. 210-285). He was well versed in pulse-taking, and was the author of the *Mai Jing* (脉经), or *The Pulse Classic*, the earliest comprehensive book on sphygmology now extant in China. He perfected and systemized the art of pulse-taking, yet emphasized the use of all other available methods of diagnosis as well, as long as they could provide useful information. He re-edited Zhang Zhongjing's *Treatise on Cold Damage and Miscellaneous Diseases*, making it an acceptable version for later generations and thus contributed significantly to the heritage of that important medical classic.

王叔和 [wáng shū hé]
Wang Shuhe: another name for Wang Xi (王熙)

皇甫谧 [huáng fǔ mì]
Huangfu Mi: also called Huangfu Shi'an (皇甫士安) (215-282), who suffering from rheumatism, studied medicine and became a famous acupuncturist. He compiled the *Zhen Jiu Jia Yi Jing* (针灸甲乙经), or *The ABC Classic of Acupuncture and Moxibustion*, the first monograph exclusively on the subject of acupuncture and moxibustion, in which detailed explanations are provided.

皇甫士安 [huáng fǔ shì ān]
Huangfu Shi'an: another name for Huangfu Mi (皇甫谧)

葛洪 [gě hóng]
Ge Hong: physician and alchemist (283-343), popularly known as Ge Zhichuan (葛稚川) or Bao Pu Zi (抱朴子), the author of the *Bao Pu Zi* (抱朴子), a treatise on alchemy, dietetics and magical practices,

and the *Zhou Hou Bei Ji Fang* (肘后备急方), or *A Handbook of Prescriptions for Emergencies*, the latter of which includes many valuable descriptions and records of diseases

葛稚川 [gě zhì chuān]
Ge Zhichuan: another name for Ge Hong (葛洪)

抱朴子 [bào pǔ zǐ]
Bao Pu Zi: alias of Ge Hong (葛洪)

龚庆宣 [gōng qìng xuān]
Gong Qingxuan: practitioner of external medicine in the Northern and Southern Dynasties (in the late 5th century) and compiler of the *Liu Juanzi Gui Yi Fang* (刘涓子鬼遗方), or *Liu Juanzi's Ghost-Bequeathed Prescriptions*, the earliest extant Chinese book on external medicine

陶弘景 [táo hóng jǐng]
Tao Hongjing: also called Tao Tongming (陶通明) (456-536), a Taoist, who specialized in the study of medicinal herbs. He compiled the *Ben Cao Jing Ji Zhu* (本草经集注), or *Commentary on Sheng Nong's Herbal*, one of the most valuable books on materia medica in China, describing 730 varieties of medical substances, including vegetable, animal and mineral drugs. Tao was also the author of the *Yang Xing Yan Ming Lu* (养性延命录), or *Records of the Art of Health and Life Preservation*.

陶通明 [táo tōng míng]
Tao Tongming: another name for Tao Hongjing (陶弘景)

徐之才 [xú zhī cái]
Xu Zhicai: physician, also called Xu Shimao (徐士茂) (505-572). He was especially proficient in the preparation of medicinal drugs, and wrote the *Yao Dui* (药对), or *Pharmacy and Compatibility* on the basis of *Lei's Pharmacy and Compatibility* (雷公药对)

徐士茂 [xú shì mào]
Xu Shimao: another name for Xu Zhicai (徐之才)

雷敩 [léi xiào]
Lei Xiao: pharmacist and the author of the *Lei Gong Pao Zhi Lun* (雷公炮炙论), or *Lei's Treatise on Medicinal Processing* (c. 500), establishing standards for the processing of medicinal drugs

甄权 [zhēn quán]
Zhen Quan (c. 540-643)**:** Tang Dynasty physician, leading expert on acupuncture and author of the *Zhen Fang* (针方), or *Needling Prescriptions*, and the *Ming Tang Ren Xing Tu* (明堂人形图) , or *Figures of the Human Body*

巢元方 [cháo yuán fāng]
Chao Yuanfang (550-630)**:** imperial physician of Emperor Yangdi (炀帝) of the Sui Dynasty and compiler of the *Zhu Bing Yuan Hou Zong Lun* (诸病源候总论), or *Treatise on the Causes and Manifestations of Diseases*, the first Chinese work on etiology and still a valuable reference book

杨上善 [yáng shàng shàn]
Yang Shangshan (585-670)**:** physician at the end of the Sui and beginning of the

Tang dynasties, imperial physician during 605-616 and one of the earliest physicians to compile notes and commentaries on the *Internal Classic* or *Canon of Medicine*. He was also the author of *Huangdi Nei Jing Tai Su* (黄帝内经太素), or *Fundamentals of Huangdi's Internal Classic*, an important reference book for studying the *Internal Classic*.

孙思邈 [sūn sī miǎo]

Sun Simiao (581-682)**:** physician of the Tang Dynasty and author of the *Qian Jin Yao Fang* (千金要方), or *Essential Prescriptions Worth a Thousand Pieces of Gold* (652) and the *Qian Jin Yi Fang* (千金翼方), or *Supplement to the Essential Prescriptions Worth a Thousand Pieces of Gold* (682), which together summarized the medical achievements made in China before the 7th century

苏敬 [sū jìng]

Su Jing (599-674)**:** court official of the Tang Dynasty, also known as Su Gong (苏恭). He was ordered by the emperor to review traditional herbals, leading a team of 22 scholars and physicians. In 659, they published the *Xin Xiu Ben Cao* (新修本草), or *Newly Revised Materia Medica (of Tang),* also called *Tang Ben Cao* (唐本草), or *The Tang Materia Medica*, the first Chinese pharmacopoeia.

苏恭 [sū gōng]

Su Gong: another name for Su Jing (苏敬 [sū jìng])

孟诜 [mèng shēn]

Meng Shen (621-713)：herbalist of the Tang Dynasty and author of the *Shi Liao Ben Cao* (食疗本草), or *A Dietetic Materia Medica.* The original version of the book has been lost, but the contents of the book can be found in the *Lei Zheng Ben Cao* (类证本草), or *Classified Materia Medica.*

鉴真 [jiàn zhēn]

Jian Zhen (688-763)**:** Buddhist monk and physician, who introduced Chinese medicine to Japan

王焘 [wáng tāo]

Wang Tao (c. 670-755)**:** physician of the Tang Dynasty. His mother's sickness made him decide to study medicine during his childhood, hoping to find a cure for her suffering. During his 20 years working in the imperial library, where he had access to various kinds of medical books, he assiduously studied each and every branch of medicine available at the time, and finally wrote a book of his own, titled *Wai Tai Mi Yao* (外台秘要), or *Arcane Essentials from the Imperial Library* (752), which is considered to contain the essence of each branch of medicine up to that time.

陈藏器 [chén cáng qì]

Chen Cangqi: herbalist of the 8th century, who compiled the *Ben Cao Shi Yi* (本草拾遗) , or *A Supplement to Materia Medica*

王冰 [wáng bīng]

Wang Bing (c. 710-805)**:** physician specializing in the art of healing and health preservation. He spent 12 years re-editing and revising the *Su Wen* (素问), or *Plain Questions*, one of the two components of *Yellow Emperor's Internal Classic*, into 24 volumes, with notes, commentaries and supplements.

昝殷 [zǎn yīn]

Zan Yin (c. 797-860)**:** specialist in women's diseases and obstetrics and the author of the *Jing Xiao Chan Bao* (经效产宝), or *Tested Treasures of Obstetrics*, written in the period 852-856 as one of China's earliest books on obstetrics

王维一 [wáng wéi yī]

Wang Weiyi (c. 987-1067)**:** acupuncturist of the Northern Song Dynasty, who sponsored the casting of two life-sized, hollow bronze figures, on the surface of which were marked the courses of the meridians/channels and the exact locations of the acupuncture points. He also compiled the *Tong Ren Shu Xue Zhen Jiu Tu Jing* (铜人俞穴针灸图经), or *Illustrated Manual of Acupoints on the Bronze Figure* (published in 1027), which is an excellent visual aid for locating acupuncture points and teaching acupuncture.

王惟德 [wáng wéi dé]

Wang Weide: another name for Wang Weiyi (王维一)

苏颂 [sū sòng]

Su Song (1020-1101)**:** official who compiled the *Tu Jing Ben Cao* (图经本草), or *Illustrated Herbal* (1062) in 21 volumes, with appended pictures of medicinal herbs collected from different regions in China by order of the emperor, the first series that visually illustrated the complete details of each medicament

沈括 [shěn kuò]

Shen Kuo (1030-1095)**:** also called Shen Cunzhong (沈存中). Though better known as a scientist in general, Shen was quite renowned in medical circles for the *Su Shen Liang Fang* (苏沈良方), or *Best Formulas Collected*, a treatise on therapeutics and medicine, co-authored with Su Shi.

沈存中 [shěn cún zhōng]

Shen Cunzhong: another name for Shen Kuo (沈括)

苏轼 [sū shì]

Su Shi: scholar and physician, co-author with Shen Kuo of the *Su Shen Liang Fang* (苏沈良方), or *Best Collected Formulas*

钱乙 [qián yǐ]

Qian Yi (c. 1032-1113)**:** also called Qian Zhong-yang (钱仲阳), appointed court physician in 1090. His experiences of more than 40 years in pediatrics were summed up by his student Yan Xiaozhong (阎孝忠) in the *Xiao Er Yao Zheng Zhi Jue* (小儿药证直诀), or *Key to the Therapeutics of Children's Diseases* (1119), one of the earliest and most influential books on the subject of pediatrics in ancient China. Qian established valuable methods for identifying and treating measles, scarlatina, chickenpox and smallpox, and was the first to point out the peculiar features of pediatrics.

钱仲阳 [qián zhòng yáng]

Qian Zhongyang: another name for Qian Yi (钱乙)

庞安时 [páng ān shí]

Pang Anshi (c. 1043-1100)**:** physician known for several medical works, among which the most widely accepted was a detailed and comprehensive treatise on various kinds of fever under the title *Shang Han Zong Bing Lun* (伤寒总病论), or *General Discourse on Cold Damage Diseases* (1100)

寇宗奭 [kòu zōng shì]
Kou Zongshi (12th century)**:** expert on materia medica of the Song Dynasty and author of the *Ben Cao Yan Yi* (本草衍义), or *Amplification on Materia Medica* (1116). He stood against the idea of administering vermilion pills for longevity, and addressed their proper use in the treatment of diseases.

刘昉 [liú fǎng]
Liu Fang (c. 1080-1150)**:** official of the Southern Song Dynasty, interested in the art of healing, especially pediatrics, and research into old prescriptions and remedies. Together with Wang Li (王历), he compiled the *You You Xin Shu* (幼幼新书), or *New Book of Pediatrics* (1132), one of the earliest monographs on the subject of pediatrics, with substantial contents.

唐慎微 [táng shèn wēi]
Tang Shenwei: also called Tang Shenyuan (唐审元), physician especially proficient in therapeutics, who declined the offer of an official post, devoting his life to practicing medicine and collecting folk recipes. He wrote the *Jing Shi Zheng Lei Bei Ji Ben Cao* (经史证类备急本草), or *Classic Classified Materia Medica for Emergencies* (1108), a work in 31 volumes, and submitted it to the emperor, who changed the book title to *Da Guan Ben Cao* (大观本草), or *Daguan Herbal.*

唐审元 [táng shěn yuán]
Tang Shenyuan: another name for Tang Shenwei (唐慎微)

成无己 [chéng wú jǐ]
Cheng Wuji (1066-1155?)**:** physician of the Jin Dynasty, known for his assiduous study of and explicit commentary on the *Treatise on Cold Damage and Miscellaneous Diseases*, a Chinese medical classic authored by Zhang Zhongjing. His *Zhu Jie Shang Han Lun* (注解伤寒论), *Commentary on the Treatise on Cold Damage Diseases* (1142), is considered the earliest of its kind in Chinese medical literature.

许叔微 [xǔ shū wēi]
Xu Shuwei (1079-1154?)**:** physician of the Song Dynasty and a disciple of Zhang Zhongjing. He designed and drew graphic illustrations of 36 typical pulse conditions based upon the relevant work previously done by his mentor Zhang Zhongjing, and propounded the theory of using medicinals in relation to the intensity of a disease. Xu was the author of several medical publications, among which the *Lei Zheng Pu Ji Ben Shi Fang* (类证普济本事方) or *Classified Effective Prescriptions for Universal Relief* (1132?) in 10 volumes has been widely accepted.

陈言 [chén yán]
Chen Yan (12th century)**:** physician of the Song Dynasty, also called Chen Wuze (陈无择), author of the *San Yin Ji Yi Bing Zheng Fang Lun* (三因极一病证方论), or *Treatise on the Three Categories of Pathogenic Factors and Prescriptions*, a work in 18 volumes published in 1174, in

which causes of diseases are classified into three categories in accordance with Zhang Zhongjing's theory

陈无择 [chén wú zé]
Chen Wuze: another name for Chen Yan (陈言)

王执中 [wáng zhí zhōng]
Wang Zhizhong (12-13th century**):** physician of the Song Dynasty skilled in acupuncture and moxibustion, author of the *Zhen Jiu Zi Sheng Jing* (针灸资生经) or *Classic of Nourishing Life with Acupuncture and Moxibustion* (1220)

齐仲甫 [qí zhòng fǔ]
Qi Zhongfu: physician of the Southern Song Dynasty with rich experience in treating women's diseases, author of the very popular medical work *Nü Ke Bai Wen* (女科百问) or *Hundred Questions on Women's Diseases* (1220)

张元素 [zhāng yuán sù]
Zhang Yuansu: physician of the 12th century, also called Zhang Jiegu (张洁古). His unique view on medicine was considered bold, that newly evolved diseases could not be treated by known methods, in other words, new diseases could not be treated with old methods. He discarded obsolete traditional formulas and devised a system of his own. Most of the doctors of the Jin-Yuan period (1115-1368) were influenced by his philosophy, which was illustrated in the *Zhen Zhu Nang* (珍珠囊), or *The Pearl Bag* and others of his medical works. Among his disciples were such eminent doctors as Li Gao (李杲) and Wang Haogu (王好古).

张洁古 [zhāng jié gǔ]
Zhang Jiegu: another name for Zhang Yuansu (张元素)

刘完素 [liú wán sù]
Liu Wansu: also called Liu Shouzhen (刘守真) (c.1120-1200). He propounded the theory that most diseases were caused by excessive heat in the body, and advocated the use of medicines of cold nature for treatment, thereby founding the Cold School of Medicine. He was the author of the *Su Wen Xuan Ji Yuan Bing* (素问玄机原病) or *Etiology Based on Plain Questions* and some other medical works, and exerted significant influence on the School of Epidemic Febrile Diseases in the Ming and Qing Dynasties.

刘守真 [liú shǒu zhēn]
Liu Shouzhen: another name for Liu Wansu (刘完素)

张从正 [zhāng cóng zhèng]
Zhang Congzheng: also called Zhang Zihe (张子和) (c. 1156-1228), once a court physician, with rich experience in various branches of medicine. He viewed a disease as a foreign substance in an organism, and advocated the use of drastic medicinals, such as diaphoretics, emetics and purgatives, as the best choice to remove foreign substances out. As the founder of the Attack or Purgation School, he authored the *Ru Men Shi Qin* (儒门事亲), or *Confucians' Duties to Their Parents*, which was completed by his disciple Ma Zhiji (麻知己).

张子和 [zhāng zǐ hé]
Zhang Zihe: another name for Zhang

Congzheng (张从正)

李杲 [lǐgǎo]

Li Gao: also called Li Mingzhi (李明之) or Li Dongyuan (李东垣) (1180-1251), a disciple of Zhang Yuansu, who held that diseases, apart from external changes, were mainly caused by internal injury to the spleen and stomach (i.e., by intemperance in drinking and eating or overwork) and advocated cure by regulating the spleen and the stomach and nourishing the original *qi*. He was considered to be the founder of the School of Strengthening the Spleen and Stomach. His masterpiece was the *Pi Wei Lun* (脾胃论), or *Treatise on the Spleen and Stomach.*

李东垣 [lǐ dōng yuán]

Li Dongyuan: another name for Li Gao (李杲)

李明之 [lǐ míng zhī]

Li Mingzhi: another name for Li Gao (李杲)

宋慈 [sòng cí]

Song Ci: also called Song Huifu (宋惠父) (1186-1249), author of the *Xi Yuan Ji Lu* (洗冤集录), or *Instructions to Coroners*, a treatise on forensic medicine written on the basis of his personal experience as a judge and his profound knowledge of previous works on the subject, which exerted a great influence on Chinese jurisprudence

宋惠父 [sòng huì fù]

Son Huifu: another name for Song Ci (宋慈)

陈自明 [chén zì míng]

Chen Ziming: also called Chen Liangfu (陈良甫) (c. 1190-1270), distinguished gynecologist from a family of medical practitioners for many generations and author of two important books – *Fu Ren Da Quan Liang Fang* (妇人大全良方), or *The Complete Book of Effective Prescriptions for Women* and *Wai Ke Jing Yao* (外科精要), or *Essence of External Medicine*

陈良甫 [chén liáng fǔ]

Chen Liangfu: another name for Chen Ziming (陈自明)

陈文中 [chén wén zhōng]

Chen Wenzhong: noted pediatrist of the 13th century, and author of the *Chen Shi Xiao Er Dou Zhen Fang* (陈氏小儿痘疹方), or *Chen's Prescriptions for Smallpox and Measles in Children* (1241), and *Xiao Er Bing Yuan Fang Lun* (小儿病源方论), or *Treatise on the Etiology of Children's Diseases* (1253)

严用和 [yán yòng hé]

Yan Yonghe: physician (c. 1206-1268), author of *Yan's Ji Sheng Fang* (严氏济生方), or *Yan's Prescriptions for Succouring the Sick* or *Ji Sheng Fang* (济生方) *Prescriptions for Succouring the Sick* for short

危亦林 [wēi yì lín]

Wei Yilin: also called Wei Dazhai (危达斋) (1277-1347), specialized in bone-setting. Based on his own experience and the findings of his ancestors, he compiled a large number of prescriptions in his book titled *Shi Yi De Xiao Fang* (世医得效方),

or *Effective Prescriptions Handed down for Generations.*

危达斋 [wēi dá zhāi]
Wei Dazhai: another name for Wei Yilin (危亦林)

齐德之 [qí dé zhī]
Qi Dezhi: court academician and surgeon of the Imperial Academy in the Yuan Dynasty. He emphasized taking the organism as a whole while treating carbuncles and sores and authored *Wai Ke Jing Yi* (外科精义), or *Essentials of External Medicine.*

罗天益 [luó tiān yì]
Luo Tianyi: also called Luo Qianfu (罗谦甫) (13th century), a physician of the Yuan Dynasty who studied medicine under Li Gao (李杲) for more than ten years and was once an imperial doctor. On the basis of Li Gao's theories and those of other schools, as well as his own experience, he authored the *Wei Sheng Bao Jian* (卫生宝鉴), or *The Precious Mirror of Hygiene*.

罗谦甫 [luó qiān fǔ]
Luo Qianfu: another name for Luo Tianyi (罗天益)

王好古 [wáng hào gǔ]
Wang Haogu: physician in the 13th century, also called Wan Jinzhi (王进之), or Wang Haizang (王海藏), whose chief contributions included elucidation of yin syndromes/patterns and the use of warming tonics in the treatment of cold damage diseases in the later stage. Five of his publications are extant, including the *Tang Ye Ben Cao* (汤液本草), or *Materia Medica for Decoctions* (1289).

王进之 [wáng jìn zhī]
Wang Jinzhi: another name for Wang Haogu (王好古)

王海藏 [wáng hǎi zàng]
Wang Haizang: another name for Wang Haogu (王好古)

曾世荣 [zēng shì róng]
Zeng Shirong: specialist in children's diseases with over fifty years of experience, author of *Huo You Kou Yi* (活幼口议), or *Discussions on Saving the Lives of Infants and Children* (1283) and the *Huo You Xin Shu* (活幼新书), or *A New Book for Saving the Life of Infants and Children* (1294). His special contribution to pediatrics lay in the skill in grouping different natures and forms of what was in fact a single disease, thus aiding diagnosis.

朱震亨 [zhū zhèn hēng]
Zhu Zhenheng: also called Zhu Danxi (朱丹溪) (1282-1358), who took indulgence as the root of all troubles and stressed the value of tonics in making up the deficit yin. He advocated the theory that yang was always in excess while yin was often deficient, and thus belonged to the Yin-Nourishing School. He was the author of the *Ge Zhi Yu Lun* (格致余论), or *Supplementary Treatise on Knowledge from Practice*, and the *Ju Fang Fa Hui* (局方发挥), or *Expounding on the Formularies of the Bureau of Pharmacy*.

朱丹溪 [zhū dān xī]
Zhu Danxi: another name for Zhu Zhenheng (朱震亨)

忽思慧 [hū sī huì]
Hu Sihui: dietitian of Mongolian nationality in the 14th century. He had been an imperial chef in the Yuan Dynasty for more than ten years before he compiled the *Yin Shan Zheng Yao* (饮膳正要), or *Principles of Correct Diet.*

滑寿 [huá shòu]
Hua Shou: also called Hua Boren (滑伯仁) (1304-1386), author of a treatise on acupuncture titled *Shi Si Jing Fa Hui* (十四经发挥), or *Elucidation of the Fourteen Meridians/Channels*. Hua was good at differential diagnosis and particularly skillful in acupuncture. His study of the meridians/channels and points contributed much to the development of acupuncture.

滑伯仁 [huá bó rén]
Hua Boren: another name for Hua Shou (滑寿)

葛乾孙 [gě qián sūn]
Ge Qiansun: also called Ge Kejiu (葛可久) (1305-1353), physician who was versed in herbal medicines, needling and massage. He was the author of the *Shi Yao Shen Shu* (十药神书), or *Miraculous Book on Ten Recipes*, a record of diagnosis and treatment of pulmonary tuberculosis.

葛可久 [gě kě jiǔ]
Ge Kejiu: another name for Ge Qiansun (葛乾孙)

倪维德 [ní wéi dé]
Ni Weide: also called Ni Zhongxian (倪仲贤) (1307-1377), eye specialist and author of the *Yuan Ji Qi Wei* (元机启微), or *Revealing the Mystery of the Origin*, a valuable book on the causes and mechanisms of eye diseases

倪仲贤 [ní zhòng xián]
Ni Zhongxian: another name for Ni Weide (倪维德)

楼英 [lóu yīng]
Lou Ying: also called Lou Gongshuang (楼公爽) or Lou Quanshan (楼全善) (1332-1402), author of the *Yi Xue Gang Mu* (医学纲目), or *Compendium of Medicine*, in which diseases were classified on the basis of the theories of yin-yang and visceral organs. This system of classification has been proven to be very helpful in diagnosis and treatment.

楼公爽 [lóu gōng shuǎng]
Lou Gongshuang: another name for Lou Ying (楼英)

戴思恭 [dài sī gōng]
Dai Sigong: also called Dai Yuanli (戴原礼) (1324-1405), court physician of the Ming Dynasty and president of the Imperial College of Physicians, author of the *Zheng Zhi Yao Jue* (证治要诀), or *Principles of Diagnosis and Treatment*, and *Zheng Zhi Yao Jue Lei Fang* (证治要诀类方), or *Classified Prescriptions According to the Principles of Diagnosis and Treatment*, in which he well expounded his mentor Zhu Zhenheng's theory of nourishing yin

戴原礼 [dài yuán lǐ]
Dai Yuanli: another name for Dai Sigong (戴思恭)

熊宗立 [xióng zōng lì]

Xiong Zongli: also called Xiong Daoxuan (熊道轩) (1415-1487), physician of the Ming Dynasty, author of the *Ming Fang Lei Zheng Yi Shu Da Quan* (名方类证医书大全), or *Complete Medical Work of Proven Recipes*, also called *Yi Shu Da Quan* (医书大全), or *Complete Work of Medical Books* (1446)

熊道轩 [xióng dào xuān]
Xiong Daoxuan: another name for Xiong Zongli (熊宗立)

寇平 [kòu píng]
Kou Ping: pediatrician of the 15th century, author of the *Quan You Xin Jian* (全幼心鉴), or *Directions in Pediatrics* (1451), in which indigestion or unsuitable food is held to be the main pathogenic factor for children's illnesses

虞抟 [yú tuán]
Yu Tuan: also called Yu Tianmin (虞天民) (1438-1517), revised over 30 precious medical works and edited his own *Yi Xue Zheng Zhuan* (医学正传), or *Orthodox Commentary of Medicine*

虞天民 [yú tiān mín]
Yu Tianmin: another name for Yu Tuan (虞抟)

韩懋 [hán mào]
Han Mao: physician of the Ming Dynasty, author of the *Han Shi Yi Tong* (韩氏医通), or *Han's Book of Medicine* (1522), in which the importance of diagnosis in the treatment of disease is stressed and improvements in case recording with more comprehensive regulations are shown

薛铠 [xuē kǎi]
Xue Kai: also called Xue Liangwu (薛良武), imperial physician, especially well-known in pediatrics, author of the *Bao Ying Cuo Yao* (保婴撮要), or *Essentials for the Care of Infants* (1556), in which he stresses the importance of varying dosages of medicinals according to age, and recommends the severing of the umbilical cord by cautery

薛良武 [xuē liáng wǔ]
Xue Liangwu: another name for Xue Kai (薛铠)

王纶 [wáng lún]
Wang Lun: physician who wrote the *Ming Yi Za Zhu* (明医杂著), or *Collection of Physicians' Experiences in the Ming Dynasty* (1549)

汪机 [wāng jī]
Wang Ji: also called Wang Xingzhi (汪省之) (1463-1539), author of *Zhen Jiu Wen Da* (针灸问答), or *Catechism on Acupuncture and Moxibustion*, which is clear, simple and keeps to essentials, and is very handy for beginners, as well as several other medical works, such as the *Wai Ke Li Li* (外科理例), or *External Medicine with Illustrations*, and *Yi Xue Yuan Li* (医学原理, or *Principles of Medicine*

汪省之 [wāng xǐng zhī]
Wang Xingzhi: another name for Wang Ji (汪机)

薛己 [xuē jǐ]
Xue Ji: also called Xue Xinfu (薛新甫) (c. 1487-1559), son of Xue Kai (薛铠). A physician versed in various branches

of medicine, he compiled a number of medical works, such as *Nü Ke Cuo Yao* (女科撮要), or *Essentials of Obstetrics and Gynecology* and *Wai Ke Shu Yao* (外科枢要), or *Essentials of External Medicine*. His and his father's medical practice records were edited by Wu Guan (吴琯) and published under the title *Xue Shi Yi An* (薛氏医案), or the *Xues' Medical Records*.

薛新甫 [xuē xīn fǔ]

Xue Xinfu: another name for Xue Ji (薛己)

卢和 [lú hé]

Lu He: herbalist of the 16th century, author of the *Shi Wu Ben Cao* (食物本草), or *Dietary Materia Medica*, in which health benefits, including the laxative value, of vegetables are elucidated, and a vegetable-based diet with a spare amount of meat is recommended

沈之问 [shěn zhī wèn]

Shen Zhiwen: expert in the diagnosis and treatment of leprosy in the 16th century, compiler of the *Jie Wei Yuan Sou* (解围元薮), or *Source of Relief* (1550), a monograph on leprosy

孙一奎 [sūn yī kuí]

Sun Yikui: also called Sun Wenyuan (孙文垣) or Sun Dongsu (孙东宿) (1520-1600), author of the *Chi Shui Xuan Zhu* (赤水玄珠), or *Black Pearl of the Red River*, *Yi Zhi Xu Yu* (医旨绪余), or *Supplement to the Principles of Medicine*, and *Yi An* (医案), or *Medical Records*, all of which were collected by his descendants. In these books, Sun advocates combination of various schools and maintains that a doctor should be conversant with all the theories in order to master the art of healing.

孙文垣 [sūn wén yuán]

Sun Wenyuan: another name for Sun Yikui (孙一奎)

孙东宿 [sūn dōng sù]

Sun Dongsu: another name for Sun Yikui (孙一奎)

徐春甫 [xú chūn fǔ]

Xu Chunfu: also called Xu Ruyuan (徐汝元), author of the *Gu Jin Yi Tong Da Quan* (古今医统大全), or *A Complete Work of Ancient and Modern Medicine* (1556), in which rich and valuable materials from various fields of medicine are collected. Xu warns that healthy people should avoid having close contact with patients suffering from consumptive diseases, particularly pulmonary tuberculosis.

徐汝元 [xú rǔ yuán]

Xu Ruyuan: another name for Xu Chunfu (徐春甫)

李梴 [lǐ yán]

Li Yan: also called Li Jianzhai (李健斋), physician of the 16th century who summarized the prescriptions used during that period and classified them into 18 categories. Li was the author of the *Yi Xue Ru Men* (医学入门), or *Introduction to Medicine* and the *Xi Yi Gui Ge* (习医规格), or *Rules for Medical Study*.

李濂 [lǐ lián]

Li Lian: literary man of the Ming Dynasty, official in Shanxi Province known for his exceptional command of ancient Chinese language and literature. The earliest biographer of ancient medical professionals, Li wrote the *Yi Shi* (医史), or *History of Medicine* (1513), which records the lives of distinguished physicians.

万全 [wàn quán]

Wan Quan: also called Wan Mizhai (万密斋) (c. 1495-1585), pediatrist from a family of physicians for three generations. With rich clinical experiences inherited from his family, especially in pediatrics, Wan believed that a child should be frequently exposed to sunlight and fresh air, trained to resist cold and protected from being frightened, and not overfed or given too much medicinal treatment. He was the author of the *Dou Zhen Shi Yi Xin Fa* (痘疹世医新法), or *Experiences in the Treatment of Smallpox and Rashes Handed Down through Generations*, *You Ke Fa Hui* (幼科发挥), or *Expounding on Pediatrics* and *Yu Ying Jia Mi* (育婴家秘), or *Family Secrets in Child Care.*

万密斋 [wàn mì zhāi]

Wan Mizhai: another name for Wan Quan (万全)

李时珍 [lǐ shí zhēn]

Li Shizhen: also called Li Dongbi (李东壁) or Li Binhu (李濒湖) (1518-1593), physician and naturalist, whose father Li Yanwen (李言闻) was an accomplished medical practitioner. Inheritance of his father's medical expertise, assiduous study of medicine and his talent in the field made Li's medical skill widely recognized among his contemporaries. He wrote a dozen medical works, among which *Ben Cao Gang Mu* (本草纲目), or *Compendium of Materia Medica* is the best known. His other works include the *Bin Hu Mai Xue* (濒湖脉学), or *Binhu's Sphygmology* and *Qi Jing Ba Mai Kao* (奇经八脉考), or *A Study of the Eight Extra Meridians.*

李濒湖 [lǐ bīn hú]

Li Binhu: another name for Li Shizhen (李时珍)

李东壁 [lǐ dōng bì]

Li Dongbi: another name for Li Shizhen (李时珍)

马莳 [mǎ shì]

Ma Shi: physician of the Ming Dynasty, author of the *Huangdi Nei Jing Su Wen Zhu Zheng Fa Wei* (黄帝内经素问注证发微), or *An Elaboration on the Spiritual Pivot of Yellow Emperor's Internal Classic* and the *Huangdi Nei Jing Ling Shu Zhu Zheng Fa Wei* (黄帝内经灵枢注证发微), or *An Elaboration and Commentary on the Spiritual Pivot of Yellow Emperor's Internal Classic* (1589)

张三锡 [zhāng sān xī]

Zhang Sanxi: physician of the Ming Dynasty, who emphasized the six aspects of medical practice, i.e., meridians/channels, diagnostic methods, pathogenesis, principles and methods of treatment, materia medica, and *qi* circulation. He wrote the *Yi Xue Liu Yao* (医学六要), or *Six Essentials of Medicine* (1609), which exerted a great influence on medical professionals of later generations.

杨继洲 [yáng jì zhōu]

Yang Jizhou: also called Yang Jishi (杨济时) (1522-1620), physician specialized in acupuncture, whose grandfather had been an imperial physician. He compiled the *Zhen Jiu Da Cheng* (针灸大成), or *Great Compendium of Acupuncture and Moxibustion* (1601), the most comprehensive and practical work at the time.

杨济时 [yáng jì shí]
Yang Jishi: another name for Yang Jizhou (杨继洲)

王肯堂 [wáng kěn táng]
Wang Kentang: also called Wang Yutai (王宇泰) or Wang Sun'an (王损庵) (1549-1639). Having served as a court official for some years, Wang returned to his hometown and devoted himself to the study of medicine. He was the author of the *Liu Ke Zheng Zhi Zhun Sheng* (六科证治准绳), or *Standards of Syndrome/Pattern Identification and Treatment in Six Branches of Medicine*, which had the largest circulation of all medical books in the 17th century in China.

王宇泰 [wáng yǔ tài]
Wang Yutai: another name for Wang Kentang (王肯堂)

王损庵 [wáng sǔn ān]
Wang Sun'an: another name for Wang Kentang (王肯堂)

李中立 [lǐ zhōng lì]
Li Zhongli: also called Li Zhengyu (李正宇), author of the *Ben Cao Yuan Shi* (本草原始), or *Origin of Materia Medica* (1612), a practical book for pharmacists. Li prepared all the illustrations of the medicinal substances on his own, including detailed descriptions of properties and methods of preparation. His book may be considered one of the earliest works in the field of pharmacognosy.

李正宇 [lǐ zhèng yǔ]
Li Zhengyu: another name for Li Zhongli (李中立)

高武 [gāo wǔ]
Gao Wu: also called Gao Meigu (高梅孤) (16th century), acupuncturist of the Ming Dynasty who compiled the *Zhen Jiu Jie Yao* (针灸节要), or *Extracts of the Principles of Acupuncture and Moxibustion*, and the *Zhen Jiu Ju Ying* (针灸聚英), or *A Collection of Gems of Acupuncture and Moxibustion*. To help locate the acupoints, he had three bronze models – of a man, a woman and a child respectively – cast.

高梅孤 [gāo méi gū]
Gao Meigu: another name for Gao Wu (高武)

赵献可 [zhào xiàn kě]
Zhao Xianke: also called Zhao Yangkui (赵养葵), physician of the Ming Dynasty in the 16th century and the author of the *Yi Guan* (医贯), or *Key Link of Medicine*. He developed the "life gate" theory, and stressed the significance of reinforcing the fire of the "life gate".

赵养葵 [zhào yǎng kuí]
Zhao Yangkui: another name for Zhao Xianke (赵献可)

陈实功 [chén shí gōng]

Chen Shigong: also called Chen Yuren (陈毓仁) (1555-1636), doctor of external medicine, whose 40-year practical experience is summarized in his book *Wai Ke Zheng Zong* (外科正宗), or *Orthodox Manual of External Medicine*

陈毓仁 [chén yù rén]

Chen Yuren: another name for Chen Shigong (陈实功)

缪希雍 [miào xī yōng]

Miao Xiyong: also called Miao Zhongchun (缪仲淳) (1556-1627?), physician of the Ming Dynasty who often treated the poor free of charge. An expert on materia medica, Miao was the author of the *Shen Nong Ben Cao Jing Shu* (神农本草经疏), or *Annotations on Sheng Nong's Herbal*, and the *Xian Xing Zhai Yi Xue Guang Bi Ji* (先醒斋医学广笔记), *or Miao's Extensive Notes on Medicine*, which impressed the readers with his rich knowledge and clinical experience in internal medicine, external medicine, gynecology and pediatrics.

缪仲淳 [miào zhòng chún]

Miao Zhongchun: another name for Miao Xiyong (缪希雍)

龚廷贤 [gōng tíng xián]

Gong Tingxian: also called Gong Yunlin (龚云林), physician of the Ming Dynasty in the 16th century, author of the *Wan Bing Hui Chun* (万病回春), or *Recovery from All Ailments*, and *Shou Shi Bao Yuan* (寿世保元), or *Longevity and Life Preservation*. Gong was also a massotherapist and the author of the *Xiao Er Tui Na Mi Zhi* (小儿推拿秘旨), or *Recondite Principles of Child Massotherapy*.

龚云林 [gōng yún lín]

Gong Yunlin: another name for Gong Tingxian (龚廷贤)

张介宾 [zhāng jiè bīn]

Zhang Jiebin: also called Zhang Jingyue (张景岳) (c. 1563-1640), author of several books covering diverse subjects such as sphygmology, gynecology, pediatrics and external medicine. Being especially versed in the *Internal Classic*, Zhang re-edited it and authored the *Lei Jing* (类经), or *Systematic Compilation of the Internal Classic*. A collection of his complete works, known as the *Jing Yue Quan Shu* (景岳全书), or *Jing Yue's Complete Works*, appeared in 1624.

张景岳 [zhāng jǐng yuè]

Zhang Jingyue: another name for Zhang Jiebin (张介宾)

吴有性 [wú yǒu xìng]

Wu Youxing: also called Wu Youke (吴又可) (1582-1652), pioneer epidemiologist, author of the *Wen Yi Lun* (温疫论), or *Treatise on Pestilence* (1642), a book focused on several epidemic diseases then prevalent in many regions of China. Wu put forward a theory of pestilential factors, and made a great contribution to the development of knowledge about epidemic infectious diseases.

吴又可 [wú yòu kě]

Wu Youke: another name for Wu Youxing (吴有性)

喻昌 [yù chāng]

Yu Chang: also called Yu Jiayan (喻嘉言) (c. 1585-1664), medical practitioner and author of the *Shang Lun Zhang Zhong Jing Shang Han Lun* (尚论张仲景伤寒论), or *A Critical Study of Zhang Zhongjing's Treatise on Cold Damage Diseases* (simply called *Shang Lun Pian* (尚论篇), *or Critical Study*) and the *Yi Men Fa Lü* (医门法律), or *Principles and Prohibitions of Medical Profession*, in which cold damage diseases are re-categorized and Yu's original ideas on some subjects, such as autumn dryness, are expounded

喻嘉言 [yù jiā yán]

Yu Jiayan: another name for Yu Chang (喻昌)

武之望 [wǔ zhī wàng]

Wu Zhiwang: also called Wu Shuqing (武叔卿) (?-1629 A.D.), physician who compiled the *Ji Yin Gang Mu* (济阴纲目), or *Compendium of Therapies for Women's Diseases* (1620), which was circulated widely. He also wrote the *Ji Yang Gang Mu* (济阳纲目), or *Compendium of Therapies for Men's Diseases*.

武叔卿 [wǔ shū qīng]

Wu Shuqing: another name for Wu Zhiwang (武之望)

陈司成 [chén sī chéng]

Chen Sicheng: also called Chen Jiushao (陈九韶), physician of the Ming Dynasty in the 17th century, specialized in treating syphilis and wrote the *Mei Chuang Mi Lu* (霉疮秘录), or *Recondite Records of Syphilis* (1632), the first monograph on syphilology in China, which not only summed up the experiences of his physician ancestors but also provided new case studies on diagnosis and treatment of syphilis

陈九韶 [chén jiǔ sháo]

Chen Jiushao: another name for Chen Sicheng (陈司成)

李中梓 [lǐ zhōng zǐ]

Li Zhongzi: also called Li Shicai (李士材) (1588-1655), physician who wrote or compiled a number of books, such as the *Nei Jing Zhi Yao* (内经知要) or *Essentials of the Internal Classic*, and *Yi Zong Bi Du* (医宗必读) or *Essential Readings for Medical Professionals*, which were written on the basis of the *Internal Classic* and *Treatise on Cold Damage Diseases*, respectively, with references to works by other physicians and without neglecting his own experience in clinical practice

李士材 [lǐ shì cái]

Li Shicai: another name for Li Zhongzi (李中梓)

傅仁宇 [fù rén yǔ]

Fu Renyu: also called Fu Yunke (傅允科), oculist of the Ming Dynasty in the 17th century and author of the *Shen Shi Yao Han* (审视瑶函), or *A Precious Work of Ophthamology*, also known as the *Yan Ke Da Quan* (眼科大全), or *A Complete Book of Ophthalmology* (1644), which contains detailed descriptions of the symptoms, diagnosis and treatment of eye diseases

傅允科 [fù yǔn kē]

Fu Yunke: another name for Fu Renyu (傅仁宇)

傅山 [fù shān]

Fu Shan: also called Fu Qingzhu (傅青主) (1607-1684), poet, painter, calligrapher and physician. In the field of medicine, he authored such books as the *Bian Zheng Lu* (辨证录) or *Notes on Diagnosis*, *Shi Shi Mi Lu* (石室秘录) or *Recondite Records of the Stone House*, and *Dong Tian Ao Zhi* (洞天奥旨) or *Mysterious Teachings in a Cave*. After the fall of the Ming Dynasty (1644), Fu devoted himself to fighting against the newly established Qing regime. Since he was persecuted by the new government, his real name was not made known. The above-mentioned books were re-edited by Chen Shiduo (陈士铎) and republished under the name of Xian Shou (仙授), or Divine Teaching in the Qing Dynasty. Certain parts of the book were extracted, compiled and published as a new series in the middle of the 19th century, titled *Fu Qing Zhu Nü Ke* (傅青主女科), *Fu Qingzhu's Works on Women's Diseases* or *Fu Qingzhu's Obstetrics and Gynecology*, and *Fu Qing Zhu Nan Ke* (傅青主男科), or *Fu Qingzhu's Works on Men's Diseases*.

傅青主 [fù qīng zhǔ]

Fu Qingzhu: another name for Fu Shan (傅山)

汪昂 [wāng áng]

Wang Ang: also called Wang Ren'an (汪讱安) (1615-?), physician of the Qing Dynasty who wrote a number of medical books such as the *Yi Fang Ji Jie* (医方集解), or *Collection of Prescriptions with Exposition*, and *Tang Tou Ge Jue* (汤头歌诀), or *Prescriptions in Rhymes*. Wang held an open-minded and welcoming attitude toward Western medicine coming into China at the end of the Ming Dynasty, and wrote that it was the brain, not the heart that was the seat of mental activities.

汪讱安 [wāng rèn ān]

Wang Ren'an: another name for Wang Ang (汪昂)

张璐 [zhāng lù]

Zhang Lu: also called Zhang Luyu (张路玉) or Zhang Shiwan (张石顽) (1617-1699), author of a number of medical works, the most popular of which, the *Yi Tong* (医通), or *Treatise on General Medicine* (1695), consisting of 16 volumes, took him 50 years to complete. In it, various methods of vaccination or variolation and ideas for nationwide implementation of this practice were provided in detail. Zhang emphasized the good points of the Warm Tonic School, and was one of its chief protagonists.

张路玉 [zhāng lù yù]

Zhang Luyu: another name for Zhang Lu (张璐)

张石顽 [zhāng shí wán]

Zhang Shiwan: another name for Zhang Lu (张璐)

张志聪 [zhāng zhì cōng]

Zhang Zhicong: also called Zhang Yin'an (张隐庵) (1610-1674), author of the *Huangdi Nei Jing Su Wen Ji Zhu* (黄帝内经素问集注), or *Variorum of the Plain Questions of the Internal Classic* (1670)

张隐庵 [zhāng yǐn ān]

Zhang Yin'an: another name for Zhang

Zhicong (张志聪)

李惺庵 [lǐ xīng ān]
Li Xing'an: also called Li Yongcui (李用粹) or Li Xiuzhi (李修之) (17th century), who compiled the *Zheng Zhi Hui Bu* (证治汇补), or *Supplement to Diagnosis and Treatment*, a book noted for its limpid style and practical value

李用粹 [lǐ yòng cuì]
Li Yongcui: another name for Li Xing'an (李惺庵)

李修之 [lǐ xiū zhī]
Li Xiuzhi: another name for Li Xing'an (李惺庵)

萧赓六 [xiāo gēng liù]
Xiao Gengliu: physician of the Qing Dynasty, author of the *Nü Ke Jing Lun* (女科经纶), or *Principles of Gynecology and Obstetrics* (1684)

柯琴 [kē qín]
Ke Qin: also called Ke Yunbo (柯韵伯) (1662-1735), physician of the beginning of the Qing Dynasty, who wrote the *Shang Han Lun Zhu* (伤寒论注), or *Annotations of the Treatise on Cold Damage Diseases*, *Shang Han Lun Yi* (伤寒论翼), or *Supplementary Treatise on Cold Damage Diseases*, and *Shang Han Fu Yi* (伤寒附翼), or *Additions to the Treatise on Cold Damage Diseases*. The three books combined are called *Shang Han Lai Su Ji* (伤寒来苏集), or *Renewal of the Treatise on Cold Damage Diseases*.

柯韵伯 [kē yùn bó]
Ke Yunbo: another name for Ke Qin (柯琴)

魏之琇 [wèi zhī xiù]
Wei Zhixiu: also called Wei Liuzhou (魏柳洲) (1722-1772), physicain of the Qing Dynasty, compiler of the *Xu Ming Yi Lei An* (续名医类案), or *Supplement to the Classified Medical Records of Distinguished Physicians*, which contains medical records of many distinguished physicians of the early Qing Dynasty. He was also the author of the *Liu Zhou Yi Hua* (柳州医话), *Liuzhou's Medical Essays*, published in the middle of the 19th century.

魏柳洲 [wèi liǔ zhōu]
Wei Liuzhou: alias of Wei Zhixiu (魏之琇)

叶桂 [yè guì]
Ye Gui: also called Ye Tianshi (叶天士) or Ye Xiangyan (叶香岩) (1667-1746), physician renowned for his methods of diagnosis and treatment, and a recognized leader of the School of Epidemic Febrile Diseases, advocating the scheme of four-aspect syndrome/pattern (defense, *qi*, nutrient, and blood) differentiation. Ye also introduced the use of aromatic stimulants for the treatment of epidemic fevers with great success. His lectures and teachings were edited by his disciples in a book titled *Wen Re Lun* (温热论), or *Treatise on Warm-Heat Diseases* (1746).

叶天士 [yè tiān shì]
Ye Tianshi: another name for Ye Gui (叶桂)

叶香岩 [yè xiāng yán]
Ye Xiangyan: alias of Ye Gui (叶桂)

尤怡 [yóu yí]
You Yi: also called You Zaijing (尤在泾) (?-1749 A.D.), physician of the

Qing Dynasty, who conducted detailed studies of the *Treatise on Cold Damage Diseases* and *Synopsis of Prescriptions of the Golden Chamber*, and wrote the *Shang Han Guan Zhu Ji* (伤寒贯珠集), or *A String of Beads from the Treatise on Cold Damage Diseases*, *Jin Gui Yi* (金匮翼), or *Supplements to the Commentaries on the Synopsis of the Golden Chamber*, etc. The medical records of his patients were systematically compiled by his descendants into a book titled *Jing Xiang Lou Yi An* (静香楼医案), or *Medical Case Records by the Master of the Quiet Fragrant Chamber*.

尤在泾 [yóu zài jīng]

You Zaijing: another name for You Yi (尤怡)

陈复正 [chén fù zhèng]

Chen Fuzheng: also called Chen Feixia (陈飞霞) (c. 1736-1795), physician of the Qing Dynasty, who studied Taoism and the art of medicine, and excelled as a pediatrist. He was particularly good at treating contagious eruptive fevers and infantile convulsions. He was the author of the *You You Ji Cheng* (幼幼集成), or *Collection of Works on Pediatrics*, with a comprehensive description of children's diseases and a collection of simple and useful prescriptions.

陈飞霞 [chén fēi xiá]

Chen Feixia: another name for Chen Fuzheng (陈复正)

薛雪 [xuē xuě]

Xue Xue: also called Xue Shengbai (薛生白) (1681-1770), who was as reputable a physician as his contemporary Ye Tianshi (叶天士) and specially skilled at treating epidemic febrile diseases. He was the author of the *Shi Re Tiao Bian* (湿热条辨), or *Detailed Analysis of Dampness-Heat*, a major contribution to the study of epidemic febrile diseases.

薛生白 [xuē shēng bái]

Xue Shengbai: another name for Xue Xue (薛雪)

徐大椿 [xú dà chūn]

Xu Dachun: also called Xu Lingtai (徐灵胎) or Xu Daye (徐大业) (1693-1771), the author of numerous books, such as the *Nan Jing Jing Shi* (难经经释), or *Explanation of Difficult Classics*, *Yi Guan Bian* (医贯砭), or *A Critique on Key Link of Medicine*, and *Yi Xue Yuan Liu Lun* (医学源流论), or *On the Origin and Source of Medicine*. He did not cling to conventional methods, and opposed the abuse of drastic medicinals, including those hot in nature and pungent in flavor, as tonics.

徐灵胎 [xú líng tāi]

Xu Lingtai: another name for Xu Dachun (徐大椿)

徐大业 [xú dà yè]

Xu Daye: another name for Xu Dachun (徐大椿)

何梦瑶 [hé mèng yáo]

He Mengyao: also called He Xichi (何西池) (1693-1763), an official as well as a literary man and physician, author of a number of books, including the *Yi Bian* (医碥), or *Fundamentals of Medicine*, *Ben Cao Yun Yu* (本草韵语), or *Herbals*

Rhymed, *Shen Xiao Jiao Qi Mi Fang* (神效脚气秘方), or *Recondite Recipes for Beriberi*, *Fu Ke Liang Fang* (妇科良方), or *Prescriptions for Gynecology*, *You Ke Liang Fang* (幼科良方), or *Prescriptions for Pediatrics*, and *Dou Zhen Liang Fang* (痘疹良方), or *Prescriptions for Poxes and Measles*

何西池 [hé xī chí]

He Xichi: alias of He Mengyao (何梦瑶)

程国彭 [chéng guó péng]

Cheng Guopeng: also called Cheng Zhongling (程钟龄) (1679-?), physician and author of the *Yi Xue Xin Wu* (医学心悟), or *Comprehension of Medicine*, a concise and practical reference book for medical practitioners. Cheng was also the author of the *Wai Ke Shi Fa* (外科十法), or *Ten Methods of External Medicine*.

程钟龄 [chéng zhōng líng]

Cheng Zhongling: another name for Cheng Guopeng (程国彭)

沈金鳌 [shěn jīn áo]

Shen Jin'ao: also called Shen Qianlü (沈芊绿) (1717-1776), author of the *Shen Shi Zun Sheng Shu* (沈氏尊生书), or *On the Importance of Life Preservation*, a popular book which covers various branches of medicine including *qigong* therapy

沈芊绿 [shěn qiān lǜ]

Shen Qianlü: another name for Shen Jin'ao (沈金鳌)

赵学敏 [zhào xué mǐn]

Zhao Xuemin: (1719-1805), also called Zhao Shuxuan (赵恕轩) (1719-1805), a physician and renowned pharmacist, author of the *Ben Cao Gang Mu Shi Yi* (本草纲目拾遗), or *Supplement to the Compendium of Materia Medica* (1765), in which all the known medicinals developed since the Ming Dynasty were listed. He also documented and analyzed the medical experiences of folk practitioner Zhao Boyun (赵伯云), leading to the publication of the *Chuan Ya Nei Bian* (串雅内编), or *Treatise on Folk Medicine* and *Chuan Ya Wai Bain* (串雅外编), or *Extra Treatise on Folk Medicine*.

赵恕轩 [zhào shù xuān]

Zhao Shuxuan: another name for Zhao Xuemin (赵学敏)

郑宏纲 [zhèng hóng gāng]

Zheng Honggang: also called Zheng Meijian (郑梅涧) (c.1727-1787), laryngologist. His book of *Chong Lou Yu Yao* (重楼玉钥) or *Jade Key to the Secluded Chamber*, a monograph on laryngology has been widely accepted in the medical field. Its contents include discussions on the physiology and pathology of the larynx and pharynx, as well as diagnosis, treatment and prognosis of laryngological diseases. The treatment sections encompass needling, massage, gargling, topical insufflation, and external application.

郑梅涧 [zhèng méi jiàn]

Zheng Meijian: another name for Zheng Honggang (郑宏纲)

郑瀚 [zhèng hàn]

Zheng Han: also called Zheng Ruoxi (郑若溪) (c. 1746-1813), son of Zheng

Honggang (郑宏纲), also expert in laryngology, who compiled the *Chong Lou Yu Yao Xu Bian* (重楼玉钥续编) or *Sequel to the Jade Key to the Secluded Chamber*

郑若溪 [zhèng ruò xī]
Zheng Ruoxi: another name for Zheng Han (郑瀚)

余霖 [yú lín]
Yu Lin: physician of the Qing Dynasty in the 18th century, experienced in the treatment of epidemic febrile diseases. He compiled the *Zhen Yi Yi De* (疹疫一得), or *A View of Epidemic Febrile Diseases with Rashes* (1785). He made the first attempt to use a large dose of gypsum in a recipe, with success.

陈念祖 [chén niàn zǔ]
Chen Nianzu: also called Chen Xiuyuan (陈修圆) or Chen Shenxiu (陈慎修) (c1753-1823). He compiled a number of works popular among both professionals and laymen, such as the *Shang Han Lun Qian Zhu* (伤寒论浅注), or *Simplified Commentary on the Treatise on Cold Damage Diseases*, *Yi Xue San Zi Jing* (医学三字经), or *The A.B.C. of Medicine*, *Jin Gui Yao Lue Qian Zhu* (金匮要略浅注), or *Simplified Commentary on the Synopsis of the Golden Chamber*, *Chang Sha Fang Ge Kuo* (长沙方歌括), or *Formulas by Zhang Zhongjing in Verse*, and *Shi Fang Ge Kuo* (时方歌括), or *Popular Prescriptions in Verse.*

陈修圆 [chén xiū yuán]
Chen Xiuyuan: another name for Chen Nianzu (陈念祖)

陈慎修 [chén shèn xiū]
Chen Shenxiu: another name for Chen Nianzu (陈念祖)

吴瑭 [wú táng]
Wu Tang: also called Wu Jutong (吴鞠通) (1758-1836), authority on acute epidemic febrile diseases, author of the *Wen Bing Tiao Bian* (温病条辨), or *Analysis of Warm Diseases* (1798), in which he summarizes his own experience in the treatment of epidemic febrile diseases, makes distinctions among different fevers, and devises new methods of treatment

吴鞠通 [wú jū tōng]
Wu Jutong: another name for Wu Tang (吴瑭)

王清任 [wáng qīng rèn]
Wang Qingren: also called Wang Xunchen (王勋臣) (1768-1831). He raised the awareness of the importance of studying the internal organs at the physiological level. In his book of *Yi Lin Gai Cuo* (医林改错), or *Corrections of Errors in Medical Works*, he drew sketches of the internal organs and corrected a number of mistakes, based upon his personal observation of exposed bodies in public cemeteries. The book also includes quite a few novel conceptions in the understandings of the human body and some effective formulas for moving *qi*, activating blood and removing stasis.

王勋臣 [wáng xūn chén]
Wang Xunchen: another name for Wang Qingren (王清任)

章楠 [zhāng nán]
Zhang Nan: physician of the Qing Dynasty and author of the *Yi Men Bang*

He (医门棒喝), or *Medical Alarms* (1825), a significant contribution to the theory and treatment of epidemic febrile diseases

林佩琴 [lín pèi qín]
Lin Peiqin: also called Lin Yunhe (林云和) or Lin Xitong (林羲桐) (1772-1839). Taking advantage of the positive aspects of various medical schools in accordance with his own clinical experience, Lin compiled the *Lei Zheng Zhi Cai* (类证治裁), or *Classified Syndromes and Treatment*, in which he emphasizes the importance of syndrome differentiation or pattern identification for treatment. The cited theories of different medical schools are well selected and are of practical value.

林云和 [lín yún hé]
Lin Yunhe: another name for Lin Peiqin (林佩琴)

林羲桐 [lín xī tóng]
Lin Xitong: another name for Lin Peiqin (林佩琴)

吴其浚 [wú qí jùn]
Wu Qijun: also called Wu Yuezhai (吴瀹斋) (1789-1847), official as well as botanist. Having devoted his whole life to the study of plants, he compiled the *Zhi Wu Ming Shi Tu Kao* (植物名实图考), or *An Illustrated Book of Plants*. This book served as a supplement to Li Shizhen's *Compendium of Materia Medica* which is considered a worldwide contribution to the study of medicinal plants and general botany.

吴瀹斋 [wú yuè zhāi]
Wu Yuezhai: another name for Wu Qijun (吴其浚)

王泰林 [wáng tài lín]
Wang Tailin: also called Wang Xugao (王旭高) (1798-1862), treating wounds in the early years of his career and practicing internal medicine afterwards, during which he made a detailed study of liver problems. Wang was the author of *Yi Fang Zheng Zhi Hui Bian* (医方证治汇编), or *A Collection of Classified Prescriptions with Diagnosis and Treatment*, and *Yi Xue Chu Yan* (医学刍言), or *Preliminary Remarks on Medicine*. His case records were collected by his disciples in the book titled *Wang Xugao Yi An* (王旭高医案), or *Medical Case Records of Wang Xugao*.

王旭高 [wáng xù gāo]
Wang Xugao: another name for Wang Tailin (王泰林)

朱沛文 [zhū pèi wén]
Zhu Peiwen: physician of the 19th century who advocated the complementarity of traditional Chinese and Western medicine. He compiled the *Hua Yang Zang Fu Tu Xiang Yue Zuan* (华洋脏腑图象约纂), or *A Brief Account of Chinese and Western Anatomy* (1892), in which some knowledge of Western medicine is introduced and comments on the *Canon of Medicine* are made from anatomical and physiological perspectives.

吴尚先 [wú shàng xiān]
Wu Shangxian: also called Wu Shiji (吴师机) or Wu Anye (吴安业) (c. 1806-1886), who recommended external therapies, such as ointment and plaster application, hydrotherapy, and kerotherapy as substitutes for corresponding oral medications that could be expensive or repugnant to some patients. He was the

author of the *Li Yue Pian Wen* (理瀹骈文), or *A Rhymed Discourse on External Therapeutics* (1870).

吴师机 [wú shī jī]
Wu Shiji: another name for Wu Shangxian (吴尚先)

吴安业 [wú ān yè]
Wu Anye: another name for Wu Shangxian (吴尚先)

王士雄 [wáng shì xióng]
Wang Shixiong: also called Wang Mengying (王孟英) (1808-1866), specialist in epidemic febrile diseases. He compiled the *Wen Re Jing Wei* (温热经纬), or *An Outline of Warm-Heat Diseases*, and the *Huo Luan Lun* (霍乱论), or *On Diseases with Sudden Vomiting and Diarrhea*, and collected all the case records of his patients in his *Wang Shi Yi An* (王氏医案), or *Wang's Medical Case Records*.

王孟英 [wáng mèng yīng]
Wang Mengying: another name for Wang Shixiong (王士雄)

张筱衫 [zhāng xiǎo shān]
Zhang Xiaoshan: also called Zhang Zhenjun (张振鋆), physician and massotherapist of the Qing Dynasty, and author of the *Li Zheng An Mo Yao Shu* (厘正按摩要术), or *Revised Techniques of Massage* (1898)

张振鋆 [zhāng zhèn jūn]
Zhang Zhenjun: another name for Zhang Xiaoshan (张筱衫)

陆懋修 [lù mào xiū]
Lu Maoxiu: also called Lu Jiuzhi (陆九芝) (1818-1886), physician who wrote the *Shi Bu Zhai Yi Shu* (世补斋医书), or *A Book on Medicine*, clung closely to the old tradition, particularly to the doctrine of Zhang Zhongjing

陆九芝 [lù jiǔ zhī]
Lu Jiuzhi: another name for Lu Maoxiu (陆懋修)

唐宗海 [táng zōng hǎi]
Tang Zonghai: also called Tang Rongchuan (唐容川) (1847-1897), physician at the end of the Qing Dynasty, who was among the pioneers in the field of integration of traditional Chinese and Western medicine, and the author of the *Zhong Xi Hui Tong Yi Jing Jing Yi* (中西汇通医经精义), or *Essentials of Confluent Traditional Chinese and Western Medicine.* Tang made efforts to prove that traditional Chinese medicine was not unscientific, and pointed out that the Chinese and Western systems of medicine had their own advantages. He also wrote the *Xue Zheng Lun* (血证论), *or Treatise on Blood Syndromes*, in which some special methods of treating hemorrhagic diseases are recommended.

唐容川 [táng róng chuān]
Tang Rongchuan: another name for Tang Zonghai (唐宗海)

何炳元 [hé bǐng yuán]
He Bingyuan: also called He Lianchen (何廉臣) (1861-1929). He studied both traditional Chinese and Western medicine. Comparing the two, he came to the conclusion that Western medicine was not perfect, and that traditional

Chinese medicine should not be neglected. He was the author of a number of books, such as the *Zhong Feng Xin Quan* (中风新诠), or *A New Exposition of Apoplexy*, *Xin Yi Zong Bi Du* (新医宗必读), or *A New Selection of Required Readings for Medical Professionals*, *Nei Ke Zheng Zhi Quan Shu* (内科证治全书), or *A Complete Book of Diagnosis and Treatment of Internal Medicine*, and *Quan Guo Ming Yi Yan An Lei Bian* (全国名医验案类编), or *A Classified Collection of Successful Medical Case Records of Noted Chinese Physicians*.

何廉臣 [hé lián chén]

He Lianchen: another name for He Bingyuan (何炳元)

陆以湉 [lù yǐ tián]

Lu Yitian: physician of the late Qing Dynasty, author of the *Leng Lu Yi Hua* (冷庐医话), or *Deserted House Medical Talks* (1897)

雷丰 [léi fēng]

Lei Feng: also called Lei Shaoyi (雷少逸), physician at the end of the Qing Dynasty and early 20th century, specialized in treating epidemic febrile diseases. He wrote the *Shi Bing Lun* (时病论), or *Treatise on Seasonal Diseases*, which was widely accepted because the recommended methods of treatment proved highly effective.

雷少逸 [léi shào yì]

Lei Shaoyi: another name for Lei Feng (雷丰)

丁甘仁 [dīng gān rén]

Ding Ganren: also called Ding Zezhou (丁泽周) (1865-1926). He set up the Shanghai Institute of Traditional Chinese Medicine in 1916, Women's Institute of Traditional Chinese Medicine, and Guangyi Hospital of Traditional Chinese Medicine, and made great contributions to the training of traditional Chinese medical doctors. He was the author of the *Hou Sha Zheng Zhi Gai Yao* (喉痧证治概要), or *An Outline of Diagnosis and Treatment of Scarlet Fever*. The *Ding Gan Ren Yi An* (丁甘仁医案), or *Ding Ganren's Medical Case Records* was compiled by his students.

丁泽周 [dīng zé zhōu]

Ding Zezhou: another name for Ding Ganren (丁甘仁)

张锡纯 [zhāng xī chún]

Zhang Xichun: also called Zhang Shoufu (张寿甫) (1860-1933), who after extensive research into medical literature advocated the combination of traditional Chinese and Western medicine. He was the author of a popular book titled *Yi Xue Zhong Zhong Can Xi Lu* (医学衷中参西录), or *Records of Traditional Chinese and Western Medicine in Combination*.

张寿甫 [zhāng shòu fǔ]

Zhang Shoufu: another name for Zhang Xichun (张锡纯)

张寿颐 [zhāng shòu yí]

Zhang Shouyi: also called Zhang Shanlei (张山雷) (1872-1934), physician during the modern period, versed in treating internal and external diseases, and author of a series of books on various medical subjects, such as *Zhong Feng Jiao Quan*

(中风斠诠), or *Treatise on Stroke*, and *Yang Ke Gang Yao* (疡科纲要), or *An Outline of Traumatology*. He was also an educationist of traditional Chinese medicine.

张山雷 [zhāng shān léi]
Zhang Shanlei: another name for Zhang Shouyi (张寿颐)

恽铁樵 [yùn tiě qiáo]
Yun Tieqiao: also called Yun Shujue (恽树珏) (1878-1935). He was a student of literature, but his poor health and the death of his children due to sickness completely changed his career orientation. He turned to studying medicine, and became a physician in the fields of both Chinese and Western medicine. Yun ran medical schools and took part in the campaign of opposing defamation and extermination of tradtional Chinese medicine. He advocated supplementing Chinese medicine with Western medical theories. He wrote more than 20 books, such as the *Qun Jing Jian Zhi Lu* (群经见智录), or *Wisdom Exposed in the Medical Classics*, *Shang Han Lun Yan Jiu* (伤寒论研究), or *Research into Treatises on Cold Damage Diseases*, and *Mai Xue Fa Wei* (脉学发微), or *Detailed Study of Pulse Lore*.

恽树珏 [yùn shù jué]
Yun Shujue: another name for Yun Tieqiao (恽铁樵)

谢观 [xiè guān]
Xie Guan: modern physician (1878-1950) who compiled the *Zhong Guo Yi Xue Da Ci Dian* (中国医学大词典), or *Dictionary of Chinese Medicine* (1921), and *Zhong Yi Yi Xue Yuan Liu Lun* (中医医学源流论), or *Origin and Development of Traditional Chinese Medicine*

陆渊雷 [lù yuān léi]
Lu Yuanlei: modern physician (1894-1955) and educationalist of traditional Chinese medicine, who, being influenced by the school of integrative traditional Chinese and Western medicine, tried to find evidence in Western medicine to support ancient Chinese medical theories

承淡安 [chéng dàn ān]
Cheng Dan'an: acupuncturist (1899-1957) who set up an institute of acupuncture research and a special school for training acupuncturists. His chief writings include the *Zhong Guo Zhen Jiu Zhi Liao Xue* (中国针灸治疗学), or *Chinese Acupuncture-Moxibustion Therapy*, *Zhen Jiu Jing Hua* (针灸精华), or *Quintessence of Acupuncture and Moxibustion*, and *Zhong Guo Zhen Jiu Xue* (中国针灸学), or *Chinese Acupuncture and Moxibustion.*

名著 Leading Chinese Medical Works

黄帝内经 [huáng dì nèi jīng]

Huang Di Nei Jing*; *Huangdi's Internal Classic*; *Yellow Emperor's Canon of Medicine: the oldest and greatest medical classic extant in China, with its authorship ascribed to the legendary Yellow Emperor Huangdi (2698-2589 B.C.), but actually completed by a number of unknown authors in the Warring States Period (475-221 B.C.). The book consists of two parts: *SuWen* (素问), or *Plain Questions*, and *Ling Shu* (灵枢), or *Spiritual Pivot* or *Divine Axis*, the latter of which is also known as the *Canon of Acupuncture.*

内经 [nèi jīng]

Nei Jing*; *Internal Classic*; *Canon of Medicine: abbreviation for *Huangdi's Internal Classic or Yellow Emperor's Canon of Medicine*

黄帝内经素问 [huáng dì nèi jīng sù wèn]

Huang Di Nei Jing Su Wen*; *Plain Questions of Huangdi's Internal Classic*; *Plain Questions of Yellow Emperor's Canon of Medicine: also called *Su Wen*, or *Plain Questions* for short, one of the two parts of the *Canon of Medicine*, originally consisting of 9 volumes, with 81 articles, but only 8 volumes extant. In the Tang Dynasty, Wang Bing (王冰) added notes and commentaries to the book, rewrote missing articles, and recompiled the book into 24 volumes. In the Northern Song Dynasty, Lin Yi (林亿) et al. proofread and made notes on it again, and all later extant editions were based on Lin's version. The book covers diverse subjects, such as human anatomy and physiology, causes of disease, pathology, diagnosis, syndrome differentiation, methods of treatment, disease prevention, health preservation, man and nature, and the philosophical bases of traditional Chinese medicine, including yin-yang theory, the theory of the five elements/phases, and the *qi* theory. The book has benefited medical practitioners of all generations since.

素问 [sù wèn]

Su Wen*; *Plain Questions: abbreviation for *Huang Di Nei Jing Su Wen* (黄帝内经素问), or *Plain Questions of Huangdi's Internal Classic*, or *Plain Questions of Yellow Emperor's Canon of Medicine*

黄帝内经灵枢经 [huáng dì nèi jīng líng shū jīng]

Huang Di Nei Jing Ling Shu Jing*; *Spiritual Pivot of Huangdi's Internal Classsic*; *Spiritual Pivot of Yellow Emperor's Canon of Medicine: also called *Ling Shu* (灵枢), *Spiritual Pivot* or *Divine Axis* for short, also titled *Zhen Jing* (针经), or *Canon of Acupuncture*, one of the two parts of the *Canon of Medicine*. The subjects discussed in the *Spiritual Pivot* are similar to those in the *Plain Questions*, but the former provides more information from the practical perspective, while the latter focuses more on the theoretical aspect. The two books are complementary.

灵枢 [líng shū]

***Ling Shu*; *Spiritual Pivot*; *Divine Axis*:** abbreviation for *Huang Di Nei Jing Ling Shu Jing*, or *Spiritual Pivot of Huangdi's Internal Classsic*, or *Spiritual Pivot of Yellow Emperor's Canon of Medicine*

黄帝内经素问注证发微 [huáng dì nèi jīng sù wèn zhù zhèng fā wēi]

***Huang Di Nei Jing Su Wen Zhu Zheng Fa Wei*; *An Elaboration on Plain Questions of Huangdi's Internal Classic* (1586):** also called *An Elaboration on Plain Questions* for short, by Ma Shi (马莳) of the Ming Dynasty

黄帝内经灵枢注证发微 [huáng dì nèi jīng líng shū zhù zhèng fā wēi]

***Huang Di Nei Jing Ling Shu Zhu Zheng Fa Wei*; *An Elaboration on the Spiritual Pivot of Huangdi's Internal Classic*; *An Elaboration on the Spiritual Pivot of Yellow Emperor's Canon of Medcine* (1586):** also called *An Elaboration on the Spiritual Pivot* for short, by Ma Shi (马莳) of the Ming Dynasty

类经 [lèi jīng]

***Lei Jing*; *Classified Classic*; *Systematic Compilation of the Internal Classic* (1624):** a rearrangement of the *Nei Jing* or *Internal Classic*, compiled by Zhang Jiebin (张介宾). This book consists of 12 categories, including hygiene, yin-yang, visceral manifestations, pulses, meridians/channels, theories of treatment, and acupuncture. It is considered as one of the most important reference books for the study of the *Nei Jing*, or *Internal Classic*.

类经图翼 [lèi jīng tú yì]

***Lei Jing Tu Yi*; *Illustrated Supplement to the Classified Classic* (1624):** a supplement to the *Classified Classic* with illustrations, compiled by Zhang Jiebin (张介宾)

内经知要 [nèi jīng zhī yào]

***Nei Jing Zhi Yao*; *Essentials of the Internal Classic*; *Essentials of the Canon of Medicine* (1642):** compiled by Li Nian'e (李念莪). This book is divided into 8 parts, including yin-yang, pulses, meridians/channels, and principles of treatment. Combining the basic and clinical theories, the author takes extracts from and makes expositions of the *Internal Classic*. The book is written clearly and well organized.

难经 [nàn jīng]

***Nan Jing*; *Classic of Difficulies*:** a book which appeared in the 1st or 2nd century B.C., with authorship ascribed to Qin Yueren (秦越人) without historic evidence. It deals with fundamental medical theories, and expounds the main points of the *Nei Jing*, or *Internal Classic*, in the form of questions and answers. Topics concerning acupuncture and moxibustion, method of needling, physiological and pathological conditions in relation to meridians/channels and collaterals, and method of pulse-taking are all discussed.

难经本义 [nàn jīng běn yì]

***Nan Jing Ben Yi*; *The Genuine Meaning of the Classic of Difficulties* (1366):** compiled by Hua Shou (滑寿), a most influential book among commentaries on the *Nan Jing*, or *Classic of Difficulties*

伤寒杂病论 [shāng hán zá bìng lùn]
***Shang Han Za Bing Lun*; *Treatise on Cold Damage and Miscellaneous Diseases*:** a book written by Zhang Zhongjing (张仲景) at the beginning of the 3rd century, in which diagnosis and treatment of fevers and other miscellaneous diseases are dealt with. The book was rearranged by Wang Shuhe (王叔和) in the Jin Dynasty, and later in the Song Dynasty it was divided by Jiao Zheng Yi Shu Ju (校正医书局), or Bureau for Rectifying and Pubilishing Medical Books into two parts: *Shang Han Lun* (伤寒论), or *Treatise on Cold Damage Diseases*, and *Jin Gui Yao Lue Fang Lun* (金匮要略方论), or *Synopsis of Prescriptions of the Golden Chamber.*

伤寒论 [shāng hán lùn]
***Shang Han Lun*; *Treatise on Cold Damage Diseases*:** a new edition of Zhang Zhongjing's (张仲景) *Treatise on Cold Damage and Miscellaneous Diseases*, re-edited by Wang Shuhe (王叔和), consisting of 10 volumes, in which acute febrile diseases induced by cold are analyzed and differentiated in accordance with the theory of the six meridians/channels. This book has been one of the most influential works in the history of Chinese medicine.

伤寒总病论 [shāng hán zǒng bìng lùn]
Shang Han Zong Bing Lun*; *General Discussion of Cold Damage Diseases (1100)**:** by Pang Anshi (庞安时) of the Song Dynasty, which contains new prescriptions for treating cold damage diseases. Some of the prescriptions were proposed according to the author's own experience while others were selected from those used by the contemporary experts.

伤寒明理论 [shāng hán míng lǐ lùn]
Shang Han Ming Li Lun*; *Concise Exposition of Cold Damage Diseases (1156)**:** by Cheng Wuji (成无己) of the Jin Dynasty, a concise reference book for beginners to study the *Treatise on Cold Damage Diseases* in which compatibility of ingredients is stressed

伤寒来苏集 [shāng hán lái sū jí]
Shang Han Lai Su Ji*; *Renewal of the Treatise on Cold Damage Diseases (1674)**:** in 8 volumes, compiled by Ke Qin (柯琴) of the Qing Dynasty, a collection of commentaries on the *Treatise on Cold Damage Diseases*

伤寒论直解 [shāng hán lùn zhí jiě]
Shang Han Lun Zhi Jie*; *Direct Explanation of the Treatise on Cold Damage Diseases (1712)**:** by Zhang Xiju (张锡驹), explains the *Treatise on Cold Damage Diseases* with the theories cited from the *Internal Classic*, or *Canon of Medicine*

伤寒类方 [shāng hán lèi fāng]
Shang Han Lei Fang*; *Classified Prescriptions from the Treatise on Cold Damage Diseases (1759)**:** by Xu Dachun (徐大椿) of the Qing Dynasty, in which the 113 prescriptions recommended in the *Treatise on Cold Damage Diseases* are classified into 12 categories and discussed on their indications

伤寒指掌 [shāng hán zhǐ zhǎng]
Shang Han Zhi Zhang*; *Thorough Understanding of Cold Damage (1796)**:**

by Su Kun'an (吴昆安) of the Qing Dynasty, in which differentiation between warm diseases and cold damage diseases is discussed in detail

伤寒贯珠集 [shāng hán guàn zhū jí]
Shang Han Guan Zhu Ji*; *A String of Beads from the Treatise on Cold Damage Diseases (1810)**:** compiled by You Yi (尤怡) of the Qing Dynasty, a new edition of the *Treatise on Cold Damage Diseases* classified in the order of the six pairs of meridians/channels

金匮要略方论 [jīn guì yào lüè fāng lùn]
***Jin Gui Yao Lue Fang Lun*; *Synopsis of Prescriptions of the Golden Chamber*:** simply *Jin Gui Yao Lue*, or *Synopsis of the Golden Chamber*, by Zhang Zhongjing (张仲景) at the beginning of the 3rd century. It was re-edited by Wang Shuhe (王叔和) in three volumes, addressing mainly the issues of miscellaneous diseases of internal medicine, as well as some external and women's diseases. The book contains 25 chapters, with a total of 262 prescriptions.

金匮要略 [jīn guì yào lüè]
***Jin Gui Yao Lue*; *Synopsis of the Golden Chamber*:** same as *Jin Gui Yao Lue Fang Lun*, or *Synopsis of Prescriptions of the Golden Chamber*

金匮要略心典 [jīn guì yào lüè xīn diǎn]
Jin Gui Yao Lue Xin Dian*; *Commentaries on the Synposis of the Golden Chamber (1729)**:** written by You Yi (尤怡) of the Qing Dynasty, in which his comments on *Synopsis of the Golden Chamber* are brief and to the point, and the relevant theories and major problems are clearly explained. While some mistakes which appeared in the original text are corrected, unintelligible statements remain untouched rather than wrongly interpreted.

金匮翼 [jīn guì yì]
Jin Gui Yi*; *Supplements to Commentaries on the Synopsis of the Golden Chamber (1768)**:** a book written by You Yi (尤怡) to supplement the *Jin Gui Yao Lue Xin Dian*, or *Commentaries on the Synopsis of the Golden Chamber*. Succinctly worded, it addresses exclusively the issues of internal medicine in 48 topics, and the prescriptions chosen are of practical value.

脉经 [mài jīng]
***Mai Jing*; *Pulse Classic*:** a book written by Wang Shuhe (王叔和) of the 3rd century, generally acknowledged as the standard work on the subject of pulse taking and the earliest comprehensive book on sphygmology extant

诊家枢要 [zhěn jiā shū yǎo]
Zhen Jia Shu Yao*; *Essentials for Diagnosticians (1359)**:** a monograph on pulse taking by Hua Shou (滑寿), in which 30 pulse patterns with their corresponding diseases are described

濒湖脉学 [bīn hú mài xué]
Bin Hu Mai Xue*; *Binhu's Sphygmology (1564) by Li Shizhen (李时珍)**:** a monograph on pulse taking in which 27 pulse patterns and their diagnostic values are given in detail. Written in lucid verses, the book has been popular for centuries.

四诊抉微 [sì zhěn jué wēi]
Si Zhen Jue Wei*; *The Essentials of

Four Diagnostic Examinations (1723): an influential monograph on diagnostics written by Lin Zhihan (林之翰)

诸病源侯总论 [zhū bìng yuán hóu zǒng lùn]
Zhu Bing Yuan Hou Zong Lun*; *Treatise on Causes and Manifestations of Diseases (610): compiled by Chao Yuanfang (巢元方) et al., in 50 volumes, with detailed discussions on the etiology and symptomology of various diseases, in which 1,720 entries of manifestations are grouped in 67 categories of causes. This book was frequently cited by experts of later generations.

三因极一病证方论 [sān yīn jí yī bìng zhèng fāng lùn]
San Yin Ji Yi Bing Zheng Fang Lun*; *Treatise on the Three Categories of Pathogenic Factors and Prescriptions (1174): a book written by Chen Yan (陈言), which classifies the causes of diseases into external, internal and miscellaneous (neither external nor internal) ones

神农本草经 [shén nóng běn cǎo jīng]
Shen Nong Ben Cao Jing*; *Shen Nong's Materia Medica*; *Shen Nong's Herbal: China's earliest materia medica, believed to be a product of the 1st century B.C., with its authorship attributed to the ancient emperor "Patron of Agriculture" or Shen Nong, in which 365 kinds of medicinal substances are listed and divided into three classes: superior, common and inferior

名医别录 [míng yī bié lù]
Ming Yi Bie Lu*; *Miscellaneous Records of Famous Physicians (5th century): a book on pharmaceutics compiled on the basis of *Shen Nong's Herbal* by Tao Hongjing (陶弘景), who expounded on *Shen Nong's Herbal*, and supplemented it with an additional 365 kinds of medicinal substances

本草经集注 [běn cǎo jīng jí zhù]
Ben Cao Jing Ji Zhu*; *Variorum of the Classic of Materia Medica (5th century): another book expounding on *Shen Nong's Herbal* by Tao Hongjing (陶弘景)

食疗本草 [shí liáo běn cǎo]
Shi Liao Ben Cao*; *Materia Medica of Diet Therapy (7th century): a monograph on herbs valuable as both food and medicine, by Meng Shen (孟诜) of the Tang Dynasty. The original version has been lost, but its contents can be found in Lei Zheng Ben Cao (类证本草) or *Classified Materia Medica* and *Ishinpo* (医心方) by Yasuriri Tanba (丹波康赖 912-995), a noted Japanese physician.

唐本草 [táng běn cǎo]
Tang Ben Cao*; *The Tang Materia Medica (659): also called *Xin Xiu Ben Cao* (新修本草) or *Newly Revised Materia Medica* (*of Tang*), compiled by Su Jing (苏敬) and 22 other scholars. Containing 844 entries of medicinal substances, and sponsored by the Tang imperial government, it is considered to be the earliest pharmacopoeia both nation- and worldwide.

新修本草 [xīn xiū běn cǎo]
***Xin Xiu Ben Cao*; *Newly Revised Materia Medica* (*of Tang*)**: another name for *Tang Ben Cao*, or *The Tang Materia Medica*

本草拾遗 [běn cǎo shí yí]

Ben Cao Shi Yi*; *A Supplement to the Materia Medica: a book in 10 volumes, by Chen Cangqi (陈藏器) of the Tang Dynasty (8th century), which mainly adds medicinal substances not included in the *Xin Xiu Ben Cao*, or *Newly Revised Tang Materia Medica*

经史证类备急本草 [jīng shǐ zhèng lèi bèi jí běn cǎo]

Jing Shi Zheng Lei Bei Ji Ben Cao*; *Classical Classified Materia Medica for Emergencies: also called *Zheng Lei Ben Cao* (证类本草) or *Classified Materia Medica* for short, compiled by Tang Shenwei (唐慎微) at the end of the 11th century, which lists 1,746 kinds of medicinal substances with directions for use and preparation, as well as many new prescriptions. The book is considered a milestone in the development of Chinese materia medica.

证类本草 [zhèng lèi běn cǎo]

Zheng Lei Ben Cao*; *Classified Materia Medica: abbreviation for *Jing Shi Zheng Lei Bei Ji Ben Cao* (经史证类备急本草) or *Classical Classified Materia Medica for Emergencies*

重修政和经史证类备急本草 [chóng xiū zhèng hé jīng shǐ zhèng lèi bèi jí běn cǎo]

Chong Xiu Zheng He Jing Shi Zheng Lei Bei Ji Ben Cao*; *Revised Zhenghe Classical Classified Materia Medica for Emergencies (1116): revised edition of *Jing Shi Zheng Lei Bei Ji Ben Cao* (经史证类备急本草), or *Classical Classified Materia Medica for Emergencies* compiled by the Northern Song government in the Zhenghe reign period (1111-1118)

政和本草 [zhèng hé běn cǎo]

Zheng He Ben Cao*; *Zhenghe Materia Medica: abbreviation for *Chong Xiu Zheng He Jing Shi Zheng Lei Bei Ji Ben Cao* (重修政和经史证类备急本草), or *Revised Zhenghe Classical Classified Materia Medica for Emergencies*

本草衍义 [běn cǎo yǎn yì]

Ben Cao Yan Yi*; *Amplification on Materia Medica (1116): a book complied by Kou Zongshi (寇宗奭), which lists 460 commonly used medicinal substances with valuable records of identification, pharmacology, and process of preparation

汤液本草 [tāng yè běn cǎo]

Tang Ye Ben Cao*; *Materia Medica for Decoctions (1289): by Wang Haogu (王好古), with a list of 238 medicinal substances, in which the flavor, taste and therapeutic properties as well as the compatibility issues are discussed in detail

救荒本草 [jiù huāng běn cǎo]

Jiu Huang Ben Cao*; *Materia Medica for Relief of Famine: compiled by Zhu Su (朱橚) in 1406, listing 414 plants which might be used as food in times of famine

本草纲目 [běn cǎo gāng mù]

Ben Cao Gang Mu*; *Compendium of Materia Medica: compiled by Li Shizhen (李时珍) and published in 1596, the most comprehensive Chinese medical work, in 52 volumes, which took the author 30 years to complete. It lists 1,892

medicinal substances, and contains more than 1,000 illustrations and over 10,000 prescriptions with detailed descriptions of the appearance, property, and method of collection, preparation and use for each substance. Far more than a compendium in the field of pharmaceutics, it is also a textbook of botany, zoology, mineralogy and metallurgy.

本草备要 [běn cǎo bèi yào]
Ben Cao Bei Yao*; *Essentials of Materia Medica: compiled by Wang Ang (王昂), published in 1694, a concise but valuable book on materia medica, listing 470 commonly used medicinal substances with over 400 illustrations, explaining the nature, property, taste, usage and indication in each case

本草纲目拾遗 [běn cǎo gāng mù shí yí]
Ben Cao Gang Mu Shi Yi*; *A Supplement to the Compendium of Materia Medica: compiled by Zhao Xuemin (赵学敏) in 1765, listing 716 medicinal substances not included in Li Shizhen's *Compendium of Materia Medica*

珍珠囊药性赋 [zhēn zhū náng yào xìng fù]
Zhen Zhu Nang Yao Xing Fu*; *Nature of the Drugs of the Pearl Bag in Songs: also known as *Lei Gong Yao Xing Fu* or *Lei's Nature of Drugs in Songs*, by Yuan Shan Dao Ren (元山道人) of the early Ming Dynasty, which describes in detail the indications and cautions for the use of 90 kinds of common medicinals, and introduces 1,406 medicinal substances in the form of songs and notes

雷公药性赋 [léi gōng yào xìng fù]
Lei Gong Yao Xing Fu*; *Lei's Nature of Drugs in Songs: another name for *Zhen Zhu Nang Yao Xing Fu*, or *Nature of the Drugs of the Pearl Bag in Songs*

用药法象 [yòng yào fǎ xiàng]
Yong Yao Fa Xiang*; *Rules for the Use of Drugs: a monograph by Li Gao (李杲) of the 13th century, in which medicinals are classified according to their therapeutic properties into four categories: ascending, descending, floating and sinking

雷公炮炙论 [léi gōng páo zhì lùn]
Lei Gong Pao Zhi Lun*; *Lei's Treatise on Medicinal Processing: by Lei Xiao (雷敩) of the 5th century, in which the fundamental processes of preparing drugs are documented and discussed. It is one of the earliest extant books on this subject.

炮炙大全 [páo zhì dà quán]
Pao Zhi Da Quan*; *A Complete Handbook of Medicinal Processing (1622): compiled by Miao Xiyong (缪希雍) and Zhuang Jiguang (庄继光), an updated version of Lei Xiao's work on the subject, in which some new processing methods are added. This book has been quite popular.

饮膳正要 [yǐn shàn zhèng yào]
Yin Shan Zheng Yao*; *Principles of Correct Diet (1330): a book written by Hu Sihui (忽思慧), which describes the daily recipes of the royal family and the nobility, as well as the nature, taste and indications of about 200 medicinal herbs which can be used as food.

植物名实图考 [zhí wù míng shí tú kǎo]
Zhi Wu Ming Shi Tu Kao*; *An illustrated

Book of Plants (1848): by Wu Qijun (吴其浚), in 38 volumes, a book on botany which includes 1,714 plant species. The author gives comparatively detailed descriptions of the shape, color, nature, taste, uses and habitats of the plants, with vivid and accurate drawings.

植物名实图考长编 [zhí wù míng shí tú kǎo cháng biān]

Zhi Wu Ming Shi Tu Kao Chang Bian*; *A Lengthy Compilation of Plants with Illustrations: a book compiled by Wu Qijun (吴其浚), in 22 volumes, on the basis of data from ancient literature, as a complement to the *Zhi Wu Ming Shi Tu Kao*, or *An Illustrated Book of Plants*, with 788 plant substances listed

全国中草药汇编 [quān guó zhōng cǎo yào huì biān]

Quan Guo Zhong Cao Yao Hui Bian*; *A Compilation of Chinese Medicinal Herbs (1975): a book compiled in two volumes, with a list of approximately 2,200 herbal medicines. The name, source, morphology, environment, cultivation, collection and preparation, chemistry, pharmacology, nature, taste, uses, indications and administration of each medicinal herb are given in detail, with illustrations of the living plants.

肘后备急方 [zhǒu hòu bèi jí fāng]

Zhou Hou Bei Ji Fang*; *A Handbook of Prescriptions for Emergencies: a book written by Ge Hong (葛洪 283-343), in which the prescriptions recorded are simple to prepare, and the medicinal ingredients are both commonly available and effective. In addition, many other valuable descriptions of diseases and treatments are recorded.

备急千金要方 [bèi jí qiān jīn yào fāng]

Bei Ji Qian Jin Yao Fang*; *Essential Prescriptions Worth a Thousand Pieces of Gold for Emergencies: also called *Qian Jin Yao Fang* (千金要方), or *Essential Prescriptions Worth a Thousand Pieces of Gold* for short, compiled by Sun Simiao (孙思邈) at the end of the 7th century in 30 volumes, which includes a general introduction, and prescriptions of various clinical branches, diet, pulse-taking, acupuncture, etc.

千金要方 [qiān jīn yào fāng]

Qian Jin Yao Fang*; *Essential Prescriptions Worth a Thousand Pieces of Gold: abbreviation for *Bei Ji Qian Jin Yao Fang*, or *Essential Prescriptions Worth a Thousand Pieces of Gold for Emergencies*

千金翼方 [qiān jīn yì fāng]

Qian Jin Yi Fang*; *Supplement to the Essential Prescriptions Worth a Thousand Pieces of Gold: compiled by Sun Simiao (孙思邈) at the end of the 7th century, in 30 volumes, including knowledge of various medical branches such as herbal lore, febrile diseases, obstetrics and gynecology, pediatrics, miscellaneous diseases of internal medicine, pulse-taking, acupuncture and diet, which, together with the *Qian Jin Yao Fang*, or *Essential Prescriptions Worth a Thousand Pieces of Gold*, is considered a compendium of the medical achievements made before the Tang Dynasty

外台秘要 [wài tái mì yào]

Wai Tai Mi Yao*; *Arcane Essentials from

the Imperial Library (752): compiled by Wang Tao (王焘), in 40 volumes, in which a comprehensive and exhaustive study of medicine is made, with 1,104 medical problems discussed and over 6,000 prescriptions recorded

太平圣惠方 [tài píng shèng huì fāng]
Tai Ping Sheng Hui Fang; ***Taiping Holy Benevolent Prescriptions*** (992): simply *Sheng Hui Fang*, or *Holy Benevolent Prescriptions*, compiled by Wang Huaiyin (王怀隐) in 10 volumes, recording 16,834 prescriptions from various medical branches with discussions on the diagnosis and pathology of various diseases

圣惠方 [shèng huì fāng]
Sheng Hui Fang; ***Holy Benevolent Prescriptions***: abbreviation for *Tai Ping Sheng Hui Fang*, or *Taiping Holy Benevolent Prescriptions*

苏沈良方 [sū shěn liáng fāng]
Su Shen Liang Fang; ***Best Prescriptions Collected by Su Shi and Shen Kuo*** (1075): a combined edition of the *Su Xue Shi Fang* or *Scholar Su's Prescritions* by Su Shi (苏轼) and the *Liang Fang* or *Best Prescriptions* by Shen Kuo (沈括), in which a number of simple but effective prescriptions are recorded

太平惠民和剂局方 [tài píng huì mín hé jì jú fāng]
Tai Ping Hui Min He Ji Ju Fang; Formulary of the Bureau of People's Welfare Pharmacy (1151): simply *He Ji Ju Fang*, or *Formulary of the Bureau of Pharmacy*, compiled by Chen Shiwen (陈师文) et al. in 10 volumes, containing 788 prescriptions in 14 categories which were found to be both popular and effective. Most of the medicines are in pill or powder form, ready for use and storage

和剂局方 [hé jì jú fāng]
He Ji Ju Fang; ***Formulary of the Bureau of Pharmacy***: abbreviation for *Tai Ping Hui Min He Ji Ju Fang*, or *Formulary of the Bureau of People's Welfare Pharmacy*

普济本事方 [pǔ jì běn shì fāng]
Pu Ji Ben Shi Fang; ***Effective Prescriptions for Universal Relief*** (1132): also called *Ben Shi Fang*, or *Effective Prescriptions* for short, a book in 10 volumes, by Xu Shuwei (许叔微) of the Southern Song Dynasty. It mainly addresses the issues of common diseases related to internal medicine, listing 23 categories of diseases with more than 300 prescriptions, to each of which are attached proven case records.

本事方 [běn shì fāng]
Ben Shi Fang; ***Effective Prescriptions***: abbreviation for the *Pu Ji Ben Shi Fang*, or *Effective Prescriptions for Universal Relief*

济生方 [jì shēng fāng]
Ji Sheng Fang; ***Prescriptions for Succoring the Sick*** (1253): also called *Yan Shi Ji Sheng Fang* or *Yan's Prescriptions for Succoring the Sick*, a book in 10 volumes, by Yan Yonghe (严用和). It consists of 79 articles which address diverse categories of diseases including those of internal medicine, external medicine and gynecology. It also collects over 450 prescriptions, all of

which were proven clinically effective by the author.

严氏济生方 [yán shì jì shēng fāng]
***Yan Shi Ji Sheng Fang*; *Yan's Prescriptions for Succoring the Sick*:** the full name of the *Ji Sheng Fang*, or *Prescriptions for Succoring the Sick*

世医得效方 [shì yī dé xiào fāng]
Shi Yi De Xiao Fang*; *Effective Prescriptions Handed Down for Generations (1345)**:** compiled by Wei Yilin (危亦林) on the basis of the author's family experiences as physicians for five successive generations, in which are listed prescriptions for children's diseases, internal medicine, ophthalmology, oral diseases, dentistry, bone-setting, war wounds, ulcers and carbuncles

局方发挥 [jú fāng fā huī]
***Ju Fang Fa Hui*; *An Expounding of the Formulary of the Bureau of Pharmacy*:** written by Zhu Zhenheng (朱震亨) of the 14th century. Zhu pointed out and criticized the mechanical and indiscriminate use of the formularies of the Bureau of the People's Welfare Pharmacy which were popular at that time.

普济方 [pǔ jì fāng]
Pu Ji Fang*; *Prescriptions for Universal Relief (1406)**:** a comprehensive collection of prescriptions (61,739 prescriptions and 239 illustrations) in 168 volumes by Teng Hong (滕弘) et al. under the patronage of Zhu Su (朱橚)

奇效良方 [qí xiào liáng fāng]
Qi Xiao Liang Fang*; *Wonderful Well-tried Prescriptions (1470)**:** a book in 69 volumes with authorship ascribed to Dong Su (董宿) and Fang Xian (方贤). It contains more than 7,000 prescriptions and methods of needling and bone-setting, chiefly passed down during the Song and Ming Dynasties. These methods of treatment are divided into 64 families according to the principles of treatment, such as wind, cold, and heat, and then subdivided into still smaller groups.

医方考 [yī fāng kǎo]
Yi Fang Kao*; *Investigations of Medical Prescriptions (1584)**:** compiled by Wu Kun (吴昆). It lists more than 700 prescriptions, classified into 44 categories, with explanations of ingredient combinations for each prescription.

医方集解 [yī fāng jí jiě]
Yi Fang Ji Jie*; *Collection of Prescriptions with Expositions (1682)**:** authored by Wang Ang (汪昂). It lists approximately 700 prescriptions divided into 21 classes, such as tonifying, exterior-releasing, vomiting-inducing, harmonizing, *qi*-regulating, blood-regulating, etc., and describes in detail the combinations of ingredients, properties, and indications of each recipe with reference to the theories of various schools

汤头歌诀 [tāng tóu gē jué]
Tang Tou Ge Jue*; *Prescriptions in Rhymes (1694)**:** written by Wang Ang (汪昂). Over 300 prescriptions are presented in the form of more than 200 songs. To each song are appended simple notes to make it easier for beginners to learn them by heart. The book was very popular.

串雅内、外编 [chuàn yǎ nèi、wài biān]
Chuan Ya Nei Wai Bian*; *Bound Volume of Treatises on Folk Medicine (1759): a joint edition of the two books titled *Treatise on Folk Medicine* and *Extra Treatise on Folk Medicine*, respectively, written by Zhao Xuemin (赵学敏) on the basis of recipes employed by folk healers and reference materials in medical works. Each consists of four volumes of simple, handy, cheap yet effective prescriptions, as well as methods of making medicinals and of treating diseases of animals and plants.

时方歌括 [shí fāng gē kuò]
Shi Fang Ge Kuo*; *Popular Prescriptions in Verse (1801): written by Chen Nianzu (陈念祖) of the Qing Dynasty with 108 popular and practical prescriptions recorded in verse

医方论 [yī fāng lùn]
Yi Fang Lun*; *Treatise on Medical Prescriptions (1865): by Fei Boxiong (费伯雄), a book of commentaries on Wang Ang's (汪昂) *Yi Fang Ji Jie*, or *Collection of Prescriptions with Expositions*

理瀹骈文 [lǐ yuè pián wén]
Li Yue Pian Wen*; *A Rhymed Discourse on External Therapeutics (1870): written by Wu Shangxian (吴尚先) who was noted for practicing folk medicine and advocating external therapies such as ointment and plasters, hydrotherapy, breathing therapy, cautery and moxibustion

温疫论 [wēn yì lùn]
Wen Yi Lun*; *Treatise on Pestilence (1642): authored by Wu Youke (吴又可), a study of the etiology and pathology of epidemic febrile diseases. The author points out that it is pestilential factors that cause epidemic febrile diseases, and that pestilential factors may get into the human body through the mouth and nose.

温热论 [wēn rè lùn]
Wen Re Lun*; *Treatise on Warm-heat Diseases (1746): comprising lectures by Ye Tianshi (叶天士) and edited by his disciple Gu Jingwen (顾景文), a book on the diagnosis and treatment of epidemic febrile diseases in which development and transmission of such diseases are expounded on the basis of the concepts of four aspects, namely, superficial defense, *qi*, nutrient and blood

温病条辨 [wēn bìng tiáo biàn]
Wen Bing Tiao Bian*; *Analysis of Warm Diseases (1798): by Wu Tang (吴瑭), a development of Ye Tianshi's *Treatise on Warm-heat Diseases*, in which differential diagnosis of diseases according to pathological changes of the triple energizer was proposed and elucidated in detail

温热经纬 [wēn rè jīng wěi]
Wen Re Jing Wei*; *An Outline of Warm-heat Diseases (1852): by Wang Mengying (王孟英), in five volumes, shedding light on the causes of epidemic febrile diseases, their signs and symptoms, and methods of treatment based on the theories expounded in the *Internal Classic* and *Treatise on Cold Damage and Miscellaneous Diseases*, and with reference to the views of distinguished physicians of the Qing Dynasty such as Ye Gui (叶桂), Xue Xue (薛雪), Chen Pingbo (陈平伯), and Yu Shiyu (余师愚)

时病论 [shí bìng lùn]
Shi Bing Lun*; *Treatise on Seasonal Diseases (1882)**:** by Lei Feng (雷丰), a book of practical value, mainly dealing with febrile diseases of the four seasons, describing the causes, symptoms and treatment of the diseases and introducing the author's own prescriptions

霍乱论 [huò luàn lùn]
Huo Luan Lun*; *Treatise on Choleric Turmoil (1838)**:** a monograph by Wang Shixiong (王士雄), discussing the clinical manifestations, prevention and treatment of cholera and the like, with illustration of case records

脾胃论 [pí wèi lùn]
Pi Wei Lun*; *Treatise on the Spleen and Stomach (1249)**:** a book authored by Li Gao (李杲). Based on the nutritional viewpoint expressed in the *Internal Classic*, the author emphasizes and explains the importance of nourishing the spleen and stomach. Li also recommends some novel remedies to solve the problems of the spleen and stomach caused by improper diet or fatigue, which include Bu Zhong Yi Qi Tang, or Decoction for Reinforcing the Middle and Replenishing Qi and Sheng Yang Yi Wei Tang, or Decoction for Activating Yang and Replenishing the Stomach.

十药神书 [shí yào shén shū]
Shi Yao Shen Shu*; *A Miraculous Book of Ten Recipes (1348)**:** by Ge Qiansun (葛乾孙), containing 10 recipes – three recipies for hemoptysis, three for cough, one hypnotic and three nutrients. All the recipes are said to be effective for treating consumption, especially pulmonary tuberculosis.

证治汇补 [zhèng zhì huì bǔ]
***Zheng Zhi Hui Bu*; *Supplement to Diagnosis and Treatment*:** in eight volumes by Li Yongcui (李用粹) and published in 1687, mainly dealing with miscellaneous diseases of internal medicine, recording more than 80 categories of diseases with their diagnoses, methods of treatment and prescriptions

类证治裁 [lèi zhèng zhì cái]
Lei Zheng Zhi Cai*; *Classified Syndromes and Treatment (1839)**:** a book authored by Lin Peiqin (林佩琴). The author differentiates and analyzes various diseases, including the ones related to internal medicine, gynecology and external medicine, according to their causes and clinical manifestations, and introduces concrete therapeutic methods. To the descriptions of many diseases are appended case records for reference. This book collects and combines the positive aspects of various schools, and has exerted a positive impact on medical circles.

血证论 [xuè zhèng lùn]
Xue Zheng Lun*; *Treatise on Blood Syndromes (1884)**:** a book authored by Tang Rongchuan (唐容川). This book addresses the diagnosis and treatment of various blood problems, including a general introduction and descriptions of over 170 diseases. The author breaks fresh ground in the field of blood syndromes.

经效产宝 [jīng xiào chǎn bǎo]
Jing Xiao Chan Bao*; *Tested Treasures of

Obstetrics: simply *Chan Bao*, or *Treasures of Obstetrics*, by Zan Yin (昝殷). Written in 852-856, it is the earliest Chinese book on obstetrics, in which diagnosis and treatment of the diseases occurring during pregnancy, in parturition and after delivery are discussed.

产宝 [chǎn bǎo]

Chan Bao*; *Treasure of Obstetrics: abbreviation for the *Jing Xiao Chan Bao*, or *Tested Treasures of Obstetrics*

卫生家宝产科备要 [wèi shēng jiā bǎo chǎn kē bèi yào]

***Wei Sheng Jia Bao Chan Ke Bei Yao*; *Essentials of Obstetrics from the Treasury of Household Hygiene* (1184)**: a valuable book on obstetrics compiled by Zhu Duanzhang (朱端章). The author pools knowledge of obstetrics and infant nursing from all previous medical works.

女科百问 [nǚ kē bǎi wèn]

***Nü Ke Bai Wen*; *One Hundred Questions on Women's Diseases* (1220)**: compiled by Qi Zhongfu (齐仲甫) of the Song Dynasty, in which the main problems of gynecology and obstetrics are discussed in the form of questions and answers

妇人大全良方 [fù rén dà quán liáng fāng]

Fu Ren Da Quan Liang Fang*; *The Complete Book of Effective Prescriptions for Women: simply *Fu Ren Liang Fang*, or *Effective Prescriptions for Women* (1237) by Chen Ziming (陈自明), the first and most important book on gynecology and obstetrics in Chinese medicine

妇人良方 [fù rén liáng fāng]

Fu Ren Liang Fang*; *Effective Prescriptions for Women: abbreviation for *Fu Ren Da Quan Liang Fang*, or *The Complete Book of Effective Prescriptions for Women*

万氏女科 [wàn shì nǚ kē]

***Wan Shi Nü Ke*; *Wan's Gynecology and Obstetrics* (1549)**: by Wan Quan (万全) of the Ming Dynasty, with discussions on gynecological and obstetric diseases

济阴纲目 [jì yīn gāng mù]

Ji Yin Gang Mu*; *Compendium of Therapies for Women's Diseases: a book on obstetrics and gynecology, first edition in 5 volumes by Wu Zhiwang (武之望) and published in 1620, second edition in 14 volumes by Wang Qi (汪琪) and published in 1665 with additional commentaries. Problems concerning menstruation, leukorrhea, pregnancy and parturition are discussed, together with prescriptions of practical value.

女科经纶 [nǚ kē jīng lún]

***Nü Ke Jing Lun*; *Principles of Gynecology and Obstetrics* (1684)**: a book compiled by Xiao Gengliu (萧庚六) of the Qing Dynasty, substantial in content, with notes and annotations attached

傅青主女科 [fù qīng zhǔ nǚ kē]

Fu Qing Zhu Nü Ke*; *Fu Qingzhu's Obstetrics and Gynecology: also known as *Nü Ke* (女科) or *Obstetrics and Gynecology*, a book in 2 volumes by Fu Shan (傅山) in the 17th century and first published in 1827. The book consists of 77 articles discussing diagnosis and treatment of diseases of obstetrics and gynecology in a concise way. It also provides practical prescriptions. The author also wrote the *Chan Hou Bian* (产后编), or *Postpartum Care*, on the diagnosis and treatment of 43 categories of obstretic diseases. The combined edition of the two books appeared later, titled *Fu Shi Nü Ke Da Quan* (傅氏女科大全) or *Fu's Complete Works of Obstetrics and Gynecology*.

小儿药证直诀 [xiǎo ér yào zhèng zhí jué]
Xiao Er Yao Zheng Zhi Jue*; *Key to the Therapeutics of Children's Diseases (1119): a book compiled by Qian Yi (钱乙), generally acknowledged as the greatest pediatrist in Chinese medicine. It was edited and published by his disciple Yan Jizhong (阎季忠) in three volumes addressing three different issues in each volume, namely diagnosis, case recording and prescriptions. The author recognizes and emphasizes the peculiarities of pediatrics such as the characteristics of children's physiology and pathology.

幼幼新书 [yòu yòu xīn shū]
You You Xin Shu*; *A New Book of Pediatrics (1132): a comprehensive treatise on children's diseases in 40 volumes compiled by Liu Fang (刘昉), Wang Li (王历) and Wang Shi (王湜), discussing etiology, diagnosis and therapies of various kinds of children's diseases, child care, etc.

小儿痘疹方论 [xiǎo ér dòu zhěn fāng lùn]
Xiao Er Dou Zhen Fang Lun*; *Treatise on Smallpox and Measles in Children (1241): by Chen Wenzhong (陈文中), a noted pediatrist of the 13th century

幼科铁镜 [yòu kē tiě jìng]
***You Ke Tie Jing*; *Iron Mirror of Pediatrics* (1695):** a book on pediatrics by Xia Ding (夏鼎) of the Qing Dynasty, in which the diagnosis and treatment of common diseases of children are discussed and massotherapy recommended

幼幼集成 [yòu yòu jí chéng]
You You Ji Cheng*; *Collection of Works on Pediatrics (1750): by Chen Fuzheng (陈复正), who collected and revised the main contents of ancient books on pediatrics, adding his own views on some theoretical issues concerning the therapeutic methods of treating certain diseases, e.g., infantile convulsions

小儿推拿秘旨 [xiǎo ér tuī ná mì zhǐ]
Xiao Er Tui Na Mi Zhi*; *Secret Principles of Massotherapy for Children: written by Gong Yunlin (龚云林) of the Ming Dynasty and edited with a supplement and published by Yao Guozhen (姚国桢) in 1604. It is one of the earliest Chinese works on pediatric massotherapy.

小儿推拿广意 [xiǎo ér tuī ná guǎng yì]
Xiao Er Tui Na Guang Yi*; *Elucidation of Massotherapy for Children (c. 1676): also called *Tui Na Guang Yi*, or *Elucidation of Massotherapy* for short, by Xiong Yingxiong (熊应雄) of the Qing Dynasty

推拿广意 [tuī ná guǎng yì]
Tui Na Guang Yi*; *Elucidation of Massotherapy: abbreviation for *Xiao Er Tui Na Guang Yi*, or *Elucidation of Massotherapy for Children*

刘涓子鬼遗方 [liú juān zǐ guǐ yí fāng]
Liu Juanzi Gui Yi Fang*; *Liu Juanzi's Ghost-Bequeathed Prescriptions (496-499): the earliest Chinese work on external medicine, by Gong Qingxuan (龚庆宣), addressing mainly the treatment of traumatic wounds, carbuncles, mastitis, burns, eczema, and scabies, with insightful remarks on surgical nursing, drainage and sterilization. The use of the phrase "ghost-bequeathed" in the title was aimed to emphasize the marvelous effect of the prescriptions.

理伤续断秘方 [lǐ shāng xù duàn mì fāng]
Li Shang Xu Duan Mi Fang*; *Secrets of Treating Wounds and Rejoining Fractures (846): also called *Xian Shou Li Shang Xu Duan Mi Fang*, or *Secrets of Treating Wounds and Rejoining Fractures Handed Down by an Immortal*, the earliest Chinese book on bone-setting, by Taoist priest Lin Daoren (蔺道人), with comments on traction, reunion, and fixation of fractured and dislocated bones

仙授理伤续断秘方 [xiān shòu lǐ shāng xù duàn mì fāng]
Xian Shou Li Shang Xu Duan Mi Fang*; *Secrets of Treating Wounds and Rejoining Fractures Handed Down by an Immortal: full name of *Li Shang Xu Duan Mi Fang*, or *Secrets of Treating Wounds and Rejoining Fractures*

外科精要 [wài kē jīng yào]
Wai Ke Jing Yao*; *Essence of External Medicine (1263): by Chen Ziming (陈自明), one of the earliest Chinese books on external medicine with discussions on differential diagnosis and treatment of furuncles, carbuncles, gangrene, ulcers and wounds

外科精义 [wài kē jīng yì]
Wai Ke Jing Yi*; *Essentials of External Medicine (1335): by Qi Dezhi (齐德之) of the Yuan Dynasty, consisting of 35 articles on external medicine, 145 prescriptions for making decoctions, boluses, plasters and pills, the processes of preparing medicines, and the main indications of single-item recipes

解围元薮 [jiě wéi yuán sǒu]
Jie Wei Yuan Sou*; *Source of Relief: a monograph on leprosy, written by Shen Zhiwen (沈之问) in 1550, which discusses the causes and manifestations of leprosy, and their relations to meridians/channels, and lists 249 prescriptions

疮疡经验全书 [chuāng yáng jīng yàn quán shū]
Chuang Yang Jing Yan Quan Shu*; *Complete Manual of Experiences in the Treatment of Sores: publicly attributed to Dou Hanqing (窦汉卿) but actually written by Dou's grandson. The book appeared in 1569, which deals with all the diseases requiring surgical treatment, classified according to the regions of the body.

外科启玄 [wài kē qǐ xuán]
Wai Ke Qi Xuan*; *Revealing the Mystery of External Medicine: written by Shen Gongchen (申拱宸) and published in 1604. It begins with a general introduction to various forms of therapy, and then discusses the cases requiring surgical treatment with illustrations

外科正宗 [wài kē zhèng zōng]

***Wai Ke Zheng Zong*; *Orthodox Manual of External Medicine*:** by Chen Shi-gong (陈实功) on the basis of his 40 years of personal experience, in which each disease is discussed from the perspectives of diagnosis, therapeutic method and operation with case records and prescriptions attached. It was published in 1617, and has ever since been one of the most influential books in China on external medicine.

外科大成 [wài kē dà chéng]

***Wai Ke Da Cheng*; *A Complete Book on External Medicine*:** written by Qi Kun (祁坤) in 1665. It gives a complete description of diagnoses and treatment of external diseases and is the book upon which *Yi Zong Jin Jian Wai Ke Xin Fa Yao Jue* (医宗金鉴外科心法要诀) or *Golden Mirror of Medicine: Essentials of External Diseases* is based.

外科证治全生集 [wài kē zhèng zhì quán shēng jí]

Wai Ke Zheng Zhi Quan Sheng Ji*; *Life-saving Manual of Diagnosis and Treatment of External Diseases (1740)**:** by Wang Weide (王惟德) of the Qing Dynasty, emphasizing the use of the elimination method in treating ulcers and carbuncles

伤科补要 [wài kē bǔ yào]

Shang Ke Bu Yao*; *Supplement to Traumatology (1803)**:** by Qian Xiuchang (钱秀昌) of the Qing Dynasty, including treatment of trauma and bone-setting with tested prescriptions. The contents are presented in rhymed form.

伤科汇纂 [shāng kē huì zuǎn]

Shang Ke Hui Zuan*; *Compilation of Traumatology (1817)**:** by Hu Tingguang (胡廷光) of the Qing Dynasty, discussing differential diagnosis and treatment of fractures and dislocation of bones

银海精微 [yín hǎi jīng wēi]

***Yin Hai Jing Wei*; *Essence of the Silvery Sea*:** a book on ophthalmology in two volumes, which appeared in the 13th century with authorship attributed to Sun Simiao (孙思邈). "Silvery sea" is a metaphorical expression for the eyes.

秘传眼科龙木论 [mì chuán yǎn kē lóng mù lùn]

***Mi Chuan Yan Ke Long Mu Lun*; *Long Mu's Recondite Treatise on Ophthalmology*:** by an anonymous author, in 10 volumes, appeared in the 13th century. It covers 72 categories of eye diseases, with the focus on glaucoma and cataracts.

原［元］机启微 [yuán jī qǐ wēi]

Yuan Ji Qi Wei*; *Revealing the Mystery of the Origin (of Eye Diseases) (1370)**:** by Ni Weide (倪维德), which gives a systematic elucidation of eye diseases. In Ni's opinion, an eye disease is not just a local affliction but rather the result of defective functioning of the whole body, and its onset is often due to an unhygienic environment.

审视瑶函 [shěn shì yáo hán]

***Shen Shi Yao Han*; *A Precious Work on Ophthalmology*:** also titled *Yan Ke Da Quan*, or *A Complete Book on Ophthalmology*, a comprehensive monograph on eye diseases by Fu Yunke (傅允科), which appeared in

1644 in seven volumes, listing 108 eye diseases and their treatment

眼科大全 [yǎn kē dà quán]
Yan Ke Da Quan*; *A Complete Book of Ophthalmology: another name for *Shen Shi Yao Han*, or *A Precious Work on Ophthalmology*

针灸甲乙经 [zhēn jiǔ jiǎ yǐ jīng]
Zhen Jiu Jia Yi Jing*; *The ABC Classic of Acupuncture and Moxibustion (c. 259): by Huangfu Mi (皇甫谧), the earliest systematic Chinese monograph of acupuncture and moxibustion, in which the names and number of points of each meridian/channel and their exact locations are defined. It also addresses such issues as the properties and indications of each point and the methods of needle manipulation.

铜人俞穴针灸图经 [tóng rén shù xué zhēn jiǔ tú jīng]
Tong Ren Shu Xue Zhen Jiu Tu Jing*; *Illustrated Manual of Acupoints on the Bronze Figure: by Wang Weiyi (王惟一), first published in 1027 in three volumes, in which a total of 657 points on the famous bronze figure are marked

针灸资生经 [zhēn jiǔ zī shēng jīng]
Zhen Jiu Zi Sheng Jing*; *Classic of Nourishing Life with Acupuncture and Moxibustion (1220): by Wang Zhizhong (王执中), a systematic presentation of acupuncture and moxibustion, including the locations of meridians/channels and points along with 46 illustrations, based on the author's clinical experience

十四经发挥 [shí sì jīng fā huī]
Shi Si Jing Fa Hui*; *Elucidation of the Fourteen Meridians/ Channels (1341): by Hua Shou (滑寿), a marked development in meridian/channel theory

针灸聚英 [zhēn jiǔ jù yīng]
Zhen Jiu Ju Ying*; *A Collection of Gems of Acupuncture and Moxibustion (1529): by Gao Wu (高武), in which the author brings together the theories of various schools of acupuncture and moxibustion

针灸问对 [zhēn jiǔ wèn duì]
Zhen Jiu Wen Dui*; *Catechism on Acupuncture and Moxibustion (1530): by Wang Ji (汪机), in which the theories and principles of acupuncture and moxibustion are expounded

针灸问答 [zhēn jiǔ wèn dá]
Zhen Jiu Wen Da*; *Catechism on Acupuncture and Moxibustion: same as *Zhen Jiu Wen Dui* (针灸问对)

针灸大成 [zhēn jiǔ dà chéng]
Zhen Jiu Da Cheng*; *Great Compendium of Acupuncture and Moxibustion (1601): by Yang Jizhou (杨继洲), in which clarification of confusion over points and meridians/channels is provided along with an attempt to unify various divergent views

针刺麻醉 [zhēn cì má zuì]
Zhen Ci Ma Zui*; *Acupuncture Anesthesia: published in 1972, a comprehensive book on acupuncture anesthesia which includes an introduction to its history, characteristic features, theories, and methods, as well as detailed descriptions of the points most commonly used in the field, operations and electro-acupuncture devices. It is

a preliminary summary report of the achievements in this field.

洗冤集录 [xǐ yuān jí lù]
Xi Yuan Ji Lu*; *Instructions to Coroners (1247): a book on forensic medicine by Song Ci (宋慈), originally in 10 volumes, but only 4 extant since the Ming Dynasty. It systematically sums up the achievements made before the Song Dynasty in the field of forensic medicine, and introduces poisoning tests, and measures for emergency treatment in case of poisoning. It also addresses anatomy, pathology, bone-setting, surgical operations, etc. The book is of great value, and has been translated into different languages.

周易参同契 [zhōu yì cān tóng qì]
Zhou Yi Can Tong Qi*; *Analogism of the Principles of Changes Formulated in the Zhou Dynasty: by Wei Boyang (魏伯阳) of the Han Dynasty, in which along with teachings about making elixirs (pills) of immortality through alchemy, the art of internal exercise for immortality is discussed. The part of the human body where *qi* was believed to be stored has thus been called *dantian* (elixir field), analogous to the furnace in alchemy.

养性延命录 [yǎng xìng yán mìng lù]
Yang Xing Yan Ming Lu*; *Recordings of the Art of Health and Life Preservation: by Tao Hongjing (陶弘景) of the Jin Dynasty, in which many forms of *qigong* exercise are recorded

黄庭经 [huáng tíng jīng]
Huang Ting Jing*; *Classic of the Yellow Yard: a book on *qigong* exercise by Wei Huacun (魏华存) of the Jin Dynasty, in which concentration on the "yellow yard", breathing and swallowing of saliva are stressed in *qigong* exercise. The "yellow yard" is equivalent to *dantian* (the elixir field), the location in the human body on which the mind should be concentrated during *qigong* exercise.

修习止观坐禅法要 [xiū xí zhǐ guān zuò chán fǎ yào]
Xiu Xi Zhi Guan Zuo Chan Fa Yao*; *Principles of Buddhist Cultivation: compiled by Zhi Kai (智顗), a leading Bhuddist monk of the Sui Dynasty, in which methods of adjustment of posture, breathing and mentality are described

内功图说 [nèi gōng tú shuō]
Nei Gong Tu Shuo*; *Illustrated Internal Qigong Exercise: compiled by Wang Zuyuan (王祖源) of the Qing Dynasty, in which several forms of *qigong* exercise are described, with illustrations

中藏经 [zhōng zàng jīng]
Zhong Zang Jing*; *Treasured Classic: a comprehensive book on medicine, with authorship ascribed to Hua Tuo (华佗) but most probably by an unknown author during the Six Dynasties period (220-589). The book includes 49 articles on diagnosis and treatment, pulse, internal organs, deficiency and excess syndromes/patterns, cold and heat syndromes/patterns, etc., as well as a list of prescriptions.

扁鹊心书 [biǎn què xīn shū]
Bian Que Xin Shu*; *Precious Writings of Bianque (1146): a comprehensive book on medicine by Dou Cai (窦材) of the

Song Dynasty. The book is distinguished by its recording of the method of herbal anesthesia.

儒门事亲 [rú mén shì qīn]
Ru Men Shi Qin*; *Confucians' Duties to Their Parents (1228): written by Zhang Zihe (张子和), in which classification of diseases based on Liu Wansu's (刘完素) theory of six exogenous pathogenic factors is presented along with the three solutions, namely, diaphoresis, emesis and purgation

兰室秘藏 [lán shì mì cáng]
Lan Shi Mi Cang*; *Book Hidden in the Orchid Chamber (1276): a comprehensive book on medicine written by Li Gao (李杲), which deals with 21 categories of diseases. The author's opinions on the diseases of the spleen and stomach presented in the book have been appreciated by physicians of later generations. It is worth noticing that the prescriptions listed were mostly invented by the author himself.

玉机微义 [yù jī wēi yì]
Yu Ji Wei Yi*; *Subtle Meaning of the Jade Swivel (1396): a comprehensive book on medicine by Xu Yanchun (徐彦纯) and supplemented by Liu Zonghou (刘宗厚). The book deals with 33 categories of diseases covering various fields of clinical medicine.

丹溪心法 [dān xī xīn fǎ]
Dan Xi Xin Fa*; *Danxi's Experiential Therapy: written by Zhu Zhenheng (朱震亨) of the Yuan Dynasty, but edited by his disciples. In 1481, the book was re-edited with supplements and corrections by Cheng Chong (程充), with six treatises on medical theories at the beginning followed by 100 articles dealing with various diseases, most of which are concerned with internal medicine. The author's opinion that "yang is ever excessive and yin ever deficient" is the main theme of the book.

格致余论 [gé zhì yú lùn]
Ge Zhi Yu Lun*; *Supplementary Treatise on Knowledge from Practice (1347): a monograph written by Zhu Zhenheng (朱震亨), in which the theory of "ever excessive yang with deficient yin" is expounded to a greater extent

韩氏医通 [hán shì yī tōng]
Han Shi Yi Tong*; *Han's General Medicine (1522): by Han Mao (韩懋) of the Ming Dynasty, a comprehensive medical book dealing with the diagnosis and treatment of various diseases. The author stresses the role of the four examinations in differential diagnosis, introduces the Three-Seed Filial Devotion Decoction, and discusses the clinical experience of the use of tonics.

明医杂著 [míng yī zá zhù]
Ming Yi Za Zhu*; *Collection of Physicians' Experiences in the Ming Dynasty (1549): compiled by Wang Lun (王纶) and annotated by Xue Ji (薛己) of the Ming Dynasty

医门法律 [yī mén fǎ lǜ]
Yi Men Fa Lü*; *Principles and Prohibitions of the Medical Profession (1658): by Yu Chang (喻昌). It explains the principles of diagnosis and treatment based on syndrome differentiation or pattern identification, points out common errors, and suggests prohibitions in order to prevent making those errors, hence the title.

医林改错 [yī lín gǎi cuò]

Yi Lin Gai Cuo*; *Corrections of Errors in Medical Works (1830)**:** written by Wang Qingren (王清任), who insisted on making anatomical observations and spent years on the study of the internal organs. In this book the author corrects some mistakes concerning the internal organs by previous generations of physicians, and suggests new methods for treating blood stasis and hemiplegia. His method of activating the blood and removing stasis is still of practical value.

冷庐医话 [lěng lú yī huà]

Leng Lu Yi Hua*; *Deserted House Medical Talks (1897)**:** written by Lu Yitian (陆以湉), including informal essays, short sketches and notes to address medical problems

医学衷中参西录 [yī xué zhōng zhōng cān xī lù]

***Yi Xue Zhong Zhong Can Xi Lu*; *Records of Traditional Chinese and Western Medicine in Combination*:** written by Zhang Xichun (张锡纯) and published in 1918–1934. There were altogether 30 volumes in seven issues. The revised edition consists of five parts, viz., prescriptions, medical substances, medical theories, notes and case records. The author attempted to integrate traditional Chinese medicine with Western medicine.

名医类案 [míng yī lèi àn]

***Ming Yi Lei An*; *Classified Medical Records of Distinguished Physicians*:** compiled by Jiang Guan (江瓘) and his son and completed in 1552, revised later by Wei Zhixiu (魏之琇). It deals with acute and chronic infectious diseases, and miscellaneous diseases connected with internal medicine, external medicine, gynecology, pediatrics, etc., with detailed medical records and specially selected methods of treatment and prescriptions. Occasional notes and commentaries have been contributed by the authors.

续名医类案 [xù míng yī lèi àn]

Xu Ming Yi Lei An*; *Supplement to the Classified Medical Records of Distinguished Physicians (1770)**:** compiled by Wei Zhixiu (魏之琇), a sequel to the *Ming Yi Lei An*, or *Classified Medical Records of Distinguished Physicians* by Jiang Guan (江瓘) of the Ming Dynasty, with a supplement of case records from distinguished physicians of the early Qing Dynasty, most of which deal with acute infectious diseases

古今医案按 [gǔ jīn yī àn àn]

Gu Jin Yi An An*; *Comments on Ancient and Modern Medical Records (1776)**:** a collection of case records of various physicians, compiled by Yu Zhen (俞震), with comments and notes attached

医贯 [yī guàn]

***Yi Guan*; *Key Link of Medicine*:** a book of medical theories, written in 1687 by Zhao Xianke (赵献可), who supported Xue Ji's (薛己) views. In the book, the author advocates that the "life gate fire" controls the health of the whole body, and also emphasizes the importance of "genuine fire" and "genuine water". It is an important reference book on the subject of the "life gate".

临证指南医案 [lín zhèng zhǐ nán yī àn]

Lin Zheng Zhi Nan Yi An*; *Medical Records

as a Guide to Clinical Practice (1766): compiled by Ye Gui (叶桂) in 10 volumes, re-edited by Hua Xiuyun (华岫云) et al., which include eight volumes on diseases of internal medicine, one on gynecology and one on pediatrics

圣济总录 [shèng jì zǒng lù]
Sheng Ji Zong Lu*; *Complete Record of Sacred Benevolence: a work in 200 volumes (only 26 volumes extant) compiled by a staff of physicians under imperial orders and completed around 1111-1117, a monumental achievement. It covers every branch of the healing arts, with around 20,000 prescriptions recorded.

医学正傳 [yī xué zhèng zhuàn]
Yi Xue Zheng Zhuan*; *Orthodox Commentary of Medicine (1515): a comprehensive medical book compiled by Yu Tuan (虞抟), at the beginning of which are listed 51 medical problems that require elucidation. The book was written in the light of various medical works of previous generations as well as the author's own experience.

万密斋医学全书 [wàn mì zhāi yī xué quán shū]
Wan Mi Zhai Yi Xue Quan Shu*; *Complete Series of Medical Books from Wan Mizhai's Studio (1549): ten medical books compiled by Wan Quan (万全), among which the *You Ke Fa Hui* (幼科发挥) or *Elucidation of Pediatrics* enjoyed great popularity, for the author specialized in pediatrics

古今医统 [gǔ jīn yī tǒng]
Gu Jin Yi Tong*; *Ancient And Modern Medicine: compiled by Xu Chunfu (徐春甫) and completed in 1556. It sums up and classifies the contents of more than 100 medical and related works of the previous generations

古今医统大全 [gǔ jīn yī tǒng dà quán]
Gu Jin Yi Tong Da Quan*; *A Complete Work of Ancient and Modern Medicine: the full name of the *Gu Jin Yi Tong*, or *Ancient and Modern Medicine*

医学入门 [yī xué rù mén]
Yi Xue Ru Men*; *Introduction to Medicine (1575): compiled by Li Yan (李梴), a comprehensive book on various branches of medicine. It not only presents the views of various schools, but also expounds the author's own ideas.

万病回春 [wàn bìng huí chūn]
Wan Bing Hui Chun*; *Recovery from All Ailments (1587): a comprehensive book of medicine compiled by Gong Tingxian (龚廷贤). The book collects all the major achievements of the previous generations.

寿世保元 [shòu shì bǎo yuán]
Shou Shi Bao Yuan*; *Longevity and Health Preservation (1615): compiled by Gong Tingxian (龚廷贤) in 10 volumes, mainly discussing syndrome differentiation (pattern identification) and treatment of diseases in various branches of clinical medicine. Most of the prescriptions presented in this book are of practical use, with case records appended.

证治准绳 [zhèng zhì zhǔn shéng]
Zheng Zhi Zhun Sheng*; *Standards of Syndrome/Pattern Identification and

Treatment (1602): compiled by Wang Kentang (王肯堂), which gives a detailed description of symptoms and treatment methods. Six branches of medicine are covered, namely miscellaneous diseases of internal medicine, cold damage diseases, ulcers and boils, pediatrics, gynecology, and classified prescriptions. The work sums up the rich medical experience of the previous generations, and circulated widely in the 17th century.

六科证治准绳 [liù kē zhèng zhì zhǔn shéng]

Liu Ke Zheng Zhi Zhun Sheng*; *Standards of Syndrome/Pattern Identification and Treatment in Six Branches of Medicine: the full name of the *Zheng Zhi Zhun Sheng*, or *Standards of Syndrome/Pattern Identification and Treatment*

景岳全书 [jǐng yuè quán shū]

Jing Yue Quan Shu*; *Complete Works of Jingyue (1624): compiled in 64 volumes, by Zhang Jiebin (张介宾), styled Jingyue (景岳). The book includes the studies of theories, pulse taking, cold damage diseases, internal medicine, gynecology, pediatrics, external medicine, materia medica, modern prescriptions, and ancient prescriptions. The author extracted the essence of various schools, and made a systematic analysis of the diagnosis and treatment of diseases based on syndrome differentiation (pattern identification). Advocating the theory that "yang is ever in excess and yin never sufficient", he recommended using warm tonifying medicinals and spent two volumes in introduction of new prescriptions.

医宗必读 [yī zōng bì dú]

Yi Zong Bi Du*; *Essential Readings for Medical Professionals (1637): compiled by Li Zhongzi (李中梓) in 10 volumes, one of the most influential introductory books of medicine, including medical history, physiology, *zang-fu* organs, diagnostic methods, materia medica, syndrome differentiation (pattern identification) and treatment of various internal diseases

张氏医通 [zhāng shì yī tōng]

Zhang Shi Yi Tong*; *Zhang's Treatise on General Medicine (1695): comprehensive medical work by Zhang Lu (张璐), on diagnosis and treatment of diseases of various branches of medicine, with case records and prescriptions attached

古今图书集成医部全录 [gǔ jīn tú shū jí chéng yī bù quán lù]

Gu Jin Tu Shu Ji Cheng Yi Bu Quan Lu*; *Collection of Ancient and Modern Books, Medicine Section (1726): in 520 volumes, compiled by Jiang Tingxi (蒋廷锡) et al. It includes the *Internal Classic* and over 100 other major medical works completed before the early Qing Dynasty, with sections of commentaries, diagnosis and treatment, biographies of physicians, etc.

医学心悟 [yī xué xīn wù]

Yi Xue Xin Wu*; *Comprehension of Medicine (1732): one of the most influential Chinese books of clinical medicine, compiled by Cheng Guopeng (程国彭) in five volumes, including diagnostic methods, eight principles of syndrome differentiation (pattern identification), eight therapeutic methods, and syndrome differentiation and treatment of internal diseases, external diseases, women's diseases, diseases of sense organs, etc.

医宗金鉴 [yī zōng jīn jiàn]

Yi Zong Jin Jian*; *Golden Mirror of Medicine (1742): in 90 volumes, one of the best Chinese treatises on general medicine, by a staff of 80 authors headed by Wu Qian (吴谦) in compliance with an imperial order. A considerable part of the book is alloted for extracts, revisions and corrections of previous works.

陈修圆医书十六种 [chén xiū yuán yī shū shí liù zhǒng]

Chen Xiu Yuan Yi Shu Shi Liu Zhong*; *Sixteen Medical Works by Chen Xiuyuan (1865): a series of practical medical works compiled by Chen Nianzu (陈念祖), styled Xiuyuan (修圆), also known as *Nan Ya Tang Yi Shu Quan Ji*, or *Complete Medical Books of Nan Ya Tang*

南雅堂医书全集 [nán yǎ táng yī shū quán jí]

Nan Ya Tang Yi Shu Quan Ji*; *Complete Medical Books of Nan Ya Tang: another title of the *Chen Xiu Yuan Yi Shu Shi Liu Zhong*, or *Sixteen Medical Works of Chen Xiuyuan*

中国医学大辞典 [zhōng guó yī xué dà cí diǎn]

Zhong Guo Yi Xue Da Ci Dian*; *Dictionary of Chinese Medicine: compiled by Xie Guan (谢观) et al. and published in 1921, which contains more than 37,000 entries

中国药学大辞典 [zhōng guó yào xué dà cí diǎn]

Zhong Guo Yao Xue Da Ci Dian*; *Dictionary of Chinese Pharmaceutics: published in 1935, and recording all the medicinal substances which appeared in the medical literature of previous generations

珍本医书集成 [zhēn běn yī shū jí chéng]

Zhen Ben Yi Shu Ji Cheng*; *Collection of Precious Medical Works: a collection of medical books compiled by Qiu Qingyuan (裘庆元) and published in 1936. Of more than 3,000 books on medicine available at the time, the author selected 90 only, and compiled them under 12 subject headings, viz., medical classics, herbals, pulse, cold damage diseases, internal medicine, external medicine, gynecology, pediatrics, general treatment, prescriptions, medical case records and miscellaneous.

中国医学大成 [zhōng guó yī xué dà chéng]

Zhong Guo Yi Xue Da Cheng*; *A Great Collection of Chinese Medical Works (1936): compiled by Cao Bingzhang (曹炳章), on the basis of 128 prominent medical works. The collection covers 13 subjects, including medical classics, medicinal substances, diagnoses, prescriptions, general treatment, various clinical subjects, medical case records and miscellaneous topics, with abstracts and notes attached to each chapter.

附录
Appendix

中医名词术语中常用字的字义、英译及例证
Commonly Used Chinese Characters in TCM Terminologies: Their Meanings, English Translations and Examples

A

阿 [ā] 吴方言中表示询问的语助，“阿是”意为“是吗?”“是不是?” In the Wu* dialect, 阿 [ā] is an auxiliary word that is equivalent to an interrogative particle in English, and 阿是 [ā shì] means “isn’t it?” or “yes or no?” (* Wu refers to the region covering southern Jiangsu and northern Zhejiang provinces.)
阿是穴 *Ashi* (acu) point; “Yes-no” (acu) point

癌［喦］[ái]（名词）恶性肿瘤，凹凸不平，形如岩石 malignant tumor with unsmooth surface resembling that of a piece of rock, namely cancer (cf. 岩 [yán])
癌 cancer
肾癌 penial cancer

嗳 [ǎi]（动词）打嗝 to belch
嗳气 belching
嗳腐 putrid belching

艾 [ài]（名词）①草本植物，叶有香气，供灸疗用，亦可入药 *Artemisia Argyi*, Chinese mugwort, a herbaceous plant with scented leaves, usually used for moxibustion, as well as an ingredient in herbal formula
艾叶 *Folium Artemisiae Argyi*, wormwood leaf
②由艾叶制成的柔软如绒的可燃物质，称艾绒 soft wooly combustible mass prepared from wormwood, called moxa
艾绒 moxa (floss)
艾炷 moxa cone
艾炷灸 moxa-cone moxibustion
艾条灸 moxa-stick moxibustion
艾卷灸 moxa-roll moxibustion

安 [ān]（动词）①使之平安 to make safe
安胎 making the fetus safe → **preventing miscarriage**
②使安宁、安静 to calm; to quiet
安神 calming the mind; tranquilizing
安蛔 quieting the ascaris
③用药物使安静（镇静）to tranquilize; to sedate
安神药 tranquilizer; sedative

按 [àn]（动词）①按压 to push down or press
按法 pressing
喜按 preference for pressing
拒按 refusal of pressing
腹痛拒按 abdominal pain with refusal of pressing → **abdominal pain with tenderness**
②触按 to palpate (*n.* palpation)
按诊 palpation
按尺肤 palpation of the forearm
按胸腹 palpation of the chest and abdomen
按脘腹 palpation of the epigastrium and abdomen
按腧穴 acupoint palpation
（名词）按摩 pressing and rubbing → massage
按摩 massage
按摩疗法 massotherapy
按摩手法 manipulation of massage

暗 [àn]（形容词）① 昏暗 dark
暗红舌 dark red tongue
② 不显露的 latent
暗经 latent menstruation

熬 [áo]（动词）久煮 to cook something slowly in water that is gently boiling with low fire, or to simmer
熬 simmering

懊 [ào]（动词）烦恼 to vex (*n.* vexation)
懊侬 vexation

B

八 [bā]（数词）八 eight
八纲辨证 eight-principle syndrome differentiation; eight-principle pattern identification
八法 eight therapeutic methods
八卦步 eight-diagram walking
八段锦 eight-section brocade (*baduanjin* exercise)

拔 [bá]（动词）① 用手拽拉 to pull
拔伸牵引 pulling, stretching and traction
拔伸复位 pulling-extending reduction
拔伸捏正 pulling-kneading reduction
拔伸法 pulling-stretching manipulation
② 吸出 to suck off or draw out
拔罐 drawing blood to the surface of the body by a partially vacuumized cup → **cupping**
拔毒 drawing out toxins

白 [bái]（形容词）白色的 white; alba (*prefix*: leuko-)
白苔 white (tongue) coating
白腻苔 white greasy (tongue) coating
白睛（白珠、白仁）the white part of the eye → **white of the eye** (referring to the bulbar conjunctiva and sclera)
白睛发黄 yellow discoloration of the white of the eye
白痦 miliaria alba
白带 leukorrhea
（名词）白色：按五行学说白为金之色，肺属金，故白可为肺之代称。White color: According to the theory of five elements/phases, white is the color of metal, the element to which the lung also pertains, and thus used as a byword for the lung.
宣白 ventilating the lung
泻白 purging the lung
（动词）变白 to whiten
须发早白 premature whitening of the hair

百 [bǎi]（数词）十个十 hundred
百晬内嗽 cough occurring in a newborn within one hundred days after its birth → **neonatal cough**
（形容词）众多，所有 a large number of; all
百骸 all the bones in a human body → **skeleton**

摆 [bǎi]（动词）来回摇动 to wag
青龙摆尾法 method of "blue dragon wagging its tail"

败 [bài]（动词）打败 to defeat
败毒 toxin-defeating → **antitoxic, antiphlogistic**
（形容词）败坏的，腐烂的 deteriorated, putrid
败血冲心 putrid-blood-induced heart crisis

扳 [bān]（动词）用手拉 to pull
扳法 pulling manipulation
扳颈椎法 cervical pulling manipulation
扳胸椎法 thoracic pulling manipulation
扳腰椎法 lumbar pulling manipulation
斜扳腰椎法 oblique lumbar pulling manipulation

斑 [bān]（名词）与周围组织形状或颜色不同的斑点 a spot differing in color and structure from the surrounding tissues → macule; patch
斑 macule
斑疹 maculo-papule; skin eruption

斑秃 hair loss in patches → **alopecia areata**

瘢 [bān]（名词）伤疤 a scar (留下瘢痕 to scar)
瘢痕灸 scarring moxibustion

板 [bǎn]（名词）成片的硬物 a piece of solid material, such as a bar, board, or splint
刮痧板 scraping bar
托板 supporting board
夹板固定 splintage

半 [bàn]（形容词）二分之一 half (*prefixes*: hemi-; semi-)
半表半里 half-exterior half-interior
半身无汗 hemilateral anhidrosis
半身汗出 hemilateral sweating → **hemihidrosis**
半身不遂 hemiplegia
半卧式 semi-recumbent posture

绊 [bàn]（动词）行动时加以牵制 to restrict movement
绊舌 restricted movement of the tongue → **ankyloglossia**

棒 [bàng]（名词）棍子 a rod
棒击法 rod beating

傍 [bàng]（名词）邻近 to be near in distance or to be proximate
傍针刺 proximate needling

包 [bāo]（动词）用纸、布等把东西裹起来 to cover something completely in paper or cloth, to wrap
包煎 to be decocted with wrapping → **wrap-decoct**

胞 [bāo]（名词）①子宫 the uterus (*adj.* uterine)
胞宫；胞脏 uterus
胞门 parous vaginal orifice
胞脉 uterine vessel
胞络 uterine collateral vessel
胞寒不孕 uterus-coldness infertility
②胞衣 afterbirth; placenta and fetal membrane
人胞 placenta
胞衣先破 premature rupture of fetal membrane
胞衣不下 detention of the afterbirth
③眼睑 the eyelid
胞睑；目胞 eyelid; palpebra
胞睑下垂；上胞下垂 drooping of the (upper) eyelid → **blepharoptosis**
胞生痰核 a phlegm node in the eyelid → **chalazion**
胞轮振跳 tic of the eyelid
胞虚如球 ball-like swelling of the eyelid → **edema of the eyelid**
④胞通脬（膀胱）same as 脬 [pāo] the bladder cf. 胞 [pāo]

薄 [báo]（形容词）厚度小的 having a very small distance between two flat surfaces that are opposite to each other, namely thin
薄苔 thin (tongue) coating/fur
薄白苔 thin white (tongue) coating/fur
薄黄苔 thin yellow (tongue) coating/fur
另见：薄 [bó]；薄 [pò]

保 [bǎo]（动词）保护，维护 to preserve; 保重 to take care of
保健 health preservation; health care
保健功 health-preserving exercise
保健球 health(-preserving) ball
保健球按摩 health-ball massage

报 [bào]（动词）接连反复进行 to perform successively
报刺 successive trigger needling

抱 [bào]（动词）①用手臂围住 to hold in one's arms
抱球式 ball-holding posture
抱骨垫 bone-holding pad
抱膝器 an appliance for holding the patella → **peripatellapexor**
②环绕 to surround
抱头火丹 erysipelas surrounding the head

→ **head erysipelas** or **facial erysipelas**

抱踝手法 manipulation on the tissues surrounding the ankle → **peri-ankle manipulation**

抱轮红赤；白睛抱红；赤带抱轮 redness surrounding the ciliary body → **ciliary hyperemia**

豹 [bào]（名词）一种身上有黑斑的猛兽 a carnivore with yellow fur and black spots, i.e., leopard

豹文刺 leopard-spot needling

暴 [bào]（形容词）强大而突然来的 coming on suddenly with great severity; fulminant

暴聋 sudden deafness

暴盲 sudden blindness

暴崩 sudden flooding → **metrorrhagia**

暴泻 fulminant diarrhea

暴痫 fulminant epilepsy

暴发火眼 fulminant conjunctivitis

背 [bēi]（动词）人用背驮东西 to carry on the back

背法 back-carrying manipulation

悲 [bēi]（名词）悲哀 sorrow

悲 sorrow

悲伤肺 sorrow impairing the lung

背 [bèi]（名词）脊背 the back

背痛 back pain

背部穴 points on the back

心痛彻背 precordial pain radiating to the back

含胸拔背 shrinking the chest and straightening the back

（形容词）①背部的 on or connected with one's back, dorsal, or posterior

腹背配穴法 ventro-dorsal point combination

耳背 dorsal surface of the auricle

②听觉减退的 hard of hearing

耳背 hard of hearing

焙 [bèi]（动词）用微火烘烤 to heat over a slow fire or to bake

烘焙 baking

奔 [bēn]（动词）奔跑 to run

奔豚 "running piglet"

贲 [bēn]（动词）同"奔"，奔跑之意 same as 奔 which means "to run"

贲门 opening through which food runs into the stomach → upper opening of the stomach → **pylorus**

本 [běn]（名词）草木之根 root → base, foundation (*adj.* radical, basic; fundamental)

本草 root and grass (for medicinal use) → **materia medica**

本节 basic (digital) joint

治病求本 treating disease from the root

治本 treating the fundamental; radical treatment

扶正固本 reinforcing the healthy and strengthening the base

崩 [bēng]（名词）原意是山体倒塌，作为中医妇科的专用名词，则是指子宫大出血，犹如英语中的 flooding（用洪水爆发指子宫大出血）。崩 [bēng] originally means collapse of a mountain. When used as a gynecological term in Chinese medicine, it refers to profuse uterine bleeding, which is nicknamed as flooding in English language.

崩漏 flooding and spotting; metrorrhagia and metrostaxis

血崩 flooding; metrorrhagia

崩中 uterine flooding

暴崩 sudden flooding

崩证 flooding syndrome; metrorrhagic syndrome

鼻 [bí]（名词）鼻子 the nose（*adj.* nasal）

鼻根 root of the nose → **radix nasi**

鼻翼 wing of the nose → **ala nasi**

鼻孔（鼻洞） opening of the nasal cavity → **nostril**

鼻涕 nasal discharge

鼻衄；鼻出血 **nosebleed; epistaxis**
鼻渊 excessive turbid discharge from the nose → **sinusitis**

闭 [bì]（动词）原意为关门，引申为堵塞或终止 Its original meaning is to shut or close, and its extended meaning to block or end.
闭经（经闭）abnormal ending or block of menstruation → **amenorrhea**
气闭 *qi* blockage
热闭心包 heat blocking the pericardium
风热闭肺 wind-heat blocking the lung
暑闭气机 summer-heat blocking the *qi* activity

痹 [bì]（名词）①中医病名，指风寒湿邪侵袭经络、闭阻气血，引起以肢体关节疼痛为主症的一类疾病，也泛指闭阻肢体、经络、脏腑所致的各种疾病 a technical term used in Chinese medicine, referring to a group of diseases caused by pathogenic wind, cold and/or dampness leading to impediment of *qi*-blood flow in the meridian, manifested by pain in the limbs and joints (hence translated as "arthralgia"), also referring to any other disease, in a broader sense, characterized by *qi*-blood impediment (hence translated as "impediment diseasses")
痹；痹病 (1) impediment disease; (2) arthralgia
行痹 migratory impediment; migratory arthralgia
心痹 heart impediment
尪痹 lame impediment; ankylosing arthralgia
喉痹 throat impediment; pharyngitis
帘珠喉痹 granular pharyngitis
②麻痹 paralysis
小儿麻痹 infantile paralysis; poliomyelitis

辟 [bì]（动词）通"避"，躲开的意思。Same as 避 [bì] which means "to avoid" or "to keep away from".
辟谷 avoiding food intake → **fasting**
辟谷功 fasting exercise

蔽 [bì]（动词）遮挡 to lie or spread over something, namely to cover
白膜蔽睛 white membrane covering the eye → pannus
湿蔽清阳 dampness covering the clear yang (Here, yang refers to the head instead of the sun.) → **dampness beclouding the head**

壁 [bì]（名词）墙壁 wall
壁观 looking at a wall (for meditation)
面壁 facing a wall (while meditating)

避 [bì]（动词）躲开 to avoid (*n.* avoidance)
避年 avoidance of menses for as long as a year → **annual menstruation**

髀 [bì]（名词）下肢从膝到髋的部分，即大腿 the top part of the leg between the knee and the hip, namely, the thigh
髀 thigh
髀骨 thighbone; femur
髀枢 trochanter (of the thigh)

臂 [bì]（名词）上肢从肩到腕的部位，即胳膊，但有时只指前臂 the upper limb, the part from the shoulder to the wrist, namely, the arm, but sometimes only referring to the upper limb from the elbow to the wrist, or the forearm
臂内廉 inner aspect of the arm (or forearm)
臂外廉 outer aspect of the arm (or forearm)
肩臂酸痛 aching shoulder and arm
肩臂功 shoulder-arm exercise; acromiobrachial functional training

砭 [biān]（名词）古代用以治病的石针 a collective term for stone needles used for healing in ancient times
砭石 healing stone; stone needle

扁 [biǎn]（形容词）物体平而薄 flat and thin
扁瘊 flat wart; verruca planna

变 [biàn] ①（动词）改变 to change（名词）变化 a change

变蒸 sensation of steaming due to body change (growth, development, etc.) → **growth fever**
传变 transmission and change
②（动词）变坏 to deteriorate
变证 deteriorated syndrome
脓耳变证 deteriorated otopyorrhea → complications of suppurative otitis media

便 [biàn]（名词）粪便或尿液 stool or urine
溏便 sloppy stool
脓血便 purulent and bloody stool
小便黄赤 deep-colored urine
小便清长 long voiding of clear urine
（动词）①排出粪便 to discharge feces from the bowels (to defecate)
便秘；大便秘结 abnormally delayed discharge of dry hardened stools → **constipation**
通便 relaxing the bowels
便血 discharge of blood in the feces → **hematochezia**
大便难 difficulty in defecation → **dyschezia**
②排出尿液 to discharge urine; to urinate (*n.* urination)
小便频数 frequent urination
小便不利 inhibited urination
小便涩痛 difficult painful urination
小便淋漓 dribbling urination

辨 [biàn]（动词）区别、辨认 to differentiate, to identify (*n.* differentiation; identification)
辨病 disease differentiation; disease identification
辨证 syndrome differentiation; pattern identification
辨证施治；辨证论治 syndrome differentiation and treatment; pattern identification and treatment
辨证选穴法 point selection according to syndrome differentiation; point selection according to pattern identification

标 [biāo]（名词）本义为树木的末端，引申为表面的、非根本的或表面现象以与根本的或根本原因相对应。标 [biāo] originally meant the tip of a tree, and is extended to mean "superficiality" or "manifestations (symptoms)" in contrast to the radical cause
标 tip
标本兼治；标本同治 treating the incidental and radical simultaneously

瘭 [biāo]（名词）瘭是中医学专用字，瘭疽是指趾末节软组织的急性化脓性炎症，相当于英文中的whitlow或felon。"瘭 [biāo]" is a character specially used in Chinese medicine; "瘭疽 [biāo jū]" refers to acute suppurative inflammation of the finger or toe near the end, equivalent to whitlow or felon in English.
瘭疽 felon; whitlow

表 [biǎo]（名词）①外面，与"里"相对 exterior, in contrast to the interior
表里 exterior and interior
表证 exterior syndrome/pattern
表虚里实 exterior deficiency and interior excess
表里出入 entering the interior and exiting to the exterior
表里双解 releasing both the exterior and interior
②表面 surface; superficies
湿郁肌表 dampness stagnating in the superficies
补气固表 tonifying *qi* to strengthen the superficies
敛汗固表 arresting sweating and strengthening the superficies

别 [bié]（动词）分离 to separate
泌别清浊 separating the clear from the turbid
（形容词）分叉岔开的 separating and going in different directions, divergent
别络 divergent collateral vessel
（名词）岔开的分支 divergence

经别 **meridian/channel divergence**
十二经别 **twelve meridian/channel divergences**
（副词）单独地，分别地 separately
别煮 **to be decocted separately**

髌 [bìn]（名词）髌骨 patella (*adj.* patellar)
髌骨 **patella**
髌骨骨折 **patellar fracture**

禀 [bǐng]（名词）禀赋 endowment
胎禀 **fetal endowment**

并 [bìng]（动词）把两个合在一起；重叠 to combine two into one; to overlap (*n.* overlap)
并病 **overlap of diseases**
二阳并病 **overlap of two yang diseases**
并月 menstruating every two months → **bimonthly menstruation**

病 [bìng]（名词）疾病 disease (*prefix*: patho-)
病因 **cause of disease**
病机 **mechanism of disease; pathomechanism**
病能 **pathological state of disease**
并病 **overlap of diseases**
合病 **combination of diseases**
（形容词）有病的 connected with disease → **morbid**
病色 **morbid complexion**
病脉 **morbid pulse**

拨 [bō]（动词）①用手指反复拨动 to push something with a finger quickly and repeatedly, namely to poke at
拨法 **poking (manipulation)**
拨络法 **collateral-poking (manipulation)**
②拨开 to push aside
金针拨障术 manipulation of treating cataract by pushing the lens aside with a needle → **needle couching**

剥 [bō]（动词）去掉某物的外皮 to remove the outer layer from something, namely, to peel
剥苔 **peeling (tongue) coating**
光剥舌 **peeled tongue**

薄 [bó] 同薄 [báo] same as 薄 [báo]
另见：薄 [báo]；薄 [pò]

晡 [bū]（名词）午后三时至五时 3-5 p.m. or late afternoon
日晡潮热 **late afternoon (tidal) fever**
日晡发热 **late afternoon fever**

补 [bǔ]（动词）补虚、补益、补养，在药物治疗中指用补益药治疗虚证，一般情况用 to tonify（由补药 tonic 一词衍生而来），针对气虚、阳虚也常用 to replenish，针对阴虚、血虚常用 to nourish; 在针灸治疗中指扶助正气的手法，与泻相对。to tonify, to replenish, to nourish (In herbal medicine, 补 [bǔ] refers to treating deficiency syndromes with tonics, and is generally translated into "to tonify" which is derived from the word tonic, drug that increases body tone and resistance. In cases of *qi* deficiency and yang deficiency, 补 [bǔ] can also be translated into "to replenish", while in cases of yin deficiency and blood deficiency "to nourish" is the preferable translation. In non-herbal therapies such as acupuncture, 补 [bǔ] means "to reinforce (*qi*)" in contrast to 泻 [xiè] which means "to reduce (*qi*)".)
补法 **(1) tonifying method; tonification** (in herbal medicine); **(2) reinforcement** (in acupuncture)
补气固表 **tonifying *qi* to strengthen the superficies**
补益心气 **tonifying and replenishing heart *qi***
补心益气 **tonifying the heart and replenishing *qi***
补脾益肺 **tonifying the spleen to replenish the lung**
补养心血 **nourishing heart blood**
补气养血 **tonifying *qi* and nourishing blood**
补泻法 **method of reinforcement and**

reduction
提插补泻 lifting-thrusting reinforcement and reduction
捻转补泻 twirling reinforcement and reduction
平补平泻 neutral reinforcement and reduction

哺 [bǔ]（动词）喂食 to give food to a person; to feed
哺乳 secretion of milk by the breasts to feed a baby → **lactation**
哺乳疳 lactational malnutrition

不 [bù]（副词）否定词 used to negate the sentence, phrase or word it modifies; not (*prefixes*: non-; in-; *suffix*: -less)
不内外因 non-exo-endogenous cause
不仁 insensitivity
不寐 sleeplessness
不得偃卧 inability to lie flat
不传 non-transmission

布 [bù]（动词）分布 to distribute
布气 distributing *qi*
肺津不布 lung failing to distribute fluid
（名词）棉麻织物 cloth
布托牵引 cloth-wrapping traction

步 [bù]（名词）脚步 step
弓步 bow step
（动词）行走 to walk
太极步 *taiji* walking
八卦步 eight-diagram walking

部 [bù]（名词）部位 position
三部九候 three positions and nine pulse-takings

C

擦 [cā]（动词）摩搓 to rub
擦法 rubbing manipulation
擦丹田 rubbing *Dantian*
掌擦法 palm rubbing manipulation
鱼际擦法 eminence rubbing manipulation

踩 [cǎi]（动词）用脚登在上面 to press something with the foot, i.e., to tread
踩法 treading
踩跷法 treading-stamping

蚕 [cán]（名词）桑蚕 silkworm
目下有卧蚕 "sleeping silkworm beneath the eye" → **swollen lower eyelids**

苍 [cāng]（形容词）①苍白的 pale
面色苍白 pale complexion
②青色的 blue
苍龙摆尾法 "blue dragon wagging its tail"

藏 [cáng]（动词）贮藏 to store (*n.* storage)
五脏所藏 storage of the five *zang* organs
封藏失职 dysfunction in essence storage

糙 [cāo]（形容词）粗糙的 rough
糙苔 rough (tongue) coating

嘈 [cáo]（形容词）（名词）杂乱 upset
嘈杂 gastric upset

槽 [cáo]（名词）牙槽 tooth socket
骨槽风；牙槽风 tooth socket wind → **maxillary osteomyelitis**

草 [cǎo]（名词）中医学中"草"常是指药用植物。In Chinese medicine, 草 the meaning of which matches "grass", "straw" or "plant" in a general sense is translated into herb, referring to a plant valued for its medicinal qualities
草药 herbal medicinal
中草药 Chinese herbal medicinal; Chinese herbal medicine
本草 materia medica

侧 [cè]（形容词）侧面的 of (or relating to) the side of something, lateral
侧卧式 lateral recumbent posture
侧擦法 side rubbing manipulation
颈椎侧旋复位法 laterally-rotating reduction

of cervical vertebra

叉 [chā]（形容词）交叉的 contralateral, i.e., occurring or acting on the opposite side of the body
交叉选穴法 contralateral point selection

差 [chā]（名词）偏差 deviation
气功偏差 deviation of *qigong*

插 [chā]（动词）扎进去 to thrust
插入法 thrusting insertion
提插法 lifting-thrusting method
提插补泻 lifting-thrusting reinforcement and reduction
重插轻提 forceful thrusting and light lifting
重提轻插 forceful lifting and light thrusting

茶 [chá]（名词）用茶叶或其他植物沏成的饮料 a hot drink made by pouring boiling water onto the dried leaves of a particular plant; tea
茶 tea
茶剂 medicated tea

察 [chá]（动词）仔细查看 to look at something carefully; to examine
察目 examining the eye; examination of the eye

差 [chà]（形容词）交错的 crossed
差经 crossed menstruation

禅 [chán]（佛教名词）静思；全神贯注 meditation; concentration
禅定 meditating fixation
一指禅式 single-finger meditation gesture
一指禅导气 conducting *qi* with single-finger meditation
一指禅推法 *qi*-concentrated single-finger pushing manipulation

缠 [chán]（动词）缠绕，围绕 to wind one thing around another; entwine
缠喉风 throat-entwined wind; acute laryngitis
缠腰火丹（缠腰蛇丹）herpes zoster around the waist

镵 [chán]（名词）头大末锐的器具 an instrument with a big head and sharp tip, such as a pair of shears
镵针 a needle looking like a pair of shears in miniature → **shear needle**

产 [chǎn]（名词）生孩子，分娩 childbirth, delivery, labor
产难；难产 difficult labor; dystocia
早产 premature delivery; premature birth
产后病 diseases occurrrng after childbirth → **postpartum diseases**
流产 delivery of a fetus during the first 12 weeks of gestation → **abortion**
小产 delivery of a fetus which has not yet been viable → **miscarriage**

颤 [chàn]（动词）抖动，（使）抖动 to tremble, to vibrate
颤动舌 trembling tongue
手足颤动 trembling of the extremities
颤法 vibrating (method)
（名词）颤抖 tremor
颤震（颤振）tremor

长 [cháng]（形容词）长度大的，与"短"相反 long, the opposite of short
长脉 long pulse
长针 long needle
尿清长（小便清长）long voiding of clear urine

肠 [cháng]（名词）消化道的一部分，上端连胃，下端通肛门，分小肠和大肠两部分 intestines, the part of the alimentary canal between the stomach and anus, consisting of small and large intestines
大肠津亏 large intestinal fluid depletion
绞肠痧；搅肠痧 colicky intestinal turmoil
肠痹 intestinal impediment
肠痈 intestinal abscess → **(1) acute appendicitis; (2) periappendicular abscess**

（其他）
小肠气 hernia
肠痔 perianal abscess
交肠 rectovesical fistula
子肠 vagina

常 [cháng]（形容词）①正常的 normal
常色 normal color; normal complexion
常脉 normal pulse
②一般的 moderate
常毒 moderately poisonous medicinal

潮 [cháo]（名词）潮汐 tide (*adj.* tidal)
潮热 tidal fever
午后潮热 afternoon tidal fever
日晡潮热 late afternoon tidal fever
阴虚潮热 yin-deficiency tidal fever

炒 [chǎo]（动词）把东西放在锅里搅拌着加热 to heat things in a pan while stirring them; to stir-bake
炒爆 stir-baking to cracking
炒黄 stir-baking to yellowish
炒焦 stir-baking to brown
炒炭 stir-baking to charcoal
清炒 stir-baking without adjuvant

扯 [chě]（动词）拉扯 to pull
扯法 pulling (manipulation)
扯痧 pulling to congestion

掣 [chè]（动词）拽，用力拉 to pull with effort; to drag
掣痛 pulling pain; dragging pain

尘 [chén]（形容词）灰暗的 greyish and not bright, namely, dusty
面尘 dusty complexion

臣 [chén]（名词）君主时代的官吏 minister (in ancient times)
臣药 minister medicinal → minister ingredient (in a prescription)

沉 [chén]（动词）①没入水中，与“浮”相反 to sink, the opposite of float
沉脉 sunken pulse
伸腰沉跨 stretching the waist and keeping the hips sunken
升降浮沉 ascending, descending, floating, and sinking
②向下移动 to move downwards → **to droop**
沉肩 drooping shoulders

成 [chéng]（形容词）已定形的 planned and fixed → set
成方 set formula

眵 [chī]（名词）俗称眼粪 eye gum
眵（目眵）eye gum
眵泪 eye gum and tears
眵泪胶粘 sticky eye gum and tears

痴 [chī]（名词）智力减退 loss of intellectual ability → demantia
痴呆 dementia

迟 [chí]（形容词）缓慢的 slow
迟脉 slow pulse
（名词）延迟 retardation
立迟 retardation of standing
行迟 retardation of walking
发迟 retardation of hair growing
齿迟 retardation of tooth eruption
语迟 retardation of speaking

持 [chí]（动词）拿着 to hold
夹持进针法 hand-holding needle insertion

锃 [chí]（名词）按《康熙字典》，“锃”即“匙”字 spoon
锃针 spoon-like needle

尺 [chǐ]（名词）长度单位，十寸等于一尺，约与前臂长度相当 *chi*, a unit for measuring length, equal to 10 *cun* or roughly the length of the forearm (cubitus)
按尺肤 palpation of the forearm
（其他）脉诊中，关之后（肘端）为尺 *chi* or cubit, the area proximal to *guan* or bar for pulse taking

寸、关、尺 ***cun, guan, chi*; inch, bar and cubit**

齿 [chǐ]（名词）牙齿 tooth (*adj.* dental)

齿迟 retardation of tooth eruption

齿龂 teeth grinding

齿龋 dental caries

龋齿 carious tooth

齿蠹 dental decay

齿摇 looseness of teeth

叩［扣］齿 tapping the teeth

齿痕舌 teeth-marked tongue

齿龈 the flesh in which the teeth are fixed → **gum**

齿龈肿痛 painful swollen gum

齿龈结瓣 petaloid gum

齿衄 gum bleeding

赤 [chì]（形容词）红色的 red

赤白肉际 border of the red and white flesh → **dorso-ventral boundary (of the hand or foot)**

白睛红赤 redness of the white of eye → congestion of the bulbar conjunctiva

瘛［瘈］[chì]（名词）肌肉挛缩 muscle spasm

瘛［瘈］疭 alternating contracting and relaxing of the muscles → **clonic convulsion**

冲 [chōng]（动词）用热水冲泡 to infuse (*n.* infusion)

冲服 to be taken infused

冲剂；冲服剂 infusion granules

（名词）通行的大道 the main road through a place → thoroughfare

冲脉 thoroughfare vessel

冲任失调；冲任不调 disorder of the thoroughfare and conception vessels

冲任不固 insecurity of the thoroughfare and conception vessels

热伏冲任 heat lodging in the thoroughfare and conception vessels

虫 [chóng]（名词）①昆虫 insect

虫兽咬伤 insect or animal bite

②寄生虫；蠕虫 parasite; worm

虫积 worm accumulation; intestinal parasitosis

虫积腹痛 parasitic abdominal pain

虫痫 parasitic epilepsy

驱虫药 worm-expelling medicinal/drug; anthelmintic

重 [chóng]（形容词）成双的 double

重舌 double tongue

重身 double body (having a body in the body) → **gravidity**

另见：重 [zhòng]

抽 [chōu]（动词）①从中取出一部分 to take something out

釜底抽薪 taking away firewood from under the cauldron (a metaphor for the therapeutic method of clearing heat or fire by way of purgation)

②抽吸气体或液体 to suck air or liquid (*n.* suction)

抽气罐 suction cup

③手足痉挛或抽动 to convulse or become spasmodic (*n.* convulsion; spasm)

抽筋 spasm

抽搐 convulsion

臭 [chòu]（名词）气味 odor

腋臭 armpit odor; hircismus

狐臭 foxy odor

不闻香臭 inability to differentiate odors → **anosmia**

（形容词）气味难闻的 foul- or offensive-smelling; fetid or stink

鼻臭证 disease of the nose characterized by a foul-smelling nasal discharge → **ozena**

腥臭气 stink

口臭 fetid breath → **halitosis**

口气臭秽 offensive breath smell

带下臭秽 fetid vaginal discharge

出 [chū]（动词）①出来，从里面到外面，与“入”相反 to come out, to exit, the

opposite of enter
升降出入 ascending, descending, exiting, and entering
表里出入 entering the interior and exiting to the exterior
乳汁自出 milk coming out spontaneously (irrespective of nursing) → **galactorrhea**
出血 blood going out (of the vessel) → **bleeding**
鼻出血 nosebleed; epistaxis
经间期出血 intermenstrual bleeding
交接出血 copulative bleeding
②发生 to occur
出偏 (occurring of *qigong*) **deviation**
③取出 to withdraw (*n.* withdrawal)
出针 withdrawing the needle; needle withdrawal

初 [chū]（形容词）刚开始的 having just developed, not existing before
初生儿 newborn
初生不啼 failure to cry in the newborn; asphyxia neonatorum
初生不乳 failure to suck in the newborn

除 [chú]（动词）清除，解除 to remove; to relieve
除烦止渴 relieving vexation and thirst
祛风除湿 dispelling wind and removing dampness
清热除湿 clearing heat and removing dampness
消积除胀 removing accumulation and relieving distension

搐 [chù]（动词）搐鼻：用药末吹鼻使嚏以开窍 to insufflate medicinal powder into the nostril to induce sneezing for resuscitation
搐鼻 insufflating into the nose

揣 [chuǎi]（动词）揣测 to conjecture (*n.* conjecture)
司外揣内 inspection of the exterior leading to conjecture of the interior

传 [chuán]（动词）①传播 to transmit (*n.* transmission)
传染 transmission of a disease by contact → **contagion**
热邪传里 transmission of pathogenic heat into the interior
传经 meridian/channel transmission
传变 transmission and change
循经感传 transmission of sensation along the meridian/channel
②传递 to convey (*n.* conveyance)
传导之官 organ of conveyance
传化之腑 *fu* organs of conveyance and transformation
大肠传导失职 dysfunction of the large intestine in conveyance

喘 [chuǎn]（名词）①呼吸急促，气喘吁吁 quick breathing with short noisy breaths, i.e., panting ②呼吸困难费力 difficult or labored respiration, i.e., dyspnea
喘逆 dyspnea with reversed flow of *qi*
喘促；喘急 panting
喘鸣 wheezing dyspnea
喘证 dyspnea syndrome
宣肺止咳平喘 ventilating the lung to relieve cough and dyspnea

疮 [chuāng]（名词）①体表上局部发生溃烂的疾病 a localized sore spot on the body surface with its tissues ruptured, i.e., a sore (including boil, ulcer and other localized skin infections)
②皮肉外伤 a wound
疮 (1)sore; (2)wound
疮疡 sore and ulcer
发际疮 hairline boil
疮毒内陷 inward invasion of sore toxin
热疮 heat sore; herpes febrillis

吹 [chuī]（动词）合拢嘴唇用力出气 to send out a current of air from the mouth, i.e., to blow
吹药 blowing powdered medicine (to some part of the body, usually to the throat) →

insufflation of a drug

垂 [chuí]（动词）低下来 to hang down
垂肘 down-hanging elbows

捶 [chuí]（动词）用拳头或工具敲打 to hit with a fist or tool, namely, to hammer
捶法 hammering
捶腰背 hammering the lower back

春 [chūn]（名词）一年四季的第一季，即春季 the season of the year between winter and summer, namely, spring
春温 spring warmth
春温病 spring warmth disease

纯 [chún]（形容词）专一不杂的，纯粹的 not mixed with anything else, i.e., pure
纯阳之体 pure yang constitution

唇 [chún]（名词）口周围的肌肉组织，即嘴唇 the two fleshy folds which surround the opening of the mouth, namely, the lips
唇裂；口唇干裂 cracked lips
唇疮 lip sore
唇疔 lip pustule
唇疽 lip abscess

差 [cī]（形容词）不齐的 uneven or unequal
差颓［癞］ unilateral swollen testicle

磁 [cí]（名词）磁石 magnet
（形容词）有磁性的 magnetic
磁珠疗法 magnetic bead therapy
磁穴疗法 acupoint magnetic therapy

刺 [cì]（动词）①用尖锐的东西扎 to make a small hole in something or to injure somebody using an object with a sharp point, i.e., to pierce or to stab
刺痛 stabbing pain
点刺 fast piercing → **pricking**
挑刺法 piercing method
②用针扎 to pierce with a needle, i.e., to puncture or to needle
刺法 puncturing (technique)
刺灸法 puncturing and moxibustion
刺手 needling hand
刺络 collateral puncture
透刺 penetration needling
③把针扎进 to let a needle penetrate into something, i.e., to insert (a needle) (*n.* insertion)
直刺 perpendicular insertion
斜刺 oblique insertion
横刺 transverse insertion
平刺 horizontal insertion
④刺破 to prick
刺血拔罐 bloodletting pricking and cupping
刺络拔罐 collateral pricking and cupping

聪 [cōng]（动词）使听觉灵敏 to make the sense of hearing sharp
聪耳 improving the hearing

从 [cóng]（介词）由，起于 from
寒从中生 generation of cold from the interior
（动词）①依从 to be congruent with (*n.* congruity)
脉从四时 congruity of pulses with the seasons
②和……一起做，作为副手 to do something with someone else with less responsibility (*prefix*: co-)
从治 co-acting treatment

丛 [cóng]（动词）聚集，丛生 to cluster; to grow in clusters
丛毛 clustered hair

腠 [còu]（名词）皮肤肌肉之间的空隙，包括汗孔 the interstice between the skin and muscles, including the sweat pores
腠［凑］理 (1) interstitial striae; (2) subcutaneous interstice

粗 [cū]（形容词）①与“细”相反 the opposite of thin, i.e., thick (*v.* to make thick → to thicken)
筋粗 musculotendinous thickening

②（声音）粗重的 heavy
呼吸气粗 heavy breathing

卒 [cù]（形容词）忽然的 sudden
卒病 sudden onset of disease
卒中 sudden onset of apoplexy → **stroke**
卒聋 sudden deafness
卒喑［瘖］sudden hoarseness or aphonia
卒喉痹 sudden onset of throat impediment; acute pharyngitis

促 [cù]（形容词）（用于脉象）数疾而时有一止的 (for pulse condition) rapid with pauses from time to time
促脉 irregular rapid pulse

窜 [cuàn]（动词）急跑，乱跑 to scurry
窜痛；走窜痛 scurrying pain

催 [cuī]（动词）促使事物的发生或提前 to encourage an activity to begin, namely to stimulate; or to make something happen faster or sooner, namely, to hasten or to expedite
催生 expediting child delivery
催乳 stimulating lactation
催吐药 a drug that stimulates vomiting → **emetic**
催气法 *qi*-hastening method

脆 [cuì]（形容词）干脆的 crisp
咳声清脆 clear crisp cough

淬 [cuì]（动词）把物体加热后放入冷水中急速冷却 to cool a red-hot substance rapidly in cold water; to quench
淬 quenching
煅淬 calcining and quenching

焠 [cuì] 同"淬"the same as 淬 [cuì]
焠刺 red-hot needling

存 [cún]（动词）保存，保留 to preserve, to retain (*n.* preservation)
存想 preservation of the thought; imaginary concentration
存神 preservation of the mind
存泥丸 preservation of the mind in *dantian*
急下存津 emergency purgation to preserve fluid
烧存性 burning with the original property retained

寸 [cùn]（名词）①长度单位，同身寸的简称 *cun*, a unit of length, abbreviation for body *cun* or body inch
寸 *cun*
同身寸 body *cun*; body inch
中指同身寸 middle finger body-*cun*; middle body-inch
拇指同身寸 thumb body-*cun*; thumb body-inch
横指同身寸 finger-breadth body-*cun*; finger-breath body-inch
②寸口的简称，腕部桡动脉的诊脉部位 *cun*, abbreviation for *cunkou*, the area of the wrist where the radial pulsation can be easily felt
寸、关、尺 *cun, guan*, and *chi*; inch, bar, and cubit
寸口 *cunkou*
寸口脉 wrist artery; wrist pulse

搓 [cuō]（动词）用手掌反复揉擦 to twist and rub with the hand repeatedly
搓法 twisting-rubbing; foulage
搓腰 rubbing the waist
搓内肾 rubbing the inner kidney
搓柄法 handle-twisting method

撮 [cuō]（动词）①聚拢 to bring together
撮口（口撮）mouth with the lips brought together tightly → **pursed mouth**
②用手指捏住拿起来 to take up with the fingers
撮法 taking up with the fingers

挫 [cuò]（动词）擦碰 to bruise
挫伤 bruising → **contusion**
碾挫伤 crushing-contusion

莝 [cuò]（名词）铡碎的草cut or chopped grass（陈莝 stale hay）
去菀陈莝 eliminating the stale and the stagnant

错 [cuò] ①（形容词）不正确的 wrong
错语 aphasia in which the patient uses wrong words → **paraphasia**
②（动词）交错 to cross
错经 crossed menstruation

D

搭 [dā]（动词）
①架起 to build
搭鹊桥 building the magpie bridge
②接触 to touch
搭手 carbuncle occurring on the back that can be touched with a hand by the sufferer → **lumbodorsal carbuncle**

达 [dá]（动词）透散 to expel
达邪 expelling pathogens

打 [dǎ]（名词）击打 knock
跌打损伤 (injury from) knocks and falls

大 [dà]（形容词）①与小相对 large or big, the opposite of small or little
大肠 large intestine
大肠热结 large intestinal heat accumulation
大肠湿热 large intestinal dampness-heat
大脉 large pulse
大针 large needle
②大量的 profuse
大汗 profuse sweating
③主要的，与次要的相对 major, the opposite of minor
大结胸 major chest bind; major thoracic accumulation

呆 [dāi]（名词）呆傻 unsoundness of mind, moronism
痴呆 loss of intellectual ability and unsoundness of mind → **dementia**
（形容词）呆滞的 dull
纳呆 dullness in food intake → **anorexia**

代 [dài]（形容词）脉来动而时止的 regularly intermittent (referring to the pulse)
代脉 regularly intermittent pulse

带 [dài]（名词）①用皮、布等制成的围于腰部的长条物 a band of leather, cloth etc., that is worn around the waist, namely, a belt
带脉 belt vessel
带脉病证 belt vessel syndrome
②阴道流出的黏液，白带的简称 mucous discharge from the vagina, an abbreviation for leukorrhea
带下 leukorrhea
带下病 leukorrheal disease
带下臭秽 fetid vaginal discharge
固崩止带 arresting metrorrhagia and leukorrhagia

丹 [dān]（名词）①红色 red (*prefix*: eryth-)
丹痧 an infection characterized by erythematous rash → **scarlatina; scarlet fever**
烂喉丹痧 erosion of the throat with erythema → **scarlatina**
丹毒；火丹 an infection characterized by local redness of the skin → **erysipelas**
赤游丹 wandering erysipelas
②依成方制成的颗粒状的中药 a medicated preparation in the form of small particles, usually called pellet
丹；丹剂 pellet
③仙丹 elixir
丹田 elixir field; *dantian*

单 [dān]（形容词）①单一的，单个的 only one, single (*adv.* alone)
单按 pulse taking with a single finger → **individual palpation**
单盘坐 single cross-legged sitting
单手进针法 single-handed needle insertion
单煎 to be decocted alone

②单边的，一侧的 unilateral
单蛾 unilateral tonsillitis
③单纯的，简单的 simple
单腹胀 simple abdominal distension
单方 simple formula/prescription

胆 [dǎn]（名词）胆囊 gallbladder
胆气 gallbladder *qi*
胆气虚 gallbladder *qi* deficiency
胆虚气怯 gallbladder insufficiency with timidity
胆胀 gallbladder distension

疸 [dǎn]（名词）黄疸 jaundice
黄疸 jaundice
胎疸 neonatal jaundice

掸 [dǎn]（动词）轻擦 to brush, to make a quick light touch
掸拂法 brushing and whisking

旦 [dàn]（名词）早晨 morning
平旦服 to be taken in the early morning

但 [dàn]（副词、形容词）只，唯一的 only
但热不寒 (only) **fever without chills**
但寒不热 (only) **chills without fever**
但欲寐 desire only to sleep

淡 [dàn]（形容词）①浅颜色的 light in color, pale
淡红舌 light red tongue
淡白舌（舌淡）pale tongue
②味道不浓的 not having a strong taste, bland
口淡 bland taste in the mouth
淡渗利湿 draining dampness with bland diuretics
淡渗祛湿 expelling dampness with bland diuretics

膻 [dàn]（名词）胸腔 thorax
膻中 thoracic center

刀 [dāo]（名词）刀子 knife
小针刀 a small needle-knife (in combination) → **acupotome**
小针刀疗法 acupotomy

导 [dǎo]（动词）①导致 to induce
导便；导法 inducing defecation; inducing evacuation
消导药 digestant and evacuant medicinal/drug
（针灸）**导气 inducing *qi***
②引导 to conduct
导引 *daoyin*; conducting (exercise)
（气功）**导气 conducting *qi***

捣 [dǎo]（动词）多次捶打 to hit many times, to pound
（推拿）**捣法；捣击法 pounding** (in *tuina*)
（针灸）**捣法 repeated lifting-thrust method** (in acupuncture)

倒 [dào]（形容词）上下或前后颠倒的 reverted or back to front
倒经 reverted menstruation → **vicarious menstruation**
倒睫（睫毛倒入）turning inward of eyelashes → **trichiasis**

盗 [dào]（动词）偷窃 to steal
（名词）窃贼 thief
盗汗 sweating during sleeping as if a thief steals things when the victim is sleeping → **night sweat**

得 [dé]（动词）①得到 to obtain
得气 obtaining *qi*；arrival of *qi*
②有，存在 to be present (*n.* presence)
得神 presence of vitality
③能，可以 to be able to (*n.* ability)
不得眠 inability to sleep
④适合 to match
形气相得 well-matched physique and *qi*; equilibrium between physique and *qi*

瞪 [dèng]（动词）睁大眼睛注视 to gaze fixedly, with eyes wide open, namely, stare
瞪目直视 staring straight ahead

低 [dī]（形容词）低矮的 low
高低垫 high-low pad
语声低微 faint low voice

滴 [dī]（动词）液体一点一点地下落 to drip
（名词）一点一点下落的液体 drop
滴丸 dripping pill
滴酒法 a cupping procedure which involves igniting a few drops of alcohol spread at the bottom of the cup → **alcohol fire cupping**

涤 [dí]（动词）洗涤；冲洗 to wash; to flush
漱涤 washing by gargling
涤痰 flushing phlegm away

抵 [dǐ]（动词）顶住 to stick
舌抵上腭 sticking the tongue against the palate

骶 [dǐ]（名词）腰椎下面尾骨上面的部分 the region between the lumbar vertebrae and the coccyx, namely the sacrum (combining form: sacro-)
尾骶 sacrococcygeal region
尾骶骨 sacrococcyx

地 [dì]（名词）①大地，地球 earth, geo-
地支 earthly branches
地图舌 geographic tongue
②地区，地点 place or region, location
因地制宜 taking measures that are suited to the place
道地药材 geo-authentic materia medica

蒂 [dì]（名词）花或瓜果与枝茎相连的部分 the base of a fruit or flower, pedicel (In Chinese medicine, 蒂 refers to the tissue looking like a pedicel.)
蒂中（蒂丁） the fleshy lobe in the middle of the posterior border of the soft palate looking like a pedicel → **uvula**

颠 [diān]（名词）颠疾或巅疾，癫痫的另名 颠疾 [diān jí] or 巅疾 [diān jí], synonymous with 癫痫 [diān xián], i.e., epilepsy
颠疾 epilepsy

巅 [diān]（名词）山顶 top of a mountain
巅；巅顶 top of the head→ **vertex cranii; vertex**

癫 [diān]（名词）①神志痴呆、情绪抑郁的病 a mental disorder characterized by severe depression
癫 depression
癫病 depressive psychosis
癫狂 depressive-manic psychosis
②指痫病 referring to epilepsy
癫痫 epilepsy
（形容词）疯狂的 rabid
癫狗咬伤 rabid dog bite

点 [diǎn]（名词）①斑点 spot
点刺舌 spotted tongue
舌有瘀点 tongue with purple spots
②一个小点 a small dot or a point
泪点 lacrimal point; lacrimal punctum
点法 point pressing
点击法 point-hitting (in massage)
点穴疗法 digital point pressure therapy
（动词）①使液体滴落 to make the liquid fall in drops, i.e., to drop
点眼 eye dropping
②一落一起的动作 to move in followed by immediate removal
点刺 quick pricking (in acupuncture)

电 [diàn]（名词）电 electricity (*prefix*: electro-)
电针 electro-acupuncture; galvano-acupuncture
电针仪 electric stimulator
电针疗法 electro-acupuncture therapy
电灸；电热灸 electric moxibustion
电光伤目 electric ophthalmia; flash ophthalmia

垫 [diàn]（名词）垫子 pad
平垫 flat pad
分骨垫 bone-separating pad
合骨垫 bone-combining pad

大头垫 megacaput pad

掉 [diào]（动词）摇动；振动 to shake; to tremble
掉眩 dizziness with shaking
振掉 trembling

跌 [diē]（动词）跌倒 to leave a standing position suddenly; to fall
（名词）跌倒 fall
跌打损伤 (injury from) knocks and falls
踠跌 fracture from fall

丁 [dīng]（名词）①"丁"为象形字，本义是钉子。"丁", a pictograph, originally means nail.
丁奚疳 infantile malnutrition with the body as thin as a nail or looking like the Chinese character "丁" → **T-shaped (infantile) malnutrition**
②小块东西 a small piece of something
蒂丁 a small piece of flesh looking like a pedicel → **uvula**

疔 [dīng]（名词）根深的疮疡 deep-rooted boil
疔 deep-rooted boil
疔疮走黄 deep-rooted boil with pyosepticemia
鼻疔 nasal boil
耳疔 ear boil
黑疔 black boil

耵 [dīng]（名词）耳垢 earwax; cerumen
耵聍 earwax; cerumen
耵耳 impacted cerumen

顶 [dǐng]（名词）头顶 top of the head, i.e., vertex
顶中线 middle line of vertex (MS 5)
顶颞前斜线 anterior oblique line of vertex-temporal (MS 6)
顶颞后斜线 posterior oblique line of vertex-temporal (MS 7)
顶旁1线 lateral line 1 of vertex
（动词）①用头负重 to carry on the top of the head
头如顶物 keeping the head upright (as if carrying something on the top)
②推拱 to push
膝顶 pushing with the knee; knee-pushing (reduction)
膝顶扳胸椎法 knee-pushing thoracic pulling manupilation

鼎 [dǐng]（名词）古代煮食物的器物，有三足 a utensil with three legs used for cooking in ancient times → tripod
鼎式夹板 tripod-shaped splint
鼎式夹板固定 tripod-shaped splint fixation

定 [dìng]（动词）①稳定 to stabilize
安神定志 calming and stabilizing the mind
②停止 to arrest
熄［息］风定痉 extinguishing wind to arrest convulsions
熄［息］风定痫 extinguishing wind to arrest epilepsy
③固定 to fix (*n.* fixation)
禅定 meditating fixation
固定痛 fixed pain
经行先后无定期 menstruation with no fixed cycle → **irregular periods; irregular menstrual cycle**

锭 [dìng]（名词）药物制成的小块状固体 a small solid piece of medicated material, called pastil, troche or lozenge
锭（锭剂）pastil; lozenge

冬 [dōng]（名词）四季的第四季，即冬季 the season after autumn and before spring, i.e., winter
冬温 winter warm (disease)

动 [dòng]（动词）①移动 to move
口动 moving mouth
胎动不安 continuous moving of the fetus → **threatened abortion**

②使某物移动 to make something move, to stir
血热动血 blood heat stirring blood
热盛风动 exuberant heat stirring up wind
肝风内动 internal stirring of liver wind
相火妄动 frenetic stirring of the ministerial fire
动脉 stirred pulse
（形容词）①动态的 dynamic
动功 dynamic *qigong*
动静相兼功 static-dynamic *qigong*
②有动作的 in motion or action → **active**
动留针法 retaining of the needle at an acupoint with repeated needle manipulation **→ active needle retention**
（名词）运动 motion
动中有静 quiescence within motion

冻 [dòng]（动词）液体遇冷凝结 to freeze
冻疮（冻风） sore caused by freezing → **chilblain; frostbite**

洞 [dòng]（名词）孔洞 opening
鼻洞 opening of the nasal cavity; nostril

抖 [dǒu]（动词）使振动 to shake
抖法 shaking manipulation

豆 [dòu]（名词）豆子bean or bean-shaped thing
风轮赤豆 wind-orbiculus red bean; fascicular keratitis

痘 [dòu]（名词）出豆状疱疹的疾病，古指天花 a contagious disease marked by pea-like skin sores, referring to small pox in ancient times
痘 pox; small pox
痘疮 variola; small pox
水痘 varicella; chicken pox

督 [dū]
（动词）监管 to supervise; to govern (*n.* one who rules → governor)
督脉 governor vessel (GV)

毒 [dú]（名词）①有毒的物质 a poisonous substance → toxin ②有毒物质所致的疾病 a pathological condition caused by action of a toxin → toxicosis
时毒 (1) seasonal toxin; (2) seasonal toxicosis
温毒 warm toxin
麻毒 measles toxin
瘴毒 miasmic toxin
胎毒 (1) fetal toxin; (2) fetal toxicosis
（形容词）有毒的 toxic, poisonous, venomous
疫毒痢 epidemic toxic dysentery
毒蛇咬伤venomous snake bite
毒虫咬伤 poisonous insect bite

独 [dú]（副词）独自 to oneself
独语 talking to oneself → **soliloquy**

妒 [dù]（名词）嫉妒 jealousy
嫉妒不孕 infertility due to jealousy

蠹 [dù]（名词） 蛀蚀 decay
齿蠹 dental decay

端 [duān]（动词）用手捧着 to hold, to carry
端法 hold-carrying
提按端挤 lifting, pressing, holding, and squeezing
端提捺正 holding, lifting, and restoring to the right location
（名词）事物的一头，也指尖端 one end of something, also called tip if pointed
舌端 tip of the tongue

短 [duǎn]（形容词）长度小，与“长”相反 short, the opposite of long (*n.* shortness; *v.* shorten)
短脉 short pulse
短气 shortness of breath
短缩舌（舌短）shortened tongue; contracted tongue

断 [duàn]（动词）①折断 to make something separate into two or more pieces, to break
断针 breaking of the needle
骨断（骨折） breaking of bone → **fracture**

断骨接整 reduction of fracture
断端移位 displacement of fractured ends
②断裂 to tear apart of a tissue → to rupture (*n.* rupture)
断裂伤 rupture; ruptured wound
筋断 musculotendinous rupture
③断绝，不继续 to stop doing something, to discontinue
断乳 (1) stopping feeding a baby on its mother's milk → **weaning;** (2) terminating lactation → **delactation**
断经，经断 the time when a woman stops menstruating → **menopause**
断经前后诸证 menopausal syndromes

煅 [duàn]（动词）把药石放在火里烧 to heat or burn a mineral medicinal, to calcine (*n.* calcination)
煅 calcination
煅淬 calcining and quenching

对 [duì]（形容词）方向相反的 opposite (*prefix*: anti-) (*n.* opposition)
阴阳对立 yin-yang opposition
对耳轮 ridge opposite to the helix → **antihelix**
对耳轮上脚 superior crus of antihelix
对耳轮下脚 inferior crus of antihelix
（介词）对于 according to
对症选穴法 point selection according to symptoms

兑 [duì]（动词）交换；交流 to exchange; interact (*n.* exchange; interaction)
塞兑反听 blocking the interaction with the outside and listening to the inside → **blocking the ears and inward listening**

炖 [dùn]（动词）"炖"一般是指用文火慢慢煨煮，在中药学"炖"是把药材加入液体辅料后放在容器中隔水加热或在蒸汽中加热。Generally, 炖 [dùn] means to cook something slowly in a liquid, namely, to simmer. But in Chinese pharmaceutics, 炖 refers to a particular process in which an airtight container filled with a medicinal substance and some fluid adjuvant is heated in a water bath or steam.
炖 simmering (in a bath)

顿 [dùn]（名词）量词，用于服药的次数 a measure word for the number of times of administration
顿服 to be taken in one single dose
（副词）忽然，一下子 suddenly, at a time (*adj.* sudden)
顿咳 (a disease marked by) sudden repeated cough → **whooping cough**

多 [duō]（形容词）①大量的 produced in large quantity → profuse
痰多 profuse sputum
多汗 profuse sweating
多梦 profuse dreaming; dreamfulness
②比适宜的数量大 more than what is reasonable or appropriate → excessive (prefix poly- or hyper-)
多汗 excessive sweating; hyperhidrosis
多尿 polyuria
多食善饥 polyphagia with frequent hunger

夺 [duó]（动词）原意为丧失。Its original meaning is to lose. (*n.* loss)
夺血 loss of blood

堕 [duò]（动词）掉下，脱落 to fall down; to fall off
堕胎 falling-off of the fetus → **abortion**

E

鹅 [é]（名词）一种像鸭但较鸭大的家禽 a domestic foul that is similar to but larger than a duck, namely, goose
鹅口疮 a disease marked by white patches in the mouth making it look like the mouth of a goose → **thrush**
鹅掌风 ringworm affecting the palmar surfaces of the hands, making the latter looking like the palms of a goose → **tinea**

manuum

鹅爪风 ringworm affecting the nails and causing them opaque, white, thickened and brittle, making them look like the nails of a goose → **tinea unguium**

蛾 [é]（名词）飞蛾　moth

乳蛾 milky moth → **tonsillitis** (An inflammed tonsil is accompanied by yellowish-white secretion, resembling a moth with milky-colored wings.)

喉蛾 throat moth → **tonsillitis**

单蛾 unilateral moth → **unilateral tonsillitis**

石蛾 stony moth → **hypertrophy of the tonsil**

额 [é]（名词）前额 forehead

额；额颅 forehead

额角 forehead corner

额汗 sweating forehead

额中线 middle line of forehead

额旁线 lateral line of forehead

恶 [ě] 只用于恶心，急迫欲呕的感觉

恶心 [ě xīn] is an urge to vomit.

恶心 nausea

另见：恶 [è]；恶 [wù]

扼 [è]（动词）用手抓紧 to hold tight

扼法 holding tight

呃 [è]（拟声词）打嗝时胃气上冲发出的声音 an onomatopoeia that imitates the noise made by the uprush of the stomach *qi* during hiccupping

呃逆 hiccup; hiccough

恶 [è]（形容词）①令人厌恶的 nasty

恶露 nasty discharge (from the uterus following delivery) → **lochia**

恶露不下 retention of lochia

恶露不绝 lochiorrhea

恶露不止 incessant discharge of lochia

②恶性的 pernicious

恶阻 pernicious vomiting of pregnancy → **morning sickness; hyperemesis gravidarum**

③恶劣的，不好的 unfavorable

恶色 unfavorable complexion

④有害的 malign; noxious

恶气 malign *qi*

中恶 attack of noxious factor

另见：恶 [ě]；恶 [wù]

遏 [è]（动词）遏制 to depress

卫阳被遏 defense yang being depressed

腭 [è]（名词）口腔的上膛 the roof of the mouth; palate

腭裂 cleft palatte

舌抵上腭 sticking the tongue against the palate

頞 [è]（名词）①鼻梁 nose stem ②两目内眦间的鼻梁部分 that part of the nose stem between the inner canthi, the root of the nose

頞 (1)nose stem; (2) nose root; radix nasi

儿 [ér]（名词）①儿童child (*pl.* children)

小儿暑温 epidemic summer fever in children

小儿诸热 fevers in children

②幼儿 infant (*adj.* infantile)

小儿哮喘 infantile asthma

小儿多涎 infantile slobbering

小儿泄泻 infantile diarrhea

耳 [ěr]（名词）耳朵 ear

耳廓（耳壳） the outer part of the ear → **auricle**

耳膜 eardrum

耳道；耳窍 the canal from the ear hole to the eardrum → **external acoustic meatus**

耳门 the small fleshy projection at the front of the external meatus of the ear → **tragus**

耳轮 the incurved rim of the ear → **helix**

二 [èr]（数词）二；第二 two; second

二阴 (1) two yin；two private parts (2)

the second yin
二阳 the second yang
二阳并病 overlap of two yang diseases

F

发 [fā]（动词）①放出 to emit (*n.* emission)
发热 emission of heat → **fever**
发热恶寒 fever with chills
发气 emission of *qi*
发功 emission of trained *qi*
②变成 to become or to turn to
发黄 becoming yellow in color → **yellow discoloration**
（名词）病势严重的体表痈疽 severe case of suppurative inflammation of subcutaneous tissue, such as cellutitis, phlegmon, and carbuncle
发 cellulitis: phlegmon
发背 dorsal carbuncle
手发背 phlegmon of the dorsum of the hand
足发背 phlegmon of the dorsum of the foot
发颐 suppurative parotitis
另见：发 [fà]

法 [fǎ]（名词）方法 method
诊法 diagnostic method
下法 purgative method; purgation
和法 harmonizing method
吐法 emetic method; emesis
外治法 external therapeutic method → **external therapy**

发 [fà]（名词）头发 hair
发际 hairline
发际疮 hairline boil
发迟 retardation of hair-growing
另见：发 [fā]

翻 [fān]（动词）翻转或内外移位 to turn over: either to turn inside out or to turn outside in, namely, to invert (*n.* inversion) or to evert (*n.* eversion), respectively
内翻 inversion
外翻 eversion
肾岩翻花 carcinoma of the penis with ulceration
睥翻粘睑 cicatrical ectropion of eyelid

烦 [fán]（动词）烦恼 to vex (*n.* vexation)
烦热 vexing fever
烦渴 vexing thirst
烦躁 vexation and agitation
躁烦 agitated vexation
五心烦热 vexing heat in the chest, palms and soles

燔 [fán]（动词）焚烧 to burn, to blaze
燔针 burnt needle
气营两燔 blazing in both *qi* and nutrient
气血两燔 blazing in both *qi* and blood

反 [fǎn]（形容词）相反的、反向的 opposite, reverse
反胃；胃反 bringing the stomach contents in the reverse direction → **regurgitation**
反酸 acid regurgitation
反关脉 bar pulse on the reverse side → **pulse on the back of the wrist**
反治 treating in the reverse way → **paradoxical treatment**
反佐 use of medicinals with property opposite to that of the principal ingredient → **use of corrigents**
（动词）相反作用 to act in opposition, to antagonize
相反 antagonizing relationship; incompatibility
十八反 eighteen antagonisms

犯 [fàn]（动词）侵犯 to invade (*n.* invasion)
温邪犯肺 warm pathogen invading the lung
肝气犯胃 liver *qi* invading the stomach
风热犯肺 wind-heat invading the lung
瘀血犯头证 syndrome/pattern of static blood invading the head

泛 [fàn]（动词）泛滥，水向外漫流 to overflow, to flood (*n.* overlow; flood)

泛酸 overflow of acid → **acid regurgitation**

泛恶 nausea with outflow of saliva from the mouth → **slobbery nausea**

阳虚水泛 yang deficiency with water flood; edema due to yang deficiency

方 [fāng]（名词）方剂，药方 formula, prescription, recipe

方；方剂；药方 formula; prescription

单方 simple formula/prescription

复方 compound formula/prescription

祖传秘方 secret formula handed down in a family

偏方 special but irregular recipe

芳 [fāng]（形容词）芳香的 aromatic (*n.* aromatic)

芳香化湿 resolving dampness with aromatics

芳香化湿药 aromatic dampness-resolving medicinal/drug

芳香开窍 opening the orifices with aromatics; inducing resuscitation with aromatics

芳香开窍药 aromatic orifice-opening medicinal/drug → **aromatic stimulant**

房 [fáng]（名词）房间 room（房事指人性交之事。"Bedroom activity" is a euphemism for sexual activity.）

房事过度 excess of sexual activity

房事不节 intemperance in sexual life

房劳 sexual consumption

放 [fàng]（动词）解除约束 to release constraints（"放松"意为由紧变松。"放松 [fàng sōng]" means to release constraints to become less tight or to give more space, i.e., to relax) (*n.* relaxation)

放松功 relaxation exercise

飞 [fēi]（动词）在空中行动 to move through the air, to fly

蝇影飞越 flying fly shadow

飞扬喉 up-flying inflammation of the throat → **diffuse palatitis**

（名词）古与"扉"通，扉即门扇 In archaic Chinese, the character "飞" was used identically to "扉", meaning a door leaf.

飞门 two-leaved door → **lip**

非 [fēi]（副词、动词）不；不是 not; to be not (*prefix*: non-)

非化脓灸 non-pustulating moxibustion

肥 [féi]（形容词）肥胖的 fat（名词）肥肉；肥胖 fat; obesity

肥疮 fat sore; tinea favosa; favus

肥胖不孕 obesity infertility

减肥功 exercise for reducing body fat → **slimming exercise**

腓 [féi]（名词）腿肚子 calf

腓腨 calf

肺 [fèi]（名词）肺脏 lung

肺气 lung *qi*

肺系 (1) lung system; (2) lung tract

肺气上逆 upward counterflow of lung *qi*

肺痈 lung abscess

肺痨；肺劳 lung phthisis; pulmonary tuberculosis

废 [fèi]（形容词）残废的 invalid

睑废 invalid eyelid

沸 [fèi]（动词）沸腾 to change from liquid to gaseous state, with production of bubbles rising to the surface, namely, to boil

釜沸脉 bubble-rising pulse

痱 [fèi]（名词）痱子 prickly heat

痱（痱子）prickly heat; miliaria

分 [fēn]（名词）分界 boundary

分肉 muscle boundary

分刺 intermuscular needling

（动词）分开，使分离 to separate

分筋 tendon-separating 分

骨垫 bone-separating pad
（其他）
分娩 delivery; childbirth; parturition
另见：分 [fèn]

分 [fèn]（名词）分别的方面 one part of a thing that has many parts, i.e., aspect
卫分 defense aspect
气分 *qi* aspect
营分 nutrient aspect
血分 blood aspect
另见：分 [fēn]

粉 [fěn]（名词）粉末 powder
粉瘤 tumor containing powdered sebum → **sebaceous cyst**
粉刺 pimple containing powdered sebum → **acne**

风 [fēng]（名词）风（病因、证名、病名等）wind (as a pathogenic factor, syndrome name, disease name, etc.)
风寒湿邪 pathogenic wind-cold-dampness
风热表证 wind-heat exterior syndrome/pattern
风寒感冒 wind-cold common cold
风水 wind edema
风疹；风痧 wind rash; rubella
风牵偏视 wind-induced squint; paralytic strabismus

封 [fēng]（动词）①封藏 to store (*n.* storage)
封藏失职 dysfunction in essence storage
②封闭 to block (*n.* block)
穴位封闭 acupoint block

锋 [fēng]（名词）兵器的锋利尖端 sharp end of a metallic weapon
锋针 sharp pointed needle → **lance needle**

佛 [fó]（名词）佛教 Buddhism
佛家气功 Buddhist *qigong*

肤 [fū]（名词）皮肤 skin (*adj.* dermal)
皮肤针 dermal needle
着肤灸 skin-contact moxibustion → **direct contact moxibustion**
折骨列肤 fracture with split skin → open fracture
血虚肤燥生风证 syndrome/pattern of blood deficiency with dryness of skin and generation of wind

趺 [fū]（名词）同"跗"，脚背 same as 跗, instep
趺阳脉 artery (or pulse) at the instep → **anterior tibial artery; anterior tibial pulse**

跗 [fū]（名词）脚背 the upper surface of the foot, i.e., the instep
跗；足跗 instep
跗骨 instep bones → **metatarsal bones**
跗肿 instep edema

敷 [fū]（动词）涂搽（药物）to apply (medicine) (*n.* application)
敷；外敷 external application

伏 [fú]（动词）隐藏 to hide
热伏冲任 heat hiding in the thoroughfare and conception vessels
（形容词）潜伏的 latent
伏热在里 latent heat in the interior
伏气温病 latent-*qi* warm disease
伏暑病 latent summerheat disease
伏饮 latent fluid retention

扶 [fú]（动词）扶助 to give support to; to reinforce
扶正 reinforcing healthy *qi*
扶正固本 reinforcing the healthy and strengthening the base
扶正祛邪 reinforcing the healthy and eliminating the pathogenic
扶阳 reinforcing yang

拂 [fú]（动词）轻轻擦掉 to move something away with a quick light sweeping movement; to whisk
拂法 whisking
掸拂法 brushing and whisking

服 [fú]（动词）①适应 to acclimatize (*n.* acclimatization)
水土不服 non-acclimatization (to a new environment)
②吃（药）to take (medicine)
服药法 method of taking medicines; administration
冲服 to be taken infused
空腹服 to be taken on an empty stomach
顿服 to be taken at a draught
服药食忌 dietary prohibitions during medication

浮 [fú]（动词）停留在液体表面上，与沉相对 to stay on the surface of a liquid, the opposite of sink → to float
浮脉 floating pulse
升降浮沉 ascending, descending, floating and sinking
蛛丝飘浮 floaters; muscae volitantes
（形容词）①在表面上的 superficial
浮刺 superficial needling
浮络 superficial collateral vessel
②空虚不实的 not fully stuffed
浮肿 unstuffed swelling → pitting edema

府 [fǔ]（名词）府邸 house
元神之府 house of the original spirit
髓之府 house of marrow
血之府 house of blood

釜 [fǔ]（名词）古代烹饪用的金属圆形大锅 a large round metal pot used for cooking over a fire in ancient times → cauldron
釜底抽薪 "taking away firewood from under the cauldron"
釜沸脉 pulse felt like bubbles rising in the cauldron → **bubble-rising pulse**

辅 [fǔ]（动词）辅助 to assist
辅骨 assisting bones (the radius and fibula)
外辅骨 the outer assisting bone →**fibula**
（名词）辅助者 one that helps or facilitates → adjunvant
辅料 adjuvant
加辅料炒 stir-baking with adjuvant
主辅佐引 principal, adjuvant, auxiliary and conductant

腑 [fǔ]（名词）传化物而不藏的内脏器官，包括胃、大小肠、胆、膀胱和三焦 internal organs that receive, contain and transmit food and drink, including the stomach, small and large intestines, gallbladder, bladder and triple energizer. (Since no English equivalent can be found, transliteration is preferred.)
腑 *fu* organ
腑气 *fu*-organ *qi*
脏腑 *zang-fu* organs
传化之腑 *fu* organs of conveyance and transformation

腐 [fǔ]（形容词）①凝乳状的 curdy
腐苔 curdy (tongue) coating/fur
②腐臭的 fetid; putrid
呕吐酸腐 vomiting of sour fetid matter
嗳腐 putrid belching
（名词）腐烂 putridity
化腐 resolving putridity
提脓去腐 drawing out pus and removing putridity
蚀疮去腐 corroding wounds and removing putridity

附 [fù]（动词）附着 to attach
附骨疽 bone-attached abscess → **suppurative osteomyelitis**

复 [fù]（动词）①恢复 to bring back
复位 to bring displaced or broken parts back to their normal positions → **reduction**
坐式复位 sitting reduction
拔伸复位 pulling-extending reduction
平整复元 correction and reduction
（动词）②往复 to alternate
阴阳胜复 alternating preponderance of yin and yang
（副词）再；又 again (*prefix*: re-)

劳复 sick again due to fatigue → **relapse due to fatigue**
食复 **relapse due to diet**
女劳复 **relapse due to sex**
离而复合 **reunion after separation**
（形容词）复合的 compound
复方 **compound formula/prescription**

腹 [fù]（名词）肚子 abdomen (*adj.* abdominal)
腹痛 **abdominal pain**
腹鸣 a rumbling sound in the abdomen → **borborygmus**
腹满 **abdominal fullness**
腹胀 **abdominal distension**
腹中硬块 **hard mass in the abdomen**
（形容词）腹侧的ventral (*prefix*: ventro-)
腹背配穴法 **ventro-dorsal point combination**
（其他）
空腹服 **to be taken on an empty stomach**

G

干 [gān]（形容词）①干燥的 dry
干咳 **dry cough**
口干不欲饮 **dryness in the mouth with no desire to drink**
干霍乱 **dry choleraic turmoil**
干癣 **dry ringworm**
干聋 **dry deafness**
②只具形式的 only in the form of
干呕 only making effort to vomit → **retching**
（其他）
天干 **heavenly stems**
纳干法 **day-prescription of points**

甘 [gān]（形容词）甜的 sweet
口甘 **sweet taste in the mouth**
甘温除热 **relieving fever with sweet-warm** (drugs)
甘寒生津 **engendering fluid with sweet-cold** (drugs)
甘寒润燥 **moistening (dryness) with sweet-cold** (drugs)

肝 [gān]（名词）肝脏 liver
肝阳上亢 **ascendant hyperactivity of liver yang**
肝火上炎 **up-flaming of liver fire**
肝气犯胃 **liver *qi* invading the stomach**
肝胃不和 **liver-stomach disharmony**
肝胆湿热 **liver-gallbladder dampness-heat**

疳 [gān]（名词）①小儿慢性营养障碍 infantile malnutrition
食疳 **feeding malnutrition**
蛔疳 **(infantile) malnutrition due to ascariasis**
②一种疮名 a kind of sore
下疳 **chancre**

感 [gǎn]（动词）①感受 to be affected (*n.* affection)
感暑 **summerheat affection**
感暑眩晕 dizziness due to summerheat affection → **summerheat dizziness**
②感染 to contract (*n.* contraction)
外感 **external contraction**
新感 **recent contraction**
（名词）感觉 sensation
针感 **needling sensation**
气感 **sensation of *qi***
（其他）
感冒 **common cold; colds**

骭 [gàn]（名词）小腿骨 shinbone
骭骨 **shinbone; tibia**

刚 [gāng]（形容词）坚硬的，柔的反义词 rigid, an antonym of soft
刚痉 convulsion accompanied by rigidity of the neck and back → **tonic convulsion**

肛 [gāng]（名词）肛门；肛肠 anus; anorectum
肛门 **anus**
脱肛 **prolapse of the rectum**
肛漏（肛瘘）**anal fistula**
肛裂 **anal fissure**

肛痈 anorectal abscess

杠 [gàng]（名词）粗棍子 a rigid bar (杠杆：a rigid bar that pivots at some point used for lifting a thing by placing it on one end and pushing down on the other → lever)
杠杆支撑 propping with a lever

高 [gāo]（形容词）①从下向上距离大的 having a long upward or vertical distance, i.e., high
高低垫 high-low pad
②突出的 protruding
高骨 protruding bone → **(1) styloid process of the radius; (2) lumbar vertebra**
（其他）
高风内障 pigmentary retinopathy
高风雀目 pigmentary retinopathy

睾 [gāo]（名词）睾丸 testis (*adj.* testicular)
睾 testis; testicle
睾丸萎缩 testicular atrophy
睾丸肿痛 painful swollen testis
控睾 radiated testicular pain

膏 [gāo]（名词）①内服的膏剂和外用的药膏的总称 a general term for soft extract, ointment and adhesive plaster, usually called paste
膏；膏剂 paste
煎膏；膏滋 soft extract
膏药 adhesive plaster
膏摩疗法 massage therapy with ointment
膏药风 plaster dermatitis
②乳糜 chyle (*adj.* chylous)
膏淋 chylous stranguria

槁 [薹] [gǎo]（动词）枯槁；萎缩 wither; atrophy
鼻槁 [薹] atrophied nose → **atrophic rhinitis**
大骨枯槁 cachexia with withering bones
齿槁 withered teeth

革 [gé]（名词）去毛的兽皮，用于制鼓时称鼓革 material made by removing the hair or fur from an animal skin (i.e., leather), also called drumskin when used for making a drum
革脉 drumskin pulse; tympanic pulse

格 [gé]（动词）格拒，排斥 to repulse, to repel
格阴 repelling yin
阳盛格阴 exuberant yang repelling yin
格阳 repelling yang
阴阳格拒 yin-yang repulsion
关格 blockage and repulsion

鬲 [gé]（名词）同"膈" same as 膈, the diaphragm
鬲 diaphragm

隔 [gé]（动词）使介入两者之间 to put something between two other things, namely, to interpose
隔物灸；间隔灸 interposed moxibustion
隔姜灸 ginger-interposed moxibustion
隔蒜灸 garlic-interposed moxibustion
隔盐灸 salt-interposed moxibustion
（名词）阻塞不通（常写作膈，见"膈"）obstruction (usually written as 膈, cf. 膈 [gé])

膈 [gé]（名词）①胸腔和腹腔之间的膜状肌肉 the membraneous muscle that separates the chest and abdominal cavities, namely, the diaphragm
膈 diaphragm
②通"隔"，阻塞不通 synonym for 隔 [gé] which means obstruction
膈噎 obstruction that leads to difficulty in swallowing → **dysphagia**
上膈 upper obstruction
下膈 lower obstruction

根 [gēn]（名词）物体的基部 the base part of a thing, namely, the root
鼻根 root of the nose; radix nasi
舌根 root of the tongue

胃、神、根 stomach *qi*, vitality, and root
针根 needle root
无根苔 rootless (tongue) coating/fur
（动词）植根于 to root
阴阳互根 mutual rooting of yin and yang
有根苔 rooted (tongue) coating/fur

鲠 [gěng]（动词）（鱼骨）卡在嗓子里 (of a fishbone) to get stuck in the throat
骨鲠 bone stuck in the throat

弓 [gōng]（名词）射箭的器械，弧形的长木条两端系有坚韧的弦 a weapon for shooting arrows, consisting of a long curved piece of wood with a tight string joining its ends, namely, a bow
弓步 bow step

功 [gōng]（名词）①练功 exercise
内功 internal exercise
外功 external exercise
②气功的简称 abbreviation for *qigong*
静功 static *qigong*
动功 dynamic *qigong*

攻 [gōng]（动词）①（病机）攻击；侵袭 to attack; to invade (*n.* invasion)
麻毒内攻 inward invasion of measles
热毒攻喉 heat toxin attacking the throat
风热攻目 wind-heat attacking the eye
风火攻目 wind-fire attacking the eye
②（治则）攻除 to eliminate (*n.* elimination)
攻补兼施 simultaneous elimination and reinforcement
先攻后补 elimination followed by reinforcement
寓攻于补 reinforcemnt for elimination
③（治则）攻逐 to expel
攻逐水饮 expelling retained water
（名词）进攻 offense (*adj.* offensive)
攻下 (offensive) **purgation**
攻下药 offensive purgative (medicinal/drug)
（其他）
攻溃 promoting suppuration
攻毒 counteracting toxins
以毒攻毒 combating poison with poison

肱 [gōng]（名词）上臂 the upper arm
肱 upper arm

宫 [gōng]（名词）原意为帝王居住的房屋，用于中医指胎儿或心脏所居之处，即子宫或心包。 Its original meaning is palace, i.e., the house where a king lives. In Chinese medicine (by metaphor) it refers to either the uterus that houses the embryo or the pericardium that houses the heart (the sovereign organ).
胞宫 uterus
宫冷不孕 uterus coldness infertility
暖宫 warming the uterus
清宫 clearing the pericardium

垢 [gòu]（名词）脏东西 dirt
垢胎 appearance of dirt during pregnancy **→ menstruation during pregnancy**

孤 [gū]（形容词）单独的 solitary
孤阳上越 solitary yang floating upward

谷 [gǔ]（名词）①粮食的总称 a collective term for grains → food
水谷 water and grain; food and drink
水谷之海 reservoir of food and drink
谷气 food *qi*
水谷精微 food essence
下利清谷 diarrhea with undigested food
②山谷 valley
合谷刺 joined valley needling

股 [gǔ]（名词）大腿，自胯至膝盖的部分 the top part of the leg or the part of leg between the hip and the knee, i.e., the thigh
股 thigh
股疽 thigh cellulitis
股阴疽 cellulitis on the medial aspect of the thigh

股阳疽 cellulitis on the lateral aspect of the thigh

骨 [gǔ]（名词）体内支持人体的坚硬组织 the hard tissue that forms the frame of a human body, viz., the bone

骨空 "bony space" → **(1) interosseous space; (2) bone marrow cavity; (3) articular cavity**

骨解 the part where two bones meet → **joint**

骨蒸热 bone-steaming fever; consumptive fever

骨折 (bone) **fracture**

骨度法 bone measurement

蛊 [gǔ]（名词）腹中虫 parasitic infestation

蛊毒 parasitic toxin

臌 [gǔ]（名词）腹部胀起的疾病 a disease characterized by abdominal distension

臌胀 abdominal distension

气臌 abdominal distension caused by accumulation of gas → **tympanites**

水臌 abdominal distension caused by accumulation of fluid → **ascites**

血臌 abdominal distension with varicose veins and vascular spiders → **ascites with engorgement**

瞽 [gǔ]（名词）盲也，无目曰瞽 blindness due to loss of the eye

瞽症 blindness in ophathalmosteresis

固 [gù]（形容词）①牢固的 secure (*n.* security)

表气不固 insecurity of exterior *qi*

卫气不固 insecurity of defense *qi*

肾气不固 insecurity of kidney *qi*

脬气不固 insecurity of bladder *qi*

冲任不固 insecurity of the thoroughfare and conception vessels

②固定的 fixed

固定痛 fixed pain

（动词）①巩固 to strengthen; to consolidate

固表止汗 consolidating the superficies and checking sweating

固表止汗药 superficies-consolidating anhidrotic

固肾 strengthening the kidney

固肾涩精 strengthening the kidney to arrest emission

②固涩 to astringe; to arrest discharge

固涩药 astringent (medicinal/drug)

固精 arresting emission

固崩止血 arresting blood flooding

固冲止血 astringing the thoroughfare vessel to stop bleeding

痼 [gù]（形容词）经久难治愈的 not easily cured, or obstinate

痼疾 obstinate disease

瓜 [guā]（名词）蔓生植物的果实 fruit of vining plants, usually referring to melons（瓜藤 melon vine）

瓜藤缠 cutaneous tender nodules winding like melon vine → **erythema nodosum**

刮 [guā]（动词）用硬物将物体表面的东西去掉 to remove something from a surface, using a sharp and hard thing, i.e., to scrape

刮痧 scraping (the skin) **to congestion**

刮痧疗法 scraping therapy

刮痧板 scraping bar

刮柄法 handle-scrapng method

挂 [guà]（动词）悬挂 to hang

挂线疗法 method for treating anal fistula whereby the fistula is ligated with a medicated thread which is hung at the site until the tensile strength of the thread causes tissue degeneration and eventually breakage of the fistula → **threaded ligation therapy**

怪 [guài]（形容词）反常的 paradoxical

七怪脉 seven paradixical pulses

关 [guān]（名词）①来往经过的关口 pass

喉关 throat pass → **faucial isthmus**

喉关痈 (1) faucial abscess; (2) peritonsillar abscess
②关节 joint
关刺 joint needling
（动词）闭塞不通 to block (*n.* blockage)
关格 blockage and repulsion
关格病 blockage-repulsion disease

光 [guāng]（副词）一点不剩 completely
光剥舌 (completely) **peeled tongue**

归 [guī]（动词）①回到原处 to go back to the original place
引火归原 conducting fire back to its origin
②取向 to orient
归经 involuntary orientation to certain meridian or meridians → **meridian/channel tropism**

鬼 [guǐ]（名词）鬼魂 ghost (古通“魄”，肺藏魄，肺气通于皮毛，汗从皮肤而出，称“魄汗”，汗孔称“鬼门”。In ancient Chinese literature, the characters 鬼 [guǐ] and 魄 [pò] are interchangeable, both signifying corporeal soul. The lung holds corporeal soul and in the meanwhile lung *qi* communicates with the skin and promotes secretion of sweat from the skin. Therefore, sweat is called 魄汗 [pò hàn] or corporeal-soul sweat and the sweat pore is called 鬼门 [guǐ mén] or ghost gate.)
鬼门 “ghost gate” → **sweat pore**
开鬼门 opening the “ghost gate” → **inducing perspiration**
鬼胎 “ghost fetus” → **pseudopregnancy**

滚 [gǔn]（动词）旋转着移动 to move by turning over and over, i.e., to roll
滚刺筒 needle roller
滚刺疗法 roller needle therapy
滚法 rolling (manipulation)

腘 [guó]（名词）膝部后方屈膝时的凹处 the depression in the posterior region of the knee
腘；膝腘 popliteal fossa

H

虾 [há]（名词）虾蟆（蛤蟆）toad or frog
虾蟆瘟 toad-like infection → **erysipelas facialis**
另见：虾 [xiā]

骸 [hái]（名词）人的骨头 bones of the human body
百骸 all bones of the human body → **skeleton**

海 [hǎi]（名词）①海洋 sea ②储水的地域 place where water is collected and stored → reservoir
髓海 sea of marrow
血海 sea of blood; reservoir of blood
水谷之海 reservoir of food and drink

含 [hán]（动词）①把东西放在嘴里，不咽下，也不吐出 to hold something in the mouth
含漱 washing the mouth and throat by holding a liquid in the mouth and keeping it in motion→ **gargling**
②藏在里面 to hide inside
含胸拔背 shrinking the chest and straightening the back

寒 [hán]（名词）①寒（病因、证名、病名等，与“热”相对）
cold (as a pathogenic factor, syndrome name, disease name, etc., the opposite of heat)
寒湿 cold-dampness
寒滞肝脉 cold stagnating in the liver meridian/channel
寒热 (1) cold and heat; (2) chills and fever
寒证 cold syndrome/pattern
寒饮停胃证 syndrome/pattern of cold-fluid retention in the stomach

寒哮 cold wheezing
②寒冷，寒意 a feeling of coldness, chill
寒战 tremor caused by a chill → **rigor**
寒热往来 alternating chills and fever

汗 [hàn]（名词）汗液 sweat
汗 sweat
汗出如油 oily sweat
（动词）①出汗 to sweat
汗证 sweating syndrome
汗病 sweating disease
②使出汗 to induce sweating
汗法 method of inducing sweating → **diaphoretic method**

颔 [hàn]（名词）下巴 chin
颔 chin

颃 [háng]（名词）颃颡指咽后壁上的后鼻道　颃颡 [háng sǎng] refers to the upper part of the pharynx continuous with the nasal passages.
颃颡 nasopharynx

毫 [háo]（名词）纤细的毛 fine hair
毫毛 fine hair of the skin → **down**
（形容词）纤细如丝的 filiform
毫针 filiform needle

耗 [hào]（动词）消耗 to consume (*n.* consumption)
心营过耗 over-consumption of heart nutrient
神光耗散 spirit-consumed eyes → **spiritless eyes**

合 [hé]（动词）①结合，组合 to combine (*n.* combination)
合邪 combined pathogen
合病 combination of diseases
太阳(与)少阳合病 combination of greater yang and lesser yang diseases
合骨垫 bone-combining pad
②再结合 to reunite (*n.* reunion)
筋合 tendon reunion
③汇合 to flow together
合穴 the place where two rivers flow together → **confluent point;** the place where all rivers flow together → **sea point**
下合穴 lower confluent point; lower sea point
（其他）
合骨 internal malleolus
合谷刺 multi-directional needling
合金针 alloy needle

和 [hé]（动词）协调 to harmonize (*n.* harmony)
和法；和解法 harmonizing method
和解少阳 harmonizing *shaoyang* meridian/channel; harmonizing lesser yang meridian/channel
和胃 harmonizing the stomach
肝胃不和 liver-stomach disharmony

核 [hé]（名词）果实中的坚硬部分（医学中表示像核的东西，例如结节）the large hard seed in some fruits, i.e., the pit, and in medicine something resembling a pit such as node or nodule
核骨 the bone with an expanded projection like a pit → **external malleolus**
结核 subcutaneous node
乳中结核 nodule in the breast
乳核 breast nodule

颌 [hé]（名词）构成口腔上部和下部的骨头和肌肉组织 either of the upper and lower bony and muscular structures that border the mouth, i.e., the jaw or mandible
颌 jaw
颌下痈 submandibular abscess

阖 [hé]（动词）关闭 to close
开阖补泻 open-closed reinforcement and reduction

黑 [hēi]（形容词）①像煤那样的颜色 having the color like that of coal, namely, black
黑色 black discoloration

黑苔 black (tongue) coating/fur
黑疔 black boil
②暗 dark
黑睛 dark of the eye
面黑；面色黎黑 darkish complexion
耳轮青黑 bluish dark helices

痕 [hén]（名词）①痕迹 mark (*v.* to mark)
齿痕舌 tooth-marked tongue
②瘢痕 scar (*v.* to scar)
瘢痕灸 scarring moxibustion

横 [héng]（形容词）横向的 transverse
横骨 transverse bone → **(1) pubic bone; (2) *henggu* (KI 11)**
上横骨 upper transverse bone → **manubrium of the sternum**
肝气横逆 transverse counterflow of liver *qi*
横刺 transverse insertion
横透 transverse penetration
横垫 transverse pad
（副词）横着地 sideways
横目斜视 staring sideways
（名词）横宽 breadth
横指同身寸 finger-breadth body-*cun*; finger-breath body-inch

胻 [héng]（名词）脚胫 shank
胻骨 shank bone

烘 [hōng]（动词）用火烤 to heat over fire, i.e., to bake
烘焙 baking
热烘 warming over fire

红 [hóng]（形容词）红色的 red
红舌；舌红 red tongue
红丝疔 redstreaked boil; acute lymphangitis
红膜 red membrane → pannus
红霞映日 red clouds shining on the cornea → **keratic pannus**
红蝴蝶疮 (a disease marked by) red butterfly rash → **lupus erythematosus**
（名词）红色 redness
白睛抱红 redness of the bulbar conjunctiva surrounding the ciliary body → **ciliary hyperemia**
消肿退红 relieving swelling and redness
（动词）变红 to redden
面红 reddened complexion

虹 [hóng]（名词）古代认为虹是彩龙，雨过天晴时现身。In ancient China, a rainbow (虹) was considered to be a colorful dragon that appears when the sky just turns bright and clear right after a rain. → colorful substance
虹膜 colorful membrane in the eye → **iris**

洪 [hóng]（形容词）洪波状的 surging
洪脉 surging pulse

喉 [hóu]（名词）①喉咙；嗓子 throat
喉关 throat passage → **faucial isthmus**
喉底 back of the throat → **retropharynx**
喉核 prominent mass on the side of the throat → **tonsil**
喉痧；烂喉痧 throat infection with erythema → **scarlatina**
喉蛾 throat moth → **tonsillitis**
②喉咙；嗓音 voice
喉喑［瘖］hoarseness of voice or aphonia

瘊 [hóu]（名词）疣的通称 wart, a common name for verruca
瘊子 wart
扁瘊 flat wart; verruca plana
线瘊 filiform wart; verruca filiformis

后 [hòu]（形容词）①（空间上）后面的，与前面的相对 posterior (the opposite of anterior)
后发际 posterior hairline
后阴 posterior yin → **anus**
后侧夹板 posterior splint
②（时间上）以后的 occurring after an event
后天之气 *qi* acquired after birth → **acquired *qi*; postnatal *qi***

后天之精 acquired essence
后天失调 lack of proper care after birth
（副词）后来 later
后下 to be added (for decoction) later
（其他）
后伸扳腰法 lumbar extending-counter-pulling manipulation

厚 [hòu]（形容词）①扁平物上下两面距离大的 having a larger distance between two opposite surfaces than normal, namely thick
厚苔 thick (tongue) coating/fur
②（味道）浓的 giving a strong flavor
膏粱厚味 rich and flavored food

候 [hòu]（动词）等待 to await
候气 awaiting *qi*
行针候气 manipulating the needle to await *qi*
留针候气 retaining the needle to await *qi*
（名词）事物变化的情况或表现 condition or manifestation of the change of a thing
征候 objective evidence of a disease condition → **sign**
惊风八候 eight signs of infantile convulsions
证候 syndrome/pattern manifestation
（其他）
三部九候 three positions and nine pulse-takings

呼 [hū]（动词）呼出 to exhale（呼吸 to breathe; to respire）
呼吸 breathing; respiration
呼吸之气 breathed air
呼吸气粗 heavy breathing
呼吸气微 feeble breathing
呼吸补泻 respiratory reinforcement and reduction

狐 [hú]（名词）①狐狸 fox
狐臭 bad odor (from the ampit) like that of the gas from a fox → **armpit odor**
②中医专用，蚀于阴为狐，蚀于喉为惑。In traditional Chinese medicine, 狐 [hú] signifies erosion of the genitalia, and 惑 [huò], erosion of the throat.
狐惑 throat-anus-genital syndrome

葫 [hú]（名词）葫芦 calabash gourd
葫芦垫 calabash pad

糊 [hú]（动词）粘合 to paste
糊丸 pasted pill

虎 [hǔ]（名词）老虎 tiger
虎口 "tiger's mouth"; thumb web

互 [hù]（形容词）互相的 mutual
精气互化 mutual transformation of essence and *qi*
阴阳互根 mutual rooting of yin and yang; yin-yang interdependence
阴阳互损 mutual impairment between yin and yang
痰瘀互结证 (mutually) **combined syndrome/pattern of phlegm and static blood**

户 [hù]（名词）门户 door
户门 entrance doors → **teeth**
阴户 door of the female genital organ → **vulva**

花 [huā]（名词）花瓣 petal
花翳白陷 petaloid nebula with a sunken center → **ulcerative keratitis**

滑 [huá]（形容词）光滑的 slippery
滑苔 slippery (tongue) coating/fur
（动词）滑动，用于医学表示容易流出 to slide easily, and in medicine, to flow out easily
滑精 outflowing of semen without copulation → **spermatorrhea; spontaneous seminal emission**
滑泄 diarrhea with uncontrolled fecal outflow → **efflux diarrhea**
滑胎 frequent outflowing of the embryo or

fetus → **habitual abortion**
血虚滑胎 habitual abortion due to blood deficiency

化 [huà]（动词）①变化 to transform (*n.* transformation)
化热 transformation into heat
化火 transformation into fire
化风 transformation into wind
化燥 transformation into dryness
化脓 transformation into pus → **pustulation**
②化解 to resolve
化痰宣肺 resolving phlegm to ventilate the lung
化饮解表 resolving retained fluid and releasing the exterior
化湿 resolving dampness
化瘀药 stasis-resolving medicinal/drug
化痰止咳平喘药 phlegm-resolving, cough-stopping and asthma-relieving medicinal/drug
③溶化 to dissolve
化石 dissolving calculi

踝 [huái]（名词）①腿与脚之间的关节 the joint between the leg and the foot, namely, the ankle
抱踝手法 peri-ankle manipulation
②脚踝左右两侧的突起 bony projection at each side of the ankle, namely, the malleolus
内踝 internal malleolus; medial malleolus
外踝 external malleolus; lateral malleolus

缓 [huǎn]（形容词）①缓和的 moderate or mild ②松弛的 relaxed ③缓慢的 slow
缓脉 (1) moderate pulse; (2) relaxed pulse
缓下 inducing mild bowel movement → **laxation**
缓方 slow-acting formula
胃缓 relaxed stomach → **gastroptosis**

肓 [huāng]（名词）心下膈上的部位 the space below the heart and above the diaphragm
膏肓 infracardio-supradiaphragmatic space

黄 [huáng]（形容词）黄色的 yellow
黄苔 yellow (tongue) coating/fur
黄疸 yellow discoloration of the body → **jaundice**
黄水疮 yellow-water sore; impetigo
黄仁 yellow kernel; iris
黄油障；黄油证 yellowish creamy patch of proliferative substance on the bulbar conjunctiva → **pinguecula**

㿠 [huàng]（形容词）虚浮的 puffy
面色㿠白 pale puffy complexion

灰 [huī]（形容词）灰色的 gray
灰苔 gray (tongue) coating/fur

恢 [huī]（动词）恢复 to recover
恢刺 needling for recovering (from muscular contracture) → **relaxing needling**

回 [huí]（动词）①使回复 to restore
回阳 restoring yang
回阳救逆 restoring yang from collapse
温经回阳 warming the meridians/channels and restoring yang
②回绝；终止 to reject; to terminate
回乳 terminating lactation
③盘旋；使回旋 to circle; to rotate
回旋灸 circling moxibustion
回旋 reverse rotation
（其他）
回光返照 "last radiance of the setting sun"

蛔 [huí]（名词）蛔虫 ascaris
蛔厥 ascariasis syncope; syncope due to ascariasis
蛔疳 ascariasis malnutrition; malnutrition due to ascariasis
安蛔定痛 quieting ascaris to relieve pain

会 [huì]（动词）会合 to join（厌：遮盖 to

cover）（会厌：会厌者，喉间之薄膜也，周围会合，…… 咽喉食息之道得以不乱者，赖其遮厌，故谓之会厌。The so-called 会厌 [huì yàn] is a lamella that joins with the surrounding tissues in the throat and serves to cover the glottis during the act of swallowing.）

会厌 epiglottis

秽 [huì]（名词）污浊 filth (*adj.* filthy)

暑秽 summerheat filth

暑秽病 summer filth disease

秽气气感 sensation of filthy *qi*

昏 [hūn]（名词）① 神志障碍 impaired consciousness

神昏 clouded consciousness

昏蒙；神志昏愦；神识昏溃 clouded consciousness with confusion → **mental confusion**

昏厥 sudden loss of consciousness → **fainting**

昏迷 profound unconsciousness → **coma**

② 视物模糊 blurred vision

视瞻昏渺；瞻视昏渺 blurring of vision

混 [hún]（形容词）混浊的 turbid; murky

混睛障；混睛外障；混障症 murky nebula; interstitial keratitis

白睛混赤 turbid redness of the white of the eye → **hyperemia of the bulbar conjunctiva**

魂 [hún]（名词）灵魂 soul（魂与魄的区别：魂是离开肉体、纯属精神的灵魂；魄是依附肉体的魄力。The difference between 魂 [hún] and 魄 [pò]: The former is purely the spiritual part of soul apart from the body, namely, ethereal soul, while the latter is attached to the body, namely, corporeal soul.）

魂 ethereal soul

活 [huó]（动词）使活动 to activate

活血化瘀 activating blood and resolving stasis

活血调经 activating blood to regulate menstruation

活血通络 activating blood to unblock collaterals

活血止痛 activating blood to relieve pain

舒筋活络 relaxing tendons and activating collaterals

火 [huǒ]（名词）① 火为五行之一。生理性的火为生命的动力，病理性的火为功能亢进的表现，火又为六淫之一。Fire is one of the five elements/phases. In physiological context, fire refers to dynamic energy that supports all life activities, while in pathological one, it signifies diverse manifestations of hyperfunction. In addition, fire also means one of the six pathogenic factors.

火生土 fire generating earth

火克金 fire restricting metal

火毒 fire toxin

火扰心神证 syndrome/pattern of fire harassing the mind

火丹 a reddened inflammatory skin lesion that gives the patient a burning sensation → **erysipelas 火疳；火疡 fire ulcer (of the eye); episcleritis**

② 物体燃烧所发出的火焰 fire: heat and flame produced when something burns

火制 fire processing

文火 mild fire

火针 fire needle

火罐法 fire cupping

火伤 fire-caused injury → **burn**

霍 [huò]（副词）霍然 suddenly（霍乱：其病剧烈吐泻，"挥霍之间，便致扰乱"。霍乱 [huò luàn] is a disease characterized by severe vomiting and diarrhea which cause bodily turmoil in a sudden, usually referring to cholera and the like.）

霍乱 cholera or choleraic turmoil

干霍乱 dry choleraic turmoil

寒霍乱 cold choleraic turmoil
霍乱转筋 systremma in choleraic turmoil

豁 [huò]（动词）清除 to eliminate
豁痰 eliminating phlegm
豁痰开窍 eliminating phlegm to induce resuscitation
豁痰醒脑 eliminating phlegm to arouse the brain

J

击 [jī]（动词）击打 to strike
拍击法 patting-striking manipulation
拳击法 fist-striking manipulation
掌击法 palm-striking manipulation
棒击法 rod-striking manipulation

饥 [jī]（动词、名词）饿 hunger
饥不欲食 no desire to eat despite hunger
多食善饥 polyphagia with frequent hunger
消谷善饥 swift digestion with rapid hungering

肌 [jī]（名词）肌肉 muscle
肌腠；肌凑 muscular striae
肌痹 muscle impediment
（其他）肌肤，主要指皮肤 muscle and skin, in most occasions referring to the skin
肌肤甲错 encrusted skin
肌肤麻木 numbness of the skin
肌肤不仁 insensitivity of the skin

鸡 [jī]（名词）chicken
鸡胸 chicken breast
鸡眼 small area of hard thickened skin on the foot resembling the eye of a chicken → **clavus; corn**

奇 [jī]（形容词）单数的，与偶相对 odd-numbered, the opposite of even-numbered
奇方 odd-numbered formula/prescription

积 [jī]（动词）积聚；积滞 to accumulate; to retain (*n.* accumulation; retention)
积聚 accumulation-aggregation
积证 accumulation syndrome
食积 food retention → **dyspepsia; indigestion**
乳积 milk retention → **infantile dyspepsia**
积吐 food-retention vomiting

激 [jī]（动词）激发 to stimulate
激经 stimulated menses; menstruation during pregnancy

急 [jí]（名词）紧急情况 emergency
产后三急 three postpartum emergencies
急下 emergency purgation
急下存阴 emergency purgation to preserve yin
急下存津 emergency purgation to preserve fluid
（形容词）①急性的 acute
急惊风 acute infantile convulsion
急喉喑［瘖］acute hoarseness or aphonia
急喉风 acute throat wind; acute throat infection
急喉痹 acute throat impediment; acute pharyngitis
②快速而且猛烈的 rapid and strong
急火 strong fire
急方 quick-acting formula
急黄 jaundice with sudden onset and rapid deterioration → **fulminant jaundice**

疾 [jí]（名词）疾病 disease; illness; sickness
疾；疾病 disease; illness; sickness
宿疾 old disease
固［痼］疾 stubborn disease
隐疾 occult disease
（形容词）迅速的 quick; rapid; swift
疾脉 swift pulse
疾徐补泻 quick-slow reinforcement and reduction

嫉 [jí]（名词）嫉妒 jealousy
嫉妒不孕 infertility due to jealousy

己 [jǐ]（代词）自己 oneself
练己 cultivating oneself

挤 [jǐ]（动词）用手指挤压 to press something forcefully with fingers, namely, to squeeze
挤法 squeezing
提按端挤 lifting, pressing, holding, and squeezing
夹挤分骨 separate bones by squeezing

脊 [jǐ]（名词）脊椎 spine
捏脊 pinching along the spine
夹脊 pressing the spine

忌 [jì]（动词、名词）禁戒 to prohibit; prohibition; taboo
忌口 food taboo
食忌 dietary prohibitions
服药食忌 dietary prohibitions during medication

季 [jì]（形容词）（在伯仲叔季序列中）排行最末的 last (in the sequence of 伯 [bó] 仲 [zhòng] 叔 [shū]季 [jì])
季肋；季胁 region overlying the costal cartilages of the lowest ribs → **hypochondrium**

剂 [jì]（名词）①配制成的药 prepared medicine
剂量 the quantity of a prepared medicine to be taken → **dosage**
剂型 preparation form
丸剂 (medicine prepared in the form of) **pills**
②药物的配方 medicinal formula
方剂 formula

济 [jì]（动词）协调 to coordinate (*n.* coordination)
水火相济 water-fire coordination

悸 [jì]（动词）①因害怕而心跳 (of the heart) to beat rapidly because of fear → to palpitate or throb (*n.* palpitations)
心悸 palpitations
心下悸 palpitations below the heart
心动悸 throbbing palpitations
②强烈而有节奏地搏动 to beat with strong force and a regular rhythm, namely, to throb
脐下悸 throbbing below the umbilicus

加 [jiā]（介词）添加；与……在一起 plus; with
加辅料炒 stir-baking with adjuvant

夹 [jiā]（动词）①夹着；从两个相对方面施加压力，使物体固定不动 to compress and hold; to immobilize with forces opposite in direction
夹持进针法 hand-holding needle insertion
夹板 boards designed to immobilize (broken bones) → **splint**
夹板固定 splintage
②夹杂 to mingle with; to be complicated by (*n.* complexity)
虚中夹实 deficiency complicated by excess
虚实夹杂 deficiency-excess in complexity
夹惊吐 vomiting (mingled) **with fright**
慢惊夹痰 chronic convulsion (mingled) **with phlegm**

痂 [jiā]（名词）痂块；嘎渣 crust; scab
痂 crust

家 [jiā]（名词）①学派 school of thought (*suffixes*: -ian; -ist)
儒家气功 Confucian *qigong*
道家气功 Taoist *qigong*
佛家气功 Buddhist *qigong*
②一类的人或事物，例如胃家指胃及大小肠等 a group of people or things, e.g., 胃家 (“the stomach group”) refering to the stomach and intestines collectively
胃家实 excessiveness in the stomach and intestines

颊 [jiá]（名词）脸的两侧 the lateral aspect of the face, namely, the cheek
颊 cheek
颊车 cheek cart, the site of the cheekbone where the molars are located like a cart loaded with goods → **mandibular angle**

曲颊 mandibular arch

甲 [jiǎ]（名词）①指甲 nail

透关射甲；通关射甲 shooting through the passes to the nail; extension through the passes toward the nail

②甲壳 shell (concha)

耳甲 concha auricularis; concha

耳甲腔 cavity of the concha; cavitas concha

③天干第一位 first of the heavenly stems

纳甲法 day-prescription of points

（形容词）有硬壳覆盖的 having a hard outer covering

肌肤甲错 encrusted skin

胛 [jiǎ]（名词）肩胛 scapula (*adj*. scapular)

肩胛疽 scapular cellulitis

假 [jiǎ]（形容词）不真实的 false (*prefix*: pseudo-)

假神 false vitality

假寒 false cold; pseudo-cold

假热 false heat; pseudo-heat

架 [jià]（名词）架子 a framework or shelf for supporting objects, namely, a rack

架火法 fire-rack cupping (method)

坚 [jiān]（形容词）坚硬的 rigid (*n*. rigidity)

心下坚 rigidity below the heart; epigastric rigidity

溃坚 promoting rupture (of the rigid)

间 [jiān]（介词）之间 between

肾间动气 motive *qi* between the kidneys

屏间切迹 depression between the tragus and antitragus → **intertragic notch**

（形容词）两者之间的 intermediate

间气 intermediate *qi*

肩 [jiān]（名词）肩膀 shoulder

肩胛 shoulder blade; scapula

肩臂酸痛 aching shoulder and arm

肩不举 inability to lift the shoulder and arm

肩臂功 shoulder-arm exercise; functional training of the shoulder and arm

兼 [jiān]（动词）兼有 to have both or more simultaneously

相兼脉象 pulse having two or more features simultaneously → **multi-featured pulse**

攻补兼施 simultaneous elimination and reinforcement

（介词）和……在一起 with

扶正兼祛邪 reinforcing the healthy with elimination of the pathogenic

祛邪兼扶正 eliminating the pathogenic with reinforcement of the healthy

煎 [jiān]（动词）把东西放在水里煮，使所含的成分进入水中 to extract the active ingredients by boiling, i.e., to decoct

煎药法 method of decocting medicinal(s) → **method of making a decoction**

先煎 to be decocted first

包煎 to be decocted with wrapping; wrap-decoct

煎膏 semisolid preparation made by concentrating a decoction → **soft extract**

茧 [jiǎn]（名词）蚕茧 silkworm cocoon

茧唇 cocoon-like neoplasia of the lip → **lip cancer**

趼 [jiǎn]（名词）因摩擦而生成的硬皮，即老茧 thickened hard part of the skin caused by rubbing, namely, callus

趼子 callus

减 [jiǎn]（动词）减少 to reduce

减肥功 fat-reducing exercise → **slimming exercise**

睑 [jiǎn]（名词）眼睑 eyelid; palpebra

睑弦 palpebral margin

睑皮垂缓 drooping of the upper eyelid → **blepharoptosis**

睑废 invalid eyelid → **serious blepharoptosis**

睑粘睛珠 adhesion between an eyelid and the eyeball → **symblepharon**

謇［蹇］[jiǎn]（名词）言辞不顺利 sluggish speech
舌謇［蹇］sluggish tongue

间 [jiàn]（动词）使介入两者之间 to interpose
间隔灸 interposed moxibustion
（形容词）间接的 indirect
间接灸 indirect moxibustion

剑 [jiàn]（名词）一种兵器，长条形，一端尖，两边有刃，安有短柄 a weapon consisting of a long pointed double-edged blade and a handle, i.e., a sword
剑针 sword needle
剑决式 sword-thrusting gesture

健 [jiàn]（动词）使强健 to invigorate
健脾 invigorating the spleen
健脾止泻 invigorating the spleen to arrest diarrhea
健脾益气 invigorating the spleen and replenishing *qi*
健胃 invigorating the stomach
健胃止呕 invigorating the stomach to stop vomiting
（副词）多，善于 often, recurrently
健忘 recurrently forgetting things → **forgetfulness; amnesia**

渐 [jiàn]（形容词）逐渐发生的 progressive
渐聋 progressive deafness

楗 [jiàn]（名词）股骨 thighbone
楗 thighbone; femur

箭 [jiàn]（名词）箭矢 arrow
箭头针arrow-headed needle
血箭痔 hemorrhoid with spurting of blood like a shooting arrow → **blood-spurting hemorrhoid**

姜 [jiāng]（名词）生姜 ginger
隔姜灸 ginger-interposed moxibustion
姜炙 stir-baking with ginger

浆 [jiāng]（名词）浆液 fluid
承浆 place where fluid excreted from the mouth is held → **middle of the mentolabial groove**
沥浆产；沥浆生untimely dribbling of amniotic fluid during delivery → **premature amniotic rupture**

降 [jiàng]（动词）①下降 to descend
升、降、出、入 ascending, descending, exiting and entering
胃气不降 stomach *qi* failing to descend
②使下降；抑制 to direct something (to move) downward; to suppress
降气化痰 directing *qi* downward and resolving phlegm
降气平喘 directing *qi* downward to relieve dyspnea
降逆下气 suppressing upward perversion of *qi*
降逆止呕 suppressing upward perversion of *qi* to stop vomiting

绛 [jiàng]（形容词）略带紫的深红色的 deep purplish red; crimson
绛舌；舌绛 crimson tongue

强 [jiàng]（形容词）僵硬的 stiff or rigid
强硬舌 stiff tongue
舌强 stiff tongue
项强 rigidity of the neck
头项强痛 headache and painful stiff neck
另见：强 [qiáng]

交 [jiāo]（动词）①连接 to join together (*n.* union)
交骨 union bone → **(1) the sacrococcygeal joint; (2) the pubic bone**
交骨不开fixation of the union bone → **fixation of the pubic cartilage**
②交互作用 to interact (*n.* interaction)
阴阳交感 yin-yang interaction
心肾相交 heart-kidney interaction
心肾不交 heart-kidney non-interaction
③使相互配合 to coordinate

交通心肾 coordinating the heart and kidney
④相交 to meet and pass, i.e., to cross
交会穴 crossing point
交会选穴法 crossing point selection
（形容词）与病侧交叉的 contralateral (pertaining to or situated on the side opposite to the site of a disease)
交叉选穴法 contralateral point selection

胶 [jiāo]（名词）用动物皮/骨等熬制而成的黏性物质 a sticky substance obtained by boiling animal skins or bones in water, namely, glue or gelatine
胶 glue
胶囊剂 medicinal preparation in a small gelatine container→ **capsule**
（形容词）胶粘的 sticky
眵泪胶粘 sticky eye gum and tears

椒 [jiāo]（名词）花椒 Chinese prickly ash
椒疮 prickly-ash sore (of the eye) → **trachoma**

焦 [jiāo]（形容词）①焦干的 parched
齿焦 parched teeth
②焦黄的 brown
炒焦 stir-baking to brown
（名词）同"膲"，体腔之意 interchangeable with 膲 [jiāo], meaning the body cavity
三焦 three portions of the body cavity → **triple energizer**
下焦 lower portion of the body cavity → **lower energizer**
三焦气化 activity of the triple energizer
热结下焦 heat accumulation in the lower energizer

角 [jiǎo]（名词）①动物头上的角 horn
角弓反张 hyperextension of the body like an inversely stretched horn-decked bow → **opisthotonus**
②物体边缘相接的地方 the point at which two surfaces meet, namely, the corner
额角 forehead corner
口角流涎 drooping from the corner of the mouth

绞 [jiǎo]（动词）扭，拧紧 to wring, to twist
绞痛 pain in an organ as if the organ were twisted → **colicky pain; colic**
绞肠痧 colicky intestinal turmoil

脚 [jiǎo]（名词）本义是小腿，引申为腿的下端。 脚 [jiǎo] originally means the calf of the leg, and is extended to mean the foot.
脚弱 leg weakness
脚气 leg *qi*: (1) leg flaccidity; (2) beriberi
脚气冲心 beriberi involving the heart
脚湿气；脚气疮 athlete's foot; tinea pedis
脚肿 swollen feet

搅 [jiǎo]（动词）搅动 to stir
搅舌 stirring the tongue
赤龙搅海 "red dragon stirring the sea"; tongue-stirring exercise
搅肠痧 "intestine-stirring turmoil"; colicky intestinal turmoil

叫 [jiào]（动词）喊叫 to call loudly（叫化子是乞丐的口语。叫化子 [jiào huā zi] is a colloquialism of beggar.）
叫化功 beggar's exercise

疖 [jiē]（名词）疖子 boil; furuncle
疖病 furunculosis
暑疖 summer boil
蝼蛄疖 mole cricket boil
耳疖 ear furuncle
消痈散疖 dispersing abscesses and boils

接 [jiē]（动词）连接 to rejoin; to reunite
接法 rejoining; (bone-)setting
接骨续筋 reunion of the bone, muscle and ligament

节 [jié]（名词）①关节 joint
百节 all joints

通利关节 easing the joint
指节拍法 method of patting with finger joints → **knuckle-patting manipulation**
②节制 control
房事不节 lack of control over oneself in sexual life → **intemperance in sexual life**
③规律性 regularity
饮食不节 dietary irregularities

洁 [jié]（动词）弄干净 to clean
洁净府 "cleaning the bladder" (treating edema by diuresis)
（形容词）干净的 clean
饮食不洁 unclean food; contaminated food

结 [jié]（动词）系；束 to tie; to bind (*n.* bind: an annoying situation)
结扎 to tie with ligature → **ligate**
结扎疗法 ligation therapy
结舌 tongue-tie; ankyloglossia
结胸 chest bind; thoracic accumulation
寒结 cold bind; cold constipation
（名词）用绳索打成的结，用于医学指体表或组织中的圆形突起 knot; in medicine, prominence on body surface or swelling in the tissue resembling a knot → tubercle, nodule or node
结喉 laryngeal prominence; the Adam's apple
耳轮结节 helix tubercle
结核 (subcutaneous) node
乳中结核 nodule in the breast
消痈散结 dispersing abscesses and nodules
（其他）结膜 conjunctiva
结膜红赤 conjunctival hyperemia

睫 [jié]（名词）睫毛 eyelash
睫毛倒入；倒睫 turning inward of the eyelashes → **trichiasis**
倒睫拳毛 trichiasis and entropion

截 [jié]（动词）中断 to interrupt
截疟 interrupting malaria

竭 [jié] (动词)耗尽 to exhaust (*n.* exhaustion)
天癸竭 (1) exhaustion of the sex-stimulating essence; (2) menopause
阴竭阳脱 yin exhaustion and yang collapse
经气衰竭 exhaustion of meridian/channel *qi*

解 [jiě]（动词）①释放 to release
解表 releasing the exterior
解表清热 releasing the exterior and clearing heat
解肌 releasing the flesh
解表透疹 releasing the exterior to promote eruption
解表药 exterior-releasing medicinal/drug
②解除 to remove
解毒 removing toxins; detoxication
解酒毒 removing alcoholic toxins
解毒消肿 removing toxins and promoting subsidence of swelling
解毒透疹 removing toxins to promote eruption
③把绕在一起的绳索解开 to undo a twined rope, namely, to untwine
解索脉 untwining rope pulse
（形容词）分解开的，未连接在一起的 ununited
解颅 ununited skull; hydrocephalus

疥 [jiè]（名词）疥疮 scabies
疥疮；疥癞 scabies

金 [jīn]（名词）①五行之一的金 metal, one of the five elements/phases
金克木 metal restricting wood
金寒水冷 coldness of metal and water
金井 metallic well → pupil (The pupil resembles a well and aqueous humor at the bottom seems like water in the well, and the "well" has never been dried as if there were a water generator. Since metal generates water according to the five-element theory, the pupil is thus called metallic well.)

金疳；金疡 metallic ulcer (of the eye) → ulcer (of the eye) caused by lung (metal) fire → **phlyctnular conjunctivitis**
②金属 metal
金针 metal needle
金针拨障法 (metal) **needle couching; cataractopiesis with needle**
金疮；金创；金疡 wound made by a metalic cutting tool → **incised wound**
金疮痉 spasm in the case of incised wound → **tetanus**

津 [jīn]（名词）①津液 fluid
津液 body fluids
津亏血燥 fluid depletion with blood dryness
津枯肠燥 fluid exhaustion with intestinal dryness
津液亏虚证 fluid deficiency syndrome/pattern
津亏热结证 syndrome/pattern of fluid depletion with retained heat
②唾液 saliva
津窍 orifice of saliva

筋 [jīn]（名词）①肌腱 sinew; tendon
筋之府 house of sinews/tendons → knee
筋痿 sinew atrophy-flaccidity
筋断 musculotendinous rupture
筋正 tendon restoration
筋合 tendon reunion
②肌肉 muscle (*adj.* muscular)
筋惕肉瞤 muscular twitching
筋缩 (1) muscle contracture; (2) ***jinsuo*** **(GV 8)**
筋痿 (1) muscle flaccidity; (2) impotence
③皮下可见的静脉 visible vein beneath the skin
筋瘿 goiter with varicose veins
④泛指人体的皮肤、皮下筋膜、肌肉、肌腱、韧带、关节囊、周围神经及血管等软组织 a collective term referring to the skin and subcutaneous soft tissues of the human body, including ligaments, muscles, tendons, peripheral nerves and blood vessels
筋伤 soft tissue injury

紧 [jǐn]（形容词）①绷紧的，与"松"相反 tight or tense, the opposite of loose
紧脉 tight pulse; tense pulse
②紧急的，与"缓慢的"相反 swift, the opposite of slow
紧按慢提 swift thrusting and slow lifting
紧提慢按 swift lifting and slow thrusting
（动词）收紧 to contract; to constrict (*adj.* constrictive)
紧喉风 constrictive throat wind; constrictive throat infection
瞳神紧小 contraction of the pupil → **miosis**

锦 [jǐn]（名词）锦缎 brocade
八段锦 eight-section brocade

进 [jìn]（动词）使进入 → 插入 to introduce something into the body → to insert (*n.* insertion)
进针 needle insertion
单手进针法 single-handed needle insertion
指切进针法 fingernail-pressing needle insertion
夹持进针法 hand-holding needle insertion
舒张进针法 skin-spreading needle insertion
提捏进针法 pinching needle insertion

近 [jìn]（形容词）距离短的 near; proximal
近血 proximal bleeding
近视；能近怯远症 nearsightedness; myopia

浸 [jìn]（动词）把东西泡在液体里 to soak or to immerse
浸淫疮 exudate-soaked skin lesion → **exudative eczema**

禁 [jìn]（动词）禁止 to prohibit
禁针穴 needling-prohibited point
禁灸穴 moxibustion-prohibited point
禁例 the case in which the use of a certain medicine is prohibited → **contraindication**

发汗禁例 contraindications of diaphoresis
（名词）控制，尤常用于排泄的控制 control, especially that of the evacuative functions
小便失禁 urinary incontinence
大便失禁 fecal incontinence
（形容词）禁止外传的 prohibiting others from knowing, i.e., secrete
禁方 secrete formula

噤 [jìn]（词素）闭口不张 inability to open the mouth
噤风；口噤 lockjaw
噤口痢 food-denial dysentery

茎 [jīng]（名词）阴茎 penis
茎；阴茎 penis
茎垂 penis and testes

经 [jīng]（名词）①体内大的脉络 the main vessels in the body, usually translated into meridians or channels
经络 meridian/channel and collateral
经脉 meridians; channels
经别 meridian/channel divergence
经气 meridian/channel *qi*
经络辨证meridian/channel syndrome differentiation; meridian/channel pattern identification
经穴(1) meridian/channel points; (2) river points
经外穴 points away from meridians → **extra points**
②月经 menstruation; period (*adj.* menstrual)
经带胎产 menstrual disorders, leukorrheal diseases, gravid troubles, and parturition problems
经水先期；经行先期 early periods; shortened menstrual cycles
经乱 irregular periods
经崩 menstrual flooding; menorrhagia
经漏 menstrual dripping
（形容词）经典的 classical
经方 classical formula

惊 [jīng]（名词）①惊吓 fright
惊悸 fright palpitation
惊痫 fright epilepsy
惊疳 fright (infantile) malnutrition
惊热 fever by fright
惊吐 fright vomiting
②惊风 convulsion (*adj.* convulsive)
惊风病 infantile convulsive disease
急惊风 acute infantile convulsion
惊风抽搐 infantile convulsive seizure
（其他）
惊震内障 traumatic cataract

晶 [jīng]（名词）晶体 crystal（形容词）晶状的 crystalline
晶珠 crystalline lens
晶瘖 miliaria crystalline; sudamina

睛 [jīng]（名词）眼睛；眼球 eye; eyeball
睛珠 eyeball
黑睛 dark of the eye
睛帘 the membrane suspended in front of the lens of the eye → **iris**
睛高突起 suddenly protruding eyeball
睛胀 distension of the eyebal

精 [jīng]（名词）①精华 essence (*adj.* essential)
精气 essential *qi*
精气互化 mutual transformation of essence and *qi*
精室 essence chamber
精血 essence-blood
精微 refined essence
②精明 intelligence
精明之府 house of intelligence
③精子 semen (*adj.* seminal)
精冷；精寒 cold semen
精浊 seminal turbidity
滑精 spontaneous seminal emission; spermatorrhea
精窍 the external orifice from which semen is discharged → **male urinary meatus**

（形容词）精炼的 refined
精汁 refined juice
（其他）
精神 spirit
精珠 lens

井 [jǐng]（名词）水井 a well
井穴 well points

颈 [jǐng]（名词）颈项 neck; cervix (*adj.* cervical)
颈痈 cervical abscess
颈项功 neck exercise
颈椎单人旋转复位法 single-handed rotating reduction of cervical vertebra
颈椎角度复位法 angular reduction of cervical vertebra

净 [jìng]（形容词）干净的 clean
净府 clean *fu*-viscus → **bladder**
洁净府 cleaning the clean *fu*-viscus→ **cleaning the bladder**

胫 [jìng]（名词）小腿 shin
胫 shin
胫骨 shinbone; tibia

痉 [jìng]（名词）痉挛；抽搐 spasm; convulsion (*adj.* convulsive)
痉病 convulsive disease
刚痉 tonic convulsion
金疮痉 convulsions associated with an incised wound → **tetanus**
止痉 relieving spasms; arresting convulsions

静 [jìng]（形容词）安静不动，与“动”相反 static or actionless, the opposite of dynamic
静留针法 actionless needle retention
静功 static *qigong*
（名词）静止状态 quiescence
静中有动 motion within quiescence
入静 entering quiescence; falling into static state

镜 [jìng]（名词）镜子 a mirror
镜面舌 mirror tongue

鸠 [jiū]（名词）斑鸠一类的鸟 turtle dove
鸠尾 the lowest division of the sternum resembling the tail of a turtle dove → **xiphoid process**

揪 [jiū]（动词）用力拉拽 to drag
揪法 dragging
揪痧 dragging to congestion

九 [jiǔ]（数词）九 nine
九窍 nine orifices
九针 nine classical needles
九刺 nine needling methods
九九阳功 double-nine yang exercise

久 [jiǔ]（形容词）时间长的 lasting for a long time; chronic
久嗽；久咳 chronic cough
久泄；久泻 chronic diarrhea
久痢 chronic dysentery
久疟 chronic malaria
久流浊涕 chronic turbid nasal discharge

灸 [jiǔ]（名词）用艾叶烧灼的热刺激人体的治疗方法 a method of therapeutic procedure whereby heat generated by moxa combustion is applied to the body as a stimulus（moxa + combustion → moxibustion）
灸法；灸疗法 moxibustion
针灸 acupuncture and moxibustion
艾条灸 moxa-stick moxibustion; moxibustion with moxa stick
艾卷灸 moxa-roll moxibustion
雀啄灸 bird-pecking moxibustion; pecking moxibustion

酒 [jiǔ]（名词）含乙醇的饮料 a collective term for alcoholic drinks such as brandy and wine
酒剂；药酒 medicinal wine
酒醴 vinum (Latin for wine)
酒癖 alcohol addiction
酒皶鼻 brandy nose; rosacea
（其他）

酒刺 acne

臼 [jiù]（名词）关节 joint
脱臼 displacement of a bone from a joint **→dislocation; luxation**
入臼 joint reduction

救 [jiù]（动词）拯救；救援 to save; to rescue
救脱 saving from collapse
救阳 rescuing yang

拘 [jū]（动词）拘挛 to contract (*n.* contracture; contraction)
拘挛 contracture
拘急 contraction

居 [jū]（动词）停留 to stop over
居经 menstruation with three-months' stop-over → **tri-monthly menstruation**

疽 [jū]（名词）发于肌肉筋骨间的疮肿，创面浅者为痈，创面深者为疽 purulent inflammation infiltrated into the subcutaneous tissue: The superficial one is called 痈 [yōng] (carbuncle), and the deep-rooted one called 疽 [jū] (phlegmon).
疽 phlegmon; cellulitis

局 [jú]（形容词）局部的 local
局部选穴法 selection of local points

举 [jǔ]（动词）向上抬，用于脉诊时意为轻按 to lift, and to touch lightly in pulse-taking
肩不举 inability to lift the shoulder and arm
举、按、寻 touching, pressing, and searching
举法 touching (inpulse taking)

拒 [jù]（动词）拒绝 to refuse (*n.* refusal)
拒按 refusal of pressure

俱 [jù]（形容词）两者 both
表里俱热 heat in both the exterior and interior
表里俱虚 deficiency in both the exterior and interior
脉阴阳俱浮 floating pulse at both yin and yang
（动词）相一致 to harmonize (*n.* harmony)
形与神俱 harmony between physique and spirit

聚 [jù]（动词）积聚；聚集 to aggregate; to cluster (*n.* aggregation)
聚证 accumulation syndrome
积聚 aggregation-accumulation
聚星障 star-clustered nebula; superficial punctate keratitis

卷 [juǎn]（动词）把东西弯转裹成卷 to form into a curl, or to curl
舌卷囊缩 curled tongue and retracted testicles
（名词）弯转裹成的筒形物 anything rolled up in cylindrical form, namely, a roll
艾卷 moxa roll
艾卷灸 moxa-roll moxibustion

倦 [juàn]（名词）疲倦 fatigue
劳倦 overstrain (and fatigue)
饮食劳倦 improper diet and overstrain

绝 [jué]（动词）①停断 to pause
经绝 menopause
绝经前后诸病 menopausal diseases
②（生命）终结 to expire (*n.* expiry); to die (*adj.* dying, moribund)
绝汗 expiry sweating
七绝脉 seven moribund pulses

厥 [jué]（名词）①突然昏倒 temporary loss of consciousness, namely, syncope
厥证 syncope
气厥 *qi* syncope
痰厥 phlegm syncope
②四肢逆冷 reversed cold limbs (cold limbs due to reversed *qi* flow)

手足厥冷 **reversed cold of hands and feet**

厥心痛 heart pain with cold limbs

（形容词）向相反方向转化的 reverting

厥阴 reverting yin

厥阴病 reverting yin disease

君 [jūn]（名词）君主 sovereign

君火 sovereign fire

君臣佐使 sovereign, minister, adjuvant and courier; chief, associate, assistant and guide

君药 sovereign ingredient; chief ingredient

菌 [jūn]（名词）菌类，例如蘑菇 fungus, e.g., mushroom (In traditional Chinese medicine, a benign mass of tissue resembling a mushroom refers to polyp, and a malignant one refers to cancer.)

耳菌 ear polyp

鼻菌 nasal polyp

舌菌 tongue cancer

喉菌 throat cancer

皲 [jūn]（名词）皲裂 chap; rhagas

皲裂疮 rhagades

峻 [jùn]（形容词）峻烈的 drastic

峻下 drastic purgation

峻下逐水药 drastic hydragogue

K

咯 [kǎ]（动词）使东西从咽喉或气管出来 to expel from the throat or respiratory tract

咯血 expectoration of blood from the respiratory tract → **hemoptysis**

开 [kāi]（动词）①打开 to open

开鬼门 opening the "devil's gates"; opening sweat pores

开窍 opening the orifices → inducing resuscitation

芳香开窍药 aromatic orifice-opening medicinal/drug → aromatic stimulant

开阖补泻 open-closed reinforcement and reduction

②散开 to disperse (*n.* dispersion)

辛开苦泄 dispersion with the pungent and purgation with the bitter

开泄 dispersion and purgation

③挖开 to dredge

开达膜原；开达募原 dredging the pleura-diaphragmatic space

（其他）

开胃 improving appetite

亢 [kàng]（形容词）亢盛的 hyperactive (*n.* hyperactivity)

阴虚阳亢 yin deficiency with yang hyperactivity

肝阳上亢 ascendant hyperactivity of liver yang

肝阳亢盛 hyperactivity of liver yang

心火亢盛 exuberance of heart fire

肾火偏亢 hyperactive kidney fire

尻 [kāo]（名词）尾骶部 sacral region

尻骨 sacrum

靠 [kào]（动词）依着 to lean against

靠坐 leaning sitting

颗 [kē]（名词）颗粒 granule (*adj.* granular)

颗粒剂 granules

颗粒型皮内针 granular intradermal needle

髁 [kē]（名词）髁即髋 hip

髁骨 hipbone

咳 [ké]（动词）咳嗽 to cough (*n.* cough)

咳声重浊 deep dull cough

咳声清脆 clear crisp cough

咳声不扬 muffled cough

咳如犬吠 barking cough

渴 [kě]（名词）口渴 thirst

口渴引饮 thirst with frequent drinking

口渴喜冷 thirst with preference for cold drinks

克 [kè]（动词）克制 to restrict (*n.* restriction)

五行相克 **restriction among the five elements/phases**

木克土 **wood restricting earth**

土克水 **earth restricting water**

客 [kè]（名词）宾客 guest

客运 **guest circuit**

客气 **guest *qi***

（动词）由外面侵入 to intrude

客邪 **intruding pathogen**

客忤 **intruding fright seizure**

客忤夜啼 **night crying due to** (intruding) **fright**

（形容词）不同于主要的；不期而至的 varied from normal; coming from time to time

客色 **varied normal complexion**

客热 **irregular recurrent fever**

空 [kōng]（形容词）空的 empty

空痛 **empty pain**

空腹服 **to be taken on an empty stomach**

孔 [kǒng]（名词）孔洞 opening; hole

孔窍 outer opening in the body → **orifice**

鼻孔 opening of the nose → **nostril**

耳孔 **ear-hole**

廷孔 opening of the urethra on female body surface → **external urethral orifice (of the female)**

恐 [kǒng]（名词）恐惧 fear

恐 **fear**

控 [kòng]（动词）牵涉 to involve

控睾 pain involving the testicle → **referred testicular pain**

（其他）

控脑砂 **rhinorrhea with turbid discharge; sinusitis**

抠 [kōu]（动词）用手指挖 to dig with the finger

抠法 **digging (manipulation)**

芤 [kōu]（名词）古代称葱为芤 archaic name for scallion

芤脉 a pulse felt like touching a scallion stalk → **hollow pulse**

口 [kǒu]（名词）嘴 mouth

口眼㖞斜 **deviated eye and mouth**

口噤 inability to open the mouth → **lockjaw; trismus**

口疮；口疳 small ulcer in the mouth → **aphtha**

口中和 normal taste in the mouth → **harmony in the mouth**

口淡 **bland taste in the mouth**

口苦 **bitter taste in the mouth**

叩［扣］[kòu]（动词）轻轻敲打 to tap

叩［扣］法 **tapping** (manipulation)

叩［扣］齿 tapping the upper and lower teeth on each other → **clicking the teeth**

枯 [kū]（动词）①枯槁 to wither

荣枯老嫩 **luxuriant, withered, tough and tender-soft**

枯痔法 method of treating hemorrhoids by making them withered → **necrotizing therapy for hemorrhoids**

偏枯 withering (or functional loss) of one side of the body → **hemiplegia**

②枯竭 to be exhausted

津枯肠燥 **fluid exhaustion with intestinal dryness**

苦 [kǔ]（形容词）苦味的 bitter

辛开苦泄 **dispersion with the pungent and purgation with the bitter**

苦寒清热 **clearing heat with the bitter-cold**

苦寒泻火 **discharging fire with the bitter-cold**

苦温燥湿 **drying dampness with the bitter-warm**

（动词）为某种事物所苦 to suffer from something

苦夏 suffering from (harsh climate conditions of) summer → **summer affliction**

胯 [kuà]（名词）腰和大腿之间的部分 the area of the body between the top of the leg and the waist, namely, the hip
胯骨 hipbone
伸腰沉胯 stretching the waist and keeping the hips sunken
胯腹痈 abscess at the ventral side of the part of the body between the thighs → **inguinal abscess**

宽 [kuān]（动词）①宽松 to loosen
宽解衣带 loosening clothes
②宽舒 to soothe
行气宽胸 moving *qi* to soothe the chest
宽胸散结 soothing the chest and dissipating stagnation
宽中散结 soothing the middle and dissipating stagnation

髋 [kuān]（名词）同"胯" same as 胯 [kuà], i.e., the hip or the part between the top of the leg and the waist
髋骨 hipbone

狂 [kuáng]（名词）躁狂 mania
狂；躁狂 mania
狂言 manic raving
狂病 manic psychosis

溃 [kuì]（动词）①破溃 to rupture (*n.* rupture)
溃坚 promoting rupture
②溃烂 to ulcerate
溃疡 ulcerating sore → **ulcer**

L

拉 [lā]（动词）牵拉；拖 to pull; to drag
拉法；牵拉法 the way of pulling → **traction**
牵拉肩 dragged shoulder
拉腿手法 leg-pulling manipulation

蜡 [là]（名词）制作蜡烛的物质 material used in making candles, namely, wax
蜡丸 wax-coated pill; waxed pill

癞 [lài]　（名词）①麻风病 leprosy
癞病 leprosy
②皮肤病引起的毛发脱落或表皮凹凸不平 hair loss or occurrence of unsmoothed skin surface due to skin disease
疥癞 scabies (with unsmoothed skin)

阑 [lán]（名词）《说文》门遮也 screen
阑门 screen gate → **ileocecal conjunction**
阑尾 tail growing out of the screen gate → **vermiform appendix**

蓝 [lán]（形容词）蓝色的 blue (*v.* to make blue → to blue)
白睛青蓝 blueing the white of the eye

烂 [làn]（名词）糜烂；溃烂 erosion; ulceraton (*adj.* ulcerated, ulcerative)
烂喉痧；烂喉丹痧 erosion of the throat with erythema → **scarlatina angionosa**
烂疔 ulcerated gangrene; gas gangrene
睑弦糜烂 ulceration of the palpebral margin; ulcerative marginal blepharitis
眦帷赤烂 erosion of the canthal eyelid; blepharitis angularis

劳 [láo]（名词）①虚劳 consumption (*adj.* consumptive)
劳咳；劳嗽 consumptive cough
虚劳（病）consumptive disease
肺劳 (1) lung consumption; (2) lung phthisis
房劳 sexual consumption
②劳倦 overstrain
饮食劳倦 improper diet and overstrain
劳淋 overstrain stranguria
劳复 relapse due to overstrain
③通"痨" same as phthisis
劳［痨］瘵 phthisis

牢 [láo]（形容词）牢固 firm
牢脉 firm pulse

痨 [láo]（名词）痨病 phthisis
痨病 phthisic disease; phthisis
痨瘵 phthisis
肺痨；肺劳 lung phthisis

老 [lǎo]（形容词）与“嫩”相反 tough, the opposite of tender-soft
荣枯老嫩 luxuriant, withered, tough and tender-soft

烙 [lào]（动词）烧灼（伤口）to burn (a wound); to cauterize (*n.* cauterization)
烙法 cauterization

雷 [léi]（名词）打雷 thunder (*adj.* thunderous)
雷头风 thunder head wind
腹中雷鸣 thunderous borborygmus
雷火神针 thunder fire miraculous moxibustion

肋 [lèi]（名词）肋骨 rib
季肋 region overlying the lowest ribs → **hypochondrium**

泪 [lèi]（名词）眼泪 tear; lacrima (Latin for tear) (*adj.* lacrimal)
泪泉 lacrimal gland
泪窍 lacrimal punctum
迎风流泪 lacrimination induced by wind
流泪证 morbid secretion of tears → **dacryorrhea syndrome**
不时泪溢 excessive secretion of tears from time to time → **epiphora**

类 [lèi]（动词）类似 to resemble
类中风 disease resembling wind stroke → **apoplectic wind stroke; apoplexy**
类中 apoplectic stroke

棱 [léng]（名词）①边缘 edge
三棱针 three-edged needle
②物体表面上的条状突起 a raised narrow strip on the surface of something, namely, ridge
眉棱骨 supra-orbital ridge

冷 [lěng]（形容词）寒冷的 cold
冷汗 cold sweats
冷痛 cold pain
贪食生冷 overindulgence in raw and cold food
冷瘴 cold miasmic malaria 冷服 to be taken cold

离 [lí]（动词）分开 to separate (*n.* separation)
阴阳离决 separation of yin and yang
离而复合 reunion after separation
欲合先离 separation before reunion
离体周天 heavenly circuit running separately from the body → **extracorporeal cosmic cycle**

里 [lǐ]（名词，形容词）①内部；内部的 interior
里寒 interior cold
里热 interior heat
里急后重 interior distress with ineffectual urge to evacuate → **tenesmus**
里虚寒证 interior deficiency cold syndrome/pattern
里实证 interior excess syndrome
②后面；后面的 back (*prefix*: retro-)
里喉痈 retropharyngeal abscess

理 [lǐ]（动词）调理 to regulate
理中 regulating the middle
理气和血 regulating *qi* and harmonizing blood
理气止痛 regulating *qi* to relieve pain
理血药 blood-regulating medicinal/drug
理筋手法 tendon-regulating manipulation; therapeutic manipulation for tendon injury

历 [lì]（形容词）遍历 multiple
历节风 multiple arthralgia

立 [lì]（动词）站立 to stand
立迟 retardation of standing

利 [lì]（动词）①通利 to drain; to promote draining
利湿 draining dampness

利湿药 dampness-draining medicinal/drug
利胆退黄药 bile-draining anti-icteric (medicinal/drug)
②利尿 to increase the excretion of urine (*n.* diuresis; *adj.* diuretic)
利水渗湿 inducing diuresis to drain dampness
利水消肿 inducing diuresis to alleviate edema
利水渗湿药 dampness-draining diuretic (medicinal/drug)
利尿逐水药 diuretic hydragogue (medicinal/drug)
③清利，通畅 to disinhibit
利气 disinhibiting *qi*
利咽 disinhibiting the throat → **relieving sore throat**

沥 [lì]（动词）液体一滴一滴地落下 to dribble
鼻沥血 dribbling of blood from the nose → **nosebleed**
余沥不尽 dribbling after voiding
沥血腰痛 lumbago caused supposedly by blood dribbling into the lumbar region → **blood-stasis lumbago**
沥浆产；沥浆生；沥胞生 untimely dribbling of amniotic fluid during delivery → **premature amniotic rupture**

疠 [lì]（名词）①疫疠 pestilence (*adj.* pestilential)
疠气；戾气；疫疠之气 pestilential *qi*; epidemic pathogen
②麻风病 leprosy
疠风 leprosy

戾 [lì]（名词）疫疠 pestilence (*adj.* pestilential)
戾气 pestilential *qi*; epidemic pathogen
时行戾气 seasonal epidemic pathogen

栗 [lì]（动词）发抖 to shiver (*n.* shiver)
战栗 shiver

粒 [lì]（名词）①颗粒 granule (*adj.* granular)
颗粒剂 granules
颗粒型皮内针 granular intradermal needle
②谷粒 grain
麦粒灸 wheat-grain-sized cone moxibustion
麦粒型皮内针 wheat-grain intradermal needle

痢 [lì]（名词）痢疾 dysentery
湿热痢 dampness-heat dysentery
疫毒痢 epidemic toxic dysentery
噤口痢 food-denial dysentery
休息痢 intermittent dysentery
迁延痢 protracted dysentery

连 [lián]（动词）粘连 to adhere
连舌 adhered tongue → **ankyloglossia**
（形容词）连续不断的 incessant
目连劄 incessant blinking; frequent nictitation

莲 [lián]（名词）莲花即荷花 lotus
莲花舌 lotus tongue

廉 [lián]（名词）某方面的侧边 side facing towards a certain direction, i.e., aspect
臂内廉 inner aspect of the arm
臂外廉 outer aspect of the arm

臁 [lián]（名词）胫的两侧 lateral aspect of the shank
臁疮 shank sore

敛 [liǎn]（动词）收敛；遏制 to astringe; to arrest
敛汗 arresting sweating
敛汗固脱 arresting sweating to prevent collapse
敛肺止咳 astringing the lung to stop coughing
敛汗固表药 sweating-arresting and superficies-strengthening medicinal/drug
敛肺止咳剂 lung-astringing antitussive formula

练 [liàn]（动词）锻炼；训练 to practice; to train
练功 practicing *qigong*
练气 training *qi*
练神 training of the mind

炼 [liàn]（动词）修炼 to cultivate
炼气 cultivating *qi*
炼神 cultivating the mind
炼精化气 cultivating essence to become *qi*
炼气化神 cultivating *qi* to become mentality
（其他）
炼丹 (1) alchemy; (2) physiological alchemy

良 [liáng]（形容词）良好的 good
良方 a medicinal formula that gives good therapeutic effect → **effective formula**

凉 [liáng]（形容词）稍冷，微寒 cool
凉燥证 cool-dryness syndrome/pattern
辛凉轻剂 mild pungent-cool formula
辛凉平剂 moderate pungent-cool formula
辛凉重剂 drastic pungent-cool formula
（动词）变凉，使变凉 to cool
凉血散瘀 cooling the blood and dissipating stasis
凉血止血 cooling the blood to stop bleeding
滋阴凉血 replenishing yin and cooling blood
凉肝熄风 cooling the liver to extinguish wind

两 [liǎng]（数词）二 two
两眼无光 (two) **lusterless eyes**
（代词）两者 both
两眼翻上 upward rotation of both eyes → **supraduction**
气营两燔 blazing of both *qi* and nutrient
气血两亏 insufficiency of both *qi* and blood
气血两虚 deficiency of both *qi* and blood
心脾两虚 deficiency in both the heart and spleen
（形容词）双重的 dual
阴阳两虚 dual deficiency of yin-yang

量 [liàng]（名词）数量 amount
剂量 amount of medicine to be taken at one time → **dosage**

疗 [liáo]（动词）治疗 to treat (*n.* 疗法 therapy: treatment of illness, especially without using drugs)
牵引疗法 traction therapy
结扎疗法 ligation therapy
挂线疗法 threaded ligation therapy
药捻疗法 medicated spill therapy
一指禅推拿疗法 *qi*-concentrated single-finger pushing therapy

髎 [liáo]（名词）骨节之间 intra-articular space
脱髎 displacement of a bone or bones from a joint → **dislocation; luxation**

裂 [liè]（名词）裂缝，裂隙 fissure
裂纹舌 fissured tongue
舌裂 fissure of the tongue
肛裂 anal fissure
（动词）裂开 cleave
腭裂 cleft palate

临 [lín]（动词）就要做某事 to be going to
临睡前服 to be taken before bed-time
临产 going to delivery → **labor; parturition**
临产病 parturient diseases

鳞 [lín]（名词）鱼鳞 scale (*adj.* scaly)
白陷鱼鳞 scaly nebula with sunken center; ulcerative keratitis

淋 [lìn]（名词）小便涩痛，滴沥不尽 a slow and painful, drop-by-drop discharge of urine, viz., stranguria
淋；淋证 stranguria
淋浊 stranguria with turbid discharge
（其他）
淋病 gonorrhea

凌 [líng]（动词）侵袭 to attack; to invade
水气凌心 **retained fluid attacking the heart**
风湿凌目证 **syndrome/pattern of wind-dampness invading the eye**
流金凌木 flow of metal (the bulbar conjunctiva) invading wood (the cornea) → **pseudopterygium**

另 [lìng]（副词）另行 separately
另煎 **to be decocted separately**

留 [liú]（动词）停留 to retain
留针 **retaining the needle; needle retention**
留针候气 **retaining the needle to await *qi***
留罐 **retained cupping**
留针拔罐 **cupping with retaining of needle**

流 [liú]（动词）流动 to flow
流涎 flowing of saliva from the mouth → **drooling**
流注 an abscess with the pus flowing from another place → **metastatic abscess**
流泪证 overabundant flow of tear → **dacryorrhea syndrome**
流金凌木 flow of metal (bulbar conjunctiva) invading wood (cornea) → **pseudopterygium**

瘤 [liú]（名词）肿瘤 tumor
气瘤 *qi* tumor → **neurofibroma**
血瘤 blood tumor → **hemangioma**
肉瘤 flesh tumor → **lipoma**
筋瘤 sinew tumor → **varix**
脂瘤 fat tumor → **sebaceous cyst**

六 [liù]（数词）六 six
六腑 **six *fu* organs; six bowels**
六经辨证 **six-meridian/channel syndrome differentiation; six-meridian/channel pattern identification**
六经病 **diseases of the six meridians/channels**
六阴脉 **six yin meridians/channels**
六阳脉 **six yang meridians/channels**

龙 [lóng]（名词）传说中的神异动物 dragon or loong, a legendary creature
龙衔式 **dragon-mouth gesture**
苍龙摆尾法 **method of "dark dragon wagging its tail"**
赤龙搅海 **"red dragon stirring the sea"**

聋 [lóng]（形容词）耳聋的 deaf (*n.* deafness)
耳聋 **deafness**
暴聋；卒聋 **sudden deafness**
渐聋 **progressive deafness**
耳聋口哑 **deaf-mutism**

癃 [lóng]（名词）小便不利 reduction in the flow of urine; ischuria
癃闭 **ischuria**
精癃 **prostatic hypertrophy** (with ischuria)

蝼 [lóu]（名词）蝼蛄 mole cricket
蝼蛄疖 **mole cricket boil; folliculitis abscedens et suffodiens**

瘘 [lòu]（名词）瘘管 fistula
耳瘘 **ear fistula**
肛瘘 **anal fistula**

漏 [lòu]（动词）①渗漏 to leak
漏汗 **leaking sweating**
屋漏脉 **roof-leaking pulse**
②子宫不正常的小量出血 to bleed abnormally in small amounts from the uterus, namely, to spot
崩漏 **flooding and spotting; metrorrhagia and metrostaxis**
漏下 **spotting; metrostaxis**
（名词）①瘘管 fistula
脐漏 **umbilical fistula**
乳漏 **mammary fistula**
肛漏 **anal fistula**
②外流 outflow
漏睛；漏睛眼；漏睛脓出 outflow of pus from the canthus → **dacryopyorrhea; chronic dacryocystitis**
漏睛疮 acute inflammation of the lacrimal

sac with outflow of pus → **dacryocyst sore; acute dacryocystitis**

颅 [lú]（名词）头颅 skull
头颅骨 skull; cranium
解颅 ununited skull → **hydrocephalus**

露 [lù]（名词）药物加水蒸馏而得的液体 liquid product condensed from vapor during distillation, namely distillate
露；露剂 distillate
（动词）显露 to show; to be visible
昏睡露睛 lethargic sleeping with the eyes open (with the eyeballs visible)

鹭 [lù]（名词）鹭鸶 egret
鹭鸶咳 egret's cough; pertussis

绿 [lǜ]（形容词）绿色的 green; greenish
绿风；绿风内障 greenish glaucoma

挛 [luán]（动词）挛缩 to contract (*n.* contracture)
拘挛 contracture

乱 [luàn]（名词）①混乱 disorder
神乱 mental disorder
②紊乱 derangement
经气逆乱 derangement of meridian/channel *qi*
③动乱 turmoil
霍乱 (1) choleraic turmoil; (2) cholera
霍乱转筋 cramp in choleraic turmoil
转筋霍乱 choleraic turmoil with cramp
寒气霍乱 cold-*qi* choleraic turmoil
（形容词）不规则的 irregular
经乱 irregular periods

轮 [lún]（名词）轮状结构 a wheel-like structure such as orbiculus or helix
五轮 five orbiculi
耳轮 helix
轮屏切迹 helix notch

瘰 [luǒ]（名词）瘰疬，即颈淋巴结结核 scrofula or tuberculosis of lymph nodes in the neck
瘰疬 scrofula

络 [luò]（名词）络脉 collateral
络脉 collateral vessel
络刺 collateral needling
（动词）联络 to connect
络穴 connecting points

落 [luò]（动词）①掉落 to lose (*n.* loss)
发落 loss of hair → **alopecia**
齿落 loss of teeth → **dedentition**
②脱落 to peel
舌苔脱落 peeling of the tongue coating/fur

捋 [lǚ]（动词）用手指抹过去，使物体顺溜 to move the hand over something to make it smooth, i.e., to stroke
顺骨捋筋 tendon-stroking along the bone

M

麻 [má]（名词）①麻木 numbness
麻木 numbness
②麻疹 measles
麻毒 measles toxin
麻毒陷肺 measles toxin penetrating into the lung
麻疹顺证 favorable syndrome/pattern of measles
麻疹逆证 unfavorable syndrome/pattern of measles
麻疹险证 critical case of measles
（其他）
奶麻 roseola infantum; exathema subitum
麻风 leprosy

马 [mǎ]（名词）畜名 horse
马脾风 horse-spleen wind → sudden dyspnea due to wind attacking the heart and spleen (Horse is used as a byword for the heart hearby, since both the animal horse and the organ heart pertain to fire according to the five-element theory.) → **acute asthmatic attack**

马牙 eruption of yellowish nodules on the gums of a newborn like the teeth erupton of a horse → **gingival eruption**

走马牙疳；走马疳 an ulcerative gingivitis that develops as rapidly as a horse runs → **noma; cancrum oris**

（其他）

马桶癣 chamber-pot dermatitis

埋 [mái]（动词）埋藏 to embed

埋针疗法 needle-embedding therapy

穴位埋线疗法 acupoint catgut-embedding therapy

麦 [mài]（名词）通常指小麦 wheat

麦粒型皮内针 wheatgrain intradermal needle

麦粒灸 wheat-grain-sized cone moxibustion

脉 [mài]（名词）①脉搏 pulse

切脉 pulse taking

脉象 pulse manifestation; pulse condition

脉诊 pulse diagnosis

脉从四时；脉应四时 congruity of pulse with the seasons

脉悬绝 extremely abnormal pulse

脉症合参 comprehensive analysis of the pulse and symptoms

②脉管 vessel

脉口 "vessel opening"

脉痿 vessel atrophy-flaccidity

脉痹 vessel impediment

满 [mǎn]（形容词）全部充实，没有余地的 containing as much as possible leaving no empty space, namely full (*n.* fullness)

腹满 abdominal fullness

腹满腹胀 abdominal fullness and distension

少腹硬满 lower abdominal rigidity and fullness

痞满 stuffiness and fullness

心下满 fullness below the heart; epigastric fullness

慢 [màn]（形容词）①缓慢的 slow

慢火 slow fire

紧按慢提 swift thrusting and slow lifting

②慢性的 chronic; gradual

慢惊风 chronic infantile convulsion

慢脾风 chronic convulsion due to spleen disorder

慢惊自汗 chronic convulsion with incessant sweating

慢喉喑［瘖］chronic hoarseness or aphonia

慢性复位 gradual reduction

芒 [máng]（名词）芒刺 prickle

舌起芒刺 prickles on the tongue

芒刺舌 prickly tongue

盲 [máng]（形容词）眼睛的 blind (*n.* blindness)

盲；目盲 blindness

暴盲 sudden blindness

青盲 bluish blindness

雀盲 sparrow's blindness; night blindness; nyctalopia

猫 [māo]（名词）一种家畜名 cat

猫眼疮 sores resembling a cat's eyes → **erythema multiforme**

毛 [máo]（名词）动植物表皮上生长的丝状物 a filamentous outgrowth of the epidermis of an animal or plant, namely the hair

毛际 border of the region where the pubic hair grows → **suprapubic margin**

鼻毛 the hair growing in the nasal cavity → **vibrissa**

皮毛 skin and body hair

毫毛 fine hair of the skin → **down**

丛毛 clustered hair

（形容词）浮浅的 superficial

毛刺 superficial needling

冒 [mào]（动词）感受 to be afflicted（*n.* affliction）

冒暑 summerheat affliction

冒湿 dampness affliction

眉 [méi]（名词）眉毛 eyebrow
眉棱骨 bony prominence at the site of the eyebrow → **supra-orbital ridge**
眉心 center of the eyebrows; glabella
拧眉心 pinching the glabella

梅 [méi]（名词）一种植物名 plum
梅花针 plum-blossom needle
梅核气 "plum-stone *qi*"; globus hystericus

寐 [mèi]（动词）睡觉 to sleep (*n.* sleep)
不寐 sleeplessness
但欲寐 desire only to sleep

门 [mén]（名词）①大门 gate
命门 life gate
温补命门 warming and tonifying the life gate
开鬼门 opening the "ghost gates"; opening sweat pores
吸门 "breath gate"; epiglottis
贲门 "rushing gate"; cardia
②房门 door
户门 "entrance doors"; teeth
飞门 "flying door"; lip
③门口（出入口）opening; orifice
玉门 virginal vaginal orifice
龙门 nulliparous vaginal orifice
胞门 parous vaginal orifice
产门 parturient vaginal orifice
畜门 opening of smelling → **nostril**
咽门 opening of the pharynx

闷 [mèn]（形容词）①满闷；懑闷 stuffy; oppressed
闷痛 stuffy pain
胸闷 thoracic oppression
②晕闷 drowsy
闷痧 drowsy filthy attack

蒙 [méng]（动词）①使蒙眬；使糊涂 to cloud; to confuse
痰蒙心神 phlegm clouding the mind
痰蒙心包 phlegm clouding the pericardium
昏蒙 mental confusion
②变昏暗 to dim
徇蒙招尤 dizziness with dimmed vision and shaking

猛 [měng]（形容词）来势凶险的 ominous
猛疽 ominous (throat) abscess

梦 [mèng]（名词）寐中所见事形 a series of images or scenes passing through mind during sleep, namely, dream
梦遗 dream emission; nocturnal emission
多梦 profuse dreaming; dreamfulness

迷 [mí] (动词) 使模糊不清 to mist
痰迷心窍 phlegm misting the heart orifices
（名词）昏迷 coma
中风昏迷 apoplectic coma

糜 [mí]（动词）糜烂；溃疡 to erode (*n.* erosion); to ulcerate (*n.* ulceration; ulcer)
口唇糜烂 erosion of the lips
口糜 oral erosion; ulcerative stomatitis
经行口糜 menstrual oral ulcer; oral ulcer during menstruation
睑弦糜烂 ulceration of the palpebral margin

秘 [mì]（形容词）秘密的 secret
秘方 secret formula
祖传秘方 secret formula handed down in a family

蜜 [mì]（名词）蜂蜜 honey
蜜炙 stir-baking with honey
蜜丸 honeyed pill

棉 [mián]（名词）棉花 cotton
棉枕固定 fixation with cotton-pad
贴棉法 cotton-burning cupping

面 [miàn]（名词）①脸 face (*adj.* facial)
面色 (facial) complexion
面浮 puffy face
面针 facial acupuncture
面游风 (facial) **seborrhea; seborrheic dermatitis**

②面色 complexion
面色皖白 bright pale complexion
面黄肌瘦 sallow complexion with emaciation
面红 reddened complexion
面尘 dusty complexion
③粉末 powder
药面 medicinal powder
（动词）面对 to face
面壁 facing a wall

苗 [miáo]（名词）苗头 sign or signal
苗窍 signal orifices
审苗窍 inspection of the signal orifices

眇 [miǎo] (名词) 一只眼睛瞎 blindness in one eye
眇目 monocular blindness

名 [míng]（名词）名称 name
无名肿毒 toxic swelling without a name **→ innominate toxic swelling**
同名经配穴法 combination of points from the meridians/channels with the same name

明 [míng]（形容词）①明亮的 bright
明堂 "bright hall"; (euphemism for) **apex of the nose**
②直白的 direct
明灸 direct moxibustion
（名词）光亮 light
羞明；畏明；羞明畏日 fear of light → **photophobia**
（其他）明目 to improve vision
清热明目 clearing heat to improve vision
清肝明目clearing the liver to improve vision
退翳明目 removing nebula to improve vision

鸣 [míng]（动词）发出声音 to produce sound; to ring
鸣天鼓 "sounding the celestial drum"
喘鸣 dyspnea with sound (produced in the airway) → **wheezing dyspnea**
肠鸣 sound produced in the intestines → **borborygmus**
耳鸣 ringing in the ear; tinnitus

瞑 [míng]（名词）视物昏花 dim vision or dimness of vision
瞑眩 dimness of vision

命 [mìng]（名词）生命 life
命门 life gate
命门之火 life gate fire
命火 life fire
命关 life pass

摸 [mō]（动词）用手接触或抚摸 to touch or palpate
摸法 palpating
手摸心会 comprehending (or perceiving) **by touching**

膜 [mó]（名词）体内像薄皮的组织 a thin layer of tissue inside the body, namely, the membrane
耳膜 tympanic membrane; eardrum
白膜蔽睛 white membrane covering the eye → pannus
黄膜上冲 upsurging of the yellow membrane → hypopyon
（其他）
膜原 pleurodiaphragmatic interspace
开达膜原 dredging the pleurodiaphragmatic space

摩 [mó]（动词）摩擦 to rub in a circular motion
摩法 circular rubbing (manipulation)
摩颈项 rubbing the neck
摩腹 rubbing the abdomen
摩脐 rubbing the navel
掌摩法 palmar circular rubbing manipulation

抹 [mǒ]（动词）擦抹 to wipe
抹法 wiping (with the palm or thumb)
抹前额 wiping the forehead (with fingers)

沫 [mò]（名词）泡沫 froth (*adj.* frothy)
痰如泡沫 frothy sputum

母 [mǔ]（名词）母亲 mother
母气 mother (element/phase) *qi*
子母补泻法 mother-son reinforcing and reducing method

牡 [mǔ]（形容词）雄性的 male
牡脏 male *zang* organs; male viscera

拇 [mǔ]（名词）拇指 thumb
拇指同身寸 thumb body-*cun*; thumb body-inch

木 [mù]（名词）①五行之一的木 wood, one member of the five elements/phases
木生火 wood generating fire
木克土 wood restricting earth
木乘土 wood overrestricting earth
木火刑金 wood fire tormenting metal
木形之人 wood-featured person
②麻木 numbness
肌肤麻木 numbness of the skin
（形容词）木头似的 wooden
木舌 wooden tongue

目 [mù]（名词）眼睛 eye
目胞；目裹 eyelid; palpebra
目上弦 margin of the upper eyelid
目眶骨 bones forming the eye socket → **orbit bone**
目连劄；目劄 involuntary frequent closing and opening the eye → **frequent nictitation**
目偏视 inability of one eye to attain binocular vision with the other → **squint; strabismus**

募 [mù]（名词）与"膜"通，常指肋膜和膈膜 same as 膜 [mó], membrane, usually referring to pleura and diaphragm
募原 pleurodiaphragmatic space
开达募原 dredging the pleurodiaphragmatic space

暮 [mù]（名词）傍晚 evening
暮食朝吐 vomiting in the morning of food eaten in the previous evening
朝食暮吐 vomiting in the evening of food eaten in the morning

N

拿 [ná]（动词）用手抓住 to grasp
拿法 grasping manipulation
拿捏法 grasping and pinching
拿颈项 grasping the neck and nape
拿合谷 grasping *Hegu* (LI 4)

纳 [nà]（动词）①接受 to receive or to take (*n.* reception)
纳呆 no interest in taking food → **anorexia**
纳气 receiving air → **inspiration**
纳气平喘 improving *qi* reception to relieve asthma
吐纳 expelling and receiving air → **breathing in and out**
②采纳 to adopt (*n.* adoption)
纳甲法；纳干法 selection of acupoints by adoption of the heavenly stems → **day-prescription of points**
纳子法；纳支法 selection of acupoints by adoption of the earthly branches → **hour-prescription of points**
③放进 to put something into
纳入原位 putting (a dislocated bone) into its normal position → **manual restoration**

捺 [nà]（动词）用手按 to press with the hand
捺法 pressing-grasping
端提捺正 holding, lifting, and (pressing for) **restoring to the right location**
捺正 manual correction

奶 [nǎi]（名词）乳汁 milk
奶癣 milk lichen; infantile eczema
（形容词）哺乳婴儿的 infantile
奶麻 roseola infantum; exathema subitum

难 [nán]（形容词）困难的，与易相对

difficult, the opposite of easy
难产；产难 difficult labor; dystocia

囊 [náng]（名词）口袋，医学上常指阴囊 bag, in medicine usually referring to one that contains the testicles, namely, the scrotum (*adj.* scrotal)
囊痈 scrotal abscess
肾囊风 scrotal eczema
舌卷囊缩 curled tongue and retracted testicles

挠 [náo]（动词）用手指甲搔抓 to rub the skin with the nails, namely, to scratch
挠法 scratching

脑 [nǎo]（名词）脑髓 brain
脑漏 brain leakage → rhinorrhea with turbid discharge → **sinusitis**
脑衄 severe epistaxis as if the brain were bleeding → **severe epistaxis**
脑风 brain wind; chronic or recurrent headache
醒脑 arousing the brain; inducing resuscitation

臑 [nào]（名词）肩下肘上的肱部 the region of the arm below the shoulder and above the elbow, namely, the humeral region
臑 humeral region
臑骨 humerus

内 [nèi]（形容词）①里面 internal; within (*prefix*: intra-)
内燥证 internal dryness syndrome/pattern
内消 elimination from within
内托 expulsion from within
皮内针 intradermal needle
②向里面 inward
内陷 inward invasion

嫩 [nèn]（形容词）柔嫩的，与“老”相反 tender-soft, the opposite of tough
荣枯老嫩 luxuriant, withered, tough and tender-soft

能 [néng]（动词）能够 to be able to (*n.* ability)
能近怯远症 ability to see things clearly only at a short distance → **nearsightedness; myopia**
能远怯近症 better vision for distant than for near objects → **farsightedness; hyperopia**
另见：能 [tài]

泥 [ní]（名词）泥土 mud
泥丸 mud ball; upper *dantian* or *Baihui* (GV 20)
存泥丸 preserving the mud ball → **rubbing the forehead to the top**

逆 [nì]（形容词）①反向的，不利的 adverse
逆传 adverse transmission
逆传心包 adverse transmission to the pericardium
②倒转的 inverted
逆经 inverted menstruation → **vicarious menstruation**
③不顺利的 unfavorable
麻疹逆证 unfavorable syndrome/pattern of measles
④与环境不协调的 incongruous (*n.* incongruity)
脉逆四时 incongruity of pulses with the seasons
⑤对抗作用的 counteracting
逆治 counteracting treatment
（动词）反向而行；颠倒 counterflow; reverse (*n.* counterflow; reversal)
气逆 *qi* counterflow
肝气横逆 transverse counterflow of liver *qi*
肺气上逆 upward counterflow of lung *qi*
咳逆上气 cough with reversed ascent of *qi*
喘逆 dyspnea with reversed flow of *qi*
（其他）
逆流挽舟 “rowing upstream”
逆腹式呼吸 antidromic abdominal breathing

腻 [nì]（形容词）油腻的；黏腻的 greasy; slimy
腻苔 greasy (tongue) coating/fur; slimy (tongue) coating/fur
口黏腻 sticky slimy sensation in the mouth

年 [nián]（名词）① 日历年 (calendar) year (*adj*. annual: happening once every year)
避年 annual menstruation
② 年纪 age
天年 maximum age (of a human) endowed by nature → **natural life span**

捻 [niǎn]（动词）捻转 to twirl; to twist
捻法 twisting
捻转法 twirling
捻转补泻 twirling reinforcement and reduction
（名词）纸捻 a piece of twisted paper, namely a spill
药捻疗法 medicated spill therapy
（其他）
捻衣摸床 floccillation

碾 [niǎn]（动词）轧碎 to crush
碾挫伤 crushing-contusion

尿 [niào]（名词）尿液 urine
尿清长 profuse clear urine
尿短赤 scanty dark urine
尿赤 deep-colored urine
尿血 presence of blood in the urine → **hematuria**
尿浊 turbid urine
（动词）排尿 to urinate (*n*. urination)
尿频 frequent urination

捏 [niē]（动词）用拇指和别的手指夹住 to press something tightly with the thumb and finger, i.e., to pinch
捏法 pinching (manipulation)
合指捏法 finger-combining pinching manipulation
屈指捏法 bent-finger pinching anipulation
捏脊 pinching along the spine

颞 [niè]（名词）前额两侧的部位 the region on either side of the forehead, namely the temple (*adj*. temporal)
颞颥 anterior temple
颞前线 anterior temporal line (MS 10)
颞后线 posterior temporal line (MS 11)

宁 [níng]（形容词）安宁的 restful (*ant*. restless)
心气不宁 restlessness of heart *qi*
（动词）使安宁 to calm
化饮宁心 resolving retained fluid to calm the heart
益肾宁神 replenishing the kidney to calm the mind

拧 [nǐng]（动词）① 用手指夹住扭转 to hold tightly between the thumb and finger and turn, i.e., to pinch
拧法 pinching and lifting
拧眉心 pinching the glabella
② 拧转 to turn over
拧拳反掌式 clenching a fist, turning over and opening the hand

凝 [níng]（动词）凝结 to congeal
凝脂翳 fat-congealed nebula → purulent keratitis
寒凝痛经 cold congealing dysmenorrhea
寒凝气滞 *qi* stagnation due to cold congealing

牛 [niú] 畜名 ox
牛皮癣 oxhide lichen → **neurodermatitis**

扭 [niǔ]（动词）扭动 to twist
扭伤 damage by sudden twisting → **sprain**
扭痧 twisting to congestion

浓 [nóng]（形容词）浓缩的 concentrated
浓缩丸 concentrated pill

脓 [nóng]（名词）化脓性炎症所形成的

黄白色汁液 yellowish-white fluid matter formed by suppuration, namely, pus
脓疱 a small circumscribed elevation of the skin containing pus → **pustule**
排脓 expelling pus
提脓拔毒 drawing out pus and toxins
黄脓上冲 upsurging of the yellowish pus → **hypopyon**
（形容词）脓性的；化脓的 purulent; suppurative
脓血便 purulent and bloody stool
脓毒证 purulent toxin syndrome/pattern
脓耳 purulent discharge from the ear → **otopyorrhea; suppurative otitis media**

弄 [nòng]（动词）摆弄 to waggle
弄舌 waggling tongue
吐弄舌 protruding and waggling of tongue
（其他）
弄胎 agitated fetus; false labor

努 [nǔ]（动词）按压拨动 to press and flick
努法 shaft-flicking method

胬 [nǔ]（名词）胬肉 polyp 翼状胬肉 pterygium
胬肉攀睛；胬肉扳睛；胬肉侵睛 pterygium

怒 [nù] 愤怒 anger
怒 anger

女 [nǚ]（名词）女性 female
女子胞 uterus; womb (of the female)
女劳复 relapse due to sex

衄 [nǜ] (名词) 出血，尤指鼻出血 bleeding, especially nosebleed
鼻衄 nosebleed; epistaxis
齿衄 gum bleeding
经行吐衄 menstrual hematemesis and epistaxis
经行衄血 menstrual epistaxis; epistaxis during menstruation
乳衄 bleeding from the nipple → **thelorrhagia**

暖 [nuǎn]（动词）使温暖 to warm
暖宫 warming the uterus
温经暖宫 warming the meridians/channels and the uterus

疟 [nüè]（名词）疟疾 malaria (*adj.* malarial)
瘴疟 miasmic malaria
正疟 ordinary malaria
疟母 malarial mass
疟痞 malarial lump
疟积 malarial accumulation

挪 [nuó]（动词）挪动 to move or to shift
挪法 shifting

O

呕 [ǒu]（动词）呕吐 to vomit
妊娠呕吐 vomiting of pregnancy; hyperemesis gravidarum
呕乳 vomiting of milk
干呕 trying to vomit but without vomitus → **retching**

偶 [ǒu]（形容词）①偶数的 even-numbered
偶方 even-numbered formula/prescription
②成双成对的 paired
偶刺 needling with a pair of needles → **paired needling**

P

拍 [pāi]（动词）用手掌轻轻地打 to repeatedly strike somebody or something gently with the hand flat, i.e., to pat
拍法 patting (manipulation)
拍击法 patting-striking manipulation
指节拍法 knuckle-patting manipulation

排 [pái]（动词）排出；排空；排除 to expel; to evacuate; to get rid of
排脓托毒 evacuating pus and expelling toxins
排脓消肿 evacuating pus and eliminating swelling
托里排脓 evacuating pus from within

排石 expelling calculi
排除杂念 getting rid of mental distractions

攀 [pān]（动词）用手抓住向上爬 to grasp or hold something with hands for climbing
攀索叠砖 holding rope and standing on a pile of bricks
双手攀足式 grasping the feet with both hands

盘 [pán]（名词）盘子 plate（托盘 tray）
托盘疔 tray-like palmar infection; palmar pustule
（动词）回旋地绕 to circle; to surround
盘法；盘旋法 circular needling method
盘肠气痛 *qi* colic surrounding the intestines → **intestinal *qi* colic**
（其他）（盘腿 to be cross-legged）
盘坐 cross-legged sitting
单盘坐 single cross-legged sitting
双盘坐 double cross-legged sitting

旁 [páng]（名词）旁侧 side
舌旁 side of the tongue
（形容词）旁侧的 lateral
额旁1线 lateral line 1 of the forehead (MS 2)
顶旁1线 lateral line 1 of the vertex (MS 8)
枕下旁线 lower-lateral line of the occiput (MS 14)

膀 [páng]（名词）膀胱 (urinary) bladder
膀胱 bladder
膀胱不利 inhibited bladder
膀胱气闭 blockage of bladder *qi*
膀胱失约 failure of bladder retention
膀胱湿热 bladder dampness-heat; dampness-heat in the bladder

胖 [pàng]（名词）肥胖 obesity
肥胖不孕 obesity infertility
（形容词）①丰腴的 plump
舌胖 plump tongue
舌体胖大 plump (enlarged) **tongue body**
胖大舌 (plump) **enlarged tongue**
②肿胀的 puffy
黄胖 yellowish puffiness
黄胖病 yellowish puffy disease

脬 [pāo]（名词）膀胱 (urinary) bladder
脬气不固 insecurity of bladder *qi*

胞 [pāo]（名词）通脬，即膀胱 same as 脬 [pāo] bladder
胞痹 bladder impediment

炮 [páo]（动词）用烘、炒等方法加工制造中药 to treat or prepare by baking, frying, etc. in the manufacturing of Chinese medicinals, namely to process
炮制；炮炙 processing (of materia medica)
药材炮制 processing of medicinal substances

泡 [pào]（名词）①皮肤表面上隆起的水泡 a vesicle on the surface of the skin, containing watery matter, namely a blister
发泡 the process of causing blister formation → **vesiculation**
发泡灸 vesiculating moxibustion
②气泡 bubble
泡腾片a tablet that dissolves in water, giving off gas bubbles → **effervescent tablet**
（动词）浸泡 to soak
泡 soaking; maceration

疱 [pào]（名词）疱 small circumscribed elevation of the skin containing liquid, usually referring to vesicle
疱疹 vesicle
脓疱 small circumscribed elevation of the skin containing pus → **pustule**
水疱 (1) small circumscribed elevation of the skin containing watery liquid → **vesicle; (2) chickenpox**

培 [péi]（动词）（在植物根部或墙根部）增加土 to bank up
培土 banking up earth

培土生金 banking up earth to benefit metal
培土抑木 banking up earth and supressing wood

配 [pèi]（动词）使结合或组合 to combine (*n.* combination)
配方 to combine ingredients according to prescription → **dispense a prescription**
方剂配伍 ingredient combination in a formula/prescription
配穴法 point combination
上下配穴法 upper-lower point combination
左右配穴法 right-left point combination
腹背配穴法 ventro-dorsal point combination

铍 [pī]（名词）针灸用的长针，其形如剑 a long acupuncture needle with the appearance of a sword, namely, a stiletto needle
铍针 stiletto needle

劈 [pī]（动词）由纵面破开 to strike vertically with the intention to split
劈法 vertical palm striking manipulation

皮 [pí]（名词）皮肤 skin
皮毛 skin and body hair
皮痹 skin impediment; skin numbness
皮水 skin edema
（形容词）皮肤的 dermal; cutaneous
皮肤针dermal needle
皮内针 intradermal needle
十二皮部 twelve cutaneous regions

脾 [pí]（名词）脾脏 spleen
脾气虚 spleen *qi* deficiency
脾失健运 dysfunction of the spleen in transportation
脾不统血 spleen failing to control blood
脾胃阳虚 spleen-stomach yang deficiency
脾气下陷证 spleen *qi* sinking syndrome/pattern

痞 [pǐ]（名词）①胸腹部痞满，按之不痛 a non-tender sensation of stuffinesss in the chest or abdomen
痞满 stuffiness and fullness
虚痞 stuffiness of deficiency type
胸痞 thoracic stuffiness
心下痞硬 stuffiness and rigidity below the heart → **epigastric stuffiness and rigidity**
理气消痞 regulating *qi* to relieve stuffiness
②胸腹部的痞块 a mass or lump in the chest or abdomen with a sensation of stuffiness
痞块 stuffy lump; mass
消痞 eliminating mass

癖 [pǐ]（名词）①嗜好 addiction
癖嗜 addiction
酒癖 alcohol addiction
②癖通痞 癖 [pǐ] and 痞 [pǐ] are interchangeable, meaning mass or lump
癖热 fever with hypochondriac mass
乳癖 presence of masses in the breast → **mammary hyperplasia**

睥 [pì]（名词）眼睑 eyelid
睥生痰核 phlegm node of the eyelid → **chalazion**
睥翻粘睑 cicatrical ectropion of eyelid
睥肉粘轮 adhesion between the eyelid and bulbar conjunctiva → **symblepharon**
睥虚如球 ball-like eyelid swelling
睥轮振跳 tic of the eyelid

偏 [piān]（形容词）①偏离的 deviated
偏斜瞻视；目偏视 deviation of the eye → **squint; strabismus**
风牵偏视 squint caused by attack of wind → **paralytic strabismus**
②偏向的 partial
偏嗜 partiality; predilection
饮食偏嗜 dietary partiality
嗜偏食 food partiality
③偏于一侧的 affecting one side (of the body) → hemilateral
偏头痛 hemilateral headache; migraine
偏头风 hemilateral head wind; migraine

偏枯 hemilateral paralysis; hemiplegia
（名词）偏差 deviation
气功偏差 deviation of *qigong*
出偏 deviation (of *qigong*)
（其他）
偏方 special but irregular recipe

胼 [pián]（名词）手脚上的老茧 an area of thick hard skin on the hand or foot, namely, callus
胼胝 callus; callosity

片 [piàn]（名词）①药片 tablet
片；片剂 tablet
②薄片 slice
切片 cutting into slices → **slicing**

频 [pín]（形容词）频繁的 frequent
尿频；小便频数 frequent urination
频服 to be taken frequently

品 [pǐn]（名词）等级 grade
三品 three grades of medicinals
上品 top-grade medicinal
中品 medium-grade medicinal
下品 inferior-grade medicinal

牝 [pìn]（形容词）雌性的 female
牝脏 female *zang* organs; yin viscera
牝疟 yin malaria

平 [píng]（形容词）①平常的 normal
平气 normal circuit *qi*
平息 normal breathing
平脉 normal pulse
②平素的，简单的 plain
平坐 plain sitting
③水平的 horizontal
平刺 horizontal insertion
④不偏不倚的 neutral
平补平泻 neutral reinforcement and reduction
⑤平稳的 steady
平稳出针法 steady withdrawal of the needle
⑥扁平的 flat
平掌式 flat-palm gesture
平垫 flat pad
（动词）①使平静 to pacify
平肝潜阳 pacifying the liver and subduing yang
平肝熄风 pacifying the liver to extinguish wind
平肝熄风药 liver-pacifying and wind-extinguishing medicinal/drug
②平整，矫正 to correct (*n.* correction)
平整复元 correction and reduction
（副词）接近地 close
平旦 close to the daytime → **early morning**
平旦服 to be taken in the early morning

屏 [píng]（名词）耳屏 tragus
对耳屏 antitragus
屏上切迹 supratragic notch
屏间切迹 intertragic notch

迫 [pò]（动词）窘迫 to distress
热迫大肠 heat distressing the large intestine

破 [pò]（动词）破坏 to break
破气 breaking stagnant *qi*
破血；破瘀 breaking blood stasis
破瘀消癥 breaking blood stasis and eliminating masses
破瘀生新 breaking blood stasis and promoting regeneration
破伤风 a disease caused by toxic wind pathogen introduced through a broken wound → **tetanus**

魄 [pò]（名词）依附形体而存在的精神 the part of soul attached to the body
魄 corporeal soul
魄门 "corporeal-soul gate"; anus

薄 [pò]（形容词）通"迫"，急促的 薄 [pò] and 迫 [pò] are interchangeable, meaning sudden
薄厥 sudden syncope
另见：薄 [báo]；薄 [bó]

扑 [pū]（动词）扑敷 to apply (*n.* application)

扑粉 application of medicinal powder

葡 [pú]（名词）葡萄 grape
葡萄胎 abnormal fetus resembling a bunch of grapes → **hydatidiform mole**

Q

七 [qī]（数词）七 seven
七窍 seven orifices
七情 seven emotions
七死脉；七绝脉 seven moribund pulses
七星针 seven-star needle
七星功 seven-star exercise

漆 [qī]（名词）用漆树汁液制成的涂料 paints derived from lacquer trees, also called lacquer
漆疮 lacquer dermatitis

奇 [qí]（形容词）特殊的 extraordinary
奇恒之腑 extraordinary organs
奇经八脉 eight extra meridians/channels

脐 [qí]（名词）肚脐 navel; umbilicus
脐腹 the part of the abdomen around the navel → **peri-umbilical abdomen**
脐风 convulsions due to unhygienic dressing of the umbilical stump → **neonatal tetanus**
脐疮 umbilical sore → omphalelcosis
脐湿 umbilical dampness → omphalorrhea
脐血 umbilical bleeding → omphalorrhagia

骑 [qí]（动词）两腿跨坐 to sit with legs open; 骑马 to sit on a horse
骑马式 horseman's stance

起 [qǐ]（动词）①开始 to begin (*n.* beginning; onset)
问起病 inquiry about the onset of illness
②发生 to form
舌起芒刺 prickles (formed) **on the tongue**
③把东西拿开或取走 to remove; to withdraw (*n.* removal; withdrawal)
起罐 cup removal
起针 needle withdrawal
快速起针法 quick withdrawal of the needle

气 [qì]（名词）气 *qi*
气机 *qi* movement; *qi* activity
气化 *qi* transformation
气轮 *qi* orbiculus → white of the eye
气郁 *qi* depression
气滞 *qi* stagnation
气逆 *qi* counterflow
气陷 *qi* sinking
（其他）
气色 complexion
气味 property and flavor

器 [qì]（名词）①器官 organ
阴器 yin organ → **external genitals**
阴器痛 genital pain
②器具 device
温灸器 moxa-burning device → **moxa burner**
温灸器灸 moxa-burner moxibustion
电灸器 electric moxibustion device
③器械 appliance
抱膝器 appliance for patellapexy → **peripatellapexor**

掐 [qiā]（动词）用指甲按 to press with a fingernail
掐法 fingernail pressing (manipulation)

髂 [qià]（名词）髂骨 ilium (iliac bone)
髂窝 iliac fossa
髂窝流注 metastatic abscess of the iliac fossa

迁 [qiān]（动词）迁延 to last a long time, especially longer than usual, i.e., to protract
迁延痢 protracted dysentery

牵 [qiān]（动词）牵拉 to pull; to drag
牵引；牵拉法 action of pulling → **traction**
牵推法 pulling-pushing manipulation
牵引疗法 traction therapy
牵拉肩 dragged shoulder

前 [qián]（形容词）前面的，与后相对 anterior, the opposite of posterior
前后配穴法 anterior-posterior point combination
前发际 anterior hairline
前阴 anterior yin

潜 [qián]（动词）制伏 to subdue
潜阳 subduing yang
潜阳熄风 subduing yang and extinguishing wind
（形容词）潜在的 latent
潜呼吸 latent breathing

浅 [qiǎn]（形容词）从表面到底距离小的，深的反面 having a small distance between the surface and the bottom, namely shallow, the opposite of deep
浅刺 shallow insertion

腔 [qiāng]（名词）身体中空的部分 a hollow space within the body, namely a cavity
耳甲腔 cavity of the concha; cavitas conchae

强 [qiáng]（动词）使变强 to strengthen
强筋健骨 strengthening the muscles and bones
（形容词）起强壮作用的 roborant
强壮功 roborant exercise

跷 [qiāo]（动词）重踩 to put the foot down heavily, namely, to stamp
跷法 stamping

壳 [qiào]（名词）外壳 shell
耳壳 shell-like portion of the ear → **auricle**
耳壳流痰 auricular pseudocyst

窍 [qiào]（名词）孔窍 orifice
窍漏 orifice pyorrhea → **dacryopyorrhea**

切 [qiē]（动词）切割；切开 to cut; to incise (*n.* cut; incision)
切片 cutting into slices → **slicing**
切开埋线法 catgut-embedding by incision
切迹 a V-shaped cut → **notch**
屏间切迹 intertragic notch
轮屏切迹 helix notch

切 [qiè]（动词）（诊病时）触摸 to give someone a medical examination by touch, namely to palpate (*n.* palpation)
切诊 palpation
切脉 palpation of pulse; pulse taking

侵 [qīn]（动词）入侵 to invade
赤脉侵睛 red vessels invading the eye → **angular conjunctivitis**
胬肉侵睛 fleshy mass invading the eye → **pterygium**
白膜侵睛 white membrane invading the eye → **phlyctenular kerato-conjunctivitis**
风热侵喉 [咽]证 syndrome/pattern of wind-heat invading the throat

噙 [qín]（动词）含在嘴里 to hold in the mouth
噙化 to be dissolved in the mouth

揿 [qìn]（动词）用手指按 to press with the thumb or a finger (揿钉 a short pin with a large flat top for pressing, called thumbtack)
揿针 thumbtack needle

青 [qīng]（形容词）蓝色的或绿色的 blue or green; bluish
青紫舌 bluish purple discoloration of the tongue → **cyanotic tongue**
青蛇毒 blue snake toxin sore; superficial thrombophlebitis
青盲 bluish blindness
青风内障；青风 bluish glaucoma

轻 [qīng]（形容词）①作用轻的 mild
轻下 mild purgation
②重量轻的 light; lightweighted
轻剂 light (diaphoretic) formula
轻宣外燥剂 formula for dispersing

exogenous dryness with lightweighted medicinals → **exogenous-dryness-dispersing formula**
③动作轻的 gentle
轻捻出针法 withdrawal of the needle with gentle twirling
轻重徐疾补泻法 reinforcement-reduction by varying the force and speed

清 [qīng]（形容词）清新的 clear (*n.* clarity)
清气 clear *qi*
清阳 clear yang
清浊 clarity and turbidity
（动词）清除 to clear
清法 (heat-) **clearing method**
清热解毒 clearing heat and resolving toxins
清肝明目 clearing the liver to improve vision
清心安神 clearing the heart and calming the mind
清肺利咽 clearing the lung to soothe the throat
（副词）单独地 alone or without
清炒 stir-baking without adjuvant

情 [qíng]（名词）情志 emotion
七情 seven emotions
经行情志异常 abnormal emotions during menstruation → **moodiness during menstruation; menstrual mental disorder**

丘 [qiū]（名词）土丘 hill
丘疹 small hill-like eruption of the skin → **papule**

秋 [qiū]（名词）一年四季的第三季，即秋季 the season of the year between summer and winter, namely autumn
秋燥 autumn dryness
秋燥病 autumn dryness disease

鼽 [qiú]（名词）鼻塞久涕 a chronic running and stuffy nose
鼻鼽 sniveling nose → **allergic rhinits**
鼽嚏 sniveling nose with sneezing → **allergic rhinits**

曲 [qū]（形容词）弯曲的 curved
曲颊；曲牙 curved junction of the posterior and lower borders of the lower jaw → **mandibular angle**
曲骨 curved bone → **(1) pubic symphysis; (2) *qugu* (CV 2)**
（名词）粬的简体字 simplified Chinese character of 粬 (leaven)
曲 leaven

驱 [qū]（动词）驱逐 to expel
驱虫 expelling worms
驱虫消积 expelling intestinal worms and dissipating accumulation
驱虫药 worm-expelling medicinal/drug; anthelmintic

屈 [qū]（动词）弯曲 to flex or to bend
屈法 flexing (manipulation)
屈伸法 flexing-stretching (manipulation)
屈指捏法 bent-finger pinching (manipulation)

祛 [qū]（动词）①祛除 to dispel
祛风 dispelling wind
祛风止痒 dispelling wind to relieve itching
祛寒化痰 dispelling cold and resolving phlegm
祛湿剂 dampness-dispelling formula
祛瘀生新 dispelling stasis to promote regeneration
②消除，扶助的对立 to eliminate, the opposite of reinforce
祛邪 eliminating the pathogenic factors
扶正祛邪 reinforcing the healthy and eliminating the pathogenic
祛邪兼扶正 eliminating the pathogenic with reinforcement of the healthy

取 [qǔ]（动词）选取 to select (*n.* selection)
左病右取，右病左取 treating diseases of the left with points (selected) **on the right, and vice versa**

取穴法 selection of points

龋 [qǔ]（名词）牙齿受侵蚀 decay in teeth, i.e., caries (*adj.* carious)
龋齿 carious tooth
齿龋 dental caries
龋齿牙痛 carious toothache
龋脱 carious odontoptosis

去 [qù]（动词）去掉；消除 to remove; to eliminate (*n.* removal; elimination)
去菀陈莝 eliminating the stale and the stagnant
去腐肉 removing necrotic tissue
提脓去腐 drawing out pus and removing putridity
去火毒 removal of fire toxin
去油 removing fat or oil → **defatting**

全 [quán]（形容词）完全的 complete
全不产 complete loss of reproductive capacity → **primary infertility**

泉 [quán]（名词）水源 source of water
泪泉 source of tears → **lacrimal gland**
（其他）
在泉 terrestrial effect; affecting Earth

拳 [quán]（名词）拳头 fist
拳击法 rapping with fist; fist-striking manipulation
拳揉法 fist-kneading manipulation

踡［蜷］[quán]（动词）踡伏 to lie with the knees drawn up
踡［蜷］卧缩足 lying on one's side with the knees drawn up

颧 [quán]（名词）颊骨的突出部分 the prominence of the cheekbone, namely, malar eminence
颧 malar eminence

缺 [quē]（动词）缺乏； 缺失 to lack; to lose
缺乳 lacking milk secretion → **oligogalactia; hypogalactia**
产后缺乳 postpartum oligogalactia; postpartum hypogalactia
瞳神干缺；瞳人干缺；瞳神缺陷 loss of normal shape of the pupil → **pupillary metamorphosis**

却 [què]（动词）拒绝 to refuse
却谷食气 refusing food but feeding on *qi*; **feeding on *qi* instead of food**

雀 [què]（名词）麻雀，泛指小鸟 a sparrow or a little bird
雀啄脉 bird-pecking pulse
雀斑 spots on the skin resembling sparrow eggs → **freckle**
雀盲；雀目；雀目内障 sparrow's blindness; sparrow's vision; sparrow's cataract → **night blindness; nyctalopia**
雀啄灸 bird-pecking moxibustion; pecking moxibustion

鹊 [què]（名词）喜鹊 magpie
鹊桥 magpie bridge
搭鹊桥 building the magpie bridge

阙 [què]（名词）眉间中点 mid-point in between the eyebrows, i.e., the ophryon
阙；阙中 ophryon
阙上 supra-ophryon area

R

染 [rǎn]（动词）染色；染污 to dye; to stain
染苔 stained (tongue) coating/fur

扰 [rǎo]（动词）侵扰 to harass (*n.* harassment)
痰火扰心 phlegm-fire harassing the heart
热扰心神 heat harassing the mind
痰热内扰证 syndrome/pattern of internal harassment of phlegm-heat

热 [rè]（名词）① 中医病因、病机、辨证中的"热" "heat" in etiology, pathogenessis and syndrome/pattern diagnosis of Chinese medicine

热邪 pathogenic heat; heat pathogen
热入营血 heat entering nutrient-blood
热盛伤津 exuberant heat damaging fluid
热极生风 extreme heat producing wind
热扰心神证 syndrome/pattern of heat harassing the mind
热疮 heat sore; herpes febrilis
②发热 fever
夜热 fever at night
惊热 fever due to fright
客热 irregular recurrent fever
血热 (1) blood fever; (2) fever at blood aspect
骨蒸热 bone-steaming fever; consumptive fever
（形容词）①热的 hot
热汗 hot sweats
热因热用 heating for the hot
热罨 hot compression
热服 to be taken hot
②发热的 febrile
热病 febrile disease
热甚发痉 febrile convulsion
（动词）使温暖 to warm
热剂 warming formula

人 [rén]（名词）①人 human
人胞 (human) **placenta**
人中 (1) philtrum; (2) ***renzhong*** **(GV 26)**（天食人以五气，天气通于鼻，地食人以五味，地气通于口。该处正当鼻下口上，亦天之下，地之上，取人在其中，因名人中。人中 [rén zhōng] literally means human in the middle. The heaven feeds the human with five *qi* (five odors) that all pass through the nose. The earth feeds the human with five flavors that all pass through the mouth. (So the nose and the mouth can be taken as the representatives of the heaven and the earth, respectively.) The philtrum lies underneath the nose and above the mouth, as the human stands under the sky (heaven) and on the earth, or the human stands in the middle.)
人迎脉 (1) common carotid artery; (2) carotid pulse（在古汉语中"迎"与"亢"是通假字，"亢"是"人颈"的象形字。In archaic Chinese, the charcters "迎" and "亢" are interchangeable, and the latter is a pictographic character that depicts the human neck.)
②个人 individual
因人制宜 treatment according to individual

仁 [rén]（名词）果核的最内部分 the innermost part of a seed or nut, namely, the kernel
白仁 white kernel → **white of the eye**
黄仁 yellow kernel → **iris**
（形容词）感觉灵敏的 sensitive (不仁 *adj.* insensitive; numb *n.* insensitivity; numbness)
不仁 insensitivity
肌肤不仁 insensitivity of the skin; numbness of the skin
小腹不仁 lower abdominal numbness
口不仁 numbness of the mouth

任 [rèn]（名词）古汉语中"任"与"妊"相通，妊娠之意 In archaic Chinese, 任 [rèn] and 妊 [rèn] are interchangeable, meaning conception.
任脉 conception vessel (CV)

妊 [rèn]（名词）妊娠 pregnancy
妊娠恶阻 nausea and vomiting during pregnancy → **morning sickness**
妊娠眩晕 vertigo in pregnancy
妊娠失音aphonia of pregnancy
妊娠肿胀 edema of pregnancy
妊娠禁忌药 medicinals contraindicated during pregnancy

日 [rì]（名词）白天 day
日晡 3–5 p.m. (in the day) → **late afternoon**
日晡发热 late afternoon fever
日晡潮热 late afternoon tidal fever

溶 [róng]（动词）溶解 to dissolve (*n.* disolution)

溶化 disolution

柔 [róu] （动词）使柔润 to emolliate

柔肝 emolliating the liver

养血柔肝 nourishing blood and emolliating the liver

柔肝药 liver-emolliating medicinal/drug

揉 [róu]（动词）用手来回搓摸 to rub and press with the hand to and fro, i.e., to knead

揉腰眼 kneading the sides of the small of the back

揉肩 kneading the shoulders

揉膝 kneading the knees

指揉法 finger kneading manipulation

掌揉法 palm-kneading manipulation

肉 [ròu]（名词）人体皮骨之间的软物质，包括肌肉和脂肪 the soft substances between the skin and bones of human bodies, namely, flesh, including muscle and fat

肉瘿 fleshy goiter

肉瘤 fat tumor; lipoma

肉轮 flesh orbiculus → eyelid

肉痿 flesh atrophy-flaccidity

（其他）

肉刺 clavus; corn

儒 [rú]（名词）儒家，遵循孔子教诲的学派 Confucian, an adherent of the teachings of Confucius

儒家气功 Confucian *qigong*

濡 [rú]（形容词）湿软的 wet and soft, namely soggy

濡脉 soggy pulse

濡泻 soggy diarrhea

乳 [rǔ]（名词）①乳房 breast

乳痈 acute pyogenic inflammation of the breast → **acute mastitis**

乳发 pyogenic inflammation of the breast with abscess formation → **phlegmonous mastitis**

乳中结核；乳核 nodule in the breast; breast nodule

乳疬 (1) excessive development of the breast in males → **gynecomastia; (2)** enlargement of the breast in children → **mastauxy in children**

乳头 the protuberance of a breast from which milk is drawn → **nipple**

乳头破碎 cracked nipple

乳头风 nipple wind

乳衄 bleeding from the nipple → **thelorrhagia**

②乳汁 milk

乳汁自出；乳溢 spontaneous flow of milk → **galactorrhea**

乳积 milk indigestion; infantile dyspepsia

乳汁不行；乳汁不通 no milk secretion after childbirth → **agalactia**

乳膏 a thick lipuid (containing medicinals) looking like the fatty part of milk that rises to the surface when standing → **cream**

乳蛾 milky moth → tonsillitis

③泌乳 lactation

催乳 stimulating lactation

下乳 promoting lactation

回乳 terminating lactation

断乳 (1) terminating lactation; (2) stopping feeding a baby its mother's milk → **weaning**

（形容词）乳房的 mammary

乳疽 intramammary abscess

乳痨 mammary phthisis

乳漏 mammary fistula

乳癖 mammary hyperplasia

乳岩 mammary cancer

入 [rù]（动词）①进入，与出相对 to enter, the opposite of exit

表里出入 entering the interior and exiting to the exterior

由表入里 entering the interior from the exterior

入里化热 conversion into heat after entering the interior

热入营血 heat entering nutrient-blood
入静 (in meditation) **entering quiescence; falling into static state**
②插入 to insert
插入法 thrusting insertion
飞入法 needle-flying insertion
弹入法 flicking-in insertion

蓐 [rù]（名词）产妇的床铺 obstetric bed → 产褥期 puerperium (*adj.* puerperal)
蓐劳 puerperal phthisis
蓐风 puerperal tetanus

褥 [rù]（名词）床上的铺垫物 bed clothes
褥疮 bedsore; decubitus ulcer

软 [ruǎn]（形容词）柔软的，与硬相对 soft, the opposite of hard
软脉 soft pulse
软膏 a soft medicinal substance for rubbing into the skin → **ointment**
软气功 soft *qigong*

锐 [ruì]（形容词）尖锐的 sharp
锐发 hair growing on the sharp area before the ear → **sideburn**
锐眦；目锐眦 the sharper corner of the eye → **lateral canthus**

瞤 [rún]（动词）颤动 to twitch
筋惕肉瞤 muscular twitching
身瞤动 twitching of the body

润 [rùn]（形容词）湿润的 moist
润苔 moist (tongue) coating/fur
（动词）使湿润；使润滑 to moisten; to lubricate (*adj.* lubricant)
润燥 moistening (dryness)
润肺止咳 moistening the lung to relieve cough
润肠通便 moistening the intestines to loose the bowels; moistening the intestines to relieve constipation
润下 lubricant laxation
润下药 (lubricant) laxative (medicinal/drug)

弱 [ruò]（形容词）虚弱的，与"强"相反 weak, the opposite of strong
弱脉 weak pulse
卫弱营强 weak defense *qi* with strong nutrient
卫强营弱 strong defense *qi* with weak nutrient

S

腮 [sāi]（名词）面颊的下半部 the lower part of the cheek
腮肿 swollen cheek
痄腮 mumps; epidemic parotitis

塞 [sāi]（动词）①塞满，填满 to stuff (*adj.* stuffy), to fill
塞因塞用 filling for the stuffed
鼻塞 stuffy nose; nasal congestion
②塞入 to insert (*n.* insertion)
塞法 insertion method
另见：塞 [sè]

三 [sān]（数词）①三 three (*prefix*: tri-)
三角窝 triangular fossa
三消 three types of wasting-thirst; three types of diabetes
三部九候 three positions and nine pulse-takings
三品 three grades of medicinals
三棱针 three-edged needle
②第三 third
三阴 (1) the three yin; (2) the third yin
三阳 (1) the three yang; (2) the third yang
（形容词）有三部分的 triple
三焦 triple energizer
三焦虚寒 triple energizer deficiency cold; deficiency cold in the triple energizer
三焦气化 activity of the triple energizer

散 [sǎn]（名词）药末 powder
散；散剂 powder

（形容词）分散的 scattered
散脉 scattered pulse
散刺 scattered needling

散 [sàn]（动词）使消散 to dissipate
散寒 dissipating cold
散寒化饮 dissipating cold and resolving retained fluid

色 [sè]（名词）①颜色 color
青色 bluish discoloration
黄色 yellow discoloration
五色主病 diagnostic significance of the five colors
②面色 complexion
望色 inspection of the complexion
常色normal complexion
病色 morbid complexion
善色 favorable complexion
色脉合参 comprehensive analysis of the pulse and complexion

涩 [sè]（形容词）不光滑的 unsmooth
涩脉 unsmooth pulse; choppy pulse
（动词）收涩；阻止 to astringe (*adj.* astringent); to check
涩精 checking emission
涩肠止泻 astringing the intestines to check diarrhea
涩剂 astringent formula
涩精止遗剂 semen-astringing enuresis-arresting formula

塞 [sè]（动词）堵塞 to block
塞兑反听 blocking the ears and inward listening
另见：塞 [sāi]

杀 [shā]（动词）①杀死 to kill
杀虫 killing the worms
②遏抑 to suppress
相杀 suppressing relationship; neutralizing

砂 [shā] (名词) ①砂子 sand (*adj.* sandy)
白砂苔 white sandy (tongue) coating/fur
②细小的石粒 small pieces of stone
砂淋；砂石淋 stranguria characterized by passing of urinary stones → **urolithic stranguria**
（其他）
控脑砂 rhinorrhea with turbid discharge

痧 [shā]（名词）①皮疹 rash ②感受秽浊之气 filthy attack
痧 (1) rash; exanthema; (2) filthy attack
小儿发痧 filthy attack in children
闷痧 drowsy filthy attack; filthy attack with mental confusion

山 [shān]（名词）①山岳 mountain
山岚瘴气 mountainous miasma
烧山火 "burning the mountain"; mountain-burning manipulation
②像山的东西 something that looks like a mountain, referring to the nose in Chinese medicine
山根 root of the nose; radix nasi

闪 [shǎn]（动词）闪耀 to flash
闪火法 flash-fire cupping

疝 [shàn]（名词）①脏器通过周围组织而凸出 a protrusion of an organ through its surrounding tissue, namely, a hernia
疝；疝气 hernia
脐疝 umbilical hernia
②外生殖器的疾病 external genital disease
水疝 a protrusion due to accumulation of fluid in the testicle → **hydrocele**
③腹部的绞痛 abdominal colic
盘疝 periumbilical colic

善 [shàn]（形容词）①良好的 favorable
善色 favorable complexion
②时常的 frequent
善太息 frequent sighing
善忘 frequently forgetting things → **forgetfulness**
多食善饥 polyphagia with frequent hunger

潬 [shàn]（动词）用沸水烫 to put into boiling

water for a short time, i.e., to blanch
潬 blanching

伤 [shāng]（名词）①损伤 damage
伤津 damage to fluid
伤寒 cold damage
伤暑 summerheat damage
伤食 food damage; dyspepsia (indigestion)
伤食泻 indigestion diarrhea
②（对躯体）的损伤 injury
伤产 injury-induced labor
③外伤 trauma
伤科 traumatology

上 [shàng]（形容词）①上面的 upper
上焦 upper energizer
上虚下实 upper deficiency and lower excess
上病下取 treating the lower for the upper
上下配穴法 upper-lower point combination
上胞下垂 drooping of the upper eyelid → **blepharoptosis**
②最上面的 top
上品 top-grade medicinal
（动词、名词）上升 ascend; ascent
上气 (1) ascent of *qi*; (2) upper *qi*

烧 [shāo]（动词）燃烧 to burn
烧伤 burn
烧心 heartburn
烧存性 burning with the original property retained
烧针burnt needle
烧山火 "burning the mountain"

少 [shǎo]（动词）缺少 to lack; to be short of
少气 shortage of *qi*
少神 lack of vitality
（形容词）缺少的 scant
精少 scant semen
月经过少 scant menorrhea; hypomenorrhea
月经涩少 scant inhibited menorrhea
另见：少 [shào]

少 [shào]（形容词）①较下面的 lower
少腹 (1) lateral lower abdomen; (2) lower abdomen
少腹拘急 lower abdominal cramp
少腹硬满 lower abdominal rigidity and fullness
②较少的 lesser
少阳病证 lesser yang disease pattern/syndrome
少阳病机 pathogenesis of *shaoyang* (lesser yang) disease
少阴寒化 cold transformation of lesser yin
少阴热化 heat transformation of lesser yin
足少阴肾经 kidney meridian/channel of foot lesser yin; kidney meridian/channel (KI)
另见：少 [shǎo]

舌 [shé]（名词）舌头 tongue
舌象 tongue manifestations
舌绛 crimson tongue
舌胖 plump tongue
舌战 trembling tongue
舌卷囊缩 curled tongue and retracted testicles

折 [shé]（动词）折断 to break
折针 breaking of the needle

蛇 [shé]（名词）长虫 snake
蛇眼疔 snake-eye whitlow; snake-eye felon
蛇头疔 snake-head whitlow; snake-head felon
蛇肚疔 snake-body whitlow; snake-body felon
蛇串疮；缠腰蛇丹；蛇丹 eruptive disease with a girdle-like distribution of clustered vesicles (around the waist) as if a snake wrapped around the waist → **herpes zoster**
青蛇毒 blue snake toxin sore → **superficial thrombophlebitis**

舍 [shě]（动词）舍弃 to disregard
舍脉从症 disregarding the pulse condition and only looking into symptoms when making a diagnosis → **precedence of**

symptoms over pulse

舍症从脉 precedence of pulse over symptoms

舍 [shè]（名词）住所 abode

神不守舍 failure of the mind to keep to its abode

射 [shè]（动词）①射出 to shoot

通关射甲 shooting through the passes to the nail

②射击 to attack

水寒射肺 water-cold attacking the lung

③注射 to inject (*n.* injection)

穴位注射 acupoint injection

摄 [shè]（动词）①固摄 to control; to constrain

气虚不摄 *qi* deficiency failing to control the blood

气不摄血 failure of *qi* to control the blood

摄唾 constraining spittle

②擦搓 to rub

摄领疮 skin lesion aggravated by rubbing with the collar → **cervical neurodermatitis**

伸 [shēn]（动词）舒展 to stretch

伸法 stretching (manipulation)

伸腰沉胯 stretching the waist and keeping the hips sunken

旋转屈伸 rotating, bending and stretching

身 [shēn]（名词）身体 body

身瞤动 twitching of the body

身热 heat all over the body → **(generalized) fever**

身热不扬 unsurfaced fever

同身寸 body *cun*; body inch

深 [shēn]（形容词）从表面到底距离大的，浅的反面 having a large distance between the surface and the bottom, namely, deep, the opposite of shallow

深刺 deep insertion

神 [shén]（名词）①精神 spirit

神 spirit; mind; vitality

神光耗散 spiritless eyes

②心神 mind (*adj.* mental)

神不守舍 failure of the mind to keep to its abode

神乱 mental disorder

神识昏溃 mental confusion

安神 calming the mind

③活力 vitality (vital *qi*)

望神 inspection of vitality

得神 presence of vitality

神气不足；少神 insufficiency of vital *qi*; lack of vitality

失神 loss of vitality

④神志 consciousness

神昏 clouded consciousness

神志不清 unconsciousness

（其他）

神水 (1) aqueous humor; (2) tears

神膏 vitreous

审 [shěn]（动词）①审查 to inspect

审苗窍 inspection of the signal orifices → inspection of the sensory organs

审证求因 cause seeking from (the inspected) **symptoms**

②审定 to determine (*n.* determination)

审因施治；审因论治 cause determination and treatment

肾 [shèn]（名词）①肾脏 kidney

肾之府 house of the kidney

肾气不足 kidney *qi* insufficiency

肾不纳气 kidney failing to receive *qi*

肾虚水泛 kidney deficiency with water flooding

肾阴虚证 kidney yin deficiency syndrome/pattern

②男性生殖器，包括睾丸和阴茎 male gentitalia, including testis and penis

肾子 testis

肾囊 external pouch that contains testes → **scrotum**

肾岩翻花 carcinoma of the penis with

ulceration

胂 [shèn]（名词）高起丰满的肌肉群 a group of prominent muscles
胂 prominent muscles → **(1) the paravertebral muscle; (2) the muscle below the iliac crest**

渗 [shèn]（动词）使流走 to make liquid flow away, i.e., to drain
渗湿 draining dampness
淡渗利湿 draining dampness with bland diuretics
利水渗湿 inducing diuresis to drain dampness

升 [shēng]（不及物动词）上升 to ascend
升、降、出、入 ascending, descending, exiting and entering
升降失常 disturbance in ascending and descending
（及物动词）升举 to raise; to elevate
升提中气 elevating the middle *qi*
升举中气 raising the middle *qi*
升阳举陷 elevating yang to cure drooping

生 [shēng]（动词）①产生 to generate; to engender
生化 generation and transformation
甘寒生津 engendering fluid with sweet-cold
热极生风 extreme heat engendering wind
②再生 to regenerate (regeneration)
生肌 promoting tissue regeneration
生肌敛疮 promoting tissue regeneration and wound healing
生肌收口 promoting tissue regeneration and closing the wound
③生殖 to reproduce (*n.* reproduction; *adj.* reproductive)
生殖之精 reproductive essence

声 [shēng]（名词）①声音 sound
闻声音 listening to sounds → **auscultation**
②语声 voice
语声重浊；声重 deep turbid voice
语声低微 faint low voice
声嗄 deep turbid voice → **hoarseness**

胜 [shèng]（动词）占优势 to predominate; to preponderate (*n.* predominance; preponderance)
形胜气 physique predominating *qi*
气胜形 *qi* predominating physique
阴阳胜复 alternate preponderance of yin and yang

盛 [shèng]（动词）兴盛 to exuberate (*n.* exuberance; *adj.* exuberant)
阳虚阴盛 yang deficiency with yin exuberance
阴盛阳衰 yin exuberance with yang debilitation
阳盛格阴 exuberant yang repelling yin
邪正盛衰 exuberance and debilitation between pathogenic and healthy *qi*
（形容词）丰盛的 abundant
痰盛 abundant expectoration

失 [shī] （动词）丧失 to lose (*n.* loss)
失音 loss of voice → aphonia
失禁 loss of the ability to control evacuative functions → **incontinence**
失音 loss of voice; aphonia
失语 loss of the ability of expression by speech → **aphasia**
失血 loss of blood; hemorrhage

湿 [shī]（名词）湿（病因、证名、病名等）dampness (as a pathogenic factor, syndrome name, disease name, etc.)
湿热 dampness-heat
湿邪困脾 dampness (pathogen) encumbering the spleen
湿热下注 downpour of dampness-heat
湿困脾阳证 syndrome/pattern of dampness encumbering spleen yang
湿温病 dampness-warmth disease
湿热带下 dampness-heat leukorrhagia
（动词）使湿润 to moisten

湿剂 moistening formula

十 [shí]（数词）十 ten
十问 ten questions
十四经 fourteen meridians/channels
十五络脉 fifteen collateral vessels
十八反 eighteen antagonisms
十九畏 nineteen incompatibilities

石 [shí]（名词）①石头 stone (*adj.* stony)
石瘿 stony goiter
石蛾 stony moth → **hypertrophy of the tonsil**
砭石 healing stone; stone needle
②结石 calculus
石淋；砂石淋 painful and difficult urination caused by calculi → **urolithic stranguria**
排石 expelling calculi
睑内结石 calculus of conjunctiva

时 [shí]　（名词）①时间 time
因时制宜 treatment according to time; taking measures that are suited to the time
②季节 season
时毒 (1) seasonal toxin; (2) seasonal toxicosis
时病；时令病 seasonal diseases
时疫 seasonal epidemic
时疫痢 (seasonal) **epidemic dysentery**
（形容词）当时的 updated
时方 updated formula

实 [shí]（名词）邪气盛则实 "实" refers to excess of pathogenic factors, which is abbreviated as excess
实寒 excess cold
实证 excess syndrome/pattern
实脉 (1) pulse of excess type; (2) replete pulse
实热证 excess heat syndrome/pattern
实秘 constipation of excess type
（形容词）真实的 real
实按灸 (real) **pressing moxibustion**

食 [shí]（名词）①食物；饮食 food; diet (*adj.* dietary)
食积 food accumulation; dyspepsia; indigestion
食疗；食治 diet therapy
食忌 dietary prohibitions
食复 relapse due to diet
②一顿饭 meal
食远服 to be taken (a long time) apart from meal → **to be taken between meals**
（动词）①吃 to eat
食已即吐 vomiting right after eating
食厥 syncope due to overeating → **crapulent syncope**
②通 "蚀"，侵蚀 same as "蚀", meaning to erode
食床 erosion of the gum → **gingival recession**
③另见：食 [sì]

蚀 [shí]（动词）侵蚀 to corrode
蚀疮去腐 corroding wounds and removing putridity
（其他）月蚀 eclipse of the moon
月蚀疮 eclipsed lunar sore → **peri-auricular eczema**

矢 [shǐ]（名词）同 "屎" same as "屎", feces (*adj.* fecal)
吐矢 vomiting fecal matter

使 [shǐ]（名词）信使 courier
使药 courier ingredient → **guide ingredient**
君臣佐使 sovereign, minister, adjuvant and courier → **chief, associate, assistant and guide**

事 [shì]（名词）事情 matter
月事 "monthly matter" → menstruation
房事 "bedroom matter" → sexual intercourse

试 [shì]（动词）在正式进行前试探 to test earlier than formal action
试胎；试月 testing labor

试水 early leakage of amniotic fluid

视 [shì]（名词）视力 vision

视瞻昏渺 blurring of vision

视物易色 disturbance of vision in which colorless objects appear colored → **chromatopsia**

视直为曲 disturbance of vision characterized by distortion in shape → **metamorphopsia**

（动词）注视 to stare

瞪目直视 staring straight ahead

横目斜视 staring sideways

室 [shì]（名词）房室 chamber

血室 blood chamber → **(1) uterus; (2) thoroughfare vessel; (3) liver**

精室 essence chamber

嗜 [shì]（动词）嗜好 to like for something special or excessively

嗜睡；嗜卧 excessive sleepiness → **somnolence**

嗜偏食 special likening for some unusual food → **food partiality**

收 [shōu]（动词）①合上 to close

生肌收口 promoting tissue regeneration and closing the wound

止血收口 arresting bleeding and closing cut

②阻止 to arrest

收涩药 discharge-arresting medicinal/drug → **astringent**

收敛止血药 astringent hemostatic (medicinal/drug)

③结束 to close

收功 closing form

④收缩 to contract

收臀松膝 contracting the buttocks and relaxing the knees

手 [shǒu]（名词）手 hand

手足汗 sweating hands and feet

手阳明大肠经 large intestine meridian/channel of hand yang brightness

手针疗法 hand acupuncture therapy

手心 inner surface of the hand → **palm**

手足心热 feverish sensation in the palms and soles

守 [shǒu]（动词）保持 to keep

守气 keeping *qi*

神不守舍 failure of the mind to keep to its abode

兽 [shòu]（名词）野兽 animal

虫兽伤 insect or animal bite

瘦 [shòu]（形容词）瘦薄的 thin

瘦薄舌 thin tongue

枢 [shū]（名词）户枢 hinge

髀枢 hinge of the thigh → **trochanter**

梳 [shū]（动词）梳理（头发）to comb

梳法 combing (in massage)

舒 [shū]（动词）①舒缓 to relax

舒筋通络 relaxing tendons and unblocking collaterals

舒筋活络 relaxing tendons and activating collaterals

舒筋止痛 relaxing tendons to relieve pain

舒腰松腹 keeping the waist and abdomen relaxed

②展开 to spread

舒张进针法 skin-spreading needle insertion

疏 [shū]（动词）①疏散 to make something move apart in different directions, i.e., to disperse

疏风 dispersing wind

疏散风热 dispersing wind-heat

疏风清热 dispersing wind and clearing heat

疏风止痒 dispersing wind to relieve itching

②去掉郁滞 to relieve depression and stagnation or to soothe

疏肝 soothing the liver
疏肝和胃 soothing the liver and harmonizing the stomach
疏肝理脾 soothing the liver and regulating the spleen
疏肝明目功 liver-soothing and vision-improving exercise

输 [shū]（名词）①运输 transport
输刺 transport needling
五输穴 five transport points
五输配穴法 five-transport-points combination
②通"腧" interchangeable with "腧", referring to acupoint
输穴 acupoints; stream points
（其他）五输穴之一，在手部或足部接近腕踝部 one of the five transport points on the hand or foot, close to the wrist or ankle, namely stream point

暑 [shǔ]（名词）暑热 summerheat
暑证 summerheat syndrome/pattern
暑湿证 summerheat-dampness syndrome/pattern
中暑 summerheat stroke; heat stroke
暑厥 summerheat syncope
暑入阳明 summerheat entering *yangming* (yang brightness)

鼠 [shǔ]（名词）老鼠 mouse
鼠乳 "mouse nipple" (a chronic skin disease characterized by formation of small nodules with a central opening and secretion of contents resembling a lactating mouse nipple) → **molluscum contagiosum**

数 [shǔ]（动词）数数 to count
数吸 breath counting

术 [shù]（名词）技艺 art
武术气功 martial-art *qigong*
内丹术 inner elixir art

束 [shù]（动词）束缚 to fetter
风寒束表 wind-cold fettering the exterior
寒邪外束 cold pathogen fettering the exterior
风寒束肺 wind-cold fettering the lung

俞 [shù]（名词）① 身体上的穴位 acupuncture point
俞穴 acupuncture point; acupoint
②运输 transport
背俞穴 back transport points
俞募配穴法 transport-alarm point combination

腧 [shù]（名词）身体上的穴位 acupuncture point
腧穴 acupuncture point; acupoint

漱 [shù]（动词）含水荡洗口腔 to clean the inside of the mouth by blowing air through water or an aqueous medicine in the mouth, i.e., to gargle
漱津 gargling with saliva
漱涤 washing by gargling

腨 [shuàn]（名词）小腿肚 calf
腨 calf
腓腨 calf

双 [shuāng]（形容词）成双的；两者 double; both (*prefix*: bi-)
双手进针法 double-handed needle insertion
双盘坐 double cross-legged sitting
双蛾 bilateral tonsillitis
双手托天式 pushing upwards with both hands

霜 [shuāng]（名词）冰霜 frost
制霜 making (a medicinal) into a frost-like powder → **frosting**

爽 [shuǎng]（形容词）痛快的 gratifying
泻下不爽 ungratifying diarrhea

水 [shuǐ]（名词）① 水液 water (*prefix*: hydro-)
水不涵木 water failing to nourish wood
水火相济 water-fire coordination

水轮 water orbiculus → the pupil
水土 water and earth → **natural environment**
水土不服 failure to acclimatize to unfamiliar natural environments → **non-acclimatization**
水飞 refining with water → elutriation
②饮物 drink
水谷 food and drink
水谷之海 reservoir of food and drink
水谷精微 essence of food and drink → **food essence**
③液体 fluid
水肿 fluid-induced → **edema**
水疱 small epidermal elevation containing fluid → **vesicle**
水痘；水疱；水花；水疮 an epidemic disease marked by fever and formation of vesicles → **chickenpox; varicella**
水臌（病） abdominal distension with fluid accumulation → **ascites**
水饮 fluid retention; retained fluid

睡 [shuì]（动词）睡眠 to sleep
嗜睡 inclination to sleep → **somnolence**
昏睡露睛 lethargic sleeping with the eyes open
临睡前服 to be taken before going to sleep → **to be taken before bed-time**

顺 [shùn]（动词）①理顺 to arrange
顺气 arranging *qi*
②顺应 to adapt to
顺应四时 adaptation to seasonal changes
（形容词）①顺序的 sequential
顺传 sequential transmission
②顺利的 favorable
麻疹顺证 favorable syndrome/pattern of measles
③顺向的 orthodromic
顺腹式呼吸 orthodromic abdominal breathing
（介词）顺着 along
顺骨捋筋 tendon-stroking along the bone

数 [shuò]（形容词）快的 rapid
数脉 rapid pulse

司 [sī]（动词）主管 to control (*n.* control)
司天 controlling Heaven; celestial control

丝 [sī]（名词）细线；一丝一缕 thread; streak
血丝痰 blood-streaked sputum
丝状疣 a wart with thread-like projections → **verruca filiformis**
红丝疔 red-streaked boil; acute lymphangitis

撕 [sī]（动词）用手使东西裂开 to pull apart or in pieces by hands, i.e., to tear
撕裂伤 a torn and ragged wound → **laceration; lacerated wound**

嘶 [sī] (形容词）嘶哑的 hoarse (*n.* hoarseness)
嘶嗄 hoarseness

死 [sǐ]（动词）to die (*n.* death; *adj.* dead, moribund)
七死脉 seven pulse patterns indicating impending death → **seven moribund pulses**
子死腹中 dead fetus in the uterus
死胎 dead fetus
死胎不下；胎死不下 retention of a dead fetus in the uterus → **missed labor**

四 [sì]（数词）四 four
四时不正之气 abnormal weather in the four seasons
四诊合参 comprehensive analysis of the four examinations
四气五味 four natures and five flavors
四弯风 four-articular eczema → **cubito-popliteal eczema**

似 [sì]（动词）看起来像 to resemble
阴证似阳 yin syndrome/pattern resembling yang
阳证似阴 yang syndrome/pattern resembling yin

阴极似阳 extreme yin resembling yang
阳极似阴 extreme yang resembling yin

食 [sì]（动词）通 "饲" same as "饲", meaning to feed
食疳 feeding malnutrition

松 [sōng]（动词）放松 to relax (*n.* relaxation)
放松功 relaxation exercise
舒腰松腹 keeping the waist and abdomen relaxed
收臀松膝 contracting the buttocks and relaxing the knees
（名词）松树 pine
松皮癣 pine-bark lichen → psoriasis

送 [sòng]（动词）送服 to take with fluid
送服 to be taken with fluid

溲 [sōu]（名词）小便 urine
溲血 bloody urine → **hematuria**
失溲 incontinence of urine → **enuresis**

嗽 [sòu]（名词）咳嗽 cough
咳嗽 cough
风燥咳嗽 wind-dryness cough
久嗽 chronic cough
劳嗽 consumptive cough

速 [sù]（形容词）迅速的 quick
迅速出针法；快速起针法 quick withdrawal of the needle

宿 [sù]（形容词）①旧有的；长久有的 old; chronic
宿疾 old disease; long illness
宿翳 chronic corneal opacity
②过夜的 retained overnight
宿食 food retention
呕吐宿食 vomiting of retained food

粟 [sù]（名词）小米 millet
粟疮 millet sore → **follicular conjunctivitis**

酸 [suān]（名词）酸 acid
泛酸 acid regurgitation
吐酸 acid vomiting
吞酸 acid swallowing
（形容词）①酸味的 sour
呕吐酸腐 vomiting of sour fetid matter
口酸 sour taste in the mouth
酸甘化阴 transformation of the sour-sweet into yin
②微痛无力的 aching
酸痛；痠痛 aching pain

随 [suí]（动词）①跟随 to follow
气随血脱 (*qi*) collapse following blood loss
血随气陷 bleeding following sinking of *qi*
随息 following one's own breathing
②伴随 to do something together with
随咳进针法 needle insertion during coughing

髓 [suǐ]（名词）骨髓 marrow
髓 marrow
髓海 sea of marrow; brain
髓之府 house of marrow; bone

孙 [sūn]（名词）第三代 the third generation → third in order (tertiary)
孙络 tertiary collateral vessel

飧 [sūn]（名词）夕食（晚饭）meal taken in the evening → food
飧泄；飧泻 diarrhea characterized by the passage of undigested food → **lienteric diarrhea**

锁 [suǒ]（动词）用锁锁住 → 堵住 to fasten something with a lock, namely, to lock → to block
锁喉痈 throat-blocking abscess
锁喉毒 throat-blocking infection
锁肚 locked abdomen

T

溻 [tā]（动词）浸没 to immerse (*n.* immersion)

溻浴 medicated immersion

踏 [tà]（动词）踩踏 to step
踏跳法 rhythmic stepping

苔 [tāi]（名词）舌苔 tongue coating
舌苔 tongue coating; tongue fur
苔色 tongue coating/fur color

胎 [tāi]（名词）胎儿 fetus (*adj.* fetal)
胎毒 fetal toxin
胎衣 clothes of the fetus → **afterbirth**
胎水 fetus fluid (fluid in the amnion where the fetus is suspended) → **amniotic fluid**
胎动不安 abnormal movement of the fetus → **threatened miscarriage**
胎患内障 cataract contracted by the fetus → **congenital cataract**
（形容词）（与胎儿期有关的）新生儿的 (fetus-related) neonatal
胎黄；胎疸；胎黄病 neonatal jaundice; icterus neonatorum
胎痫 neonatal epilepsy

太 [tài]（形容词）比大还大的 greater
太阳之人 person of greater yang
太阴病机 pathogenesis of *taiyin* (greater yin) disease
太阳经证 greater yang meridian/channel syndrome/pattern
太阳伤寒 greater yang cold damage
太阳蓄血证 greater yang blood retention syndrome/pattern
（动词）太息即叹气 to sigh
太息 sighing
善太息 frequent sighing

能 [tài]（名词）古通態［态］In archaic Chinese, characters 能 and 態 [态 tài] are interchangeable, the latter of which means condition or state.
病能 pathological state of disease
另见：能 [néng]

贪 [tān]（动词）贪食 to eat too much → to overindulge (*n.* overindulgence)
贪食生冷 overindulgence in raw and cold food

弹 [tán]（动词）①用手指快速地轻弹 to hit something with a sudden quick movement, using the thumb and finger together, namely, to flick
弹石脉 flicking stone pulse
弹法 flicking manipulation
弹击法 flicking (in *tuina*)
弹入法 flicking-in insertion
弹柄法 handle-flicking method (in acupuncture)
②弹拨（琴弦）to pluck (at the strings)
弹筋 tendon-plucking
弹筋法 tendon-plucking manipulation
（其他）弹响（啪的一声作响）to snap
弹响指 snapping finger

痰 [tán]（名词）①呼吸道疾病的病理产物 pathological secretions of the diseased respiratory tract, namely, sputum
痰稀白 thin white sputum
痰如泡沫 frothy sputum
痰多 profuse sputum
痰中带血 blood-stained sputum
②能在体内聚集引起多种疾病的黏稠混浊的病理产物 the viscous turbid pathological product that can accumulate in the body, causing a variety of diseases, customarily translated as phlegm
痰湿 phlegm-dampness
痰迷心窍 phlegm misting the heart orifices
痰热闭肺 phlegm-heat blocking the lung
痰饮 phlegm-fluid retention
痰火耳鸣 phlegm-fire tinnitus

炭 [tàn]（名词）①碳素 carbon
制炭 carbonization
②木炭 charcoal
炒炭 stir-baking to charcoal

探 [tàn]（动词）①试探；诱使 to induce
探吐 mechanical induction of vomiting

②伸展 to spread
探爪式 spreading-claw gesture (in *qigong*)

汤 [tāng]（名词）汤剂 decoction
汤药；汤剂 decoction
汤头 decoction formula
汤头歌 formulas in rhyme

溏 [táng]（形容词）稀溏的 loose; sloppy
溏便 loose stool; sloppy stool
便溏 loose bowels
溏结不调 stools sometimes loose and sometimes bound

糖 [táng]（名词）食糖 sugar
糖浆 (concentrated) sugar solution (aqueous and with the addition of medicinal substance) → **syrup**

螳 [táng]（名词）螳螂 mantis
螳螂子 something like a mantis egg → **corpus adiposum bucca**

烫 [tàng]（动词）烫伤 to burn with very hot liquid, i.e., to scald (*n.* scald)
烫火伤 scald and burn

桃 [táo]（名词）桃子 peach
胞肿如桃 peach-like eyelid swelling

陶 [táo]（名词）陶器 pottery
陶罐 pottery cup

特 [tè]（形容词）特定的 specific
特定穴 specific points

腾 [téng]（动词）腾跃 to move quickly with exaggerated steps, i.e., to prance
腾跃爆发导气 prancing to conduct *qi* in burst

提 [tí]（动词）①提起，抬高 to lift
提插补泻法 lifting-thrusting reinforcemen-treduction method (in acupuncture)
提伸法 lifting and stretching (in massage)
提肛呼吸 anus-lifting breathing (in *qigong*)
提按端挤 lifting, pressing, holding, and squeezing (in bone-setting)
②提取，抽出 to draw out
提脓拔毒 drawing out pus and toxins
提脓去腐 drawing out pus and removing putridity

体 [tǐ]（名词）①人的身体 body (*adj.* bodily; corporeal)
形体 general appearance and condition of a person's body → **physique**
意守体外 concentration on something outside the body
离体周天 extracorporeal heavenly circuit; extracorporeal cosmic cycle
②人的体质 constitution
纯阳之体 pure yang constitution
③物体的主要部分 main mass of a thing, namely body
舌体 tongue body
针体 body of the needle

涕 [tì]（名词）鼻涕 nasal discharge; snivel
鼻涕 nasal discharge
鼻流清涕 thin nasal discharge
久流浊涕 chronic turbid nasal discharge

惕 [tì]（动词）颤动 to twitch
筋惕肉瞤 muscular twitching

嚏 [tì]（动词）打喷嚏 to sneeze
鼽嚏 running nose with sneezing

天 [tiān]（名词）①天空，与地相对 heaven, the opposite of earth
天干 heavenly stems
司天 controlling the heaven → **celestial control**
周天 heavenly circuit; cosmic cycle
②自然界 nature (*adj.* natural)
天人相应 correspondence between human and nature
天年 natural life span
天灸 natural moxibustion

③出生 birth
先天 existing before birth → **inborn; innate**
先天之精 innate essence
先天不足 imperfection existing before birth → **congenital defect**
后天 developed or originating after birth → **acquired**
后天之精 acquired essence
后天失调 lack of proper care after birth
（形容词）①面向天的 facing the sky → upward
天钓 upward-staring convulsion
②天行的；流行的 epidemic; prevalent
天行时疫 prevalent seasonal epidemic
天行赤眼；天行赤目 epidemic red eye; epidemic conjunctivitis
天行暴赤 epidemic fulminant red eye
天行赤眼暴翳；天行赤目暴翳 epidemic red eye with fulminant nebula; epidemic kerato-conjunctivitis
③天然的 natural
天受 caused by natural substances → (1) air- or water-borne; (2) air- or water-borne infection
（其他）
天癸 *tiangui*: (1) sex-stimulating substance (2) menstruation
天癸竭 (1) exhaustion of *tiangui*; exhaustion of the sex-stimulating essence; (2) cease of menstruation; menopause
天花 smallpox
天白蚁 throat tinea with moth-eaten holes

田 [tián]（名词）田地 field
丹田 *dantian*; elixir fields
上丹田 upper *dantian*; upper elixir field
意守丹田 concentration on *dantian*

甜 [tián]（形容词）甜味的 sweet
口甜 sweet taste in the mouth

填 [tián]（动词）填满鼓起 to bulge
囟填 bulging fontanel

调 [tiáo]（动词）①调和；调理 to harmonize (*n.* harmony); to regulate
阴阳调和 yin-yang harmony
阴阳失调 yin-yang disharmony
调和营卫 harmonizing the nutrient and defense
调理气血 regulating *qi* and blood
调经 regulating menstruation
②调控 to manage (*n.* management)
调息 management of breath
调气 management of *qi*

龆 [tiáo]（名词）儿童 child
龆龀 seven- or eight-year-old children

挑 [tiǎo]（动词）挑刺 to prick
挑刺法 pricking method

铁 [tiě]（名词）金属铁 iron
铁裆功 iron-crotch exercise

听 [tīng]（动词）聆听 to listen
听息 breath listening
塞兑反听 blocking the ears and inward listening
（名词）听力 hearing
重听 hearing impairment

廷 [tíng]（名词）宫廷 palace (euphemistically referring to the uterus and vagina)
廷孔 (1) vaginal orifice; (2) external urethral orifice (of the female)

停 [tíng]（动词）①停留 to retain (*n.* retention)
停食 food retention; indigestion
水停证 water retention syndrome/pattern
寒饮停肺 cold-fluid retention in the lung
胃寒饮停 stomach cold with fluid retention
②停止 to cease
停经 ceasing of menstruation
③暂停 to pause (*n.* pause)
停息 breathing with pause

聤 [tíng]（名词）耳病流脓 ear disease characterized by purulent discharge

聤耳 otopyorrhea; suppurative otitis media

挺 [tǐng]（动词）①挺直 to straighten

挺腿拔伸 leg-straightening traction

②凸出 to stick out

阴挺 that which sticks out from the vagina → **prolapse of the uterus**

耳挺 that which sticks out from the ear → **ear protuberance**

齿挺 out-sticking of tooth → **exposure of dental root**

（其他）

振挺 small wooden stick

通 [tōng]（动词）①疏通 to unblock

通里 unblocking the interior

通阳 unblocking yang

通经活络 unblocking the meridian/channel and activating the collateral

通络止痛 unblocking collaterals to relieve pain

②使通畅流动 to free the flow

通气 freeing *qi*

通乳 freeing milk flow

③通便 to relieve constipation or to relax the bowels, namely, to purge (*n.* purgation)

通便 relaxing the bowels

通腑泄热 relaxing the bowels and purging heat

通泄 relaxing and purging

通下 purgation

通因通用 purging for the diarrhetic

（其他）

通脉 invigorating the pulse

同 [tóng]（形容词）①相同的 same

同病异治 different treatments for the same disease

异病同治 same treatment for different diseases

②相称的 proportional

同身寸 a unit for measuring length proportional to the body → **body *cun*; body inch**

瞳 [tóng]（名词）瞳孔 pupil

瞳神紧小；瞳神细小；瞳神缩小 contraction of the pupil → **miosis**

瞳神散大 dilatation of the pupil → **mydriasis**

瞳神干缺；瞳人干缺；瞳神缺陷 pupillary metamorphosis

统 [tǒng]（动词）统摄 to control

脾不统血 spleen failing to control blood

痛 [tòng]（形容词）疼痛的 painful; agonizing (causing great pain)

痛经 painful menstruation → dysmenorrheal

痛痹 agonizing impediment; agonizing arthralgia

偷 [tōu]（动词）偷看 to steal a glance

偷针 stye; hordeolum (an eye disease which was once supposed to be due to stealing a glance at what one ought not to look at)

头 [tóu]（名词）脑袋 head

头颅骨 bone structure of the head → **skull; cranium**

头项强痛 headache and painful stiff neck

头重脚轻 heavy head and light feet

头如顶物 keeping the head upright as if carrying something on the top

头皮针；头针 scalp acupuncture

（其他）

汤头 decoction formula

汤头歌 formulas in rhyme

投 [tóu]（动词）投入 to insert (*n.* insertion)

投火法 fire-insertion cupping

透 [tòu]（动词）①通过；通过……排出 to go through; to expel something through

透关射甲 extension through the passes toward the nail

透表 expelling pathogens through the exterior
透泄 expelling through the exterior and removing from the interior
透邪 expelling pathogens
②穿透 to penetrate (*n.* penetration)
透刺 penetration needling
直透 perpendicular penetration
横透 transverse penetration
③使达到充分的程度 to help something develop fully, i.e., to promote
透疹 promoting eruption
解表透疹 releasing the exterior to promote eruption
透斑 promoting eruption of macules
（其他）
透天凉 "cooling the sky"

秃 [tū]（形容词）秃头的 bald
秃疮 bald scalp sore
白秃疮 white bald scalp sore; tinea alba; white ringworm
白秃 white bald
斑秃 baldness in defined areas → **alopecia areata**

突 [tū]（动词）突出 to protrude (*n.* protrusion)
突起睛高；睛高突起 sudden protrusion of the eyeball
眼球突出 protrusion of the eyeball; exophthalmos
脐突 umbilical protrusion

图 [tú]（名词）图画 drawing (图钉 drawing pin → thumbtack*) (*drawing pin 为英式英语，thumbtack为美式英语)
图钉型皮内针 thumbtack intradermal needle

徒 [tú]（副词）仅仅 alone（徒手 using the hands alone → manual）
徒手整复 manual reduction

土 [tǔ]（名词）五行之一的土 earth, one of the five elements/phases
土生金 earth generating metal
土克水 earth restricting water
土虚木乘 wood overrestricting asthenic earth
土不制水 earth failing to control water
土虚水侮 reversed restriction of water on asthenic earth
（形容词）民间的 folk
土方 folk recipe/formula
土法 folk treatment
（其他）
土疡；土疳 stye; hordeolum

吐 [tǔ]（动词）①从口中伸出 to extend or protrude out of the mouth
吐舌 protruding tongue
吐弄舌 protruding and waggling of tongue
②把东西吐出 to expel something out of the mouth or to spit
吐血 spitting of blood
（其他）
吐纳 breathing in and out
吐字呼吸 word-articulating breathing

吐 [tù]（动词）呕吐 to vomit
上吐下泻 simultaneous vomiting and diarrhea
吐酸 acid vomiting
吐血vomiting of blood → **hematemesis**
吐法 method to induce vomiting → **emetic method; emesis**

兔 [tù]（名词）兔子 hare
兔唇 harelip

推 [tuī]（动词）推动 to push
推罐 pushing a cup to and fro → **glide cupping**
推拿 (1) *tuina*; (2) pushing and kneading
一指禅推法 single-finger meditation pushing
推扳手法 pushing-pulling

腿 [tuǐ]（名词）腿脚的腿 leg

腿功 leg training
拉腿手法 leg-pulling manipulation
挺腿拔伸 leg-straightening traction

退 [tuì]（动词）①退出 to retreat
退法 needle-retreating method
②使消退；去掉 to eliminate; to remove
退黄 eliminating jaundice
退目翳 removing nebula
退翳明目 removing nebula to improve vision

吞 [tūn] （动词）吞咽 to take in without chewing; to swallow
吞酸 acid swallowing
吞服 to be swallowed

臀 [tún]（名词）臀部 buttock
臀痈 inflammation of the buttock characterized by abscess formation → **gluteal abscess**
收臀松膝 contracting the buttocks and relaxing the knees

托 [tuō]（动词）①推 to expel (*n.* expulsion)
内托 expulsion from within
托法 expulsion method
托毒 expelling toxin
托疮 expelling pus of sores
②用手掌承受 to support with the palm of the hand
托提法 supporting and lifting
托盘疔 palmar pustule
托板 supporting board
双手托天式 supporting the sky with both hands → **pushing upwards with both hands**

脱 [tuō]（名词）①虚脱 collapse
脱阳；阳脱 yang collapse
血脱气脱 blood loss with (*qi*) collapse
中风脱证 collapse pattern of wind stroke
②脱垂（体内器官从其原有位置脱出下垂）prolapse (a condition in which an organ of the body slips down from its normal position)
脱肛 prolapse of the rectum
（动词）①脱落 to peel
舌苔脱落 peeling of the tongue coating/fur
②脱失 to lose (*n.* loss)
龋脱 loss of teeth due to caries → **carious odontoptosis**
脱疽 a sore which ends in local death (loss) of soft tissues → **digital gangrene**
脱位 loss of normal position → **dislocation; luxation**

唾 [tuò]（名词）唾液 spittle; saliva
唾 spittle; (thick) saliva
摄唾 constraining spittle; checking salivation

W

歪 [wāi]（形容词）偏斜的 deviated
歪斜舌；舌歪 deviated tongue

㖞 [wāi] (形容词) 不正的；偏斜的 wry; deviated
㖞僻不遂 hemiplegia with wry mouth
口㖞 wry mouth
口眼㖞斜 deviated eye and mouth

外 [wài]（形容词）①外界的、外面的、外来的 external (happening outside, situated or being outside, coming from without)
外邪 external pathogen
外感 external contraction
外治法 external therapy
外感腰痛 externally contracted lumbago
外障 external ophthalmopathy
②外侧的 outer
外眦；目外眦 outer canthus
外辅骨 outer shank bone → **fibula**
③向外的 outward
外翻 turning outward → **eversion**
④额外的 extra
经外穴 extra points

弯 [wān]（动词）弯曲 to bend
弯针 bending of the needle
（名词）肢体弯曲形成的窝，四弯指左右手肘窝和腘窝 弯 [wān] refers to fossa formed by bending of the extremities. "The four fossae" is a collective term referring to the right and left cubital and popliteal fossae
四弯风 cubito-popliteal eczema

丸 [wán]（名词）丸药 pill
水丸 watered pill
蜜丸 honeyed pill
蜡丸 (1) waxed pill；(2) wax-coated pill
糊丸 pasted pill

完 [wán]（形容词）完整的 intact or unchanged
完谷不化 undigested food (in stool)

顽 [wán]（形容词）久治不愈的；顽固的 stubborn; obstinate
顽癣 stubborn lichen → **neurodermatitis**
顽痰 obstinate phlegm

脘 [wǎn]（名词）胃腔 stomach cavity
脘；胃脘 stomach cavity
脘痛；胃脘痛 pain in the stomach; epigastric pain

踠 [wǎn]（名词）足胫相连的弯曲部位 the curved region between the foot and the leg, roughly referring to the ankle
踠跌 (ankle) **fracture from fall**

尪 [wāng]（形容词）瘸的，跛的 unable to walk well or lame
尪痹［病］ lame impediment → **ankylosing arthralgia**

亡 [wáng]（动词）耗尽 to exhaust
亡阴 yin exhaustion
亡阳 yang exhaustion
亡津液 fluid exhaustion

往 [wǎng]（动词）去 to go（往来 to alternate）
寒热往来 alternating chills and fever

望 [wàng]（动词）审视，查看 to look closely at something and to check that everything is satisfactory, i.e., to inspect (*n.* inspection)
望神 inspection of vitality
望色 inspection of the complexion
望形体 inspection of the physical build
望姿态 inspection of the posture

微 [wēi]（形容词）①轻微的 mild
微热 mild fever
微炒 stir-baking mildly → **stir-baking to dryness**
②微弱的 faint
微脉 faint pulse
③微小的 very small or minute; micro-
微丸 minute pill
微波针灸 microwave acumoxibustion
微波针灸疗法 microwave acupuncture therapy

煨 [wēi]（动词）在带火的灰里把东西烧熟 to roast in hot ashes
煨 roasting (in hot ashes)
（其他）煨脓 to promote suppuration
煨脓长肉 promoting suppuration to regenerate flesh

尾 [wěi]（名词）①尾巴 tail
鸠尾 the pointed process of cartilage resembling the tail of a turtle dove → **xiphoid process**
②尾骨 tailbone → **coccyx**
尾闾骨 coccyx
尾骶 sacrococcygeal region
尾骶骨 sacrococcyx

委 [wěi]（动词）弯曲 to bend
委中 middle of the region of the leg where the knee bends → **middle of the popliteal fossa**
委中毒 popliteal sore

痿 [wěi]（名词）萎软；萎缩 flaccidity; atrophy (*adj.* flaccid, atrophic)
痿软舌；舌痿 flaccid tongue

痿病 **atrophy-flaccidity disease**
骨痿 **bone atrophy-flaccidity**
痿躄 **atrophic crippling**

卫 [wèi]（名词）保卫 defense
卫气营血 **defense, *qi*, nutrient and blood**
卫气不固 **insecurity of defense *qi***
卫强营弱 **strong defense *qi* with weak nutrient**
卫分证 **defense aspect syndrome/pattern**
卫气同病证 **syndrome/pattern of both defense and *qi* aspects**

畏 [wèi]（名词）畏惧 fear
畏寒 fear of cold → **intolerance of cold**
畏明 fear of light → **photophobia**
（其他）
相畏 **restraining relationship**
十九畏 **nineteen incompatibilities**

胃 [wèi]（名词）①胃 stomach (*adj.* gastric)
胃津 **stomach fluid**
胃热消谷 **stomach heat with accelerated digestion**
胃阴不足 **stomach yin insufficiency**
胃气上逆 **upward counterflow of stomach *qi***
胃火炽盛证 **intense stomach fire syndrome/pattern**
②胃肠道 gasto-intestinal tracts (stomach and intestines)
胃家实 **excessiveness in the stomach and intestines**

温 [wēn]（名词）多种热病的总称 general term for febrile diseases, usually translated as warm diseases, and abbreviated to warmth or warm
温热 **(1) warmth-heat; (2) warm-heat disease**
温邪 **pathogenic warmth; warmth pathogen**
温邪犯肺 **attack of warm pathogen on the lung**
温下寒积 **warm purgation of cold accumulation**
（动词）使温暖 to warm
温中和胃 **warming the middle and harmonizing the stomach**
温胃止呕 **warming the stomach to stop vomiting**
温经暖宫 **warming the meridians/channels and the uterus**
温经止痛 **warming the meridians/channels to relieve pain**
温补命门 **warming and tonifying the life gate**
（形容词）温热的 warm
温服 **to be taken warm**

瘟 [wēn]（名词）流行性急性传染病 epidemic acute infectious disease; pestilence
瘟疫 **pestilence**
大头瘟 epidemic swollen-head infection → **erysipelas facialis**
虾蟆瘟 epidemic toad-like infection → **erysipelas facialis**

文 [wén]（形容词）柔和，不猛烈 mild, not strong
文火 **mild fire**

纹 [wén]（名词）①纹理，指浅表的静脉 superficial vein or venule
望指纹 **inspection of finger venules**
②裂纹 fissure (*v.* fissure)
裂纹舌 **fissured tongue**

闻 [wén]（动词）①听 to listen ②嗅 to smell
闻诊 listening and smelling examination → **auscultation and olfaction**
闻声音 listening to sounds → **auscultation**
不闻香臭 loss of the sense of smell → **anosmia**

吻 [wěn]（名词）口之角 corner of the mouth
吻 **corner of the mouth**

口吻疮 sore at the corner of the mouth → **angular stomatitis**

问 [wèn]（动词）询问 to inquire (*n.* inquiry)
问诊 **inquiry**
问起病 **inquiry about the onset of illness**
问现证 **inquiry about the present illness**
问口味 **inquiry about taste in the mouth**
问妇女经带 **inquiry about menstruation and leukorrhea**

窝 [wō]（名词）洼陷的地方 (1) a hollow place → fossa; (2) a hollow place into which something fits → socket
髂窝流注 **metastatic abscess of the iliac fossa**
三角窝 **triangular fossa**
眼窝凹陷 **sunken eye sockets**

卧 [wò]（动词）①躺下 to lie
卧式 **lying posture**
仰卧式 lying on the back → **supine posture**
侧卧式 lying on the side → **lateral recumbent posture**
踡卧缩足 **lying on one's side with the knees drawn up**
不得偃卧 **inability to lie flat**
②睡觉 to sleep
不得卧 inability to sleep → **insomnia**

乌 [wū]（动词）使变黑 to make something black, i.e., to blacken
乌须发 **blackening the hair and beard**

屋 [wū]（名词）房屋 house（屋漏 The house leaks. → The roof leaks.）
屋漏脉 **roof-leaking pulse**

无 [wú]（动词，副词，介词）没有 not, not have (be absent), without (*prefix*: non-, in-; *suffix*: -less)
无形之痰 phlegm that cannot be seen → **invisible phlegm**
无根苔 tongue coating/fur without root → **rootless (tongue) coating/fur**
无汗 **absence of sweating; anhidrosis**
无瘢痕灸 **non-scarring moxibustion**
无名肿毒 toxic swelling without a specific name → **innominate toxic swelling**
无头疽 abscess with no change of the skin surface → **deep abscess**

五 [wǔ]（数词）①五 five
五行 **five elements/phases**
五行归类 **categorization according to the five elements/phases**
五运六气 **five circuits and six *qi***
五官 **five (sense) organs**
五迟 **five kinds of retardation**
五软 **five types of flaccidity**
②第五 fifth
五更咳 **fifth-watch cough**
五更泻；五更泄 **fifth-watch diarrhea**

午 [wǔ]（名词）中午，午时 midday or noon (from 11 a.m. to 1 p.m.)
午后潮热 **afternoon tidal fever**
子午流注 **midnight-midday ebb flow**

武 [wǔ]（形容词）①猛烈的 strong
武火 **strong fire**
②军事的 martial
武术气功 **martial-art *qigong***

侮 [wǔ]（动词）反克 to restrict reversely (*n.* counter-restriction)
五行相侮 **counter-restriction among the five elements/phases**
土虚水侮 **reversed restriction of water on asthenic earth**

物 [wù]（名词）物体 thing or body (physical object)
物损真睛 some physical object causing injury to the eyeball → **traumatic injury to the eyeball**
隔物灸 moxibustion performed by placing something between the moxa cone and the skin → **interposed moxibustion**

误 [wù]（副词）错误地 erroneously
误下 **erroneous administration of**

purgatives

恶 [wù]（动词）厌恶 to be averse to (*n.* aversion)

恶热 aversion to heat

恶寒 aversion to cold; chill

恶风 aversion to wind

恶寒发热 aversion to cold with fever; chill and fever

雾 [wù]（名词）雾气 fog

云雾移睛 fog floating before the eye → **vitreous opacity**

X

吸 [xī]（动词）吸入 to inhale (*n.* inhalation)

吸入 inhalation

呼吸 exhaling and inhaling → **breathing**

呼吸之气 breathed air

吸门 "breath gate" → **epiglottis**

息 [xī]（名词）①呼吸 breath

平息 normal breathing

调息 management of breath

太息 taking a deep breath followed by letting it out audibly → **sighing**

善太息 frequent sighing

②停歇 the state of being kept in a place, viz., detention

息胞 detention of the afterbirth

（形容词）多余的 more than what is needed, viz., surplus

息肉 surplus flesh → **polyp**

息肉痔 rectal polyp

熄 [xī]（动词）熄灭 to extinguish

熄风 extinguishing wind

熄风化痰 extinguishing wind and resolving phlegm

熄风解痉 extinguishing wind to relieve convulsions

熄风定痫 extinguishing wind to arrest epilepsy

膝 [xī]（名词）大腿和小腿之间的关节 the joint between the thigh and the lower leg, namely, the knee

膝 knee

膝髌 kneecap; patella

膝腘 post-patellar fossa

膝顶扳胸椎法 knee-pushing thoracic pulling manipulation

洗 [xǐ]（动词）用水去掉污垢 to make clean using water, i.e., to wash

洗手 wringing the hands (as if washing the hands with water) (in auto-massage)

熏洗疗法 fuming-washing therapy

喜 [xǐ]（名词）欢喜 joy

喜 joy

喜脉 pulse of joy → **pregnancy pulse**

（动词）喜欢 to prefer (*n.* preference)

喜按 preference for pressing

细 [xì]（形容词）细的，纤细的，细微的 thin, thready, fine

细脉 thin pulse; thready pulse; fine pulse

郄 [xì]（名词）间隙 cleft

郄穴 cleft point

虾 [xiā]（名词）小虾 shrimp

虾游脉 shrimp-darting pulse

另见：虾 [há]

下 [xià]（形容词）①下面的 lower

下元不固 insecurity of lower origin

下焦病证 lower-energizer syndrome/pattern

下焦湿热证 lower-energizer dampness-heat syndrome/pattern

下丹田 lower *dantian*; lower elixir field

下消 lower wasting-thirst

②级别低的 inferior

下品 inferior-grade medicinal

（副词）向下 downward

下陷 falling, dropping, or descending gradually to a lower level → **sinking**

中气下陷 sinking of the middle *qi*

下按式 downward-pressing posture

下按式站桩功 hand- (downward-) **pressing postural stake-standing**

（动词）①泻下 to discharge fluid stools → to have diarrhea

下利 (1) diarrhea; (2) dysentery

下利清谷 diarrhea with undigested food

下利［痢］脓血 dysentery with purulent and bloody stools

②使泻下 to purge (*adj.* purgative)

下法 purgative method

③使下行 to direct something to move downward

下气 directing *qi* downward

下气消痰 directing *qi* downward and eliminating phlegm

下乳 "directing milk downward" → **promoting lactation**

（介词、副词）在下面 below

心下痞 stuffiness below the heart; epigastric stuffiness

心下硬 rigidity below the heart; epigastric rigidity

下坠 straining below (at stool); tenesmus

夏 [xià]（名词）四季的第二季，即夏季 the season between spring and autumn, namely, summer

夏季热 summer fever

夏季热病 summer fever disease

苦夏 summer affliction

疰夏 summer non-acclimation

先 [xiān]（形容词）①时间在前的 existing or happening before

先天 existing before birth → **inborn, innate or prenatal; congenital** (usually referring to a disease or medical condition)

先天之火 inborn fire

先天之气 innate *qi*; prenatal *qi*

先天之精 innate essence

先天不足 congenital defect

合先离 separation before reunion

②提前的 early (done before the usual) or premature

月经先期；经行先期；经水先期 early periods; polymenorrhea

胞衣先破 premature rupture of fetal membrane

（副词）首先 first (before anything else)

先煎 to be decocted first

弦 [xián]（名词）①弓弦 string

弦脉 string-like pulse, wiry pulse

②边缘 margin

睑弦 palpebral margin

目弦 margin of the eyelid

涎 [xián]（名词）口水 drool; thin saliva

流涎 drooling

口角流涎 drooling from the corner of the mouth

小儿多涎 excessive discharge of saliva in infancy → **infantile slobbering**

痫 [xián]（名词）癫痫；惊厥发作 epilepsy; convulsive attack

痫病 epilepsy (disease)

惊痫 fright epilepsy

痰痫 phlegm epilepsy

妊娠痫证 convulsive attack in pregnancy → **eclampsia of pregnancy**

险 [xiǎn]（形容词）危险的 critical

麻疹险证 critical case of measles

线 [xiàn]（名词）①细线；细丝 thread; filament

挂线疗法 threaded ligation therapy

线瘊 filiform wart → verruca filiformis

②线条 line

头穴线 scalp acupuncture lines

额中线 middle line of forehead

顶中线 middle line of vertex

相 [xiāng]（副词）①互相 mutually (*adj.* mutual)

风湿相搏 mutual contention of wind and dampness

风火相煽 mutual incitement of wind

and fire
相兼脉象 multi-featured pulse
②之间 between or among
五行相生 generation among the five elements/phases
正邪相争 struggle between healthy *qi* and pathogenic *qi*
形气相得 equilibrium between physique and *qi*
形气相失 disequilibrium between physique and *qi*
③表示一方对另一方的动作 a word showing the action of one object over the other → state or relationship (between two objects)
相使 assisting relationship
相畏 restraining relationship
相恶 inhibiting relationship; counteracting
相杀 suppressing relationship; neutralizing
相反 antagonizing relationship; incompatibility

项 [xiàng]（名词）颈的后部 the back part of the neck, namely, the nape (The meaning of the word neck includes both the anterior and posterior parts of the neck.)
项强 rigidity of the neck
头项强痛 headache and painful stiff neck
按揉颈项 pressing and kneading the neck
颈项功 neck exercise
项功 nape exercise

相 [xiàng]（名词）大臣 minister (*adj.* ministerial)
相火 ministerial fire
相火妄动 frenetic stirring of the ministerial fire
清泄相火 clearing and purging ministerial fire

消 [xiāo]（动词）①消化（食物）to digest (*n.* digestion; *adj.* digestant)
消食 promoting digestion
消谷善饥 swift digestion with rapid hunger
消食药 digestant (medicinal/drug)
消食剂 digestant formula
②（使）消散 to disperse
消痈散疖 dispersing abscesses and boils
消肿止痛 dispersing swelling to relieve pain
③消除 to remove
消积 removing accumulation
消积除胀 removing accumulation and relieving distension
④消解 to resolve; to relieve
消法 resolving method; resolution
消痞 (1) relieving stuffiness; (2) eliminating mass
消胀 relieving distension
消肿 relieving swelling
⑤消溶 to dissolve
消骨鲠 dissolving fish bone (that gets stuck in the throat)
⑥疾病引起消瘦虚弱 to become thin and weak due to illness, i.e., to waste
消渴［病］wasting thirst → diabetes
消肌 muscle-wasting diabetes
消浊 turbid diabetes
⑦亏缺 to wane
阴阳消长 waxing and waning of yin and yang

小 [xiǎo]（形容词）①小的 small; little
小舌 "little tongue" → palatine uvula
小肠 small intestine
小腹 smaller part of the abdomen → **lower abdomen**
小周天 small heavenly circuit; microcosmic cycle
②微小的 tiny
小针刀 a therapeutic instrument bearing a metal head with an appearance of both a needle and a tiny surgical knife → **acupotome**
小针刀疗法 acupotomy
③相对小的 minor
小结胸 minor chest bind; minor thoracic accumulation
小方 minor formula; mild formula

④轻微的 slight

小毒 slightly poisonous

（其他）①小便 urine (*adj.* urinary); 排小便 to urinate; to void (the bladder) (*n.* urination)

小便频数 frequent urination

小便清长 long voiding of clear urine

小便短赤 short voiding of dark urine

小便涩痛 difficult painful urination

小便淋漓 dribbling urination

小便失禁 urinary incontinence

②小儿 child; infant (*adj.* infantile)

小儿多涎 infantile slobbering

小儿暴泻 sudden infantile diarrhea

小儿麻痹 infantile paralysis; poliomyelitis

小儿遗尿 enuresis in children; bed-wetting

③小产 miscarriage

哮 [xiào]（动词）喘鸣 to breathe with difficulty and a whistling sound, namely, to wheeze

哮病 wheezing disease

寒哮 cold wheezing

冷哮 cold wheezing

热哮 heat wheezing

哮喘 dyspnea with wheezing → **asthma**

邪 [xié]（形容词）致病的 pathogenic（名词）致病的邪气 pathogenic factor; pathogen

邪气 pathogenic *qi*; pathogen

邪正盛衰 exuberance and debilitation between pathogenic *qi* and healthy *qi*

邪正消长 rise and decline between pathogenic and healthy *qi*

邪热壅肺 accumulation of pathogenic heat in the lung

胁 [xié]（名词）侧胸部 lateral pectoral region

胁 lateral pectoral region

季胁 hypochondrium; hypochondriac region

胁痛［病］lateropectoral or **hypochondriac pain**

胁下痛 hypochondriac pain

挟 [xié]（动词）夹杂 to be complicated

血虚挟瘀 blood deficiency complicated by stasis

斜 [xié]（形容词）①倾斜的 oblique

斜飞脉 oblique-running pulse

斜刺 oblique insertion

斜扳腰椎法 oblique lumbar pulling manipulation

②弯曲的 twisted

斜颈 twisting of the neck to one side → **torticollis**

泄 [xiè]（动词）①排出液体 to discharge liquid

早泄 discharging semen before the proper time → **premature ejaculation**

②清除 to purge (*adj.* purgative)

泄热 purging heat

泄热存津 purging heat to preserve fluids

泄火 purging fire

泄剂 purgative formula

（名词）泄泻 discharging fluid stools from the bowels → diarrhea

泄泻 diarrhea

泄注 pouring diarrhea

泄注赤白 watery diarrhea with blood and mucus

泻 [xiè]（动词）①清洗 to rid of the unwanted, i.e., to purge

泻肝 purging the liver

泻心 purging the heart

泻肺平喘 purging the lung to relieve dyspnea

②通便泻下 to cause evacuation from the bowels, i.e., to purge (*n.* purgation; *adj.* purgative)

泻下 purgation

泻下逐饮 expelling retained fluid by purgation

泻下药 purgative (medicinal/drug)

泻下剂 purgative formula
（名词）泄泻 diarrhea
水泻 watery diarrhea
泻下不爽 ungratifying diarrhea
热泻 heat diarrhea
寒泻 cold diarrhea

蟹 [xiè]（名词）螃蟹 crab
蟹目；蟹珠；蟹睛病 crab's eye (disease) → **corneal perforation with irridoptosis**

龂 [xiè]（动词）牙齿相磨 to grind the teeth
龂齿；齿龂 teeth grinding

心 [xīn]（名词）①心脏 heart
心血不足 insufficiency of heart blood
心阳不振 decline of heart yang
心肾不交 heart-kidney non-interaction
心移热于小肠 heart shifting heat to the small intestine
心下痞硬 stuffiness and rigidity below the heart; epigastric stuffiness and rigidity
心火炽［亢］盛证 intense heart-fire syndrome/pattern
②中心 center
眉心 center of the eyebrows; glabella
舌心 center of the tongue
（形容词）心前部的 precordial
心汗 precordial sweating
心痛彻背 precordial pain radiating to the back
（其他）
心烦 vexation
心慌 flusteredness

辛 [xīn]（形容词）辛辣的 pungent
辛温解表 releasing the exterior with pungent-warm (medicinals)
辛凉清热 clearing heat with pungent-cool (medicinals)
辛开苦泄 dispersion with the pungent and purgation with the bitter
辛凉轻剂 mild pungent-cool formula
辛凉重剂 drastic pungent-cool formula

新 [xīn]（形容词）①新近的 recent
新病 recent illness
新感 recent contraction
②新发的 fresh
新翳 fresh nebula
（名词）重新再生 regeneration
祛瘀生新 dispelling stasis to promote regeneration
和营生新 harmonizing the nutrient to promote regeneration

囟 [xìn]（名词）婴儿头顶骨未合缝的地方 the space remaining in the incompletely ossified skull of an infant, which is called fontanel
囟；囟门 fontanel
囟填 bulging fontanel
囟陷 sunken fontanel

星 [xīng]（名词）①星星 star
七星针 seven-star needle
七星功 seven-star exercise
②星星点点 dot
星翳 dotted nebula
聚星障 dot-clustered nebula → **superficial punctate keratitis**

腥 [xīng]（名词）腥臭 a strong, very unpleasant smell, or stink
腥臭气 stink

行 [xíng]（动词）①移动 to move
行气 moving *qi*
行气止痛 moving *qi* to relieve pain
行气宽胸 moving *qi* to soothe the chest
行气化痰 moving *qi* and resolving phlegm
行气活血 moving *qi* and activating blood; moving *qi* to activate blood
②（使）运行 to conduct (*n.* conduction)
行气法 *qi*-conducting method
指压行气法 finger-pressure conduction of *qi*
针向行气法 needle-direction conduction of *qi*

③操作 to manipulate
行针 manipulating the needle; needle manipulation
行针候气 manipulating the needle to await *qi*
④行走 to walk
行迟 retardation of walking
（形容词）移动的 migratory
行痹 migratory impediment; migratory arthralgia
（名词）①元素element ②变化的阶段 phase
五行 five elements/phases
五行学说 five-element/phase theory

形 [xíng]（名词）形体 physique
形气 physique and *qi*
形气相得 equilibrium between physique and *qi*
形气相失 imbalance between physique and *qi*
形气转化 conversion between physique and *qi*
形与神俱 harmony between physique and spirit

醒 [xǐng]（动词）①唤醒 to arouse
醒神 arousing from unconsciousness
醒脑 arousing the brain
②使有活力 to enliven
醒脾 enlivening the spleen

性 [xìng]（名词）性质 property
性味 property and flavor
药性 medicinal properties
四性 four properties
烧存性 burning with the original property retained

胸 [xiōng]（名词）胸部 chest; thorax (*adj.* pectoral; thoracic)
胸痛 chest pain
胸闷 thoracic oppression
胸痞 thoracic stuffiness
结胸 chest bind; thoracic accumulation
胸痹 chest impediment

休 [xiū]（动词）停歇 to have a rest or pause
休息痢 dysentery with pauses → **intermittent dysentery**

修 [xiū]（动词）加工处理 to process
修治；修事 processing (of materia medica)

羞 [xiū]（动词）怕见 to fear of seeing
羞明；羞明畏日 an abnormal fear of light → **photophobia**

畜 [xiù]（动词）古文"畜"同"嗅" In archaic Chinese, "畜" and "嗅" (to smell) are interchangeable
畜门 "opening of smelling" → nostril

嗅 [xiù]（动词）用鼻子闻 to smell
嗅气味 smelling odors

须 [xū]（名词）胡须 beard
须发早白 premature whitening of the hair and beard
乌须发 blackening the hair and beard
（动词）加强 to reinforce (*n.* reinforcement)
相须 reinforcing relationship; mutual reinforcement

虚 [xū]（名词）①不足 deficiency; insufficiency (*adj.* deficient; insufficient)
虚邪 deficiency-exploiting pathogen
虚实夹杂 deficiency-excess in complexity
虚热 (1) deficiency heat; (2) fever of deficiency type
虚中夹实 deficiency complicated by excess
虚热证 deficiency heat syndrome/pattern
虚胀 abdominal distension of deficiency type
②虚弱 asthenia (*adj.* asthenic)
小儿虚热 asthenic fever in children
土虚木乘 wood overrestricting asthenic earth
土虚水侮 reversed restriction of water on asthenic earth

虚阳上浮 asthenic yang floating upward
③虚损 consumption (*adj.* consumptive)
虚劳(病) consumptive disease
（形容词）虚弱的；空虚的 feeble and void or vacuous
虚脉 feeble pulse; vacuous pulse

徐 [xú]（形容词）徐缓的 slow
疾徐补泻 quick-slow reinforcement and reduction
疾徐补泻法 quick-slow reinforcing-reducing method

续 [xù]（动词）再连接to reunite (*n.* reunion)
续筋接骨 reunion of fractured bone and tendon

蓄 [xù]（动词）集聚 to accumulate (*n.* accumulation)
蓄血 blood accumulation
太阳蓄水证 greater yang water accumulation syndrome/pattern
太阳蓄血证 greater yang blood accumulation syndrome/pattern

宣 [xuān]（动词）①宣散 to disperse (*n.* dispersion)
肺气不宣 lung *qi* failing in dispersion
宣剂 dispersing formula
②宣通（空气的出入）to allow air to enter and move, namely to ventilate
宣肺；宣白 ventilating the lung
宣肺化痰 ventilating the lung and resolving phlegm
宣肺止咳平喘 ventilating the lung to relieve cough and dyspnea
宣肺降气 ventilating the lung and directing *qi* downward
③显露 to expose (*n.* exposure)
牙宣 exposure of dental root; gingival recession
（其他）
宣痹通阳 removing impediment and unblocking yang

玄 [xuán]（形容词）暗色的 dark
玄府 residence of dark-colored fluid (sweat) → **sweat pore**

悬 [xuán]（动词）悬挂 to suspend; to hang
悬灸；悬起灸 suspended moxibustion
悬雍垂 the fleshy mass hanging from the palate → **(palatine) uvula**
悬雍肿 swollen uvula; uvulitis
悬饮 fluid suspended (in the pleural space) → **pleural fluid retention**

旋 [xuán]（动词）①旋转 to rotate; to revolve
旋转屈伸 rotating, bending and stretching
旋耳 revolving the ears (in massage)
②迅速旋转 to whirl
风火内旋 wind-fire whirling internally
③盘旋 to circle (*adj.* circular)
盘旋法 circular needling method
回旋灸 circling moxibustion
（介词）在…周围 around (*prefix*: peri-)
旋耳疮 peri-auricular sore → **auricular eczema**

选 [xuǎn]（动词）选择 to select (*n.* selection)
选穴法 selection of points
局部选穴法 selection of local points
远道选穴法 selection of distant points
交叉选穴法 contralateral point selection
会选穴法 crossing point selection

癣 [xuǎn]（名词）凡皮肤增厚伴有鳞屑或有渗液的皮肤病，统称为癣 any of the skin diseases characterized by skin thickening along with the appearance of scales or exudates, including lichen, tinea, and ringworm
圆癣 round ringworm; tinea circinata
松皮癣 pine-bark lichen
奶癣 milk lichen; infantile eczema
风癣 tinea corporis
股癣 tinea cruris
喉癣 tinea-like erosion of the throat

眩 [xuàn]（名词）头晕眼花 dizziness and

dimmed vision
眩晕 (1) dizziness; (2) vertigo
瞑眩 dimness of vision
眩冒 dizziness with dimmed vision
掉眩 dizziness with shaking

穴 [xué]（名词）穴位，人体可以施行针灸的部位 points on the body surface that are suitable for the application of acupuncture and moxibustion, namely, acupoints
穴位注射 acupoint injection
穴位封闭 acupoint block
耳穴 ear acupoints

雪 [xuě]（名词）雪 snow
雪口 snow-white mouth → **thrush**

血 [xuè]（名词）血液 blood (*prefix*: hemo-)
血室 blood chamber
血脉 blood vessel
血瘀 blood stasis
血热妄行 heat enabling frenetic movement of blood
血精 hemospermia
（形容词）带血的 bloody
血痰 bloody sputum
血尿 bloody urine
（其他）
血崩 flooding; metrorrhagia
血缕 vascular spider; spider nevus
血翳包睛 keratic pannus

熏 [xūn]（动词）冒气 to fume
熏蒸 fuming and steaming
熏洗疗法 fuming-washing therapy

寻 [xún]（动词）寻找 to search
寻法 searching (in pulse-taking)
举、按、寻 touching, pressing, and searching

循 [xún]（动词）①顺着……进行 to go along
循按法；循法 massage along the meridian/channel
循经感传 transmission of sensation along the meridian/channel
循经选穴法 selection of points along the affected meridian/channel
②追寻 to trace
循法 tracing (in pulse taking)
③通"揗"，抚摸，对于危重病人而言是瞎摸的意思。循 [xún] is the same as揗 [xún] which means to fondle in the general sense. However, when either of the characters is used to describe the behavior of a critically illed patient, it means to fumble.
循衣摸床 semiconscious fumbling and picking at the clothes and the bed → **floccillation**

徇 [xùn]（副词）猝然 suddenly (*adj.* sudden)
徇蒙招尤 sudden dizziness with dimmed vision and shaking

Y

压 [yā]（动词）施加压力 to press (*n.* pressure)
压力垫；压垫 pressure pad
指压行气法 finger-pressure conduction of *qi*
指压疗法 finger-pressure therapy
指压麻醉 finger-pressure anesthesia

押 [yā]（动词）按压 **to press**
押手 pressing hand

牙 [yá]（名词）牙齿 tooth（形容词）牙齿的 dental
牙痛 toothache
牙宣 exposure of dental root → **gingival recession**
（其他）牙龈 gingiva (*adj.* gingival)
牙痈 gingival abscess
牙鲛［咬］痈 distal gingival abscess
牙疳 ulcerative gingivitis
风热牙疳 wind-heat ulcerative gingivitis

哑 [yǎ]（形容词）哑巴的 mute (*n.* mutism)
耳聋口哑 deaf-mutism

咽 [yān]（名词）口腔与食道之间的通道 the passage between the mouth and the esophagus, namely, the pharynx (*adj.* pharyngeal)
咽底 retropharynx
咽痹 pharynx impediment; pharyngitis
咽后痈 retropharyngeal abscess
咽喉 laryngopharynx; throat

延 [yán]（动词）延长；拖延 to prolong; to protract
经期延长 prolonged menstruation; menostaxis
迁延痢 protracted dysentery

言 [yán]（名词）说话；语言 talk; speech
狂言 mentally deranged wild talk → **manic raving**
语言謇涩 sluggish speech

岩 [yán]（名词）"岩"通"癌"，硬如岩石的恶性肿瘤 malignant tumor as hard as rock, i.e., cancer or carcinoma (interchangeable with 癌, cf. 癌 [ái])
舌岩 carcinoma of the tongue
乳岩 mammary cancer
肾岩翻花 carcinoma of the penis with ulceration
喉岩 throat cancer; carcinoma of the throat

炎 [yán] (动词) 燃起火焰 to flame
肝火上炎 up-flaming of liver fire
肝火上炎证 syndrome/pattern of up-flaming liver fire
虚火上炎 deficiency fire flaming upward

盐 [yán]（名词）食盐 salt
隔盐灸 salt-interposed moxibustion

颜 [yán]（名词）脸面 face (*adj.* facial)
颜面疔疮 deep-rooted facial boil

眼 [yǎn]（名词）眼睛；眼球 eye; eyeball (*adj.* ocular)
眼带 extra-ocular muscles
眼系 ocular connector
眼珠牵斜 involutary deviation of the eye → **strabismus; squint**
眼球突出 protrusion of the eyeball; exophthalmos
火眼 inflammed eye; conjunctivitis

偃 [yǎn]（动词）偃卧 to lie flat
不得偃卧 inability to lie flat

罨 [yǎn]（名词）覆盖（医疗方法）compression
罨 compression
冷罨 cold compression
热罨 hot compression

厌 [yàn]（动词）厌恶 to be tired of
厌食 "being tired of food" → **anorexia**

验 [yàn]（形容词）经检验证实的 proven (tested and shown to be true)
验方 proven formula

燕 [yàn]（名词）燕子 swallow
燕口疮；燕口 inflamed mouth angles with fissuring making the mouth look like that of a swallow → **angular stomatitis; perlèche**

羊 [yáng]（名词）绵羊或山羊 sheep or goat
羊痫风 convulsion with an aura like the sound that sheep or goats make → **"bleating convulsion" → epilepsy**

阳 [yáng]（名词）①阴阳学说中的阳 Yang in yin-yang theory
阳中之阳 yang within yang
阳虚阴盛 yang deficiency with yin exuberance
阳证似阴 yang syndrome/pattern resembling yin
阳明腑证 yang brightness *fu*-organ syndrome/pattern

阳跷脉 yang heel vessel (YangHV)
阳黄 yang jaundice
②男性生殖器 male genitalia
阳痿［病］inability to initiate or maintain an erection in sexual intercourse → **impotence**

杨 [yáng]（名词）杨梅 strawberry
杨莓舌 strawberry tongue

疡 [yáng]（名词）①"身伤曰疡"（身体受伤，皆可称疡）any trauma of the body
疡 (1) trauma; (2) ulcer; (3) surgical conditions (on the body surface)
疡医 traumato-orthopedist
折疡 trauma and fracture
②溃疡 ulcer
溃疡 ulcer
疮疡 sore and ulcer
金疡 metal ulcer (of the eye); phlyctenular conjunctivitis
火疡 fire ulcer (of the eye); episcleritis

烊 [yáng]（动词）融化 to melt
烊化 melting

仰 [yǎng]（形容词）仰卧的 supine
仰卧伸足 lying supine with the legs stretched
仰卧式 supine posture

养 [yǎng]（动词）滋养 to nourish
养心 nourishing the heart
养胃生津 nourishing the stomach to produce fluid
养阴润燥 nourishing yin to moisten dryness
养血柔肝 nourishing blood and emolliating the liver
养心安神药 heart-nourishing tranquilizing medicinal/drug; heart-nourishing tranquilizer
（其他）
养生 health preservation

痒 [yǎng]（动词）发痒 to itch (*n.* itching; pruritus)
风瘙痒 wind pruritus
目痒 eye itching
身痒 generalized itching
阴痒 itching of the vulva → **pruritus vulvae**

腰 [yāo]（名词）①身体的中部，在胯上胁下 the area around the middle of the body between the ribs and hips, i.e., the waist
腰部功 waist exercise
伸腰沉胯 stretching the waist and keeping the hips sunk
舒腰松腹 keeping the waist and abdomen relaxed
②后背的下部 the lower part of the back, i.e., the lumbus or lower back
腰骨 lumbar bone
腰痛 lumbar pain; lumbago
腰酸；腰痠 lumbar aching

摇 [yáo]（动词）①摇摆 to rock
摇摆触碰 rocking and tapping
②摇动 to rotate; to waggle
摇法 rotating manipulation
摇柄法 handle-waggling method
③松动 to loosen (*n.* looseness)
齿摇 looseness of teeth

咬 [yǎo]（动词）用牙齿把东西夹断或夹碎 to cut or crush with teeth, or to bite (*n.* bite)
癫狗咬伤 rabid dog bite
咬骨疽 suppurative inflammaton of bone with local separation of tissues as if crushed by teeth → **medial suppurative osteomyelitis**

药 [yào]（名词）药物 medicinal; drug
中药 Chinese medicinals; Chinese drugs
草药 herbal medicinals; herbal drugs
药味 (1) taste or flavor of a medicinal; (2) medicinal ingredients (in a prescription)
（形容词）①药物的 medicinal
药材 medicinal substance; materia medica

药材炮制 processing of medicinal substances
药性 medicinal properties
药面 medicinal powder
药引子 "medicinal guide"; extra conductant ingredient
②药制的 medicated
药酒 medicated wine
药捻疗法 medicated spill therapy
药线疗法 medicated thread therapy
药罐 medicated cupping

噎 [yē]（名词）吞咽困难 difficulty in swallowing; dysphagia
噎嗝；膈噎 dysphagia

夜 [yè]（名词）夜晚 night
夜啼 night crying
热夜啼 night crying due to heat
寒夜啼 night crying due to cold
客忤夜啼 night crying due to fright
夜热 fever at night

液 [yè]（名词）液体 liquid
液 (thick) liquid
阴液 yin liquid
液脱 liquid collapse
黄液上冲 upsurging of the yellow liquid → **hypopyon**

一 [yī]（数词）一；第一 one; first
一夫法 the breadth of (one) palm as measuring unit → **palm measurement**
一垫固定法 fixation with one pad
一次性针 needle intended to be used for one time only → **disposable needle**
一阴 first yin
一阳 first yang
（形容词）单一的 single
一指禅功 single-finger meditation manipulation
一指禅推拿 single-finger meditation *tuina*; single-finger meditation massage
一指禅导气 conducting *qi* with single-finger meditation
一指禅式 single-finger meditation gesture

医 [yī]（名词）医学 medicine (*adj*. medical)
医用气功 medical *qigong*

遗 [yí]（动词）不自觉地排出尿液或精液 to discharge urine or semen involuntarily
遗尿 involuntary discharge of urine→ **enuresis; bed-wetting**
遗精 involuntary discharge of semen → **seminal emission**

颐 [yí]（名词）下颌 lower cheek
颐 lower cheek
滞颐 dribbling with wet cheeks

以 [yǐ]（介词）用以 by means of, with
以毒攻毒 combating poison with poison

异 [yì]（形容词）①不同的 different
异病同治 same treatment for different diseases
同病异治 different treatments for the same disease
②另外的 other
异经选穴法 selection of points on other meridians/channels
③异常的 abnormal
异气 abnormal *qi*
（其他）异物 foreign body
异物入目 foreign body entering the eye

呓 [yì]（名词）梦话 the act of talking in one's sleep
呓语 talking while asleep → **somniloquy**

易 [yì]（形容词）容易 liable (*n*. liability)
易虚易实 liability to change from excess to deficiency and vice versa
易寒易热 liability to change from heat to cold and vice versa
（动词）①改变 to transform
易筋功 sinew-transforming exercise
②染易 to transmit (disease) (*n*. transmission)

阴阳易 yin-yang transmission

疫 [yì]（名词）瘟疫；流行性急性传染病 pestilence (*adj.* pestilential); acute epidemic infectious disease

疫疠之气；疠气；戾气 pestilential *qi*; epidemic pathogen

疫痢 epidemic dysentery

疫喉痧；疫痧 epidemic throat disease with eruption → **scarlet fever**

疫咳 epidemic cough → **pertussis**

疫疔 pestilent boil → **cutaneous anthrax**

益 [yì]（动词）补益 to replenish

益气 replenishing *qi*

益气解表 replenishing *qi* and releasing the exterior

益阴 replenishing yin

益气生津 replenishing *qi* and engendering fluid

益气安神 replenishing *qi* to calm the mind

益肾宁神 replenishing the kidney to calm the mind

意 [yì]（名词）思想；思考 thought; mind

意呼吸 breathing in the mind → **imaginary breathing**

意守自身 concentration (of the mind) **on oneself**

意守丹田 concentration (of the mind) **on *dantian***

意守体外 concentration (of the mind) **on something outside the body**

溢 [yì]（动词）溢出 to overflow

溢饮 overflowing of fluid (under the skin) → **subcutaneous fluid retention**

溢乳 milk overflowing (the stomach) → **milk regurgitation**

翳 [yì]（名词）角膜上遮蔽视线的班块 opacity of the cornea that impairs the vision, i.e., nebula

翳 nebula

新翳 fresh nebula

宿翳 chronic corneal opacity

星翳 dotted nebula

臆 [yì]（名词）胸肉 pectoral muscle

臆 pectoral muscle

因 [yīn]（名词）原因 cause

病因 cause of disease

外因 exogenous cause; external cause

内因 endogenous cause; internal cause

不内外因 non-exo-endogenous cause; cause neither internal nor external

（介词）按照 according to

因时制宜 treatment according to time

因地制宜 treatment according to place

因人制宜 treatment according to individual

阴 [yīn]（名词）①阴阳学说中的阴 yin in yin-yang theory

阴阳学说 yin-yang theory

阴阳交感 yin-yang interaction

阴阳互根 mutual rooting of yin and yang; yin-yang interdependence

阴阳对立 yin-yang opposition

阴阳消长 waxing and waning of yin and yang

阴虚火旺 yin deficiency with effulgent fire

②生殖器 genitalia

阴户 vaginal orifice; vulva

阴挺 prolapse of the uterus

阴囊 scrotum

阴痒 pruritus vulvae

阴器痛 genital pain

喑［瘖］[yīn]（名词）声哑；失音 hoarseness; aphonia

子喑［瘖］gravidic aphonia; aphonia of pregnancy

喉喑［瘖］hoarseness or aphonia

淫 [yín]（名词）过度 excess (*adj.* excessive)

六淫 six excesses

淫气 excessive *qi*

龈 [yín]（名词）牙龈 gum (*adj.* gingival)

龈 gum
齿龈肿痛 painful swelling of gums
齿龈结瓣 petaloid gum
齿龈宣露 gingival recession

引 [yǐn]（动词）①引导；指引 to conduct; to direct
引火归原 conducting fire back to its origin
引经报使 directing to the affected meridian/channel or site
药引子 extra conductant ingredient; medicinal guide
②用手拉 to pull
引伸法 pulling and stretching
③拔出来 to withdraw
引针 withdrawing of the needle

饮 [yǐn]（名词）①水液停留的病证 disease due to fluid retention
饮 fluid retention; retained fluid
②冷服的汤剂 decoction to be taken cold
饮 cold decoction
（动词）喝 to drink
口渴引饮 thirst with frequent drinking
口干不欲饮 dryness in the mouth with no desire to drink
（其他）饮食 food; diet (*adj.* dietary)
饮食劳倦 improper diet and overstrain
饮食不节 dietary irregularties
饮食不洁 contaminated food

隐 [yǐn]（形容词）①不明显的，隐隐约约的 not intense enough to be apparent, but indistinctly sensible → dull
隐痛 dull pain
②隐匿的 hidden from view
隐疹 eruption which becomes hidden from view quickly → **urticaria; hives**
③隐秘不公开的 not divulged; occult
隐疾 occult disease

婴 [yīng]（名词）婴儿 infant (*adj.* infantile)
婴儿瘛疭 infantile clonic convulsion
婴儿湿疮 infantile eczema

膺 [yīng]（名词）胸 chest
膺 chest; pectoral muscle

迎 [yíng]（动词）对着，向着 to meet in the opposite direction or to be against
迎随补泻 directing the needle insertion along or against the run of meridian/channel for reinforcement or reduction respectively → **directional reinforcing-reducing method**
迎风流泪 shedding tears when looking against the wind → **lacrimination induced by wind**
迎风冷泪 cold tear shedding induced by wind
迎风热泪 warm tear shedding induced by wind

荥 [yíng]（名词）绝小水也 the very beginning of a river → spring
荥穴 spring points

营 [yíng]（名词）养分 nutrient
营气 nutrient *qi*
营阴 nutrient yin
营血 nutrient-blood
营卫不和 disharmony between nutrient and defense *qi*

蝇 [yíng]（名词）苍蝇 fly
蝇影飞越 flying fly shadow → **vitreous opacity**
蝇翅黑花 fly-wing-like shadow → **vitreous opacity**

瘿 [yǐng]（名词）颈瘤也，通常指甲状腺肿大 tumor of the neck, more often referring to enlargement of the thyroid gland (goiter)
瘿 goiter
气瘿 *qi* goiter
肉瘿 fleshy goiter
石瘿 stony goiter
筋瘿 goiter with varicose veins
瘿痈 thyroiditis

硬 [yìng]（形容词）①坚硬的 hard
硬气功 hard *qigong*
硬肿症 chronic hardening and thickening of the skin → **sclerederma (neonatorum)**
②僵硬的 rigid (*n.* rigidity)
心下硬 rigidity below the heart; epigastric rigidity
心下痞硬 stuffiness and rigidity below the heart; epigastric stuffiness and rigidity

痈 [yōng]（名词）皮肤深层脓肿；内脏的脓肿 deep-rooted abscess or carbuncle; visceral abscess
痈 abscess; carbuncle
肺痈 lung abscess
肠痈 intestinal abscess → **acute appendicitis or periappendicular abscess**

涌 [yǒng]（动词）水从下向上冒出来 to bring up fluid from below (涌吐 inducing vomiting → emetic)
涌吐药 emetic (medicinal/drug)
涌吐禁例 contraindications for emesis

忧 [yōu]（名词）忧虑 anxiety
忧 anxiety

幽 [yōu]（形容词）幽静的 serene
幽门 "serene gate"; pylorus

由 [yóu]（介词）从 from
由表入里 entering the interior from the exterior
由里出表 exiting to the exterior from the interior

油 [yóu]（名词）油脂 oil; fat (*adj.* oily; fatty)
油汗；汗出如油 oily sweat
去油 defatting
黄油障 yellowish fatty proliferation blocking the vision → **pinguecula**
（其他）
油风 sudden patchy loss of hair → **alopecia**

疣 [yóu]（名词）瘊子 wart
疣 wart; verruca
疣目 wart eye; verruca vulgaris
跖疣 plantar wart; verruca plantaris
丝状疣 thread-shaped wart → **verruca filiformis**

游 [yóu]（动词）①在水里行动 to move through water: (fish) to swim, (shrimp) to dart
虾游脉 shrimp-darting pulse
②游走 to wander
游走痛 wandering pain
赤游丹 wandering erysipelas
面游风 facial wandering wind → **seborrhea; seborrheic dermatitis**

有 [yǒu]（动词）表示存在 to have (having → with)
有头疽 phlegmon with heads → **headed phlegmon; carbuncle**
有根苔 a tongue coating/fur with root → **rooted (tongue) coating/fur**
（其他）
有形之痰 visible phlegm

瘀 [yū]（名词）血瘀 (blood) stasis (*adj.* static)
血瘀 blood stasis
瘀血 static blood
瘀血犯头 static blood invading the head
瘀阻脑络证 syndrome/pattern of static blood obstructing the brain collateral
化瘀药 stasis-resolving medicinal/drug
（形容词）瘀滞的 stagnant
瘀热 stagnant heat

余 [yú]（形容词）剩余的 residual
余沥不尽 residual dribbling → **dribbling after voiding**
余热未清证 residual heat syndrome/pattern

鱼 [yú]（名词）生活在水中的鱼 fish
鱼翔脉 fish-swimming pulse
（其他）

鱼际 **thenar eminence**
鱼络 collateral vessel in the thenar eminence **→ thenar collateral vessel**
鱼际擦法 (thenar) **eminence rubbing manipulation**

语 [yǔ]（动词）说话 to speak (*n.* speech)
语迟 **retardation of speaking**
语言謇涩 **sluggish speech**
语声 sounds formed by speaking → **voice**
语声重浊 **deep turbid voice**
语声低微 **faint low voice**

玉 [yù]（名词）玉石 jade
玉枕骨 jade pillow bone → **occipital bone**
玉门 jade gate → **virginal vaginal orifice**

郁 [yù]（形容词）①抑郁的 depressive (*n.* depression)
郁病 **depressive disease; depression**
产后郁冒 **postpartum depression and dizziness**
气郁 ***qi* depression**
气郁化火 **depressed *qi* transforming into fire**
②郁滞的 stagnant (*n.* stagnation; *v.* stagnate)
郁火 **stagnant fire**
湿郁肌表 **dampness stagnating in the superficies**
湿郁化热 **stagnant dampness transforming into heat**

育 [yù]（动词）①生育 to give birth to offspring
不育 inability to give birth to offspring → **sterility**
②养育 to nourish
育阴 **nourishing yin**

欲 [yù]（动词）期望 to desire（*n.* desire）
口干不欲饮 **dryness in the mouth with no desire to drink**
饥不欲食 **no desire to eat despite hunger**
但欲寐 **desire only to sleep; somnolence**

寓 [yù]（动词）寄托 to repose in
寓攻于补 reposing elimination in reinforcement **→ reinforcemnt for elimination**
寓补于攻 reposing reinforcement in elimination **→ elimination for reinforcement**

元 [yuán]（名词）本原 origin (*adj.* original)
元气 **original *qi***
下元不固 **insecurity of lower origin**
元阳亏虚 **original yang insufficiency**
真元亏虚 **genuine origin insufficiency**
胎元 **fetal origin**

原 [yuán]（名词）①本原 origin
原气 **original *qi***
纳入原位 restoring the dislocated bone to its original position (with the hands) → **(manual) restoration**
引火归原 **conducting fire back to its origin**
②发源 source
原穴 **source points**
原络配穴法 **source-connecting point combination**

圆 [yuán]（形容词）圆形的 round
圆癣 **round ringworm; tinea circinata**
圆翳 round nebula → **cataract**
圆翳内障 round nebula impairing vision **→ cataract**
圆针 **round-pointed needle**
圆利针 **round-sharp needle**

远 [yuǎn]（副词）空间或时间的距离长 a long distance or long time, i.e., far or long
远血 bleeding into the alimentary tract far from the anus → **distal bleeding**
远视 **farsightedness; hyperopia**
食远服 to take (medicine) at a long time from meal → **to be taken midway between meals**
（形容词）远处的 distant
远道选穴法 **selection of distant points**

远道刺 distant needling

月 [yuè]（名词）①月亮 the moon (*adj.* lunar)
月蚀疮 eclipsed lunar sore → **peri-auricular eczema**
②计时单位，一年分为十二个月 one of the twelve periods of time that a year is divided into, namely month
月经；月信；月事；月水 cyclic discharge of blood from the womb, usually once a month → **menstruation**
月经不调；月水不调 menstrual irregularities
月经过多；月水过多 abnormally profuse menstrual flow → **hypermenorrhea; menorrhagia**
月经提前；月经先期 advanced menstruation; early periods
月经错后；月经后期 late periods

越 [yuè]（动词）跳过 to skip over
越经传 skip-over meridian/channel transmission

晕 [yūn]（形容词）眩晕的 dizzy (*n.* dizziness; vertigo)
眩晕 (1) dizziness; (2) vertigo
子晕 gravid vertigo
另见：晕 [yùn]

云 [yún]（名词）云雾 fog
云雾移睛 fog floating before the eye → **vitreous opacity**

孕 [yùn]（动词）怀胎 to become pregnant
不孕 inability to become pregnant → **infertility**

运 [yùn]（名词）环行 circuit
运气学说 theory of the circuits and *qi*
运气 (1) circuit-*qi*; (2) moving of *qi*
主运 dominant circuit
客运 guest circuit
运法 circular kneading (in massage)
（动词）①使运行，启动 to activate
运脾 activating the spleen
②运作 to manipulate (*n.* manipulation)
运针 needle manipulation

晕 [yùn]（动词）晕倒 to faint
晕针 fainting during acupuncture
晕灸 fainting during moxibustion
另见：晕 [yūn]

熨 [yùn]（动词）用热物压敷 to compress with a piece of hot pad
熨法 hot compression (with rubbing)
熨目 compressing the eyes (with the hot palms)
熨药 hot-compressing medicinal

Z

扎 [zā]（动词）①包扎 to bind
扎带 cloth ribbon for binding (a splint) → **bandage**
②结扎 to ligate (*n.* ligation)
结扎疗法 ligation therapy

杂 [zá]（形容词）①各种各样的 miscellaneous
杂病 miscellaneous diseases
②混杂不纯的 impure
杂气 impure *qi*
（名词）紊乱 upset
嘈杂 gastric upset

脏 [zàng]（名词）内脏器官 *zang* organ; viscus (*pl.* viscera; *adj.* visceral)
脏象 visceral manifestation
脏腑 *zang-fu* organs; viscera and bowels
脏气 *qi* of *zang* organs; visceral *qi*
脏腑辨证 visceral syndrome differentiation; visceral pattern identification
脏躁 visceral agitation → **hysteria**

早 [zǎo]
（形容词）提前的 early; premature
早泄 premature ejaculation
经早 early periods

燥 [zào]（形容词）干燥的 dry

燥苔 dry (tongue) coating/fur

（名词）干燥 dryness

燥热 dryness-heat

燥火 dryness-fire

燥伤肺气 dryness damaging lung *qi*

燥化 dryness transformation

燥结 dryness accumulation

燥痰证 dryness-phlegm syndrome/pattern

（动词）使变干；使干燥 to dry; to dessicate

燥湿 drying dampness

燥湿化痰 drying dampness and resolving phlegm

燥湿健脾 drying dampness to invigorate the spleen

燥湿止痒 drying dampness and relieving itching

燥剂 desiccating formula

躁 [zào]（动词）躁动不安 to agitate (*n.* agitation)

躁狂 mental disorder characterized by agitation and hyperexicitability → **mania**

躁烦 agitated vexation

烦躁 vexation and agitation

脉躁 agitated pulse

脏躁 visceral agitation → **hysteria**

择 [zé]（动词）选择 to choose

择向补泻法 reinforcement-reduction by choosing direction

贼 [zéi]（形容词）偷偷的 stealthy

贼风 stealthy wind

增 [zēng]（动词）增加 to increase

增液通下 increasing fluid to induce laxation

憎 [zēng]（动词）憎恶 to abhore (*n.* abhorrence)

憎寒 abhorrence of cold

痄 [zhà]（名词）痄腮 mumps

痄腮 mumps; epidemic parotitis

谵 [zhān]（名词）说胡话 disordered or delirious speech

谵妄 mental confusion with disordered speech → **delirium**

谵语 delirious speech

战 [zhàn]（动词）颤抖 to tremble; to shiver (*n.* shiver)

战栗 shiver

战汗 shiver sweating

寒战 shiver caused by a chill → **rigor**

舌战 trembling tongue

掌 [zhǎng]（名词）手掌 palm (*adj.* palmar)

掌心毒 palmar infection; palmar pustule

掌揉法 palm-kneading manipulation

掌推法 palm-pushing manipulation

掌摩法 palmar circular rubbing manipulation

鹅掌风 ringworm affecting the palmar surface of the hand → **tinea manuum**

胀 [zhàng]（动词）肿胀 to distend (*n.* distension)

胀痛 distending pain

腹胀 abdominal distension

臌胀（病）abdominal distension (disease)

虚胀 abdominal distension of deficiency type

实胀 abdominal distension of excess type

障 [zhàng]（名词）障碍视力的眼病 any vision-impairing eye disease, e.g., nebula, cataract, and glaucoma; ophthalmopathy

内障 internal ophthalmopathy

青风内障 bluish glaucoma; simple glaucoma

黄风内障 yellowish glaucoma (glaucoma characterized by yellow-discoloration of the pupil)

金针拨障法 needle cataractopiesis

瘴 [zhàng]（名词）瘴气 miasma (*adj.* miasmic)

瘴疟 miasmic malaria
热瘴 heat miasmic malaria
寒瘴 cold miasmic malaria
瘴毒 miasmic toxin

招 [zhāo]（动词）掉摇不定 to shake
徇蒙招尤 sudden dizziness with dimmed vision and shaking

朝 [zhāo]（名词）早晨 morning
朝食暮吐 vomiting in the evening of food eaten in the morning
暮食朝吐 vomiting in the morning of food eaten in the previous evening

着 [zháo]（动词）接触 to contact (*n.* contact)
着肤灸 direct contact moxibustion

折 [zhé]（动词）①折断 to break
骨折 breaking of a bone → **fracture**
折疡 trauma and fracture
折骨列肤 fracture with split skin; open fracture
折骨绝筋 fracture with broken tendon
②折返 to turn back
折顶 turning to the opposite

针 [zhēn]（名词）①在身体上针刺治病 puncturing the body with a needle to cure disease → acupuncture (prefix denoting relationship to a needle: acu-)
针灸 acupuncture-moxibustion
针灸师 acupuncturist
针刺疗法 acupuncture therapy
针法 acupuncture; needling (technique)
②针灸用的针 needle for acupuncture
针尖 tip of the needle
针柄 handle of the needle
针感 needling sensation
针向行气法 needle-direction conduction of *qi*
③缝纫用的针 needle for sewing
针眼 a small furuncle appearing on the eyelid resembling the eye of a needle → **stye; hordeolum**

真 [zhēn]（形容词）①真正的，其反义词是“人造的” genuine, the opposite of manmade
真水 genuine water
真阴 genuine yin
真阳 genuine yang
真火 genuine fire
真气气感 sensation of genuine *qi*
②真的，其反义词是假的 true, the opposite of false
真脏色 true visceral color; visceral exhaustion color
真脏脉 true visceral pulse; visceral exhaustion pulse
真实假虚 true excess with false deficiency
真寒假热 true cold with false heat
③真实的，其反义词是虚构的 real, the opposite of fantastical
真心痛 real heart pain
真头痛 real headache; true headache
真中风 real wind stroke; true wind stroke
真中 real stroke; true stroke
（其他）
真牙 wisdom tooth; third molar tooth
真睛破损 ruptured wound of the eyeball

诊 [zhěn]（动词）诊查 to examine (*n.* examination)
四诊 four examinations
诊断 the process of identifying a disease by examination, as well as the decision reached via such a process → **diagnosis**
诊断学 diagnostics
诊法 diagnostic method
诊病 disease identification
诊籍 the record of a patient's diagnosis and treatment → **case record**

枕 [zhěn]（名词）枕部 occiput
枕上正中线 upper-middle line of occiput (MS 12)
枕上旁线 upper-lateral line of occiput (MS 13)

枕下旁线 lower-lateral line of occiput (MS 14)

疹 [zhěn]（名词）①皮疹 rash
②麻疹的简称 measles
疹 (1) rash; (2) measles

振 [zhèn]（动词）①使振动 to vibrate
振法 vibrating (manipulation of massage)
振挺 a stick used to pat an injured area → **patting stick**
②震动 to tremble
振掉 trembling

震 [zhèn]（动词）震动 to tremble
震颤法 trembling method (in acupuncture)（其他）
震桩式 pile-driving standing posture (in *qigong*)

镇 [zhèn]（动词）①使平静 to settle
镇惊安神 settling fright and calming the mind
镇心安神 settling the heart and calming the mind
镇肝熄风 settling the liver to extinguish wind
②镇静 to sedate
镇静安神 inducing sedation and calming the mind

争 [zhēng]（动词）斗争 to struggle (*n.* struggle)
正邪相争；正邪分争 struggle between healthy and pathogenic *qi*

征 [zhēng]（名词）征象 sign
征候 sign

怔 [zhēng]（形容词）惶恐不安的 fearful
怔忡 fearful throbbing; severe palpitations
产后怔忡 postpartum palpitations

蒸 [zhēng]（动词）用蒸汽加热 to heat by steam, or to steam
劳蒸 consumptive steaming → **consumptive fever**
变蒸 growth steaming → **growth fever**
骨蒸热 bone-steaming fever; consumptive fever
湿热蒸舌 dampness-heat steaming the tongue
熏蒸 fuming and steaming

癥 [zhēng]（名词）腹内结块，坚硬不能移动者 abdominal mass, hard and immovable
癥瘕 abdominal mass
癥瘕积聚 aggregation-accumulation masses
破瘀消癥 breaking blood stasis and eliminating masses

整 [zhěng]（形容词）整体的 holistic (*n.* holism)
整体观念 concept of holism
（动词）恢复原位 to reduce (*n.* reduction)
整复 reduction

正 [zhèng]（形容词）①健康的，与邪相对 healthy, the opposite of pathogenic
正气 healthy *qi*
正邪相争；正邪分争 struggle between healthy and pathogenic *qi*
正虚邪实 insufficiency of healthy *qi* and excessiveness of pathogenic *qi*
②合乎常规的；通常的；正规的 routine; ordinary; regular
正治 routine treatment
正经 regular meridians/channels
正疟 ordinary malaria
正水 regular edema; typical edema
（动词）矫正 to set right
正骨 bone setting
正骨手法 bone setting manipulation

证 [zhèng]（名词）症候的综合；症候的模式 syndrome; pattern
证 syndrome; pattern
辨证 syndrome differentiation; pattern identification
证型 syndrome/pattern type
证候 syndrome/pattern manifestation

郑 [zhèng]（形容词）重复的 repeated (*n.* repetition)
郑声 repeated sounding → **unconscious murmuring** (with repetition)

支 [zhī]（名词）分支 branch
地支 earthly branches
（动词）支撑 to sustain
支饮 sustained retention of excess fluid (in the chest) → **thoracic fluid retention**

脂 [zhī]（名词）脂肪；脂质 fat; lipid
脂瘤 a tumor filled with lipid-rich debris → **sebaceous cyst**
颊脂垫 buccal fat pad → corpus adiposum bucca
凝脂翳 fat-congealed nebula → purulent keratitis
脂塞不孕 fat infertility

直 [zhí]（形容词）① 直的（不弯曲的）straight (not bending)
瞪目直视 staring straight ahead
② 垂直的 perpendicular
直刺 perpendicular insertion
直透 perpendicular penetration
③ 直接的 direct
直中 direct attack
直针刺 direct needling
直接灸 direct moxibustion

跖 [zhí]（名词）① 脚面上接近脚趾的部分 the part of the foot between the tarsus and phalanges, namely metatarsus
跖 metatarsus
② 脚掌 sole of the foot
跖疣 wart on the sole of the foot → **plantar wart; verruca plantaris**

止 [zhǐ]（动词）① 使停止 to stop
止血 stopping bleeding; hemostasis
止呃 stopping hiccups
② 阻止 to arrest; to check
止呕 arresting vomiting
止遗尿 arresting enuresis
止汗 checking sweating
止血药 a medicinal that arrests bleeding → **hemostatic (medicinal/drug)**
止血剂 a formula for arresting bleeding → **styptic formula**
③ 缓解 to relieve
止咳化痰 relieving cough and resolving phlegm
止痛 relieving pain
止痒 relieving itching
止痉 relieving spasm
止咳平喘药 a medicinal that relieves cough and asthma → **antitussive and antasthmatic (medicinal/drug)**
④ 止（渴）to quench (thirst)
止渴 quenching thirst

指 [zhǐ]（名词）手指 finger
指切进针法 fingernail-pressing needle insertion
指揉法 finger kneading manipulation
指推法 finger-pushing manipulation
指节拍法 patting with the dorsal side of the finger joints → **knuckle-patting manipulation**

志 [zhì]（名词）神志；情志；意志 mind; emotion; will
志 (1) will; (2) emotion; (3) mind
五志 five minds; five emotions
五志过极 five emotions/minds in excess
五志化火 transformation of the five emotions/minds into fire

制 [zhì]（动词）① 制作 to make
制炭 making (a medicinal substance) carbonized → **carbonization**
制霜 making (a medicinal substance) into a frost-like powder → **frosting**
② 抑制 to inhibit
五行制化 inhibition and generation among the five elements/phases

质 [zhì]（名词）① 质地 texture
舌质 tongue texture

②体质 constitution
阴阳平和质 balanced yin-yang constitution
偏阴质 yin-preponderant constitution
偏阳质 yang-preponderant constitution

炙 [zhì]（动词）把药材加辅料同炒 to stir-bake a medicinal substance with a fluid adjuvant
炙 stir-baking with fluid adjuvant
蜜炙 stir-baking with honey
酒炙 stir-baking with wine
姜炙 stir-baking with ginger
醋炙 stir-baking with vinegar

治 [zhì]（动词）治疗 to treat (*n.* treatment)
治病求本 treating disease from the root
治本 treating the fundamental
治标 treating the incidental
治未病 treating a disease before its onset → **preventive treatment**
正治 routine treatment
反治 paradoxical treatment

栉 [zhì]（动词）梳头 to comb
栉头 combing the head

痔 [zhì]（名词）①孔窍中的小肉突起皆曰痔 any small lump protruding from an orifice in the body
鼻痔 nasal polyp
耳痔 ear pile; nodular vegetation of the ear
息肉痔 rectal polyp
②痔疮 hemorrhoid; pile
内痔 internal hemorrhoid
外痔 external hemorrhoid
内外痔 mixed hemorrhoid
血箭痔 blood-spurting hemorrhoid
枯痔法 necrotizing therapy for hemorrhoids
（其他）
肠痔 perianal abscess

滞 [zhì]（动词）①停滞 to stagnate (*n.* stagnation)
气滞 *qi* stagnation
气机郁滞 depression and stagnation of *qi* movement
气滞血瘀 *qi* stagnation and blood stasis; blood stasis due to *qi* stagnation
②难以移动 difficult to move, namely, to stick
滞针 sticking of the needle
（其他）
滞颐 dribbling with wet cheeks

稚 [zhì]（形容词）幼稚的 immature
稚阴稚阳 immature yin-yang
（其他）
稚子 ten-year-old children

中 [zhōng]（名词）中间；中部 interior; middle
中精之腑 *fu* organ with refined juice (in the interior)
中清之腑 *fu* organ with clear juice (in the interior)
中渎之腑 *fu* organ for water communication (in the interior)
中满 middle fullness
（形容词）①中国的 Chinese
中药学 Chinese pharmaceutics
中药 Chinese medicinals; Chinese drugs
中草药 Chinese herbal medicinal
②中间的 middle
中脘 middle stomach cavity
中焦 middle energizer
中指同身寸 middle finger body-*cun*; middle finger body-inch
中气不足 insufficiency of middle *qi*
中阳不振 devitalized middle yang
③中等的 medium
中品 medium-grade medicinal
另见：中 [zhòng]

肿 [zhǒng]（名词）皮肉浮胀 abnormal enlargement of a body part, namely, swelling
肿胀舌 swollen tongue
舌肿 swelling of the tongue
消肿 relieving swelling

肿疡 swelling (sore)
肿毒 toxic swelling

踵 [zhǒng]（名词）脚后跟 the back part of the foot below the ankle, namely, the heel
踵 heel

中 [zhòng]（名词）突然袭击 a sudden and serious attack, i.e., stroke
中恶 attack of noxious factor
中暑 summerheat stroke; heatstroke
中风病 wind stroke disease
中风闭证 blockage pattern of wind stroke
中风脱证 collapse pattern of wind stroke
（其他）
中毒 poisoning
另见：中 [zhōng]

重 [zhòng]（形容词）①沉重的 heavy
重痛 heavy pain
重镇安神 calming the mind with heavy settling (medicinals)
重镇安神药 (heavy) **settling tranquilizer; settling tranquilizing medicinal/drug**
重剂 heavy formula
②强有力的 forceful
重插轻提 forceful thrusting and light lifting
重提轻插 forceful lifting and light thrusting
③费力的 hard (*n.* hardness)
重听 hardness of hearing

周 [zhōu]（名词）环绕一圈 circuit
周天 heavenly circuit; cosmic cycle
周天功 heavenly circuit exercise
小周天功 small heavenly circuit exercise
大周天功 large heavenly circuit exercise
周天自转功 automatic *qi* circulation exercise

肘 [zhǒu]（名词）胳膊肘 elbow
肘揉法 elbow-kneading manipulation
肘推法 elbow pushing manipulation
肘按法 elbow-pressing manipulation
坠肘 dropping elbows
垂肘 down-hanging elbows

侏 [zhū]（形容词）身材矮小的 dwarf
侏儒 dwarfism

珠 [zhū] (名词) ①珠子 bead
磁珠疗法 magnetic bead therapy
②球形的物体，如眼球 ball, e.g., eyeball
目珠；眼珠 eyeball
眼珠干涩 dryness and discomfort of the eye(ball)s
眼珠牵斜 deviation of the eye(ball) → **strabismus; squint**
眼珠塌陷 sunken eye(ball)s
精珠；晶珠 the clear portion inside the eyeball → **lens**

诸 [zhū]（形容词）众多的 various or all kinds of
诸阳之会 confluence of all the yang meridians/channels
诸虫 (various) **parasitic worms**

蛛 [zhū]（名词）蜘蛛 spider
蛛丝飘浮 image of spider's threads floating before the eyes → **floaters; muscae volitantes**

竹 [zhú]（名词）竹子 bamboo
竹罐 bamboo cup

逐 [zhú]（动词）驱逐 to expel
逐水 expelling water; hydrogogue therapy
逐水药 hydragogue
逐水剂 hydragogue formula
泻下逐水 expelling water by catharsis
泻下逐饮 expelling retained fluid by catharsis

主 [zhǔ]（名词）主角 principal
主辅佐引 principal, adjuvant, auxiliary and conductant
（形容词）占支配地位的 dominant
主运 dominant circuit
主气 dominant *qi*

（动词）掌管 to be in charge of

五脏所主 charges of the five *zang* organs

（其他）

主色 individual's normal complexion

五色主病 diagnostic significance of the five colors

煮 [zhǔ]（动词）①煮沸 to boil

煮 boiling

煮罐法 cup-boiling method

②煎煮 to decoct

别煮 to be decocted separately

助 [zhù]（动词）扶助 to support

助阳 supporting yang

助阳解表 supporting yang and releasing the exterior

补肾助阳 tonifying the kidney and supporting yang

注 [zhù]（动词）倾泻 to pour

注泄；泄注 pouring diarrhea

柱 [zhù]（名词）柱子或柱状物 column or something like a column such as a stem

鼻柱 nose stem → **(1) dorsum of the nose; (2) nasal septum**

（形容词）柱形的 columnar

柱骨 columnar bone → **(1) the clavicle; (2) the cervical vertebra**

（动词）支撑 to prop

舌柱上腭 tongue propping the palate

柱舌 tongue propping

疰 [zhù]（名词）病也 illness

疰夏 illness due to non-acclimation to the hot weather in summer → **summer non-acclimation**

抓 [zhuā]（动词）用手握住 to grasp

抓法（推拿）grasping with the whole hand

爪 [zhuǎ]（名词）①爪子 claw

探爪式 spreading-claw gesture

②爪甲 nail

鹅爪风 goose-claw nail wind → **tinea unguium**

转 [zhuàn]（动词）旋转 to rotate (*n.* rotation)

转筋 rotation of the muscle due to spasmodic contraction → **cramp**

霍乱转筋 cramps in choleraic turmoil

转筋霍乱 choleraic turmoil with cramps

壮 [zhuàng]（名词）艾灸的计数单位，每燃烧一个艾柱为一壮 cone, the time taken for burning a moxa cone, as a unit of measuring the treatment amount of moxibustion

壮 cone

（动词）增强；充实 to invigorate; to supplement

壮阳 invigorating yang

补火壮阳 supplementing fire and invigorating yang

壮水制阳 supplementing water to inhibit yang

状 [zhuàng]（形容词）相似的 alike (*suffix*: -like)

丝状疣 wart with threadlike projections → **verruca filiformis**

撞 [zhuàng]（动词）碰撞；撞击 to knock; to strike

撞击伤目 eye injury due to a knock or strike → **ocular contusion**

椎 [zhuī]（名词）椎骨 vertebra

扳颈椎法 pulling to restore a dislocated cervical vertebra → **cervical pulling manipulation**

扳胸椎法 thoracic (vertebral) **pulling manipulation**

扳腰椎法 lumbar (vertebral) **pulling manipulation**

坠 [zhuì]（动词）①垂下 to drop

坠肘 dropping elbows
②下垂 to sag
偏坠 hemilateral sagging (of the testis)
（其他）
下坠 straining at stool; tenesmus

灼 [zhuó]（动词）①烧灼 to burn
灼热 burning fever
小便灼热 burning sensation during urination
灼痛 burning pain
②烧坏 scorch
热灼肾阴 heat scorching kidney yin

浊 [zhuó]（形容词）污浊的 turbid (*n.* turbidity)
浊气 turbid *qi*
清浊 clarity and turbidity
浊邪 turbid pathogen
痰浊 phlegm turbidity
秽浊 filthy turbidity

啄 [zhuó]（动词）鸟类啄食 (birds) to move the beak forward quickly and bite something, i.e., to peck
啄法；啄击法 pecking manipulation
雀啄脉 bird-pecking pulse
雀啄灸 bird-pecking moxibustion; pecking moxibustion

着 [zhuó]（形容词）执着的 persistent → fixed
着痹 fixed impediment; fixed arthralgia

姿 [zī]（名词）姿态 posture
望姿态 inspection of the posture
姿式 posturization (in *qigong*)

滋 [zī]（动词）滋补；滋养 to replenish; to nourish
滋水涵木 replenishing water and/to moisten wood
滋阴清热 replenishing yin and clearing heat
滋阴降火 replenishing yin and reducing fire
滋阴抑阳 replenishing yin to suppress yang
滋阴润燥剂 yin-replenishing moistening formula

子 [zǐ]（名词）①儿子 son
子母配穴法 mother-son point combination
子母补泻法 mother-son reinforcing and reducing method
②未出生的子嗣 a baby before it is born, i.e., fetus
子宫；子脏 the viscus that holds the fetus → **uterus**
子门 the orifice through which a baby is delivered → **cervical orifice**
子肠 the tube through which a baby is delivered → **vagina**
子满 excess amount of amniotic fluid → **hydramnios**
子死腹中 dead fetus in the uterus
③男子的生殖器官如睾丸、附睾 male reproductive organs such as testicle and epididymis
子痈 testicular abscess
子痰 tuberculosis of epididymis
④子时（午夜）midnight
子午流注 midnight-midday ebb flow
子午流注针法 midnight-midday ebb flow acupuncture
（形容词）怀有未出生子嗣的，即怀孕的 of a woman having a baby developing inside her body, i.e., pregnant, gravid or gravidic
子痫；子冒 convulsions late in pregnancy → **eclampsia**
子晕 gravid vertigo
子淋 gravid stranguria
子喑 gravidic aphonia
子肿 gravidic edema

紫 [zǐ]（形容词）紫色的 purple; violet (bluish purple)

紫舌 purple tongue
紫斑 purpura
紫白癜风 multiple macular patches varying from white in pigmented skin to purplish in pale skin → **tinea versicolor**
紫外线穴位照射疗法 acupoint ultraviolet irradiation therapy

自 [zì]（形容词）① 自发的 spontaneous
自汗 spontaneous sweating
乳汁自出 spontaneous flow of milk → **galactorrhea**
阴阳自和 spontaneous harmonization of yin and yang
② 自然的 natural
自然站式 natural standing posture
自然呼吸 natural breathing
自然站桩功 natural stake-standing
（前缀）自己的或自己做的 of or by oneself, viz., auto-
自我按摩 automassage

眦 [zì]（名词）上下眼睑的结合处 corner of the eye formed by the meeting of upper and lower eyelids, namely canthus (*adj.* canthal)
眦；目眦 canthus
目锐眦；锐眦 lateral canthus
眦帷赤烂 erosion of the canthal eyelid
眦漏 canthus pyorrhea

宗 [zōng]（名词）祖宗 ancestor (*adj.* ancestral)
宗气 ancestral *qi*; pectoral *qi*
宗筋 ancestral sinew (either a collective term for the sinews that control the articular movement or an euphemism for penis)
宗筋之会 confluence of ancestral sinews (an euphemism for male genitals)

总 [zǒng]（形容词）全部的 all
总按 palpating the pulses on all three sections simultaneously → **simultaneous palpation; pulse-taking with three fingers**

走 [zǒu]（动词）① 行走 to walk
走式 walking posture
② 移动 to move; to change location
走罐 cupping with a moving cup → **slide cupping**
走窜痛 a pain which repeatedly changes its location → **scurrying pain**
③ 扩散 to spread
走黄；癀走 wide spreading of heat toxin (in the body) →**pyosepticemia**
④ 跑 to run
走马牙疳；走马疳 "horse-running" ulcerative gingivitis → noma; cancrum oris
（其他）
走火入魔 evil reactions; deviation of *qigong*

足 [zú]（名词）脚 foot
足跗 the top part of the foot → **instep**
足跟痛 pain in the back part of the foot below the ankle → **heel pain**
足底疔 inflammation of the sole of the foot with pustule formation → **plantar pustule**
足发背 phlegmon of the dorsum of the foot
足三阳经 three yang meridians/channels of the foot

阻 [zǔ]（动词）阻塞 to obstruct (*n.* obstruction)
热邪阻肺 heat pathogen obstructing the lung
痰浊阻肺 phlegm-turbidity obstructing the lung
湿阻中焦 dampness obstructing the middle energizer
心血瘀阻 heart blood stasis (and obstruction)

祖 [zǔ]（名词）祖先 ancestor
祖传秘方 secret formula handed down in a family

醉 [zuì]（名词）麻醉 anesthesia

针刺麻醉 acupuncture anesthesia

电针麻醉 electro-acupuncture anesthesia

指压麻醉 finger-pressure anesthesia

撙 [zǔn]（动词）挫也（按下）to press or knead

撙令平正 kneading restoration

撙捺皮相 observation via kneading-pressing

撙捺相近 kneading-pressing (the fractured ends) close

左 [zuǒ]（形容词）左边的，右的反义词 left, the opposite of right

左右配穴法 right-left point combination

左病右取，右病左取 treating disease of the left with points on the right, and vice versa

佐 [zuǒ]（形容词）辅佐的 adjuvant; assistant

佐药 adjuvant ingredient; assistant ingredient

君臣佐使 sovereign, minister, adjuvant and courier; chief, associate, assistant and guide

坐 [zuò]（动词）①以臀着物而止息 to rest with the weight supported by the buttocks, namely, to sit

坐式 sitting posture

盘坐 cross-legged sitting

坐忘 sitting in forgetfulness

静坐 silent sitting

坐式复位 sitting reduction

②停留不动 to retain

坐罐 retained cupping

索引
Indices

中文笔画索引 Chinese Character Stroke Index

一画

一夫法 / 445
一次性针 / 452
一阳 / 400
一阴 / 399
一贯煎 / 373
一指禅功 / 482
一指禅式 / 504
一指禅导气 / 503
一指禅推法 / 482，648
一指禅推拿 / 490
一指禅推拿疗法 / 648
一垫固定法 / 641

二画

［一］

二十八脉 / 160
二仙汤 / 373
二白 / 442
二母宁嗽丸［片］ / 382
二阳 / 400
二阳并病 / 178
二阴 / 48，399
二间 / 409
二陈汤 / 380
二垫固定法 / 641
十二节 / 52
十二皮部 / 407
十二刺 / 461
十二剂 / 360
十二经 / 398
十二经别 / 407
十二经脉 / 398
十二经筋 / 406
十七椎 / 441
十八反 / 359
十九畏 / 359
十五络脉 / 407
十四剂 / 360
十四经 / 400
十四经发挥 / 699
十全大补丸 / 388
十全大补汤 / 372
十问 / 142
十枣汤 / 365
十剂 / 359
十药神书 / 694
十宣 / 443
丁甘仁 / 681
丁泽周 / 681
丁香 / 318
丁香柿蒂汤 / 376
丁奚疳 / 580
七死脉 / 163
七冲门 / 40
七怪脉 / 163
七厘散 / 396
七星功 / 503
七星针 / 450
七绝脉 / 163
七窍 / 38
七情 / 69

［丿］

八风 / 443
八正散 / 380
八邪 / 442
八会穴 / 439
八纲 / 168
八纲辨证 / 168
八卦步 / 496
八法 / 225
八珍丸 / 388
八珍汤 / 372
八珍益母丸 / 395
八段锦 / 502
八脉交会穴 / 439
八廓 / 44，607
八溪 / 52
人中 / 46
人迎 / 412
人迎脉 / 160
人参 / 340
人参再造丸 / 391
人参养荣丸 / 391
人参健脾丸 / 388
人胞 / 555
入臼 / 642
入里化热 / 83
入静 / 493
儿茶 / 356
九九阳功 / 503
九针 / 451
九刺 / 460
九味羌活汤 / 361
九香虫 / 327
九窍 / 38

［乛］

刀豆 / 328

三画

［一］

三七 / 328
三因 / 62
三因极一病证方论 / 687
三关 / 138
三阳 / 399
三阳合病 / 178
三阳络 / 427
三阴 / 399
三阴交 / 415
三角针埋线法 / 478

三角窝 / 472
三间 / 409
三板推拿疗法 / 486
三法 / 225
三宝 / 2
三垫固定法 / 641
三点求圆导气 / 504
三点拉线导气 / 504
三品 / 279
三圆式 / 496
三圆站桩功 / 502
三部九候 / 159
三消 / 551
三接式 / 495
三黄片 / 384
三棱 / 334
三棱针 / 449
三棱针疗法 / 449
三焦 / 24
三焦气化 / 27
三焦实热 / 215
三焦咳 / 525
三焦俞 / 420
三焦虚寒 / 214
三焦湿热证 / 181
三焦辨证 / 181
三痹 / 540
三颗针 / 307
干血痨 / 530
干呕 / 152
干咳 / 142，525
干咳嗽 / 525
干姜 / 317
干疳 / 580
干疳证 / 580
干陷 / 595
干聋 / 625
干霍乱 / 522
干癣 / 605
土不制水 / 14
土牛膝 / 313
土方 / 357
土生金 / 11
土形之人 / 73
土克水 / 12
土疡 / 613
土法 / 357
土荆皮 / 355
土茯苓 / 309
土疳 / 613
土虚木乘 / 13
土虚水侮 / 14
土鳖虫 / 333
下元亏损 / 112
下元不固 / 112
下巨虚 / 414
下气 / 254
下气消痰 / 253
下丹田 / 497
下耳根 / 473
下合穴 / 439
下关 / 411
下极俞 / 441
下利 / 150，545
下利［痢］脓血 / 150
下利清谷 / 150，545
下坠 / 156
下乳 / 268
下肢功 / 501
下肢穴 / 443
下法 / 235
下按式 / 496
下按式站桩功 / 502
下品 / 280
下消 / 551
下窍 / 38
下陷 / 94
下脘 / 24，436
下睑 / 609
下焦 / 24
下焦实热 / 215
下焦病证 / 181
下焦虚寒 / 215
下焦湿热证 / 182
下廉 / 410
下膈 / 543
下髎 / 421
寸 / 444
寸、关、尺 / 158
寸口 / 159
寸口脉 / 160
大山楂丸 / 387
大巨 / 413
大气 / 53
大风 / 605
大方 / 357
大节 / 52
大包 / 416
大头垫 / 641
大头瘟 / 520
大肉陷下 / 126
大汗 / 144
大汗淋漓 / 144
大芸 / 346
大针 / 452
大肠 / 24
大肠传导失职 / 110
大肠实热 / 111
大肠咳 / 525
大肠俞 / 420
大肠津［液］亏 / 111
大肠津［液］亏证 / 208
大肠津亏 / 81
大肠热结 / 110
大肠热结证 / 208
大肠虚寒 / 111
大肠虚寒证 / 208
大肠湿热 / 111
大肠湿热证 / 208
大肠寒结 / 110
大肠寒结证 / 208
大迎 / 411
大补大泻法 / 458
大补阴丸 / 389
大青叶 / 311
大杼 / 419

大枣 / 341
大周天 / 500
大周天功 / 502
大泻刺 / 460
大承气汤 / 364
大毒、常毒、小毒、无毒 / 279
大骨空 / 442
大骨枯槁 / 126
大钟 / 424
大便秘结 / 149
大脉 / 162
大炷灸 / 465
大活络丸［丹］/ 392
大结胸 / 519
大都 / 415
大柴胡汤 / 366
大陵 / 426
大黄 / 352
大黄牡丹汤 / 364
大黄附子汤 / 364
大眦 / 608
大眦脓漏 / 615
大椎 / 434
大厥 / 538
大敦 / 432
大蓟 / 328
大腹 / 48
大腹皮 / 321
大赫 / 424
大横 / 416
万氏女科 / 695
万全 / 670
万病回春 / 703
万密斋 / 670
万密斋医学全书 / 703
［丨］
上下配穴法 / 447
上巨虚 / 414
上气 / 141，526
上丹田 / 496
上火 / 519
上耳根 / 473
上吐下泻 / 150
上关 / 428
上迎香 / 440
上肢穴 / 442
上实下虚 / 84
上实下虚证 / 172
上星 / 435
上品 / 279
上胞下垂 / 614
上热下寒 / 91
上热下寒证 / 172
上病下取，下病上取 / 221
上消 / 551
上窍 / 38
上盛下虚 / 84
上虚下实 / 84
上虚下实证 / 172
上脘 / 23，436
上睑 / 608
上焦 / 24
上焦实热 / 215
上焦病证 / 181
上焦虚寒 / 214
上焦湿热证 / 181
上寒下热 / 91
上寒下热证 / 171
上廉 / 410
上膈 / 543
上横骨 / 47
上髎 / 421
小儿水气肿 / 590
小儿水肿 / 590
小儿火泻 / 587
小儿发痧 / 583
小儿多涎 / 578
小儿呕吐 / 586
小儿卒利 / 587
小儿泄泻 / 587
小儿药证直诀 / 696
小儿热泻 / 587
小儿哮喘 / 577
小儿消渴 / 589
小儿浮肿 / 590
小儿诸热 / 582
小儿推拿广意 / 696
小儿推拿疗法 / 486
小儿推拿秘旨 / 696
小儿虚热 / 583
小儿麻痹 / 590
小儿暑温 / 582
小儿遗尿 / 590
小儿痘疹方论 / 696
小儿寒湿泻 / 587
小儿湿热泻 / 587
小儿感冒冲剂 / 381
小儿腹胀 / 588
小儿腹痛 / 588
小儿暴泻 / 587
小儿瘳气 / 589
小方 / 357
小舌 / 40，628
小产 / 569
小针刀 / 451
小针刀疗法 / 451
小肠 / 24
小肠气 / 554
小肠实热 / 101
小肠实热证 / 202
小肠咳 / 525
小肠俞 / 420
小肠虚寒 / 101
小青龙汤 / 361
小金丸［丹］/ 395
小周天 / 500
小周天功 / 501
小建中汤 / 370
小承气汤 / 364
小茴香 / 318
小骨空 / 442
小便不利 / 151
小便失禁 / 151
小便灼热 / 151
小便涩痛 / 151
小便黄赤 / 151

小便清长 / 150
小便淋漓 / 151
小便短赤 / 151
小便频数 / 150
小炷灸 / 465
小活络丸［丹］/ 392
小结胸 / 519
小柴胡汤 / 365
小海 / 417
小眦 / 608
小蓟 / 328
小蓟饮子 / 377
小腹 / 48
小腹不仁 / 154
小腹满 / 154
口 / 39
口干 / 149
口干不欲饮 / 149
口不仁 / 155
口中无味 / 154
口中和 / 154
口气 / 142
口气臭秽 / 142
口气酸臭 / 142
口甘 / 155
口禾髎 / 411
口动 / 136
口吻疮 / 580
口角流涎 / 136
口苦 / 155
口齿科（学）/ 632
口咸 / 155
口疮 / 579，633
口唇干裂 / 136
口唇青紫 / 137
口唇糜烂 / 136
口振 / 136
口㖞 / 127，537
口眼㖞斜 / 127
口臭 / 142
口疳 / 580，633
口甜 / 155
口黏腻 / 155
口淡 / 154
口渴 / 148
口渴引饮 / 149
口渴喜冷 / 149
口酸 / 155
口撮 / 136
口僻 / 136，537
口噤 / 136，537
口糜 / 579，633
山豆根 / 313
山岚瘴气 / 72
山茱萸 / 343
山药 / 341
山根 / 626
山楂 / 351
山慈菇 / 300

［丿］

千年健 / 315
千金子 / 355
千金要方 / 690
千金翼方 / 690
川木通 / 321
川贝母 / 302
川贝枇杷糖浆 / 382
川牛膝 / 331
川乌 / 314
川芎 / 330
川芎嗪注射液 / 394
川楝子 / 328
久疟 / 521
久泄［泻］/ 545
久咳 / 142
久流浊涕 / 130
久痢 / 522
久嗽 / 142
丸 / 280
丸剂 / 280

［丶］

广豆根 / 313
广藿香 / 319
亡阳 / 80
亡阳证 / 173
亡阴 / 80
亡阴证 / 173
亡津液 / 81

［乛］

弓步 / 496
卫 / 55
卫气 / 54
卫气不固 / 85
卫气同病 / 86
卫气同病证 / 179
卫气营血 / 55
卫气营血辨证 / 179
卫分 / 55
卫分证 / 179
卫生家宝产科备要 / 695
卫阳 / 54
卫阳被遏 / 85
卫弱营强 / 86
卫营同病 / 86
卫营同病证 / 179
卫强营弱 / 86
女子胞 / 25，556
女贞子 / 344
女劳复 / 71
女科百问 / 695
女科经纶 / 695
飞入法 / 453
飞门 / 39
飞扬喉 / 631
飞阳 / 423
子 / 13
子门 / 49，555
子午流注 / 459
子午流注针法 / 459
子气 / 13
子母补泻法 / 458
子母配穴法 / 448
子死腹中 / 567
子肠 / 555
子肿 / 568
子冒 / 567

子宫 / 441，555
子晕 / 566
子脏 / 25，556
子痈 / 599
子烦 / 567
子悬 / 567
子淋 / 567
子喑 / 568
子痫 / 566
子痰 / 599
子满 / 567
子嗽 / 568
马牙 / 579
马齿苋 / 309
马勃 / 313
马莳 / 670
马钱子 / 316
马桶癣 / 605
马兜铃 / 303
马脾风 / 586
马鞭草 / 334

四画

［一］

丰隆 / 414
王士雄 / 680
王不留行 / 333
王执中 / 664
王旭高 / 679
王冰 / 661
王宇泰 / 671
王好古 / 666
王进之 / 666
王纶 / 668
王叔和 / 659
王肯堂 / 671
王孟英 / 680
王勋臣 / 678
王泰林 / 679
王损庵 / 671
王海藏 / 666
王焘 / 661
王惟德 / 662
王清任 / 678
王维一 / 662
王熙 / 659
开达膜［募］原 / 238
开泄 / 229
开胃 / 246
开鬼门 / 229
开窍 / 266
开窍药 / 293
开阖补泻 / 457
开阖补泻法 / 457
井穴 / 437
天人相应 / 17
天干 / 18
天门冬 / 343
天井 / 427
天仙子 / 303
天白蚁 / 629
天冬 / 343
天年 / 18
天行 / 514
天行赤目 / 616
天行赤目暴翳 / 616
天行赤眼 / 616
天行赤眼暴翳 / 616
天行时疫 / 514
天行暴赤 / 616
天冲 / 429
天池 / 425
天花 / 585
天花粉 / 300
天灸 / 466
天枢 / 413
天钓 / 575
天竺黄 / 300
天受 / 514
天府 / 408
天宗 / 418
天南星 / 298
天柱 / 419
天泉 / 426
天庭 / 43
天突 / 437
天癸 / 556
天癸竭 / 556
天容 / 418
天符 / 18
天麻 / 338
天麻丸 / 393
天麻钩藤饮 / 378
天鼎 / 411
天窗 / 418
天溪 / 416
天牖 / 427
天髎 / 427
元气 / 53
元阳 / 23
元阳亏虚 / 113
元阴 / 22
元府 / 41
元胡 / 332
元胡止痛片 / 393
元神之府 / 25
无头疽 / 595
无名肿毒 / 594
无汗 / 145
无形之痰 / 71
无根苔 / 136
无瘢痕灸 / 465
云门 / 408
云雾移睛 / 620
扎带 / 642
木火刑金 / 13
木生火 / 11
木瓜 / 314
木瓜丸 / 392
木舌 / 134，579
木形之人 / 73
木克土 / 12
木旺乘土 / 13
木香 / 326
木香顺气丸 / 387
木贼 / 305

木乘土 / 13
木通 / 321
木蝴蝶 / 303
五子衍宗丸 / 389
五气 / 14
五水 / 549
五仁丸 / 364
五化 / 14
五方 / 14
五心烦热 / 144
五处 / 419
五加皮 / 316
五行 / 11
五行归类 / 11
五行母子相及 / 13
五行制化 / 12
五行学说 / 11
五行相生 / 11
五行相克 / 12
五行相侮 / 13
五行相乘 / 12
五色 / 125
五色主病 / 126
五运 / 17
五运六气 / 17
五志 / 26，69
五志化火 / 70
五志过极 / 70
五声 / 14
五劳 / 529
五更泄［泻］/ 545
五更咳 / 526
五时 / 14
五灵脂 / 332
五迟 / 577
五苓散 / 379
五枢 / 430
五刺 / 459
五轮 / 43，607
五软 / 578
五味 / 279
五味子 / 350
五味所入 / 26，280
五味偏嗜 / 70
五官 / 14，38
五倍子 / 348
五脏 / 20
五脏化液 / 58
五脏所主 / 26
五脏所恶 / 26
五脏所藏 / 26
五痞 / 580
五趾抓地 / 494
五淋 / 552
五液 / 58
五硬 / 578
五禽戏 / 502
五输穴 / 437
五输配穴法 / 448
支正 / 417
支饮 / 528
支沟 / 427
不内外因 / 62
不仁 / 148
不孕 / 565
不传 / 116
不更衣 / 149
不时泪溢 / 611
不育 / 553
不省人事 / 124
不闻香臭 / 626
不容 / 412
不得卧 / 535
不得眠 / 155
不得偃卧 / 141
不锈钢针 / 452
不寐 / 155
太乙 / 413
太子参 / 340
太平圣惠方 / 691
太平惠民和剂局方 / 691
太白 / 415
太冲 / 432
太阳 / 43，440
太阳（与）少阳合病 / 178
太阳（与）阳明合病 / 178
太阳之人 / 74
太阳中风 / 175
太阳中风证 / 175
太阳伤寒 / 176
太阳伤寒证 / 175
太阳经证 / 175
太阳经病 / 175
太阳病 / 175
太阳病机 / 115
太阳病证 / 175
太阳腑证 / 176
太阳腑病 / 176
太阳蓄水证 / 176
太阳蓄血证 / 176
太阴之人 / 74
太阴病 / 177
太阴病机 / 115
太阴病证 / 177
太极步 / 496
太息 / 141
太渊 / 409
太溪 / 424
历节风 / 540
尤在泾 / 676
尤怡 / 675
车前子 / 320
车前草 / 320
巨刺 / 460
巨骨 / 410
巨阙 / 436
巨髎 / 411
牙宣 / 633
牙疳 / 633
牙痈 / 633
牙痛 / 632
牙龄［咬］痈 / 633
切开埋线法 / 478
切片 / 276
切诊 / 158
切脉 / 158

瓦松 / 330
瓦楞子 / 350

[丨]

止血 / 257
止血行瘀 / 271
止血收口 / 271
止血剂 / 377
止血药 / 291
止血敛疮 / 271
止汗 / 261
止呕 / 267
止呃 / 267
止咳化痰 / 264
止咳平喘药 / 292
止咳药 / 301
止晕 / 267
止痉 / 268
止痒 / 267
止遗尿 / 268
止痛 / 267
止渴 / 267
止嗽散 / 361
少气 / 141，526
少冲 / 417
少阳之人 / 74
少阳病 / 177
少阳病机 / 115
少阳病证 / 177
少阴之人 / 74
少阴热化 / 116
少阴热化证 / 177
少阴病 / 177
少阴病机 / 115
少阴病证 / 177
少阴寒化 / 115
少阴寒化证 / 177
少尿 / 150
少府 / 417
少泽 / 417
少神 / 123
少海 / 416
少商 / 409
少腹 / 48
少腹拘急 / 154
少腹硬满 / 154
日月 / 430
日晡发热 / 519
日晡潮热 / 144，519
中气 / 56
中气下陷 / 94
中气下陷证 / 206
中气不足 / 108
中风 / 536
中风后遗症 / 537
中风闭证 / 536
中风阳闭 / 536
中风阴闭 / 536
中风昏迷 / 537
中风病 / 536
中风脱证 / 536
中丹田 / 496
中冲 / 426
中阳不振 / 108
中极 / 435
中枢 / 433
中国医学大成 / 705
中国医学大辞典 / 705
中国药学大辞典 / 705
中府 / 408
中注 / 424
中经 / 537
中毒 / 72
中封 / 432
中指同身寸 / 444
中指独立式 / 505
中草药 / 275
中药 / 275
中药学 / 275
中品 / 279
中泉 / 442
中庭 / 436
中络 / 537
中都 / 432
中恶 / 72
中脏 / 536
中消 / 551
中脘 / 23，436
中清之腑 / 27
中渚 / 426
中渎 / 431
中渎之腑 / 27
中暑 / 517
中暑眩晕 / 533
中焦 / 24
中焦实热 / 215
中焦病证 / 181
中焦虚寒 / 215
中焦湿热 / 106
中焦湿热证 / 181，207
中腑 / 537
中湿 / 66
中寒 / 64，91
中寒泻 / 588
中魁 / 442
中满 / 154
中膂俞 / 421
中精之腑 / 27
中藏经 / 700
中髎 / 421
内气 / 500
内风 / 64
内丹 / 498
内丹功 / 498
内丹术 / 499
内功 / 491
内功图说 / 700
内功推拿 / 490
内外配穴法 / 448
内外痔 / 599
内托 / 269
内因 / 62
内伤 / 69
内伤头痛 / 533
内伤发热 / 530
内伤咳嗽 / 526
内伤腰痛 / 553

内关 / 426
内吹 / 596
内吹乳痈 / 596
内迎香 / 440
内固定 / 642
内钓 / 575
内视 / 493
内经 / 683
内经知要 / 684
内毒 / 69
内科杂病 / 524
内庭 / 414
内养功 / 500
内痈 / 593
内消 / 269
内陷 / 94，595
内眦 / 44，608
内痔 / 599
内景 / 493
内湿 / 65
内寒 / 64
内障 / 612
内踝 / 50
内踝尖 / 443
内膝眼 / 443
内燥 / 66
内燥证 / 197
内翻 / 656
水土不服 / 72
水丸 / 280
水飞 / 276
水不化气 / 93
水不涵木 / 14
水牛角 / 306
水气 / 66，548
水气证 / 189
水气凌心 / 101
水气凌心证 / 202
水分 / 436
水火共制 / 276
水火相济 / 27
水生木 / 12
水红花子 / 332
水形之人 / 74
水花 / 585
水克火 / 12
水针 / 470
水谷 / 53
水谷之气 / 53
水谷之海 / 26
水谷之精 / 57
水谷精微 / 57
水饮 / 527
水饮内停证 / 187
水沟 / 435
水轮 / 44，607
水制 / 276
水肿 / 138，548
水肿病 / 548
水胀 / 548
水疝 / 599
水泻 / 150
水泉 / 424
水疮 / 585
水突 / 412
水疱 / 139，585
水停证 / 189
水蛭 / 333
水痘 / 584
水道 / 413
水寒射肺 / 103
水寒射肺证 / 205
水臌（病）/ 547
［ 丿 ］
午后潮热 / 144，519
牛皮癣 / 602
牛西西 / 330
牛黄 / 335
牛黄上清丸 / 384
牛黄降压丸 / 384
牛黄清心丸［片］/ 384
牛黄解毒丸［片］/ 384
牛蒡子 / 297
牛膝 / 344
手三阳经 / 399
手三阴经 / 399
手三里 / 410
手五里 / 410
手太阳小肠经 / 402
手太阳小肠经穴 / 417
手太阴肺经 / 400
手太阴肺经穴 / 408
手少阳三焦经 / 404
手少阳三焦经穴 / 426
手少阴心经 / 402
手少阴心经穴 / 416
手心毒 / 592
手发背 / 594
手阳明大肠经 / 400
手阳明大肠经穴 / 409
手足心汗 / 145
手足心热 / 144
手足汗 / 145
手足逆冷 / 538
手足厥冷 / 538
手足颤动 / 127
手足蠕动 / 127
手针 / 478
手针疗法 / 478
手法牵引 / 642
手骨 / 47
手厥阴心包经 / 404
手厥阴心包经穴 / 425
手摸心会 / 638
气 / 2，53
气口 / 160
气门 / 41
气不摄［统］血证 / 186
气不摄血 / 95
气化 / 2，56
气化无权 / 93
气化不利 / 93
气分 / 56
气分证 / 179
气户 / 412
气功 / 491

气功疗法 / 492
气功偏差 / 505
气穴 / 424
气机 / 2，56
气机不利 / 93
气机失调 / 93
气机郁滞 / 93
气至 / 456
气血双补剂 / 372
气血失调 / 95
气血两亏 / 96
气血两虚 / 96
气血两虚证 / 186
气血两虚质 / 75
气血两燔 / 86
气血两燔证 / 180
气血虚弱痛经 / 560
气血瘀滞证 / 186
气血辨证 / 182
气色 / 124
气闭 / 94
气闭证 / 182
气闭神厥证 / 202
气冲 / 413
气关 / 138
气阴亏虚证 / 184
气阴两虚证 / 183
气郁 / 93
气郁化火 / 93
气郁血崩 / 562
气郁证 / 182
气轮 / 44，607
气味 / 278
气舍 / 412
气胜形 / 126
气逆 / 94
气逆证 / 182
气鬲 / 586
气积腹痛 / 588
气秘 / 544
气疳 / 581
气海 / 25，435
气海俞 / 420
气陷 / 94
气陷血崩 / 561
气陷证 / 182
气营两燔 / 86
气营两燔证 / 180
气虚 / 92
气虚不摄 / 94
气虚中满 / 95
气虚水停证 / 183
气虚气滞证 / 183
气虚外感证 / 183
气虚头痛 / 534
气虚发热证 / 183
气虚耳窍失充证 / 183
气虚自汗 / 531
气虚血瘀 / 95，96
气虚血瘀证 / 186
气虚证 / 182
气虚经行先期 / 557
气虚咳嗽 / 526
气虚眩晕 / 532
气虚崩漏 / 561
气虚湿阻［困］证 / 183
气虚滑胎 / 569
气虚感冒 / 516
气虚鼻窍失充证 / 183
气脱 / 93
气脱证 / 182
气淋 / 552
气随血脱 / 96
气随血脱证 / 186
气厥 / 538
气街 / 48
气痞 / 542
气滞 / 93
气滞水停证 / 188
气滞血瘀 / 96
气滞血瘀证 / 186
气滞证 / 182
气滞经行后期 / 558
气滞胃痛颗粒 / 387
气滞痛经 / 560
气滞腰痛 / 554
气滞腹痛 / 546
气滞痰凝咽喉证 / 186
气感 / 505
气管炎丸 / 383
气端 / 444
气瘤 / 598
气瘿 / 597
气翳 / 619
气臌（病）/ 547
毛冬青 / 334
毛际 / 48
毛刺 / 460
升、降、出、入 / 2
升阳 / 247
升阳举陷 / 247
升剂 / 360
升降失常 / 94
升降浮沉 / 279
升举中气 / 246
升麻 / 298
升麻葛根汤 / 363
升提中气 / 246
长针 / 452
长脉 / 162
长强 / 433
片 / 282
片剂 / 282
片姜黄 / 331
仆参 / 423
化风 / 92
化火 / 92
化石 / 272
化饮 / 259
化饮宁心 / 259
化饮宽胸 / 259
化饮解表 / 230
化热 / 92
化脓灸 / 465
化湿 / 259
化湿和胃剂 / 379

化湿药 / 289
化瘀止血药 / 291
化瘀药 / 292
化痰 / 258
化痰开窍 / 267
化痰止咳平喘药 / 292
化痰药 / 292
化痰宣肺 / 228
化腐 / 269
化橘红 / 327
化燥 / 92
反关脉 / 163
反佐 / 221，358
反治 / 220
反胃 / 152，543
反酸 / 153
从治 / 220
分肉 / 41
分刺 / 460
分骨垫 / 641
分娩 / 568
分筋 / 647
公孙 / 415
仓公 / 658
月水 / 157，556
月水不调 / 557
月水过多 / 157，561
月事 / 157，556
月季花 / 332
月经 / 157，556
月经不调 / 557
月经过少 / 157，558
月经过多 / 157，560
月经先后无定期 / 558
月经先期 / 157，557
月经后期 / 157，557
月经病 / 557
月经涩少 / 558
月经提前 / 157
月经错后 / 157
月信 / 157，556
月蚀疮 / 623
风 / 64
风门 / 419
风中血脉 / 89
风中经络证 / 191
风水 / 549
风水相搏证 / 188
风火 / 67
风火牙痛 / 632
风火内旋 / 89
风火攻目证 / 193
风火相煽 / 89
风火眼 / 615
风火眼痛 / 616
风市 / 431
风邪 / 64
风邪犯表证 / 191
风邪外袭证 / 191
风邪袭络证 / 191
风团 / 603
风关 / 138
风池 / 430
风赤疮疾 / 614
风赤疮痍 / 614
风轮 / 44，607
风轮赤豆 / 619
风府 / 434
风弦赤烂 / 613
风毒证 / 199
风牵偏视 / 622
风胜行痹证 / 191
风热 / 67
风热牙疳 / 633
风热牙痛 / 632
风热犯目证 / 193
风热犯头证 / 193
风热犯耳证 / 193
风热犯肺 / 110
风热犯肺证 / 193，203
风热犯鼻证 / 193
风热外袭证 / 192
风热头痛 / 533
风热耳鸣 / 624
风热邪气 / 67
风热闭肺证 / 193
风热攻目证 / 193
风热证 / 192
风热表证 / 192
风热乳蛾 / 628
风热咳嗽 / 525
风热侵喉［咽］证 / 193
风热疮 / 602
风热眩晕 / 532
风热眼 / 616
风热喉痹 / 629
风热感冒 / 516
风热腰痛 / 553
风疹 / 583
风袭表疏证 / 191
风痒 / 602
风痫 / 589
风痧 / 584
风湿 / 68
风湿犯头证 / 194
风湿外袭证 / 194
风湿头痛 / 533
风湿邪气 / 68
风湿证 / 193
风湿相搏 / 89
风湿凌目证 / 194
风湿袭表证 / 194
风湿腰痛 / 553
风温 / 67，516
风温邪气 / 67
风温病 / 516
风寒 / 67
风寒牙痛 / 632
风寒犯头证 / 192
风寒头痛 / 533
风寒邪气 / 67
风寒束表 / 88
风寒束肺 / 110
风寒束肺证 / 203
风寒证 / 191
风寒表证 / 192

风寒咳嗽 / 525
风寒眩晕 / 532
风寒袭表证 / 192
风寒袭肺 / 109
风寒袭肺证 / 192，203
风寒袭络证 / 192
风寒袭喉［咽］证 / 192
风寒袭鼻证 / 192
风寒喉痹 / 629
风寒湿 / 68
风寒湿邪 / 68
风寒湿阻证 / 192
风寒感冒 / 516
风寒腰痛 / 553
风痹 / 540
风痰 / 64
风痰头痛 / 534
风痰证 / 189
风痰眩晕 / 532
风瘙痒 / 603
风瘾疹 / 603
风燥 / 64，68
风燥咳嗽 / 526
风燥袭表证 / 194
风癣 / 604
丹 / 281
丹田 / 42，497
丹剂 / 281
丹参 / 331
丹毒 / 593
丹痧 / 520，585
丹溪心法 / 701
乌鸡白凤丸 / 394
乌药 / 326
乌须发 / 271
乌贼骨 / 350
乌梢蛇 / 315
乌梅 / 349

［丶］

六一散 / 369
六气 / 17，62
六阳脉 / 400
六阴脉 / 400
六郁 / 70
六味地黄丸 / 389
六味地黄汤 / 372
六经 / 399
六经病 / 175
六经病机 / 115
六经病证 / 175
六经辨证 / 175
六科证治准绳 / 704
六神丸 / 395
六淫 / 62
六腑 / 20
文火 / 283
方 / 356
方上 / 38
方剂 / 356
方剂配伍 / 358
火 / 66
火不生土 / 13
火丹 / 593
火生土 / 11
火邪 / 66
火邪经闭 / 559
火伤 / 605
火伤血络 / 90
火形之人 / 73
火扰心神证 / 201
火克金 / 12
火针 / 450
火针疗法 / 450
火制 / 276
火疡 / 617
火毒 / 68
火毒内陷证 / 198
火毒攻舌证 / 199
火毒攻喉证 / 199
火毒证 / 198
火带疮 / 600
火热炽盛证 / 173
火疳 / 617
火陷 / 596
火眼 / 616
火麻仁 / 352
火痰 / 528
火罐法 / 468
户门 / 40
心 / 20
心下支结 / 156
心下坚 / 156
心下急 / 156
心下逆满 / 156
心下悸 / 151
心下硬 / 156
心下痞 / 156，542
心下痞硬 / 156
心下痛 / 152
心下满 / 156
心中懊侬 / 124
心水 / 549
心气 / 21，54
心气（亏）虚证 / 200
心气不宁 / 99
心气不收 / 99
心气不足 / 99
心气不固 / 99
心气血两虚证 / 200
心气虚 / 99
心气虚不得卧 / 535
心火 / 21
心火上炎 / 101
心火上炎证 / 201
心火内炽 / 101
心火内焚 / 101
心火亢盛 / 101
心火炽［亢］盛证 / 201
心包 / 23
心包络 / 23
心动悸 / 151
心血 / 21
心血（亏）虚证 / 200
心血不足 / 99
心血虚 / 99
心血虚不得卧 / 535

心血瘀阻 / 99
心血瘀阻证 / 200
心汗 / 145
心阳 / 21
心阳（亏）虚证 / 200
心阳不足 / 100
心阳不振 / 100
心阳虚 / 100
心阳虚脱证 / 200
心阳暴脱 / 100
心阳暴脱证 / 200
心阴 / 21
心阴（亏）虚证 / 201
心阴不足 / 100
心阴虚 / 99
心劳 / 529
心肾不交 / 101
心肾不交证 / 202
心肾相交 / 27
心经咳嗽 / 524
心咳 / 524
心俞 / 419
心脉痹阻证 / 201
心神失养 / 100
心疳 / 581
心病辨证 / 200
心烦 / 124
心营过耗 / 100
心虚 / 99
心虚经闭 / 559
心移热于小肠 / 101
心移热小肠证 / 202
心移热膀胱证 / 202
心悸 / 151，530
心脾两虚 / 101
心脾两虚证 / 202
心痛 / 530
心痛彻背 / 151
心慌 / 151
心痹 / 541
心痿 / 539

［→］

尺泽 / 409
引火归原 / 251
引针 / 462
引伸法 / 485
引经报使 / 358
巴豆 / 355
巴豆霜 / 324
巴戟天 / 347
孔窍 / 38
孔最 / 409
以毒攻毒 / 270
双手托天式 / 654
双手进针法 / 453
双手捏法 / 652
双手攀足式 / 653
双黄连口服液 / 383
双盘坐 / 495
双蛾 / 628

五画

［一］

玉门 / 555
玉机微义 / 701
玉竹 / 343
玉米须 / 323
玉枕 / 419
玉枕骨 / 46
玉屏风口服液 / 383
玉屏风散 / 371
玉堂 / 436
玉液 / 440
击下肢 / 489
击头 / 487
击法 / 484，649
正水 / 549
正气 / 54
正邪分争 / 78
正邪相争 / 78
正疟 / 520
正治 / 220
正经 / 398
正骨（科）/ 635
正骨八法 / 638
正骨手法 / 638
正营 / 429
正虚邪实 / 78
扑粉 / 273
去火毒 / 278
去油 / 278
去菀陈莝 / 237
去腐肉 / 269
甘汞 / 354
甘松 / 326
甘草 / 340
甘遂 / 324
甘温除热 / 244
甘寒生津 / 264
甘寒润燥 / 263
世医得效方 / 692
艾 / 463
艾叶 / 318
艾条 / 464
艾条灸 / 464
艾附暖宫丸 / 394
艾卷 / 464
艾卷灸 / 464
艾炷 / 463
艾炷灸 / 464
艾绒 / 463
古今医统 / 703
古今医统大全 / 703
古今医案按 / 702
古今图书集成医部全录 / 704
本 / 219
本节 / 52
本事方 / 691
本经配穴法 / 447
本草 / 275
本草纲目 / 688
本草纲目拾遗 / 689
本草备要 / 689
本草经集注 / 687
本草拾遗 / 688
本草衍义 / 688

本神 / 429
左右配穴法 / 447
左归丸 / 372
左病右取，右病左取 / 221
厉兑 / 414
石门 / 435
石韦 / 323
石水 / 549
石关 / 425
石决明 / 339
石菖蒲 / 335
石斛 / 343
石斛夜光丸 / 396
石淋 / 552
石蛾 / 629
石榴皮 / 349
石膏 / 304
石瘿 / 597
右归丸 / 373
布气 / 504
龙门 / 555
龙齿 / 337
龙虎草 / 324
龙骨 / 337
龙胆 / 308
龙胆泻肝汤 / 368
龙胆草 / 308
龙眼肉 / 342
龙衔式 / 505
龙葵 / 312
平贝母 / 302
平气 / 18
平旦服 / 284
平坐 / 495
平肝 / 265
平肝抑阳药 / 293
平肝息［熄］风药 / 293
平肝熄［息］风 / 266
平肝潜阳 / 265
平补平泻 / 458
平补平泻法 / 458
平刺 / 454
平垫 / 641
平胃散 / 379
平脉 / 160
平息 / 159
平掌式 / 504
平喘药 / 303
平稳出针法 / 462
平熄内风剂 / 377
平整复元 / 638

［丨］

北豆根 / 313
北沙参 / 343
北鹤虱 / 353
卢和 / 669
归来 / 413
归经 / 279
归脾汤 / 372
目 / 43
目下有卧蚕 / 128
目下网 / 608
目下纲 / 608
目下肿 / 128
目下弦 / 45，609
目下胞 / 45，609
目上网 / 608
目上纲 / 608
目上弦 / 45，609
目上胞 / 44，608
目内眦 / 44，608
目功 / 506
目本 / 610
目外眦 / 608
目连劄 / 614
目系 / 45，610
目纲 / 44，608
目盲 / 612
目弦 / 44，608
目胞 / 607
目胞浮肿 / 128
目珠 / 610
目眶 / 43，608
目眶骨 / 608
目眦 / 44，607
目眵 / 610
目偏视 / 622
目痒 / 622
目锐眦 / 44，607
目痛 / 610
目窗 / 429
目窠上微肿 / 128
目窠肿 / 128
目劄 / 614
目裹 / 607
叶天士 / 675
叶香岩 / 675
叶桂 / 675
申脉 / 423
电光伤目 / 621
电针 / 470
电针仪 / 470
电针疗法 / 470
电针麻醉 / 470
电灸 / 467
电灸器 / 467
电热灸 / 467
由里出表 / 83
由表入里 / 82
由实转虚 / 84
由虚转实 / 84
叫化功 / 502
叩［扣］齿 / 488
叩［扣］法 / 484
叩齿 / 505
另煎 / 283
四气 / 279
四白 / 411
四时不正之气 / 63
四诊 / 123
四诊合参 / 165
四诊抉微 / 686
四君子汤 / 371
四物汤 / 371
四性 / 279
四弯风 / 603

四逆 / 538
四逆汤 / 370
四逆散 / 366
四神丸 / 374
四神聪 / 439
四海 / 25
四渎 / 427
四满 / 424
四缝 / 443

［ 丿 ］

生化 / 2
生化汤 / 376
生地 / 306
生肌 / 270
生肌收口 / 270
生肌敛疮 / 270
生脉饮 / 389
生姜 / 295
生津 / 264
生殖之精 / 57
失血 / 549
失荣 / 598
失音 / 140，524
失音病 / 524
失语 / 537
失神 / 123
失眠 / 155，535
失溲 / 151
禾髎 / 411
丘疹 / 591
丘墟 / 431
代脉 / 162
代赭石 / 339
仙灵脾 / 346
仙茅 / 346
仙授理伤续断秘方 / 697
仙鹤草 / 328
白及 / 328
白仁 / 45，609
白丑 / 324
白术 / 341
白头翁 / 308
白头翁汤 / 369
白芍 / 342
白色 / 126
白芷 / 295
白花蛇舌草 / 312
白芥子 / 299
白芥子灸 / 467
白豆蔻 / 319
白秃 / 604
白秃疮 / 604
白疕 / 602
白附子 / 299
白驳风 / 602
白环俞 / 421
白苔 / 134
白茅根 / 307
白矾 / 354
白虎汤 / 367
白虎摇头法 / 458
白果 / 301
白带 / 158，564
白砒 / 354
白砂苔 / 135
白前 / 301
白扁豆 / 341
白珠 / 609
白珠俱青 / 617
白涩症 / 617
白涩病 / 617
白屑风 / 602
白陷鱼鳞 / 618
白硇砂 / 355
白淫 / 552
白喉 / 585
白痢 / 522
白睛 / 45，609
白睛发黄 / 129
白睛色诊 / 129
白睛红赤 / 129，611
白睛赤肿 / 611
白睛虬脉 / 618
白睛青蓝 / 617
白睛抱红 / 611
白睛浮壅 / 611
白睛涩痛 / 611
白睛混赤 / 611
白睛溢血 / 617
白睛暴赤 / 611
白腻苔 / 134
白痦 / 139
白缠喉 / 585
白蔹 / 312
白膜侵睛 / 617
白膜蔽睛 / 617
白鲜皮 / 308
白僵蚕 / 338
白薇 / 307
白癜风 / 602
他经选穴法 / 446
瓜蒌 / 299
瓜蒌薤白半夏汤 / 375
瓜藤缠 / 601
丛毛 / 52
用药法象 / 689
印堂 / 43，440
外气 / 500
外风 / 64
外风证 / 191
外功 / 492
外丘 / 431
外台秘要 / 690
外耳门 / 473
外邪 / 62
外因 / 62
外关 / 427
外劳宫 / 442
外吹 / 596
外吹乳痈 / 596
外证 / 591
外固定 / 640
外治 / 272
外治法 / 272
外经 / 400
外科大成 / 698

外科正宗 / 698
外科证治全生集 / 698
外科启玄 / 697
外科精义 / 697
外科精要 / 697
外痈 / 593
外陵 / 413
外辅骨 / 51
外眦 / 44，608
外痔 / 599
外湿 / 65
外寒 / 64
外感 / 62，519
外感头痛 / 533
外感咳嗽 / 525
外感腰痛 / 553
外障 / 612
外敷 / 272
外踝 / 50
外踝尖 / 443
外燥 / 66
外燥证 / 197
外翻 / 656
冬瓜皮 / 321
冬虫夏草 / 348
冬葵果 / 322
冬温 / 519
包煎 / 283
饥不欲食 / 153

［丶］

主气 / 18
主色 / 124
主运 / 18
主应配穴法 / 448
主辅佐引 / 358
立迟 / 577
玄明粉 / 353
玄府 / 41
玄参 / 306
闪火法 / 468
兰室秘藏 / 701
半边莲 / 312
半身无汗 / 145
半身不遂 / 537
半身汗出 / 145
半表半里 / 83
半表半里证 / 171
半枝莲 / 312
半卧式 / 495
半刺 / 459
半夏 / 298
半夏泻心汤 / 366
半夏厚朴汤 / 375
头风 / 146，533
头正 / 493
头穴线 / 471
头皮针 / 470
头皮针疗法 / 471
头汗 / 145
头如顶物 / 493
头针 / 470
头针疗法 / 471
头项强痛 / 146
头面功 / 500
头临泣 / 429
头重 / 146
头重脚轻 / 146
头窍阴 / 429
头颅骨 / 42
头颈部穴 / 439
头维 / 412
头痛 / 146，533
穴位注射 / 470
穴位封闭 / 470
穴位埋线疗法 / 478
穴位磁疗法 / 478

［一］

司天 / 18
尻 / 51
尻骨 / 51
出针 / 462
出针法 / 462
出偏 / 505
奶麻 / 584
奶癣 / 604
加味乌药汤 / 375
加味逍遥丸 / 386
加辅料炒 / 277
加减葳蕤汤 / 363
皮内针 / 450
皮内针疗法 / 450
皮水 / 549
皮毛 / 41
皮肤针 / 449
皮肤针疗法 / 450
皮痹 / 541，602
发 / 594
发气 / 504
发气手势 / 504
发功 / 504
发汗禁例 / 229
发汗解表 / 225
发汗解表药 / 287
发芽 / 278
发迟 / 578
发际 / 42
发际疮 / 592
发表药 / 287
发放外气 / 504
发泡 / 273
发泡灸 / 466
发背 / 594
发热 / 143
发热恶寒 / 143
发黄 / 139，523
发蛀脱发 / 602
发散风热药 / 287
发散风寒药 / 287
发落 / 602
发颐 / 594
发酵 / 278
圣济总录 / 703
圣惠方 / 691
对耳轮 / 472
对耳轮下脚 / 472
对耳轮上脚 / 472

对耳轮体 / 472
对耳屏 / 473
对应选穴法 / 446
对症选穴法 / 446
对掌推拉导气 / 503
母 / 13
母气 / 13
幼幼集成 / 696
幼幼新书 / 696
幼科铁镜 / 696
丝瓜络 / 316
丝竹空 / 428
丝状疣 / 600

六画

[一]

动中有静 / 492
动功 / 492
动脉 / 162
动留针法 / 462
动静相兼功 / 492
托里排脓 / 269
托板 / 640
托法 / 269
托毒 / 269
托疮 / 269
托盘疔 / 592
托提法 / 484
老鹳草 / 316
地五会 / 431
地支 / 18
地仓 / 411
地龙 / 339
地机 / 415
地图舌 / 579
地肤子 / 322
地骨皮 / 306
地黄 / 306
地黄丸 / 389
地榆 / 329
地锦草 / 309
耳 / 45
耳门 / 45，428
耳孔 / 45
耳功 / 501，505
耳甲 / 473
耳甲艇 / 473
耳甲腔 / 473
耳穴 / 473
耳穴推拿疗法 / 490
耳穴探测仪 / 477
耳尖 / 440
耳后发 / 625
耳后附骨痈 / 624
耳舟 / 473
耳闭 / 623
耳壳 / 45
耳壳流痰 / 623
耳针 / 472
耳针疗法 / 472
耳疔 / 623
耳疖 / 623
耳轮 / 45，472
耳轮干枯 / 129
耳轮甲错 / 129
耳轮红肿 / 129
耳轮尾 / 472
耳轮青黑 / 129
耳轮结节 / 472
耳轮萎缩 / 129
耳轮脚 / 472
耳轮淡白 / 129
耳鸣 / 624
耳垂 / 45，473
耳和髎 / 428
耳胀 / 623
耳挺 / 625
耳科（学）/ 623
耳疮 / 623
耳屏 / 473
耳根毒 / 624
耳根痈 / 624
耳眩晕 / 625
耳痔 / 625
耳窍 / 45
耳菌 / 625
耳聋 / 624
耳聋口哑 / 625
耳聋左慈丸 / 397
耳痔 / 625
耳道 / 45
耳廓 / 45
耳膜 / 45
耳瘘 / 625
耳蕈 / 625
芒刺舌 / 133
芒硝 / 352
臣药 / 358
再造丸 / 391
西红花 / 330
西河柳 / 298
西洋参 / 343
西黄丸 / 384
压力垫 / 641
压垫 / 641
厌食 / 582
在泉 / 18
百日咳 / 586
百节 / 52
百虫窝 / 443
百会 / 434
百合 / 302
百合病 / 534
百部 / 302
百晬内嗽 / 577
百骸 / 50
有头疽 / 594
有形之痰 / 71
有根苔 / 136
存泥丸 / 487
存神 / 498
存息 / 498
存想 / 499
夺血 / 549
灰苔 / 135
达邪 / 229

列缺 / 409
死胎 / 567
死胎不下 / 567
成无己 / 663
成方 / 356
夹板固定 / 640
夹板固定疗法 / 640
夹持进针法 / 453
夹挤分骨 / 638
夹脊 / 441，506
夹惊吐 / 587
扬刺 / 461
邪 / 62
邪气 / 62
邪火 / 70
邪正消长 / 78
邪正盛衰 / 78
邪热壅肺 / 102
邪热壅肺证 / 204
至阳 / 434
至阴 / 423
[|]
光明 / 431
光剥舌 / 136
当归 / 342
当归丸 / 394
当归四逆汤 / 370
当归补血汤 / 372
当阳 / 439
早泄 / 156
早泄（病）/ 552
吐矢 / 544
吐舌 / 134
吐血 / 152，550
吐字呼吸 / 497
吐弄舌 / 134
吐纳 / 497
吐法 / 267
吐酸 / 543
虫吐 / 587
虫咬皮炎 / 603
虫积 / 582
虫积（证）/ 547
虫积证 / 199
虫积经闭 / 559
虫积腹痛 / 546，588
虫兽伤 / 71
虫痫 / 590
曲 / 282
曲牙 / 46
曲池 / 410
曲泽 / 426
曲垣 / 418
曲骨 / 48，435
曲泉 / 432
曲差 / 419
曲频 / 46
曲鬓 / 429
同名经配穴法 / 448
同身寸 / 444
同病异治 / 218
因人制宜 / 218
因地制宜 / 17，218
因时、因地、因人制宜 / 218
因时制宜 / 17，218
吸入 / 272
吸门 / 41
岁会 / 18
岁运 / 17
回光返照 / 123
回阳 / 240
回阳救逆 / 240
回阳救逆剂 / 370
回乳 / 268
回旋 / 639
回旋灸 / 464
刚痉 / 127
肉 / 41
肉人 / 75
肉苁蓉 / 346
肉豆蔻 / 349
肉刺 / 601
肉轮 / 44，607
肉果 / 350
肉桂 / 317
肉痿 / 539
肉瘤 / 598
肉瘿 / 597
[丿]
朱丹溪 / 666
朱沛文 / 679
朱砂 / 336
朱砂安神丸 / 380，385
朱震亨 / 666
先天之气 / 53
先天之火 / 27
先天之精 / 57
先天不足 / 73
先攻后补 / 220
先补后攻 / 220
先煎 / 283
牝疟 / 521
牝脏 / 20
廷孔 / 49
舌 / 39
舌下脉络 / 131
舌下痰包 / 634
舌中 / 130
舌心 / 131
舌功 / 505
舌本 / 131
舌边 / 39，130
舌有齿痕 / 132
舌有瘀点 / 132
舌有瘀斑 / 132
舌尖 / 39，130
舌色 / 131
舌红 / 131
舌形 / 132
舌体 / 131
舌体胖大 / 132
舌疔 / 634
舌诊 / 130
舌青紫 / 132
舌抵上腭 / 494
舌苔 / 134

舌苔脱落 / 135
舌态 / 133
舌岩 / 598
舌的分部 / 130
舌质 / 131
舌肿 / 133
舌卷囊缩 / 134
舌柱上腭 / 494
舌战 / 133
舌胖 / 132
舌疮 / 634
舌神 / 131
舌绛 / 131
舌起芒刺 / 132
舌根 / 131
舌痈 / 634
舌旁 / 39
舌菌 / 598，634
舌象 / 130
舌淡 / 131
舌裂 / 133
舌短 / 134
舌强 / 133
舌痿 / 133
舌端 / 39
舌謇［蹇］ / 133
竹叶 / 305
竹叶石膏汤 / 367
竹茹 / 300
竹罐 / 467
迁延痢 / 522
传化之腑 / 26
传导之官 / 27
传导之腑 / 27
传变 / 116
传经 / 116
传染 / 514
休息痢 / 522
伏气 / 63，515
伏气温病 / 515
伏龙肝 / 349
伏邪 / 64
伏饮 / 528
伏兔 / 413
伏脉 / 160
伏热 / 88
伏热在里 / 88
伏暑 / 518
伏暑病 / 518
延胡索 / 332
任脉 / 406
任脉穴 / 435
伤风鼻塞 / 626
伤产 / 569
伤阳 / 81
伤阴 / 80
伤乳 / 577
伤乳吐 / 587
伤科 / 635
伤科汇纂 / 698
伤科补要 / 698
伤食 / 543
伤食吐 / 587
伤食证 / 543
伤食泄泻 / 545
伤食泻 / 588
伤食腹胀 / 589
伤津 / 81
伤暑 / 517
伤湿 / 518
伤湿止痛膏 / 396
伤寒 / 515
伤寒杂病论 / 685
伤寒论 / 685
伤寒论直解 / 685
伤寒来苏集 / 685
伤寒明理论 / 685
伤寒贯珠集 / 686
伤寒指掌 / 685
伤寒类方 / 685
伤寒总病论 / 685
伤寒眼 / 616
华山参 / 304
华佗 / 659
华佗再造丸 / 394
华莠 / 659
华盖 / 436
仰卧式 / 495
仰卧伸足 / 127
自汗 / 144，531
自我按摩 / 486
自然呼吸 / 497
自然站式 / 495
自然站桩功 / 502
自然铜 / 335
伊贝母 / 302
血 / 56
血亏经闭 / 559
血之府 / 25
血不归经 / 95
血不养筋 / 95
血不循经 / 95
血气 / 56
血分 / 56
血分证 / 180
血分热毒 / 87
血分瘀热 / 88
血丝痰 / 138
血余炭 / 329
血证 / 549
血证论 / 694
血尿 / 550
血轮 / 44，607
血府逐瘀汤 / 376
血枯经闭 / 559
血脉 / 56
血室 / 26，555
血结胸 / 520
血热 / 95，583
血热化燥 / 87
血热化燥证 / 180
血热风盛 / 87
血热风盛证 / 180
血热动血 / 87
血热动血证 / 180
血热妄行 / 95

血热证 / 185
血热经行先期 / 557
血热崩漏 / 561
血热滑胎 / 569
血脂宁丸 / 385
血脏 / 556
血海 / 25，415
血虚 / 95
血虚不孕 / 565
血虚内热证 / 184
血虚月经过少 / 558
血虚风燥证 / 184
血虚生风 / 88
血虚生［动］风证 / 184
血虚外感证 / 184
血虚头痛 / 534
血虚发热 / 530
血虚证 / 184
血虚肤燥生风证 / 185
血虚经行后期 / 558
血虚挟瘀证 / 184
血虚眩晕 / 532
血虚滑胎 / 569
血虚寒凝证 / 184
血虚感冒 / 516
血虚腰痛 / 554
血崩 / 561
血脱 / 95，550
血脱气脱 / 96
血脱证 / 184
血淋 / 552
血随气逆 / 96
血随气陷 / 96
血厥 / 538
血滞不孕 / 565
血滞月经过少 / 558
血寒 / 95
血寒证 / 185
血寒经行后期 / 558
血寒凝滞证 / 185
血缕 / 601
血痹 / 542
血瘀 / 95
血瘀不孕 / 565
血瘀水停证 / 186
血瘀风燥证 / 185
血瘀舌下证 / 185
血瘀证 / 185
血瘀质 / 75
血瘀经闭 / 559
血瘀崩漏 / 561
血瘀痛经 / 560
血瘀腰痛 / 554
血瘀腹痛 / 546
血痰 / 137
血竭 / 355
血精 / 552
血箭痔 / 599
血瘤 / 598
血翳包睛 / 619
血臌（病）/ 547
血燥生风 / 88
囟 / 42
囟门 / 42
囟会 / 435
囟陷 / 577
囟填 / 576
后下 / 283
后天之气 / 53
后天之精 / 57
后天失调 / 73
后发际 / 42
后阴 / 48
后伸扳腰法 / 653
后顶 / 434
后侧夹板 / 640
后溪 / 417
行气 / 252
行气止痛 / 253
行气化痰 / 253
行气剂 / 374
行气法 / 459
行气药 / 291
行气活血 / 253
行气消痞 / 253
行气宽中 / 253
行气宽胸 / 253
行气通络 / 254
行针 / 454
行针候气 / 456
行间 / 432
行迟 / 578
行痹 / 540
全不产 / 565
全虫 / 338
全国中草药汇编 / 690
全鹿丸 / 390
全蝎 / 338
会厌 / 40
会阳 / 421
会阴 / 48，435
会宗 / 427
合穴 / 438
合邪 / 63
合阳 / 422
合欢皮 / 336
合欢花 / 336
合谷 / 410
合谷刺 / 460
合金针 / 452
合指捏法 / 652
合骨 / 50
合骨垫 / 641
合病 / 178
合掌震桩导气 / 503
杀虫 / 272
肌 / 41
肌肤不仁 / 147
肌肤甲错 / 139
肌肤麻木 / 147
肌腠［凑］/ 41
肌痹 / 541
杂气 / 63
杂病 / 524
危达斋 / 666
危亦林 / 665

名医别录 / 687
名医类案 / 702
多汗 / 144
多尿 / 150
多食善饥 / 153
多梦 / 155
色脉合参 / 165
壮 / 464
壮水制阳 / 250
壮阳 / 251
壮热 / 143
冲门 / 415
冲任不固 / 114
冲任不固证 / 215
冲任失［不］调 / 114
冲任失［不］调证 / 215
冲任损伤 / 114
冲阳 / 414
冲服 / 283
冲服剂 / 282
冲剂 / 282
冲脉 / 406
冰片 / 335
冰硼散 / 396

［丶］

刘守真 / 664
刘完素 / 664
刘昉 / 663
刘涓子鬼遗方 / 697
齐仲甫 / 664
齐刺 / 461
齐德之 / 666
交叉选穴法 / 447
交会穴 / 439
交会经配穴法 / 448
交会选穴法 / 447
交肠 / 599
交骨 / 49
交骨不开 / 570
交信 / 424
交通心肾 / 239
交接出血 / 564
次髎 / 421
产门 / 48，555
产后三冲 / 570
产后三急 / 570
产后三病 / 570
产后三脱 / 570
产后大便难 / 571
产后小便不通 / 571
产后小便失禁 / 571
产后水肿 / 572
产后头痛 / 571
产后发热 / 571
产后自汗 / 571
产后血晕 / 571
产后血崩 / 571
产后身痛 / 571
产后尿血 / 571
产后郁冒 / 571
产后乳汁自出 / 573
产后胁痛 / 572
产后怔忡 / 571
产后恶露不绝 / 570
产后缺乳 / 572
产后病 / 570
产后病痉 / 572
产后病温 / 571
产后痉证 / 572
产后痉病 / 572
产后盗汗 / 571
产后腰痛 / 572
产后腹胀 / 572
产后腹痛 / 572
产后痹证 / 572
产宝 / 695
产难 / 569
决明子 / 304
闭经 / 157，559
问二便 / 149
问大便 / 149
问口味 / 154
问小便 / 150
问头身 / 146
问汗 / 144
问妇女经带 / 156
问诊 / 142
问现证 / 142
问起病 / 142
问胸腹 / 151
问渴饮 / 148
问寒热 / 142
问睡眠 / 155
羊痫风 / 535
并月 / 556
并病 / 178
关门 / 413
关元 / 435
关元俞 / 420
关木通 / 321
关冲 / 426
关刺 / 460
关格 / 544
关格病 / 544
米壳 / 350
灯心草 / 323
汗 / 58
汗出如油 / 146
汗证 / 531
汗法 / 225
汗病 / 531
汤头 / 358
汤头歌 / 358
汤头歌诀 / 692
汤剂 / 282
汤药 / 281
汤液本草 / 688
守气 / 456
安胎 / 268
安宫牛黄丸 / 392
安神 / 264
安神补心丸 / 385
安神剂 / 380
安神定志 / 264
安神药 / 293
安息香 / 335

安蛔 / 271
安蛔定痛 / 271
许叔微 / 663

［一］

寻法 / 159
迅速出针法 / 462
导气 / 455，503
导引 / 491
导赤散 / 368
导法 / 273
导便 / 273
异气 / 63
异物入目 / 621
异经选穴法 / 446
异病同治 / 218
孙一奎 / 669
孙文垣 / 669
孙东宿 / 669
孙思邈 / 661
孙络 / 407
阳 / 5
阳中之阳 / 5
阳中之阴 / 5
阳水 / 548
阳气 / 55
阳白 / 429
阳邪 / 63
阳交 / 431
阳汗 / 145
阳池 / 426
阳极似阴 / 7
阳谷 / 417
阳证 / 168
阳证似阴 / 174
阳纲 / 422
阳明（与）少阳合病 / 178
阳明经证 / 176
阳明经病 / 176
阳明病 / 176
阳明病机 / 115
阳明病证 / 176
阳明虚寒 / 115
阳明腑证 / 177
阳明腑实 / 115
阳明腑病 / 177
阳明燥热 / 115
阳和汤 / 370
阳经 / 399
阳络 / 407
阳损及阴 / 7
阳热质 / 74
阳脏 / 20
阳衰 / 79
阳病 / 515
阳病治阴 / 221
阳陵泉 / 431
阳黄 / 523
阳萎 / 156
阳盛 / 78
阳盛格阴 / 79
阳辅 / 431
阳虚 / 79
阳虚水泛 / 86
阳虚发热 / 530
阳虚自汗 / 531
阳虚阴盛 / 78
阳虚证 / 173
阳虚质 / 75
阳虚感冒 / 516
阳脱 / 80
阳脱证 / 173
阳维脉 / 406
阳维脉病证 / 216
阳斑 / 139
阳暑 / 517
阳痫 / 535，589
阳跷脉 / 406
阳跷脉病证 / 216
阳痿（病） / 552
阳溪 / 410
收功 / 505
收涩 / 261
收涩药 / 294
收敛止血药 / 291
收臀松膝 / 494
阴 / 5
阴门 / 49
阴中之阳 / 5
阴中之阴 / 5
阴水 / 549
阴气 / 55
阴户 / 49，555
阴包 / 432
阴市 / 414
阴邪 / 63
阴交 / 436
阴汗 / 145
阴阳 / 5
阴阳五态人 / 74
阴阳不和 / 6
阴阳互损 / 7
阴阳互根 / 5
阴阳平和质 / 73
阴阳平衡 / 6
阴阳失调 / 6
阴阳对立 / 6
阴阳自和 / 6
阴阳交感 / 5
阴阳并补剂 / 373
阴阳两虚 / 80
阴阳转化 / 6
阴阳易 / 553
阴阳乖戾 / 6
阴阳和平之人 / 74
阴阳学说 / 5
阴阳胜复 / 7
阴阳格拒 / 79
阴阳配穴法 / 447
阴阳离决 / 6
阴阳消长 / 6
阴阳调和 / 6
阴阳偏胜［盛］ / 6
阴阳偏衰 / 6
阴阳辨证 / 168
阴极似阳 / 7
阴谷 / 424

阴证 / 168
阴证似阳 / 173
阴茎 / 49
阴刺 / 462
阴郄 / 416
阴经 / 399
阴挺 / 564
阴结 / 545
阴络 / 407
阴都 / 425
阴损及阳 / 7
阴脏 / 20
阴衰 / 79
阴病 / 514
阴病治阳 / 221
阴陵泉 / 415
阴黄 / 523
阴盛 / 79
阴盛阳衰 / 78
阴盛格阳 / 80
阴虚 / 79
阴虚内热证 / 172
阴虚风动 / 103
阴虚火旺 / 79
阴虚火旺证 / 172
阴虚发热 / 530
阴虚动风证 / 210
阴虚阳亢 / 79
阴虚证 / 173
阴虚质 / 75
阴虚肺燥 / 102
阴虚肺燥证 / 204
阴虚咽喉失濡证 / 203
阴虚盗汗 / 532
阴虚感冒 / 516
阴虚潮热 / 519
阴脱 / 80，81
阴脱证 / 173
阴痒 / 147
阴液 / 58
阴液亏虚证 / 173
阴维脉 / 406
阴维脉病证 / 216
阴斑 / 139
阴暑 / 517
阴痫 / 535，589
阴道 / 555
阴寒质 / 75
阴跷脉 / 406
阴跷脉病证 / 216
阴廉 / 433
阴竭阳脱 / 80
阴器 / 49
阴器痛 / 147
阴囊 / 49
防己 / 317
防风 / 295
防风通圣丸 / 382
防风通圣散 / 366
如意金黄散 / 396
妇人大全良方 / 695
妇人良方 / 695
妇科十味片 / 395
红外线灸 / 467
红丝疔 / 592
红舌 / 131
红花 / 330
红芪 / 340
红膜 / 612
红蝴蝶疮 / 601
红霞映日 / 619

七画

[一]

寿世保元 / 703
弄舌 / 134
弄胎 / 569
麦门冬 / 343
麦门冬汤 / 378
麦冬 / 343
麦芽 / 351
麦味地黄丸 / 390
麦粒灸 / 465
麦粒型皮内针 / 450
形 / 2，57
形与神俱 / 3
形气 / 3
形气转化 / 3
形气相失 / 3，126
形气相得 / 3，126
形体 / 57
形胜气 / 126
形脏 / 24
进针 / 452
进针法 / 452
吞服 / 284
吞酸 / 153，543
远血 / 550
远志 / 336
远近配穴法 / 448
远视 / 621
远道刺 / 460
远道选穴法 / 446
运气 / 17，503
运气学说 / 17
运针 / 454
运法 / 483
运脾 / 245
扶正 / 219
扶正固本 / 220
扶正祛邪 / 219
扶正兼祛邪 / 219
扶正培本 / 220
扶正解表 / 230
扶正解表剂 / 363
扶阳 / 250
扶突 / 411
抠法 / 481
扼法 / 484
拒按 / 166
扯法 / 483
扯痧 / 486
走马牙疳 / 633
走马疳 / 633
走火入魔 / 505
走式 / 496

走黄 / 595
走窜痛 / 148
走罐 / 469
攻下 / 236
攻下药 / 289
攻下逐瘀 / 238
攻补兼施 / 220
攻毒 / 270
攻逐水饮 / 237
攻溃 / 270
赤小豆 / 323
赤石脂 / 349
赤龙搅海 / 506
赤白肉际 / 52
赤白带 / 564
赤白带下 / 158
赤白痢 / 522
赤丝虬脉 / 617
赤芍 / 306
赤色 / 126
赤带抱轮 / 611
赤脉传睛 / 611
赤脉贯睛 / 612
赤脉侵睛 / 612
赤眼 / 616
赤痢 / 522
赤游丹 / 594
赤鼻 / 601
赤膜 / 612
赤膜下垂 / 619
折针 / 463
折顶 / 639
折疡 / 635
折骨列肤 / 635
折骨绝筋 / 635
抓法 / 483
抓痧疗法 / 470
扳法 / 485，652
扳胸椎法 / 652
扳颈椎法 / 652
扳腰椎法 / 653
扳腿推拿手法 / 485
投火法 / 468
抖法 / 651
志 / 58
志室 / 422
扭伤 / 646
扭痧 / 486
声重 / 140
声嗄 / 140
报刺 / 461
却谷食气 / 503
芫花 / 324
芸香草 / 304
花椒 / 318
花蕊石 / 329
花翳白陷 / 618
苍术 / 319
苍龙摆尾法 / 458
苍耳子 / 296
芡实 / 349
芳香开窍 / 266
芳香开窍药 / 293
芳香化浊 / 259
芳香化湿 / 259
芳香化湿药 / 290
严氏济生方 / 692
严用和 / 665
苎麻根 / 329
芦荟 / 353
芦根 / 305
劳伤 / 71
劳疟 / 521
劳咳 / 526
劳复 / 71
劳宫 / 426
劳倦 / 71
劳淋 / 552
劳［痨］瘵 / 529
劳蒸 / 530
劳嗽 / 526
扎脉 / 162
苏子 / 303
苏木 / 333
苏合香 / 335
苏合香丸 / 392
苏沈良方 / 691
苏恭 / 661
苏轼 / 662
苏颂 / 662
苏敬 / 661
杠杆支撑 / 639
杜仲 / 347
杏苏散 / 378
极泉 / 416
杞菊地黄丸 / 389
李士材 / 673
李中立 / 671
李中梓 / 673
李正宇 / 671
李东垣 / 665
李东壁 / 670
李用粹 / 675
李时珍 / 670
李杲 / 665
李明之 / 665
李修之 / 675
李梴 / 669
李惺庵 / 675
李濒湖 / 670
李濂 / 669
杨上善 / 660
杨济时 / 671
杨莓舌 / 585
杨继洲 / 671
更年安 / 395
束骨 / 423
豆蔻 / 319
两目垂帘内视 / 494
两面针 / 333
两眼无光 / 128
两眼翻上 / 129
医门法律 / 701
医方考 / 692
医方论 / 693
医方集解 / 692

医用气功 / 492
医林改错 / 702
医和 / 658
医学入门 / 703
医学心悟 / 704
医学正傳 / 703
医学衷中参西录 / 702
医宗必读 / 704
医宗金鉴 / 705
医贯 / 702
尪痹 / 541
尪痹颗粒 / 393
连舌 / 579
连翘 / 310

[丨]

步廊 / 425
时方 / 357
时方歌括 / 693
时令病 / 514
时邪 / 62
时行 / 514
时行戾气 / 63，514
时行感冒 / 515
时毒 / 514
时疫 / 514
时疫痢 / 522
时病 / 514
时病论 / 694
吴又可 / 672
吴有性 / 672
吴师机 / 680
吴安业 / 680
吴其浚 / 679
吴尚先 / 679
吴茱萸 / 318
吴茱萸汤 / 370
吴瑭 / 678
吴鞠通 / 678
吴瀹斋 / 679
助阳 / 250
助阳解表 / 230
里水 / 549
里证 / 169
里实 / 82
里实证 / 171
里急后重 / 150
里热 / 82
里热证 / 170
里虚 / 82
里虚热证 / 171
里虚寒证 / 170
里喉痈 / 629
里寒 / 82
里寒证 / 170
呓语 / 140
呕吐 / 542
呕吐清涎 / 152
呕吐宿食 / 152
呕吐酸腐 / 152
呕血 / 152
呕乳 / 577，587
呃逆 / 153，543
足三阳经 / 399
足三阴经 / 399
足三里 / 414
足五里 / 433
足太阳膀胱经 / 403
足太阳膀胱经穴 / 418
足太阴脾经 / 401
足太阴脾经穴 / 414
足少阳胆经 / 404
足少阳胆经穴 / 428
足少阴肾经 / 403
足少阴肾经穴 / 423
足发背 / 594
足阳明胃经 / 401
足阳明胃经穴 / 411
足针 / 478
足针疗法 / 478
足底疔 / 592
足临泣 / 431
足窍阴 / 432
足通谷 / 423
足厥阴肝经 / 405
足厥阴肝经穴 / 432
足跗 / 51
足跟痛 / 147
足蹬 / 639
串雅内、外编 / 693
听会 / 428
听宫 / 418
听息 / 498
吻 / 46
吹药 / 273
别络 / 407
别煮 / 283
岐伯 / 658

[丿]

针尖 / 449
针向行气法 / 459
针体 / 449
针灸 / 444
针灸大成 / 699
针灸甲乙经 / 699
针灸师 / 444
针灸问对 / 699
针灸问答 / 699
针灸疗法 / 444
针灸学 / 444
针灸资生经 / 699
针灸铜人 / 452
针灸聚英 / 699
针刺疗法 / 444
针刺麻醉 / 470，699
针法 / 444
针柄 / 449
针根 / 449
针眼 / 612
针麻诱导 / 470
针感 / 456
牡丹皮 / 306
牡脏 / 20
牡蛎 / 338
牡蛎散 / 374
利小便，实大便 / 261
利水 / 260

利水除湿 / 260
利水消肿 / 261
利水消肿药 / 290
利水渗湿 / 260
利水渗湿药 / 290
利气 / 252
利尿 / 260
利尿逐水药 / 290
利尿通淋药 / 290
利咽 / 271
利胆退黄药 / 290
利湿 / 260
利湿药 / 290
利湿退黄药 / 290
秃疮 / 604
体质 / 73
体质学说 / 73
何西池 / 677
何首乌 / 344
何炳元 / 680
何梦瑶 / 676
何廉臣 / 681
佐药 / 358
但热不寒 / 143
但欲寐 / 155
但寒不热 / 143
伸法 / 485
伸筋草 / 316
伸腰沉胯 / 494
身法 / 493
身柱 / 434
身重 / 147
身热 / 143
身热不扬 / 144
身痒 / 147
身瞤动 / 127
身痛 / 147
皂角刺 / 333
佛手 / 326
佛家气功 / 492
近血 / 550
近视 / 621
余沥不尽 / 151
余热未清证 / 180
余霖 / 678
坐式 / 494
坐式复位 / 642
坐忘 / 498
坐板疮 / 592
坐罐 / 469
谷气 / 53
谷芽 / 351
谷精草 / 304
含胸拔背 / 494
含漱 / 273
邻近选穴法 / 446
肝 / 21
肝水 / 549
肝气 / 21，54
肝气（亏）虚证 / 209
肝气上逆 / 98
肝气不足 / 96
肝气不和 / 97
肝气不舒 / 97
肝气犯胃 / 97，103
肝气犯胃证 / 210
肝气犯脾 / 98，104
肝气犯脾证 / 210
肝气郁结 / 97
肝气郁结证 / 210
肝气胁痛 / 531
肝气虚 / 96
肝气横逆 / 97
肝风 / 103
肝风内动 / 103
肝风内动证 / 210
肝火 / 103
肝火上炎 / 98
肝火上炎证 / 210
肝火不得卧 / 535
肝火犯头证 / 209
肝火耳鸣 / 624
肝火证 / 209
肝火炽盛 / 98
肝火炽盛证 / 209
肝火眩晕 / 532
肝火燔耳证 / 209
肝血 / 21
肝血（亏）虚证 / 209
肝血不足 / 97
肝血虚 / 97
肝阳 / 21
肝阳（亏）虚证 / 209
肝阳上亢 / 98
肝阳上亢证 / 209
肝阳化风 / 103
肝阳化风证 / 210
肝阳化火 / 98
肝阳亢盛 / 98
肝阳亢盛证 / 210
肝阳头痛 / 534
肝阳眩晕 / 532
肝阳虚 / 97
肝阴 / 21
肝阴（亏）虚证 / 209
肝阴不足 / 97
肝阴虚 / 97
肝劳 / 529
肝郁 / 103
肝郁不孕 / 565
肝郁证 / 210
肝郁胁痛 / 531
肝郁脾虚 / 104
肝郁脾虚证 / 211
肝肾阴虚 / 104
肝肾阴虚证 / 211
肝经风热 / 98
肝经风热证 / 211
肝经郁热 / 98
肝经实火 / 98
肝经咳嗽 / 524
肝经湿热 / 99
肝经湿热证 / 211
肝胃不和 / 103
肝胃不和证 / 210
肝胃气痛 / 542

肝咳 / 524
肝俞 / 420
肝胆病辨证 / 208
肝胆湿热 / 104
肝胆湿热证 / 211
肝热 / 103
肝疳 / 581
肝虚寒 / 97
肝虚寒证 / 209
肝脾不和 / 104
肝脾不和证 / 211
肝寒 / 103
肝寒证 / 209
肝痹 / 541
肝痿 / 539
肛门 / 49
肛痈 / 599
肛裂 / 599
肛瘘 / 599
肛漏 / 599
肘尖 / 442
肘后备急方 / 690
肘按法 / 651
肘推法 / 648
肘揉法 / 648
肘髎 / 410
肠鸣 / 153
肠痈 / 546
肠痔 / 599
肠痹 / 542
肠燥津亏证 / 187
龟甲 / 345
龟板 / 345
龟背 / 578
龟胸 / 578
龟鹿二仙胶 / 373
龟龄集 / 390
狂 / 534
狂言 / 140
狂病 / 534
角弓反张 / 127
角孙 / 428
鸠尾 / 47，436
条口 / 414
灸 / 463
灸疗法 / 463
灸忌 / 467
灸法 / 463
灸禁 / 467
迎风冷泪 / 611
迎风热泪 / 611
迎风流泪 / 611
迎香 / 411
迎随补泻 / 457
迎随补泻法 / 457
迎随顺逆补泻法 / 491
饮 / 72，282，527
饮片 / 282
饮证 / 188，528
饮食不节 / 70
饮食不洁 / 70
饮食有节 / 507
饮食劳倦 / 70
饮食偏嗜 / 153
饮停心包证 / 188
饮停胸胁证 / 188
饮膳正要 / 689

［丶］

冻风 / 606
冻疮 / 605
库房 / 412
疔 / 592
疔疮走黄 / 595
疖 / 591
疖病 / 592
冷心痛 / 531
冷汗 / 145
冷庐医话 / 702
冷服 / 284
冷泪 / 615
冷哮 / 527
冷秘 / 544
冷痛 / 148
冷罨 / 272
冷瘴 / 521
辛开苦泄 / 229
辛夷 / 296
辛凉平剂 / 362
辛凉轻剂 / 362
辛凉重剂 / 362
辛凉清热 / 225
辛凉解表 / 225
辛凉解表剂 / 362
辛凉解表药 / 288
辛温解表 / 225
辛温解表剂 / 361
辛温解表药 / 288
肓门 / 422
肓俞 / 425
间气 / 18
间使 / 426
间接灸 / 465
间隔灸 / 465
闷痧 / 583
闷痛 / 147
羌活 / 313
兑端 / 435
灼热 / 143
灼痛 / 148
汪切安 / 674
汪机 / 668
汪昂 / 674
汪省之 / 668
沥血腰痛 / 554
沥胞生 / 569
沥浆生 / 569
沥浆产 / 569
沙苑子 / 344
沙棘 / 301
泛恶 / 152
泛酸 / 543
没药 / 334
沈之问 / 669
沈芊绿 / 677
沈存中 / 662
沈金鳌 / 677

沈括 / 662
沉肩 / 493
沉香 / 327
沉脉 / 160
怀牛膝 / 344
忧 / 69
快速起针法 / 463
完谷不化 / 149
完骨 / 46，429，623
宋惠父 / 665
宋慈 / 665
牢脉 / 162
良方 / 357
良附丸 / 375
证 / 168
证治汇补 / 694
证治准绳 / 703
证型 / 122，168
证类本草 / 688
证候 / 122，168
诃子 / 349
启脾丸 / 387
补中益气 / 246
补中益气丸 / 388
补中益气汤 / 371
补气 / 244
补气止血 / 258
补气生血 / 247
补气固表 / 244
补气剂 / 371
补气药 / 293
补气养血 / 247
补气摄血 / 258
补火生土 / 251
补火壮阳 / 251
补心丹 / 385
补心阴 / 248
补心益气 / 244
补血 / 247
补血剂 / 371
补血药 / 294
补阳 / 250
补阳还五汤 / 376
补阳剂 / 373
补阳药 / 293
补阴 / 248
补阴剂 / 372
补阴药 / 294
补肝阴 / 248
补肾 / 249
补肾安神 / 264
补肾阳药 / 293
补肾阴 / 250
补肾助阳 / 251
补肾纳气 / 251
补肾固精 / 250
补肾健骨 / 251
补肾益气 / 249
补肾益肺 / 251
补肺 / 247
补肺阴 / 249
补肺益气 / 247
补剂 / 360
补法 / 244
补泻法 / 456
补胃阴 / 249
补骨脂 / 347
补养心血 / 247
补养心阴 / 248
补养安神剂 / 380
补养肺阴 / 249
补养药 / 293
补益中气 / 246
补益气血 / 247
补益心气 / 244
补益心脾 / 247
补益肝肾 / 248
补益肾气 / 249
补益肺气 / 247
补益剂 / 371
补益药 / 293
补脾 / 245
补脾益气 / 246
补脾益肺 / 247
初生不乳 / 574
初生不啼 / 574
诊法 / 123
诊病 / 122
诊家枢要 / 686
诊断 / 122
诊断学 / 122
诊籍 / 122

［乛］

君火 / 21
君臣佐使 / 358
君药 / 358
灵台 / 434
灵芝 / 337
灵枢 / 684
灵道 / 416
灵墟 / 425
尿血 / 151，550
尿赤 / 151
尿浊 / 551
尿清长 / 150
尿短赤 / 150
尿频 / 150
尾闾骨 / 51
尾骶 / 51
尾骶骨 / 51
迟脉 / 160
局方发挥 / 692
局部选穴法 / 446
张三锡 / 670
张山雷 / 682
张子和 / 664
张元素 / 664
张介宾 / 672
张从正 / 664
张氏医通 / 704
张石顽 / 674
张机 / 658
张仲景 / 659
张寿甫 / 681
张寿颐 / 681
张志聪 / 674

张洁古 / 664
张振鋆 / 680
张隐庵 / 674
张景岳 / 672
张路玉 / 674
张锡纯 / 681
张筱衫 / 680
张璐 / 674
忌口 / 284
陆九芝 / 680
陆以湉 / 681
陆渊雷 / 682
陆懋修 / 680
阿是穴 / 444
阿胶 / 342
陈九韶 / 673
陈飞霞 / 676
陈无择 / 664
陈文中 / 665
陈司成 / 673
陈皮 / 325
陈自明 / 665
陈言 / 663
陈良甫 / 665
陈念祖 / 678
陈实功 / 672
陈复正 / 676
陈修圆 / 678
陈修圆医书十六种 / 705
陈慎修 / 678
陈毓仁 / 672
陈藏器 / 661
附子 / 317
附子饼灸 / 466
附子理中丸 / 387
附分 / 421
附骨疽 / 595，656
坠肘 / 493
妊娠 / 564
妊娠小便淋痛 / 567
妊娠心烦 / 567
妊娠失音 / 568
妊娠呕吐 / 566
妊娠肿胀 / 568
妊娠咳嗽 / 568
妊娠恶阻 / 566
妊娠眩晕 / 566
妊娠病 / 566
妊娠痫证 / 566
妊娠禁忌药 / 284
妊娠腹痛 / 566
努法 / 455
忍冬藤 / 310
鸡内金 / 352
鸡血藤 / 332
鸡骨草 / 308
鸡胸 / 578
鸡眼 / 601
驱虫 / 271
驱虫药 / 294
驱虫消积 / 271
纯阳之体 / 574
纳入原位 / 640
纳干法 / 459
纳子法 / 459
纳支法 / 459
纳气平喘 / 242
纳甲法 / 459
纳呆 / 153

八画

[一]

环跳 / 430
环跳疽 / 595
武之望 / 673
武火 / 283
武术气功 / 492
武叔卿 / 673
青木香 / 321
青风 / 620
青风内障 / 620
青风藤 / 317
青龙摆尾法 / 458
青皮 / 325
青舌 / 132
青色 / 125
青灵 / 416
青果 / 313
青盲 / 620
青蛇毒 / 606
青葙子 / 304
青紫舌 / 132
青蒿 / 307
青蒿鳖甲汤 / 369
青黛 / 311
表气不固 / 85
表里 / 169
表里双解 / 230
表里双解剂 / 366
表里出入 / 82
表里同病 / 83
表里传 / 116
表里经配穴法 / 447
表里选穴法 / 446
表里配穴法 / 447
表里俱实 / 85
表里俱热 / 83
表里俱虚 / 85
表里俱寒 / 83
表里病机 / 81
表里虚实 / 82
表里寒热 / 82
表里辨证 / 169
表证 / 169
表实 / 82
表实里虚 / 84
表实里虚证 / 171
表实证 / 170
表热 / 82
表热传里 / 83
表热里寒 / 83
表热里寒证 / 171
表热证 / 170
表虚 / 82
表虚里实 / 83
表虚里实证 / 171

表虚证 / 170
表湿证 / 196
表寒 / 82
表寒里热 / 83
表寒里热证 / 171
表寒证 / 170
抹法 / 482
抹前额 / 487
拔伸法 / 653
拔伸牵引 / 638
拔伸复位 / 640
拔伸捏正 / 640
拔毒 / 269
拔罐 / 467
拔罐疗法 / 274，467
拔伸法 / 653
拔伸牵引 / 638
拔伸复位 / 640
拔伸捏正 / 640
拔毒 / 269
拔罐 / 467
拔罐疗法 / 274，467
坤草 / 334
押手 / 453
抽气罐 / 468
抽气罐法 / 468
抽葫芦 / 323
抽筋 / 127
抽搐 / 539
拍击法 / 649
拍法 / 483
顶中线 / 471
顶旁1线 / 471
顶旁2线 / 471
顶颞后斜线 / 471
顶颞前斜线 / 471
拘急 / 127
拘挛 / 127
抱头火丹 / 594
抱朴子 / 660
抱轮红赤 / 611
抱骨垫 / 641
抱球式 / 496
抱踝手法 / 648
抱膝器 / 641
拉法 / 639
拉腿手法 / 486
拧法 / 481
拧眉心 / 487
拧拳反掌式 / 654
拂法 / 483
拨法 / 485
拨络法 / 485
择向补泻法 / 491
拇指同身寸 / 445
耵耳 / 625
耵聍 / 625
取穴法 / 446
苦杏仁 / 301
苦参 / 308
苦夏 / 582
苦温平燥 / 244
苦温燥湿 / 244，260
苦寒泄热 / 231
苦寒泻火 / 231
苦寒清气 / 231
苦寒清热 / 230
苦寒燥湿 / 260
苦楝皮 / 353
苗窍 / 38
苘麻子 / 322
直中 / 116
直针刺 / 461
直刺 / 454
直透 / 454
直接灸 / 465
茎 / 49
茎垂 / 49
苔色 / 134
林云和 / 679
林佩琴 / 679
林羲桐 / 679
枇杷叶 / 301
板蓝根 / 310
板蓝根冲剂 / 381
松 / 493
松皮癣 / 602
枕下旁线 / 472
枕上正中线 / 471
枕上旁线 / 472
枕骨 / 46
卧式 / 495
刺五加 / 341
刺手 / 453
刺血拔罐 / 469
刺灸法 / 444
刺法 / 444
刺络 / 449
刺络拔罐 / 469
刺痛 / 148
刺蒺藜 / 339
郁火 / 70
郁李仁 / 352
郁金 / 331
郁病 / 549
奔豚 / 535
奔豚气 / 535
奇方 / 356
奇经八脉 / 405
奇恒之腑 / 24
奇效良方 / 692
转筋 / 127
转筋霍乱 / 523
轮屏切迹 / 473
软气功 / 492
软脉 / 161
软膏 / 281

[丨]

非化脓灸 / 465
齿 / 39
齿更 / 632
齿迟 / 578
齿挺 / 633
齿衄 / 137，550
齿痕舌 / 132
齿落 / 632

齿焦 / 137
齿摇 / 137
齿槁 / 137
齿龈肿痛 / 137，634
齿龈宣露 / 633
齿龈结瓣 / 634
齿龋 / 632
齿燥 / 137
齿龄 / 632
齿蠹 / 632
虎口 / 52
虎杖 / 309
虎步功 / 502
肾 / 22
肾亏 / 111
肾之府 / 27
肾不纳气 / 113
肾不纳气证 / 213
肾气 / 55
肾气（亏）虚证 / 212
肾气丸 / 373
肾气不足 / 111
肾气不固 / 112
肾气不固证 / 212
肾气虚 / 111
肾火偏亢 / 111
肾水 / 22，549
肾水亏虚证 / 212
肾水不足 / 112
肾阳 / 23
肾阳不足 / 113
肾阳衰微 / 111，113
肾阳虚 / 112
肾阳虚证 / 213
肾阳虚衰 / 113
肾阴 / 22
肾阴不足 / 112
肾阴虚 / 112
肾阴虚火旺证 / 212
肾阴虚证 / 212
肾劳 / 529
肾间动气 / 54
肾岩 / 598
肾岩翻花 / 598
肾经咳嗽 / 525
肾经寒湿证 / 213
肾咳 / 525
肾俞 / 420
肾疳 / 581
肾消 / 551
肾虚 / 111
肾虚不孕 / 565
肾虚水泛 / 113
肾虚水泛证 / 213
肾虚月经过少 / 558
肾虚耳鸣 / 624
肾虚证 / 212
肾虚泄泻 / 545
肾虚泻 / 588
肾虚经闭 / 559
肾虚带下 / 564
肾虚眩晕 / 532
肾虚崩漏 / 561
肾虚痛经 / 560
肾虚滑胎 / 570
肾虚腰痛 / 554
肾痹 / 541
肾痿 / 540
肾膀胱病辨证 / 212
肾精 / 57
肾精亏虚证 / 212
肾精不足 / 112
肾癌 / 598
肾囊 / 49
肾囊风 / 603
昆仑 / 423
昆布 / 300
国公酒 / 393
明目 / 271
明医杂著 / 701
明矾 / 354
明堂 / 625
易虚易实 / 574
易筋功 / 503
易寒易热 / 574
固冲止血 / 262
固冲止带 / 263
固表止汗 / 261
固表止汗剂 / 374
固表止汗药 / 294
固肾 / 262
固肾止带 / 262
固肾涩精 / 262
固肾缩尿 / 262
固定垫 / 641
固定痛 / 148
固经止血 / 262
固〔痼〕疾 / 524
固涩 / 261
固涩剂 / 373
固涩药 / 294
固崩止血 / 262
固崩止带 / 263
固精 / 262
固精丸 / 374
呼吸 / 140
呼吸之气 / 53
呼吸气粗 / 140
呼吸气微 / 140
呼吸补泻 / 457
呼吸补泻法 / 457
鸣天鼓 / 488
岩 / 598
罗天益 / 666
罗布麻叶 / 305
罗汉针 / 450
罗汉果 / 301
罗谦甫 / 666
败血冲心 / 570
败血冲肺 / 570
败血冲胃 / 571
败毒散 / 363
败酱片 / 385
败酱草 / 312
图钉型皮内针 / 450

〔丿〕

制川乌 / 314
制何首乌 / 344
制炭 / 276
制霜 / 278
垂肘 / 494
垂帘翳 / 619
垂盆草 / 309
知母 / 304
知柏地黄丸 / 390
物损真睛 / 621
刮法 / 481
刮柄法 / 455
刮眼眶 / 487
刮痧 / 481
刮痧疗法 / 469
刮痧板 / 469
和中 / 238
和血止痛 / 239
和血安胎 / 239
和血调经 / 239
和血熄风 / 239
和剂局方 / 691
和法 / 238
和胃 / 238
和营 / 239
和营止痛 / 240
和营生新 / 240
和营活血 / 240
和解少阳 / 238
和解少阳剂 / 365
和解表里 / 238
和解剂 / 365
和解法 / 238
和髎 / 428
委中 / 421
委中毒 / 593
委阳 / 421
季肋 / 48
季胁 / 48
季胁痛 / 547
季经 / 556
秉风 / 418
使君子 / 353
使药 / 358
侠白 / 409
侠溪 / 432
侧卧式 / 495
侧柏叶 / 329
侧擦法 / 651
侏儒 / 590
佩兰 / 319
征候 / 122
所生病 / 408
舍脉从症 / 165
舍症从脉 / 165
金门 / 423
金井 / 609
金不换膏 / 395
金生水 / 11
金创 / 605，635
金形之人 / 74
金克木 / 12
金针 / 452
金针拨障法 / 479
金疡 / 617，635
金沸草 / 299
金疮 / 605
金疮痉 / 605
金津 / 440
金钱白花蛇 / 315
金钱草 / 322
金铃子散 / 375
金疳 / 617
金匮肾气丸 / 373
金匮要略 / 686
金匮要略方论 / 686
金匮要略心典 / 686
金匮翼 / 686
金银花 / 310
金银藤 / 310
金锁固精丸 / 374
金寒水冷 / 14
金樱子 / 351
金礞石 / 301
命门 / 23，433
命门之火 / 27
命门火旺 / 111
命门火衰 / 113
命火 / 27
命关 / 138
郄门 / 426
郄穴 / 438
乳中 / 412
乳中结核 / 597
乳汁不行 / 573
乳汁不通 / 573
乳汁自出 / 573
乳头风 / 596
乳头破碎 / 596
乳发 / 596
乳岩 / 598
乳房疼痛 / 147
乳香 / 334
乳食内积证 / 199
乳疬 / 597
乳核 / 597
乳根 / 412
乳积 / 582
乳衄 / 597
乳疽 / 597
乳痈 / 596
乳痨 / 597
乳蛾 / 628
乳痰 / 597
乳溢 / 573
乳膏 / 281
乳漏 / 597
乳癖 / 597
贪食生冷 / 70
肺 / 22
肺卫气虚（不固）证 / 202
肺气 / 22，55
肺气上逆 / 109
肺气不足 / 109
肺气不利 / 109
肺气不宣 / 109

肺气虚 / 109
肺气虚证 / 202
肺气虚寒 / 109
肺风痰喘 / 585
肺水 / 549
肺火 / 102
肺火证 / 204
肺失清肃 / 109
肺阳 / 22
肺阳虚 / 109
肺阳虚证 / 203
肺阴 / 22
肺阴不足 / 109
肺阴虚 / 109
肺阴虚证 / 203
肺劳 / 529
肺系 / 40
肺肾气虚 / 102
肺肾气虚证 / 205
肺肾阳虚 / 102
肺肾阳虚证 / 205
肺肾阴虚 / 102
肺肾阴虚证 / 204
肺肾两虚 / 102
肺胀 / 528
肺炎喘嗽 / 586
肺实 / 102
肺经咳嗽 / 525
肺咳 / 525
肺俞 / 419
肺津 / 22
肺津亏损 / 81
肺津不布 / 109
肺络损伤 / 110
肺热 / 102
肺热炽盛 / 102
肺热炽盛证 / 204
肺疳 / 581
肺病辨证 / 202
肺痈 / 528
肺消 / 551
肺萎［痿］ / 528
肺虚 / 102
肺虚咳嗽 / 526
肺虚热证 / 203
肺虚寒证 / 203
肺痨 / 529
肺痹 / 541
肺燥 / 102
肺燥肠闭证 / 204
肺燥津伤证 / 187
肱 / 47
肿胀 / 138
肿胀舌 / 132
肿疡 / 591
肿毒 / 591
胀痛 / 147
股 / 49
股阳疽 / 595
股阴疽 / 595
股肿 / 606
股疽 / 594
股癣 / 604
肥人 / 75
肥胖不孕 / 565
肥疮 / 604
肥膏肉人 / 75
服药法 / 283
服药食忌 / 284
胁 / 47
胁下痛 / 547
胁痛 / 146
胁痛病 / 546
周天 / 500
周天功 / 501
周天自转功 / 502
周易参同契 / 700
周荣 / 416
昏厥 / 538
昏蒙 / 123
昏睡露睛 / 129
鱼际 / 409
鱼际擦法 / 650
鱼络 / 407
鱼翔脉 / 163
鱼腰 / 440
鱼腥草 / 311
兔唇 / 590
狐臭 / 605
狐惑 / 547
忽思慧 / 667
狗脊 / 347
备急千金要方 / 690
炙 / 277
炙甘草 / 341
饴糖 / 342

［ 丶 ］

变证 / 116
变蒸 / 583
京大戟 / 324
京门 / 430
京骨 / 423
庞安时 / 662
夜交藤 / 336
夜热 / 582
夜啼 / 577
府舍 / 415
疟 / 520
疟母 / 521
疟积 / 521
疟病 / 520
疟疾 / 520
疟痞 / 521
疠气；戾气 / 63
疠风 / 605
疝 / 554
疝气 / 554
疡 / 591，635
疡医 / 635
剂型 / 280
剂量 / 280
卒中 / 536
卒心痛 / 531
卒病 / 515
卒聋 / 624
卒喉痹 / 630

卒喑［瘖］/ 630
盲 / 612
放松功 / 500
育阴 / 248
郑声 / 140
郑宏纲 / 677
郑若溪 / 678
郑梅涧 / 677
郑瀚 / 677
卷柏 / 332
单一脉象 / 163
单手进针法 / 453
单方 / 356
单按 / 159
单盘坐 / 495
单蛾 / 628
单腹胀 / 547
单煎 / 283
炖 / 278
炒 / 277
炒炭 / 277
炒黄 / 277
炒焦 / 277
炒爆 / 277
炉甘石 / 355
浅刺 / 454
泄剂 / 360
泄注 / 150
泄注赤白 / 150
泄泻 / 149
泄泻（病）/ 545
泄热存津 / 231
河车大造丸 / 389
泪 / 58
泪点 / 609
泪泉 / 609
泪窍 / 43，609
泪堂 / 609
油风 / 603
油汗 / 145
泡 / 276
泡腾片 / 280
注泄 / 150
泻下 / 236
泻下不爽 / 149
泻下剂 / 363
泻下药 / 289
泻下逐水 / 237
泻下逐饮 / 237
泻水逐饮 / 237
泻心 / 234
泻心火 / 234
泻白散 / 368
泻肝 / 233
泻肺 / 235
泻肺平喘 / 235
泻肺散 / 369
泥丸 / 496
泽兰 / 334
泽泻 / 320
治风化痰 / 259
治风剂 / 377
治未病 / 219
治本 / 219
治标 / 219
治病求本 / 219
治燥剂 / 378
怔忡 / 151，530
性味 / 278
宗气 / 54
宗筋 / 49
宗筋之会 / 49
定喘 / 441
定喘丸 / 383
定喘汤 / 375
审因论治 / 218
审因施治 / 218
审证求因 / 191
审苗窍 / 128
审视瑶函 / 698
空痛 / 148
空腹服 / 284
帘珠喉痹 / 629
实中夹虚 / 84
实火 / 90
实火证 / 173，198
实证 / 170
实胀 / 589
实按灸 / 466
实脉 / 161
实热 / 90
实热证 / 173
实秘 / 544
实喘 / 527
实痞 / 542
实寒 / 90
实寒证 / 172，194
试水 / 569
试月 / 568
试胎 / 568
肩 / 46
肩井 / 430
肩不举 / 147
肩中俞 / 418
肩外俞 / 418
肩贞 / 418
肩胛 / 47
肩胛疽 / 594
肩痛 / 147
肩臂功 / 501，653
肩臂酸痛 / 147
肩髃 / 410
肩髎 / 427
房劳 / 71
房事不节 / 71
房事过度 / 71
视衣 / 610
视直为曲 / 621
视物易色 / 621
视瞻昏渺 / 620

［ㄧ］

建里 / 436
居经 / 556
居髎 / 430
屈伸法 / 653
屈法 / 485

屈指捏法 / 652
弦脉 / 162
承山 / 423
承光 / 419
承扶 / 421
承灵 / 430
承泣 / 411
承浆 / 46，437
承淡安 / 682
承筋 / 422
承满 / 412
孟诜 / 661
孤阳上越 / 80
降气 / 254
降气止呃 / 254
降气化痰 / 253
降气平喘 / 254
降气剂 / 375
降剂 / 360
降香 / 327
降逆下气 / 254
降逆止呕 / 254
降逆止呃 / 254
降逆止咳平喘 / 254
降逆平喘 / 254
弩法 / 455
参苏饮 / 363
参附注射液 / 391
参苓白术丸 / 388
参苓白术散 / 371
参茸卫生丸 / 391
参茸固本片 / 391
线瘊 / 600
练气 / 503
练功 / 499，653
练神 / 498
细辛 / 296
细脉 / 161
绊舌 / 634
经水 / 556
经水不调 / 557
经水过多 / 560
经水先期 / 557
经水后期 / 557
经水涩少 / 558
经水断绝 / 157
经气 / 55
经气郁滞 / 114
经气逆乱 / 114
经气衰竭 / 114
经气虚损 / 114
经方 / 357
经史证类备急本草 / 688
经外穴 / 439
经穴 / 408，437
经早 / 557
经血 / 556
经行口糜 / 563
经行风疹块 / 563
经行头痛 / 562
经行发热 / 562
经行吐血 / 562
经行吐衄 / 562
经行先后无定期 / 157
经行先期 / 157，557
经行后期 / 157，557
经行身痛 / 562
经行乳房胀痛 / 563
经行泄泻 / 563
经行便血 / 562
经行眩晕 / 562
经行衄血 / 562
经行浮肿 / 562
经行情志异常 / 563
经行隐疹 / 563
经行腹痛 / 158，560
经行瘖瘖 / 563
经闭 / 157，559
经来发热 / 562
经来泄泻 / 563
经别 / 407
经乱 / 558
经间期出血 / 560
经证 / 178
经迟 / 557
经刺 / 460
经带胎产 / 556
经脉 / 398
经络 / 398
经络之气 / 55
经络证候 / 408
经络学说 / 398
经络辨证 / 215，408
经绝 / 158
经效产宝 / 694
经崩 / 561
经断 / 158
经断复来 / 563
经渠 / 409
经期水肿 / 562
经期延长 / 559
经期错后 / 557
经筋 / 406
经漏 / 561
经隧 / 398
经隧失职 / 114

九画

［一］

春温 / 516
春温病 / 516
玳瑁 / 339
珍本医书集成 / 705
珍珠 / 337
珍珠母 / 337
珍珠囊药性赋 / 689
玻璃罐 / 467
毒 / 68
毒火攻口证 / 199
毒火攻唇证 / 198
毒虫咬伤 / 606
毒蛇咬伤 / 606
封藏失职 / 112
挂线疗法 / 273
项 / 46
项功 / 506

项强 / 127
挠法 / 482
政和本草 / 688
赵学敏 / 677
赵养葵 / 671
赵恕轩 / 677
赵献可 / 671
贲门 / 41
垢胎 / 566
挺腿拔伸 / 640
挑刺法 / 449
指切进针法 / 453
指节拍法 / 649
指压行气法 / 459
指压疗法 / 479
指压推拿 / 490
指压麻醉 / 479
指针法 / 481
指按法 / 651
指推法 / 648
指揉法 / 647
指摩法 / 650
挤法 / 484
按太阳 / 487
按手足 / 165
按尺肤 / 165
按目四眦 / 487
按压耳穴 / 488
按压法 / 480
按肌肤 / 165
按迎香 / 488
按诊 / 165
按法 / 159，480，651
按俞穴 / 165
按捏鼻梁 / 488
按胸腹 / 165
按捺耳窍 / 488
按脘腹 / 165
按揉风池 / 489
按揉颈项 / 488
按跷 / 480
按摩 / 480
按摩手法 / 480
按摩师 / 480
按摩足三里 / 489
按摩疗法 / 480
挪法 / 482
荆防败毒散 / 363
荆芥 / 295
荆芥炭 / 296
荆芥穗 / 296
革脉 / 162
茜草 / 328
荜拨 / 319
荜澄茄 / 318
带下 / 563
带下臭秽 / 158
带下病 / 564
带脉 / 406，430
带脉病证 / 215
草乌 / 314
草豆蔻 / 320
草果 / 320
草药 / 275
茧唇 / 598
茵陈 / 309
茵陈蒿 / 309
茵陈蒿汤 / 379
茯苓 / 320
茯神 / 337
茶 / 282
茶剂 / 282
荠菜 / 329
茺蔚子 / 334
荣枯老嫩 / 131
荥穴 / 437
胡黄连 / 308
胡椒 / 318
荔枝核 / 327
南瓜子 / 353
南沙参 / 300
南雅堂医书全集 / 705
南鹤虱 / 354
药方 / 356
药引子 / 358
药材 / 275
药材炮制 / 275
药味 / 278
药物灸 / 466
药性 / 279
药线疗法 / 274
药毒 / 603
药茶 / 507
药面 / 282
药酒 / 281，507
药捻疗法 / 274
药粥 / 507
药摩 / 490
药膳 / 507
药罐 / 469
标 / 219
标本同治 / 219
标本兼治 / 219
枯矾 / 354
枯痔法 / 273
栉头 / 486
柯琴 / 675
柯韵伯 / 675
相反 / 359
相火 / 27
相火妄动 / 112
相杀 / 359
相使 / 359
相畏 / 359
相须 / 358
相恶 / 359
相兼脉象 / 163
枳壳 / 325
枳实 / 325
柏子仁 / 337
柏子养心丸 / 385
栀子 / 310
枸杞子 / 343
柱舌 / 494
柱骨 / 50
柿蒂 / 328

威灵仙 / 314
歪斜舌 / 133
厚朴 / 325
厚朴花 / 327
厚苔 / 135
砂仁 / 319
砂（石）淋 / 552
砭石 / 451
面尘 / 125
面色 / 124
面色㿠白 / 125
面色苍白 / 125
面色萎黄 / 125
面色淡白 / 125
面色黎黑 / 125
面红 / 125
面针 / 477
面针疗法 / 478
面浮 / 125
面黄肌瘦 / 125
面黑 / 125
面游风 / 602
面壁 / 499
牵牛子 / 323
牵引疗法 / 642
牵正散 / 377
牵拉法 / 639
牵拉肩 / 646
牵推法 / 642
轻下 / 237
轻剂 / 360
轻重徐疾补泻法 / 491
轻宣外燥剂 / 378
轻粉 / 354
轻捻出针法 / 462
鸦胆子 / 308

［丨］

韭子 / 348
韭菜子 / 348
背法 / 653
背俞穴 / 439
背部穴 / 441
背痛 / 147
战汗 / 145，531
战栗 / 143
点击法 / 481
点穴疗法 / 490
点刺 / 449
点刺舌 / 132
点法 / 481
点眼 / 273
临产 / 568
临产病 / 569
临证指南医案 / 702
临睡前服 / 284
是动病 / 408
眇目 / 622
哑门 / 434
冒暑 / 516
冒湿 / 518
星翳 / 612
畏明 / 610
畏寒 / 143
胃 / 23
胃、神、根 / 164
胃不和 / 108
胃中热 / 108
胃气 / 24，55
胃气上逆 / 108
胃气不和 / 108
胃气不降 / 108
胃气虚 / 107
胃气虚证 / 207
胃反 / 152，543
胃仓 / 422
胃火 / 108
胃火上炎 / 108
胃火牙痛 / 632
胃火证 / 208
胃火炽盛 / 108
胃火炽盛证 / 208
胃失和降 / 108
胃阳 / 24
胃阳虚 / 107
胃阳虚证 / 207
胃阴 / 24
胃阴不足 / 107
胃阴虚 / 107
胃阴虚证 / 207
胃肠病辨证 / 207
胃实寒 / 107
胃实寒证 / 207
胃咳 / 525
胃俞 / 420
胃津 / 24
胃津亏损 / 81
胃热 / 107
胃热化火 / 92
胃热呕吐 / 586
胃热消［杀］谷 / 108
胃热消谷 / 92
胃热壅盛 / 108
胃热壅盛证 / 208
胃消 / 551
胃家实 / 523
胃虚 / 107
胃虚汗 / 586
胃虚寒 / 107
胃虚寒证 / 207
胃脘 / 23
胃脘下俞 / 441
胃脘痛 / 152
胃脘痛（病） / 542
胃痞 / 542
胃痛 / 152
胃寒 / 107
胃寒饮停证 / 188
胃缓 / 546
胃燥津亏证 / 187
虹彩 / 609
虾游脉 / 163
虾蟆瘟 / 520
虻虫 / 333
思 / 69
咽 / 40
咽门 / 40

咽后痈 / 629
咽底 / 40
咽喉 / 40
咽喉肿痛 / 629
咽喉科学 / 628
咽痹 / 629
哕 / 543
咯血 / 137，550
咬骨疽 / 595
咳血 / 137，550
咳如犬吠 / 142
咳声不扬 / 141
咳声重浊 / 141
咳声清脆 / 141
咳逆 / 526
咳逆上气 / 141，526
咳嗽 / 141，524
贴棉法 / 468
骨 / 25
骨伤科（学）/ 635
骨折 / 635
骨空 / 52
骨度分寸定穴法 / 445
骨度法 / 445
骨疳 / 581
骨病 / 654
骨痨 / 596，656
骨蒸 / 529
骨蒸热 / 583
骨碎补 / 347
骨错缝 / 646
骨解 / 52
骨痹 / 541
骨痿 / 539
骨槽风 / 633
骨鲠 / 631
骨瘤 / 598
幽门 / 41，425

［丿］

钩藤 / 338
选穴法 / 445
香加皮 / 317
香连丸 / 386
香附 / 326
香砂六君丸 / 388
香砂养胃丸 / 387
香橼 / 326
香薷 / 296
香薷散 / 361
秋燥 / 518
秋燥病 / 518
重舌 / 133，633
重听 / 624
重身 / 564
重剂 / 360
重修政和经史证类备急本草 / 688
重提轻插 / 457
重插轻提 / 456
重痛 / 148
重楼 / 311
重镇安神 / 265
重镇安神剂 / 380
重镇安神药 / 293
复方 / 356
复方川贝精片 / 382
复方丹参片 / 393
复合手法 / 490
复位 / 642
复溜 / 424
笃击法 / 481
便血 / 550
便秘 / 149，544
便溏 / 149
顺气 / 254
顺传 / 179，515
顺应四时 / 17
顺骨捋筋 / 640
顺腹式呼吸 / 497
修习止观坐禅法要 / 700
修事 / 276
修治 / 275
保和丸 / 379
保健 / 505
保健功 / 505
保健球按摩 / 490
促脉 / 162
信石 / 354
皇甫士安 / 659
皇甫谧 / 659
鬼门 / 42
鬼胎 / 567
禹余粮 / 349
禹粮石 / 349
徇蒙招尤 / 146
须发早白 / 139
俞穴 / 408
俞府 / 425
俞原配穴法 / 448
俞募配穴法 / 448
郄会配穴法 / 448
剑决式 / 504
剑针 / 452
食已即吐 / 153
食远服 / 284
食床 / 633
食疗 / 274
食疗本草 / 687
食忌 / 284
食泻［泄］/ 588
食治 / 274
食复 / 71
食积 / 582
食积证 / 199
食积盗汗 / 586
食积寒热 / 583
食积腹痛 / 546，588
食疳 / 581
食厥 / 538
食痫 / 589
食滞 / 543
食窦 / 416
胆 / 23
胆气 / 55
胆气虚 / 104
胆气虚证 / 211

胆火证 / 212
胆胀（病）/ 547
胆南星 / 299
胆咳 / 525
胆俞 / 420
胆热 / 104
胆热证 / 211
胆虚气怯 / 104
胆虚气怯证 / 211
胆囊 / 443
胂 / 47
胞 / 555
胞门 / 555
胞生痰核 / 613
胞衣 / 555
胞衣不下 / 570
胞衣先破 / 569
胞肓 / 422
胞阻 / 566
胞轮振跳 / 614
胞肿 / 614
胞肿如桃 / 614
胞脉 / 407
胞宫 / 25，555
胞宫积热证 / 213
胞宫虚寒证 / 213
胞宫湿热证 / 214
胞络 / 407
胞脏 / 25，556
胞虚如球 / 614
胞睑 / 44，607
胞睑下垂 / 129
胞睑肿核 / 613
胞寒不孕 / 565
胖大舌 / 132
胖大海 / 303
脉 / 25
脉口 / 160
脉无胃气 / 164
脉从四时 / 164
脉有胃气 / 164
脉有神 / 164
脉有根 / 164
脉阴阳俱紧 / 164
脉阴阳俱浮 / 164
脉应四时 / 164
脉诊 / 158
脉学 / 158
脉经 / 686
脉逆四时 / 164
脉症合参 / 165
脉悬绝 / 165
脉象 / 158
脉象主病 / 158
脉痹 / 541
脉痿 / 539
脉静 / 164
脉暴出 / 164
脉躁 / 164
胫 / 50
胫骨 / 50，51
胎元 / 566
胎元不固 / 569
胎水肿满 / 567
胎气上逆 / 567
胎动不安 / 568
胎死不下 / 567
胎死腹中 / 567
胎衣 / 555
胎赤 / 576
胎怯 / 576
胎毒 / 69，576
胎食 / 494
胎热 / 568，576
胎息 / 497
胎疸 / 576
胎弱 / 576
胎黄 / 576
胎黄病 / 576
胎患内障 / 620
胎痫 / 590
胎寒 / 568，576
胎禀 / 576
胎漏 / 569
独阴 / 444
独活 / 314
独活寄生汤 / 377
独语 / 140
咎殷 / 662
急下 / 236
急下存阴 / 236
急下存津 / 237
急方 / 357
急火 / 283
急脉 / 433
急黄 / 523
急惊风 / 574
急喉风 / 630
急喉喑［瘖］/ 630
急喉痹 / 630
蚀疮去腐 / 270

［丶］

弯针 / 463
疣 / 600
疣目 / 600
疥疮 / 603
疥癞 / 603
疮 / 591
疮疡 / 591
疮疡经验全书 / 697
疮毒内陷 / 596
疮痨 / 596
疫疔 / 592
疫疠之气 / 63
疫毒 / 63
疫毒证 / 200
疫毒痢 / 522
疫咳 / 586
疫喉 / 585
疫喉痧 / 520
疫痢 / 522
疫痧 / 520，585
姿式 / 493
闻声音 / 139
闻诊 / 139
差颓［癞］/ 578

养心 / 248
养心安神 / 264
养心安神药 / 293
养心阴 / 248
养生十常 / 507
养老 / 417
养血 / 247
养血生发胶囊 / 396
养血药 / 294
养血祛风 / 228
养血柔肝 / 265
养血润肠 / 263
养血润燥 / 263
养血解表 / 230
养血熄［息］风 / 266
养血熄风 / 239
养阴 / 248
养阴药 / 294
养阴润肺 / 263
养阴润燥 / 263
养阴清肺汤 / 378
养阴清肺膏 / 383
养阴解表 / 230
养肝 / 265
养肝阴 / 248
养肺阴 / 249
养性延命录 / 700
养胃 / 249
养胃生津 / 249
养胃阴 / 249
姜炙 / 277
姜黄 / 331
送服 / 284
类中 / 536
类中风 / 536
类证治裁 / 694
类经 / 684
类经图翼 / 684
前发际 / 42
前后配穴法 / 447
前阴 / 48
前谷 / 417
前顶 / 435
前胡 / 300
首乌 / 344
首乌藤 / 336
逆传 / 179，515
逆传心包 / 85
逆治 / 220
逆经 / 560
逆流挽舟 / 230
逆腹式呼吸 / 497
总按 / 159
炼己 / 499
炼气 / 499
炼气化神 / 499
炼丹 / 498
炼神 / 499
炼精 / 499
炼精化气 / 499
炮 / 277
炮制 / 275
炮炙 / 275
炮炙大全 / 689
炮姜 / 318
烂疔 / 592
烂喉丹痧 / 520，585
烂喉痧 / 520
洁净府 / 261
洪脉 / 161
浊气 / 55
浊邪 / 72
浊阴 / 57
洗 / 276
洗手 / 489
洗冤集录 / 700
活血 / 256
活血止痛 / 256
活血止痛药 / 292
活血化瘀 / 256
活血化瘀药 / 291
活血行气 / 256
活血行气药 / 292
活血疗伤药 / 292
活血药 / 292
活血祛瘀 / 256
活血祛瘀剂 / 376
活血祛瘀药 / 291
活血调经 / 256
活血调经药 / 292
活血通经 / 256
活血通络 / 256
涎 / 58
染苔 / 135
济生方 / 691
济阴纲目 / 695
洋金花 / 303
浓缩丸 / 280
津 / 58
津亏火炽 / 81
津亏血燥 / 81
津亏证 / 187
津亏热结 / 81
津亏热结证 / 187
津气 / 54
津气亏虚证 / 187
津伤证 / 187
津枯肠燥 / 90
津脱 / 81，550
津液 / 58
津液亏损证 / 187
津液亏虚证 / 187
津液辨证 / 187
恢刺 / 461
恽树珏 / 682
恽铁樵 / 682
举、按、寻 / 158
举法 / 159
宣白 / 228
宣肺 / 228
宣肺止咳 / 228
宣肺止咳平喘 / 228
宣肺化饮 / 228
宣肺化痰 / 228
宣肺平喘 / 228
宣肺降气 / 228

宣剂 / 360
宣痹通阳 / 241
宫冷不孕 / 565
突起睛高 / 622
穿山龙 / 316
穿山甲 / 333
穿心莲 / 312
穿地龙 / 317
穿刺针埋线法 / 478
客气 / 18
客邪 / 62
客色 / 124
客运 / 18
客忤 / 577
客忤夜啼 / 577
客热 / 583
冠心苏合丸 / 393
语声 / 139
语声低微 / 140
语声重浊 / 140
语言謇涩 / 140
语迟 / 578
扁鹊 / 658
扁鹊心书 / 700
扁瘊 / 600
祛风 / 227
祛风止痒 / 228
祛风止痛 / 227
祛风化痰 / 227
祛风行水 / 228
祛风除湿 / 227
祛风除湿止痛 / 227
祛风通络 / 228
祛风清热 / 227
祛风散寒 / 227
祛风湿药 / 289
祛风湿清热药 / 289
祛风湿散寒药 / 289
祛风湿强筋骨药 / 289
祛风解表 / 227
祛风解痉 / 228
祛邪 / 219
祛邪兼扶正 / 220
祛暑化湿 / 232
祛湿 / 259
祛湿剂 / 379
祛寒化痰 / 258
祛寒剂 / 370
祛寒法 / 240
祛寒药 / 290
祛瘀止血 / 258
祛瘀生新 / 257
祛瘀活血 / 256
祛瘀消肿 / 256
祛瘀通络 / 257
祛痰 / 258
祛痰剂 / 380
祖传秘方 / 357
神 / 2，57
神门 / 417
神不守舍 / 100
神水 / 610
神气不足 / 123
神光耗散 / 128
神曲 / 351
神农本草经 / 687
神志不清 / 123
神志昏愦［溃］/ 124
神乱 / 124
神昏 / 123
神封 / 425
神庭 / 435
神堂 / 422
神道 / 434
神阙 / 48，436
神膏 / 610
神藏 / 425
误下 / 238

［一］

退目翳 / 271
退法 / 463
退黄 / 269
退翳明目 / 271
屋漏脉 / 163
屋翳 / 412
屏上切迹 / 473
屏间切迹 / 473
眉心 / 43
眉冲 / 419
眉棱骨 / 43
孩儿参 / 340
除烦止渴 / 231
怒 / 69
架火法 / 468
蚤休 / 311
柔肝 / 265
柔肝药 / 294
结扎疗法 / 273
结舌 / 579
结脉 / 162
结核 / 591
结胸 / 519
结喉 / 46
结膜红赤 / 612
绛舌 / 131
络石藤 / 315
络穴 / 438
络却 / 419
络刺 / 460
络脉 / 398
绝汗 / 145
绝经前后诸病 / 563
绞肠痧 / 522
绞痛 / 148

十画

［一］

秦艽 / 314
秦皮 / 308
秦越人 / 658
素问 / 683
素髎 / 435
振法 / 484
振挺 / 654
振掉 / 540
捏法 / 482，652

捏积 / 486
捏脊 / 486
挫伤 / 646
热 / 66
热入心包 / 86
热入［闭］心包证 / 180
热入血分 / 87
热入血室 / 87
热入血室证 / 214
热入营血 / 87
热入营血证 / 180
热化 / 92
热邪 / 67
热邪内结 / 87
热邪传里 / 83
热邪阻肺 / 86
热邪阻痹证 / 198
热吐 / 586
热因热用 / 221
热伏冲任 / 87
热伤肺络 / 110
热伤神明 / 100
热伤筋脉 / 88
热汗 / 144
热扰心神证 / 201
热极生风 / 88，103
热极生风证 / 210
热呕 / 542
热灼肾阴 / 88
热证 / 169
热迫大肠 / 86
热服 / 284
热夜啼 / 577
热剂 / 360
热泪 / 615
热泻 / 545
热参 / 304
热毒 / 68
热毒内陷证 / 198
热毒闭肺证 / 204
热毒攻舌证 / 199
热毒攻喉证 / 199
热毒证 / 198
热甚发痉 / 538
热疮 / 600
热结 / 87
热结下焦 / 87
热结肠燥 / 110
热结肠燥证 / 208
热哮 / 527
热积［结］膀胱 / 113
热积［结］膀胱证 / 213
热秘 / 544
热病 / 515
热烘 / 272
热盛风动 / 88
热盛动血证 / 180
热盛伤津 / 88
热淋 / 552
热厥 / 538
热痫 / 590
热痧 / 583
热罨 / 272
热痹 / 540
热痰 / 528
热痰证 / 189
热霍乱 / 523
热瘴 / 521
捣击法 / 481
捣法 / 455，481
顽痰 / 72，528
顽癣 / 602
起针 / 462
起针法 / 462
起罐 / 469
埋针疗法 / 450
恐 / 70
莱菔子 / 352
莲子 / 349
莲子心 / 305
莲花舌 / 634
莲须 / 349
莪术 / 331
荷叶 / 320
恶气 / 63
恶风 / 143
恶心 / 152
恶色 / 125
恶阻 / 566
恶热 / 143
恶寒 / 143
恶寒发热 / 143
恶露 / 570
恶露不下 / 570
恶露不止 / 570
恶露不绝 / 570
莨菪子 / 304
真牙 / 39，632
真元亏虚证 / 212
真中 / 536
真中风 / 536
真水 / 22
真气 / 53，500
真气气感 / 505
真火 / 23
真心痛 / 530
真头痛 / 533
真阳 / 23
真阴 / 22
真阴不足 / 112
真武汤 / 380
真实假虚 / 85
真实假虚证 / 174
真热假寒 / 92
真热假寒证 / 174
真脏色 / 126
真脏脉 / 165
真虚假实 / 85
真虚假实证 / 174
真寒假热 / 92
真寒假热证 / 174
真睛破损 / 621
桂附地黄丸 / 390
桂枝 / 295
桂枝汤 / 361
桔梗 / 299

栓剂 / 282
桃仁 / 330
格阳 / 80
格阴 / 79
格致余论 / 701
核骨 / 50
核桃仁 / 346
彧中 / 425
速效救心丸 / 394
鬲咽 / 543
配方 / 357
配穴法 / 447
唇 / 39
唇风 / 633
唇疔 / 634
唇疮 / 634
唇疽 / 634
唇菌 / 634
唇裂 / 136
唇紫 / 136
夏季热 / 582
夏季热病 / 582
夏枯草 / 305
破气 / 255
破伤风 / 605
破血 / 257
破血祛瘀 / 257
破血逐瘀 / 257
破血消癥药 / 292
破䐃脱肉 / 127
破瘀 / 257
破瘀生新 / 257
破瘀消癥 / 257
原［元］机启微 / 698
原气 / 53
原穴 / 438
原络配穴法 / 447
逐水 / 237
逐水剂 / 365
顿服 / 284
顿咳 / 586

［丨］

柴胡 / 297
柴葛解肌汤 / 362
紧按慢提 / 456
紧脉 / 162
紧提慢按 / 457
紧喉风 / 630
逍遥丸 / 386
逍遥散 / 366
党参 / 340
眩冒 / 146
眩晕 / 146，532
哮 / 141，527
哮病 / 527
哮喘 / 527
鸭跖草 / 312
哺乳疳 / 582
㖞僻不遂 / 537
晕针 / 463
晕灸 / 467
圆针 / 451
圆利针 / 452
圆翳 / 620
圆翳内障 / 620
圆癣 / 604
峻下 / 236
峻下逐水药 / 289
贼风 / 63

［丿］

钱乙 / 662
钱仲阳 / 662
铁裆功 / 502
铍针 / 452
缺乳 / 572
缺盆 / 47，412
特定穴 / 437
积吐 / 587
积证 / 548
积聚 / 548
秩边 / 422
秘方 / 357
秘传眼科龙木论 / 698
透天凉 / 458
透邪 / 229
透关射甲 / 138
透表 / 228
透表清热 / 229
透刺 / 454
透泄 / 229
透疹 / 229
透斑 / 229
倒经 / 560
倒睫 / 613
倒睫拳毛 / 613
候气 / 456
倪仲贤 / 667
倪维德 / 667
健忘 / 146，535
健胃 / 246
健胃止呕 / 246
健脾 / 245
健脾止泻 / 246
健脾止带 / 246
健脾化湿 / 245
健脾化痰 / 245
健脾利水 / 245
健脾利湿 / 245
健脾补肺 / 246
健脾和胃 / 245
健脾养血 / 246
健脾祛湿 / 245
健脾益气 / 246
健脾消食 / 245
臭梧桐叶 / 316
射干 / 313
息肉痔 / 599
息胞 / 570
徒手整复 / 491
徐士茂 / 660
徐大业 / 676
徐大椿 / 676
徐之才 / 660
徐长卿 / 317
徐汝元 / 669
徐灵胎 / 676

徐春甫 / 669
殷门 / 421
拿合谷 / 489
拿法 / 483，651
拿捏法 / 483
拿颈项 / 488
釜底抽薪 / 237
釜沸脉 / 163
豹文刺 / 459
胯骨 / 51
胯腹痈 / 593
脂人 / 75
脂塞不孕 / 566
脂瘤 / 598
胸乡 / 416
胸闷 / 156
胸胁功 / 501
胸痞 / 156
胸痛 / 146，530
胸腹部穴 / 441
胸痹 / 530
脏 / 20
脏气 / 26，54
脏象 / 20，26
脏象学说 / 20
脏厥 / 538
脏腑 / 20
脏腑相合 / 26
脏腑津亏 / 81
脏腑病机 / 96
脏腑虚损耳鸣 / 624
脏腑辨证 / 200
脏寒泻 / 588
脏躁 / 535
脐下悸 / 154
脐下悸动 / 154
脐风 / 575
脐风三证 / 575
脐血 / 578
脐呼吸 / 497
脐疝 / 578
脐带 / 566
脐疮 / 578，593，603
脐突 / 578
脐痈 / 593
脐湿 / 578
脐寒泻 / 588
脐腹 / 48
脐漏 / 593
胶 / 282
胶囊剂 / 282
脑 / 25
脑风 / 146
脑户 / 434
脑立清 / 385
脑空 / 430
脑衄 / 628
脑崩 / 627
脑渗 / 627
脑漏 / 627
胼胝 / 601
脓耳 / 623
脓耳口眼㖞斜 / 624
脓耳变证 / 623
脓耳眩晕 / 625
脓血便 / 150
脓毒证 / 199
脓疱 / 591
狼毒 / 324
留针 / 462
留针拔罐 / 469
留针候气 / 456
留罐 / 469

［丶］

凌霄花 / 332
高风内障 / 620
高风雀目 / 621
高低垫 / 641
高良姜 / 318
高武 / 671
高骨 / 51
高梅孤 / 671
席疮 / 606
症状 / 122
疳 / 580
疳气 / 580
疳气证 / 580
疳证 / 580
疳积 / 580
疳积上目 / 621
疳积证 / 580
疳病 / 580
疳眼 / 621
病机 / 78
病机十九条 / 78
病因 / 62
病因辨证 / 191
病色 / 124
病脉 / 160
病能［态］/ 78
病理体质 / 74
疽 / 594
疾脉 / 162
疾徐补泻 / 457
疾徐补泻法 / 458
疾病；疾；病 / 122
痄腮 / 585
疹 / 139，591
痈 / 593
疱疹 / 591
疰夏 / 582
疰夏病 / 582
疬 / 591
痉病 / 538
脊 / 50
脊中 / 433
离而复合 / 640
离体周天 / 500
唐本草 / 687
唐宗海 / 680
唐审元 / 663
唐容川 / 680
唐慎微 / 663
颃颡 / 40，628
凉血 / 233
凉血止血 / 258

凉血止血药 / 291
凉血止痢 / 235
凉血散瘀 / 235
凉血解毒 / 233
凉肝熄［息］风 / 266
凉燥 / 66，518
凉燥证 / 197
凉燥病 / 519
站式 / 495
站桩功 / 502
畜门 / 625
羞明 / 610
羞明畏日 / 610
拳击法 / 483，649
拳参 / 309
拳揉法 / 647
粉刺 / 601
粉萆薢 / 322
粉瘤 / 598
益气 / 244
益气生津 / 264
益气安神 / 264
益气解表 / 230
益母草 / 334
益母草膏 / 395
益阴 / 248
益肾宁神 / 264
益智仁 / 346
烘焙 / 276
烦热 / 144
烦渴 / 149
烦躁 / 124
烧山火 / 458
烧心 / 153
烧存性 / 278
烧伤 / 605
烧针 / 451
烙法 / 272
烊化 / 283
浙贝母 / 302
酒刺 / 601
酒炙 / 277
酒剂 / 281
酒皶鼻 / 601
酒癖 / 70
酒醴 / 281
娑罗子 / 327
消上 / 589
消肌 / 589
消导 / 252
消导药 / 291
消谷善饥 / 153
消肿 / 252
消肿止痛 / 271
消肿退红 / 252
消胀 / 252
消法 / 251
消泺 / 427
消骨鲠 / 271
消食 / 251
消食下气 / 252
消食化滞 / 251
消食导滞 / 251
消食和中 / 252
消食和胃 / 252
消食剂 / 379
消食药 / 291
消浊 / 589
消积 / 252
消积除胀 / 252
消痈散疖 / 270
消痈散结 / 270
消痞 / 252
消渴（病）/ 551
海马 / 348
海风藤 / 315
海金沙 / 323
海泉 / 440
海桐皮 / 316
海螵蛸 / 350
海藻 / 300
浮小麦 / 348
浮白 / 429
浮刺 / 461
浮郄 / 421
浮脉 / 160
浮络 / 407
浮萍 / 298
涤痰 / 259
流火 / 594
流金凌木 / 615
流泪证 / 614
流泪病症 / 615
流注 / 595
流涎 / 578
流痰 / 596
润 / 276
润下 / 236
润下剂 / 364
润下药 / 289
润化燥痰 / 258
润肠 / 236
润肠通便 / 237，263
润苔 / 135
润肺 / 263
润肺止咳 / 264
润肺化痰 / 258
润肺生津 / 264
润燥 / 263
润燥止痒 / 267
润燥化痰 / 258
润燥通便 / 237
涕 / 58
浸淫疮 / 603
烫火伤 / 71
涩肠止泻 / 263
涩肠止痢 / 263
涩肠固脱剂 / 374
涩剂 / 360
涩脉 / 161
涩精 / 262
涩精止遗 / 262
涩精止遗剂 / 374
涌吐药 / 294
涌吐禁例 / 267
涌泉 / 423

宽中散结 / 254
宽胸 / 254
宽胸散结 / 254
宽解衣带 / 493
窍漏 / 615
诸虫 / 72
诸阳之会 / 42
诸病源侯总论 / 687
调气 / 254，497
调心 / 498
调身 / 493
调身要领 / 493
调和气血 / 239
调和肝胃 / 239
调和肝脾 / 239
调和肝脾剂 / 365
调和营卫 / 229
调和脾胃 / 238
调和寒热剂 / 366
调服 / 283
调经 / 268
调息 / 497
调理气血 / 239

［一］

剥苔 / 135
弱脉 / 161
陶弘景 / 660
陶通明 / 660
陶道 / 434
陶罐 / 467
陷谷 / 414
通下 / 236
通天 / 419
通气 / 252
通因通用 / 221
通关射甲 / 138
通阳 / 240
通里 / 236，416
通利血脉 / 268
通利关节 / 269，654
通乳 / 268
通剂 / 359
通泄 / 237
通经 / 268
通经止痛 / 268
通经活络 / 268
通经接气配穴法 / 449
通草 / 321
通便 / 236
通脉 / 241
通宣理肺丸［片］/ 382
通络止痛 / 268
通淋 / 268
通淋药 / 290
通腑泄热 / 237
通鼻 / 271
通鼻窍 / 271
能远怯近症 / 621
能近怯远症 / 621
难产 / 569
难经 / 684
难经本义 / 684
桑叶 / 297
桑白皮 / 303
桑枝 / 315
桑菊饮 / 362
桑寄生 / 344
桑椹 / 345
桑螵蛸 / 350
验方 / 357

十一画

［一］

球后 / 440
理中 / 238
理中汤 / 369
理气 / 252
理气止痛 / 252，256
理气化湿 / 255
理气化瘀 / 256
理气化痰 / 253
理气安胎 / 256
理气导滞 / 255
理气和血 / 239
理气和胃 / 238
理气剂 / 374
理气药 / 290
理气活血 / 253
理气健脾 / 253
理气消胀 / 255
理气消痞 / 253
理气通经 / 256
理气解郁 / 255
理心功 / 501
理伤续断秘方 / 697
理血 / 256
理血剂 / 376
理血药 / 291
理肺功 / 501
理筋 / 647
理筋手法 / 647
理脾功 / 501
理瀹骈文 / 693
捺正 / 640
捺法 / 483
排石 / 272
排除杂念 / 499
排脓 / 269
排脓托毒 / 269
排脓消肿 / 269
掉眩 / 146
捶法 / 485
捶腰背 / 489
推扳手法 / 486
推法 / 159，482，648
推拿 / 480
推拿广意 / 696
推拿疗法 / 480
推拿的补泻手法 / 490
推罐 / 469
捻衣摸床 / 124
捻转补泻 / 457
捻转补泻法 / 457
捻转法 / 454
捻法 / 481
掐法 / 480

培土 / 245
培土生金 / 247
培土抑木 / 247
接法 / 639
接骨续筋 / 639
接触性皮炎 / 603
掸拂法 / 483
控脑砂 / 627
控睾 / 154
探爪式 / 504
探吐 / 267
黄土汤 / 377
黄水疮 / 604
黄仁 / 610
黄风 / 620
黄风内障 / 620
黄耳伤寒 / 624
黄色 / 125
黄汗 / 531
黄芫花 / 324
黄芩 / 307
黄芪 / 340
黄芪桂枝五物汤 / 370
黄连 / 307
黄连解毒汤 / 368
黄苔 / 134
黄油证 / 618
黄油障 / 618
黄带 / 158，564
黄药子 / 301
黄栌 / 309
黄柏 / 307
黄胖 / 139，547
黄胖病 / 547
黄庭经 / 700
黄帝内经 / 683
黄帝内经灵枢注证发微 / 684
黄帝内经灵枢经 / 683
黄帝内经素问 / 683
黄帝内经素问注证发微 / 684
黄脓上冲 / 618
黄疸 / 523
黄液上冲 / 618
黄腻苔 / 134
黄膜上冲 / 618
黄精 / 341，610
萎黄 / 125，547
萎黄病 / 547
萆薢 / 322
菟丝子 / 347
菊花 / 297
营 / 56
营卫不和 / 86
营气 / 54
营分 / 56
营分证 / 179
营血 / 56
营阴 / 54
萧赓六 / 675
梦遗 / 155，552
梅花 / 327
梅花针 / 450
梅核气 / 535，631
梳法 / 483
救阳 / 240
救荒本草 / 688
救脱 / 240
硇砂 / 355
龚云林 / 672
龚廷贤 / 672
龚庆宣 / 660
盛胎 / 566
雪口 / 579
辄筋 / 430
辅骨 / 51

［ | ］

颅息 / 428
虚中夹实 / 84
虚火 / 91
虚火上炎 / 90
虚火牙痛 / 632
虚火证 / 172
虚火乳蛾 / 629
虚火喉痹 / 629
虚邪 / 63
虚阳上浮 / 80
虚劳（病） / 529
虚里 / 47
虚证 / 170
虚肿 / 548
虚胀 / 589
虚实 / 169
虚实夹杂 / 84
虚实真假 / 84
虚实辨证 / 169
虚脉 / 161
虚损 / 529
虚热 / 90，530
虚热证 / 172
虚秘 / 544
虚烦 / 529
虚喘 / 527
虚痞 / 542
虚寒 / 90
虚寒证 / 172
虚寒泄泻 / 546
虚寒痢 / 522
虚寒腹痛 / 546
雀目 / 622
雀目内障 / 622
雀舌 / 634
雀盲 / 621
雀啄灸 / 464
雀啄脉 / 163
雀斑 / 601
常山 / 298
常色 / 124
常脉 / 160
眦 / 607
眦帷赤烂 / 614
眦漏 / 615
眵 / 610
眵泪 / 611
眵泪胶粘 / 611
眼功 / 501
眼系 / 610

眼带 / 610
眼科（学）/ 607
眼科大全 / 699
眼珠 / 610
眼珠干涩 / 128
眼珠牵斜 / 128
眼珠塌陷 / 128
眼疳 / 581
眼球突出 / 128
眼睑 / 607
眼窝凹陷 / 128
眼缘赤烂 / 613
悬灸 / 464
悬饮 / 528
悬枢 / 433
悬厘 / 429
悬钟 / 431
悬起灸 / 464
悬痈 / 630
悬颅 / 429
悬雍垂 / 40，628
悬雍肿 / 630
悬旗小舌 / 630
悬旗风 / 630
野菊花 / 311
啄击法 / 484
啄法 / 650
跰子 / 601
趺阳脉 / 160
蛊毒 / 69
蛇丹 / 600
蛇头疔 / 592
蛇串疮 / 600
蛇肚疔 / 592
蛇床子 / 355
蛇胆川贝散 / 382
蛇胆陈皮散 / 382
蛇眼疔 / 592
蛇蜕 / 315
唾 / 58
崩中 / 561
崩证 / 561
崩漏 / 561
婴儿湿疮 / 604
婴儿瘛疭 / 575
［丿］
铜人俞穴针灸图经 / 699
银花 / 310
银针 / 452
银柴胡 / 306
银海精微 / 698
银黄口服液 / 383
银翘散 / 362
银翘解毒丸［片］/ 381
秽气气感 / 505
秽浊 / 72
偶方 / 356
偶刺 / 461
偷针 / 613
停经 / 559
停食 / 543
停息 / 498
偏历 / 410
偏方 / 357
偏头风 / 146，533
偏头痛 / 146，533
偏阳质 / 73
偏阴质 / 73
偏坠 / 600
偏枯 / 537
偏斜瞻视 / 622
假神 / 123
假热 / 91
假寒 / 91
得气 / 456
得神 / 123
盘坐 / 495
盘肠气痛 / 588
盘法 / 458
盘旋法 / 458
斜飞脉 / 163
斜扳腰椎法 / 653
斜刺 / 454
敛气 / 262
敛汗 / 261
敛汗固表 / 261
敛汗固表药 / 294
敛汗固脱 / 261
敛阴 / 262
敛肺 / 262
敛肺止咳 / 262
敛肺止咳剂 / 374
敛肺平喘 / 262
敛肺涩肠药 / 294
欲合先离 / 640
脚气 / 539
脚气冲心 / 539
脚气疮 / 604
脚肿 / 138
脚弱 / 539
脚湿气 / 604
脬气不固 / 113
脱臼 / 637
脱汗 / 145，531
脱阳 / 80
脱阴 / 80
脱位 / 637
脱肛 / 599
脱骨疽 / 595
脱疽 / 595
脱骱 / 637
脱髎 / 637
脘 / 23
脘痛 / 147，152
猪苓 / 320
猫眼疮 / 601
猛疽 / 629
［丶］
减肥功 / 503
毫毛 / 41
毫针 / 449
麻子仁丸 / 365
麻木 / 148，537
麻仁丸 / 386
麻仁润肠丸 / 386
麻风 / 605

麻杏石甘汤 / 362
麻毒 / 69
麻毒入营 / 584
麻毒内攻 / 584
麻毒闭肺 / 584
麻毒攻目 / 584
麻毒陷肺 / 584
麻疹 / 584
麻疹闭证 / 584
麻疹顺证 / 584
麻疹逆证 / 584
麻疹险证 / 584
麻黄 / 295
麻黄汤 / 361
麻黄根 / 348
痔 / 598
鹿角 / 345
鹿角胶 / 346
鹿角霜 / 346
鹿茸 / 345
鹿衔草 / 345
盗汗 / 144，531
章门 / 433
章楠 / 678
商丘 / 415
商曲 / 425
商阳 / 409
商陆 / 324
旋耳 / 488
旋耳疮 / 603，623
旋转屈伸 / 638
旋复代赭汤 / 376
旋覆花 / 299
望目 / 128
望皮肤 / 138
望耳 / 129
望舌 / 130
望色 / 124
望形体 / 126
望诊 / 123
望齿 / 137
望指纹 / 138
望姿态 / 127
望神 / 123
望痰 / 137
望鼻 / 129
率谷 / 429
着肤灸 / 465
着痹 / 540
羚羊角 / 338
断针 / 463
断乳 / 268
断经前后诸证 / 563
断骨接整 / 638
断绪 / 565
断裂伤 / 646
断端移位 / 635
清开灵注射液 / 384
清气 / 55
清气分热剂 / 367
清化热痰 / 258
清化热痰药 / 292
清心 / 233
清心开窍 / 234
清心火 / 234
清心安神 / 234
清心泻火 / 234
清阳 / 55
清肝 / 233
清肝火 / 233
清肝明目 / 233
清肝泻火 / 233
清肠止泻 / 235
清肠止痢 / 235
清肠润燥 / 235
清冷渊 / 427
清肺 / 234
清肺止咳 / 234
清肺止喘 / 234
清肺化痰 / 234
清肺火 / 234
清肺利咽 / 234
清肺热 / 234
清肺润燥 / 234，263
清炒 / 277
清法 / 230
清泄相火 / 235
清相火 / 235
清胃 / 235
清胃火 / 235
清胃泄火 / 235
清胃泄热 / 235
清胃热 / 235
清胃散 / 368
清骨散 / 369
清浊 / 58
清宫 / 233
清热开窍 / 233，266
清热止血 / 258
清热止呕 / 232
清热止泻 / 232
清热止痢 / 232
清热化湿 / 259
清热化痰 / 258
清热化痰开窍 / 267
清热生津 / 231
清热导滞 / 232
清热利湿 / 231，260
清热明目 / 232
清热和中 / 232
清热和胃 / 232
清热剂 / 367
清热法 / 230
清热泻火 / 231
清热泻火药 / 288
清热泻肺 / 234
清热药 / 288
清热祛暑剂 / 369
清热祛湿 / 231
清热祛湿剂 / 379
清热除湿 / 231
清热凉血 / 233
清热凉血药 / 288
清热消食 / 232
清热排脓 / 269
清热解毒 / 231

清热解毒剂 / 368
清热解毒药 / 288
清热解暑 / 232
清热熄［息］风 / 266
清热燥湿 / 231
清热燥湿药 / 288，307
清脏腑热 / 233
清脏腑热剂 / 368
清营 / 232
清营汤 / 367
清营泄热 / 233
清营透疹 / 233
清营凉血剂 / 367
清虚热剂 / 369
清虚热药 / 288
清暑化湿 / 232
清暑利湿 / 232
清暑热 / 232
清燥润肺 / 263
清燥救肺汤 / 378
淋（证）/ 551
淋浊 / 551
淋病 / 551
渐聋 / 625
混睛外障 / 619
混睛障 / 618
混障症 / 619
渊液 / 430
淫气 / 63
淫羊藿 / 346
淳于意 / 658
液 / 58
液门 / 426
液脱 / 550
液脱证 / 187
淬 / 278
淡白舌 / 131
淡竹叶 / 305
淡红舌 / 131
淡豆豉 / 298
淡渗利湿 / 260
淡渗祛湿 / 260
深刺 / 454
梁门 / 413
梁丘 / 414
渗湿 / 260
惊 / 70
惊风 / 574
惊风八候 / 574
惊风抽搐 / 575
惊风病 / 574
惊风烦渴 / 576
惊风腹痛 / 576
惊吐 / 587
惊热 / 583
惊疳 / 581
惊悸 / 530
惊厥 / 575
惊痫 / 535，589
惊震内障 / 620
寇平 / 668
寇宗奭 / 663
宿食 / 544
宿疾 / 524
宿翳 / 612
密蒙花 / 305
皲裂 / 601
皲裂疮 / 601

［一］

弹入法 / 453
弹击法 / 484
弹石脉 / 163
弹法 / 651
弹柄法 / 455
弹响指 / 647
弹筋 / 485
弹筋法 / 651
堕胎 / 569
随咳进针法 / 454
随息 / 498
隐白 / 415
隐疾 / 524
隐痛 / 148
隐［瘾］疹 / 603
胬肉扳睛 / 615
胬肉侵睛 / 615
胬肉攀睛 / 615
颈 / 46
颈白劳 / 440
颈松 / 493
颈项功 / 501
颈骨 / 50
颈痈 / 593
颈椎角度复位法 / 652
颈椎侧旋复位法 / 652
颈椎单人旋转复位法 / 652
续名医类案 / 702
续断 / 347
续筋接骨 / 640
骑马式 / 495
维道 / 430
绵草薢 / 322
绿风 / 620
绿风内障 / 619
绿萼梅 / 327
巢元方 / 660

十二画

［一］

琥珀 / 336
斑 / 139，591
斑秃 / 602
斑疹 / 139
斑蝥 / 355
斑蝥灸 / 467
款冬花 / 301
搭手 / 594
搭鹊桥 / 494
越经传 / 116
越鞠丸 / 387
提伸法 / 485
提肛呼吸 / 497
提法 / 639
提按端挤 / 638
提捏进针法 / 453
提脓去腐 / 269

提脓拔毒 / 269
提插补泻 / 456
提插补泻法 / 456
提插法 / 455
喜 / 69
喜按 / 166
喜脉 / 163
揿针 / 450
插入法 / 453
揪法 / 483
揪痧 / 486
煮 / 278
煮罐法 / 468
搓内肾 / 506
搓法 / 484，647
搓柄法 / 455
搓腰 / 506
搅舌 / 488
搅肠痧 / 523
揉四白 / 487
揉法 / 480，647
揉肩 / 506
揉颊车 / 488
揉腰眼 / 489
揉膝 / 506
揉攒竹 / 487
期门 / 433
葫芦 / 323
葫芦巴 / 347
葫芦垫 / 641
散 / 281
散刺 / 449
散剂 / 280
散脉 / 162
散寒 / 226
散寒化饮 / 259
募穴 / 438
募合配穴法 / 448
募原 / 42
葛可久 / 667
葛洪 / 659
葛根 / 297
葛根黄芩黄连汤 / 367
葛乾孙 / 667
葛稚川 / 660
葎草 / 313
葡萄胎 / 567
葶苈子 / 303
蒂丁 / 40，628
蒂中 / 40，628
萹蓄 / 322
韩氏医通 / 701
韩懋 / 668
朝食暮吐 / 152
棒击法 / 485，650
植物名实图考 / 689
植物名实图考长编 / 690
椒疮 / 613
棉枕固定 / 640
棕榈炭 / 329
楗 / 51
粟芽 / 351
粟疮 / 613
硬气功 / 492
硬肿症 / 576
硫黄 / 354
厥 / 537
厥心痛 / 530
厥阴俞 / 419
厥阴病 / 178
厥阴病机 / 116
厥阴病证 / 177
厥证 / 537
厥热胜复 / 116
裂纹舌 / 133
雄黄 / 354
颊 / 45
颊车 / 46，411
颊脂垫 / 579

[丨]

悲 / 69
龂齿 / 579，632
紫贝齿 / 337
紫白癜风 / 605
紫外线穴位照射疗法 / 479
紫舌 / 131
紫花地丁 / 311
紫苏子 / 303
紫苏叶 / 296
紫苏梗 / 326
紫河车 / 342
紫草 / 306
紫宫 / 436
紫菀 / 299
紫硇砂 / 355
紫雪 / 392
紫斑 / 550
掌心毒 / 592
掌击法 / 649
掌按法 / 651
掌推扳胸椎法 / 652
掌推法 / 648
掌揉法 / 647
掌摩法 / 650
掌擦法 / 650
暑 / 65
暑入阳明 / 517
暑入阳明证 / 518
暑气 / 65
暑风 / 517
暑风证 / 517
暑邪 / 65
暑伤肺络证 / 204
暑伤津气证 / 195
暑闭气机证 / 196
暑疖 / 592
暑证 / 195
暑疟 / 521
暑热 / 65
暑热内郁证 / 195
暑热动风证 / 195
暑热闭神证 / 196
暑热证 / 195
暑病 / 517
暑痉 / 517
暑秽 / 516

暑秽病 / 516
暑厥 / 517
暑厥证 / 517
暑痫 / 517
暑湿 / 65
暑湿证 / 195
暑湿流注 / 516
暑湿袭表证 / 195
暑温 / 517
暑温病 / 517
暑瘵 / 517
睑内 / 45，609
睑内结石 / 614
睑皮垂缓 / 614
睑废 / 614
睑弦 / 44，608
睑弦赤烂 / 613
睑弦糜烂 / 614
睑粘睛珠 / 613
鼎式夹板固定 / 640
晶瘖 / 139
晶珠 / 610
景岳全书 / 704
跖 / 50
跖疣 / 600
跌打损伤 / 71
跗 / 51
跗阳 / 423
跗肿/139
跗骨 / 52
遗尿 / 151，590
遗尿（病）/ 553
遗精 / 552
蛔疳 / 582
蛔厥 / 538
蛛丝飘浮 / 612
蛤蚧 / 348
喘 / 140，527
喘证 / 527
喘鸣 / 141
喘促 / 141
喘急 / 141
喘逆 / 141
喘病 / 527
喉风 / 630
喉关 / 40，628
喉关痈 / 629
喉岩 / 631
喉底 / 628
喉核 / 40，628
喉疳 / 631
喉痈 / 629
喉菌 / 631
喉喑［瘖］/ 630
喉痧 / 520，585
喉蛾 / 628
喉嗌 / 628
喉痹 / 629，630
喉瘤 / 631
喉癣 / 629
喻昌 / 673
喻嘉言 / 673
喑［瘖］/ 140
黑丑 / 324
黑白丑 / 324
黑芝麻 / 345
黑色 / 126
黑疔 / 623
黑苔 / 135
黑睛 / 609
骭骨 / 51

［丿］

锁阳 / 346
锁肚 / 575
锁喉风 / 630
锁喉毒 / 593
锁喉痈 / 593
锋针 / 452
锐发 / 43
锐眦 / 608
掣痛 / 148
短气 / 141，526
短刺 / 461
短脉 / 162
短缩舌 / 133
智齿 / 632
犊鼻 / 414
程国彭 / 677
程钟龄 / 677
筑宾 / 424
筋 / 42
筋之府 / 50
筋正 / 647
筋伤 / 643
筋合 / 647
筋柔 / 643
筋结 / 643
筋疳 / 581
筋惕肉瞤 / 127
筋粗 / 643
筋断 / 643
筋痹 / 541
筋痿 / 539，643
筋缩 / 433，643
筋瘤 / 598
筋瘿 / 597
鹅口疮 / 579，634
鹅不食草 / 296
鹅爪风 / 605
鹅掌风 / 604
傅山 / 674
傅仁宇 / 673
傅允科 / 673
傅青主 / 674
傅青主女科 / 695
焦三仙 / 352
焦山楂 / 351
焦麦芽 / 351
傍针刺 / 462
循衣摸床 / 124
循法 / 159，455
循经传 / 116
循经选穴法 / 446
循经感传 / 458
循按法 / 455
舒肝丸 / 386

舒张进针法 / 453
舒筋止痛 / 257
舒筋和络 / 257
舒筋活络 / 257
舒筋通络 / 257
舒腰松腹 / 494
颌 / 46
颌下痈 / 629
番红花 / 330
番泻叶 / 352
腓腨 / 50
腘 / 50
脾 / 21
脾之大络 / 407
脾不统血 / 105
脾水 / 549
脾气 / 21，54
脾气下陷 / 94
脾气下陷证 / 206
脾气不升 / 106
脾气不足 / 105
脾气虚 / 104
脾气虚证 / 205
脾失健运 / 105
脾阳 / 22
脾阳不振 / 105
脾阳虚 / 105
脾阳虚证 / 205
脾阴 / 22
脾阴虚 / 105
脾阴虚证 / 205
脾约 / 544
脾约丸 / 365
脾劳 / 529
脾肾阳虚 / 107
脾肾阳虚证 / 207
脾肾虚寒 / 107
脾肾虚寒证 / 207
脾肺气虚 / 106
脾肺气虚证 / 207
脾肺两虚 / 106
脾肺两虚证 / 207
脾经咳嗽 / 524
脾胃论 / 694
脾胃阳虚 / 106
脾胃阳虚证 / 205
脾胃虚寒 / 106
脾胃虚寒证 / 205
脾胃湿热 / 106
脾胃湿热证 / 206
脾咳 / 525
脾俞 / 420
脾疳 / 580
脾病辨证 / 205
脾消 / 551
脾虚 / 104
脾虚气陷 / 94
脾虚气陷证 / 206
脾虚生风 / 106
脾虚生痰 / 106
脾虚动风证 / 206
脾虚证 / 205
脾虚泄泻 / 545
脾虚泻 / 588
脾虚经闭 / 559
脾虚带下 / 564
脾虚湿困 / 105
脾虚湿困证 / 206
脾虚寒证 / 205
脾虚痰湿证 / 206
脾痹 / 541
脾痿 / 539
腋汗 / 145
腋臭 / 605
腋痈 / 593
腑 / 20
腑气 / 54
腑证 / 178
腕骨 / 417
飧水泻 / 588
飧泄［泻］/ 545
然谷 / 424

［丶］

痨病 / 529
痘 / 584
痘疮 / 585
痞 / 542
痞块 / 547
痞根 / 441
痞满 / 156
痢疾 / 521
痫证 / 534，589
痫病 / 534
痧 / 583
痧子 / 584
痛无定处 / 148
痛泻要方 / 366
痛经 / 560
痛经丸 / 394
痛痹 / 540
阑门 / 41
阑尾 / 443
善太息 / 141
善色 / 124
善忘 / 535
普济方 / 692
普济本事方 / 691
普济消毒饮 / 368
道地药材 / 275
道家气功 / 492
曾世荣 / 666
焠刺 / 460
滞针 / 463
滞颐 / 579
湿 / 65
湿气 / 65
湿火 / 68
湿邪 / 65
湿邪困脾 / 89
湿困脾阳 / 105
湿困脾阳证 / 206
湿证 / 196
湿阻 / 518
湿阻中焦 / 106
湿阻中焦证 / 206
湿郁化火 / 89

湿郁化热 / 89
湿郁肌表 / 89
湿疟 / 521
湿剂 / 360
湿毒 / 69
湿毒带下 / 564
湿毒流注 / 89
湿胜着痹证 / 196
湿疮 / 603
湿浊 / 65
湿热 / 68
湿热下注 / 89
湿热下注证 / 197
湿热内蕴 / 89
湿热犯耳证 / 197
湿热阻滞精室证 / 214
湿热阻痹证 / 197
湿热泄泻 / 545
湿热带下 / 564
湿热痢 / 521
湿热痛经 / 560
湿热蒸口证 / 196
湿热蒸舌证 / 197
湿热蒸齿证 / 197
湿热蒸唇证 / 196
湿热腰痛 / 553
湿热蕴脾 / 105
湿热蕴脾证 / 197
湿病 / 518
湿疹 / 603
湿温 / 518
湿温病 / 518
湿痹 / 540
湿痰 / 72
湿痰不孕 / 565
湿痰证 / 189
湿蔽清阳 / 89
湿癣 / 604
温［瘟］疫 / 515
温下 / 236
温下剂 / 364
温下药 / 289
温下寒积 / 236
温中 / 241
温中止吐 / 242
温中止呕 / 241
温中止泻 / 242
温中止痛 / 242
温中行气 / 241
温中和胃 / 241
温中祛寒 / 241
温中祛寒剂 / 369
温中散寒 / 241
温化寒痰 / 258
温化寒痰药 / 292
温心阳 / 240
温邪 / 67，514
温邪上受 / 85
温邪犯肺 / 85
温阳 / 240
温阳行水 / 261
温阳利水 / 261
温阳利湿 / 261
温里 / 240
温里剂 / 369
温里药 / 290
温里祛寒 / 244
温里散寒 / 244
温针灸 / 466
温肝 / 240
温灸器 / 464
温灸器灸 / 466
温补肾阳 / 242
温补命门 / 251
温补胃阳 / 241
温补脾肾 / 243
温补脾胃 / 246
温肾 / 242
温肾止泻 / 242
温肾化饮 / 243
温肾化痰 / 242
温肾壮阳 / 242
温肾阳 / 242
温肾利水 / 261
温肾纳气 / 242
温肾缩尿 / 242
温和灸 / 464
温肺 / 242
温肺化饮 / 242
温肺化痰 / 242
温肺散寒 / 242
温服 / 284
温疟 / 520
温法 / 240
温经 / 243
温经止血药 / 291
温经止痛 / 244
温经回阳 / 243
温经行滞 / 243
温经扶阳 / 243
温经养血 / 244
温经活血 / 243
温经祛寒 / 243
温经通阳 / 243
温经通络 / 243
温经散寒 / 243
温经散寒剂 / 370
温经暖宫 / 243
温毒 / 514
温胃 / 241
温胃止呕 / 241
温胃降逆 / 241
温疫论 / 693
温莪术 / 332
温热 / 67
温热论 / 693
温热经纬 / 693
温病 / 515
温病条辨 / 693
温脾 / 241
温脾汤 / 364
温溜 / 410
温燥 / 66，519
温燥证 / 197
温燥病 / 519
溃坚 / 270

溃疡 / 591
滑石 / 321
滑肉门 / 413
滑寿 / 667
滑伯仁 / 667
滑苔 / 135
滑剂 / 360
滑泄 / 545
滑脉 / 161
滑胎 / 569
滑精 / 155
滑精（病）/ 552
溲血 / 151
游走痛 / 148
滋水涵木 / 248
滋阴 / 248
滋阴抑阳 / 250
滋阴利水 / 250
滋阴补血 / 250
滋阴降火 / 250
滋阴药 / 294
滋阴凉血 / 250
滋阴润肺 / 249
滋阴润燥 / 250
滋阴润燥剂 / 378
滋阴清热 / 250
滋阴解表 / 230
滋阴熄［息］风 / 266
滋阴潜阳 / 265
滋补肾阴 / 249
滋补肺肾 / 249
滋肾 / 250
滋肾阴 / 250
滋养肝肾 / 248
滋养胃阴 / 249
割治疗法 / 478
寒 / 64
寒入血室 / 91
寒下 / 236
寒下剂 / 364
寒气腹痛 / 546
寒气霍乱 / 523
寒从中生 / 91
寒邪 / 64
寒邪犯胃证 / 208
寒邪外束 / 91
寒吐 / 586
寒因寒用 / 221
寒呕 / 542
寒饮内停证 / 188
寒饮停肺证 / 188
寒饮停胃证 / 188
寒冷腹痛 / 546
寒证 / 169
寒夜啼 / 577
寒剂 / 360
寒疟 / 521
寒泻 / 546
寒毒 / 69
寒战 / 143
寒胜痛痹证 / 195
寒结 / 544
寒结胸 / 520
寒热 / 169
寒热失调 / 90
寒热转化 / 83
寒热往来 / 143
寒热真假 / 91
寒热错杂 / 91
寒热辨证 / 169
寒哮 / 527
寒厥 / 538
寒痫 / 590
寒痧 / 583
寒滞心脉证 / 194
寒滞肝脉 / 104
寒滞肝脉证 / 211
寒滞经脉证 / 195
寒滞胃肠证 / 194
寒湿 / 68
寒湿内阻证 / 196
寒湿困脾 / 105
寒湿困脾证 / 206
寒湿证 / 196
寒湿痢 / 521
寒湿腰痛 / 553
寒痹 / 540
寒痰 / 527
寒痰证 / 189
寒痰阻肺证 / 203
寒霍乱 / 523
寒瘴 / 521
寒凝气滞 / 94
寒凝血瘀证 / 194
寒凝胞宫证 / 194，213
寒凝痛经 / 560
寓攻于补 / 220
寓补于攻 / 220
窜痛 / 148
颏 / 626
禅定 / 500
谢观 / 682
［一］
犀角 / 305
犀角地黄汤 / 367
强壮功 / 500
强间 / 434
强硬舌 / 133
强筋健骨 / 251
疏风 / 226
疏风止痒 / 227
疏风和营 / 227
疏风泄热 / 226
疏风宣肺 / 227
疏风透疹 / 226
疏风消肿 / 227
疏风清肺 / 226
疏风清热 / 226
疏风散寒 / 226
疏风解肌 / 226
疏风解表 / 226
疏肝 / 255
疏肝明目功 / 502
疏肝和胃 / 255
疏肝和脾 / 255
疏肝养血 / 255

疏肝健脾 / 255
疏肝理气 / 255
疏肝理脾 / 255
疏肝解郁 / 255
疏表润燥 / 227
疏散风热 / 225
疏散外风剂 / 377
隔物灸 / 465
隔姜灸 / 465
隔盐灸 / 466
隔蒜灸 / 466
皴揭 / 601
缓下 / 236
缓方 / 357
缓脉 / 161

十三画

［一］

魂 / 57
魂门 / 422
摄唾 / 271
摄领疮 / 602
摸法 / 482
摇法 / 485，652
摇柄法 / 455
摇摆触碰 / 638
搐鼻 / 273
蒜泥灸 / 466
鹊桥 / 494
蓐风 / 572
蓐劳 / 572
蒿芩清胆汤 / 365
蒺藜 / 339
蓄血 / 550
蒲公英 / 311
蒲黄 / 332
蒲黄炭 / 333
颐 / 46
蒸 / 278
椿皮 / 308
椿根白皮 / 309
禁方 / 357
禁针穴 / 463
禁灸穴 / 467
槐米 / 329
槐花 / 329
槐角 / 329
楼公爽 / 667
楼英 / 667
甄权 / 660
感冒 / 515
感冒退热冲剂 / 381
感冒清热冲剂 / 381
感暑 / 517
感暑眩晕 / 532
硼砂 / 355
雷丸 / 353
雷丰 / 681
雷少逸 / 681
雷公 / 658
雷公药性赋 / 689
雷公炮炙论 / 689
雷火神针 / 466
雷头风 / 533
雷敩 / 660
输穴 / 437
输刺 / 460

［丨］

督俞 / 420
督脉 / 405
督脉穴 / 433
频服 / 284
龆龀 / 574
虞天民 / 668
虞抟 / 668
鉴真 / 661
睛明 / 418
睛胀 / 622
睛帘 / 609
睛高突起 / 622
睫毛倒入 / 613
睡眠十忌 / 507
睥生痰核 / 613
睥肉粘轮 / 613
睥轮振跳 / 614
睥虚如球 / 614
睥翻粘睑 / 613
嗜卧 / 155
嗜偏食 / 544
嗜睡 / 155，535
暖肝煎 / 375
暖宫 / 243
暗经 / 556
照海 / 424
跷法 / 486
路路通 / 323
蜈蚣 / 338
蜂针疗法 / 451
蜂房 / 356
蜂蜜 / 352
嗅气味 / 142
嗳气 / 153
嗳腐 / 153
嗌 / 40
罨 / 272

［丿］

错经；差经 / 562
错语 / 140
锦灯笼 / 313
锭 / 281
锭剂 / 281
矮步 / 496
稚子 / 574
稚阴稚阳 / 574
鼠乳 / 600
催气法 / 454
催生 / 268
催吐药 / 294
催乳 / 268
微丸 / 280
微炒 / 277
微波针灸 / 470
微波针灸疗法 / 470
微脉 / 161
微热 / 144
颔 / 46

颔厌 / 428
腻苔 / 135
腠［凑］理 / 41
腰 / 49
腰阳关 / 433
腰奇 / 442
腰软 / 554
腰宜 / 441
腰骨 / 50
腰俞 / 433
腰部功 / 501
腰眼 / 441
腰椎旋转复位法 / 653
腰痛 / 147，553
腰痛点 / 442
腰酸；腰痠 / 147
腥臭气 / 142
腮肿 / 585
腭裂 / 590
腨 / 50
腹 / 48
腹中硬块 / 154
腹中雷鸣 / 154
腹鸣 / 153
腹胀 / 154
腹背配穴法 / 447
腹哀 / 416
腹结 / 415
腹部功 / 501
腹通谷 / 425
腹痛 / 147，546
腹痛下坠 / 153
腹满 / 154
腹满䐜胀 / 154
腧穴 / 408
腾跃爆发导气 / 504
腿功 / 653
解肌 / 225
解肌发表 / 226
解肌透疹 / 226
解肌清热 / 226
解围元薮 / 697
解表 / 225
解表剂 / 361
解表药 / 287
解表透疹 / 226
解表清肺 / 225
解表清热 / 225
解毒 / 270
解毒透疹 / 226
解毒消肿 / 270
解索脉 / 163
解酒毒 / 270
解颅 / 577
解颅病 / 577
解溪 / 414
［丶］
痱（子）/ 601
痹（病）/ 540
痹痛 / 147
痴呆 / 536
痿 / 539
痿证 / 539
痿软舌 / 133
痿病 / 539
痿躄 / 539
瘀血 / 71
瘀血犯头证 / 185
瘀血头痛 / 534
瘀血阻滞证 / 185
瘀血痫 / 590
瘀阻胞宫证 / 214
瘀阻脑络证 / 201
瘀热 / 88
瘀痰证 / 190
痰 / 71
痰中带血 / 138
痰气互［郁］结证 / 190
痰火耳鸣 / 624
痰火扰心 / 101
痰火扰心证 / 201
痰火扰神证 / 201
痰包 / 634
痰多 / 137
痰如泡沫 / 137
痰饮 / 528
痰证 / 189
痰阻精室证 / 214
痰鸣 / 141
痰咳 / 526
痰迷心窍 / 100
痰浊 / 72
痰浊犯头证 / 190
痰浊头痛 / 533
痰浊证 / 189
痰浊阻肺 / 110
痰浊阻肺证 / 203
痰核留结证 / 190
痰热内闭证 / 190
痰热内扰证 / 190
痰热动风证 / 190
痰热闭肺 / 110
痰热闭肺证 / 204
痰热壅［蕴］肺证 / 204
痰秘 / 544
痰黄 / 137
痰盛 / 137
痰厥 / 538
痰喘 / 527
痰稀白 / 137
痰痞 / 542
痰痫 / 590
痰湿 / 72
痰湿不孕 / 565
痰湿犯耳证 / 190
痰湿阻肺 / 110
痰湿阻肺证 / 203
痰湿阻滞精室证 / 214
痰湿质 / 75
痰湿咳嗽 / 526
痰蒙心包 / 100
痰蒙心神 / 100
痰蒙心神证 / 201
痰瘀互结证 / 189
廉泉 / 437
新修本草 / 687

新病 / 515
新感 / 515
新翳 / 612
意 / 57
意守 / 499
意守丹田 / 499
意守自身 / 499
意守体外 / 499
意呼吸 / 498
意舍 / 422
阙上 / 43
阙中；阙 / 43
数吸 / 498
数脉 / 160
煎药法 / 283
煎膏 / 281
煨 / 276
煨脓长肉 / 270
煅 / 276
煅瓦楞 / 350
煅龙骨 / 350
煅牡蛎 / 350
煅淬 / 276
满山红 / 302
溻浴 / 273
滚刺［针］筒 / 452
滚刺疗法 / 452
滚法 / 481，649
滚法推拿 / 490
溏便 / 149
溏结不调 / 149
溢饮 / 528
溢乳 / 577，587
溶化 / 282
塞因塞用 / 221
塞兑反听 / 494
塞法 / 273

［乛］

辟谷功 / 503
障 / 612
嫉妒不孕 / 565
缠喉风 / 630
缠腰火丹 / 600
缠腰蛇丹 / 600

十四画

［一］

静中有动 / 492
静功 / 491
静坐 / 505
静留针法 / 462
熬 / 278
截疟 / 271
聚证 / 548
聚星障 / 618
聚泉 / 440
暮食朝吐 / 152
蔓荆子 / 297
蔻仁 / 319
蓼大青叶 / 311
榧子 / 353
槟榔 / 353
酸甘化阴 / 248
酸枣仁 / 336
酸枣仁汤 / 381
酸浆 / 313
酸［痠］痛 / 148
磁石 / 336
磁穴疗法 / 478
磁朱丸 / 380
磁珠疗法 / 478
豨莶丸 / 393
豨莶草 / 314

［丨］

䪼 / 39
䪼交 / 435
颗粒剂 / 282
颗粒型皮内针 / 450
嘈杂 / 153，543
蜡丸 / 280
蝇翅黑花 / 620
蝇影飞越 / 620
蝉衣 / 298
蝉蜕 / 298
罂粟壳 / 302，350

［丿］

锓针 / 451
熏洗疗法 / 274
熏蒸 / 272
箕门 / 415
管针进针法 / 454
鼻 / 38
鼻不闻香臭 / 130
鼻毛 / 39
鼻孔 / 38
鼻出血 / 130
鼻尖 / 38，626
鼻吸鼻呼 / 497
鼻色主病 / 130
鼻针 / 477
鼻针疗法 / 477
鼻疔 / 626
鼻沥血 / 628
鼻茎 / 39
鼻齿功 / 501
鼻柱 / 39，626
鼻柱骨 / 39
鼻科（学）/ 625
鼻疮 / 626
鼻前孔 / 626
鼻前庭 / 626
鼻洪 / 628
鼻洞 / 38
鼻根 / 39
鼻臭证 / 627
鼻息肉 / 627
鼻息肉病 / 627
鼻衄 / 130，550，627
鼻疳 / 626
鼻疳疮 / 626
鼻病 / 626
鼻准 / 38，626
鼻流浊涕 / 130
鼻流清涕 / 130
鼻涕 / 626
鼻窍 / 38
鼻窍不利 / 626

鼻菌 / 627
鼻痔 / 627
鼻渊 / 627
鼻梁 / 39，626
鼻梁骨折 / 628
鼻窒 / 627
鼻塞 / 626
鼻赘 / 627
鼻槁［藁］/ 627
鼻隧 / 39
鼻鼽 / 627
鼻燥 / 626
鼻翼 / 38，626
鼻翼煽动 / 130
魄 / 57
魄门 / 41
魄户 / 421
睾 / 49
睾丸肿痛 / 600
睾丸萎缩 / 600
膜原 / 42
膈 / 42
膈关 / 422
膈俞 / 420
膈噎 / 543
膀胱 / 24
膀胱不利 / 113
膀胱气闭 / 113
膀胱失约 / 113
膀胱咳 / 525
膀胱俞 / 420
膀胱虚寒 / 114
膀胱虚寒证 / 213
膀胱湿热 / 114
膀胱湿热证 / 214

［丶］

膏 / 281
膏人 / 75
膏肓 / 42，422
膏剂 / 281
膏药 / 281
膏药风 / 603
膏淋 / 552
膏粱厚味 / 70
膏滋 / 281
膏摩 / 273，490
膏摩疗法 / 274
腐苔 / 135
瘦薄舌 / 132
瘊子 / 600
端法 / 639
端提捺正 / 639
精 / 2，56
精、气、神 / 498
精少 / 553
精气 / 2，54
精气互化 / 2
精气学说 / 2
精汁 / 57
精血 / 56
精冷 / 553
精明之府 / 42
精浊 / 599
精室 / 49
精神 / 57
精珠 / 610
精窍 / 49
精寒 / 553
精微 / 57
精癃 / 600
精髓空虚 / 111
熄［息］风 / 265
熄［息］风止痉药 / 293
熄［息］风化痰 / 259
熄风剂 / 378
熄［息］风定痉 / 266
熄［息］风定痫 / 266
熄［息］风解痉 / 266
漆疮 / 603
漱津 / 506
漱涤 / 273
漂 / 276
滴丸 / 280
滴酒法 / 468
漏 / 591
漏下 / 561
漏汗 / 145
漏芦 / 312
漏谷 / 415
漏睛 / 615
漏睛疮 / 615
漏睛脓出 / 615
漏睛眼 / 615
慢火 / 283
慢性复位 / 642
慢惊风 / 574
慢惊夹痰 / 575
慢惊自汗 / 575
慢喉喑［瘖］/ 630
慢脾风 / 575
察目 / 128
蜜丸 / 280
蜜炙 / 277

［一］

熊宗立 / 668
熊胆 / 339
熊道轩 / 668
缩泉丸 / 374
缪仲淳 / 672
缪希雍 / 672
缪刺 / 461

十五画

［一］

璇玑 / 436
撕裂伤 / 646
撮口 / 136，575
撮法 / 484
撮痧疗法 / 469
赭石 / 339
撞击伤目 / 621
撙令平正 / 648
撙捺皮相 / 648
撙捺相近 / 648
增液通下 / 237
聤耳 / 625

聪耳 / 271
蕲蛇 / 315
横目斜视 / 129
横刺 / 454
横指同身寸 / 445
横垫 / 641
横骨 / 48，424
横透 / 454
敷 / 272
醋炙 / 277
碾挫伤 / 646
震桩式 / 503
震颤法 / 455
［丨］
暴马子皮 / 303
暴风客热 / 616
暴发火眼 / 616
暴赤生翳 / 616
暴盲 / 620
暴泻（病）/ 545
暴病 / 515
暴聋 / 624
暴崩 / 561
暴喘 / 586
暴喑［瘖］/ 630
暴痫 / 589
瞑眩 / 146
噎嗝 / 543
嘶嗄 / 140
踏跳法 / 486
踩法 / 485
踩跷法 / 486，652
踡［蜷］卧缩足 / 127
踠跌 / 635
蝼蛄 / 323
蝼蛄疖 / 592
噙化 / 284
墨旱莲 / 330
［丿］
镇心安神 / 264
镇肝熄［息］风 / 266
镇肝潜阳 / 265
镇惊 / 264
镇惊安神 / 264
镇静安神 / 265
镇潜 / 265
靠坐 / 495
稻芽 / 351
箭头针 / 451
僵蚕 / 338
膝 / 49
膝关 / 432
膝阳关 / 431
膝顶 / 639
膝顶扳胸椎法 / 653
膝眼 / 443
膝腘 / 50
膝髌 / 50
［丶］
熟地黄 / 342
摩击上肢 / 489
摩法 / 482，650
摩面 / 487
摩脐 / 489
摩颈项 / 488
摩腹 / 489
瘛脉 / 428
瘛疭 / 575
瘢痕灸 / 465
瘤 / 598
颜面疔疮 / 593
糊丸 / 280
潜阳 / 265
潜阳熄风 / 265
潜呼吸 / 497
潮热 / 144，519
潬 / 278
潼蒺藜 / 344
憎寒 / 143
额 / 43
额中线 / 471
额汗 / 145
额角 / 43
额旁1线 / 471
额旁2线 / 471
额旁3线 / 471
额颅 / 43
褥疮 / 606
鹤顶 / 443
鹤虱 / 353
鹤草芽 / 354
谵妄 / 124
谵语 / 140
譩譆 / 422
［乛］
熨目 / 487
熨法 / 272
熨药 / 642
劈法 / 649
缬草 / 337

十六画

［一］
颞后线 / 471
颞前线 / 471
颞颥 / 43
燕口 / 579
燕口疮 / 579
薤白 / 326
薛己 / 668
薛生白 / 676
薛良武 / 668
薛雪 / 676
薛铠 / 668
薛新甫 / 669
薏苡仁 / 321
薄白苔 / 134
薄苔 / 135
薄荷 / 297
薄黄苔 / 134
薄厥 / 538
颠疾 / 589
橘皮竹茹汤 / 376
橘红 / 325
橘红丸［片］/ 383
橘核 / 325

整体观念 / 218
整复 / 638
醒神 / 266
醒脑 / 266
醒脾 / 245
霍乱 / 522
霍乱论 / 694
霍乱转筋 / 523
霍乱病 / 522

［丨］

噤口痢 / 522
噤风 / 575
踵 / 50
噫气 / 153

［丿］

镜面舌 / 136
赞刺 / 462
儒门事亲 / 701
儒家气功 / 492
鼽嚏 / 627

［丶］

瘭疽 / 594
瘰疬 / 596
瘿 / 597
瘿痈 / 597
瘴气 / 72，520
瘴疟 / 520，521
瘴毒 / 72，521
癃闭 / 552
凝脂翳 / 618
辨证 / 122，168
辨证论治 / 218
辨证选穴法 / 446
辨证施治 / 218
辨病 / 122
糙苔 / 135
糖浆 / 281
燔针 / 451
濒湖脉学 / 686
激光针 / 470
激经 / 566

［乛］

壁观 / 499
避年 / 556

十七画

［一］

戴思恭 / 667
戴原礼 / 667
擦丹田 / 506
擦法 / 482，650
擦面 / 506
擦涌泉 / 490，506
擦鼻 / 506
藏红花 / 330
藁本 / 296
檀香 / 326
翳 / 612
翳风 / 428
翳明 / 440

［丨］

龋齿 / 632
龋齿牙痛 / 632
龋脱 / 633
瞳人 / 609
瞳人干缺 / 619
瞳子 / 609
瞳子髎 / 428
瞳仁 / 609
瞳神 / 609
瞳神干缺 / 619
瞳神细小 / 619
瞳神紧小 / 619
瞳神缺陷 / 619
瞳神散大 / 619
瞳神缩小 / 619
瞪目直视 / 129
螳螂子 / 579
髁骨 / 51
髀 / 51
髀关 / 413
髀枢 / 51
髀骨 / 51

［丿］

魏之琇 / 675
魏柳洲 / 675
臌胀（病）/ 547
膻中 / 47，436
臁疮 / 595
臆 / 47

［丶］

䗪虫 / 333
膺 / 47
膺窗 / 412
燥 / 66
燥干清窍 / 90
燥干清窍证 / 198
燥气 / 66
燥气化热 / 90
燥气寒化 / 90
燥化 / 92
燥火 / 66，68
燥邪 / 66
燥邪犯［伤］肺证 / 198
燥伤肺气 / 89
燥伤津液 / 90
燥苔 / 135
燥剂 / 360
燥结 / 92
燥结证 / 198
燥热 / 66，68
燥湿 / 260
燥湿止痒 / 267
燥湿化痰 / 258
燥湿健脾 / 260
燥痰证 / 189
濡脉 / 161
豁痰 / 259
豁痰开窍 / 267
豁痰醒脑 / 267

［乛］

臀痈 / 594
臂 / 47
臂内廉 / 47
臂外廉 / 47
臂臑 / 410

十八画

瞽症 / 622
藕节 / 330
覆盆子 / 351
瞿麦 / 322
瞻视昏渺 / 620
鹭鸶咳 / 586
髂窝流注 / 595
翻白草 / 310
臑 / 47
臑会 / 427
臑骨 / 47
臑俞 / 418
癖热 / 583
癖嗜 / 70

十九画

攒竹 / 419
藿香 / 319
藿香正气散 / 379
攀索叠砖 / 642
蟾酥 / 356
巅 / 42
巅顶 / 42
髋骨 / 51，443
蟹目 / 618
蟹珠 / 618
蟹睛病 / 618
颤动舌 / 133
颤法 / 484
颤震［振］/ 540
癣 / 604
鳖甲 / 345

二十画

躁狂 / 124
躁烦 / 124
癥瘕 / 548
癥瘕积聚 / 548

二十一画

露 / 281
露剂 / 281
髓 / 25
髓之府 / 25
髓海 / 25
癫 / 534
癫狂 / 534
癫狗咬伤 / 71
癫病 / 534
癫痫 / 535，589
癞病 / 605
麝香 / 335
蠡沟 / 432

二十二画以上

囊痈 / 599
镵针 / 451
颧 / 45
颧髎 / 418

中文拼音索引 Chinese Character Phonetic Index

A

ā

阿是穴 / 444

ǎi

矮步 / 496
嗳腐 / 153
嗳气 / 153

ài

艾 / 463
艾附暖宫丸 / 394
艾卷 / 464
艾卷灸 / 464
艾绒 / 463
艾条 / 464
艾条灸 / 464
艾叶 / 318
艾炷 / 463
艾炷灸 / 464

ān

安宫牛黄丸 / 392
安蛔 / 271
安蛔定痛 / 271
安神 / 264
安神补心丸 / 385
安神定志 / 264
安神剂 / 380
安神药 / 293
安胎 / 268
安息香 / 335

àn

按尺肤 / 165
按法 / 159，480，651
按肌肤 / 165
按摩 / 480
按摩疗法 / 480
按摩师 / 480
按摩手法 / 480
按摩足三里 / 489
按目四眦 / 487
按捺耳窍 / 488
按捏鼻梁 / 488
按跷 / 480
按揉风池 / 489
按揉颈项 / 488
按手足 / 165
按太阳 / 487
按脘腹 / 165
按胸腹 / 165
按压耳穴 / 488
按压法 / 480
按迎香 / 488
按俞穴 / 165
按诊 / 165
暗经 / 556

áo

熬 / 278

B

bā

八段锦 / 502
八法 / 225
八风 / 443
八纲 / 168
八纲辨证 / 168
八卦步 / 496
八会穴 / 439
八廓 / 44，607
八脉交会穴 / 439
八溪 / 52
八邪 / 442
八珍汤 / 372
八珍丸 / 388
八珍益母丸 / 395
八正散 / 380
巴豆 / 355
巴豆霜 / 324
巴戟天 / 347

bá

拔毒 / 269
拔罐 / 467
拔罐疗法 / 274，467
拔伸法 / 653
拔伸复位 / 640
拔伸捏正 / 640
拔伸牵引 / 638

bái

白 / 139
白疕 / 602
白扁豆 / 341
白驳风 / 602
白缠喉 / 585
白丑 / 324
白带 / 158，564
白癜风 / 602
白豆蔻 / 319
白矾 / 354
白附子 / 299
白果 / 301
白喉 / 585
白虎汤 / 367
白虎摇头法 / 458
白花蛇舌草 / 312
白环俞 / 421
白及 / 328
白僵蚕 / 338

白芥子 / 299
白芥子灸 / 467
白睛 / 45，609
白睛抱红 / 611
白睛暴赤 / 611
白睛赤肿 / 611
白睛发黄 / 129
白睛浮壅 / 611
白睛红赤 / 129，611
白睛混赤 / 611
白睛青蓝 / 617
白睛虬脉 / 618
白睛色诊 / 129
白睛涩痛 / 611
白睛溢血 / 617
白痢 / 522
白蔹 / 312
白茅根 / 307
白膜蔽睛 / 617
白膜侵睛 / 617
白硇砂 / 355
白腻苔 / 134
白砒 / 354
白前 / 301
白仁 / 45，609
白色 / 126
白涩病 / 617
白砂苔 / 135
白芍 / 342
白苔 / 134
白头翁 / 308
白头翁汤 / 369
白秃 / 604
白秃疮 / 604
白薇 / 307
白鲜皮 / 308
白陷鱼鳞 / 618
白屑风 / 602
白淫 / 552
白芷 / 295
白珠 / 609
白珠俱青 / 617
白术 / 341

bǎi

百部 / 302
百虫窝 / 443
百骸 / 50
百合 / 302
百合病 / 534
百会 / 434
百节 / 52
百日咳 / 586
百晬内嗽 / 577
柏子仁 / 337
柏子养心丸 / 385

bài

败毒散 / 363
败酱草 / 312
败酱片 / 385
败血冲肺 / 570
败血冲胃 / 571
败血冲心 / 570

bān

扳法 / 485，652
扳颈椎法 / 652
扳腿推拿手法 / 485
扳胸椎法 / 652
扳腰椎法 / 653
斑 / 139，591
斑蝥 / 355
斑蝥灸 / 467
斑秃 / 602
斑疹 / 139
瘢痕灸 / 465

bǎn

板蓝根 / 310
板蓝根冲剂 / 381

bàn

半边莲 / 312
半表半里 / 83
半表半里证 / 171
半刺 / 459
半身不遂 / 537
半身汗出 / 145
半身无汗 / 145
半卧式 / 495
半夏 / 298
半夏厚朴汤 / 375
半夏泻心汤 / 366
半枝莲 / 312
绊舌 / 634

bàng

棒击法 / 485，650
傍针刺 / 462

bāo

包煎 / 283
胞 / 555
胞宫 / 25，555
胞宫积热证 / 213
胞宫湿热证 / 214
胞宫虚寒证 / 213
胞寒不孕 / 565
胞肓 / 422
胞睑 / 44，607
胞睑下垂 / 129
胞睑肿核 / 613
胞轮振跳 / 614
胞络 / 407
胞脉 / 407
胞门 / 555
胞生痰核 / 613
胞虚如球 / 614
胞衣 / 555
胞衣不下 / 570
胞衣先破 / 569
胞脏 / 25，556
胞肿 / 614
胞肿如桃 / 614
胞阻 / 566

báo

薄白苔 / 134
薄黄苔 / 134
薄苔 / 135

bǎo

保和丸 / 379
保健 / 505
保健功 / 505
保健球按摩 / 490
报刺 / 461

bào

抱骨垫 / 641
抱踝手法 / 648
抱轮红赤 / 611
抱朴子 / 660
抱球式 / 496
抱头火丹 / 594
抱膝器 / 641
豹文刺 / 459
暴崩 / 561
暴病 / 515
暴赤生翳 / 616
暴喘 / 586
暴发火眼 / 616
暴风客热 / 616
暴聋 / 624
暴马子皮 / 303
暴盲 / 620
暴痫 / 589
暴泻（病） / 545
暴喑［瘖］ / 630

bēi

背法 / 653
悲 / 69

běi

北豆根 / 313
北鹤虱 / 353
北沙参 / 343

bèi

备急千金要方 / 690
背部穴 / 441
背痛 / 147
背俞穴 / 439

bēn

奔豚 / 535
奔豚气 / 535
贲门 / 41

běn

本 / 219
本草 / 275
本草备要 / 689
本草纲目 / 688
本草纲目拾遗 / 689
本草经集注 / 687
本草拾遗 / 688
本草衍义 / 688
本节 / 52
本经配穴法 / 447
本神 / 429
本事方 / 691

bēng

崩漏 / 561
崩证 / 561
崩中 / 561

bí

鼻 / 38
鼻病 / 626
鼻不闻香臭 / 130
鼻齿功 / 501
鼻臭证 / 627
鼻出血 / 130
鼻疮 / 626
鼻疔 / 626
鼻洞 / 38
鼻疳 / 626
鼻疳疮 / 626
鼻槁［藁］ / 627
鼻根 / 39
鼻洪 / 628
鼻尖 / 38，626
鼻茎 / 39
鼻菌 / 627
鼻科（学） / 625
鼻孔 / 38
鼻沥血 / 628
鼻梁 / 39，626
鼻梁骨折 / 628
鼻流清涕 / 130
鼻流浊涕 / 130
鼻毛 / 39
鼻衄 / 130，550，627
鼻前孔 / 626
鼻前庭 / 626
鼻窍 / 38
鼻窍不利 / 626
鼻鼽 / 627
鼻塞 / 626
鼻色主病 / 130
鼻隧 / 39
鼻涕 / 626
鼻吸鼻呼 / 497
鼻息肉 / 627
鼻息肉病 / 627
鼻翼 / 38，626
鼻翼煽动 / 130
鼻渊 / 627
鼻燥 / 626
鼻针 / 477
鼻针疗法 / 477
鼻痔 / 627
鼻窒 / 627
鼻柱 / 39，626
鼻柱骨 / 39
鼻赘 / 627
鼻准 / 38，626

bì

闭经 / 157，559
荜拨 / 319
荜澄茄 / 318
萆薢 / 322
痹病 / 540
痹痛 / 147
壁观 / 499
避年 / 556
髀 / 51
髀骨 / 51
髀关 / 413

髀枢 / 51
臂 / 47
臂内廉 / 47
臂臑 / 410
臂外廉 / 47

biān

砭石 / 451
萹蓄 / 322

biǎn

扁瘊 / 600
扁鹊 / 658
扁鹊心书 / 700
变蒸 / 583
变证 / 116

biàn

便秘 / 149，544
便溏 / 149
便血 / 550
辨病 / 122
辨证 / 122，168
辨证论治 / 218
辨证施治 / 218
辨证选穴法 / 446

biāo

标 / 219
标本兼治 / 219
标本同治 / 219
瘭疽 / 594

biǎo

表寒 / 82
表寒里热 / 83
表寒里热证 / 171
表寒证 / 170
表里 / 169
表里辨证 / 169
表里病机 / 81
表里出入 / 82
表里传 / 116
表里寒热 / 82
表里经配穴法 / 447
表里俱寒 / 83
表里俱热 / 83
表里俱实 / 85
表里俱虚 / 85
表里配穴法 / 447
表里双解 / 230
表里双解剂 / 366
表里同病 / 83
表里虚实 / 82
表里选穴法 / 446
表气不固 / 85
表热 / 82
表热传里 / 83
表热里寒 / 83
表热里寒证 / 171
表热证 / 170
表湿证 / 196
表实 / 82
表实里虚 / 84
表实里虚证 / 171
表实证 / 170
表虚 / 82
表虚里实 / 83
表虚里实证 / 171
表虚证 / 170
表证 / 169

biē

鳖甲 / 345

bié

别络 / 407
别煮 / 283

bīn

槟榔 / 353
濒湖脉学 / 686

bīng

冰硼散 / 396
冰片 / 335

bǐng

秉风 / 418

bìng

并病 / 178
并月 / 556
病机 / 78
病机十九条 / 78
病理体质 / 74
病脉 / 160
病色 / 124
病能［态］/ 78
病因 / 62
病因辨证 / 191

bō

拨法 / 485
拨络法 / 485
玻璃罐 / 467
剥苔 / 135

bò

薄荷 / 297

bǔ

补法 / 244
补肺 / 247
补肺益气 / 247
补肺阴 / 249
补肝阴 / 248
补骨脂 / 347
补火生土 / 251
补火壮阳 / 251
补剂 / 360
补脾 / 245
补脾益肺 / 247
补脾益气 / 246
补气 / 244
补气固表 / 244
补气剂 / 371
补气摄血 / 258
补气生血 / 247
补气养血 / 247
补气药 / 293
补气止血 / 258
补肾 / 249
补肾安神 / 264
补肾固精 / 250
补肾健骨 / 251
补肾纳气 / 251

补肾阳药 / 293
补肾益肺 / 251
补肾益气 / 249
补肾阴 / 250
补肾助阳 / 251
补胃阴 / 249
补泻法 / 456
补心丹 / 385
补心益气 / 244
补心阴 / 248
补血 / 247
补血剂 / 371
补血药 / 294
补阳 / 250
补阳还五汤 / 376
补阳剂 / 373
补阳药 / 293
补养安神剂 / 380
补养肺阴 / 249
补养心血 / 247
补养心阴 / 248
补养药 / 293
补益肺气 / 247
补益肝肾 / 248
补益剂 / 371
补益气血 / 247
补益肾气 / 249
补益心脾 / 247
补益心气 / 244
补益药 / 293
补益中气 / 246
补阴 / 248
补阴剂 / 372
补阴药 / 294
补中益气 / 246
补中益气汤 / 371
补中益气丸 / 388
哺乳疳 / 582

bù

不传 / 116
不得眠 / 155
不得卧 / 535
不得偃卧 / 141
不更衣 / 149
不寐 / 155
不内外因 / 62
不仁 / 148
不容 / 412
不省人事 / 124
不时泪溢 / 611
不闻香臭 / 626
不锈钢针 / 452
不育 / 553
不孕 / 565
布气 / 504
步廊 / 425

C

cā

擦鼻 / 506
擦丹田 / 506
擦法 / 482，650
擦面 / 506
擦涌泉 / 490，506

cǎi

踩法 / 485
踩跷法 / 486，652

cāng

仓公 / 658
苍耳子 / 296
苍龙摆尾法 / 458
苍术 / 319

cāo

糙苔 / 135

cáo

嘈杂 / 153，543

cǎo

草豆蔻 / 320
草果 / 320
草乌 / 314
草药 / 275

cè

侧柏叶 / 329
侧擦法 / 651
侧卧式 / 495

chā

插入法 / 453

chá

茶 / 282
茶剂 / 282
察目 / 128

chà

差经 / 562

chái

柴葛解肌汤 / 362
柴胡 / 297

chán

禅定 / 500
缠喉风 / 630
缠腰火丹 / 600
缠腰蛇丹 / 600
蝉蜕 / 298
蝉衣 / 298
蟾酥 / 356
镵针 / 451

chǎn

产宝 / 695
产后痹证 / 572
产后病 / 570
产后病痉 / 572
产后病温 / 571
产后大便难 / 571
产后盗汗 / 571
产后恶露不绝 / 570
产后发热 / 571
产后腹痛 / 572
产后腹胀 / 572
产后痉病 / 572
产后痉证 / 572
产后尿血 / 571
产后缺乳 / 572
产后乳汁自出 / 573
产后三病 / 570

产后三冲 / 570
产后三急 / 570
产后三脱 / 570
产后身痛 / 571
产后水肿 / 572
产后头痛 / 571
产后小便不通 / 571
产后小便失禁 / 571
产后胁痛 / 572
产后血崩 / 571
产后血晕 / 571
产后腰痛 / 572
产后郁冒 / 571
产后怔忡 / 571
产后自汗 / 571
产门 / 48，555
产难 / 569

chàn

颤动舌 / 133
颤法 / 484
颤震［振］/ 540

cháng

长脉 / 162
长强 / 433
长针 / 452
肠痹 / 542
肠鸣 / 153
肠痈 / 546
肠燥津亏证 / 187
肠痔 / 599
常脉 / 160
常色 / 124
常山 / 298

cháo

巢元方 / 660
朝食暮吐 / 152
潮热 / 144，519

chǎo

炒 / 277
炒爆 / 277
炒黄 / 277
炒焦 / 277
炒炭 / 277

chē

车前草 / 320
车前子 / 320

chě

扯法 / 483
扯痧 / 486

chè

掣痛 / 148

chén

臣药 / 358
沉肩 / 493
沉脉 / 160
沉香 / 327
陈藏器 / 661
陈飞霞 / 676
陈复正 / 676
陈九韶 / 673
陈良甫 / 665
陈念祖 / 678
陈皮 / 325
陈慎修 / 678
陈实功 / 672
陈司成 / 673
陈文中 / 665
陈无择 / 664
陈修圆 / 678
陈修圆医书十六种 / 705
陈言 / 663
陈毓仁 / 672
陈自明 / 665

chéng

成方 / 356
成无己 / 663
承淡安 / 682
承扶 / 421
承光 / 419
承浆 / 46，437
承筋 / 422
承灵 / 430
承满 / 412
承泣 / 411
承山 / 423
程国彭 / 677
程钟龄 / 677

chī

眵 / 610
眵泪 / 611
眵泪胶粘 / 611
痴呆 / 536

chí

迟脉 / 160
锓针 / 451

chǐ

尺泽 / 409
齿 / 39
齿迟 / 578
齿䘌 / 632
齿槁 / 137
齿更 / 632
齿痕舌 / 132
齿焦 / 137
齿落 / 632
齿衄 / 137，550
齿龋 / 632
齿挺 / 633
齿龂 / 632
齿摇 / 137
齿龈结瓣 / 634
齿龈宣露 / 633
齿龈肿痛 / 137，634
齿燥 / 137

chì

赤白带 / 564
赤白带下 / 158
赤白痢 / 522
赤白肉际 / 52
赤鼻 / 601
赤带抱轮 / 611
赤痢 / 522
赤龙搅海 / 506

赤脉传睛 / 611
赤脉贯睛 / 612
赤脉侵睛 / 612
赤膜 / 612
赤膜下垂 / 619
赤色 / 126
赤芍 / 306
赤石脂 / 349
赤丝虬脉 / 617
赤小豆 / 323
赤眼 / 616
赤游丹 / 594
瘛脉 / 428
瘛疭 / 575

chōng

冲服 / 283
冲服剂 / 282
冲剂 / 282
冲脉 / 406
冲门 / 415
冲任不固 / 114
冲任不固证 / 215
冲任失［不］调 / 114
冲任失［不］调证 / 215
冲任损伤 / 114
冲阳 / 414
茺蔚子 / 334

chóng

虫积 / 582
虫积（证） / 547
虫积腹痛 / 546，588
虫积经闭 / 559
虫积证 / 199
虫兽伤 / 71
虫吐 / 587
虫瘸 / 590
虫咬皮炎 / 603
重楼 / 311
重舌 / 133，633
重身 / 564
重修政和经史证类备急本草 / 688

chōu

抽搐 / 539
抽葫芦 / 323
抽筋 / 127
抽气罐 / 468
抽气罐法 / 468

chòu

臭梧桐叶 / 316

chū

出偏 / 505
出针 / 462
出针法 / 462
初生不乳 / 574
初生不啼 / 574

chú

除烦止渴 / 231

chù

搐鼻 / 273

chuān

川贝母 / 302
川贝枇杷糖浆 / 382
川楝子 / 328
川木通 / 321
川牛膝 / 331
川乌 / 314
川芎 / 330
川芎嗪注射液 / 394
穿刺针埋线法 / 478
穿地龙 / 317
穿山甲 / 333
穿山龙 / 316
穿心莲 / 312

chuán

传变 / 116
传导之腑 / 27
传导之官 / 27
传化之腑 / 26
传经 / 116
传染 / 514

chuǎn

喘 / 140，527
喘病 / 527
喘促 / 141
喘急 / 141
喘鸣 / 141
喘逆 / 141
喘证 / 527

chuàn

串雅内、外编 / 693

chuāng

疮 / 591
疮毒内陷 / 596
疮痨 / 596
疮疡 / 591
疮疡经验全书 / 697

chuī

吹药 / 273

chuí

垂帘翳 / 619
垂盆草 / 309
垂肘 / 494
捶法 / 485
捶腰背 / 489

chūn

春温 / 516
春温病 / 516
椿根白皮 / 309
椿皮 / 308

chún

纯阳之体 / 574
唇 / 39
唇疮 / 634
唇疔 / 634
唇风 / 633
唇疽 / 634
唇菌 / 634
唇裂 / 136
唇紫 / 136
淳于意 / 658

cī

差颓［癞］/ 578

cí

磁石 / 336
磁穴疗法 / 478
磁朱丸 / 380
磁珠疗法 / 478

cì

次髎 / 421
刺法 / 444
刺蒺藜 / 339
刺灸法 / 444
刺络 / 449
刺络拔罐 / 469
刺手 / 453
刺痛 / 148
刺五加 / 341
刺血拔罐 / 469

cōng

聪耳 / 271

cóng

从治 / 220
丛毛 / 52

còu

腠［凑］理 / 41

cù

促脉 / 162
醋炙 / 277

cuán

攒竹 / 419

cuàn

窜痛 / 148

cuī

催气法 / 454
催乳 / 268
催生 / 268
催吐药 / 294

cuì

淬 / 278
焠刺 / 460

cūn

皴揭 / 601

cún

存泥丸 / 487
存神 / 498
存息 / 498
存想 / 499

cùn

寸 / 444
寸、关、尺 / 158
寸口 / 159
寸口脉 / 160

cuō

搓柄法 / 455
搓法 / 484，647
搓内肾 / 506
搓腰 / 506
撮法 / 484
撮口 / 136，575
撮痧疗法 / 469

cuò

挫伤 / 646
错经 / 562
错语 / 140

D

dā

搭鹊桥 / 494
搭手 / 594

dá

达邪 / 229

dà

大包 / 416
大便秘结 / 149
大补大泻法 / 458
大补阴丸 / 389
大柴胡汤 / 366
大肠 / 24
大肠传导失职 / 110
大肠寒结 / 110
大肠寒结证 / 208
大肠津［液］亏 / 111
大肠津［液］亏证 / 208
大肠津亏 / 81
大肠咳 / 525
大肠热结 / 110
大肠热结证 / 208
大肠湿热 / 111
大肠湿热证 / 208
大肠实热 / 111
大肠虚寒 / 111
大肠虚寒证 / 208
大肠俞 / 420
大承气汤 / 364
大都 / 415
大毒、常毒、小毒、无毒 / 279
大敦 / 432
大方 / 357
大风 / 605
大腹 / 48
大腹皮 / 321
大骨空 / 442
大骨枯槁 / 126
大汗 / 144
大汗淋漓 / 144
大赫 / 424
大横 / 416
大黄 / 352
大黄附子汤 / 364
大黄牡丹汤 / 364
大活络丸［丹］/ 392
大蓟 / 328
大节 / 52
大结胸 / 519
大巨 / 413
大厥 / 538
大陵 / 426
大脉 / 162
大气 / 53
大青叶 / 311
大肉陷下 / 126
大山楂丸 / 387
大头垫 / 641
大头瘟 / 520

大泻刺 / 460
大迎 / 411
大芸 / 346
大枣 / 341
大针 / 452
大钟 / 424
大周天 / 500
大周天功 / 502
大杼 / 419
大炷灸 / 465
大椎 / 434
大眦 / 608
大眦脓漏 / 615

dài

代脉 / 162
代赭石 / 339
玳瑁 / 339
带脉 / 406，430
带脉病证 / 215
带下 / 563
带下病 / 564
带下臭秽 / 158
戴思恭 / 667
戴原礼 / 667

dān

丹 / 281
丹参 / 331
丹毒 / 593
丹剂 / 281
丹痧 / 520，585
丹田 / 42，497
丹溪心法 / 701
单按 / 159
单蛾 / 628
单方 / 356
单腹胀 / 547
单煎 / 283
单盘坐 / 495
单手进针法 / 453
单一脉象 / 163

dǎn

胆 / 23
胆火证 / 212
胆咳 / 525
胆南星 / 299
胆囊 / 443
胆气 / 55
胆气虚 / 104
胆气虚证 / 211
胆热 / 104
胆热证 / 211
胆俞 / 420
胆虚气怯 / 104
胆虚气怯证 / 211
胆胀（病）/ 547
掸拂法 / 483

dàn

但寒不热 / 143
但热不寒 / 143
但欲寐 / 155
淡白舌 / 131
淡豆豉 / 298
淡红舌 / 131
淡渗利湿 / 260
淡渗祛湿 / 260
淡竹叶 / 305

dāng

当归 / 342
当归补血汤 / 372
当归四逆汤 / 370
当归丸 / 394
当阳 / 439

dǎng

党参 / 340

dāo

刀豆 / 328

dǎo

导便 / 273
导赤散 / 368
导法 / 273
导气 / 455，503
导引 / 491
捣法 / 455，481
捣击法 / 481
倒经 / 560

dào

盗汗 / 144，531
道地药材 / 275
倒睫 / 613
倒睫拳毛 / 613
道家气功 / 492
稻芽 / 351

dé

得气 / 456
得神 / 123

dēng

灯心草 / 323

dèng

瞪目直视 / 129

dī

滴酒法 / 468
滴丸 / 280

dí

涤痰 / 259

dì

地仓 / 411
地肤子 / 322
地骨皮 / 306
地黄 / 306
地黄丸 / 389
地机 / 415
地锦草 / 309
地龙 / 339
地图舌 / 579
地五会 / 431
地榆 / 329
地支 / 18
蒂丁 / 40，628
蒂中 / 40，628

diān

颠疾 / 589
巅 / 42
巅顶 / 42

癫 / 534
癫病 / 534
癫狗咬伤 / 71
癫狂 / 534
癫痫 / 535，589

diǎn

点刺 / 449
点刺舌 / 132
点法 / 481
点击法 / 481
点穴疗法 / 490
点眼 / 273

diàn

电光伤目 / 621
电灸 / 467
电灸器 / 467
电热灸 / 467
电针 / 470
电针疗法 / 470
电针麻醉 / 470
电针仪 / 470

diào

掉眩 / 146

diē

跌打损伤 / 71

dīng

丁甘仁 / 681
丁奚疳 / 580
丁香 / 318
丁香柿蒂汤 / 376
丁泽周 / 681
疔 / 592
疔疮走黄 / 595
耵耳 / 625
耵聍 / 625

dǐng

顶颞后斜线 / 471
顶颞前斜线 / 471
顶旁1线 / 471
顶旁2线 / 471
顶中线 / 471
鼎式夹板固定 / 640

dìng

定喘 / 441
定喘汤 / 375
定喘丸 / 383
锭 / 281
锭剂 / 281

dōng

冬虫夏草 / 348
冬瓜皮 / 321
冬葵果 / 322
冬温 / 519

dòng

动功 / 492
动静相兼功 / 492
动留针法 / 462
动脉 / 162
动中有静 / 492
冻疮 / 605
冻风 / 606

dǒu

抖法 / 651

dòu

豆蔻 / 319
痘 / 584
痘疮 / 585

dū

督脉 / 405
督脉穴 / 433
督俞 / 420

dú

毒 / 68
毒虫咬伤 / 606
毒火攻唇证 / 198
毒火攻口证 / 199
毒蛇咬伤 / 606
独活 / 314
独活寄生汤 / 377
独阴 / 444
独语 / 140
犊鼻 / 414

dǔ

笃击法 / 481

dù

杜仲 / 347

duān

端法 / 639
端提捺正 / 639

duǎn

短刺 / 461
短脉 / 162
短气 / 141，526
短缩舌 / 133

duàn

断端移位 / 635
断骨接整 / 638
断经前后诸证 / 563
断裂伤 / 646
断乳 / 268
断绪 / 565
断针 / 463
煅 / 276
煅淬 / 276
煅龙骨 / 350
煅牡蛎 / 350
煅瓦楞 / 350

duì

对耳轮 / 472
对耳轮上脚 / 472
对耳轮体 / 472
对耳轮下脚 / 472
对耳屏 / 473
对应选穴法 / 446
对掌推拉导气 / 503
对症选穴法 / 446
兑端 / 435

dùn

炖 / 278
顿服 / 284
顿咳 / 586

duō

多汗 / 144

多梦 / 155
多尿 / 150
多食善饥 / 153

duó

夺血 / 549

duò

堕胎 / 569

E

ē

阿胶 / 342

é

莪术 / 331
鹅不食草 / 296
鹅口疮 / 579，634
鹅掌风 / 604
鹅爪风 / 605
额 / 43
额汗 / 145
额角 / 43
额颅 / 43
额旁2线 / 471
额旁3线 / 471
额旁1线 / 471
额中线 / 471

ě

恶心 / 152

è

扼法 / 484
呃逆 / 153，543
恶露 / 570
恶露不绝 / 570
恶露不下 / 570
恶露不止 / 570
恶气 / 63
恶色 / 125
恶阻 / 566
腭裂 / 590
頞 / 626

ér

儿茶 / 356

ěr

耳 / 45
耳闭 / 623
耳疮 / 623
耳垂 / 45，473
耳道 / 45
耳疔 / 623
耳疳 / 625
耳根毒 / 624
耳根痈 / 624
耳功 / 501，505
耳和髎 / 428
耳后发 / 625
耳后附骨痈 / 624
耳甲 / 473
耳甲腔 / 473
耳甲艇 / 473
耳尖 / 440
耳疖 / 623
耳菌 / 625
耳科（学） / 623
耳壳 / 45
耳壳流痰 / 623
耳孔 / 45
耳廓 / 45
耳聋 / 624
耳聋口哑 / 625
耳聋左慈丸 / 397
耳瘘 / 625
耳轮 / 45，472
耳轮淡白 / 129
耳轮干枯 / 129
耳轮红肿 / 129
耳轮甲错 / 129
耳轮脚 / 472
耳轮结节 / 472
耳轮青黑 / 129
耳轮尾 / 472
耳轮萎缩 / 129
耳门 / 45，428
耳鸣 / 624
耳膜 / 45
耳屏 / 473
耳窍 / 45
耳挺 / 625
耳眩晕 / 625
耳穴 / 473
耳穴探测仪 / 477
耳穴推拿疗法 / 490
耳蕈 / 625
耳胀 / 623
耳针 / 472
耳针疗法 / 472
耳痔 / 625
耳舟 / 473

èr

二白 / 442
二陈汤 / 380
二垫固定法 / 641
二间 / 409
二母宁嗽丸［片］ / 382
二十八脉 / 160
二仙汤 / 373
二阳 / 400
二阳并病 / 178
二阴 / 48，399

F

fā

发 / 594
发背 / 594
发表药 / 287
发放外气 / 504
发功 / 504
发汗解表 / 225
发汗解表药 / 287
发汗禁例 / 229
发黄 / 139，523
发酵 / 278
发泡 / 273
发泡灸 / 466
发气 / 504

发气手势 / 504
发热 / 143
发热恶寒 / 143
发散风寒药 / 287
发散风热药 / 287
发芽 / 278
发颐 / 594

fà

发迟 / 578
发际 / 42
发际疮 / 592
发落 / 602
发蛀脱发 / 602

fān

番红花 / 330
番泻叶 / 352
翻白草 / 310

fán

烦渴 / 149
烦热 / 144
烦躁 / 124
燔针 / 451

fǎn

反关脉 / 163
反酸 / 153
反胃 / 152，543
反治 / 220
反佐 / 221，358

fàn

泛恶 / 152
泛酸 / 543

fāng

方 / 356
方剂 / 356
方剂配伍 / 358
方上 / 38
芳香化湿 / 259
芳香化湿药 / 290
芳香化浊 / 259
芳香开窍 / 266
芳香开窍药 / 293

fáng

防风 / 295
防风通圣散 / 366
防风通圣丸 / 382
防己 / 317
房劳 / 71
房事不节 / 71
房事过度 / 71

fàng

放松功 / 500

fēi

飞门 / 39
飞入法 / 453
飞扬喉 / 631
飞阳 / 423
非化脓灸 / 465

féi

肥疮 / 604
肥膏肉人 / 75
肥胖不孕 / 565
肥人 / 75
腓腨 / 50

fěi

榧子 / 353

fèi

肺 / 22
肺痹 / 541
肺病辨证 / 202
肺风痰喘 / 585
肺疳 / 581
肺火 / 102
肺火证 / 204
肺津 / 22
肺津不布 / 109
肺津亏损 / 81
肺经咳嗽 / 525
肺咳 / 525
肺劳 / 529
肺痨 / 529
肺络损伤 / 110
肺气 / 22，55
肺气不利 / 109
肺气不宣 / 109
肺气不足 / 109
肺气上逆 / 109
肺气虚 / 109
肺气虚寒 / 109
肺气虚证 / 202
肺热 / 102
肺热炽盛 / 102
肺热炽盛证 / 204
肺肾两虚 / 102
肺肾气虚 / 102
肺肾气虚证 / 205
肺肾阳虚 / 102
肺肾阳虚证 / 205
肺肾阴虚 / 102
肺肾阴虚证 / 204
肺失清肃 / 109
肺实 / 102
肺水 / 549
肺萎［痿］/ 528
肺卫气虚（不固）证 / 202
肺系 / 40
肺消 / 551
肺虚 / 102
肺虚寒证 / 203
肺虚咳嗽 / 526
肺虚热证 / 203
肺炎喘嗽 / 586
肺阳 / 22
肺阳虚 / 109
肺阳虚证 / 203
肺阴 / 22
肺阴不足 / 109
肺阴虚 / 109
肺阴虚证 / 203
肺痈 / 528
肺俞 / 419
肺燥 / 102
肺燥肠闭证 / 204
肺燥津伤证 / 187

肺胀 / 528
痱子 / 601

fēn

分刺 / 460
分骨垫 / 641
分筋 / 647
分娩 / 568
分肉 / 41

fěn

粉萆薢 / 322
粉刺 / 601
粉瘤 / 598

fēng

丰隆 / 414
风 / 64
风痹 / 540
风池 / 430
风赤疮疾 / 614
风赤疮痍 / 614
风毒证 / 199
风府 / 434
风关 / 138
风寒 / 67
风寒表证 / 192
风寒犯头证 / 192
风寒感冒 / 516
风寒喉痹 / 629
风寒咳嗽 / 525
风寒湿 / 68
风寒湿邪 / 68
风寒湿阻证 / 192
风寒束表 / 88
风寒束肺 / 110
风寒束肺证 / 203
风寒头痛 / 533
风寒袭鼻证 / 192
风寒袭表证 / 192
风寒袭肺 / 109
风寒袭肺证 / 192，203
风寒袭喉［咽］证 / 192
风寒袭络证 / 192
风寒邪气 / 67
风寒眩晕 / 532
风寒牙痛 / 632
风寒腰痛 / 553
风寒证 / 191
风火 / 67
风火攻目证 / 193
风火内旋 / 89
风火相煽 / 89
风火牙痛 / 632
风火眼 / 615
风火眼痛 / 616
风轮 / 44，607
风轮赤豆 / 619
风门 / 419
风牵偏视 / 622
风热 / 67
风热闭肺证 / 193
风热表证 / 192
风热疮 / 602
风热耳鸣 / 624
风热犯鼻证 / 193
风热犯耳证 / 193
风热犯肺 / 110
风热犯肺证 / 193，203
风热犯目证 / 193
风热犯头证 / 193
风热感冒 / 516
风热攻目证 / 193
风热喉痹 / 629
风热咳嗽 / 525
风热侵喉［咽］证 / 193
风热乳蛾 / 628
风热头痛 / 533
风热外袭证 / 192
风热邪气 / 67
风热眩晕 / 532
风热牙疳 / 633
风热牙痛 / 632
风热眼 / 616
风热腰痛 / 553
风热证 / 192
风瘙痒 / 603
风痧 / 584
风胜行痹证 / 191
风湿 / 68
风湿犯头证 / 194
风湿凌目证 / 194
风湿头痛 / 533
风湿外袭证 / 194
风湿袭表证 / 194
风湿相搏 / 89
风湿邪气 / 68
风湿腰痛 / 553
风湿证 / 193
风市 / 431
风水 / 549
风水相搏证 / 188
风痰 / 64
风痰头痛 / 534
风痰眩晕 / 532
风痰证 / 189
风团 / 603
风温 / 67，516
风温病 / 516
风温邪气 / 67
风袭表疏证 / 191
风弦赤烂 / 613
风痫 / 589
风邪 / 64
风邪犯表证 / 191
风邪外袭证 / 191
风邪袭络证 / 191
风癣 / 604
风痒 / 602
风瘾疹 / 603
风燥 / 64，68
风燥咳嗽 / 526
风燥袭表证 / 194
风疹 / 583
风中经络证 / 191
风中血脉 / 89

封藏失职 / 112
锋针 / 452
蜂房 / 356
蜂蜜 / 352
蜂针疗法 / 451

fó

佛家气功 / 492
佛手 / 326

fū

趺阳脉 / 160
跗 / 51
跗骨 / 52
跗阳 / 423
跗肿 / 139
敷 / 272

fú

伏龙肝 / 349
伏脉 / 160
伏气 / 63，515
伏气温病 / 515
伏热 / 88
伏热在里 / 88
伏暑 / 518
伏暑病 / 518
伏兔 / 413
伏邪 / 64
伏饮 / 528
扶突 / 411
扶阳 / 250
扶正 / 219
扶正固本 / 220
扶正兼祛邪 / 219
扶正解表 / 230
扶正解表剂 / 363
扶正培本 / 220
扶正祛邪 / 219
拂法 / 483
服药法 / 283
服药食忌 / 284
茯苓 / 320
茯神 / 337
浮白 / 429
浮刺 / 461
浮络 / 407
浮脉 / 160
浮萍 / 298
浮郄 / 421
浮小麦 / 348

fǔ

府舍 / 415
釜底抽薪 / 237
釜沸脉 / 163
辅骨 / 51
腑 / 20
腑气 / 54
腑证 / 178
腐苔 / 135

fù

妇科十味片 / 395
妇人大全良方 / 695
妇人良方 / 695
附分 / 421
附骨疽 / 595，656
附子 / 317
附子饼灸 / 466
附子理中丸 / 387
复方 / 356
复方川贝精片 / 382
复方丹参片 / 393
复合手法 / 490
复溜 / 424
复位 / 642
傅青主 / 674
傅青主女科 / 695
傅仁宇 / 673
傅山 / 674
傅允科 / 673
腹 / 48
腹哀 / 416
腹背配穴法 / 447
腹部功 / 501
腹结 / 415
腹满 / 154
腹满膜胀 / 154
腹鸣 / 153
腹通谷 / 425
腹痛 / 147，546
腹痛下坠 / 153
腹胀 / 154
腹中雷鸣 / 154
腹中硬块 / 154
覆盆子 / 351

G

gān

干疳 / 580
干疳证 / 580
干霍乱 / 522
干姜 / 317
干咳 / 142，525
干咳嗽 / 525
干聋 / 625
干呕 / 152
干陷 / 595
干癣 / 605
干血痨 / 530
甘草 / 340
甘汞 / 354
甘寒润燥 / 263
甘寒生津 / 264
甘松 / 326
甘遂 / 324
甘温除热 / 244
肝 / 21
肝痹 / 541
肝胆病辨证 / 208
肝胆湿热 / 104
肝胆湿热证 / 211
肝风 / 103
肝风内动 / 103
肝风内动证 / 210
肝疳 / 581
肝寒 / 103

肝寒证 / 209
肝火 / 103
肝火不得卧 / 535
肝火炽盛 / 98
肝火炽盛证 / 209
肝火耳鸣 / 624
肝火燔耳证 / 209
肝火犯头证 / 209
肝火上炎 / 98
肝火上炎证 / 210
肝火眩晕 / 532
肝火证 / 209
肝经风热 / 98
肝经风热证 / 211
肝经咳嗽 / 524
肝经湿热 / 99
肝经湿热证 / 211
肝经实火 / 98
肝经郁热 / 98
肝咳 / 524
肝劳 / 529
肝脾不和 / 104
肝脾不和证 / 211
肝气 / 21，54
肝气不和 / 97
肝气不舒 / 97
肝气不足 / 96
肝气犯脾 / 98，104
肝气犯脾证 / 210
肝气犯胃 / 97，103
肝气犯胃证 / 210
肝气横逆 / 97
肝气上逆 / 98
肝气胁痛 / 531
肝气虚 / 96
肝气（亏）虚证 / 209
肝气郁结 / 97
肝气郁结证 / 210
肝热 / 103
肝肾阴虚 / 104
肝肾阴虚证 / 211
肝水 / 549
肝瘘 / 539
肝胃不和 / 103
肝胃不和证 / 210
肝胃气痛 / 542
肝虚寒 / 97
肝虚寒证 / 209
肝血 / 21
肝血不足 / 97
肝血虚 / 97
肝血（亏）虚证 / 209
肝阳 / 21
肝阳化风 / 103
肝阳化风证 / 210
肝阳化火 / 98
肝阳亢盛 / 98
肝阳亢盛证 / 210
肝阳上亢 / 98
肝阳上亢证 / 209
肝阳头痛 / 534
肝阳虚 / 97
肝阳（亏）虚证 / 209
肝阳眩晕 / 532
肝阴 / 21
肝阴不足 / 97
肝阴虚 / 97
肝阴（亏）虚证 / 209
肝俞 / 420
肝郁 / 103
肝郁不孕 / 565
肝郁脾虚 / 104
肝郁脾虚证 / 211
肝郁胁痛 / 531
肝郁证 / 210
疳 / 580
疳病 / 580
疳积 / 580
疳积上目 / 621
疳积证 / 580
疳气 / 580
疳气证 / 580
疳眼 / 621
疳证 / 580

gǎn

感冒 / 515
感冒清热冲剂 / 381
感冒退热冲剂 / 381
感暑 / 517
感暑眩晕 / 532

gàn

骭骨 / 51

gāng

刚痓 / 127
肛裂 / 599
肛瘘 / 599
肛漏 / 599
肛门 / 49
肛痈 / 599

gàng

杠杆支撑 / 639

gāo

高低垫 / 641
高风内障 / 620
高风雀目 / 621
高骨 / 51
高良姜 / 318
高梅孤 / 671
高武 / 671
睾 / 49
睾丸萎缩 / 600
睾丸肿痛 / 600
膏 / 281
膏肓 / 42，422
膏剂 / 281
膏粱厚味 / 70
膏淋 / 552
膏摩 / 273，490
膏摩疗法 / 274
膏人 / 75
膏药 / 281
膏药风 / 603
膏滋 / 281

gǎo

藁本 / 296

gē

割治疗法 / 478

gé

革脉 / 162
格阳 / 80
格阴 / 79
格致余论 / 701
鬲咽 / 543
葛根 / 297
葛根黄芩黄连汤 / 367
蛤蚧 / 348
隔姜灸 / 465
隔蒜灸 / 466
隔物灸 / 465
隔盐灸 / 466
膈 / 42
膈关 / 422
膈俞 / 420
膈噎 / 543

gě

葛洪 / 659
葛可久 / 667
葛乾孙 / 667
葛稚川 / 660

gēng

更年安 / 395

gōng

弓步 / 496
公孙 / 415
攻补兼施 / 220
攻毒 / 270
攻溃 / 270
攻下 / 236
攻下药 / 289
攻下逐瘀 / 238
攻逐水饮 / 237
肱 / 47
宫冷不孕 / 565
龚庆宣 / 660
龚廷贤 / 672
龚云林 / 672

gōu

钩藤 / 338

gǒu

狗脊 / 347
枸杞子 / 343

gòu

垢胎 / 566

gū

孤阳上越 / 80

gǔ

古今图书集成医部全录 / 704
古今医案按 / 702
古今医统 / 703
古今医统大全 / 703
谷精草 / 304
谷气 / 53
谷芽 / 351
股 / 49
股疽 / 594
股癣 / 604
股阳疽 / 595
股阴疽 / 595
股肿 / 606
骨 / 25
骨痹 / 541
骨病 / 654
骨槽风 / 633
骨错缝 / 646
骨度法 / 445
骨度分寸定穴法 / 445
骨疳 / 581
骨鲠 / 631
骨解 / 52
骨空 / 52
骨痨 / 596，656
骨瘤 / 598
骨伤科（学）/ 635
骨碎补 / 347
骨痿 / 539
骨折 / 635
骨蒸 / 529
骨蒸热 / 583
蛊毒 / 69
臌胀（病）/ 547
瞽症 / 622

gù

固［痼］疾 / 524
固崩止带 / 263
固崩止血 / 262
固表止汗 / 261
固表止汗剂 / 374
固表止汗药 / 294
固冲止带 / 263
固冲止血 / 262
固定垫 / 641
固定痛 / 148
固经止血 / 262
固精 / 262
固精丸 / 374
固涩 / 261
固涩剂 / 373
固涩药 / 294
固肾 / 262
固肾涩精 / 262
固肾缩尿 / 262
固肾止带 / 262

guā

瓜蒌 / 299
瓜蒌薤白半夏汤 / 375
瓜藤缠 / 601
刮柄法 / 455
刮法 / 481
刮痧 / 481
刮痧板 / 469
刮痧疗法 / 469
刮眼眶 / 487

guà

挂线疗法 / 273

guān

关冲 / 426

关刺 / 460
关格 / 544
关格病 / 544
关门 / 413
关木通 / 321
关元 / 435
关元俞 / 420

guǎn

管针进针法 / 454

guàn

冠心苏合丸 / 393

guāng

光剥舌 / 136
光明 / 431

guǎng

广豆根 / 313
广藿香 / 319

guī

归经 / 279
归来 / 413
归脾汤 / 372
龟板 / 345
龟背 / 578
龟甲 / 345
龟龄集 / 390
龟鹿二仙胶 / 373
龟胸 / 578

guǐ

鬼门 / 42
鬼胎 / 567

guì

桂附地黄丸 / 390
桂枝 / 295
桂枝汤 / 361

gǔn

滚刺疗法 / 452
滚刺［针］筒 / 452
滚法 / 481，649
滚法推拿 / 490

guó

国公酒 / 393
腘 / 50

H

há

虾蟆瘟 / 520

hái

孩儿参 / 340

hǎi

海风藤 / 315
海金沙 / 323
海马 / 348
海螵蛸 / 350
海泉 / 440
海桐皮 / 316
海藻 / 300

hán

含漱 / 273
含胸拔背 / 494
韩懋 / 668
韩氏医通 / 701
寒 / 64
寒痹 / 540
寒从中生 / 91
寒毒 / 69
寒霍乱 / 523
寒剂 / 360
寒结 / 544
寒结胸 / 520
寒厥 / 538
寒冷腹痛 / 546
寒凝胞宫证 / 194，213
寒凝气滞 / 94
寒凝痛经 / 560
寒凝血瘀证 / 194
寒疟 / 521
寒呕 / 542
寒气腹痛 / 546
寒气霍乱 / 523
寒热 / 169
寒热辨证 / 169
寒热错杂 / 91
寒热失调 / 90
寒热往来 / 143
寒热真假 / 91
寒热转化 / 83
寒入血室 / 91
寒痧 / 583
寒胜痛痹证 / 195
寒湿 / 68
寒湿困脾 / 105
寒湿困脾证 / 206
寒湿痢 / 521
寒湿内阻证 / 196
寒湿腰痛 / 553
寒湿证 / 196
寒痰 / 527
寒痰证 / 189
寒痰阻肺证 / 203
寒吐 / 586
寒下 / 236
寒下剂 / 364
寒痫 / 590
寒哮 / 527
寒邪 / 64
寒邪犯胃证 / 208
寒邪外束 / 91
寒泻 / 546
寒夜啼 / 577
寒因寒用 / 221
寒饮内停证 / 188
寒饮停肺证 / 188
寒饮停胃证 / 188
寒战 / 143
寒瘴 / 521
寒证 / 169
寒滞肝脉 / 104
寒滞肝脉证 / 211
寒滞经脉证 / 195
寒滞胃肠证 / 194
寒滞心脉证 / 194

hàn

汗 / 58

汗病 / 531
汗出如油 / 146
汗法 / 225
汗证 / 531
颔 / 46
颔厌 / 428

háng

颃颡 / 40，628

hāo

蒿芩清胆汤 / 365

háo

毫毛 / 41
毫针 / 449

hē

诃子 / 349

hé

禾髎 / 411
合病 / 178
合谷 / 410
合谷刺 / 460
合骨 / 50
合骨垫 / 641
合欢花 / 336
合欢皮 / 336
合金针 / 452
合邪 / 63
合穴 / 438
合阳 / 422
合掌震桩导气 / 503
合指捏法 / 652
何炳元 / 680
何廉臣 / 681
何梦瑶 / 676
何首乌 / 344
何西池 / 677
和法 / 238
和剂局方 / 691
和解表里 / 238
和解法 / 238
和解剂 / 365
和解少阳 / 238
和解少阳剂 / 365
和髎 / 428
和胃 / 238
和血安胎 / 239
和血调经 / 239
和血熄风 / 239
和血止痛 / 239
和营 / 239
和营活血 / 240
和营生新 / 240
和营止痛 / 240
和中 / 238
河车大造丸 / 389
荷叶 / 320
核骨 / 50
核桃仁 / 346
颌 / 46
颌下痈 / 629

hè

鹤草芽 / 354
鹤顶 / 443
鹤虱 / 353

hēi

黑白丑 / 324
黑丑 / 324
黑疔 / 623
黑睛 / 609
黑色 / 126
黑苔 / 135
黑芝麻 / 345

héng

横刺 / 454
横垫 / 641
横骨 / 48，424
横目斜视 / 129
横透 / 454
横指同身寸 / 445

hōng

烘焙 / 276

hóng

红蝴蝶疮 / 601
红花 / 330
红膜 / 612
红芪 / 340
红舌 / 131
红丝疔 / 592
红外线灸 / 467
红霞映日 / 619
虹彩 / 609
洪脉 / 161

hóu

喉嗌 / 628
喉痹 / 629，630
喉底 / 628
喉蛾 / 628
喉风 / 630
喉疳 / 631
喉关 / 40，628
喉关痈 / 629
喉核 / 40，628
喉菌 / 631
喉瘤 / 631
喉痧 / 520，585
喉癣 / 629
喉岩 / 631
喉喑［瘖］/ 630
喉痈 / 629
瘊子 / 600

hòu

后侧夹板 / 640
后顶 / 434
后发际 / 42
后伸扳腰法 / 653
后天失调 / 73
后天之精 / 57
后天之气 / 53
后溪 / 417
后下 / 283
后阴 / 48
厚朴 / 325
厚朴花 / 327
厚苔 / 135

候气 / 456

hū

呼吸 / 140
呼吸补泻 / 457
呼吸补泻法 / 457
呼吸气粗 / 140
呼吸气微 / 140
呼吸之气 / 53
忽思慧 / 667

hú

狐臭 / 605
狐惑 / 547
胡黄连 / 308
胡椒 / 318
葫芦 / 323
葫芦巴 / 347
葫芦垫 / 641
糊丸 / 280

hǔ

虎步功 / 502
虎口 / 52
虎杖 / 309
琥珀 / 336

hù

户门 / 40

huā

花椒 / 318
花蕊石 / 329
花翳白陷 / 618

huá

华盖 / 436
滑伯仁 / 667
滑剂 / 360
滑精 / 155
滑精（病） / 552
滑脉 / 161
滑肉门 / 413
滑石 / 321
滑寿 / 667
滑胎 / 569
滑苔 / 135
滑泄 / 545

huà

化风 / 92
化腐 / 269
化火 / 92
化橘红 / 327
化脓灸 / 465
化热 / 92
化湿 / 259
化湿和胃剂 / 379
化湿药 / 289
化石 / 272
化痰 / 258
化痰开窍 / 267
化痰宣肺 / 228
化痰药 / 292
化痰止咳平喘药 / 292
化饮 / 259
化饮解表 / 230
化饮宽胸 / 259
化饮宁心 / 259
化瘀药 / 292
化瘀止血药 / 291
化燥 / 92
华旉 / 659
华山参 / 304
华佗 / 659
华佗再造丸 / 394

huái

怀牛膝 / 344
槐花 / 329
槐角 / 329
槐米 / 329

huán

环跳 / 430
环跳疽 / 595

huǎn

缓方 / 357
缓脉 / 161
缓下 / 236

huāng

肓门 / 422
肓俞 / 425

huáng

皇甫谧 / 659
皇甫士安 / 659
黄柏 / 307
黄带 / 158，564
黄疸 / 523
黄帝内经 / 683
黄帝内经灵枢经 / 683
黄帝内经灵枢注证发微 / 684
黄帝内经素问 / 683
黄帝内经素问注证发微 / 684
黄耳伤寒 / 624
黄风 / 620
黄风内障 / 620
黄汗 / 531
黄精 / 341，610
黄连 / 307
黄连解毒汤 / 368
黄栌 / 309
黄膜上冲 / 618
黄腻苔 / 134
黄脓上冲 / 618
黄胖 / 139，547
黄胖病 / 547
黄芪 / 340
黄芪桂枝五物汤 / 370
黄芩 / 307
黄仁 / 610
黄色 / 125
黄水疮 / 604
黄苔 / 134
黄庭经 / 700
黄土汤 / 377
黄药子 / 301
黄液上冲 / 618
黄油障 / 618
黄油证 / 618
黄芫花 / 324

huī

灰苔 / 135
恢刺 / 461

huí

回光返照 / 123
回乳 / 268
回旋 / 639
回旋灸 / 464
回阳 / 240
回阳救逆 / 240
回阳救逆剂 / 370
蛔疳 / 582
蛔厥 / 538

huì

会厌 / 40
会阳 / 421
会阴 / 48，435
会宗 / 427
秽气气感 / 505
秽浊 / 72

hūn

昏厥 / 538
昏蒙 / 123
昏睡露睛 / 129

hún

混睛外障 / 619
混睛障 / 618
混障症 / 619
魂 / 57
魂门 / 422

huó

活血 / 256
活血化瘀 / 256
活血化瘀药 / 291
活血疗伤药 / 292
活血祛瘀 / 256
活血祛瘀剂 / 376
活血祛瘀药 / 291
活血调经 / 256
活血调经药 / 292
活血通经 / 256
活血通络 / 256
活血行气 / 256
活血行气药 / 292
活血药 / 292
活血止痛 / 256
活血止痛药 / 292

huǒ

火 / 66
火不生土 / 13
火带疮 / 600
火丹 / 593
火毒 / 68
火毒攻喉证 / 199
火毒攻舌证 / 199
火毒内陷证 / 198
火毒证 / 198
火疳 / 617
火罐法 / 468
火克金 / 12
火麻仁 / 352
火扰心神证 / 201
火热炽盛证 / 173
火伤 / 605
火伤血络 / 90
火生土 / 11
火痰 / 528
火陷 / 596
火邪 / 66
火邪经闭 / 559
火形之人 / 73
火眼 / 616
火疡 / 617
火针 / 450
火针疗法 / 450
火制 / 276

huò

霍乱 / 522
霍乱病 / 522
霍乱论 / 694
霍乱转筋 / 523
藿香 / 319
藿香正气散 / 379
豁痰 / 259
豁痰开窍 / 267
豁痰醒脑 / 267

J

jī

击法 / 484，649
击头 / 487
击下肢 / 489
饥不欲食 / 153
肌 / 41
肌痹 / 541
肌腠 / 41
肌肤不仁 / 147
肌肤甲错 / 139
肌肤麻木 / 147
鸡骨草 / 308
鸡内金 / 352
鸡胸 / 578
鸡血藤 / 332
鸡眼 / 601
积聚 / 548
积吐 / 587
积证 / 548
箕门 / 415
激光针 / 470
激经 / 566

jí

极泉 / 416
急方 / 357
急喉痹 / 630
急喉风 / 630
急喉喑［瘖］/ 630
急黄 / 523
急火 / 283
急惊风 / 574
急脉 / 433
急下 / 236
急下存津 / 237
急下存阴 / 236
疾病；疾；病 / 122

疾脉 / 162
疾徐补泻 / 457
疾徐补泻法 / 458
蒺藜 / 339
嫉妒不孕 / 565

jǐ

挤法 / 484
脊 / 50
脊中 / 433

jì

忌口 / 284
季经 / 556
季肋 / 48
季胁 / 48
季胁痛 / 547
剂量 / 280
剂型 / 280
荠菜 / 329
济生方 / 691
济阴纲目 / 695

jiā

加辅料炒 / 277
加减葳蕤汤 / 363
加味乌药汤 / 375
加味逍遥丸 / 386
痂 / 591
夹板固定 / 640
夹板固定疗法 / 640
夹持进针法 / 453
夹脊 / 441，506
夹挤分骨 / 638
夹惊吐 / 587

jiá

颊 / 45
颊车 / 46，411
颊脂垫 / 579

jiǎ

假寒 / 91
假热 / 91
假神 / 123

jià

架火法 / 468

jiān

间气 / 18
间使 / 426
肩 / 46
肩臂功 / 501，653
肩臂酸痛 / 147
肩不举 / 147
肩胛 / 47
肩胛疽 / 594
肩井 / 430
肩髎 / 427
肩痛 / 147
肩外俞 / 418
肩髃 / 410
肩贞 / 418
肩中俞 / 418
煎膏 / 281
煎药法 / 283

jiǎn

茧唇 / 598
趼子 / 601
减肥功 / 503
睑废 / 614
睑内 / 45，609
睑内结石 / 614
睑皮垂缓 / 614
睑弦 / 44，608
睑弦赤烂 / 613
睑弦糜烂 / 614
睑粘睛珠 / 613

jiàn

间隔灸 / 465
间接灸 / 465
建里 / 436
剑决式 / 504
剑针 / 452
健脾 / 245
健脾补肺 / 246
健脾和胃 / 245
健脾化湿 / 245
健脾化痰 / 245
健脾利湿 / 245
健脾利水 / 245
健脾祛湿 / 245
健脾消食 / 245
健脾养血 / 246
健脾益气 / 246
健脾止带 / 246
健脾止泻 / 246
健忘 / 146，535
健胃 / 246
健胃止呕 / 246
渐聋 / 625
楗 / 51
鉴真 / 661
箭头针 / 451

jiāng

姜黄 / 331
姜炙 / 277
僵蚕 / 338

jiàng

降剂 / 360
降逆平喘 / 254
降逆下气 / 254
降逆止呃 / 254
降逆止咳平喘 / 254
降逆止呕 / 254
降气 / 254
降气化痰 / 253
降气剂 / 375
降气平喘 / 254
降气止呃 / 254
降香 / 327
绛舌 / 131
强硬舌 / 133

jiāo

交叉选穴法 / 447
交肠 / 599
交骨 / 49
交骨不开 / 570
交会经配穴法 / 448

交会选穴法 / 447
交会穴 / 439
交接出血 / 564
交通心肾 / 239
交信 / 424
胶 / 282
胶囊剂 / 282
椒疮 / 613
焦麦芽 / 351
焦三仙 / 352
焦山楂 / 351

jiǎo

角弓反张 / 127
角孙 / 428
绞肠痧 / 522
绞痛 / 148
脚气 / 539
脚气冲心 / 539
脚气疮 / 604
脚弱 / 539
脚湿气 / 604
脚肿 / 138
搅肠痧 / 523
搅舌 / 488

jiào

叫化功 / 502

jiē

疖 / 591
疖病 / 592
接触性皮炎 / 603
接法 / 639
接骨续筋 / 639

jié

洁净府 / 261
结核 / 591
结喉 / 46
结脉 / 162
结膜红赤 / 612
结舌 / 579
结胸 / 519
结扎疗法 / 273
睫毛倒入 / 613
截疟 / 271

jiě

解表 / 225
解表剂 / 361
解表清肺 / 225
解表清热 / 225
解表透疹 / 226
解表药 / 287
解毒 / 270
解毒透疹 / 226
解毒消肿 / 270
解肌 / 225
解肌发表 / 226
解肌清热 / 226
解肌透疹 / 226
解酒毒 / 270
解颅 / 577
解颅病 / 577
解索脉 / 163
解围元薮 / 697
解溪 / 414

jiè

疥疮 / 603
疥癞 / 603

jīn

金不换膏 / 395
金疮 / 605
金疮痉 / 605
金创 / 605，635
金沸草 / 299
金疳 / 617
金寒水冷 / 14
金津 / 440
金井 / 609
金克木 / 12
金匮肾气丸 / 373
金匮要略 / 686
金匮要略方论 / 686
金匮要略心典 / 686
金匮翼 / 686
金铃子散 / 375
金门 / 423
金礞石 / 301
金钱白花蛇 / 315
金钱草 / 322
金生水 / 11
金锁固精丸 / 374
金形之人 / 74
金疡 / 617，635
金银花 / 310
金银藤 / 310
金樱子 / 351
金针 / 452
金针拨障法 / 479
津 / 58
津枯肠燥 / 90
津亏火炽 / 81
津亏热结 / 81
津亏热结证 / 187
津亏血燥 / 81
津亏证 / 187
津气 / 54
津气亏虚证 / 187
津伤证 / 187
津脱 / 81，550
津液 / 58
津液辨证 / 187
津液亏损证 / 187
津液亏虚证 / 187
筋 / 42
筋痹 / 541
筋粗 / 643
筋断 / 643
筋疳 / 581
筋合 / 647
筋结 / 643
筋瘤 / 598
筋柔 / 643
筋伤 / 643
筋缩 / 433，643
筋惕肉瞤/ 127

筋痿 / 539，643
筋瘿 / 597
筋正 / 647
筋之府 / 50

jǐn

紧按慢提 / 456
紧喉风 / 630
紧脉 / 162
紧提慢按 / 457
锦灯笼 / 313

jìn

进针 / 452
进针法 / 452
近视 / 621
近血 / 550
浸淫疮 / 603
禁方 / 357
禁灸穴 / 467
禁针穴 / 463
噤风 / 575
噤口痢 / 522

jīng

茎 / 49
茎垂 / 49
京大戟 / 324
京骨 / 423
京门 / 430
经崩 / 561
经闭 / 157，559
经别 / 407
经迟 / 557
经刺 / 460
经带胎产 / 556
经断 / 158
经断复来 / 563
经方 / 357
经间期出血 / 560
经筋 / 406
经绝 / 158
经来发热 / 562
经来泄泻 / 563
经漏 / 561
经乱 / 558
经络 / 398
经络辨证 / 215，408
经络学说 / 398
经络证候 / 408
经络之气 / 55
经脉 / 398
经期错后 / 557
经期水肿 / 562
经期延长 / 559
经气 / 55
经气逆乱 / 114
经气衰竭 / 114
经气虚损 / 114
经气郁滞 / 114
经渠 / 409
经史证类备急本草 / 688
经水 / 556
经水不调 / 557
经水断绝 / 157
经水过多 / 560
经水后期 / 557
经水涩少 / 558
经水先期 / 557
经隧 / 398
经隧失职 / 114
经外穴 / 439
经效产宝 / 694
经行便血 / 562
经行发热 / 562
经行风疹块 / 563
经行浮肿 / 562
经行腹痛 / 158，560
经行后期 / 157，557
经行口糜 / 563
经行痞瘤 / 563
经行衄血 / 562
经行情志异常 / 563
经行乳房胀痛 / 563
经行身痛 / 562
经行头痛 / 562
经行吐衄 / 562
经行吐血 / 562
经行先后无定期 / 157
经行先期 / 157，557
经行泄泻 / 563
经行眩晕 / 562
经行隐疹 / 563
经穴 / 408，437
经血 / 556
经早 / 557
经证 / 178
荆防败毒散 / 363
荆芥 / 295
荆芥穗 / 296
荆芥炭 / 296
惊 / 70
惊风 / 574
惊风八候 / 574
惊风病 / 574
惊风抽搐 / 575
惊风烦渴 / 576
惊风腹痛 / 576
惊疳 / 581
惊悸 / 530
惊厥 / 575
惊热 / 583
惊吐 / 587
惊痫 / 535，589
惊震内障 / 620
晶痦 / 139
晶珠 / 610
睛高突起 / 622
睛帘 / 609
睛明 / 418
睛胀 / 622
精 / 2，56
精、气、神 / 498
精寒 / 553
精冷 / 553
精瘤 / 600

精明之府 / 42
精气 / 2，54
精气互化 / 2
精气学说 / 2
精窍 / 49
精少 / 553
精神 / 57
精室 / 49
精髓空虚 / 111
精微 / 57
精血 / 56
精汁 / 57
精珠 / 610
精浊 / 599

jǐng

井穴 / 437
颈 / 46
颈白劳 / 440
颈骨 / 50
颈松 / 493
颈项功 / 501
颈痈 / 593
颈椎侧旋复位法 / 652
颈椎单人旋转复位法 / 652
颈椎角度复位法 / 652
景岳全书 / 704

jìng

胫 / 50
胫骨 / 50，51
痉病 / 538
静功 / 491
静留针法 / 462
静中有动 / 492
静坐 / 505
镜面舌 / 136

jiū

鸠尾 / 47，436
揪法 / 483
揪痧 / 486

jiǔ

九刺 / 460
九九阳功 / 503
九窍 / 38
九味羌活汤 / 361
九香虫 / 327
九针 / 451
久咳 / 142
久痢 / 522
久流浊涕 / 130
久疟 / 521
久嗽 / 142
久泄［泻］/ 545
灸 / 463
灸法 / 463
灸忌 / 467
灸禁 / 467
灸疗法 / 463
韭菜子 / 348
韭子 / 348
酒刺 / 601
酒剂 / 281
酒醴 / 281
酒癖 / 70
酒皶鼻 / 601
酒炙 / 277

jiù

救荒本草 / 688
救脱 / 240
救阳 / 240

jū

拘急 / 127
拘挛 / 127
居经 / 556
居髎 / 430
疽 / 594

jú

局部选穴法 / 446
局方发挥 / 692
桔梗 / 299
菊花 / 297
橘核 / 325
橘红 / 325
橘红丸［片］/ 383
橘皮竹茹汤 / 376

jǔ

举、按、寻 / 158
举法 / 159

jù

巨刺 / 460
巨骨 / 410
巨髎 / 411
巨阙 / 436
拒按 / 166
聚泉 / 440
聚星障 / 618
聚证 / 548

juǎn

卷柏 / 332

jué

决明子 / 304
绝汗 / 145
绝经前后诸病 / 563
厥 / 537
厥热胜复 / 116
厥心痛 / 530
厥阴病 / 178
厥阴病机 / 116
厥阴病证 / 177
厥阴俞 / 419
厥证 / 537

jūn

君臣佐使 / 358
君火 / 21
君药 / 358
皲裂 / 601
皲裂疮 / 601

jùn

峻下 / 236
峻下逐水药 / 289

K

kǎ

咯血 / 137，550

kāi

开达膜［募］原 / 238
开鬼门 / 229
开阖补泻 / 457
开阖补泻法 / 457
开窍 / 266
开窍药 / 293
开胃 / 246
开泄 / 229

kāo

尻 / 51
尻骨 / 51

kào

靠坐 / 495

kē

柯琴 / 675
柯韵伯 / 675
颗粒剂 / 282
颗粒型皮内针 / 450
髁骨 / 51

ké

咳逆 / 526
咳逆上气 / 141，526
咳如犬吠 / 142
咳声不扬 / 141
咳声清脆 / 141
咳声重浊 / 141
咳嗽 / 141，524
咳血 / 137，550

kè

客气 / 18
客热 / 583
客色 / 124
客忤 / 577
客忤夜啼 / 577
客邪 / 62
客运 / 18

kōng

空腹服 / 284
空痛 / 148

kǒng

孔窍 / 38
孔最 / 409
恐 / 70

kòng

控睾 / 154
控脑砂 / 627

kōu

抠法 / 481
芤脉 / 162

kǒu

口 / 39
口不仁 / 155
口齿科（学）/ 632
口臭 / 142
口疮 / 579，633
口唇干裂 / 136
口唇糜烂 / 136
口唇青紫 / 137
口撮 / 136
口淡 / 154
口动 / 136
口干 / 149
口干不欲饮 / 149
口甘 / 155
口疳 / 580，633
口禾髎 / 411
口角流涎 / 136
口噤 / 136，537
口渴 / 148
口渴喜冷 / 149
口渴引饮 / 149
口苦 / 155
口糜 / 579，633
口僻 / 136，537
口气 / 142
口气臭秽 / 142
口气酸臭 / 142
口酸 / 155
口甜 / 155
口㖞 / 127，537
口眼㖞斜 / 127
口吻疮 / 580
口咸 / 155
口粘腻 / 155
口振 / 136
口中和 / 154
口中无味 / 154

kòu

叩［扣］齿 / 488
叩［扣］法 / 484
叩齿 / 505
寇平 / 668
寇宗奭 / 663
蔻仁 / 319

kū

枯矾 / 354
枯痔法 / 273

kǔ

苦寒清气 / 231
苦寒清热 / 230
苦寒泄热 / 231
苦寒泻火 / 231
苦寒燥湿 / 260
苦楝皮 / 353
苦参 / 308
苦温平燥 / 244
苦温燥湿 / 244，260
苦夏 / 582
苦杏仁 / 301

kù

库房 / 412

kuà

胯腹痈 / 593
胯骨 / 51

kuài

快速起针法 / 463

kuān

宽解衣带 / 493
宽胸 / 254
宽胸散结 / 254
宽中散结 / 254
髋骨 / 51，443

kuǎn

款冬花 / 301

kuáng

狂 / 534
狂病 / 534
狂言 / 140

kuì

溃坚 / 270
溃疡 / 591

kūn

坤草 / 334
昆布 / 300
昆仑 / 423

L

lā

拉法 / 639
拉腿手法 / 486

là

蜡丸 / 280

lái

莱菔子 / 352

lài

癞病 / 605

lán

兰室秘藏 / 701
阑门 / 41
阑尾 / 443

làn

烂疔 / 592
烂喉丹痧 / 520，585
烂喉痧 / 520

láng

狼毒 / 324

láo

劳［痨］瘵 / 529
劳复 / 71
劳宫 / 426
劳倦 / 71
劳咳 / 526
劳淋 / 552
劳疟 / 521
劳伤 / 71
劳嗽 / 526
劳蒸 / 530
牢脉 / 162
痨病 / 529

lǎo

老鹳草 / 316

lào

烙法 / 272

léi

雷丰 / 681
雷公 / 658
雷公炮炙论 / 689
雷公药性赋 / 689
雷火神针 / 466
雷少逸 / 681
雷头风 / 533
雷丸 / 353
雷敩 / 660

lèi

泪 / 58
泪点 / 609
泪窍 / 43，609
泪泉 / 609
泪堂 / 609
类经 / 684
类经图翼 / 684
类证治裁 / 694
类中 / 536
类中风 / 536

lěng

冷服 / 284
冷汗 / 145
冷泪 / 615
冷庐医话 / 702
冷秘 / 544
冷痛 / 148
冷哮 / 527
冷心痛 / 531
冷罨 / 272
冷瘴 / 521

lí

离而复合 / 640
离体周天 / 500
蠡沟 / 432

lǐ

李濒湖 / 670
李东璧 / 670
李东垣 / 665
李杲 / 665
李濂 / 669
李明之 / 665
李时珍 / 670
李士材 / 673
李惺庵 / 675
李修之 / 675
李梴 / 669
李用粹 / 675
李正宇 / 671
李中立 / 671
李中梓 / 673
里寒 / 82
里寒证 / 170
里喉痈 / 629
里急后重 / 150
里热 / 82
里热证 / 170
里实 / 82
里实证 / 171
里水 / 549
里虚 / 82
里虚寒证 / 170
里虚热证 / 171
里证 / 169
理肺功 / 501
理筋 / 647
理筋手法 / 647
理脾功 / 501
理气 / 252
理气安胎 / 256
理气导滞 / 255

理气和胃 / 238
理气和血 / 239
理气化湿 / 255
理气化痰 / 253
理气化瘀 / 256
理气活血 / 253
理气剂 / 374
理气健脾 / 253
理气解郁 / 255
理气通经 / 256
理气消痞 / 253
理气消胀 / 255
理气药 / 290
理气止痛 / 252，256
理伤续断秘方 / 697
理心功 / 501
理血 / 256
理血剂 / 376
理血药 / 291
理瀹骈文 / 693
理中 / 238
理中汤 / 369

lì

历节风 / 540
历兑 / 414
立迟 / 577
利胆退黄药 / 290
利尿 / 260
利尿通淋药 / 290
利尿逐水药 / 290
利气 / 252
利湿 / 260
利湿退黄药 / 290
利湿药 / 290
利水 / 260
利水除湿 / 260
利水渗湿 / 260
利水渗湿药 / 290
利水消肿 / 261
利水消肿药 / 290
利小便，实大便 / 261
利咽 / 271
沥胞生 / 569
沥浆产 / 569
沥浆生 / 569
沥血腰痛 / 554
疠风 / 605
疠气；戾气 / 63
荔枝核 / 327
痢疾 / 521

lián

连翘 / 310
连舌 / 579
帘珠喉痹 / 629
莲花舌 / 634
莲须 / 349
莲子 / 349
莲子心 / 305
廉泉 / 437
臁疮 / 595

liǎn

敛肺 / 262
敛肺平喘 / 262
敛肺涩肠药 / 294
敛肺止咳 / 262
敛肺止咳剂 / 374
敛汗 / 261
敛汗固表 / 261
敛汗固表药 / 294
敛汗固脱 / 261
敛气 / 262
敛阴 / 262

liàn

练功 / 499，653
练气 / 503
练神 / 498
炼丹 / 498
炼己 / 499
炼精 / 499
炼精化气 / 499
炼气 / 499
炼气化神 / 499
炼神 / 499

liáng

良方 / 357
良附丸 / 375
莨菪子 / 304
凉肝熄［息］风 / 266
凉血 / 233
凉血解毒 / 233
凉血散瘀 / 235
凉血止痢 / 235
凉血止血 / 258
凉血止血药 / 291
凉燥 / 66，518
凉燥病 / 519
凉燥证 / 197
梁门 / 413
梁丘 / 414

liǎng

两面针 / 333
两目垂帘内视 / 494
两眼翻上 / 129
两眼无光 / 128

liǎo

蓼大青叶 / 311

liè

列缺 / 409
裂纹舌 / 133

lín

邻近选穴法 / 446
林佩琴 / 679
林羲桐 / 679
林云和 / 679
临产 / 568
临产病 / 569
临睡前服 / 284
临证指南医案 / 702

lìn

淋（证）/ 551
淋病 / 551
淋浊 / 551

líng

灵道 / 416
灵枢 / 684
灵台 / 434
灵墟 / 425
灵芝 / 337
凌霄花 / 332
羚羊角 / 338

lìng

另煎 / 283

liú

刘昉 / 663
刘涓子鬼遗方 / 697
刘守真 / 664
刘完素 / 664
留罐 / 469
留针 / 462
留针拔罐 / 469
留针候气 / 456
流火 / 594
流金凌木 / 615
流泪病症 / 615
流泪证 / 614
流痰 / 596
流涎 / 578
流注 / 595
硫黄 / 354
瘤 / 598

liù

六腑 / 20
六经 / 399
六经辨证 / 175
六经病 / 175
六经病机 / 115
六经病证 / 175
六科证治准绳 / 704
六气 / 17，62
六神丸 / 395
六味地黄汤 / 372
六味地黄丸 / 389
六阳脉 / 400
六一散 / 369
六阴脉 / 400
六淫 / 62
六郁 / 70

lóng

龙齿 / 337
龙胆 / 308
龙胆草 / 308
龙胆泻肝汤 / 368
龙骨 / 337
龙虎草 / 324
龙葵 / 312
龙门 / 555
龙衔式 / 505
龙眼肉 / 342
癃闭 / 552

lóu

楼公爽 / 667
楼英 / 667
蝼蛄 / 323
蝼蛄疖 / 592

lòu

漏 / 591
漏谷 / 415
漏汗 / 145
漏睛 / 615
漏睛疮 / 615
漏睛脓出 / 615
漏睛眼 / 615
漏芦 / 312
漏下 / 561

lú

卢和 / 669
芦根 / 305
芦荟 / 353
炉甘石 / 355
颅息 / 428

lù

陆九芝 / 680
陆懋修 / 680
陆以湉 / 681
陆渊雷 / 682
鹿角 / 345
鹿角胶 / 346
鹿角霜 / 346
鹿茸 / 345
鹿衔草 / 345
路路通 / 323
鹭鸶咳 / 586
露 / 281
露剂 / 281

lǜ

绿萼梅 / 327
绿风 / 620
绿风内障 / 619
葎草 / 313

lún

轮屏切迹 / 473

luó

罗布麻叶 / 305
罗汉果 / 301
罗汉针 / 450
罗谦甫 / 666
罗天益 / 666

luǒ

瘰疬 / 596

luò

络刺 / 460
络脉 / 398
络却 / 419
络石藤 / 315
络穴 / 438

M

má

麻毒 / 69
麻毒闭肺 / 584
麻毒攻目 / 584
麻毒内攻 / 584
麻毒入营 / 584
麻毒陷肺 / 584
麻风 / 605
麻黄 / 295

麻黄根 / 348
麻黄汤 / 361
麻木 / 148，537
麻仁润肠丸 / 386
麻仁丸 / 386
麻杏石甘汤 / 362
麻疹 / 584
麻疹闭证 / 584
麻疹逆证 / 584
麻疹顺证 / 584
麻疹险证 / 584
麻子仁丸 / 365

mǎ

马鞭草 / 334
马勃 / 313
马齿苋 / 309
马兜铃 / 303
马脾风 / 586
马钱子 / 316
马莳 / 670
马桶癣 / 605
马牙 / 579

mái

埋针疗法 / 450

mài

麦冬 / 343
麦粒灸 / 465
麦粒型皮内针 / 450
麦门冬 / 343
麦门冬汤 / 378
麦味地黄丸 / 390
麦芽 / 351
脉 / 25
脉暴出 / 164
脉痹 / 541
脉从四时 / 164
脉经 / 686
脉静 / 164
脉口 / 160
脉逆四时 / 164
脉痿 / 539
脉无胃气 / 164
脉象 / 158
脉象主病 / 158
脉悬绝 / 165
脉学 / 158
脉阴阳俱浮 / 164
脉阴阳俱紧 / 164
脉应四时 / 164
脉有根 / 164
脉有神 / 164
脉有胃气 / 164
脉躁 / 164
脉诊 / 158
脉症合参 / 165

mǎn

满山红 / 302

màn

蔓荆子 / 297
慢喉喑［瘖］/ 630
慢火 / 283
慢惊风 / 574
慢惊夹痰 / 575
慢惊自汗 / 575
慢脾风 / 575
慢性复位 / 642

máng

芒刺舌 / 133
芒硝 / 352
盲 / 612

māo

猫眼疮 / 601

máo

毛刺 / 460
毛冬青 / 334
毛际 / 48

mào

冒湿 / 518
冒暑 / 516

méi

眉冲 / 419
眉棱骨 / 43
眉心 / 43
梅核气 / 535，631
梅花 / 327
梅花针 / 450

mèn

闷痧 / 583
闷痛 / 147

méng

虻虫 / 333

měng

猛疽 / 629

mèng

孟诜 / 661
梦遗 / 155，552

mǐ

米壳 / 350

mì

秘传眼科龙木论 / 698
秘方 / 357
密蒙花 / 305
蜜丸 / 280
蜜炙 / 277

mián

绵萆薢 / 322
棉枕固定 / 640

miàn

面壁 / 499
面尘 / 125
面浮 / 125
面黑 / 125
面红 / 125
面黄肌瘦 / 125
面色 / 124
面色㿠白 / 125
面色苍白 / 125
面色淡白 / 125
面色黎黑 / 125
面色萎黄 / 125
面游风 / 602
面针 / 477
面针疗法 / 478

miáo

苗窍 / 38

miǎo

眇目 / 622

miào

缪希雍 / 672
缪仲淳 / 672

míng

名医别录 / 687
名医类案 / 702
明矾 / 354
明目 / 271
明堂 / 625
明医杂著 / 701
鸣天鼓 / 488
瞑眩 / 146

mìng

命关 / 138
命火 / 27
命门 / 23，433
命门火衰 / 113
命门火旺 / 111
命门之火 / 27

miù

缪刺 / 461

mō

摸法 / 482

mó

膜原 / 42
摩法 / 482，650
摩腹 / 489
摩击上肢 / 489
摩颈项 / 488
摩面 / 487
摩脐 / 489

mǒ

抹法 / 482
抹前额 / 487

mò

没药 / 334
墨旱莲 / 330

mǔ

母 / 13
母气 / 13
牡丹皮 / 306
牡蛎 / 338
牡蛎散 / 374
牡脏 / 20
拇指同身寸 / 445

mù

木乘土 / 13
木瓜 / 314
木瓜丸 / 392
木蝴蝶 / 303
木火刑金 / 13
木克土 / 12
木舌 / 134，579
木生火 / 11
木通 / 321
木旺乘土 / 13
木香 / 326
木香顺气丸 / 387
木形之人 / 73
木贼 / 305
目 / 43
目胞 / 607
目胞浮肿 / 128
目本 / 610
目眵 / 610
目窗 / 429
目纲 / 44，608
目功 / 506
目裹 / 607
目窠上微肿 / 128
目窠肿 / 128
目眶 / 43，608
目眶骨 / 608
目连劄 / 614
目盲 / 612
目内眦 / 44，608
目偏视 / 622
目锐眦 / 44，607
目上胞 / 44，608
目上纲 / 608
目上网 / 608
目上弦 / 45，609
目痛 / 610
目外眦 / 608
目系 / 45，610
目下胞 / 45，609
目下纲 / 608
目下网 / 608
目下弦 / 45，609
目下有卧蚕 / 128
目下肿 / 128
目弦 / 44，608
目痒 / 622
目劄 / 614
目珠 / 610
目眦 / 44，607
募合配穴法 / 448
募穴 / 438
募原 / 42
暮食朝吐 / 152

N

ná

拿法 / 483，651
拿合谷 / 489
拿颈项 / 488
拿捏法 / 483

nà

纳呆 / 153
纳干法 / 459
纳甲法 / 459
纳气平喘 / 242
纳入原位 / 640
纳支法 / 459
纳子法 / 459
捺法 / 483
捺正 / 640

nǎi

奶麻 / 584

奶癣 / 604

nán

南瓜子 / 353
南鹤虱 / 354
南沙参 / 300
南雅堂医书全集 / 705
难产 / 569

nàn

难经 / 684
难经本义 / 684

náng

囊痈 / 599

náo

挠法 / 482
硇砂 / 355

nǎo

脑 / 25
脑崩 / 627
脑风 / 146
脑户 / 434
脑空 / 430
脑立清 / 385
脑漏 / 627
脑衄 / 628
脑渗 / 627

nào

臑 / 47
臑骨 / 47
臑会 / 427
臑俞 / 418

nèi

内吹 / 596
内吹乳痈 / 596
内丹 / 498
内丹功 / 498
内丹术 / 499
内钓 / 575
内毒 / 69
内翻 / 656
内风 / 64
内功 / 491
内功图说 / 700
内功推拿 / 490
内固定 / 642
内关 / 426
内寒 / 64
内踝 / 50
内踝尖 / 443
内经 / 683
内经知要 / 684
内景 / 493
内科杂病 / 524
内气 / 500
内伤 / 69
内伤发热 / 530
内伤咳嗽 / 526
内伤头痛 / 533
内伤腰痛 / 553
内湿 / 65
内视 / 493
内庭 / 414
内托 / 269
内外配穴法 / 448
内外痔 / 599
内膝眼 / 443
内陷 / 94，595
内消 / 269
内养功 / 500
内因 / 62
内迎香 / 440
内痈 / 593
内燥 / 66
内燥证 / 197
内障 / 612
内痔 / 599
内眦 / 44，608

néng

能近怯远症 / 621
能远怯近症 / 621

ní

泥丸 / 496
倪维德 / 667
倪仲贤 / 667

nì

逆传 / 179，515
逆传心包 / 85
逆腹式呼吸 / 497
逆经 / 560
逆流挽舟 / 230
逆治 / 220
腻苔 / 135

niǎn

捻法 / 481
捻衣摸床 / 124
捻转补泻 / 457
捻转补泻法 / 457
捻转法 / 454
碾挫伤 / 646

niào

尿赤 / 151
尿短赤 / 150
尿频 / 150
尿清长 / 150
尿血 / 151，550
尿浊 / 551

niē

捏法 / 482，652
捏积 / 486
捏脊 / 486

niè

颞后线 / 471
颞前线 / 471
颞颥 / 43

níng

凝脂翳 / 618

nǐng

拧法 / 481
拧眉心 / 487
拧拳反掌式 / 654

niú

牛蒡子 / 297
牛黄 / 335
牛黄降压丸 / 384

牛黄解毒丸［片］/ 384
牛黄清心丸［片］/ 384
牛黄上清丸 / 384
牛皮癣 / 602
牛西西 / 330
牛膝 / 344

niǔ

扭痧 / 486
扭伤 / 646

nóng

浓缩丸 / 280
脓毒证 / 199
脓耳 / 623
脓耳变证 / 623
脓耳口眼㖞斜 / 624
脓耳眩晕 / 625
脓疱 / 591
脓血便 / 150

nòng

弄舌 / 134
弄胎 / 569

nǔ

努法 / 455
弩法 / 455
胬肉扳睛 / 615
胬肉攀睛 / 615
胬肉侵睛 / 615

nù

怒 / 69

nǚ

女科百问 / 695
女科经纶 / 695
女劳复 / 71
女贞子 / 344
女子胞 / 25，556

nuǎn

暖肝煎 / 375
暖宫 / 243

nüè

疟 / 520
疟病 / 520
疟积 / 521
疟疾 / 520
疟母 / 521
疟痞 / 521

nuó

挪法 / 482

O

ǒu

呕乳 / 577，587
呕吐 / 542
呕吐清涎 / 152
呕吐宿食 / 152
呕吐酸腐 / 152
呕血 / 152
偶刺 / 461
偶方 / 356
藕节 / 330

P

pāi

拍法 / 483
拍击法 / 649

pái

排除杂念 / 499
排脓 / 269
排脓托毒 / 269
排脓消肿 / 269
排石 / 272

pān

攀索叠砖 / 642

pán

盘肠气痛 / 588
盘法 / 458
盘旋法 / 458
盘坐 / 495

páng

庞安时 / 662
膀胱 / 24
膀胱不利 / 113
膀胱咳 / 525
膀胱气闭 / 113
膀胱失约 / 113
膀胱湿热 / 114
膀胱湿热证 / 214
膀胱俞 / 420
膀胱虚寒 / 114
膀胱虚寒证 / 213

pàng

胖大海 / 303
胖大舌 / 132

pāo

脬气不固 / 113

pào

炮 / 277
炮姜 / 318
炮制 / 275
炮炙 / 275
炮炙大全 / 689
泡 / 276
泡腾片 / 280
疱疹 / 591

péi

培土 / 245
培土生金 / 247
培土抑木 / 247

pèi

佩兰 / 319
配方 / 357
配穴法 / 447

péng

硼砂 / 355

pī

铍针 / 452
劈法 / 649

pí

皮痹 / 541，602
皮肤针 / 449
皮肤针疗法 / 450
皮毛 / 41
皮内针 / 450
皮内针疗法 / 450

皮水 / 549
枇杷叶 / 301
脾 / 21
脾痹 / 541
脾病辨证 / 205
脾不统血 / 105
脾肺两虚 / 106
脾肺两虚证 / 207
脾肺气虚 / 106
脾肺气虚证 / 207
脾疳 / 580
脾经咳嗽 / 524
脾咳 / 525
脾劳 / 529
脾气 / 21，54
脾气不升 / 106
脾气不足 / 105
脾气下陷 / 94
脾气下陷证 / 206
脾气虚 / 104
脾气虚证 / 205
脾肾虚寒 / 107
脾肾虚寒证 / 207
脾肾阳虚 / 107
脾肾阳虚证 / 207
脾失健运 / 105
脾水 / 549
脾瘘 / 539
脾胃论 / 694
脾胃湿热 / 106
脾胃湿热证 / 206
脾胃虚寒 / 106
脾胃虚寒证 / 205
脾胃阳虚 / 106
脾胃阳虚证 / 205
脾消 / 551
脾虚 / 104
脾虚带下 / 564
脾虚动风证 / 206
脾虚寒证 / 205
脾虚经闭 / 559
脾虚气陷 / 94
脾虚气陷证 / 206
脾虚生风 / 106
脾虚生痰 / 106
脾虚湿困 / 105
脾虚湿困证 / 206
脾虚痰湿证 / 206
脾虚泄泻 / 545
脾虚泻 / 588
脾虚证 / 205
脾阳 / 22
脾阳不振 / 105
脾阳虚 / 105
脾阳虚证 / 205
脾阴 / 22
脾阴虚 / 105
脾阴虚证 / 205
脾俞 / 420
脾约 / 544
脾约丸 / 365
脾之大络 / 407

pǐ

痞 / 542
痞根 / 441
痞块 / 547
痞满 / 156
癖热 / 583
癖嗜 / 70

pì

睥翻粘睑 / 613
睥轮振跳 / 614
睥肉粘轮 / 613
睥生痰核 / 613
睥虚如球 / 614
辟谷功 / 503

piān

偏方 / 357
偏枯 / 537
偏历 / 410
偏头风 / 146，533
偏头痛 / 146，533
偏斜瞻视 / 622
偏阳质 / 73
偏阴质 / 73
偏坠 / 600

pián

胼胝 / 601

piàn

片 / 282
片剂 / 282
片姜黄 / 331

piāo

漂 / 276

pín

频服 / 284

pìn

牝疟 / 521
牝脏 / 20

píng

平贝母 / 302
平补平泻 / 458
平补平泻法 / 458
平喘药 / 303
平刺 / 454
平旦服 / 284
平垫 / 641
平肝 / 265
平肝潜阳 / 265
平肝熄［息］风 / 266
平肝熄［息］风药 / 293
平肝抑阳药 / 293
平脉 / 160
平气 / 18
平胃散 / 379
平稳出针法 / 462
平息 / 159
平熄内风剂 / 377
平掌式 / 504
平整复元 / 638
平坐 / 495
屏间切迹 / 473
屏上切迹 / 473

pò

破腘脱肉 / 127
破气 / 255
破伤风 / 605
破血 / 257
破血祛瘀 / 257
破血消癥药 / 292
破血逐瘀 / 257
破瘀 / 257
破瘀生新 / 257
破瘀消癥 / 257
魄 / 57
魄户 / 421
魄门 / 41
薄厥 / 538

pū

扑粉 / 273
仆参 / 423

pú

葡萄胎 / 567
蒲公英 / 311
蒲黄 / 332
蒲黄炭 / 333

pǔ

普济本事方 / 691
普济方 / 692
普济消毒饮 / 368

Q

qī

七冲门 / 40
七怪脉 / 163
七绝脉 / 163
七厘散 / 396
七窍 / 38
七情 / 69
七死脉 / 163
七星功 / 503
七星针 / 450
期门 / 433
漆疮 / 603

qí

齐刺 / 461
齐德之 / 666
齐仲甫 / 664
岐伯 / 658
奇方 / 356
奇恒之腑 / 24
奇经八脉 / 405
奇效良方 / 692
脐疮 / 578，593，603
脐带 / 566
脐风 / 575
脐风三证 / 575
脐腹 / 48
脐寒泻 / 588
脐呼吸 / 497
脐漏 / 593
脐疝 / 578
脐湿 / 578
脐突 / 578
脐下悸 / 154
脐下悸动 / 154
脐血 / 578
脐痈 / 593
骑马式 / 495
蕲蛇 / 315

qǐ

杞菊地黄丸 / 389
启脾丸 / 387
起罐 / 469
起针 / 462
起针法 / 462

qì

气 / 2，53
气闭 / 94
气闭神厥证 / 202
气闭证 / 182
气不摄［统］血证 / 186
气不摄血 / 95
气冲 / 413
气端 / 444
气分 / 56
气分证 / 179
气疳 / 581
气感 / 505
气鬲 / 586
气功 / 491
气功疗法 / 492
气功偏差 / 505
气臌（病） / 547
气关 / 138
气管炎丸 / 383
气海 / 25，435
气海俞 / 420
气户 / 412
气化 / 2，56
气化不利 / 93
气化无权 / 93
气机 / 2，56
气机不利 / 93
气机失调 / 93
气机郁滞 / 93
气积腹痛 / 588
气街 / 48
气厥 / 538
气口 / 160
气淋 / 552
气瘤 / 598
气轮 / 44，607
气门 / 41
气秘 / 544
气逆 / 94
气逆证 / 182
气痞 / 542
气色 / 124
气舍 / 412
气胜形 / 126
气随血脱 / 96
气随血脱证 / 186
气脱 / 93
气脱证 / 182
气味 / 278

气陷 / 94
气陷血崩 / 561
气陷证 / 182
气虚 / 92
气虚崩漏 / 561
气虚鼻窍失充证 / 183
气虚不摄 / 94
气虚耳窍失充证 / 183
气虚发热证 / 183
气虚感冒 / 516
气虚滑胎 / 569
气虚经行先期 / 557
气虚咳嗽 / 526
气虚气滞证 / 183
气虚湿阻［困］证 / 183
气虚水停证 / 183
气虚头痛 / 534
气虚外感证 / 183
气虚眩晕 / 532
气虚血瘀 / 95，96
气虚血瘀证 / 186
气虚证 / 182
气虚中满 / 95
气虚自汗 / 531
气穴 / 424
气血辨证 / 182
气血两燔 / 86
气血两燔证 / 180
气血两亏 / 96
气血两虚 / 96
气血两虚证 / 186
气血两虚质 / 75
气血失调 / 95
气血双补剂 / 372
气血虚弱痛经 / 560
气血瘀滞证 / 186
气翳 / 619
气阴亏虚证 / 184
气阴两虚证 / 183
气营两燔 / 86
气营两燔证 / 180
气瘿 / 597
气郁 / 93
气郁化火 / 93
气郁血崩 / 562
气郁证 / 182
气至 / 456
气滞 / 93
气滞腹痛 / 546
气滞经行后期 / 558
气滞水停证 / 188
气滞痰凝咽喉证 / 186
气滞痛经 / 560
气滞胃痛颗粒 / 387
气滞血瘀 / 96
气滞血瘀证 / 186
气滞腰痛 / 554
气滞证 / 182

qiā

掐法 / 480

qià

髂窝流注 / 595

qiān

千金要方 / 690
千金翼方 / 690
千金子 / 355
千年健 / 315
迁延痢 / 522
牵拉法 / 639
牵拉肩 / 646
牵牛子 / 323
牵推法 / 642
牵引疗法 / 642
牵正散 / 377

qián

前顶 / 435
前发际 / 42
前谷 / 417
前后配穴法 / 447
前胡 / 300
前阴 / 48
钱乙 / 662
钱仲阳 / 662
潜呼吸 / 497
潜阳 / 265
潜阳熄风 / 265

qiǎn

浅刺 / 454

qiàn

芡实 / 349
茜草 / 328

qiāng

羌活 / 313

qiáng

强间 / 434
强筋健骨 / 251
强壮功 / 500

qiāo

跷法 / 486

qiào

窍漏 / 615

qiē

切开埋线法 / 478
切片 / 276

qiè

切脉 / 158
切诊 / 158

qín

秦艽 / 314
秦皮 / 308
秦越人 / 658
噙化 / 284

qìn

揿针 / 450

qīng

青黛 / 311
青风 / 620
青风内障 / 620
青风藤 / 317
青果 / 313
青蒿 / 307
青蒿鳖甲汤 / 369
青灵 / 416

青龙摆尾法 / 458
青盲 / 620
青木香 / 321
青皮 / 325
青色 / 125
青舌 / 132
青蛇毒 / 606
青葙子 / 304
青紫舌 / 132
轻粉 / 354
轻剂 / 360
轻捻出针法 / 462
轻下 / 237
轻宣外燥剂 / 378
轻重徐疾补泻法 / 491
清肠润燥 / 235
清肠止痢 / 235
清肠止泻 / 235
清炒 / 277
清法 / 230
清肺 / 234
清肺化痰 / 234
清肺火 / 234
清肺利咽 / 234
清肺热 / 234
清肺润燥 / 234，263
清肺止喘 / 234
清肺止咳 / 234
清肝 / 233
清肝火 / 233
清肝明目 / 233
清肝泻火 / 233
清宫 / 233
清骨散 / 369
清化热痰 / 258
清化热痰药 / 292
清开灵注射液 / 384
清冷渊 / 427
清气 / 55
清气分热剂 / 367
清热除湿 / 231
清热导滞 / 232
清热法 / 230
清热和胃 / 232
清热和中 / 232
清热化湿 / 259
清热化痰 / 258
清热化痰开窍 / 267
清热剂 / 367
清热解毒 / 231
清热解毒剂 / 368
清热解毒药 / 288
清热解暑 / 232
清热开窍 / 233，266
清热利湿 / 231，260
清热凉血 / 233
清热凉血药 / 288
清热明目 / 232
清热排脓 / 269
清热祛湿 / 231
清热祛湿剂 / 379
清热祛暑剂 / 369
清热生津 / 231
清热熄［息］风 / 266
清热消食 / 232
清热泻肺 / 234
清热泻火 / 231
清热泻火药 / 288
清热药 / 288
清热燥湿 / 231
清热燥湿药 / 288，307
清热止痢 / 232
清热止呕 / 232
清热止泻 / 232
清热止血 / 258
清暑化湿 / 232
清暑利湿 / 232
清暑热 / 232
清胃 / 235
清胃火 / 235
清胃热 / 235
清胃散 / 368
清胃泄火 / 235
清胃泄热 / 235
清相火 / 235
清泄相火 / 235
清心 / 233
清心安神 / 234
清心火 / 234
清心开窍 / 234
清心泻火 / 234
清虚热剂 / 369
清虚热药 / 288
清阳 / 55
清营 / 232
清营凉血剂 / 367
清营汤 / 367
清营透疹 / 233
清营泄热 / 233
清脏腑热 / 233
清脏腑热剂 / 368
清燥救肺汤 / 378
清燥润肺 / 263
清浊 / 58

qǐng

苘麻子 / 322

qiū

丘墟 / 431
丘疹 / 591
秋燥 / 518
秋燥病 / 518

qiú

球后 / 440
鼽嚏 / 627

qū

曲 / 282
曲鬓 / 429
曲差 / 419
曲池 / 410
曲骨 / 48，435
曲颊 / 46
曲泉 / 432
曲牙 / 46

曲垣 / 418
曲泽 / 426
驱虫 / 271
驱虫消积 / 271
驱虫药 / 294
屈法 / 485
屈伸法 / 653
屈指捏法 / 652
祛风 / 227
祛风除湿 / 227
祛风除湿止痛 / 227
祛风化痰 / 227
祛风解表 / 227
祛风解痉 / 228
祛风清热 / 227
祛风散寒 / 227
祛风湿强筋骨药 / 289
祛风湿清热药 / 289
祛风湿散寒药 / 289
祛风湿药 / 289
祛风通络 / 228
祛风行水 / 228
祛风止痛 / 227
祛风止痒 / 228
祛寒法 / 240
祛寒化痰 / 258
祛寒剂 / 370
祛寒药 / 290
祛湿 / 259
祛湿剂 / 379
祛暑化湿 / 232
祛痰 / 258
祛痰剂 / 380
祛邪 / 219
祛邪兼扶正 / 220
祛瘀活血 / 256
祛瘀生新 / 257
祛瘀通络 / 257
祛瘀消肿 / 256
祛瘀止血 / 258

qú

瞿麦 / 322

qǔ

取穴法 / 446
龋齿 / 632
龋齿牙痛 / 632
龋脱 / 633

qù

去腐肉 / 269
去火毒 / 278
去菀陈莝 / 237
去油 / 278

quán

全不产 / 565
全虫 / 338
全国中草药汇编 / 690
全鹿丸 / 390
全蝎 / 338
拳参 / 309
拳击法 / 483，649
拳揉法 / 647
踡［蜷］卧缩足 / 127
颧 / 45
颧髎 / 418

quē

缺盆 / 47，412
缺乳 / 572

què

却谷食气 / 503
雀斑 / 601
雀盲 / 621
雀目 / 622
雀目内障 / 622
雀舌 / 634
雀啄灸 / 464
雀啄脉 / 163
鹊桥 / 494
阙上 / 43
阙中；阙 / 43

R

rán

然谷 / 424

rǎn

染苔 / 135

rè

热 / 66
热痹 / 540
热病 / 515
热疮 / 600
热毒 / 68
热毒闭肺证 / 204
热毒攻喉证 / 199
热毒攻舌证 / 199
热毒内陷证 / 198
热毒证 / 198
热伏冲任 / 87
热服 / 284
热汗 / 144
热烘 / 272
热化 / 92
热霍乱 / 523
热积［结］膀胱 / 113
热积［结］膀胱证 / 213
热极生风 / 88，103
热极生风证 / 210
热剂 / 360
热结 / 87
热结肠燥 / 110
热结肠燥证 / 208
热结下焦 / 87
热厥 / 538
热泪 / 615
热淋 / 552
热秘 / 544
热呕 / 542
热迫大肠 / 86
热扰心神证 / 201
热入［闭］心包证 / 180
热入心包 / 86
热入血分 / 87
热入血室 / 87
热入血室证 / 214

热入营血 / 87
热入营血证 / 180
热痧 / 583
热伤肺络 / 110
热伤筋脉 / 88
热伤神明 / 100
热参 / 304
热甚发痉 / 538
热盛动血证 / 180
热盛风动 / 88
热盛伤津 / 88
热痰 / 528
热痰证 / 189
热吐 / 586
热痫 / 590
热哮 / 527
热邪 / 67
热邪传里 / 83
热邪内结 / 87
热邪阻痹证 / 198
热邪阻肺 / 86
热泻 / 545
热罨 / 272
热夜啼 / 577
热因热用 / 221
热瘴 / 521
热证 / 169
热灼肾阴 / 88

rén

人胞 / 555
人参 / 340
人参健脾丸 / 388
人参养荣丸 / 391
人参再造丸 / 391
人迎 / 412
人迎脉 / 160
人中 / 46

rěn

忍冬藤 / 310

rèn

任脉 / 406
任脉穴 / 435
妊娠 / 564
妊娠病 / 566
妊娠恶阻 / 566
妊娠腹痛 / 566
妊娠禁忌药 / 284
妊娠咳嗽 / 568
妊娠呕吐 / 566
妊娠失音 / 568
妊娠痫证 / 566
妊娠小便淋痛 / 567
妊娠心烦 / 567
妊娠眩晕 / 566
妊娠肿胀 / 568

rì

日晡潮热 / 144，519
日晡发热 / 519
日月 / 430

róng

荣枯老嫩 / 131
溶化 / 282

róu

柔肝 / 265
柔肝药 / 294
揉法 / 480，647
揉颊车 / 488
揉肩 / 506
揉四白 / 487
揉膝 / 506
揉腰眼 / 489
揉攒竹 / 487

ròu

肉 / 41
肉刺 / 601
肉苁蓉 / 346
肉豆蔻 / 349
肉桂 / 317
肉果 / 350
肉瘤 / 598
肉轮 / 44，607
肉人 / 75
肉痿 / 539
肉瘿 / 597

rú

如意金黄散 / 396
儒家气功 / 492
儒门事亲 / 701
濡脉 / 161

rǔ

乳蛾 / 628
乳发 / 596
乳房疼痛 / 147
乳膏 / 281
乳根 / 412
乳核 / 597
乳积 / 582
乳疽 / 597
乳痨 / 597
乳疬 / 597
乳漏 / 597
乳岫 / 597
乳癖 / 597
乳食内积证 / 199
乳痰 / 597
乳头风 / 596
乳头破碎 / 596
乳香 / 334
乳岩 / 598
乳溢 / 573
乳痈 / 596
乳汁不通 / 573
乳汁不行 / 573
乳汁自出 / 573
乳中 / 412
乳中结核 / 597

rù

入静 / 493
入臼 / 642
入里化热 / 83
蓐风 / 572
蓐劳 / 572
褥疮 / 606

ruǎn

软膏 / 281
软脉 / 161
软气功 / 492

ruì

锐发 / 43
锐眦 / 608

rùn

润 / 276
润肠 / 236
润肠通便 / 237，263
润肺 / 263
润肺化痰 / 258
润肺生津 / 264
润肺止咳 / 264
润化燥痰 / 258
润苔 / 135
润下 / 236
润下剂 / 364
润下药 / 289
润燥 / 263
润燥化痰 / 258
润燥通便 / 237
润燥止痒 / 267

ruò

弱脉 / 161

S

sāi

腮肿 / 585
塞法 / 273
塞因塞用 / 221

sān

三板推拿疗法 / 486
三宝 / 2
三痹 / 540
三部九候 / 159
三点拉线导气 / 504
三点求圆导气 / 504
三垫固定法 / 641
三法 / 225
三关 / 138
三黄片 / 384
三间 / 409
三焦 / 24
三焦辨证 / 181
三焦咳 / 525
三焦气化 / 27
三焦湿热证 / 181
三焦实热 / 215
三焦俞 / 420
三焦虚寒 / 214
三角窝 / 472
三角针埋线法 / 478
三接式 / 495
三颗针 / 307
三棱 / 334
三棱针 / 449
三棱针疗法 / 449
三品 / 279
三七 / 328
三消 / 551
三阳 / 399
三阳合病 / 178
三阳络 / 427
三因 / 62
三因极一病证方论 / 687
三阴 / 399
三阴交 / 415
三圆式 / 496
三圆站桩功 / 502

sǎn

散 / 281
散刺 / 449
散寒 / 226
散寒化饮 / 259
散剂 / 280
散脉 / 162

sāng

桑白皮 / 303
桑寄生 / 344
桑菊饮 / 362
桑螵蛸 / 350
桑椹 / 345
桑叶 / 297
桑枝 / 315

sè

色脉合参 / 165
涩肠固脱剂 / 374
涩肠止痢 / 263
涩肠止泻 / 263
涩剂 / 360
涩精 / 262
涩精止遗 / 262
涩精止遗剂 / 374
涩脉 / 161
塞兑反听 / 494

shā

杀虫 / 272
沙棘 / 301
沙苑子 / 344
砂（石）淋 / 552
砂仁 / 319
痧 / 583
痧子 / 584

shān

山慈菇 / 300
山豆根 / 313
山根 / 626
山岚瘴气 / 72
山药 / 341
山楂 / 351
山茱萸 / 343
膻中 / 47，436

shǎn

闪火法 / 468

shàn

疝 / 554
疝气 / 554
善色 / 124
善太息 / 141
善忘 / 535
潬 / 278

shāng

伤产 / 569
伤风鼻塞 / 626
伤寒 / 515
伤寒贯珠集 / 686
伤寒来苏集 / 685
伤寒类方 / 685
伤寒论 / 685
伤寒论直解 / 685
伤寒明理论 / 685
伤寒眼 / 616
伤寒杂病论 / 685
伤寒指掌 / 685
伤寒总病论 / 685
伤津 / 81
伤科 / 635
伤科补要 / 698
伤科汇纂 / 698
伤乳 / 577
伤乳吐 / 587
伤湿 / 518
伤湿止痛膏 / 396
伤食 / 543
伤食腹胀 / 589
伤食吐 / 587
伤食泄泻 / 545
伤食泻 / 588
伤食证 / 543
伤暑 / 517
伤阳 / 81
伤阴 / 80
商陆 / 324
商丘 / 415
商曲 / 425
商阳 / 409

shàng

上胞下垂 / 614
上病下取，下病上取 / 221
上丹田 / 496
上耳根 / 473
上膈 / 543
上关 / 428
上寒下热 / 91
上寒下热证 / 171
上横骨 / 47
上火 / 519
上睑 / 608
上焦 / 24
上焦病证 / 181
上焦湿热证 / 181
上焦实热 / 215
上焦虚寒 / 214
上巨虚 / 414
上廉 / 410
上髎 / 421
上品 / 279
上气 / 141，526
上窍 / 38
上热下寒 / 91
上热下寒证 / 172
上盛下虚 / 84
上实下虚 / 84
上实下虚证 / 172
上吐下泻 / 150
上脘 / 23，436
上下配穴法 / 447
上消 / 551
上星 / 435
上虚下实 / 84
上虚下实证 / 172
上迎香 / 440
上肢穴 / 442

shāo

烧存性 / 278
烧山火 / 458
烧伤 / 605
烧心 / 153
烧针 / 451

shǎo

少尿 / 150
少气 / 141，526
少神 / 123

shào

少冲 / 417
少府 / 417
少腹 / 48
少腹拘急 / 154
少腹硬满 / 154
少海 / 416
少商 / 409
少阳病 / 177
少阳病机 / 115
少阳病证 / 177
少阳之人 / 74
少阴病 / 177
少阴病机 / 115
少阴病证 / 177
少阴寒化 / 115
少阴寒化证 / 177
少阴热化 / 116
少阴热化证 / 177
少阴之人 / 74
少泽 / 417

shé

舌 / 39
舌本 / 131
舌边 / 39，130
舌疮 / 634
舌淡 / 131
舌的分部 / 130
舌抵上腭 / 494
舌疔 / 634
舌端 / 39
舌短 / 134
舌根 / 131
舌功 / 505
舌红 / 131
舌尖 / 39，130
舌謇［蹇］/ 133
舌绛 / 131
舌卷囊缩 / 134
舌菌 / 598，634
舌裂 / 133

舌旁 / 39
舌胖 / 132
舌起芒刺 / 132
舌强 / 133
舌青紫 / 132
舌色 / 131
舌神 / 131
舌苔 / 134
舌苔脱落 / 135
舌态 / 133
舌体 / 131
舌体胖大 / 132
舌痿 / 133
舌下脉络 / 131
舌下痰包 / 634
舌象 / 130
舌心 / 131
舌形 / 132
舌岩 / 598
舌痈 / 634
舌有齿痕 / 132
舌有瘀斑 / 132
舌有瘀点 / 132
舌战 / 133
舌诊 / 130
舌质 / 131
舌中 / 130
舌肿 / 133
舌柱上腭 / 494
折针 / 463
蛇串疮 / 600
蛇床子 / 355
蛇丹 / 600
蛇胆陈皮散 / 382
蛇胆川贝散 / 382
蛇肚疔 / 592
蛇头疔 / 592
蛇蜕 / 315
蛇眼疔 / 592

shě

舍脉从症 / 165
舍症从脉 / 165

shè

射干 / 313
摄领疮 / 602
摄唾 / 271
麝香 / 335

shēn

申脉 / 423
伸法 / 485
伸筋草 / 316
伸腰沉胯 / 494
身法 / 493
身热 / 143
身热不扬 / 144
身瞤动 / 127
身痛 / 147
身痒 / 147
身重 / 147
身柱 / 434
参附注射液 / 391
参苓白术散 / 371
参苓白术丸 / 388
参茸固本片 / 391
参茸卫生丸 / 391
参苏饮 / 363
深刺 / 454

shén

神 / 2，57
神不守舍 / 100
神藏 / 425
神道 / 434
神封 / 425
神膏 / 610
神光耗散 / 128
神昏 / 123
神乱 / 124
神门 / 417
神农本草经 / 687
神气不足 / 123
神曲 / 351
神阙 / 48，436
神水 / 610
神堂 / 422
神庭 / 435
神志不清 / 123
神志昏愦［溃］/ 124

shěn

沈存中 / 662
沈金鳌 / 677
沈括 / 662
沈芊绿 / 677
沈之问 / 669
审苗窍 / 128
审视瑶函 / 698
审因论治 / 218
审因施治 / 218
审证求因 / 191

shèn

肾 / 22
肾癌 / 598
肾痹 / 541
肾不纳气 / 113
肾不纳气证 / 213
肾疳 / 581
肾火偏亢 / 111
肾间动气 / 54
肾经寒湿证 / 213
肾经咳嗽 / 525
肾精 / 57
肾精不足 / 112
肾精亏虚证 / 212
肾咳 / 525
肾亏 / 111
肾劳 / 529
肾囊 / 49
肾囊风 / 603
肾膀胱病辨证 / 212
肾气 / 55
肾气不固 / 112
肾气不固证 / 212
肾气不足 / 111
肾气丸 / 373

肾气虚 / 111
肾气（亏）虚证 / 212
肾俞 / 420
肾水 / 22，549
肾水不足 / 112
肾水亏虚证 / 212
肾痿 / 540
肾消 / 551
肾虚 / 111
肾虚崩漏 / 561
肾虚不孕 / 565
肾虚带下 / 564
肾虚耳鸣 / 624
肾虚滑胎 / 570
肾虚经闭 / 559
肾虚水泛 / 113
肾虚水泛证 / 213
肾虚痛经 / 560
肾虚泄泻 / 545
肾虚泻 / 588
肾虚眩晕 / 532
肾虚腰痛 / 554
肾虚月经过少 / 558
肾虚证 / 212
肾岩 / 598
肾岩翻花 / 598
肾阳 / 23
肾阳不足 / 113
肾阳衰微 / 111，113
肾阳虚 / 112
肾阳虚衰 / 113
肾阳虚证 / 213
肾阴 / 22
肾阴不足 / 112
肾阴虚 / 112
肾阴虚火旺证 / 212
肾阴虚证 / 212
肾之府 / 27
胂 / 47
渗湿 / 260

shēng

升剂 / 360
升、降、出、入 / 2
升降浮沉 / 279
升降失常 / 94
升举中气 / 246
升麻 / 298
升麻葛根汤 / 363
升提中气 / 246
升阳 / 247
升阳举陷 / 247
生地 / 306
生化 / 2
生化汤 / 376
生肌 / 270
生肌敛疮 / 270
生肌收口 / 270
生姜 / 295
生津 / 264
生脉饮 / 389
生殖之精 / 57
声嗄 / 140
声重 / 140

shèng

圣惠方 / 691
圣济总录 / 703
盛胎 / 566

shī

失眠 / 155，535
失荣 / 598
失神 / 123
失溲 / 151
失血 / 549
失音 / 140，524
失音病 / 524
失语 / 537
湿 / 65
湿痹 / 540
湿蔽清阳 / 89
湿病 / 518
湿疮 / 603
湿毒 / 69
湿毒带下 / 564
湿毒流注 / 89
湿火 / 68
湿剂 / 360
湿困脾阳 / 105
湿困脾阳证 / 206
湿疟 / 521
湿气 / 65
湿热 / 68
湿热带下 / 564
湿热犯耳证 / 197
湿热痢 / 521
湿热内蕴 / 89
湿热痛经 / 560
湿热下注 / 89
湿热下注证 / 197
湿热泄泻 / 545
湿热腰痛 / 553
湿热蕴脾 / 105
湿热蕴脾证 / 197
湿热蒸齿证 / 197
湿热蒸唇证 / 196
湿热蒸口证 / 196
湿热蒸舌证 / 197
湿热阻痹证 / 197
湿热阻滞精室证 / 214
湿胜着痹证 / 196
湿痰 / 72
湿痰不孕 / 565
湿痰证 / 189
湿温 / 518
湿温病 / 518
湿邪 / 65
湿邪困脾 / 89
湿癣 / 604
湿郁化火 / 89
湿郁化热 / 89
湿郁肌表 / 89
湿疹 / 603
湿证 / 196
湿浊 / 65

湿阻 / 518
湿阻中焦 / 106
湿阻中焦证 / 206

shí

十八反 / 359
十二刺 / 461
十二剂 / 360
十二节 / 52
十二经 / 398
十二经别 / 407
十二经筋 / 406
十二经脉 / 398
十二皮部 / 407
十剂 / 359
十九畏 / 359
十七椎 / 441
十全大补汤 / 372
十全大补丸 / 388
十四剂 / 360
十四经 / 400
十四经发挥 / 699
十问 / 142
十五络脉 / 407
十宣 / 443
十药神书 / 694
十枣汤 / 365
石菖蒲 / 335
石蛾 / 629
石膏 / 304
石关 / 425
石斛 / 343
石斛夜光丸 / 396
石决明 / 339
石淋 / 552
石榴皮 / 349
石门 / 435
石水 / 549
石韦 / 323
石瘿 / 597
时病 / 514
时病论 / 694
时毒 / 514
时方 / 357
时方歌括 / 693
时令病 / 514
时邪 / 62
时行 / 514
时行感冒 / 515
时行戾气 / 63，514
时疫 / 514
时疫痢 / 522
实按灸 / 466
实喘 / 527
实寒 / 90
实寒证 / 172，194
实火 / 90
实火证 / 173，198
实脉 / 161
实秘 / 544
实痞 / 542
实热 / 90
实热证 / 173
实胀 / 589
实证 / 170
实中夹虚 / 84
食床 / 633
食窦 / 416
食复 / 71
食积 / 582
食积盗汗 / 586
食积腹痛 / 546，588
食积寒热 / 583
食积证 / 199
食忌 / 284
食厥 / 538
食疗 / 274
食疗本草 / 687
食痫 / 589
食泻［泄］/ 588
食已即吐 / 153
食远服 / 284
食治 / 274
食滞 / 543
蚀疮去腐 / 270

shǐ

使君子 / 353
使药 / 358

shì

世医得效方 / 692
试水 / 569
试胎 / 568
试月 / 568
视物易色 / 621
视衣 / 610
视瞻昏渺 / 620
视直为曲 / 621
柿蒂 / 328
是动病 / 408
嗜偏食 / 544
嗜睡 / 155，535
嗜卧 / 155

shōu

收功 / 505
收敛止血药 / 291
收涩 / 261
收涩药 / 294
收臀松膝 / 494

shǒu

手发背 / 594
手法牵引 / 642
手骨 / 47
手厥阴心包经 / 404
手厥阴心包经穴 / 425
手摸心会 / 638
手三里 / 410
手三阳经 / 399
手三阴经 / 399
手少阳三焦经 / 404
手少阳三焦经穴 / 426
手少阴心经 / 402
手少阴心经穴 / 416
手太阳小肠经 / 402
手太阳小肠经穴 / 417

手太阴肺经 / 400
手太阴肺经穴 / 408
手五里 / 410
手心毒 / 592
手阳明大肠经 / 400
手阳明大肠经穴 / 409
手针 / 478
手针疗法 / 478
手足颤动 / 127
手足汗 / 145
手足厥冷 / 538
手足逆冷 / 538
手足蠕动 / 127
手足心汗 / 145
手足心热 / 144
守气 / 456
首乌 / 344
首乌藤 / 336

shòu

寿世保元 / 703
瘦薄舌 / 132

shū

梳法 / 483
舒肝丸 / 386
舒筋和络 / 257
舒筋活络 / 257
舒筋通络 / 257
舒筋止痛 / 257
舒腰松腹 / 494
舒张进针法 / 453
疏表润燥 / 227
疏风 / 226
疏风和营 / 227
疏风解表 / 226
疏风解肌 / 226
疏风清肺 / 226
疏风清热 / 226
疏风散寒 / 226
疏风透疹 / 226
疏风消肿 / 227
疏风泄热 / 226
疏风宣肺 / 227
疏风止痒 / 227
疏肝 / 255
疏肝和脾 / 255
疏肝和胃 / 255
疏肝健脾 / 255
疏肝解郁 / 255
疏肝理脾 / 255
疏肝理气 / 255
疏肝明目功 / 502
疏肝养血 / 255
疏散风热 / 225
疏散外风剂 / 377
输刺 / 460
输穴 / 437

shú

熟地黄 / 342

shǔ

暑 / 65
暑闭气机证 / 196
暑病 / 517
暑风 / 517
暑风证 / 517
暑秽 / 516
暑秽病 / 516
暑疖 / 592
暑痉 / 517
暑厥 / 517
暑厥证 / 517
暑疟 / 521
暑气 / 65
暑热 / 65
暑热闭神证 / 196
暑热动风证 / 195
暑热内郁证 / 195
暑热证 / 195
暑入阳明 / 517
暑入阳明证 / 518
暑伤肺络证 / 204
暑伤津气证 / 195
暑湿 / 65
暑湿流注 / 516
暑湿袭表证 / 195
暑湿证 / 195
暑温 / 517
暑温病 / 517
暑痫 / 517
暑邪 / 65
暑瘵 / 517
暑证 / 195
鼠乳 / 600

shù

束骨 / 423
俞府 / 425
俞募配穴法 / 448
俞穴 / 408
俞原配穴法 / 448
腧穴 / 408
数脉 / 160
数吸 / 498
漱涤 / 273
漱津 / 506

shuài

率谷 / 429

shuān

栓剂 / 282

shuàn

腨 / 50

shuāng

双蛾 / 628
双黄连口服液 / 383
双盘坐 / 495
双手进针法 / 453
双手捏法 / 652
双手攀足式 / 653
双手托天式 / 654

shuǐ

水不涵木 / 14
水不化气 / 93
水疮 / 585
水道 / 413
水痘 / 584

水飞 / 276
水分 / 436
水沟 / 435
水谷 / 53
水谷精微 / 57
水谷之海 / 26
水谷之精 / 57
水谷之气 / 53
水臌（病） / 547
水寒射肺 / 103
水寒射肺证 / 205
水红花子 / 332
水花 / 585
水火共制 / 276
水火相济 / 27
水克火 / 12
水轮 / 44，607
水牛角 / 306
水疱 / 139，585
水气 / 66，548
水气凌心 / 101
水气凌心证 / 202
水气证 / 189
水泉 / 424
水疝 / 599
水生木 / 12
水停证 / 189
水突 / 412
水土不服 / 72
水丸 / 280
水泻 / 150
水形之人 / 74
水饮 / 527
水饮内停证 / 187
水胀 / 548
水针 / 470
水制 / 276
水蛭 / 333
水肿 / 138，548
水肿病 / 548

shuì

睡眠十忌 / 507

shùn

顺传 / 179，515
顺腹式呼吸 / 497
顺骨捋筋 / 640
顺气 / 254
顺应四时 / 17

sī

司天 / 18
丝瓜络 / 316
丝竹空 / 428
丝状疣 / 600
思 / 69
撕裂伤 / 646
嘶嗄 / 140

sǐ

死胎 / 567
死胎不下 / 567

sì

四白 / 411
四渎 / 427
四缝 / 443
四海 / 25
四君子汤 / 371
四满 / 424
四逆 / 538
四逆散 / 366
四逆汤 / 370
四气 / 279
四神聪 / 439
四神丸 / 374
四时不正之气 / 63
四弯风 / 603
四物汤 / 371
四性 / 279
四诊 / 123
四诊合参 / 165
四诊抉微 / 686
食痞 / 581

sōng

松 / 493
松皮癣 / 602

sòng

宋慈 / 665
宋惠父 / 665
送服 / 284

sōu

溲血 / 151

sū

苏恭 / 661
苏合香 / 335
苏合香丸 / 392
苏敬 / 661
苏木 / 333
苏沈良方 / 691
苏轼 / 662
苏颂 / 662
苏子 / 303

sù

素髎 / 435
素问 / 683
速效救心丸 / 394
宿疾 / 524
宿食 / 544
宿翳 / 612
粟疮 / 613
粟芽 / 351

suān

酸甘化阴 / 248
酸浆 / 313
酸［痠］痛 / 148
酸枣仁 / 336
酸枣仁汤 / 381

suàn

蒜泥灸 / 466

suí

随咳进针法 / 454
随息 / 498

suǐ

髓 / 25
髓海 / 25
髓之府 / 25

suì

岁会 / 18
岁运 / 17

sūn

孙东宿 / 669
孙络 / 407
孙思邈 / 661
孙文垣 / 669
孙一奎 / 669
飧水泻 / 588
飧泄［泻］/ 545

suō

娑罗子 / 327
缩泉丸 / 374

suǒ

所生病 / 408
锁肚 / 575
锁喉毒 / 593
锁喉风 / 630
锁喉痈 / 593
锁阳 / 346

T

tā

他经选穴法 / 446
溻浴 / 273

tà

踏跳法 / 486

tāi

苔色 / 134
胎禀 / 576
胎赤 / 576
胎疸 / 576
胎动不安 / 568
胎毒 / 69，576
胎寒 / 568，576
胎患内障 / 620
胎黄 / 576
胎黄病 / 576
胎漏 / 569
胎气上逆 / 567
胎怯 / 576
胎热 / 568，576
胎弱 / 576
胎食 / 494
胎水肿满 / 567
胎死不下 / 567
胎死腹中 / 567
胎息 / 497
胎痫 / 590
胎衣 / 555
胎元 / 566
胎元不固 / 569

tài

太白 / 415
太冲 / 432
太极步 / 496
太平惠民和剂局方 / 691
太平圣惠方 / 691
太息 / 141
太溪 / 424
太阳 / 43，440
太阳病 / 175
太阳病机 / 115
太阳病证 / 175
太阳腑病 / 176
太阳腑证 / 176
太阳经病 / 175
太阳经证 / 175
太阳伤寒 / 176
太阳伤寒证 / 175
太阳蓄水证 / 176
太阳蓄血证 / 176
太阳（与）少阳合病 / 178
太阳（与）阳明合病 / 178
太阳之人 / 74
太阳中风 / 175
太阳中风证 / 175
太乙 / 413
太阴病 / 177
太阴病机 / 115
太阴病证 / 177
太阴之人 / 74
太渊 / 409
太子参 / 340

tān

贪食生冷 / 70

tán

痰 / 71
痰包 / 634
痰喘 / 527
痰多 / 137
痰核留结证 / 190
痰黄 / 137
痰火耳鸣 / 624
痰火扰神证 / 201
痰火扰心 / 101
痰火扰心证 / 201
痰厥 / 538
痰咳 / 526
痰蒙心包 / 100
痰蒙心神 / 100
痰蒙心神证 / 201
痰迷心窍 / 100
痰秘 / 544
痰鸣 / 141
痰痞 / 542
痰气互［郁］结证 / 190
痰热闭肺 / 110
痰热闭肺证 / 204
痰热动风证 / 190
痰热内闭证 / 190
痰热内扰证 / 190
痰热壅［蕴］肺证 / 204
痰如泡沫 / 137
痰盛 / 137
痰湿 / 72
痰湿不孕 / 565
痰湿犯耳证 / 190
痰湿咳嗽 / 526
痰湿质 / 75
痰湿阻肺 / 110
痰湿阻肺证 / 203

痰湿阻滞精室证 / 214
痰稀白 / 137
痰痫 / 590
痰饮 / 528
痰瘀互结证 / 189
痰证 / 189
痰中带血 / 138
痰浊 / 72
痰浊犯头证 / 190
痰浊头痛 / 533
痰浊证 / 189
痰浊阻肺 / 110
痰浊阻肺证 / 203
痰阻精室证 / 214
弹柄法 / 455
弹法 / 651
弹击法 / 484
弹筋 / 485
弹筋法 / 651
弹入法 / 453
弹石脉 / 163
弹响指 / 647
檀香 / 326

tàn

探吐 / 267
探爪式 / 504

tāng

汤剂 / 282
汤头 / 358
汤头歌 / 358
汤头歌诀 / 692
汤药 / 281
汤液本草 / 688

táng

唐本草 / 687
唐容川 / 680
唐审元 / 663
唐慎微 / 663
唐宗海 / 680
溏便 / 149
溏结不调 / 149
糖浆 / 281
螳螂子 / 579

tàng

烫火伤 / 71

táo

桃仁 / 330
陶道 / 434
陶罐 / 467
陶弘景 / 660
陶通明 / 660

tè

特定穴 / 437

téng

腾跃爆发导气 / 504

tí

提按端挤 / 638
提插补泻 / 456
提插补泻法 / 456
提插法 / 455
提法 / 639
提肛呼吸 / 497
提捏进针法 / 453
提脓拔毒 / 269
提脓去腐 / 269
提伸法 / 485

tǐ

体质 / 73
体质学说 / 73

tì

涕 / 58

tiān

天白蚁 / 629
天池 / 425
天冲 / 429
天窗 / 418
天钓 / 575
天鼎 / 411
天冬 / 343
天符 / 18
天府 / 408
天干 / 18
天癸 / 556
天癸竭 / 556
天花 / 585
天花粉 / 300
天井 / 427
天灸 / 466
天髎 / 427
天麻 / 338
天麻钩藤饮 / 378
天麻丸 / 393
天门冬 / 343
天南星 / 298
天年 / 18
天泉 / 426
天人相应 / 17
天容 / 418
天受 / 514
天枢 / 413
天庭 / 43
天突 / 437
天溪 / 416
天仙子 / 303
天行 / 514
天行暴赤 / 616
天行赤目 / 616
天行赤目暴翳 / 616
天行赤眼 / 616
天行赤眼暴翳 / 616
天行时疫 / 514
天牖 / 427
天竺黄 / 300
天柱 / 419
天宗 / 418

tiáo

条口 / 414
调服 / 283
调和肝脾 / 239
调和肝脾剂 / 365
调和肝胃 / 239
调和寒热剂 / 366
调和脾胃 / 238

调和气血 / 239
调和营卫 / 229
调经 / 268
调理气血 / 239
调气 / 254，497
调身 / 493
调身要领 / 493
调息 / 497
调心 / 498
龆龀 / 574

tiǎo

挑刺法 / 449

tiē

贴棉法 / 468

tiě

铁裆功 / 502

tīng

听宫 / 418
听会 / 428
听息 / 498

tíng

廷孔 / 49
停经 / 559
停食 / 543
停息 / 498
葶苈子 / 303
聤耳 / 625

tǐng

挺腿拔伸 / 640

tōng

通鼻 / 271
通鼻窍 / 271
通便 / 236
通草 / 321
通腑泄热 / 237
通关射甲 / 138
通剂 / 359
通经 / 268
通经活络 / 268
通经接气配穴法 / 449
通经止痛 / 268
通里 / 236，416
通利关节 / 269，654
通利血脉 / 268
通淋 / 268
通淋药 / 290
通络止痛 / 268
通脉 / 241
通气 / 252
通乳 / 268
通天 / 419
通下 / 236
通泄 / 237
通宣理肺丸［片］/ 382
通阳 / 240
通因通用 / 221

tóng

同病异治 / 218
同名经配穴法 / 448
同身寸 / 444
铜人俞穴针灸图经 / 699
潼蒺藜 / 344
瞳人 / 609
瞳人干缺 / 619
瞳仁 / 609
瞳神 / 609
瞳神干缺 / 619
瞳神紧小 / 619
瞳神缺陷 / 619
瞳神散大 / 619
瞳神缩小 / 619
瞳神细小 / 619
瞳子 / 609
瞳子髎 / 428

tòng

痛痹 / 540
痛经 / 560
痛经丸 / 394
痛无定处 / 148
痛泻要方 / 366

tōu

偷针 / 613

tóu

头风 / 146，533
头汗 / 145
头颈部穴 / 439
头临泣 / 429
头颅骨 / 42
头面功 / 500
头皮针 / 470
头皮针疗法 / 471
头窍阴 / 429
头如顶物 / 493
头痛 / 146，533
头维 / 412
头项强痛 / 146
头穴线 / 471
头针 / 470
头针疗法 / 471
头正 / 493
头重 / 146
头重脚轻 / 146
投火法 / 468

tòu

透斑 / 229
透表 / 228
透表清热 / 229
透刺 / 454
透关射甲 / 138
透天凉 / 458
透邪 / 229
透泄 / 229
透疹 / 229

tū

秃疮 / 604
突起睛高 / 622

tú

图钉型皮内针 / 450
徒手整复 / 491

tǔ

土鳖虫 / 333
土不制水 / 14
土法 / 357

土方 / 357
土茯苓 / 309
土疳 / 613
土荆皮 / 355
土克水 / 12
土牛膝 / 313
土生金 / 11
土形之人 / 73
土虚木乘 / 13
土虚水侮 / 14
土疡 / 613
吐纳 / 497
吐弄舌 / 134
吐舌 / 134
吐字呼吸 / 497

tù

吐法 / 267
吐矢 / 544
吐酸 / 543
吐血 / 152，550
兔唇 / 590
菟丝子 / 347

tuī

推扳手法 / 486
推法 / 159，482，648
推罐 / 469
推拿 / 480
推拿的补泻手法 / 490
推拿广意 / 696
推拿疗法 / 480

tuǐ

腿功 / 653

tuì

退法 / 463
退黄 / 269
退目翳 / 271
退翳明目 / 271

tūn

吞服 / 284
吞酸 / 153，543

tún

臀痈 / 594

tuō

托板 / 640
托疮 / 269
托毒 / 269
托法 / 269
托里排脓 / 269
托盘疔 / 592
托提法 / 484
脱肛 / 599
脱骨疽 / 595
脱汗 / 145，531
脱骱 / 637
脱臼 / 637
脱疽 / 595
脱髎 / 637
脱位 / 637
脱阳 / 80
脱阴 / 80

tuò

唾 / 58

W

wǎ

瓦楞子 / 350
瓦松 / 330

wāi

歪斜舌 / 133
㖞僻不遂 / 537

wài

外吹 / 596
外吹乳痈 / 596
外耳门 / 473
外翻 / 656
外风 / 64
外风证 / 191
外敷 / 272
外辅骨 / 51
外感 / 62，519
外感咳嗽 / 525
外感头痛 / 533
外感腰痛 / 553
外功 / 492
外固定 / 640
外关 / 427
外寒 / 64
外踝 / 50
外踝尖 / 443
外经 / 400
外科大成 / 698
外科精要 / 697
外科精义 / 697
外科启玄 / 697
外科正宗 / 698
外科证治全生集 / 698
外劳宫 / 442
外陵 / 413
外气 / 500
外丘 / 431
外湿 / 65
外台秘要 / 690
外邪 / 62
外因 / 62
外痈 / 593
外燥 / 66
外燥证 / 197
外障 / 612
外证 / 591
外治 / 272
外治法 / 272
外痔 / 599
外眦 / 44，608

wān

弯针 / 463

wán

丸 / 280
丸剂 / 280
完谷不化 / 149
完骨 / 46，429，623
顽痰 / 72，528
顽癣 / 602

wǎn

脘 / 23
脘痛 / 147，152
踠跌 / 635

wàn

万病回春 / 703
万密斋 / 670
万密斋医学全书 / 703
万全 / 670
万氏女科 / 695
腕骨 / 417

wāng

尪痹 / 541
尪痹颗粒 / 393
汪昂 / 674
汪机 / 668
汪讱安 / 674
汪省之 / 668

wáng

亡津液 / 81
亡阳 / 80
亡阳证 / 173
亡阴 / 80
亡阴证 / 173
王冰 / 661
王不留行 / 333
王海藏 / 666
王好古 / 666
王进之 / 666
王肯堂 / 671
王纶 / 668
王孟英 / 680
王清任 / 678
王士雄 / 680
王叔和 / 659
王损庵 / 671
王泰林 / 679
王焘 / 661
王惟德 / 662
王维一 / 662
王熙 / 659
王旭高 / 679
王勋臣 / 678
王宇泰 / 671
王执中 / 664

wàng

望鼻 / 129
望齿 / 137
望耳 / 129
望目 / 128
望皮肤 / 138
望色 / 124
望舌 / 130
望神 / 123
望痰 / 137
望形体 / 126
望诊 / 123
望指纹 / 138
望姿态 / 127

wēi

危达斋 / 666
危亦林 / 665
威灵仙 / 314
微波针灸 / 470
微波针灸疗法 / 470
微炒 / 277
微脉 / 161
微热 / 144
微丸 / 280
煨 / 276
煨脓长肉 / 270

wéi

维道 / 430

wěi

尾骶 / 51
尾骶骨 / 51
尾闾骨 / 51
委阳 / 421
委中 / 421
委中毒 / 593
萎黄 / 125，547
萎黄病 / 547
痿 / 539
痿躄 / 539
痿病 / 539
痿软舌 / 133
痿证 / 539

wèi

卫 / 55
卫分 / 55
卫分证 / 179
卫气 / 54
卫气不固 / 85
卫气同病 / 86
卫气同病证 / 179
卫气营血 / 55
卫气营血辨证 / 179
卫强营弱 / 86
卫弱营强 / 86
卫生家宝产科备要 / 695
卫阳 / 54
卫阳被遏 / 85
卫营同病 / 86
卫营同病证 / 179
畏寒 / 143
畏明 / 610
胃 / 23
胃不和 / 108
胃仓 / 422
胃肠病辨证 / 207
胃反 / 152，543
胃寒 / 107
胃寒饮停证 / 188
胃缓 / 546
胃火 / 108
胃火炽盛 / 108
胃火炽盛证 / 208
胃火上炎 / 108
胃火牙痛 / 632
胃火证 / 208
胃家实 / 523
胃津 / 24
胃津亏损 / 81
胃咳 / 525

胃痞 / 542
胃气 / 24，55
胃气不和 / 108
胃气不降 / 108
胃气上逆 / 108
胃气虚 / 107
胃气虚证 / 207
胃热 / 107
胃热化火 / 92
胃热呕吐 / 586
胃热消谷 / 92
胃热消［杀］谷 / 108
胃热壅盛 / 108
胃热壅盛证 / 208
胃、神、根 / 164
胃失和降 / 108
胃实寒 / 107
胃俞 / 420
胃实寒证 / 207
胃痛 / 152
胃脘 / 23
胃脘痛 / 152
胃脘痛（病） / 542
胃脘下俞 / 441
胃消 / 551
胃虚 / 107
胃虚寒 / 107
胃虚寒证 / 207
胃虚汗 / 586
胃阳 / 24
胃阳虚 / 107
胃阳虚证 / 207
胃阴 / 24
胃阴不足 / 107
胃阴虚 / 107
胃阴虚证 / 207
胃燥津亏证 / 187
胃中热 / 108
魏柳洲 / 675
魏之琇 / 675

wēn

温病 / 515
温病条辨 / 693
温补命门 / 251
温补脾肾 / 243
温补脾胃 / 246
温补肾阳 / 242
温补胃阳 / 241
温毒 / 514
温莪术 / 332
温法 / 240
温肺 / 242
温肺化痰 / 242
温肺化饮 / 242
温肺散寒 / 242
温服 / 284
温肝 / 240
温和灸 / 464
温化寒痰 / 258
温化寒痰药 / 292
温经 / 243
温经扶阳 / 243
温经回阳 / 243
温经活血 / 243
温经暖宫 / 243
温经祛寒 / 243
温经散寒 / 243
温经散寒剂 / 370
温经通络 / 243
温经通阳 / 243
温经行滞 / 243
温经养血 / 244
温经止痛 / 244
温经止血药 / 291
温灸器 / 464
温灸器灸 / 466
温里 / 240
温里剂 / 369
温里祛寒 / 244
温里散寒 / 244
温里药 / 290
温溜 / 410
温疟 / 520
温脾 / 241
温脾汤 / 364
温热 / 67
温热经纬 / 693
温热论 / 693
温肾 / 242
温肾化痰 / 242
温肾化饮 / 243
温肾利水 / 261
温肾纳气 / 242
温肾缩尿 / 242
温肾阳 / 242
温肾止泻 / 242
温肾壮阳 / 242
温胃 / 241
温胃降逆 / 241
温胃止呕 / 241
温下 / 236
温下寒积 / 236
温下剂 / 364
温下药 / 289
温邪 / 67，514
温邪犯肺 / 85
温邪上受 / 85
温心阳 / 240
温阳 / 240
温阳利湿 / 261
温阳利水 / 261
温阳行水 / 261
温［瘟］疫 / 515
温疫论 / 693
温燥 / 66，519
温燥病 / 519
温燥证 / 197
温针灸 / 466
温中 / 241
温中和胃 / 241
温中祛寒 / 241
温中祛寒剂 / 369
温中散寒 / 241

温中行气 / 241
温中止呕 / 241
温中止痛 / 242
温中止吐 / 242
温中止泻 / 242

wén

文火 / 283
闻声音 / 139
闻诊 / 139

wěn

吻 / 46

wèn

问大便 / 149
问二便 / 149
问妇女经带 / 156
问寒热 / 142
问汗 / 144
问渴饮 / 148
问口味 / 154
问起病 / 142
问睡眠 / 155
问头身 / 146
问现证 / 142
问小便 / 150
问胸腹 / 151
问诊 / 142

wò

卧式 / 495

wū

乌鸡白凤丸 / 394
乌梅 / 349
乌梢蛇 / 315
乌须发 / 271
乌药 / 326
乌贼骨 / 350
屋漏脉 / 163
屋翳 / 412

wú

无瘢痕灸 / 465
无根苔 / 136
无汗 / 145
无名肿毒 / 594
无头疽 / 595
无形之痰 / 71
吴安业 / 680
吴鞠通 / 678
吴其浚 / 679
吴尚先 / 679
吴师机 / 680
吴瑭 / 678
吴有性 / 672
吴又可 / 672
吴瀹斋 / 679
吴茱萸 / 318
吴茱萸汤 / 370
蜈蚣 / 338

wǔ

五倍子 / 348
五迟 / 577
五处 / 419
五刺 / 459
五方 / 14
五疳 / 580
五更咳 / 526
五更泄［泻］/ 545
五官 / 14，38
五化 / 14
五加皮 / 316
五劳 / 529
五淋 / 552
五灵脂 / 332
五苓散 / 379
五轮 / 43，607
五气 / 14
五禽戏 / 502
五仁丸 / 364
五软 / 578
五色 / 125
五色主病 / 126
五声 / 14
五时 / 14
五枢 / 430
五输配穴法 / 448
五输穴 / 437
五水 / 549
五味 / 279
五味偏嗜 / 70
五味所入 / 26，280
五味子 / 350
五心烦热 / 144
五行 / 11
五行归类 / 11
五行母子相及 / 13
五行相乘 / 12
五行相克 / 12
五行相生 / 11
五行相侮 / 13
五行学说 / 11
五行制化 / 12
五液 / 58
五硬 / 578
五运 / 17
五运六气 / 17
五脏 / 20
五脏化液 / 58
五脏所藏 / 26
五脏所恶 / 26
五脏所主 / 26
五趾抓地 / 494
五志 / 26，69
五志过极 / 70
五志化火 / 70
五子衍宗丸 / 389
午后潮热 / 144，519
武火 / 283
武叔卿 / 673
武术气功 / 492
武之望 / 673

wù

物损真睛 / 621
误下 / 238
恶风 / 143
恶寒 / 143

恶寒发热 / 143
恶热 / 143

X

xī

西河柳 / 298
西红花 / 330
西黄丸 / 384
西洋参 / 343
吸门 / 41
吸入 / 272
郗会配穴法 / 448
息胞 / 570
息肉痔 / 599
犀角 / 305
犀角地黄汤 / 367
豨莶草 / 314
豨莶丸 / 393
熄［息］风 / 265
熄［息］风定痉 / 266
熄［息］风定痫 / 266
熄［息］风化痰 / 259
熄风剂 / 378
熄［息］风解痉 / 266
熄［息］风止痉药 / 293
膝 / 49
膝髌 / 50
膝顶 / 639
膝顶扳胸椎法 / 653
膝关 / 432
膝腘 / 50
膝眼 / 443
膝阳关 / 431

xí

席疮 / 606

xǐ

洗 / 276
洗手 / 489
洗冤集录 / 700
喜 / 69
喜按 / 166
喜脉 / 163

xì

郄门 / 426
郄穴 / 438
细脉 / 161
细辛 / 296

xiā

虾游脉 / 163

xiá

侠白 / 409
侠溪 / 432

xià

下按式 / 496
下按式站桩功 / 502
下丹田 / 497
下耳根 / 473
下法 / 235
下膈 / 543
下关 / 411
下合穴 / 439
下极俞 / 441
下睑 / 609
下焦 / 24
下焦病证 / 181
下焦湿热证 / 182
下焦实热 / 215
下焦虚寒 / 215
下巨虚 / 414
下利 / 150，545
下利［痢］脓血 / 150
下利清谷 / 150，545
下廉 / 410
下髎 / 421
下品 / 280
下气 / 254
下气消痰 / 253
下窍 / 38
下乳 / 268
下脘 / 24，436
下陷 / 94
下消 / 551
下元不固 / 112
下元亏损 / 112
下肢功 / 501
下肢穴 / 443
下坠 / 156
夏季热 / 582
夏季热病 / 582
夏枯草 / 305

xiān

仙鹤草 / 328
仙灵脾 / 346
仙茅 / 346
仙授理伤续断秘方 / 697
先补后攻 / 220
先攻后补 / 220
先煎 / 283
先天不足 / 73
先天之火 / 27
先天之精 / 57
先天之气 / 53

xián

弦脉 / 162
涎 / 58
痫病 / 534
痫证 / 534，589

xiàn

线瘊 / 600
陷谷 / 414

xiāng

相恶 / 359
相反 / 359
相兼脉象 / 163
相杀 / 359
相使 / 359
相畏 / 359
相须 / 358
香附 / 326
香加皮 / 317
香连丸 / 386
香薷 / 296
香薷散 / 361

香砂六君丸 / 388
香砂养胃丸 / 387
香橼 / 326

xiàng

项 / 46
项功 / 506
项强 / 127
相火 / 27
相火妄动 / 112

xiāo

逍遥散 / 366
逍遥丸 / 386
消导 / 252
消导药 / 291
消法 / 251
消谷善饥 / 153
消骨鲠 / 271
消肌 / 589
消积 / 252
消积除胀 / 252
消渴（病）/ 551
消泺 / 427
消痞 / 252
消上 / 589
消食 / 251
消食导滞 / 251
消食和胃 / 252
消食和中 / 252
消食化滞 / 251
消食剂 / 379
消食下气 / 252
消食药 / 291
消痈散疖 / 270
消痈散结 / 270
消胀 / 252
消肿 / 252
消肿退红 / 252
消肿止痛 / 271
消浊 / 589
萧赓六 / 675

xiǎo

小便不利 / 151
小便短赤 / 151
小便黄赤 / 151
小便淋漓 / 151
小便频数 / 150
小便清长 / 150
小便涩痛 / 151
小便失禁 / 151
小便灼热 / 151
小柴胡汤 / 365
小产 / 569
小肠 / 24
小肠咳 / 525
小肠气 / 554
小肠实热 / 101
小肠实热证 / 202
小肠俞 / 420
小肠虚寒 / 101
小承气汤 / 364
小儿暴泻 / 587
小儿痘疹方论 / 696
小儿多涎 / 578
小儿发痧 / 583
小儿浮肿 / 590
小儿腹痛 / 588
小儿腹胀 / 588
小儿感冒冲剂 / 381
小儿寒湿泻 / 587
小儿火泻 / 587
小儿麻痹 / 590
小儿呕吐 / 586
小儿热泻 / 587
小儿湿热泻 / 587
小儿暑温 / 582
小儿水气肿 / 590
小儿水肿 / 590
小儿推拿广意 / 696
小儿推拿疗法 / 486
小儿推拿秘旨 / 696
小儿消渴 / 589
小儿哮喘 / 577
小儿泄泻 / 587
小儿虚热 / 583
小儿药证直诀 / 696
小儿遗尿 / 590
小儿瘿气 / 589
小儿诸热 / 582
小儿卒利 / 587
小方 / 357
小腹 / 48
小腹不仁 / 154
小腹满 / 154
小骨空 / 442
小海 / 417
小茴香 / 318
小活络丸［丹］/ 392
小蓟 / 328
小蓟饮子 / 377
小建中汤 / 370
小结胸 / 519
小金丸［丹］/ 395
小青龙汤 / 361
小舌 / 40，628
小针刀 / 451
小针刀疗法 / 451
小周天 / 500
小周天功 / 501
小灶灸 / 465
小眦 / 608

xiào

哮 / 141，527
哮病 / 527
哮喘 / 527

xié

邪 / 62
邪火 / 70
邪气 / 62
邪热壅肺 / 102
邪热壅肺证 / 204
邪正盛衰 / 78
邪正消长 / 78
胁 / 47

胁痛 / 146
胁痛病 / 546
胁下痛 / 547
斜扳腰椎法 / 653
斜刺 / 454
斜飞脉 / 163
缬草 / 337

xiè

泄剂 / 360
泄热存津 / 231
泄泻 / 149
泄泻（病） / 545
泄注 / 150
泄注赤白 / 150
泻白散 / 368
泻肺 / 235
泻肺平喘 / 235
泻肺散 / 369
泻肝 / 233
泻水逐饮 / 237
泻下 / 236
泻下不爽 / 149
泻下剂 / 363
泻下药 / 289
泻下逐水 / 237
泻下逐饮 / 237
泻心 / 234
泻心火 / 234
谢观 / 682
薤白 / 326
龂齿 / 579，632
蟹睛病 / 618
蟹目 / 618
蟹珠 / 618

xīn

心 / 20
心包 / 23
心包络 / 23
心痹 / 541
心病辨证 / 200
心动悸 / 151
心烦 / 124
心疳 / 581
心汗 / 145
心慌 / 151
心火 / 21
心火炽［亢］盛证 / 201
心火亢盛 / 101
心火内炽 / 101
心火内焚 / 101
心火上炎 / 101
心火上炎证 / 201
心悸 / 151，530
心经咳嗽 / 524
心咳 / 524
心劳 / 529
心脉痹阻证 / 201
心脾两虚 / 101
心脾两虚证 / 202
心气 / 21，54
心气不固 / 99
心气不宁 / 99
心气不收 / 99
心气不足 / 99
心气（亏）虚证 / 200
心气虚 / 99
心气虚不得卧 / 535
心气血两虚证 / 200
心神失养 / 100
心肾不交 / 101
心肾不交证 / 202
心肾相交 / 27
心俞 / 419
心水 / 549
心痛 / 530
心痛彻背 / 151
心痿 / 539
心下急 / 156
心下悸 / 151
心下坚 / 156
心下满 / 156
心下逆满 / 156
心下痞 / 156，542
心下痞硬 / 156
心下痛 / 152
心下硬 / 156
心下支结 / 156
心虚 / 99
心虚经闭 / 559
心血 / 21
心血不足 / 99
心血（亏）虚证 / 200
心血虚 / 99
心血虚不得卧 / 535
心血瘀阻 / 99
心血瘀阻证 / 200
心阳 / 21
心阳暴脱 / 100
心阳暴脱证 / 200
心阳不振 / 100
心阳不足 / 100
心阳（亏）虚证 / 200
心阳虚 / 100
心阳虚脱证 / 200
心移热膀胱证 / 202
心移热小肠证 / 202
心移热于小肠 / 101
心阴 / 21
心阴不足 / 100
心阴（亏）虚证 / 201
心阴虚 / 99
心营过耗 / 100
心中懊侬 / 124
辛开苦泄 / 229
辛凉解表 / 225
辛凉解表剂 / 362
辛凉解表药 / 288
辛凉平剂 / 362
辛凉轻剂 / 362
辛凉清热 / 225
辛凉重剂 / 362
辛温解表 / 225
辛温解表剂 / 361

辛温解表药 / 288
辛夷 / 296
新病 / 515
新感 / 515
新修本草 / 687
新翳 / 612

xìn

囟 / 42
囟会 / 435
囟门 / 42
囟填 / 576
囟陷 / 577
信石 / 354

xīng

星翳 / 612
腥臭气 / 142

xíng

行痹 / 540
行迟 / 578
行间 / 432
行气 / 252
行气法 / 459
行气化痰 / 253
行气活血 / 253
行气剂 / 374
行气宽胸 / 253
行气宽中 / 253
行气通络 / 254
行气消痞 / 253
行气药 / 291
行气止痛 / 253
行针 / 454
行针候气 / 456
形 / 2，57
形气 / 3
形气相得 / 3，126
形气相失 / 3，126
形气转化 / 3
形胜气 / 126
形体 / 57
形与神俱 / 3
形脏 / 24

xǐng

醒脑 / 266
醒脾 / 245
醒神 / 266

xìng

杏苏散 / 378
性味 / 278

xiōng

胸痹 / 530
胸腹部穴 / 441
胸闷 / 156
胸痞 / 156
胸痛 / 146，530
胸乡 / 416
胸胁功 / 501

xióng

雄黄 / 354
熊胆 / 339
熊道轩 / 668
熊宗立 / 668

xiū

休息痢 / 522
修事 / 276
修习止观坐禅法要 / 700
修治 / 275
羞明 / 610
羞明畏日 / 610

xiù

畜门 / 625
嗅气味 / 142

xū

须发早白 / 139
虚喘 / 527
虚烦 / 529
虚寒 / 90
虚寒腹痛 / 546
虚寒痢 / 522
虚寒泄泻 / 546
虚寒证 / 172
虚火 / 91
虚火喉痹 / 629
虚火乳蛾 / 629
虚火上炎 / 90
虚火牙痛 / 632
虚火证 / 172
虚劳（病） / 529
虚里 / 47
虚脉 / 161
虚秘 / 544
虚痞 / 542
虚热 / 90，530
虚热证 / 172
虚实 / 169
虚实辨证 / 169
虚实夹杂 / 84
虚实真假 / 84
虚损 / 529
虚邪 / 63
虚阳上浮 / 80
虚胀 / 589
虚证 / 170
虚中夹实 / 84
虚肿 / 548

xú

徐长卿 / 317
徐春甫 / 669
徐大椿 / 676
徐大业 / 676
徐灵胎 / 676
徐汝元 / 669
徐士茂 / 660
徐之才 / 660

xǔ

许叔微 / 663

xù

续断 / 347
续筋接骨 / 640
续名医类案 / 702
蓄血 / 550

xuān

宣白 / 228

宣痹通阳 / 241
宣肺 / 228
宣肺化痰 / 228
宣肺化饮 / 228
宣肺降气 / 228
宣肺平喘 / 228
宣肺止咳 / 228
宣肺止咳平喘 / 228
宣剂 / 360

xuán

玄府 / 41
玄明粉 / 353
玄参 / 306
悬灸 / 464
悬厘 / 429
悬颅 / 429
悬旗风 / 630
悬旗小舌 / 630
悬起灸 / 464
悬枢 / 433
悬饮 / 528
悬痈 / 630
悬雍垂 / 40，628
悬雍肿 / 630
悬钟 / 431
旋耳 / 488
旋耳疮 / 603，623
旋复代赭汤 / 376
旋覆花 / 299
旋转屈伸 / 638
璇玑 / 436

xuǎn

选穴法 / 445
癣 / 604

xuàn

眩冒 / 146
眩晕 / 146，532

xuē

薛己 / 668
薛铠 / 668
薛良武 / 668
薛生白 / 676
薛新甫 / 669
薛雪 / 676

xué

穴位磁疗法 / 478
穴位封闭 / 470
穴位埋线疗法 / 478
穴位注射 / 470

xuě

雪口 / 579

xuè

血 / 56
血崩 / 561
血痹 / 542
血不归经 / 95
血不循经 / 95
血不养筋 / 95
血分 / 56
血分热毒 / 87
血分瘀热 / 88
血分证 / 180
血府逐瘀汤 / 376
血臌（病）/ 547
血海 / 25，415
血寒 / 95
血寒经行后期 / 558
血寒凝滞证 / 185
血寒证 / 185
血箭痔 / 599
血结胸 / 520
血竭 / 355
血精 / 552
血厥 / 538
血枯经闭 / 559
血亏经闭 / 559
血淋 / 552
血瘤 / 598
血轮 / 44，607
血缕 / 601
血脉 / 56
血尿 / 550
血气 / 56
血热 / 95，583
血热崩漏 / 561
血热动血 / 87
血热动血证 / 180
血热风盛 / 87
血热风盛证 / 180
血热滑胎 / 569
血热化燥 / 87
血热化燥证 / 180
血热经行先期 / 557
血热妄行 / 95
血热证 / 185
血室 / 26，555
血丝痰 / 138
血随气逆 / 96
血随气陷 / 96
血痰 / 137
血脱 / 95，550
血脱气脱 / 96
血脱证 / 184
血虚 / 95
血虚不孕 / 565
血虚发热 / 530
血虚风燥证 / 184
血虚肤燥生风证 / 185
血虚感冒 / 516
血虚寒凝证 / 184
血虚滑胎 / 569
血虚挟瘀证 / 184
血虚经行后期 / 558
血虚内热证 / 184
血虚生风 / 88
血虚生［动］风证 / 184
血虚头痛 / 534
血虚外感证 / 184
血虚眩晕 / 532
血虚腰痛 / 554
血虚月经过少 / 558
血虚证 / 184
血翳包睛 / 619

血瘀 / 95
血瘀崩漏 / 561
血瘀不孕 / 565
血瘀风燥证 / 185
血瘀腹痛 / 546
血瘀经闭 / 559
血瘀舌下证 / 185
血瘀水停证 / 186
血瘀痛经 / 560
血瘀腰痛 / 554
血瘀证 / 185
血瘀质 / 75
血余炭 / 329
血脏 / 556
血燥生风 / 88
血证 / 549
血证论 / 694
血之府 / 25
血脂宁丸 / 385
血滞不孕 / 565
血滞月经过少 / 558

xūn

熏洗疗法 / 274
熏蒸 / 272

xún

寻法 / 159
循按法 / 455
循法 / 159，455
循经传 / 116
循经感传 / 458
循经选穴法 / 446
循衣摸床 / 124

xùn

迅速出针法 / 462
徇蒙招尤 / 146

Y

yā

压垫 / 641
压力垫 / 641
押手 / 453
鸦胆子 / 308
鸭跖草 / 312

yá

牙疳 / 633
牙痛 / 632
牙宣 / 633
牙齩［咬］痈 / 633
牙痈 / 633

yǎ

哑门 / 434

yān

咽 / 40
咽痹 / 629
咽底 / 40
咽喉 / 40
咽喉科学 / 628
咽喉肿痛 / 629
咽后痈 / 629
咽门 / 40

yán

延胡索 / 332
严氏济生方 / 692
严用和 / 665
岩 / 598
颜面疔疮 / 593

yǎn

眼带 / 610
眼疳 / 581
眼功 / 501
眼睑 / 607
眼科（学）/ 607
眼科大全 / 699
眼球突出 / 128
眼窝凹陷 / 128
眼系 / 610
眼缘赤烂 / 613
眼珠 / 610
眼珠干涩 / 128
眼珠牵斜 / 128
眼珠塌陷 / 128
罨 / 272

yàn

厌食 / 582
验方 / 357
燕口 / 579
燕口疮 / 579

yáng

扬刺 / 461
羊痫风 / 535
阳 / 5
阳白 / 429
阳斑 / 139
阳病 / 515
阳病治阴 / 221
阳池 / 426
阳辅 / 431
阳纲 / 422
阳谷 / 417
阳汗 / 145
阳和汤 / 370
阳黄 / 523
阳极似阴 / 7
阳交 / 431
阳经 / 399
阳陵泉 / 431
阳络 / 407
阳明病 / 176
阳明病机 / 115
阳明病证 / 176
阳明腑病 / 177
阳明腑实 / 115
阳明腑证 / 177
阳明经病 / 176
阳明经证 / 176
阳明虚寒 / 115
阳明（与）少阳合病 / 178
阳明燥热 / 115
阳气 / 55
阳跷脉 / 406
阳跷脉病证 / 216
阳热质 / 74
阳盛 / 78

阳盛格阴 / 79
阳暑 / 517
阳衰 / 79
阳水 / 548
阳损及阴 / 7
阳脱 / 80
阳脱证 / 173
阳维脉 / 406
阳维脉病证 / 216
阳萎 / 156
阳痿（病） / 552
阳溪 / 410
阳痫 / 535，589
阳邪 / 63
阳虚 / 79
阳虚发热 / 530
阳虚感冒 / 516
阳虚水泛 / 86
阳虚阴盛 / 78
阳虚证 / 173
阳虚质 / 75
阳虚自汗 / 531
阳脏 / 20
阳证 / 168
阳证似阴 / 174
阳中之阳 / 5
阳中之阴 / 5
杨济时 / 671
杨继洲 / 671
杨莓舌 / 585
杨上善 / 660
疡 / 591，635
疡医 / 635
洋金花 / 303
烊化 / 283

yǎng

仰卧伸足 / 127
仰卧式 / 495
养肺阴 / 249
养肝 / 265
养肝阴 / 248
养老 / 417
养生十常 / 507
养胃 / 249
养胃生津 / 249
养胃阴 / 249
养心 / 248
养心安神 / 264
养心安神药 / 293
养心阴 / 248
养性延命录 / 700
养血 / 247
养血解表 / 230
养血祛风 / 228
养血柔肝 / 265
养血润肠 / 263
养血润燥 / 263
养血生发胶囊 / 396
养血熄风 / 239
养血熄［息］风 / 266
养血药 / 294
养阴 / 248
养阴解表 / 230
养阴清肺膏 / 383
养阴清肺汤 / 378
养阴润肺 / 263
养阴润燥 / 263
养阴药 / 294

yāo

腰 / 49
腰部功 / 501
腰骨 / 50
腰奇 / 442
腰软 / 554
腰俞 / 433
腰酸；腰痠 / 147
腰痛 / 147，553
腰痛点 / 442
腰眼 / 441
腰阳关 / 433
腰宜 / 441
腰椎旋转复位法 / 653

yáo

摇摆触碰 / 638
摇柄法 / 455
摇法 / 485，652

yǎo

咬骨疽 / 595

yào

药材 / 275
药材炮制 / 275
药茶 / 507
药毒 / 603
药方 / 356
药罐 / 469
药酒 / 281，507
药面 / 282
药摩 / 490
药捻疗法 / 274
药膳 / 507
药味 / 278
药物灸 / 466
药线疗法 / 274
药性 / 279
药引子 / 358
药粥 / 507

yē

噎嗝 / 543

yě

野菊花 / 311

yè

叶桂 / 675
叶天士 / 675
叶香岩 / 675
夜交藤 / 336
夜热 / 582
夜啼 / 577
液 / 58
液门 / 426
液脱 / 550
液脱证 / 187
腋臭 / 605
腋汗 / 145

腋痈 / 593

yī

一次性针 / 452
一垫固定法 / 641
一夫法 / 445
一贯煎 / 373
一阳 / 400
一阴 / 399
一指禅导气 / 503
一指禅功 / 482
一指禅式 / 504
一指禅推法 / 482，648
一指禅推拿 / 490
一指禅推拿疗法 / 648
伊贝母 / 302
医方集解 / 692
医方考 / 692
医方论 / 693
医贯 / 702
医和 / 658
医林改错 / 702
医门法律 / 701
医学入门 / 703
医学心悟 / 704
医学正傳 / 703
医学衷中参西录 / 702
医用气功 / 492
医宗必读 / 704
医宗金鉴 / 705
噫气 / 153
谚语 / 422

yí

饴糖 / 342
遗精 / 552
遗尿 / 151，590
遗尿（病）/ 553
颐 / 46

yǐ

以毒攻毒 / 270

yì

异病同治 / 218
异经选穴法 / 446
异气 / 63
异物入目 / 621
呓语 / 140
易寒易热 / 574
易筋功 / 503
易虚易实 / 574
疫疔 / 592
疫毒 / 63
疫毒痢 / 522
疫毒证 / 200
疫喉 / 585
疫喉痧 / 520
疫咳 / 586
疫疠之气 / 63
疫痢 / 522
疫痧 / 520，585
益母草 / 334
益母草膏 / 395
益气 / 244
益气安神 / 264
益气解表 / 230
益气生津 / 264
益肾宁神 / 264
益阴 / 248
益智仁 / 346
嗌 / 40
意 / 57
意呼吸 / 498
意舍 / 422
意守 / 499
意守丹田 / 499
意守体外 / 499
意守自身 / 499
溢乳 / 577，587
溢饮 / 528
薏苡仁 / 321
翳 / 612
翳风 / 428
翳明 / 440
臆 / 47

yīn

因地制宜 / 17，218
因人制宜 / 218
因时、因地、因人制宜 / 218
因时制宜 / 17，218
阴 / 5
阴斑 / 139
阴包 / 432
阴病 / 514
阴病治阳 / 221
阴刺 / 462
阴道 / 555
阴都 / 425
阴谷 / 424
阴寒质 / 75
阴汗 / 145
阴户 / 49，555
阴黄 / 523
阴极似阳 / 7
阴交 / 436
阴结 / 545
阴竭阳脱 / 80
阴茎 / 49
阴经 / 399
阴廉 / 433
阴陵泉 / 415
阴络 / 407
阴门 / 49
阴囊 / 49
阴气 / 55
阴器 / 49
阴器痛 / 147
阴跷脉 / 406
阴跷脉病证 / 216
阴盛 / 79
阴盛格阳 / 80
阴盛阳衰 / 78
阴市 / 414
阴暑 / 517
阴衰 / 79
阴水 / 549

阴损及阳 / 7
阴挺 / 564
阴脱 / 80，81
阴脱证 / 173
阴维脉 / 406
阴维脉病证 / 216
阴郄 / 416
阴痫 / 535，589
阴邪 / 63
阴虚 / 79
阴虚潮热 / 519
阴虚盗汗 / 532
阴虚动风证 / 210
阴虚发热 / 530
阴虚肺燥 / 102
阴虚肺燥证 / 204
阴虚风动 / 103
阴虚感冒 / 516
阴虚火旺 / 79
阴虚火旺证 / 172
阴虚内热证 / 172
阴虚咽喉失濡证 / 203
阴虚阳亢 / 79
阴虚证 / 173
阴虚质 / 75
阴阳 / 5
阴阳辨证 / 168
阴阳并补剂 / 373
阴阳不和 / 6
阴阳对立 / 6
阴阳格拒 / 79
阴阳乖戾 / 6
阴阳和平之人 / 74
阴阳互根 / 5
阴阳互损 / 7
阴阳交感 / 5
阴阳离决 / 6
阴阳两虚 / 80
阴阳配穴法 / 447
阴阳偏胜［盛］/ 6
阴阳偏衰 / 6
阴阳平和质 / 73
阴阳平衡 / 6
阴阳胜复 / 7
阴阳失调 / 6
阴阳调和 / 6
阴阳五态人 / 74
阴阳消长 / 6
阴阳学说 / 5
阴阳易 / 553
阴阳转化 / 6
阴阳自和 / 6
阴痒 / 147
阴液 / 58
阴液亏虚证 / 173
阴脏 / 20
阴证 / 168
阴证似阳 / 173
阴中之阳 / 5
阴中之阴 / 5
茵陈 / 309
茵陈蒿 / 309
茵陈蒿汤 / 379
殷门 / 421
喑［瘖］/ 140

yín

银柴胡 / 306
银海精微 / 698
银花 / 310
银黄口服液 / 383
银翘解毒丸［片］/ 381
银翘散 / 362
银针 / 452
淫气 / 63
淫羊藿 / 346
龈 / 39
龈交 / 435

yǐn

引火归原 / 251
引经报使 / 358
引伸法 / 485
引针 / 462
饮 / 72，282，527
饮片 / 282
饮膳正要 / 689
饮食不节 / 70
饮食不洁 / 70
饮食劳倦 / 70
饮食偏嗜 / 153
饮食有节 / 507
饮停心包证 / 188
饮停胸胁证 / 188
饮证 / 188，528
隐白 / 415
隐疾 / 524
隐痛 / 148
隐瘾疹 / 603

yìn

印堂 / 43，440

yīng

婴儿瘛疭 / 575
婴儿湿疮 / 604
罂粟壳 / 302，350
膺 / 47
膺窗 / 412

yíng

迎风冷泪 / 611
迎风流泪 / 611
迎风热泪 / 611
迎随补泻 / 457
迎随补泻法 / 457
迎随顺逆补泻法 / 491
迎香 / 411
荥穴 / 437
营 / 56
营分 / 56
营分证 / 179
营气 / 54
营卫不和 / 86
营血 / 56
营阴 / 54
蝇翅黑花 / 620
蝇影飞越 / 620

yǐng

瘿 / 597
瘿痈 / 597

yìng

硬气功 / 492
硬肿症 / 576

yōng

痈 / 593

yǒng

涌泉 / 423
涌吐禁例 / 267
涌吐药 / 294

yòng

用药法象 / 689

yōu

忧 / 69
幽门 / 41，425

yóu

尤怡 / 675
尤在泾 / 676
由表入里 / 82
由里出表 / 83
由实转虚 / 84
由虚转实 / 84
油风 / 603
油汗 / 145
疣 / 600
疣目 / 600
游走痛 / 148

yǒu

有根苔 / 136
有头疽 / 594
有形之痰 / 71

yòu

右归丸 / 373
幼科铁镜 / 696
幼幼集成 / 696
幼幼新书 / 696

yū

瘀热 / 88
瘀痰证 / 190
瘀血 / 71
瘀血犯头证 / 185
瘀血头痛 / 534
瘀血痫 / 590
瘀血阻滞证 / 185
瘀阻胞宫证 / 214
瘀阻脑络证 / 201

yú

余沥不尽 / 151
余霖 / 678
余热未清证 / 180
鱼际 / 409
鱼际擦法 / 650
鱼络 / 407
鱼翔脉 / 163
鱼腥草 / 311
鱼腰 / 440
虞天民 / 668
虞抟 / 668

yǔ

禹粮石 / 349
禹余粮 / 349
语迟 / 578
语声 / 139
语声低微 / 140
语声重浊 / 140
语言謇涩 / 140

yù

玉机微义 / 701
玉门 / 555
玉米须 / 323
玉屏风口服液 / 383
玉屏风散 / 371
玉堂 / 436
玉液 / 440
玉枕 / 419
玉枕骨 / 46
玉竹 / 343
郁病 / 549
郁火 / 70
郁金 / 331
郁李仁 / 352
育阴 / 248
彧中 / 425
欲合先离 / 640
喻昌 / 673
喻嘉言 / 673
寓补于攻 / 220
寓攻于补 / 220

yuān

渊液 / 430

yuán

元府 / 41
元胡 / 332
元胡止痛片 / 393
元气 / 53
元神之府 / 25
元阳 / 23
元阳亏虚 / 113
元阴 / 22
芫花 / 324
原［元］机启微 / 698
原络配穴法 / 447
原气 / 53
原穴 / 438
圆利针 / 452
圆癣 / 604
圆翳 / 620
圆翳内障 / 620
圆针 / 451

yuǎn

远道刺 / 460
远道选穴法 / 446
远近配穴法 / 448
远视 / 621
远血 / 550
远志 / 336

yuě

哕 / 543

yuè

月季花 / 332

月经 / 157，556
月经病 / 557
月经不调 / 557
月经错后 / 157
月经过多 / 157，560
月经过少 / 157，558
月经后期 / 157，557
月经涩少 / 558
月经提前 / 157
月经先后无定期 / 558
月经先期 / 157，557
月蚀疮 / 623
月事 / 157，556
月水 / 157，556
月水不调 / 557
月水过多 / 157，561
月信 / 157，556
越经传 / 116
越鞠丸 / 387

yún

云门 / 408
云雾移睛 / 620
芸香草 / 304

yùn

运法 / 483
运脾 / 245
运气 / 17，503
运气学说 / 17
运针 / 454
恽树珏 / 682
恽铁樵 / 682
晕灸 / 467
晕针 / 463
熨法 / 272
熨目 / 487
熨药 / 642

Z

zá

杂病 / 524
杂气 / 63

zài

再造丸 / 391
在泉 / 18

zǎn

昝殷 / 662

zàn

赞刺 / 462

zāng

脏 / 20
脏腑 / 20
脏腑辨证 / 200
脏腑病机 / 96
脏腑津亏 / 81
脏腑相合 / 26
脏腑虚损耳鸣 / 624
脏寒泻 / 588
脏厥 / 538
脏气 / 26，54
脏象 / 20，26
脏象学说 / 20
脏躁 / 535

zàng

藏红花 / 330

zǎo

早泄 / 156
早泄（病） / 552
蚤休 / 311

zào

皂角刺 / 333
燥 / 66
燥干清窍 / 90
燥干清窍证 / 198
燥化 / 92
燥火 / 66，68
燥剂 / 360
燥结 / 92
燥结证 / 198
燥气 / 66
燥气寒化 / 90
燥气化热 / 90
燥热 / 66，68
燥伤肺气 / 89
燥伤津液 / 90
燥湿 / 260
燥湿化痰 / 258
燥湿健脾 / 260
燥湿止痒 / 267
燥苔 / 135
燥痰证 / 189
燥邪 / 66
燥邪犯［伤］肺证 / 198
躁烦 / 124
躁狂 / 124

zé

择向补泻法 / 491
泽兰 / 334
泽泻 / 320

zéi

贼风 / 63

zēng

曾世荣 / 666
增液通下 / 237
憎寒 / 143

zhā

扎带 / 642

zhà

痄腮 / 585

zhān

谵妄 / 124
谵语 / 140
瞻视昏渺 / 620

zhàn

战汗 / 145，531
战栗 / 143
站式 / 495
站桩功 / 502

zhāng

张从正 / 664
张机 / 658
张洁古 / 664
张介宾 / 672

张景岳 / 672
张路玉 / 674
张璐 / 674
张三锡 / 670
张山雷 / 682
张石顽 / 674
张氏医通 / 704
张寿甫 / 681
张寿颐 / 681
张锡纯 / 681
张筱衫 / 680
张隐庵 / 674
张元素 / 664
张振鋆 / 680
张志聪 / 674
张仲景 / 659
张子和 / 664
章门 / 433
章楠 / 678

zhǎng

掌按法 / 651
掌擦法 / 650
掌击法 / 649
掌摩法 / 650
掌揉法 / 647
掌推扳胸椎法 / 652
掌推法 / 648
掌心毒 / 592

zhàng

胀痛 / 147
障 / 612
瘴毒 / 72，521
瘴疟 / 520，521
瘴气 / 72，520

zháo

着肤灸 / 465

zhào

赵恕轩 / 677
赵献可 / 671
赵学敏 / 677
赵养葵 / 671
照海 / 424

zhé

折顶 / 639
折骨绝筋 / 635
折骨列肤 / 635
折疡 / 635
辄筋 / 430

zhě

赭石 / 339

zhè

浙贝母 / 302
䗪虫 / 333

zhēn

针柄 / 449
针刺疗法 / 444
针刺麻醉 / 470，699
针法 / 444
针感 / 456
针根 / 449
针尖 / 449
针灸 / 444
针灸大成 / 699
针灸甲乙经 / 699
针灸聚英 / 699
针灸疗法 / 444
针灸师 / 444
针灸铜人 / 452
针灸问答 / 699
针灸问对 / 699
针灸学 / 444
针灸资生经 / 699
针麻诱导 / 470
针体 / 449
针向行气法 / 459
针眼 / 612
珍本医书集成 / 705
珍珠 / 337
珍珠母 / 337
珍珠囊药性赋 / 689
真寒假热 / 92
真寒假热证 / 174
真火 / 23
真睛破损 / 621
真气 / 53，500
真气气感 / 505
真热假寒 / 92
真热假寒证 / 174
真实假虚 / 85
真实假虚证 / 174
真水 / 22
真头痛 / 533
真武汤 / 380
真心痛 / 530
真虚假实 / 85
真虚假实证 / 174
真牙 / 39，632
真阳 / 23
真阴 / 22
真阴不足 / 112
真元亏虚证 / 212
真脏脉 / 165
真脏色 / 126
真中 / 536
真中风 / 536
甄权 / 660

zhěn

诊病 / 122
诊断 / 122
诊断学 / 122
诊法 / 123
诊籍 / 122
诊家枢要 / 686
枕骨 / 46
枕上旁线 / 472
枕上正中线 / 471
枕下旁线 / 472
疹 / 139，591

zhèn

振掉 / 540
振法 / 484
振挺 / 654
震颤法 / 455

震桩式 / 503
镇肝潜阳 / 265
镇肝熄［息］风 / 266
镇惊 / 264
镇惊安神 / 264
镇静安神 / 265
镇潜 / 265
镇心安神 / 264

zhēng

征候 / 122
怔忡 / 151，530
蒸 / 278
癥瘕 / 548
癥瘕积聚 / 548

zhěng

整复 / 638
整体观念 / 218

zhèng

正骨（科）/ 635
正骨八法 / 638
正骨手法 / 638
正经 / 398
正疟 / 520
正气 / 54
正水 / 549
正邪分争 / 78
正邪相争 / 78
正虚邪实 / 78
正营 / 429
正治 / 220
证 / 168
证候 / 122，168
证类本草 / 688
证型 / 122，168
证治汇补 / 694
证治准绳 / 703
郑瀚 / 677
郑宏纲 / 677
郑梅涧 / 677
郑若溪 / 678
郑声 / 140
政和本草 / 688
症状 / 122

zhī

支沟 / 427
支饮 / 528
支正 / 417
知柏地黄丸 / 390
知母 / 304
栀子 / 310
脂瘤 / 598
脂人 / 75
脂塞不孕 / 566

zhí

直刺 / 454
直接灸 / 465
直透 / 454
直针刺 / 461
直中 / 116
植物名实图考 / 689
植物名实图考长编 / 690
跖 / 50
跖疣 / 600

zhǐ

止呃 / 267
止汗 / 261
止痉 / 268
止咳化痰 / 264
止咳平喘药 / 292
止咳药 / 301
止渴 / 267
止呕 / 267
止嗽散 / 361
止痛 / 267
止血 / 257
止血剂 / 377
止血敛疮 / 271
止血收口 / 271
止血行瘀 / 271
止血药 / 291
止痒 / 267
止遗尿 / 268
止晕 / 267
指按法 / 651
指节拍法 / 649
指摩法 / 650
指切进针法 / 453
指揉法 / 647
指推法 / 648
指压疗法 / 479
指压麻醉 / 479
指压推拿 / 490
指压行气法 / 459
指针法 / 481
枳壳 / 325
枳实 / 325

zhì

至阳 / 434
至阴 / 423
志 / 58
志室 / 422
制川乌 / 314
制何首乌 / 344
制霜 / 278
制炭 / 276
炙 / 277
炙甘草 / 341
治本 / 219
治标 / 219
治病求本 / 219
治风化痰 / 259
治风剂 / 377
治未病 / 219
治燥剂 / 378
栉头 / 486
秩边 / 422
痔 / 598
智齿 / 632
滞颐 / 579
滞针 / 463
稚阴稚阳 / 574
稚子 / 574

zhōng

中藏经 / 700
中草药 / 275
中冲 / 426
中丹田 / 496
中都 / 432
中渎 / 431
中渎之腑 / 27
中封 / 432
中府 / 408
中国药学大辞典 / 705
中国医学大成 / 705
中国医学大辞典 / 705
中极 / 435
中焦 / 24
中焦病证 / 181
中焦湿热 / 106
中焦湿热证 / 181，207
中焦实热 / 215
中焦虚寒 / 215
中精之腑 / 27
中魁 / 442
中髎 / 421
中膂俞 / 421
中满 / 154
中品 / 279
中气 / 56
中气不足 / 108
中气下陷 / 94
中气下陷证 / 206
中清之腑 / 27
中泉 / 442
中湿 / 66
中枢 / 433
中庭 / 436
中脘 / 23，436
中消 / 551
中阳不振 / 108
中药 / 275
中药学 / 275
中指独立式 / 505
中指同身寸 / 444
中渚 / 426
中注 / 424

zhǒng

肿毒 / 591
肿疡 / 591
肿胀 / 138
肿胀舌 / 132
踵 / 50

zhòng

中毒 / 72
中恶 / 72
中风 / 536
中风闭证 / 536
中风病 / 536
中风后遗症 / 537
中风昏迷 / 537
中风脱证 / 536
中风阳闭 / 536
中风阴闭 / 536
中腑 / 537
中寒 / 64，91
中寒泻 / 588
中经 / 537
中络 / 537
中暑 / 517
中暑眩晕 / 533
中脏 / 536
重插轻提 / 456
重剂 / 360
重提轻插 / 457
重听 / 624
重痛 / 148
重镇安神 / 265
重镇安神剂 / 380
重镇安神药 / 293

zhōu

周荣 / 416
周天 / 500
周天功 / 501
周天自转功 / 502
周易参同契 / 700

zhǒu

肘按法 / 651
肘后备急方 / 690
肘尖 / 442
肘髎 / 410
肘揉法 / 648
肘推法 / 648

zhū

朱丹溪 / 666
朱沛文 / 679
朱砂 / 336
朱砂安神丸 / 380，385
朱震亨 / 666
侏儒 / 590
诸病源侯总论 / 687
诸虫 / 72
诸阳之会 / 42
猪苓 / 320
蛛丝飘浮 / 612

zhú

竹罐 / 467
竹茹 / 300
竹叶 / 305
竹叶石膏汤 / 367
逐水 / 237
逐水剂 / 365

zhǔ

主辅佐引 / 358
主气 / 18
主色 / 124
主应配穴法 / 448
主运 / 18
煮 / 278
煮罐法 / 468

zhù

苎麻根 / 329
助阳 / 250
助阳解表 / 230
注泄 / 150
柱骨 / 50
柱舌 / 494

疰夏 / 582
疰夏病 / 582
筑宾 / 424

zhuā

抓法 / 483
抓痧疗法 / 470

zhuàn

转筋霍乱 / 523
转筋 / 127

zhuàng

壮 / 464
壮热 / 143
壮水制阳 / 250
壮阳 / 251
撞击伤目 / 621

zhuì

坠肘 / 493

zhuó

灼热 / 143
灼痛 / 148
浊气 / 55
浊邪 / 72
浊阴 / 57
啄法 / 650
啄击法 / 484
着痹 / 540

zī

姿式 / 493
滋补肺肾 / 249
滋补肾阴 / 249
滋肾 / 250
滋肾阴 / 250
滋水涵木 / 248
滋养肝肾 / 248
滋养胃阴 / 249
滋阴 / 248
滋阴补血 / 250
滋阴降火 / 250
滋阴解表 / 230
滋阴利水 / 250
滋阴凉血 / 250
滋阴潜阳 / 265
滋阴清热 / 250
滋阴润肺 / 249
滋阴润燥 / 250
滋阴润燥剂 / 378
滋阴熄［息］风 / 266
滋阴药 / 294
滋阴抑阳 / 250

zǐ

子 / 13
子肠 / 555
子烦 / 567
子宫 / 441，555
子淋 / 567
子满 / 567
子冒 / 567
子门 / 49，555
子母补泻法 / 458
子母配穴法 / 448
子气 / 13
子死腹中 / 567
子嗽 / 568
子痰 / 599
子午流注 / 459
子午流注针法 / 459
子痫 / 566
子悬 / 567
子喑 / 568
子痈 / 599
子晕 / 566
子脏 / 25，556
子肿 / 568
紫白癜风 / 605
紫斑 / 550
紫贝齿 / 337
紫草 / 306
紫宫 / 436
紫河车 / 342
紫花地丁 / 311
紫硇砂 / 355
紫舌 / 131
紫苏梗 / 326
紫苏叶 / 296
紫苏子 / 303
紫外线穴位照射疗法 / 479
紫菀 / 299
紫雪 / 392

zì

自汗 / 144，531
自然呼吸 / 497
自然铜 / 335
自然站式 / 495
自然站桩功 / 502
自我按摩 / 486
眦 / 607
眦漏 / 615
眦帷赤烂 / 614

zōng

宗筋 / 49
宗筋之会 / 49
宗气 / 54
棕榈炭 / 329

zǒng

总按 / 159

zǒu

走窜痛 / 148
走罐 / 469
走黄 / 595
走火入魔 / 505
走马疳 / 633
走马牙疳 / 633
走式 / 496

zú

足蹬 / 639
足底疔 / 592
足发背 / 594
足跗 / 51
足跟痛 / 147
足厥阴肝经 / 405
足厥阴肝经穴 / 432
足临泣 / 431
足窍阴 / 432

足三里 / 414
足三阳经 / 399
足三阴经 / 399
足少阳胆经 / 404
足少阳胆经穴 / 428
足少阴肾经 / 403
足少阴肾经穴 / 423
足太阳膀胱经 / 403
足太阳膀胱经穴 / 418
足太阴脾经 / 401
足太阴脾经穴 / 414
足通谷 / 423
足五里 / 433
足阳明胃经 / 401
足阳明胃经穴 / 411
足针 / 478
足针疗法 / 478
卒病 / 515
卒喉痹 / 630
卒聋 / 624
卒心痛 / 531
卒喑［瘖］/ 630
卒中 / 536

zǔ

祖传秘方 / 357

zǔn

撙令平正 / 648
撙捺皮相 / 648
撙捺相近 / 648

zuǒ

左病右取，右病左取 / 221
左归丸 / 372
左右配穴法 / 447
佐药 / 358

zuò

坐板疮 / 592
坐罐 / 469
坐式 / 494
坐式复位 / 642
坐忘 / 498

引文索引 Index of Citations

二画

[一]

七情之病，看花解闷，听曲消愁，胜于服药。/ 509

[丿]

人与天地相参。/ 18
人以天地之气生，四时之法成。/ 18
人欲劳于形，百病不能成。/ 508

三画

[一]

三焦为营卫之源。/ 37
三焦有名无形。/ 37
三焦者，决渎之官，水道出焉。/ 37
土为木之所胜。/ 16
土为水之所不胜。/ 16
土生万物。/ 15
土郁夺之。/ 223
土爰稼啬。/ 14
土喜温燥。/ 15
下者举之。/ 223
下棋可忘忧，慢跑可长寿。/ 509
下焦主出。/ 37
下焦如渎。/ 37
下燥则结。/ 76
下燥治血。/ 287
大肠主传导。/ 35
大肠者，传导之官，变化出焉。/ 35
大实如羸状。/ 174
大毒治病，十去其六。/ 286
万物之生，皆禀元气。/ 3

[丨]

上工治未病。/ 222
上焦主纳。/ 37
上焦如雾。/ 37
上燥则咳。/ 76
上燥治气。/ 287
小大不利治其标；小大利治其本。/ 222
小肠化食，泌别清浊。/ 29
小肠主化物。/ 29
小肠主受盛。/ 29
小肠者，受盛之官，化物出焉。/ 29
小毒治病，十去其八。/ 286

[丿]

久热伤阴。/ 119

[乛]

子病及母。/ 16
子盗母气。/ 16
卫气者，所以温分肉，充皮肤，肥腠理，司开合者也。/ 60
卫气虚则不用。/ 119

四画

[一]

天为阳，地为阴；日为阳，月为阴。/ 7
天食人以五气，地食人以五味。/ 19
夫百病者，多以旦慧昼安，夕加夜甚。/ 19
夫精者，身之本也。/ 60
无犯胃气。/ 224
无毒治病，十去其九。/ 286
木曰曲直。/ 14
木为土之所不胜。/ 16
木为金之所胜。/ 15
木郁达之。/ 223
木喜条达。/ 15
五谷为养，五果为助，五畜为益，五菜为充。/ 510
五脏为实，藏而不泄。/ 28
五脏应四时。/ 19
五脏藏精气而不泄。/ 28

[丨]

少火生气。/ 119
少思以养神，少欲以养精。/ 508
中焦主化。/ 37
中焦如沤。/ 37
中满者，泻之于内。/ 286
中燥则渴。/ 76
中燥增液。/ 287
水曰润下。/ 15
水为土之所胜。/ 16
水为火之所不胜。/ 16
水为阴，火为阳。/ 7
水郁折之。/ 223
水性流下。/ 15
见微知著。/ 166

[丿]

气大伤人，酒多伤身。/ 510
气为血帅。/ 59
气由脏发，色随气华。/ 166
气有余便是火。/ 119
气行血行。/ 60
气始而生化，气散而有形，气布而蕃育，气终而象

变，其致一也。/ 3
气虚则寒。/ 118
气虚宜掣引之。/ 286
升降出入，无器不有。/ 3
爪为筋之余。/ 30
勿药为中医。/ 508
风为百病之长。/ 76
风胜则动。/ 76
风盛则动。/ 119
风善行而数变。/ 76
［丶］
六腑为空，泄而不藏。/ 28
六腑以降为顺。/ 36
六腑以通为用。/ 36
六腑传化物而不藏。/ 28
亢则害，承乃制。/ 15
火曰炎上。/ 14
火为水之所胜。/ 16
火为金之所不胜。/ 16
火郁发之。/ 223
火性炎上。/ 76
户枢不蠹，流水不腐，人之形体，其亦由是。/ 508
心与小肠相表里。/ 29
心开窍于舌。/ 28
心包络与三焦相表里。/ 37
心主血脉。/ 28
心主神明。/ 28
心在志为喜。/ 29
心有所忆谓之意。/ 60
心合小肠。/ 29
心者，君主之官，神明出焉。/ 28
心者，其华在面。/ 28
心脉洪。/ 167
心恶热。/ 29
心胸宽，人快活；心胸窄，忧愁多。/ 509
心属火。/ 28
心藏神。/ 28
［乛］
以动养形，以形养神。/ 508
毋逆天时，是谓至治。/ 224

五画

［一］
甘入脾。/ 285
［丨］
四变之动，脉与之上下，以春应中规，夏应中矩，秋应中衡，冬应中权。/ 19
［丿］
生之本，本于阴阳。/ 8
生之来谓之精，两精相搏谓之神。/ 3，60
失神者亡。/ 166
用温远温，用热远热，用凉远凉，用寒远寒。/ 285
外者为阳，内者为阴。/ 8
冬不欲极温，夏不欲极凉。/ 510
冬伤于寒，春必温病。/ 19
冬应中权。/ 167
饥不暴食，渴不狂饮。/ 511
［丶］
立如松，坐如钟，卧如弓。/ 510
宁可三日无粮，不可一日无茶。/ 511
必先岁气，无伐天和。/ 19
［乛］
司外揣内。/ 166
发为血之余。/ 30
母病及子。/ 16

六画

［一］
百病（皆）生于气。/ 119
有毒无毒，所治为主。/ 286
有故无殒，亦无殒也。/ 286
有胃气则生，无胃气则死。/ 224
至虚有盛候。/ 174
邪之所凑，其气必虚。/ 118
邪气盛则实。/ 174
［丨］
因志而存变谓之思。/ 61
因其轻而扬之。/ 286
因其重而减之。/ 286
因其衰而彰之。/ 286
因思而远慕谓之虑。/ 61
因虑而处物谓之智。/ 61
［丿］
先饥而食，先渴而饮；食欲数而少，不欲顿而多。/ 510
先睡心，后睡眼。/ 508
舌为心之苗。/ 28
血为气母。/ 60
血汗同源。/ 59
血实宜决之。/ 286
多思则神殆，多念则智散。/ 509
多欲则智昏，多事则劳形。/ 509
［丶］
衣着寒暖适体，勿侈华艳。/ 509
并精出入者谓之魄。/ 60
壮火食气。/ 119
壮水之主，以制阳光。/ 224
汗为心液。/ 59
［乛］
阳化气，阴成形。/ 8
阳为气，阴为味。/ 9
阳生于阴。/ 9
阳胜则热，阴胜则寒。/ 9
阳根于阴，阴根于阳。/ 8
阳盛［胜］则热。/ 118
阳虚则外寒。/ 118
阳常有余，阴常不足。/ 9
阴中有阳，阳中有阴。/ 8
阴平阳秘，精神乃治。/ 8

阴生于阳。/ 9
阴在内，阳之守也。阳在外，阴之使也。/ 8
阴阳之要，阳密乃固。/ 8
阴阳者，万物之能始也。/ 8
阴阳者，天地之道也，万物之纲纪，变化之父母，生杀之本始。/ 7
阴阳者，数之可十，推之可百，数之可千，推之可万，万之大不可胜数，然其要一也。/ 9
阴阳离决，精气乃绝。/ 8
阴胜则阳病，阳胜则阴病。/ 9
阴盛［胜］则寒。/ 118
阴虚则内热。/ 118
阴静阳躁，阳生阴长。/ 9

七画

［一］

形不足者温之以气。/ 223
劳则气耗。/ 77
劳者温之。/ 223

［丨］

坚者削之。/ 223
足要常搓，腹要常摩。/ 508

［丿］

肝与胆相表里。/ 31
肝开窍于目。/ 30
肝为风木之脏。/ 30
肝为刚脏。/ 30
肝为血海。/ 30
肝为牡脏。/ 30
肝主升发。/ 29
肝主目。/ 30
肝主怒。/ 30
肝主筋。/ 29
肝主疏泄。/ 29
肝在志为怒。/ 30
肝合胆。/ 31
肝体阴而用阳。/ 30
肝者，其华在爪。/ 29
肝者，将军之官，谋虑出焉。/ 29
肝肾同源。/ 31
肝脉弦。/ 167
肝恶风。/ 30
肝属木。/ 29
肝藏血。/ 29
肝藏魂。/ 30
饭后百步走，活到九十九。/ 508
饮食自倍，脾胃乃伤。/ 510

［丶］

辛入肺。/ 285
辛甘发散为阳，酸苦涌泄为阴。/ 10
辛散，酸收，甘缓，苦坚，咸软。/ 285
间者并行，甚者独行。/ 222
忧则气郁。/ 77
忧伤肺。/ 77

八画

［一］

其下者，引而竭之。/ 286
其下者引而竭之。/ 224
其在皮者汗而发之。/ 224
其高者，因而越之。/ 286
其高者因而越之。/ 224
苦入心。/ 285
若要安，三里常不干。/ 508

［丨］

齿为骨之余。/ 36
肾与膀胱相表里。/ 36
肾开窍于二阴。/ 36
肾开窍于耳。/ 36
肾气通于耳。/ 36
肾为气之根。/ 35
肾为水脏。/ 35
肾为先天之本。/ 35
肾主水。/ 35
肾主生殖。/ 35
肾主纳气。/ 35
肾主命门之火。/ 36
肾主骨。/ 36
肾司二阴。/ 36
肾司开阖。/ 35
肾在志为恐。/ 35
肾合膀胱。/ 36
肾者，作强之官，伎巧出焉。/ 35
肾者，其华在发。/ 36
肾其充在骨，骨充则髓实。/ 35
肾脉沉。/ 167
肾恶燥。/ 36
肾属水。/ 35
肾藏志。/ 35
肾藏精。/ 35
炅则气泄。/ 77

［丿］

所不胜，克我者也。/ 15
所胜，我所克也。/ 15
金曰从革。/ 15
金气肃降。/ 15
金为木之所不胜。/ 16
金为火之所胜。/ 15
金郁泻之。/ 223
金实不鸣。/ 15
金破不鸣。/ 15
乳贵有时，食贵有节。/ 510
贪吃贪睡，添病减岁。/ 508
肺与大肠相表里。/ 34
肺开窍于鼻。/ 34
肺为气之主。/ 33
肺为水之上源。/ 33
肺为华盖。/ 34
肺为贮痰之器。/ 34
肺为娇脏。/ 34
肺主一身之表。/ 34

肺主气，司呼吸。/ 33
肺主皮毛。/ 34
肺主行水。/ 33
肺主声。/ 34
肺主肃降。/ 33
肺主宣发。/ 33
肺主通调水道。/ 33
肺在志为忧。/ 34
肺在志为悲。/ 34
肺合大肠。/ 34
肺合皮毛。/ 33
肺者，其华在毛。/ 34
肺脉浮。/ 167
肺恶寒。/ 34
肺朝百脉。/ 33
肺属金。/ 33
肺藏魄。/ 34

［丶］

泪为肝液。/ 59
治未病。/ 507
治标不如治本。/ 222
治热以寒。/ 222
治热以寒，温而行之。/ 285
治病必求其本。/ 222
治寒以热。/ 222
治寒以热，凉而行之。/ 285
宗气积于胸中，出于喉咙，以贯心脉，而行呼吸。/ 60
实则泻之。/ 222
诗书悦心，山林逸兴，可以延年。/ 509

［乛］

孤阳不生，独阴不长。/ 9

九画

［一］

春应中规。/ 167
春夏养阳，秋冬养阴。/ 19，508
甚者从之。/ 223
荣气虚则不仁。/ 119
药补不如食补。/ 510
咸入肾。/ 285
轻可去实。/ 287
背为阳，阳中之阳，心也。/ 8
背为阳，阳中之阴，肺也。/ 8
背要常暖，胸要常护。/ 508

［丨］

胃不和，卧不安。/ 511
胃气主降。/ 33
胃为水谷之海。/ 33
胃主受纳。/ 33
胃主降浊。/ 33
胃主腐熟。/ 33
思则气结。/ 77
思伤脾。/ 77

［丿］

秋应中衡。/ 167
重可去怯。/ 287
重阴必阳，重阳必阴。/ 9
修性以保神，安心以全身。/ 508
食饱不可睡，睡则诸疾生。/ 508
胆主决断。/ 31
胆者，中正之官。/ 31
急则治标。/ 222
急者缓之。/ 223

［丶］

恬淡虚无，真气从之；精神内守，病从安来。/ 61，507
涎为脾液。/ 59
津血同源。/ 59
客者除之。/ 222

［乛］

怒则气上。/ 77
怒伤肝。/ 77
结者散之。/ 223

十画

［一］

起居有常，养其神也，不妄作劳，养其精也。/ 509
恐则气下。/ 77
恐伤肾。/ 77
莫吃空心茶，休饮卯时酒，更兼戌后饭，禁之当谨守。/ 511
真气存内，邪不可干。/ 507
根于中者，命曰神机，神去则机息。/ 3
根于外者，命曰气立，气止则化绝。/ 4
夏应中矩。/ 167
热之而寒者取之阳。/ 224
热可制寒/ 287
热极生寒。/ 119
热极似寒。/ 174
热者寒之。/ 222
热胜则肿。/ 77
热盛则肿。/ 119

［丿］

积精全神。/ 3
笑一笑，少一少；恼一恼，老一老。/ 509
笑口常开，青春常在。/ 509
脏行气于腑。/ 28
留者攻之。/ 222

［丶］

高者抑之。/ 223
病从口入。/ 510
益火之源，以消阴翳。/ 224
酒通血脉，消愁遣兴，少饮壮神，过多损命。/ 510
涕为肺液。/ 59
涩可固脱。/ 287
诸气膹郁，皆属于肺。/ 117
诸风掉眩，皆属于肝。/ 117
诸呕吐酸，暴注下迫，皆属

于热。/ 118
诸转反戾，水液混浊，皆属于热。/ 118
诸胀腹大，皆属于热。/ 117
诸逆冲上，皆属于火。/ 117
诸热瞀瘛，皆属于火。/ 117
诸病水液，澄澈清冷，皆属于寒。/ 118
诸病有声，鼓之如鼓，皆属于热。/ 118
诸病胕肿，疼酸惊骇，皆属于火。/ 118
诸痉项强，皆属于湿。/ 117
诸厥固泄，皆属于下。/ 117
诸痛痒疮，皆属于心。/ 117
诸湿肿满，皆属于脾。/ 117
诸寒之而热者取之阴，热之而寒者取之阳。/ 285
诸寒收引，皆属于肾。/ 117
诸禁鼓栗，如丧神守，皆属于火。/ 117
诸痿喘呕，皆属于上。/ 117
诸暴强直，皆属于风。/ 117
诸躁狂越，皆属于火。/ 117

十一画

[一]

菜饭宜清淡，少盐少疾患。/ 510
营气者，泌其津液，注之于脉，化以为血，以荣四末，内注五脏六腑。/ 60

[丨]

虚邪贼风，避之有时。/ 507
虚则补之。/ 222
虚者补其母，实者泻其子。/ 224
常毒治病，十去其七。/ 286
晨起三百步，睡前一盆汤。/ 510
唾为肾液。/ 59

[丿]

得神者昌。/ 166
得神者昌，失神者亡。/ 3
欲不可纵，纵欲成灾；乐不可极，乐极生灾。/ 509
欲知病色，必先知常色；欲知常色，必先知常色之变；欲知常色之变，必先知常色变中之变。/ 166
逸者行之。/ 222

[丶]

烹调有方。/ 510
望而知之谓之神，闻而知之谓之圣，问而知之谓之工，切脉知之谓之巧。/ 166
惊则气乱。/ 77
惊者平之。/ 223

[一]

随神往来谓之魂。/ 60

十二画

[一]

喜则气缓。/ 77
喜伤心。/ 77
散者收之。/ 223
揆度奇恒。/ 166
悲则气消。/ 77
脾与胃相表里。/ 32
脾开窍于口。/ 32
脾气主升。/ 31
脾为气血生化之源。/ 32
脾为生痰之源。/ 32
脾主升清。/ 31
脾主四肢。/ 32
脾主后天。/ 32
脾主肌肉。/ 32
脾主运化。/ 31
脾在志为思。/ 32
脾合胃。/ 32
脾者，其华在唇。/ 32
脾胃为后天之本。/ 32
脾胃者，仓廪之官，五味出焉。/ 31
脾脉缓。/ 167
脾统血。/ 31
脾恶湿。/ 32
脾属土。/ 31
脾藏营。/ 31
脾藏意。/ 32
腑输精于脏。/ 28

[丶]

湿易伤阳。/ 76
湿性重浊。/ 76
湿性黏滞。/ 76
湿胜则阳微。/ 76
湿胜则濡泻。/ 76
湿盛则濡泻。/ 118
湿盛阳微。/ 119
温邪上受，首先犯肺。/ 119
寒之而热者取之阴。/ 224
寒为阴邪，易伤阳气。/ 76
寒则气收。/ 77
寒极生热。/ 119
寒极似热。/ 174
寒者热之。/ 222
寒性收引。/ 76
寒性凝滞。/ 76

[一]

缓则治本。/ 222

十三画

[丿]

微者逆之。/ 223
腰为肾之府。/ 35
腹为阴，阴中之至阴，脾也。/ 8
腹为阴，阴中之阳，肝也。/ 8
腹为阴，阴中之阴，肾也。/ 8

[丶]
意之所存谓之志。/ 60
谨察阴阳所在而调之，以平为期。/ 9

十四画

[一]
歌咏所以养性情，舞蹈所以养血脉。/ 509
酸入肝。/ 285
[丿]
膀胱主藏津液。/ 36
膀胱者，州都之官。/ 36
[丶]
精不足者补之以味。/ 224
精气夺则虚。/ 174
精血同源。/ 59
精神到处文章老，学问深处意气平。/ 509

十七画

[丶]
燥者濡之。/ 223
燥胜则干。/ 76

十八画

[丨]
髓海不足，则脑转耳鸣。/ 37
髓海有余，则轻劲多力，自过其度。/ 37

英文索引 Index of Terms in English

A

A Collection of Gems of Acupuncture and Moxibustion 针灸聚英 / 699
A Compilation of Chinese Medicinal Herbs 全国中草药汇编 / 690
A Complete Book of Ophthalmology 眼科大全 / 699
A Complete Book on External Medicine 外科大成 / 698
A Complete Handbook of Medicinal Processing 炮炙大全 / 689
A Complete Work of Ancient and Modern Medicine 古今医统大全 / 703
A Great Collection of Chinese Medical Works 中国医学大成 / 705
A Handbook of Prescriptions for Emergencies 肘后备急方 / 690
A Lengthy Compilation of Plants with Illustrations 植物名实图考长编 / 690
A Miraculous Book of Ten Recipes 十药神书 / 694
A New Book of Pediatrics 幼幼新书 / 696
A Precious Work on Ophthalmology 审视瑶函 / 698
A Rhymed Discourse on External Therapeutics 理瀹骈文 / 693
A String of Beads from the Treatise on Cold Damage Diseases 伤寒贯珠集 / 686
A Supplement to the Compendium of Materia Medica 本草纲目拾遗 / 689
A Supplement to the Materia Medica 本草拾遗 / 688
abdomen 腹 / 48
abdomen exercise 腹部功 / 501
abdominal distension 腹胀，臌胀（病）/ 154，547
abdominal distension in children 小儿腹胀 / 588
abdominal distension of deficiency type 虚胀 / 589
abdominal distension of excess type 实胀 / 589
abdominal distension with indigestion 伤食腹胀 / 589
abdominal fullness 腹满 / 154
abdominal fullness and distension 腹满䐜胀 / 154
abdominal mass 癥瘕 / 548
abdominal pain 腹痛 / 147，546
abdominal pain during menstruation 经行腹痛 / 560
abdominal pain in children 小儿腹痛 / 588
abdominal pain in pregnancy 妊娠腹痛 / 566
abdominal pain with tenesmus 腹痛下坠 / 153
abhorrence of cold 憎寒 / 143
abnormal debilitation of yin or yang 阴阳偏衰 / 6
abnormal exuberance of yin or yang 阴阳偏胜［盛］/ 6
abnormal pulse; morbid pulse 病脉 / 160
abnormal *qi* 异气 / 63
abnormal rising of *qi* 上气 / 141，526
abnormal weather in the four seasons 四时不正之气 / 63
abortion 堕胎 / 569
abrupt illness 卒病 / 515
abscess 痈 / 593
absence of sweating 无汗 / 145
abundant expectoration 痰盛 / 137
accessibility of the five flavors 五味所入 / 26
accumulation-aggregation 积聚 / 548
accumulation-aggregation masses 癥瘕积聚 / 548
accumulation of dampness-heat in the spleen 湿热蕴脾 / 105
accumulation of pathogenic heat in the lung 邪热壅肺 / 102
accumulation syndrome 积证 / 548
aching pain 酸［痠］痛 / 148
aching shoulder and arm 肩臂酸痛 / 147
acid regurgitation 反酸 / 153
acid regurgitation 泛酸 / 543
acid swallowing 吞酸 / 153，543
acid vomiting 吐酸 / 543
acne 粉刺，酒刺 / 601
Aconite Middle-regulating Pills 附子理中丸 / 387
aconite-interposed moxibustion 附子饼灸 / 466

acquired essence 后天之精 / 57
acquired *qi* 后天之气 / 53
actionless needle retention 静留针法 / 462
activating blood 活血 / 256
activating blood and dispelling stasis 活血祛瘀 / 256
activating blood and moving *qi* 活血行气 / 256
activating blood and resolving stasis 活血化瘀 / 256
activating blood to regulate menstruation 活血调经 / 256
activating blood to relieve pain 活血止痛 / 256
activating blood to stimulate menstruation 活血通经 / 256
activating blood to unblock collaterals 活血通络 / 256
activating the spleen 运脾 / 245
active needle retention 动留针法 / 462
activity of the triple energizer 三焦气化 / 27
acupoint block 穴位封闭 / 470
acupoint catgut-embedding therapy 穴位埋线疗法 / 478
acupoint injection 穴位注射 / 470
acupoint magnetic therapy 磁穴疗法，穴位磁疗法 / 478
acupoint palpation 按俞穴 / 165
acupoint ultraviolet irradiation therapy 紫外线穴位照射疗法 / 479
acupoint 腧穴，输穴，俞穴 / 408，437
acupotome 小针刀 / 451
acupotomy 小针刀疗法 / 451
acupuncture 针法 / 444
acupuncture and moxibustion 针灸学 / 444
acupuncture and moxibustion therapy 针灸疗法 / 444
acupuncture anesthesia 针刺麻醉 / 470
Acupuncture Anesthesia 针刺麻醉 / 699
acupuncture-moxibustion 针灸 / 444
acupuncture point 俞穴 / 408
acupuncture therapy 针刺疗法 / 444
acupuncturist 针灸师 / 444
acute asthmatic attack in children 马脾风 / 586
acute conjunctivitis 风火眼，风热眼 / 615，616
acute dacryocystitis 漏睛疮 / 615
acute hoarseness or aphonia 急喉喑［瘖］/ 630
acute infantile convulsions 急惊风 / 574
acute kerato-conjunctivitis 暴赤生翳 / 616
acute laryngemphraxis 锁喉风 / 630
acute lymphangitis 红丝疔 / 592
acute mastitis 乳痈 / 596
acute pharyngitis 急喉痹 / 630
acute rhinitis 伤风鼻塞 / 626
acute throat impediment 急喉痹 / 630
acute throat infection 急喉风 / 630
acute throat trouble 喉风 / 630
acute throat wind 急喉风 / 630
adaptation to seasonal changes 顺应四时 / 17
addiction 癖嗜 / 70
adhered tongue 连舌 / 579
adhesive plaster 膏药 / 281
adjusting *qi* 调气 / 254
adjuvant ingredient 佐药 / 358
administration 服药法 / 283
advanced menstruation 月经提前 / 157
adverse transmission 逆传 / 179，515
adverse transmission to the pericardium 逆传心包 / 85
affecting Earth 在泉 / 18
afterbirth 胞衣，胎衣 / 555
afternoon (tidal) fever 午后潮热 / 144，5199
agalactia 乳汁不行，乳汁不通 / 573
Agastache 藿香 / 319
aggregation syndrome 聚证 / 548
agitated fetus 弄胎 / 569
agitated pulse 脉躁 / 164
agitated vexation 躁烦 / 124
Agkistrodon 蕲蛇 / 315
agonizing arthralgia 痛痹 / 540
agonizing impediment 痛痹 / 540
Agrimonia Bud 鹤草芽 / 354
Aifu Nuangong Pills 艾附暖宫丸 / 394
air 大气 / 53
air- or water-borne 天受 / 514
air- or water-borne infection 天受 / 514
Airpotato Yam 黄药子 / 301
ala nasi 鼻翼 / 38，626
ala nasi area 方上 / 38
alarm point 募穴 / 438
alarm-sea point combination 募合配穴法 / 448
Albizia Flower 合欢花 / 336
alchemy 炼丹 / 498
alcohol addiction 酒癖 / 70
alcohol fire cupping 滴酒法 / 468
all joints 百节 / 52

allergic rhinits 鼻臭证 / 627
All-inclusive Grand Tonic Decoction 十全大补汤 / 372，388
All-inclusive Grand Tonic Pills 十全大补丸 / 388
alloy needle 合金针 / 452
Aloe 芦荟 / 353
alopecia 发落，油风 / 602，603
alopecia areata 斑秃 / 602
alopecia seborrheica 发蛀脱发 / 602
Alpinia-Cyperus Pill 良附丸 / 375
alternate preponderance of yin and yang 阴阳胜复 / 7
alternating chills and fever 寒热往来 / 143
Alum 白矾 / 354
Alumen 白矾 / 354
Alumen Ustum 枯矾 / 354
Amber 琥珀 / 336
Amenarrhena-Phellodendron Rehmannia Pills 知柏地黄丸 / 390
amenorrhea 闭经，经闭 / 157，559
American Ginseng 西洋参 / 343
amnesia 健忘 / 535
Amplification on Materia Medica 本草衍义 / 688
Amur Corktree 黄柏 / 307
An Elaboration on Plain Questions of Huangdi's Internal Classic 黄帝内经素问注证发微 / 684
An Elaboration on the Spiritual Pivot of Huangdi's Internal Classic 黄帝内经灵枢注证发微 / 684
An Elaboration on the Spiritual Pivot of Yellow Emperor's Canon of Medcine 黄帝内经灵枢注证发微 / 684
An Expounding of the Formulary of the Bureau of Pharmacy 局方发挥 / 692
An illustrated Book of Plants 植物名实图考 / 689
An Outline of Warm-heat Diseases 温热经纬 / 693
anal fissure 肛裂，肛瘘，肛漏 / 599
Analogism of the Principles of Changes Formulated in the Zhou Dynasty 周易参同契 / 700
Analysis of Warm Diseases 温病条辨 / 693
anasarca in children 小儿水气肿 / 590
ancestral *qi* 宗气 / 54
ancestral sinew 宗筋 / 49
Ancient And Modern Medicine 古今医统 / 703
Angelica Cold-extremities Decoction 当归四逆汤 / 370
Angelica Blood-tonifying Decoction 当归补血汤 / 372
anger 怒 / 69
Angong Niuhuang Pills 安宫牛黄丸 / 392
angular conjunctivitis 赤脉传睛，赤脉贯睛，赤脉侵睛 / 612
angular reduction of cervical vertebra 颈椎角度复位法 / 652
angular stomatitis 口吻疮，燕口，燕口疮/ 579，580
anhidrosis 无汗 / 145
ankyloglossia 绊舌，连舌 / 634，579
ankylosing arthralgia 尫痹 / 541
annual congruence 岁会 / 18
annual menstruation 避年 / 556
anorectal abscess 肛痈 / 599
anorexia 纳呆，厌食/ 153，582
anosmia 不闻香臭 / 626
ano-urethral bleeding during menstruation 经行便血 / 562
Anshen Buxin Pills 安神补心丸 / 385
antagonizing relationship 相反 / 359
Antasthmatic Pills 定喘丸 / 383
Antelope Horn 羚羊角 / 338
anterior hairline 前发际 / 42
anterior naris 鼻前孔 / 626
anterior oblique line of the vertex-temporal (MS 6) 顶颞前斜线 / 471
anterior-posterior point combination 前后配穴法 / 447
anterior temple 颞颥 / 43
anterior temporal line (MS 10) 颞前线 / 471
anterior tibial artery 趺阳脉 / 160
anterior yin 前阴 / 48
anthelmintic 驱虫药 / 294
Anti-bruise Powder 七厘散 / 396
antidromic abdominal breathing 逆腹式呼吸 / 497
Antifeverile Dichroa Root 常山 / 298
antihelix 对耳轮 / 472
Antiphlogistic Granules for Flu 感冒退热冲剂 / 381
Antiphlogistic Powder 败毒散 / 363
Antipyretic Granules for Colds 感冒清热冲剂 / 381
antirheumatic 祛风湿药 / 289
antitragus 对耳屏 / 473

antitussive and antasthmatic (medicinal/drug) 止咳平喘药 / 292
Antitussive Powder 止嗽散 / 361
Antler 鹿角 / 345
anus 魄门，肛门 / 41，49
anus-lifting breathing 提肛呼吸 / 497
anxiety 忧 / 69
apex nasi 鼻准 / 38，626
apex of the nosei 鼻准 / 626
aphagopraxia 鬲咽 / 543
aphasia 失语 / 537
aphonia 喑［瘖］，失音，喉喑［瘖］/ 140，524，630
aphonia (disease) 失音病 / 524
aphonia of pregnancy 妊娠失音 / 568
aphtha 口疮，口疳 / 579，633
apoplectic coma 中风昏迷 / 537
apoplectic stroke 类中 / 536
apoplectic wind stroke 类中风 / 536
apoplexy 中风 / 536
Appendiculate Cremastra Pseudobulb 山慈菇 / 300
application of medicinal powder 扑粉 / 273
Apricot-seed and Perilla-leaf Powder 杏苏散 / 378
aqueous humor 神水 / 610
Arc Shell 瓦楞子 / 350
Arcane Essentials from the Imperial Library 外台秘要 / 690
Areca Peel 大腹皮 / 321
Areca Seed 槟榔 / 353
Argyi Leaf 艾叶 / 318
Argyi Wormwood Leaf 艾叶 / 318
Argyi-Cyperus Uterus-warming Pills 艾附暖宫丸 / 394
arhat needle 罗汉针 / 450
Arillus Longan 龙眼肉 / 342
Arisaema cum Bile 胆南星 / 299
arm 臂 / 47
Armand Clematis Stem 川木通 / 321
armpit odor 腋臭 / 605
armpit sweating 腋汗 / 145
Arnebia Root or Gromwell Root 紫草 / 306
aromatic dampness-resolving medicinal/drug 芳香化湿药 / 290
aromatic orifice-opening medicinal/drug 芳香开窍药 / 293
aromatic stimulant 芳香开窍药 / 293
arousing from unconsciousness 醒神 / 266
arousing the brain 醒脑 / 266
arranging *qi* 顺气 / 254
arresting bleeding and closing cut 止血收口 / 271
arresting bleeding and closing sores 止血敛疮 / 271
arresting bleeding and removing ecchymosis 止血行瘀 / 271
arresting blood flooding 固崩止血 / 262
arresting convulsion 止痉 / 268
arresting discharge 固涩，收涩 / 261
arresting emission 固精 / 262
arresting enuresis 止遗尿 / 268
arresting metrorrhagia and leukorrhagia 固崩止带 / 263
arresting sweating 敛汗 / 261
arresting sweating and consolidating the superficies 敛汗固表 / 261
arresting sweating to prevent collapse 敛汗固脱 / 261
arresting vomiting 止呕 / 267
arrival of *qi* 气至 / 456
arrow-headed needle 箭头针 / 451
Arsenic Trioxide 信石 / 354
Arsenicum Trioxidum 信石 / 354
Arteminsia-Scutellaria Gallbladder-clearing Decoction 蒿芩清胆汤 / 365
arthralgia 痹痛，痹（病）/ 147，540
ascariasis (infantile) malnutrition 蛔疳 / 582
ascariasis syncope 蛔厥 / 538
ascariasis vomiting 虫吐 / 587
ascendant hyperactivity of liver yang 肝阳上亢 / 98
ascending，descending，exiting and entering 升、降、出、入 / 2
ascending, descending, floating and sinking 升降浮沉 / 279
ascites 水臌（病）/ 547
ascites with engorgement 血臌（病）/ 547
Ash Bark 秦皮 / 308
Ashi point 阿是穴 / 444
Asiatic Cornelian Cherry Fruit 山茱萸 / 343
Asiatic Moonseed Rhizome 北豆根 / 313
Asparagus Root 天冬 / 343
asphyxia neonatorum 初生不啼 / 574
Aspongopus 九香虫 / 327
Ass-hide Glue 阿胶 / 342
assistant ingredient 佐药 / 358
assisting bone 辅骨 / 51
assisting relationship 相使 / 359
associated ingredient 臣药 / 358

asthenic fever in children 小儿虚热 / 583

asthenic yang floating upward 虚阳上浮 / 80

asthma 哮喘 / 527

Asthma-arresting Decoction 定喘汤 / 375

astringency 固涩 / 261

astringent formula 固涩剂，涩剂 / 360，373

astringent hemostatic (medicinal/drug) 收敛止血药 / 291

astringent (medicinal/drug) 固涩药 / 294

astringing menstruation and stopping bleeding 固经止血 / 262

astringing *qi* 敛气 / 262

astringing semen and checking emission 涩精止遗 / 262

astringing the intestines to check diarrhea 涩肠止泻 / 263

astringing the intestines to check dysentery 涩肠止痢 / 263

astringing the lung 敛肺 / 262

astringing the lung to relieve dyspnea 敛肺平喘 / 262

astringing the lung to stop coughing 敛肺止咳 / 262

astringing the thoroughfare vessel to stop bleeding 固冲止血 / 262

astringing yin 敛阴 / 262

Atractylodes Rhizome 苍术 / 319

atrophic crippling 痿躄 / 539

atrophic rhinitis 鼻槁［藁］/ 627

atrophy-flaccidity 痿 / 539

atrophy-flaccidity disease 痿病 / 539

atrophy-flaccidity syndrome 痿证 / 539

atrophy of the helices 耳轮萎缩 / 129

attack of noxious factor 中恶 / 72

attack of warm pathogen on the upper 温邪上受 / 85

Aucklandia Carminative Pills 木香顺气丸 / 387

Aucklandia-Coptis Pills

aural vertigo 耳眩晕 / 625

auricle 耳壳，耳廓 / 45

auricular eczema 旋耳疮 / 603

auricular point detector 耳穴探测仪 / 477

auricular pseudocyst 耳壳流痰 / 623

auscultation 闻声音 / 139

auscultation and olfaction 闻诊 / 139

automassage 自我按摩 / 486

automatic *qi* circulation exercise 周天自转功 / 502

autumn dryness 秋燥 / 518

autumn dryness disease 秋燥病 / 518

aversion to cold 恶寒 / 143

aversion to cold with fever 恶寒发热 / 143

aversion to heat 恶热 / 143

aversion to wind 恶风 / 143

aversions of the five *zang* organs 五脏所恶 / 26

awaiting *qi* 候气 / 456

axillary abscess 腋痈 / 593

B

back-carrying manipulation 背法 / 653

back pain 背痛 / 147

back transport points 背俞穴 / 439

Bafeng (EX-LE 10) 八风 / 443

Baical Skullcap Root 黄芩 / 307

Baichongwo (EX-LE 3) 百虫窝 / 443

Baidu Powder 败毒散 / 363

Baihu Decoction 白虎汤 / 367

Baihuanshu (BL 30) 白环俞 / 421

Baihui (GV 20) 百会 / 434

Baijiang Tablets 败酱片 / 385

Baitouweng Decoction 白头翁汤 / 369

Baizi Yangxin Pills 柏子养心丸 / 385

baking 烘焙 / 276

balanced yin-yang constitution 阴阳平和质 / 73

balanced yin-yang person 阴阳和平之人 / 74

bald scalp sore 秃疮 / 604

ball-holding posture 抱球式 / 496

ball-like eyelid swelling 胞虚如球，脾虚如球 / 614

bamboo cup 竹罐 / 467

Bamboo Shavings 竹茹 / 300

bandage 扎带 / 642

banking up earth 培土 / 245

banking up earth and supressing wood 培土抑木 / 247

banking up earth to benefit metal 培土生金 / 247

Banlangen Granules 板蓝根冲剂 / 381

Banxia Houpo Decoction 半夏厚朴汤 / 375

Banxia Xiexin Decoction 半夏泻心汤 / 366

Bao Pu Zi 抱朴子 / 660

Baohe Pill 保和丸 / 379

Baohuang (BL 53) 胞肓 / 422

Barbary Wolfberry Fruit 枸杞子 / 343

Barbated Skullcap Herb 半枝莲 / 312
Barberry Root 三颗针 / 307
barking cough 咳如犬吠 / 142
base of the tongue 舌本 / 131
basic (digital) joints 本节 / 52
Baxie (EX-UE 9) 八邪 / 442
Bazhen Decoction 八珍汤 / 372
Bazhen Pills 八珍丸 / 388
Bazhen Yimu Pills 八珍益母丸 / 395
Bazheng Powder八正散 / 380
Bear Gall 熊胆 / 339
Beautiful Sweetgum Fruit 路路通 / 323
bedsore 席疮，褥疮 / 606
bed-wetting 遗尿 / 590
bee sting therapy 蜂针疗法 / 451
beggar's exercise 叫化功 / 502
Bei Ji Qian Jin Yao Fang 备急千金要方 / 690
belching 噫气，嗳气 / 153
belt vessel (BV) 带脉 / 406
belt vessel syndrome/pattern 带脉病证 / 215
Belvedere Fruit 地肤子 / 322
Ben Cao Bei Yao 本草备要 / 689
Ben Cao Gang Mu 本草纲目 / 688
Ben Cao Gang Mu Shi Yi 本草纲目拾遗 / 689
Ben Cao Jing Ji Zhu 本草经集注 / 687
Ben Cao Shi Yi 本草拾遗 / 688
Ben Cao Yan Yi 本草衍义 / 688
Ben Shi Fang 本事方 / 691
bending of the needle 弯针 / 463
Benshen (GB 13) 本神 / 429
bent-finger pinching manipulation 屈指捏法 / 652
Benzoin 安息香 / 335
Benzoinum 安息香 / 335
beriberi involving the heart 脚气冲心 / 539
*Best Prescriptions Collected by Su Shi and Shen Kuo*苏沈良方 / 691
Bezoar Antihypertensive Pills 牛黄降压丸 / 384
Bezoar Detoxicant Pills [Tablets] 牛黄解毒丸［片］/ 384
Bezoar Pill 西黄丸 / 384
Bezoar Pills for Clearing the Upper 牛黄上清丸 / 384
Bezoar Resurrection Pills 安宫牛黄丸 / 392
Bezoar Sedative Pills [Tablets] 牛黄清心丸［片］/ 384
Bian Que 扁鹊 / 658
Bian Que Xin Shu 扁鹊心书 / 700
big canthus 大眦 / 608
Biguan (ST 31) 髀关 / 413
bilateral tonsillitis 双蛾 / 628
Bile Arisaema 胆南星 / 299
bile-draining anti-icteric (medicinal/drug) 利胆退黄药 / 290
bimanual pinching manipulation 双手捏法 / 652
bimonthly menstruation 并月 / 556
Bin Hu Mai Xue 濒湖脉学 / 686
Binao (LI 14) 臂臑 / 410
Bingfeng (SI 12) 秉风 / 418
Bingpeng Powder 冰硼散 / 396
Binhu's Sphygmology 濒湖脉学 / 686
Biond Magnolia Flower 辛夷 / 296
bird-pecking moxibustion 雀啄灸 / 464
bird-pecking pulse 雀啄脉 / 163
Bistort Rhizome 拳参 / 309
Bitter Apricot Seed 苦杏仁 / 301
bitter taste in the mouth 口苦 / 155
black (tongue) coating/fur 黑苔 / 135
Black and White Pharbitis Seed 黑白丑 / 324
black boil 黑疔 / 623
Black Catechu 儿茶 / 356
black discoloration 黑色 / 126
Black Nightshade Herb 龙葵 / 312
Black Pharbitis Seed 黑丑 / 324
Black Sesame 黑芝麻 / 345
Black-berrylily Rhizome 射干 / 313
Blackened Swallowwort Root 白薇 / 307
blackening the hair and beard 乌须发 / 271
Black-tailed Snake 乌梢蛇 / 315
bladder 膀胱 / 24
bladder cough 膀胱咳 / 525
bladder dampness-heat 膀胱湿热 / 114
bladder dampness-heat syndrome/pattern 膀胱湿热证 / 214
bladder deficiency cold 膀胱虚寒 / 114
bladder deficiency cold syndrome/pattern 膀胱虚寒证 / 213
bladder heat accumulation [retention] syndrome/pattern 热积［结］膀胱证 / 213
bladder meridian/channel (BL) 足太阳膀胱经 / 403
bladder meridian/channel of foot greater yang 足太阳膀胱经 / 403
blanching 潬/ 278
bland taste in the mouth 口淡 / 154

blazing in both *qi* and blood 气血两燔 / 86
blazing in both *qi* and nutrient 气营两燔 / 86
blazing liver fire 肝火炽盛 / 98
blazing liver fire syndrome/pattern 肝火炽盛证 / 209
"bleating convulsions" 羊痫风 / 535
bleeding following sinking of *qi* 血随气陷 / 96
bleeding gums 齿衄 / 137
blepharitis angularis 眦帷赤烂 / 614
blepharoptosis 胞睑下垂，睑皮垂缓，上胞下垂 / 129，614
blindness 盲，目盲 / 612
blindness in ophathalmosteresis 瞽症 / 622
Blister Beetle 斑蝥 / 355
block syndrome/pattern of measles 麻疹闭证 / 584
blockage and repulsion 关格 / 544
blockage of bladder *qi* 膀胱气闭 / 113
blockage pattern of wind stroke 中风闭证 / 536
blockage-repulsion disease 关格病 / 544
blocking the ears and inward listening 塞兑反听 / 494
blood 血 / 56
blood accumulation 蓄血 / 550
blood-activating analgesic (medicinal/drug) 活血止痛药 / 292
blood-activating and menstruation-regulating medicinal/drug 活血调经药 / 292
blood-activating and *qi*-moving medicinal/drug 活血行气药 / 292
blood-activating and stasis-dispelling medicinal/drug 活血祛瘀药 / 291
blood-activating and stasis-removing formula 活血祛瘀剂 / 376
blood-activating and stasis-resolving medicinal/drug 活血化瘀药 / 291
blood-activating and trauma-curing medicinal/drug 活血疗伤药 / 292
blood-activating medicinal/drug 活血药 / 292
blood aspect 血分 / 56
blood aspect syndrome/pattern 血分证 / 180
blood chamber 血室 / 26，555
blood chest bind 血结胸 / 520
blood cold 血寒 / 95
blood cold congealing syndrome/pattern 血寒凝滞证 / 185
blood-cold late periods 血寒经行后期 / 558
blood cold syndrome/pattern 血寒证 / 185
blood collapse 血脱 / 95，550
blood collapse syndrome/pattern 血脱证 / 184
blood-cooling hemostatic (medicinal/drug) 凉血止血药 / 291
blood deficiency 血虚 / 95
blood deficiency amenorrhea 血亏经闭 / 559
blood-deficiency common cold 血虚感冒 / 516
blood deficiency dizziness 血虚眩晕 / 532
blood deficiency engendering wind 血虚生风 / 88
blood-deficiency fever 血虚发热 / 530
blood deficiency habitual abortion 血虚滑胎 / 569
blood-deficiency headache 血虚头痛 / 534
blood deficiency hypomenorrhea 血虚月经过少 / 558
blood deficiency infertility 血虚不孕 / 565
blood-deficiency lumbago 血虚腰痛 / 554
blood deficiency syndrome/pattern 血虚证 / 184
blood deficiency vertigo 血虚眩晕 / 532
blood-deficient late periods 血虚经行后期 / 558
blood dryness engendering wind 血燥生风 / 88
blood exhaustion amenorrhea 血枯经闭 / 559
blood failing to circulate in the vessels 血不循经 / 95
blood failing to stay in the vessels 血不归经 / 95
blood fever 血热 / 583
blood heat 血热 / 95
blood-heat early periods 血热经行先期 / 557
blood heat habitual abortion 血热滑胎 / 569
blood heat metrorrhagia and metrostaxis 血热崩漏 / 561
blood heat stirring blood 血热动血 / 87
blood heat syndrome/pattern 血热证 / 185
blood heat transforming into dryness 血热化燥 / 87
blood heat with raging wind 血热风盛 / 87
blood impediment 血痹 / 542
Blood-lipid Lowering Pills 血脂

宁丸 / 385
blood loss with (*qi*) collapse 血脱气脱 / 96
Blood-nourishing Hair-growing Capsules 养血生发胶囊 / 396
blood-nourishing medicinal/drug 养血药 / 294
blood orbiculus 血轮 / 44，607
blood *qi* 血气 / 56
blood-regulating formula 理血剂 / 376
blood-regulating medicinal/drug 理血药 / 291
blood rush following counterflow of *qi* 血随气逆 / 96
blood-spurting hemorrhoid 血箭痔 / 599
blood stagnation hypomenorrhea 血滞月经过少 / 558
blood stagnation infertility 血滞不孕 / 565
blood-stained sputum 痰中带血 / 138
blood stasis 血瘀 / 95
blood-stasis abdominal pain 血瘀腹痛 / 546
blood stasis amenorrhea 血瘀经闭 / 559
blood-stasis-breaking and mass-eliminating medicinal/drug 破血消癥药 / 292
blood stasis diathesis 血瘀质 / 75
blood stasis dysmenorrhea 血瘀痛经 / 560
blood-stasis epilepsy 瘀血痫 / 590
blood-stasis headache 瘀血头痛 / 534
blood stasis infertility 血瘀不孕 / 565
blood-stasis lumbago 沥血腰痛，血瘀腰痛 / 554
blood stasis metrorrhagia and metrostaxis 血瘀崩漏 / 561
blood stasis syndrome/pattern 血瘀证 / 185
blood-streaked sputum 血丝痰 / 138
blood-tonifying formula 补血剂 / 371
blood-tonifying medicinal/drug 补血药 / 294
blood stranguria 血淋 / 552
blood syncope 血厥 / 538
blood tonic 补血药 / 294
blood tumor 血瘤 / 598
blood vessel 血脉 / 56
bloodletting pricking and cupping 刺血拔罐 / 469
bloody sputum 血痰 / 137
bloody urine 血尿 / 550
“blue dragon wagging its tail” 苍龙摆尾法，青龙摆尾法 / 458
blue snake toxin sore 青蛇毒 / 606
blue tongue 青舌 / 132
blueing the white of the eye 白睛青蓝，白珠俱青 / 617
bluish blindness 青盲 / 620
bluish dark helices 耳轮青黑 / 129
bluish discoloration 青色 / 125
bluish glaucoma 青风，青风内障 / 620
blurring of vision 视瞻昏渺，瞻视昏渺 / 620
Boat-fruited Sterculia Seed 胖大海 / 303
body *cun* 同身寸 / 444
body fluid pattern identification 津液辨证 / 187
body fluid syndrome differentiation 津液辨证 / 187
body fluids 津液 / 58
body inch 同身寸 / 444
body of the needle 针体 / 449
boil 疖 / 591
boiling 煮 / 278
Bombyx Batryticatus 僵蚕 / 338
bone 骨 / 25
bone atrophy-flaccidity 骨痿 / 539
bone-attached abscess 附骨疽 / 595，656
Bone-clearing Powder 清骨散 / 369
bone-combining pad 合骨垫 / 641
bone-holding pad 抱骨垫 / 641
bone impediment 骨痹 / 541
bone (infantile) malnutrition 骨疳 / 581
bone measurement 骨度法 / 445
bone phthisis 骨痨 / 596，656
bone-separating pad 分骨垫 / 641
(bone-)setting 接法 / 639
bone-setting manipulation 正骨手法 / 638
bone steaming 骨蒸 / 529
bone-steaming fever 骨蒸热 / 583
bone stuck in the throat 骨鲠 / 631
bone tumor 骨瘤 / 598
bony nasal septum 鼻柱骨 / 39
“bony space” 骨空 / 52
Book Hidden in the Orchid Chamber 兰室秘藏 / 701
Borax 硼砂 / 355
borborygmus 肠鸣，腹鸣 / 153
“border of the red and white flesh” 赤白肉际 / 52

border of the tongue 舌边 / 39
Borneol 冰片 / 335
Borneolum 冰片 / 335
Borneolum-Borax Powder 冰硼散 / 396
bound pulse 结脉 / 162
Bound Volume of Treatises on Folk Medicine 串雅内、外编 / 693
bow step 弓步 / 496
bowel stroke 中腑 / 537
bowel 腑 / 20
brain 脑 / 25
brain wind 脑风 / 146
brandy nose 酒皶鼻 / 601
breaking and dispelling blood stasis 破血祛瘀 / 257
breaking and expelling blood stasis 破血逐瘀 / 257
breaking blood stasis 破血，破瘀 / 257
breaking blood stasis and eliminating masses 破瘀消癥 / 257
breaking blood stasis and promoting regeneration 破瘀生新 / 257
breaking of the needle 断针，折针 / 463
breaking stagnant *qi* 破气 / 255
breast nodule 乳核 / 597
breast pain 乳房疼痛 / 147
breath counting 数吸 / 498
"breath gate" 吸门 / 41
breath listening 听息 / 498
breathed air 呼吸之气 / 53
breathing 呼吸 / 140
breathing in and out 吐纳 / 497
breathing with pause 停息 / 498
bridge of the nose 鼻茎，鼻梁 / 39，626
"bright hall" 明堂 / 625
bright pale complexion 面色㿠白 / 125
Bronchitis Pills 气管炎丸 / 383
bronze model of meridians/channels and acupoints 针灸铜人 / 452
brushing and whisking 掸拂法 / 483
bubble-rising pulse 釜沸脉 / 163
buccal fat pad 颊脂垫 / 579
Buckeye Seed 娑罗子 / 327
Buddhist *qigong* 佛家气功 / 492
Buffalo Horn 水牛角 / 306
Bugleweed Herb 泽兰 / 334
building the magpie bridge 搭鹊桥 / 494
Bulang (KI 22) 步廊 / 425
Bulbus Allii Macrostemoni 薤白 / 326
Bulbus Fritillariae Pallidiflorae 伊贝母 / 302
Bulbus Fritillariae Thunbergii 浙贝母 / 302
Bulbus Fritillarie Cirrhosae 川贝母 / 302
Bulbus Fritillarie Ussuriensis 平贝母 / 302
Bulbus Lilii 百合 / 302
bulging fontanel囟填 / 576
Bungarus Parvus 金钱白花蛇 / 315
Bupleurum-Pueraria Muscle-releasing Decoction 柴葛解肌汤 / 362
Burdock Fruit 牛蒡子 / 297
burn 火伤，烧伤 / 605
burning fever灼热 / 143
burning pain 灼痛 / 148
burning sensation during urination 小便灼热 / 151
"burning the mountain" 烧山火 / 458
burning with the original property retained 烧存性 / 278
burnt needle 燔针，烧针 / 451
Burong (ST 19) 不容 / 412
Buxin Pills 补心丹 / 385
Buyang Huanwu Decoction 补阳还五汤 / 376
Buzhong Yiqi Decoction 补中益气汤 / 371
Buzhong Yiqi Pills 补中益气丸 / 388

C

Cablin Patchouli Herb 广藿香 / 319
cachexia with withering bones 大骨枯槁 / 126
Cacumen Platycladi 侧柏叶 / 329
Cacumen Tamaricis 西河柳 / 298
Calabash Gourd 葫芦 / 323
calabash pad 葫芦垫 / 641
Calamina 炉甘石 / 355
Calamine 炉甘石 / 355
calcination 煅 / 276
Calcined Alumen 枯矾 / 354
Calcined Arc Shell 煅瓦楞 / 350
Calcined Dragon's Bone 煅龙骨 / 350
Calcined Oyster Shell 煅牡蛎 / 350
Calcined Yellow Earth 伏龙肝 / 349
calcining and quenching 煅淬 / 276
Calculus Bovis 牛黄 / 335
calculus of the conjunctiva 睑内结石 / 614
calf 腨，腓腨 / 50
callosity 胼胝 / 601

callus 跰子，胼胝 / 601
calmed pulse 脉静 / 164
calming and stabilizing the mind 安神定志 / 264
calming the mind 安神 / 264
calming the mind with heavy settling (medicinals) 重镇安神 / 265
Calomel 轻粉 / 354
Calomelas 轻粉 / 354
Calyx Kaki 柿蒂 / 328
Calyx seu Fructus Physalis 锦灯笼 / 313
cancer 岩 / 598
cancrum oris 走马牙疳 / 633
Cang Gong 仓公 / 658
Cannabis Laxative Pills 麻仁润肠丸 / 386
Cannabis-seed Pills 麻仁丸 / 386
Canon of Medicine 内经 / 683
cantharis moxibustion 斑蝥灸 / 467
canthus 目眦 / 607
canthus (of the eye) 目眦 / 44
canthus pyorrhea 眦漏 / 615
Canton Love-pea Vine 鸡骨草 / 308
Caoguo 草果 / 320
Cape-jasmine Fruit 栀子 / 310
Caper Euphorbia Seed 千金子 / 355
capsule 胶囊剂 / 282
Carapax Eretmochelydis 玳瑁 / 339
Carapax et Plastrum Testudinis 龟甲 / 345
Carapax Trionycis 鳖甲 / 345
carbonization 制炭 / 276
Carbonized Cat-tail Pollen 蒲黄炭 / 333
Carbonized Fineleaf Schizonepeta Herb 荆芥炭 / 296
Carbonized Hair 血余炭 / 329
Carbonized Windmillpalm Petiole 棕榈炭 / 329
carbuncle 痈，有头疽 / 593，594
carcinoma 岩 / 598
carcinoma of the penis 肾癌 / 598
carcinoma of the penis with ulceration 肾岩翻花 / 598
carcinoma of the throat 喉岩，喉菌 / 631
carcinoma of the tongue 舌岩 / 598
cardia 贲门 / 41
Carefree Pills 逍遥丸 / 386
Carefree Powder 逍遥散 / 366
carious odontoptosis 龋脱 / 633
carious tooth 龋齿 / 632
carious toothache 龋齿牙痛 / 632
Carrot Fruit 南鹤虱 / 354
case record 诊籍 / 122
Cassia Bark 肉桂 / 317
Cassia Seed 决明子 / 304
Cassia Twig 桂枝 / 295
Cassia-Aconite Rehmannia Pills 桂附地黄丸 / 390
Cassia-twig Decoction 桂枝汤 / 361
cataract 圆翳，圆翳内障 / 620
Catechism on Acupuncture and Moxibustion 针灸问答 / 699
Catechism on Acupuncture and Moxibustion 针灸问对 / 699
Catechu 儿茶 / 356
categorization according to the five elements/phases 五行归类 / 11
catgut-embedding by incision 切开埋线法 / 478
catgut-embedding with lumbar puncture needle 穿刺针埋线法 / 478
catgut-embedding with triangular needle 三角针埋线法 / 478
Cat-tail Pollen 蒲黄 / 332
Caulis Aristolochiae Manshuriensis 关木通 / 321
Caulis Aristolochiae Manshuriensis 木通 / 321
Caulis Bambusae in *Taeniam* 竹茹 / 300
Caulis Clematidis Armandii 川木通 / 321
Caulis Lonicerae 忍冬藤 / 310
Caulis Perillae 紫苏梗 / 326
Caulis Piperis Kadsurae 海风藤 / 315
Caulis Polygoni Multiflori 首乌藤 / 336
Caulis Sinomenii 青风藤 / 317
Caulis Spatholobi 鸡血藤 / 332
Caulis Trachelospermi 络石藤 / 315
cause determination and treatment 审因施治 / 218
cause neither internal nor external 不内外因 / 62
cause of disease 病因 / 62
cause seeking from symptoms 审证求因 / 191
cauterization 烙法 / 272
cavitas conchae 耳甲腔 / 473
cavity of the concha 耳甲腔 / 473
ceasing of menstruation 停经 / 559
celestial control 司天 / 18
cellulitis 发，疽 / 594
cellulitis at *Huantiao* (GB 30) 环跳疽 / 595
center of the eyebrows 眉心 / 43

center of the tongue 舌心 / 131
Center-regulating Decoction 理中汤 / 369
Center-tonifying *Qi*-replenishing Decoction 补中益气汤 / 371
center-warming cold-dispelling formula 温中祛寒剂 / 369
Centipede 蜈蚣 / 338
cerumen 耵聍 / 625
cervical abscess 颈痈 / 593
cervical malignancy with cachexia 失荣 / 598
cervical neurodermatitis 摄领疮 / 602
cervical orifice 子门 / 49，555
cervical pulling manipulation 扳颈椎法 / 652
Chaenomeles Pills 木瓜丸 / 392
Chai Ge Jieji Decoction 柴葛解肌汤 / 362
chalazion 胞睑肿核，睥生痰核 / 613
chalazion 胞生痰核 / 613
Chamaedaphne Leaf and Flower 黄芫花 / 324
chamber-pot dermatitis 马桶癣 / 605
Chan Bao 产宝 / 695
Changqiang (GV 1) 长强 / 433
channel passage 经隧 / 398
channel stroke 中经 / 537
channel syndrome/pattern 经证 / 178
channels 经脉 / 398
channel-warming hemostatic (medicinal/drug) 温经止血药 / 291
Chao Yuanfang 巢元方 / 660
chap 皲揭 / 601
charges of the five *zang* organs 五脏所主 / 26
Charred Germinated Barley 焦麦芽 / 351
Charred Hawthorn Fruit 焦山楂 / 351
Charred Triplet 焦三仙 / 352
checking emission 涩精 / 262
checking sweating 止汗 / 261
cheek 颊 / 45
chemosis 白睛浮壅 / 611
Chen Cangqi 陈藏器 / 661
Chen Feixia 陈飞霞 / 676
Chen Fuzheng 陈复正 / 676
Chen Jiushao 陈九韶 / 673
Chen Liangfu 陈良甫 / 665
Chen Nianzu 陈念祖 / 678
Chen Shenxiu 陈慎修 / 678
Chen Shigong 陈实功 / 672
Chen Sicheng 陈司成 / 673
Chen Wenzhong 陈文中 / 665
Chen Wuze 陈无择 / 664
Chen Xiu Yuan Yi Shu Shi Liu Zhong 陈修圆医书十六种 / 705
Chen Xiuyuan 陈修圆 / 678
Chen Yan 陈言 / 663
Chen Yuren 陈毓仁 / 672
Chen Ziming 陈自明 / 665
Cheng Dan'an 承淡安 / 682
Cheng Guopeng 程国彭 / 677
Cheng Wuji 成无己 / 663
Cheng Zhongling 程钟龄 / 677
Chengfu (BL 36) 承扶 / 421
Chengguang (BL 6) 承光 / 419
Chengjiang (CV 24) 承浆 / 437
Chengjin (BL 56) 承筋 / 422
Chengling (GB 18) 承灵 / 430
Chengman (ST 20) 承满 / 412
Chengqi (ST 1) 承泣 / 411
Chengshan (BL 57) 承山 / 423
Cherokee Rose Fruit 金樱子 / 351
chest 膺 / 47
chest bind 结胸 / 519
chest-hypochondrium exercise 胸胁功 / 501
chest impediment 胸痹 / 530
chest pain 胸痛 / 146，530
chicken breast 鸡胸 / 578
Chicken's Gizzard-skin 鸡内金 / 352
chickenpox 水痘，水疮，水花，水疱 / 585
chief, associate, assistant and guide 君臣佐使 / 358
chief ingredient 君药 / 358
chilblain 冻疮，冻风 / 605，606
child (element/phase) 子 / 13
child (element/phase) *qi* 子气 / 13
childbirth 分娩 / 568
Children's Colds Granules 小儿感冒冲剂 / 381
chill 恶寒 / 143
chills and fever 恶寒发热 / 143
chills without fever 但寒不热 / 143
Chimai (TE 18) 瘛脉 / 428
chin 颔 / 46
Chinese Angelica 当归 / 342
Chinese Angelica Pills 当归丸 / 394
Chinese Arborvitae Seed 柏子仁 / 337
Chinese Arborvitae Twig and Leaf 侧柏叶 / 329
Chinese Caterpillar Fungus 冬虫夏草 / 348
Chinese Clematis Root 威灵仙 / 314
Chinese Date 大枣 / 341
Chinese drugs 中药 / 275
Chinese Dwarf Cherry Seed 郁李仁 / 352
Chinese Eagle Wood 沉香 / 327

Chinese Gall 五倍子 / 348
Chinese Gentian 龙胆 / 308
Chinese herbal medicinals 中草药 / 275
Chinese Honeylocust Spine 皂角刺 / 333
Chinese Lobelia Herb 半边莲 / 312
Chinese Lovage 藁本 / 296
Chinese Magnoliavine Fruit 五味子 / 350
Chinese medicinals 中药 / 275
Chinese pharmaceutics 中药学 / 275
Chinese Pulsatilla Root 白头翁 / 308
Chinese Rose Flower 月季花 / 332
Chinese Silkvine Bark 香加皮 / 317
Chinese Starjasmine Stem 络石藤 / 315
Chinese Tamarisk Twig 西河柳 / 298
Chinese Thorowax Root 柴胡 / 297
Chinese Wax-gourd Peel 冬瓜皮 / 321
Chinese White Olive 青果 / 313
Chinese Wolfberry Bark 地骨皮 / 306
Chinghao and Turtle Shell Decoction 青蒿鳖甲汤 / 369
Chingma Abutilon Seed 苘麻子 / 322
Chize (LU 5) 尺泽 / 409
cholera 霍乱，霍乱病 / 522
choleraic turmoil with cramps 转筋霍乱 / 523
Chong Xiu Zheng He Jing Shi Zheng Lei Bei Ji Ben Cao 重修政和经史证类备急本草 / 688
Chongmen (SP 12) 冲门 / 415
Chongyang (ST 42) 冲阳 / 414
choppy pulse 涩脉 / 161
chorioretina 视衣 / 610
Christina Loosestrife 金钱草 / 322
chromatopsia 视物易色 / 621
chronic convulsions due to spleen disorder 慢脾风 / 575
chronic convulsions with incessant sweating 慢惊自汗 / 575
chronic convulsions with phlegm 慢惊夹痰 / 575
chronic corneal opacity 宿翳 / 612
chronic cough 久咳，久嗽 / 142
chronic dacryocystitis 漏睛 / 615
chronic diarrhea 久泄 / 545
chronic dysentery 久痢 / 522
chronic hoarseness or aphonia 喉喑［瘖］/ 630
chronic infantile convulsions 慢惊风 / 574
chronic malaria 久疟 / 521
chronic rhinitis 鼻窒 / 627
chronic turbid nasal discharge 久流浊涕 / 130
Chrysanthemum Flower 菊花 / 297
Chuan Ya Nei Wai Bian 串雅内、外编 / 693
Chuanbei Pipa Syrup 川贝枇杷糖浆 / 382
Chuang Yang Jing Yan Quan Shu 疮疡经验全书 / 697
Chuling 猪苓 / 320
Chunyu Yi 淳于意 / 658
chylous stranguria 膏淋 / 552
Ci Zhu Pill 磁朱丸 / 380
Cibot Rhizome 狗脊 / 347
Cicada Slough 蝉蜕 / 298
cicatrical ectropion of the eyelid 睥翻粘睑 / 613
Ciliao (BL 32) 次髎 / 421
ciliary hyperemia 白睛抱红，抱轮红赤，赤带抱轮 / 611
Cimicifuga-Pueraria Decoction 升麻葛根汤 / 363
Cinnabar Sedative Pills 朱砂安神丸 / 385
Cinnabar 朱砂 / 336
Cinnabaris 朱砂 / 336
Cinnabar-Magnetite Pill 磁朱丸 / 380
circling moxibustion 回旋灸 / 464
circuit of year 岁运 / 17
circuit-*qi* 运气 / 17
circular kneading 运法 / 483
circular needling method 盘法，盘旋法/ 458
circular rubbing 摩法 / 482
circular rubbing manipulation 摩法 / 650
Cirsium Decoction 小蓟饮子 / 377
Citron Fruit 香橼 / 326
clarity and turbidity 清浊 / 58
Classic of Difficulies 难经 / 684
Classic of Nourishing Life with Acupuncture and Moxibustion 针灸资生经 / 699
Classic of the Yellow Yard 黄庭经 / 700
Classical Classified Materia Medica for Emergencies 经史证类备急本草 / 688
classical formula 经方 / 357
Classified Classic 类经 / 684
Classified Materia Medica 证类本草 / 688
Classified Medical Records of

Distinguished Physicians 名医类案 / 702
Classified Prescriptions from the Treatise on Cold Damage Diseases 伤寒类方 / 685
Classified Syndromes and Treatment 类证治裁 / 694
clavus 鸡眼，肉刺 / 601
"cleaning the bladder" 洁净府 / 261
clear crisp cough 咳声清脆 / 141
clear *qi* 清气 / 55
clear yang 清阳 / 55
clearing and purging ministerial fire 清泄相火 / 235
clearing and resolving heat-phlegm 清化热痰 / 258
clearing dryness to moisten the lung 清燥润肺 / 263
clearing heart fire 清心火 / 234
clearing heat and cooling blood 清热凉血 / 233
clearing heat and dispelling dampness 清热祛湿 / 231
clearing heat and draining dampness 清热利湿 / 231，260
clearing heat and drying dampness 清热燥湿 / 231
clearing heat and evacuating pus 清热排脓 / 269
clearing heat and harmonizing the middle 清热和中 / 232
clearing heat and harmonizing the stomach 清热和胃 / 232
clearing heat and promoting digestion 清热消食 / 232
clearing heat and promoting fluid production 清热生津 / 231
clearing heat and purging fire 清热泻火 / 231
clearing heat and purging the lung 清热泻肺 / 234
clearing heat and relieving (food) stagnation 清热导滞 / 232
clearing heat and removing dampness 清热除湿，清热化湿 / 231，259
clearing heat and resolving phlegm 清热化痰 / 258
clearing heat and resolving phlegm to induce resuscitation 清热化痰开窍 / 267
clearing heat and resolving toxins 清热解毒 / 231
clearing heat to extinguish wind 清热熄［息］风 / 266
clearing heat to improve vision 清热明目 / 232
clearing heat to induce resuscitation 清热开窍，清热开窍 / 233，266
clearing heat to open the orifices 清热开窍 / 233
clearing heat to relieve dysentery 清热止痢 / 232
clearing heat to stop bleeding 清热止血 / 258
clearing heat to stop diarrhea 清热止泻 / 232
clearing heat to stop vomiting 清热止呕 / 232
clearing heat with bitter-cold 苦寒清热 / 230
clearing heat with pungent-cool (medicinals) 辛凉清热 / 225
clearing liver fire 清肝火 / 233
clearing lung fire 清肺火 / 234
clearing lung heat 清肺热 / 234
clearing ministerial fire 清相火 / 235
clearing *qi* with bitter-cold 苦寒清气 / 231
clearing stomach fire 清胃火 / 235
clearing stomach heat 清胃热 / 235
clearing summerheat 清热解暑，清暑热 / 232
clearing summerheat and draining dampness 清暑利湿 / 232
clearing summerheat and resolving dampness 清暑化湿 / 232
clearing the heart and calming the mind 清心安神 / 234
clearing the heart 清心 / 233
clearing the heart and purging fire 清心泻火 / 234
clearing the heart to open the orifices 清心开窍 / 234
clearing the heart to restore consciousness 清心开窍 / 234
clearing the intestines and moistening dryness 清肠润燥 / 235
clearing the intestines to relieve dysentery 清肠止痢 / 235
clearing the intestines to stop diarrhea 清肠止泻 / 235
clearing the liver 清肝 / 233
clearing the liver and purging fire 清肝泻火 / 233
clearing the liver to improve vision 清肝明目 / 233
clearing the lung 清肺 / 234
clearing the lung and moistening dryness 清肺润燥 / 234，263
clearing the lung and resolving phlegm 清肺化痰 / 234
clearing the lung to relieve cough 清肺止咳 / 234
clearing the lung to relieve dyspnea 清肺止喘 / 234
clearing the lung to soothe the

throat 清肺利咽 / 234
clearing the nutrient aspect 清营 / 232
clearing the nutrient aspect and promoting eruption 清营透疹 / 233
clearing the nutrient aspect and purging heat 清营泄热 / 233
clearing the pericardium 清宫 / 233
clearing the stomach 清胃 / 235
clearing the stomach and purging fire 清胃泄火 / 235
clearing the stomach and purging heat 清胃泄热 / 235
clearing *zang-fu* organ heat 清脏腑热 / 233
cleft palate 腭裂 / 590
cleft point 郄穴 / 438
cleft-influential point combination 郗会配穴法 / 448
clenching a fist，turning over and opening the hand 拧拳反掌式 / 654
clicking the teeth 叩齿 / 505
Climacteric Peace Tablets 更年安 / 395
Climbing Hop Herb 葎草 / 313
clonic convulsions 瘛疭 / 575
closing form 收功 / 505
clouded consciousness 神昏 / 123
Cloves 丁香 / 318
Cluster Mallow Fruit 冬葵果 / 322
clustered hair 丛毛 / 52
clutching the ground with the toes 五趾抓地 / 494
coacting treatment 从治 / 220
Coastal Glehia Root 北沙参 / 343
coats of the eyeball 视衣 / 610
coccyx 尾闾骨 / 51
coincidence of heavenly *qi* 天符 / 18
Coin-like White-banded Snake 金钱白花蛇 / 315
Coix Seed 薏苡仁 / 321
cold 寒 / 64
cold abdominal pain 寒冷腹痛 / 546
cold and heat 寒热 / 169
cold and heat in complexity 寒热错杂 / 91
cold arthralgia 寒痹 / 540
cold bind 寒结 / 544
cold chest bind 寒结胸 / 520
cold choleraic turmoil 寒霍乱 / 523
cold compression 冷罨 / 272
cold congealing dysmenorrhea 寒凝痛经 / 560
cold constipation 冷秘 / 544
cold dacryorrhea 冷泪 / 615
cold damage 伤寒 / 515
cold-damaged eye 伤寒眼 / 616
cold-dampness 寒湿 / 68
cold-dampness dysentery 寒湿痢 / 521
cold-dampness encumbering the spleen 寒湿困脾 / 105
cold-dampness lumbago 寒湿腰痛 / 553
cold-dampness syndrome/pattern 寒湿证 / 196
cold decoction 饮 / 282
cold diarrhea 寒泻 / 546
cold-dispelling formula 祛寒剂 / 370
cold-dispelling medicinal/drug 祛寒药 / 290
cold-dispelling method 祛寒法 / 240
cold entering the blood chamber 寒入血室 / 91
cold epilepsy 寒痫 / 590
Cold-extremities Decoction 四逆汤 / 370
cold filthy attack 寒痧 / 583
cold-heat harmonizing formula 调和寒热剂 / 366
cold heart pain 冷心痛 / 531
cold-heat pattern identification 寒热辨证 / 169
cold-heat syndrome differention 寒热辨证 / 169
cold impediment 寒痹 / 540
cold in both the exterior and interior 表里俱寒 / 83
cold in the middle (energizer) 中寒 / 91
cold malaria 寒疟 / 521
cold miasmic malaria 寒瘴，冷瘴 / 521
cold or heat of the exterior and interior 表里寒热 / 82
cold pain 冷痛 / 148
cold pathogen fettering the exterior 寒邪外束 / 91
cold phlegm 寒痰 / 527
cold-phlegm syndrome/pattern 寒痰证 / 189
cold purgation 寒下 / 236
cold purgative formula 寒下剂 / 364
cold-*qi* abdominal pain 寒气腹痛 / 546
cold-*qi* choleraic turmoil 寒气霍乱 / 523
cold semen 精寒，精冷 / 553
cold stagnating in the liver meridian/channel 寒滞肝脉 / 104
cold stroke 中寒 / 64
cold-stroke diarrhea 中寒泻 / 588
cold sweats 冷汗 / 145
cold syncope 寒厥 / 538

cold syndrome/pattern 寒证 / 169
cold syndrome of the gravida 胎寒 / 568
cold tear shedding induced by wind 迎风冷泪 / 611
cold toxin 寒毒 / 69
cold transformation of lesser yin 少阴寒化 / 115
cold transformation syndrome/pattern of lesser yin 少阴寒化证 / 177
cold vomiting 寒呕，寒吐 / 542，586
cold wheezing 寒哮，冷哮 / 527
coldness of metal and water 金寒水冷 / 14
colds 感冒 / 515
colicky intestinal turmoil 绞肠痧 / 522
colicky intestinal turmoil 搅肠痧 / 523
colicky pain 绞痛 / 148
Colla Corii Asini 阿胶 / 342
Colla Cornus Cervi 鹿角胶 / 346
collapse following blood loss 气随血脱 / 96
collapse pattern of wind stroke 中风脱证 / 536
collapse sweating 脱汗 / 145
Collateral-activating Pills (heavy recipe) 大活络丸［丹］/ 392
Collateral-activating Pills (mild recipe) 小活络丸［丹］/ 392
collateral needling 络刺 / 460
collateral-poking 拨络法 / 485
collateral pricking and cupping 刺络拔罐 / 469
collateral puncture 刺络 / 449
collateral stroke 中络 / 537
collateral vessel 络脉 / 398
Collection of Ancient and Modern Books，Medicine Section 古今图书集成医部全录 / 704
Collection of Physicians' Experiences in the Ming Dynasty 明医杂著 / 701
Collection of Precious Medical Works 珍本医书集成 / 705
Collection of Prescriptions with Expositions 医方集解 / 692
Collection of Works on Pediatrics 幼幼集成 / 696
columnar bone 柱骨 / 50
combatting poison with poison 以毒攻毒 / 270
combination of diseases 合病 / 178
combination of greater yang and lesser yang diseases 太阳（与）少阳合病 / 178
combination of greater yang and yang brightness diseases 太阳（与）阳明合病 / 178
combination of points from the meridians/channels with the same name 同名经配穴法 / 448
combination of yang brightness and lesser yang diseases 阳明（与）少阳合病 / 178
combined pathogen 合邪 / 63
Combined Spicebush Root 乌药 / 326
combined syndrome/pattern of phlegm and static blood 痰瘀互结证 / 189
combing 梳法 / 483
combing the head 栉头 / 486
Commentaries on the Synposis of the Golden Chamber 金匮要略心典 / 686
Comments on Ancient and Modern Medical Records 古今医案按 / 702
Common Andrographis Herb 穿心莲 / 312
Common Anemarrhena Rhizome 知母 / 304
Common Aucklandia Root 木香 / 326
Common Bletilla Tuber 白及 / 328
Common Burreed Tuber 三棱 / 334
common carotid artery 人迎脉 / 160
Common Carpesium Fruit 鹤虱 / 353
Common Clubmoss Herb 伸筋草 / 316
Common Cnidium Fruit 蛇床子 / 355
common cold 感冒 / 515
Common Coltsfoot Flower 款冬花 / 301
Common Curculigo Rhizome 仙茅 / 346
Common Dayflower Herb 鸭跖草 / 312
Common Ducksmeat Herb 浮萍 / 298
Common Fenugreek Seed 葫芦巴 / 347
Common Flowering-quince Fruit 木瓜 / 314
Common Knotgrass Herb 萹蓄 / 322
Common Pleione Pseudobulb 山慈菇 / 300
Common Rush 灯心草 / 323
Common Scouring Rush Herb 木贼 / 305
Common Selfheal Fruit-Spike 夏枯草 / 305
Common Yam Rhizome 山药 / 341

Compendium of Materia Medica 本草纲目 / 688
Compendium of Therapies for Women's Diseases 济阴纲目 / 695
Compilation of Traumatology 伤科汇纂 / 698
Complete Manual of Experiences in the Treatment of Sores 疮疡经验全书 / 697
Complete Medical Books of Nan Ya Tang 南雅堂医书全集 / 705
Complete Record of Sacred Benevolence 圣济总录 / 703
Complete Series of Medical Books from Wan Mizhai's Studio 万密斋医学全书 / 703
Complete Works of Jingyue 景岳全书 / 704
complexion 面色，气色 / 124
compound formula/prescription 复方 / 356
compound manipulation 复合手法 / 490
Compound Salvia Tablets 复方丹参片 / 393
Compound Tablets of Fritillary Extract 复方川贝精片 / 382
comprehending (perceiving) by touching 手摸心会 / 638
Comprehension of Medicine 医学心悟 / 704
comprehensive analysis of the four examinations 四诊合参 / 165
comprehensive analysis of the pulse and complexion 色脉合参 / 165
comprehensive analysis of the pulse and symptoms 脉症合参 / 165
compressing the eyes (with the hot palms) 熨目 / 487
compression 罨 / 272
Concentrated Motherwort Decoction 益母草膏 / 395
concentrated pill 浓缩丸 / 280
Concentrated *Yimucao* Decoction 益母草膏 / 395
concentration of the mind 意守 / 499
concentration on *dantian* 意守丹田 / 499
concentration on oneself 意守自身 / 499
concentration on something outside the body 意守体外 / 499
concept of holism 整体观念 / 218
conception vessel (CV) 任脉 / 406
Concha Arcae Usta 煅瓦楞 / 350
Concha Arcae 瓦楞子 / 350
concha auricularis 耳甲 / 473
Concha Haliotidis 石决明 / 339
Concha Margaritifera Usta 珍珠母 / 337
Concha Mauritiae 紫贝齿 / 337
Concha Ostreae 牡蛎 / 338
Concha Ostreae Usta 煅牡蛎 / 350
concha 耳甲 / 473
Concise Exposition of Cold Damage Diseases 伤寒明理论 / 685
Concretio Silicea Bambusae 天竺黄 / 300
conducting (exercise)导引 / 491
conducting fire back to its origin 引火归原 / 251
conducting *qi* 导气 / 503
conducting *qi* with pile-driving standing and palms put together 合掌震桩导气 / 503
conducting *qi* with single-finger meditation 一指禅导气 / 503
cone 壮 / 464
configuration and constitution 形体 / 57
confluence of all the yang meridians/channels 诸阳之会 / 42
confluence of ancestral sinews 宗筋之会 / 49
Confucian *qigong* 儒家气功 / 492
Confucians' Duties to Their Parents 儒门事亲 / 701
congenital cataract 胎患内障 / 620
congenital defect 先天不足 / 73
congruity of pulse with the seasons 脉从四时，脉应四时 / 164
conjunctival hyperemia 结膜红赤 / 612
conjunctivitis 火眼 / 616
connecting points 络穴 / 438
consolidating the superficies and checking sweating 固表止汗 / 261
constipation of deficiency type 虚秘 / 544
constipation of excess type 实秘 / 544
constipation 便秘，大便秘结 / 149，544
constitution 体质 / 73
constitution theory 体质学说 / 73
constraining spittle 摄唾 / 271
constraint of liver *qi* 肝气不舒 / 97
constrictive throat infection 紧

喉风 / 630
constrictive throat wind 紧喉风 / 630
consumption 虚损 / 529
consumption of meridian/channel *qi* 经气虚损 / 114
consumptive cough 劳咳，劳嗽 / 526
consumptive disease 劳（病） / 529
consumptive fever 骨蒸热 / 583
consumptive malaria 劳疟 / 521
consumptive steaming (fever) 劳蒸 / 530
contact dermatitis 接触性皮炎 / 603
contagion 传染 / 514
contaminated food 饮食不洁 / 70
contracted tongue 短缩舌 / 133
contracting the buttocks and relaxing the knees 收臀松膝 / 494
contraction 拘急，拘挛 / 127
contraindications for emesis 涌吐禁例 / 267
contraindications of diaphoresis 发汗禁例 / 229
contralateral collateral needling 缪刺 / 461
contralateral meridian/channel needling 巨刺 / 460
contralateral point selection 交叉选穴法 / 447
controlling Heaven 司天 / 18
contusion 挫伤 / 646
conversion between physique and *qi* 形气转化 / 3
conversion into heat after entering the interior 入里化热 / 83
conversion of cold and heat 寒热转化 / 83
conversion of deficiency into excess 由虚转实 / 84
conversion of excess into deficiency 由实转虚 / 84
convulsions 抽搐，惊厥 / 539，575
convulsive disease 痉病 / 538
cool dryness 凉燥 / 66，518
cool dryness disease 凉燥病 / 519
cool-dryness syndrome/pattern 凉燥证 / 197
cooling blood 凉血 / 233
cooling for the cold 寒因寒用 / 221
cooling formula 寒剂 / 360
cooling phlegm-resolving medicinal/drug 清化热痰药 / 292
cooling the blood and dissipating stasis 凉血散瘀 / 235
cooling the blood and removing toxins 凉血解毒 / 233
cooling the blood to stop bleeding 凉血止血 / 258
cooling the blood to treat dysentery 凉血止痢 / 235
cooling the liver to extinguish wind 凉肝熄［息］风 / 266
"cooling the sky" 透天凉 / 458
coordinating the heart and kidney 交通心肾 / 239
copulative bleeding 交接出血 / 564
Coral-bean Bark 海桐皮 / 316
Cordyceps 冬虫夏草 / 348
Corn Stigma 玉米须 / 323
corn 鸡眼，肉刺 / 601
corneal perforation with irridoptosis 蟹睛病，蟹目，蟹珠 / 618
corner of the mouth 吻 / 46
Cornu Bubali 水牛角 / 306
Cornu Cervi 鹿角 / 345
Cornu Cervi Degelatinatum 鹿角霜 / 346
Cornu Cervi Pantotrichum 鹿茸 / 345
Cornu Rhinoceri 犀角 / 305
Cornu Saigae Tataricae 羚羊角 / 338
Coronary Storax Pills 冠心苏合丸 / 393
corporeal soul 魄 / 57
"corporeal-soul gate" 魄门 / 41
corpus adiposum bucca 螳螂子 / 579
correction and reduction 平整复元 / 638
Corrections of Errors in Medical Works 医林改错 / 702
correspondence between nature and human 天人相应 / 17
corroding wounds and removing putridity 蚀疮去腐 / 270
Cortex Acanthopanacis 五加皮 / 316
Cortex Ailanthi 椿皮 / 308
Cortex Albiziae 合欢皮 / 336
Cortex Cinnamomi 肉桂 / 317
Cortex Dictamni 白鲜皮 / 308
Cortex Erythrinae 海桐皮 / 316
Cortex Eucommiae 杜仲 / 347
Cortex Fraxini 秦皮 / 308
Cortex Lycii 地骨皮 / 306
Cortex Magnoliae Officinalis 厚朴 / 325
Cortex Meliae 苦楝皮 / 353
Cortex Mori 桑白皮 / 303
Cortex Moutan 牡丹皮 / 306
Cortex Periplocae 香加皮 / 317
Cortex Phellodendri 黄柏 / 307
Cortex Pseudolaricis 土荆皮 / 355
Cortex Syringae 暴马子皮 / 303

Corydalis Analgesic Tablets 元胡止痛片 / 393
cosmic cycle 周天 / 500
cotton-burning cupping 贴棉法 / 468
cough 咳嗽 / 141，524
cough during pregnancy 妊娠咳嗽 / 568
Cough Pills [Tablets] with Anemarrhena and Fritillary 二母宁嗽丸［片］/ 382
cough with dyspnea 咳逆 / 526
cough with no expectoration 干咳嗽 / 525
cough with reversed ascent of *qi* 咳逆上气 / 141，526
coughing blood 咳血 / 137
counter-restriction among the five elements/phases 五行相侮 / 13
counteracting 相恶 / 359
counteracting toxins 攻毒 / 270
counteracting treatment 逆治 / 220
counterflow fullness below the heart 心下逆满 / 156
Counterflow-relieving Powder 四逆散 / 366
courier ingredient 使药 / 358
Cow-Bezoar 牛黄 / 335
Cow-herb Seed 王不留行 / 333
crab's eye disease 蟹睛病 / 618
crab's eye 蟹目，蟹珠 / 618
cracked lips 唇裂 / 136
cracked nipple 乳头破碎 / 596
cramp 转筋，抽筋 / 127
cramp in choleraic turmoil 霍乱转筋 / 523
cranium; skull 头颅骨 / 42
crapulent syncope 食厥 / 538
cream 乳膏 / 281
Creeping Euphorhia 地锦草 / 309
crimson tongue 绛舌，舌绛 / 131
Crinis Carbonisatus 血余炭 / 329
critical case of measles 麻疹险证 / 584
Crocus 西红花 / 330
cross-legged sitting 盘坐 / 495
crossed menstruation 错经；差经 / 562
crossing meridian/channel point combination 交会经配穴法 / 448
crossing point 交会穴 / 439
crossing point selection 交会选穴法 / 447
Croton Seed 巴豆 / 355
crushing-contusion 碾挫伤 / 646
crust 痂 / 591
crystalline lens 晶珠 / 610
Cuanzhu (BL 2) 攒竹 / 419
cubito-popliteal eczema 四弯风 / 603
cultivating essence 炼精 / 499
cultivating essence to become *qi* 炼精化气 / 499
cultivating oneself 炼己 / 499
cultivating *qi* 炼气 / 499
cultivating *qi* to become mentality 炼气化神 / 499
cultivating the mind 炼神 / 499
cun 寸 / 444
cun, guan, chi 寸、关、尺 / 158
cunkou 寸口 / 159
cup-boiling method 煮罐法 / 468
cup removal 起罐 / 469
cupping 拔罐 / 467
cupping therapy 拔罐疗法 / 274，467
cupping with needle retention 留针拔罐 / 469
curdy (tongue) coating/fur 腐苔 / 135
curled tongue and retracted testicles 舌卷囊缩 / 134
curtain-falling and inward vision 两目垂帘内视 / 494
cutaneous anthrax 疫疔 / 592
Cutch 儿茶 / 356
Cuttlebone 海螵蛸 / 350
cyanosis of the tongue 舌青紫 / 132
cyanotic lips 口唇青紫 / 137
cyanotic tongue 青紫舌 / 132
cymba conchae 耳甲艇 / 473
Cyperus-Amomum Six-noble Pills 香砂六君丸 / 388
Cyperus-Amomum Stomach-nourishing Pills 香砂养胃丸 / 387

D

Da Chaihu Decoction 大柴胡汤 / 366
Da Chengqi Decoction 大承气汤 / 364
Dabao (SP 21) 大包 / 416
Dabuyin Pills 大补阴丸 / 389
Dachangshu (BL 25) 大肠俞 / 420
dacryocyst sore 漏睛疮 / 615
dacryopyorrhea 漏睛，漏睛脓出 / 615
dacryopyorrheal eye 漏睛眼 / 615
dacryorrhea disease 流泪病症 / 615
dacryorrhea syndrome 流泪证 / 614
Dadu (SP 2) 大都 / 415

Dadun (LR 1) 大敦 / 432
Dagukong (EX-UE 5) 大骨空 / 442
Dahe (KI 12) 大赫 / 424
Daheng (SP 15) 大横 / 416
Dahuang Fuzi Decoction 大黄附子汤 / 364
Dahuang Mudan Decoction 大黄牡丹汤 / 364
Dahuoluo Pills 大活络丸［丹］/ 392
Dahurian Angelica Root 白芷 / 295
Dahurian Rhododendron Leaf 满山红 / 302
Dahurican Patrinia Tablets 败酱片 / 385
Dai Sigong 戴思恭 / 667
Dai Yuanli 戴原礼 / 667
Daimai (GB 26) 带脉 / 430
Daju (ST 27) 大巨 / 413
Daling (PC 7) 大陵 / 426
damage to fluid 伤津 / 81
damage to lung vessels 肺络损伤 / 110
damage to the thoroughfare and conception vessels 冲任损伤 / 114
damage to yang 伤阳 / 81
damage to yin 伤阴 / 80
damp lichen 湿癣 / 604
dampness 湿 / 65
dampness (*qi*) 湿气 / 65
dampness affliction 冒湿 / 518
dampness arthralgia 湿痹 / 540
dampness beclouding the head 湿蔽清阳 / 89
dampness damage 伤湿 / 518
dampness disease 湿病 / 518
dampness-dispelling formula 祛湿剂 / 379
dampness-draining anti-icteric (medicinal/drug) 利湿退黄药 / 290
dampness-draining diuretic (medicinal/drug) 利水渗湿药 / 290
dampness-draining medicinal/drug 利湿药 / 290
dampness encumbering spleen yang 湿困脾阳 / 105
dampness-fire 湿火 / 68
dampness-heat 湿热 / 68
dampness-heat diarrhea 湿热泄泻 / 545
dampness-heat dysentery 湿热痢 / 521
dampness-heat dysmenorrhea 湿热痛经 / 560
dampness-heat in the bladder 膀胱湿热 / 114
dampness-heat in the liver meridian/channel 肝经湿热 / 99
dampness-heat leukorrhagia 湿热带下 / 564
dampness-heat lumbago 湿热腰痛 / 553
dampness impediment 湿阻，湿痹 / 518，540
dampness malaria 湿疟 / 521
dampness obstructing the middle energizer 湿阻中焦 / 106
dampness (pathogen) encumbering the spleen 湿邪困脾 / 89
dampness-phlegm 湿痰 / 72
dampness-phlegm infertility 湿痰不孕 / 565
dampness-phlegm syndrome/pattern 湿痰证 / 189
dampness-resolving medicinal/drug 化湿药 / 289
dampness-resolving stomach-pacifying formula 化湿和胃剂 / 379
dampness stagnating in the superficies 湿郁肌表 / 89
dampness stroke 中湿 / 66
dampness syndrome/pattern 湿证 / 196
dampness toxin 湿毒 / 69
dampness turbidity 湿浊 / 65
dampness-warmth 湿温 / 518
dampness-warmth disease 湿温病 / 518
Dan Xi Xin Fa 丹溪心法 / 701
Dandelion 蒲公英 / 311
Danggui Buxue Decoction 当归补血汤 / 372
Danggui Pills 当归丸 / 394
Danggui Sini Decoction 当归四逆汤 / 370
Dangyang (EX-HN 2) 当阳 / 439
Dannang (EX-LE 6) 胆囊 / 443
Danshen Root 丹参 / 331
Danshu (BL 19) 胆俞 / 420
dantian 丹田 / 42，497
Danxi's Experiential Therapy 丹溪心法 / 701
Danzhong (CV 17) 膻中 / 436
Daochi Powder 导赤散 / 368
daoyin 导引 / 491
dark of the eye 黑睛 / 609
dark urine 小便黄赤 / 151
darkish complexion 面黑，面色黎黑 / 125
Dashanzha Pills 大山楂丸 / 387
Datura Flower 洋金花 / 303
Daying (ST 5) 大迎 / 411
day-prescription of points 纳干法，纳甲法 / 459
Dazhong (KI 4) 大钟 / 424
Dazhu (BL 11) 大杼 / 419
Dazhui (GV 14) 大椎 / 434

dead fetus 死胎 / 567
dead fetus in the uterus 胎死腹中，子死腹中 / 567
deaf-mutism 耳聋口哑 / 625
deafness 耳聋 / 624
debilitation of kidney yang 肾阳衰微，肾阳虚衰 / 111，113
debilitation of the life gate fire 命门火衰 / 113
decline of heart yang 心阳不振 / 100
decline of yang 阳衰 / 79
decline of yin 阴衰 / 79
decoction 汤药，汤剂 / 281，282
decoction formula 汤头 / 358
Decoction of Cloves and Persimon Calyx 丁香柿蒂汤 / 376
Decoction of Ephedra，Apricot Kernel, Gypsum and Liquorice 麻杏石甘汤 / 362
Decoction of Four Noble Ingredients 四君子汤 / 371
Decoction of Liquorice，Wheat and Jujube 甘麦大枣汤 / 381
Decoction of Rhinoceros Horn and Rehmannia 犀角地黄汤 / 367
Decoction of Tangerine Peel and Bamboo Shavings 橘皮竹茹汤 / 376
Decoction of Two Old Drugs 二陈汤 / 380
decubitus ulcer 褥疮 / 606
dedentition 齿落 / 632
deep abscess 无头疽 / 595
deep-colored urine 尿赤 / 151
deep dull cough 咳声重浊 / 141
deep insertion 深刺 / 454
deep pulse 沉脉 / 160
deep-rooted boil with pyosepticemia 疔疮走黄 / 595
deep-rooted boil 疔 / 592
deep-rooted facial boil 颜面疔疮 / 593
deep thrombophlebitis 股肿 / 606
deep turbid voice 语声重浊 / 140
Deer Tonic Pills 全鹿丸 / 390
Deer-horn 鹿角 / 345
Deer-horn Gelatin 鹿角胶 / 346
Defatted Croton Seed Powder 巴豆霜 / 324
defatting 去油 / 278
defense 卫 / 55
defense aspect syndrome/pattern 卫分证 / 179
defense aspect 卫分 / 55
defense *qi* 卫气 / 54
defense, *qi*, nutrient and blood 卫气营血 / 55
defense-*qi*-nutrient-blood pattern identification 卫气营血辨证 / 179
defense-*qi*-nutrient-blood syndrome differentiation 卫气营血辨证 / 179
defense yang 卫阳 / 54
defense yang being depressed 卫阳被遏 / 85
deficiency and excess 虚实 / 169
deficiency cold 虚寒 / 90
deficiency-cold abdominal pain 虚寒腹痛 / 546
deficiency-cold diarrhea 虚寒泄泻 / 546
deficiency-cold dysentery 虚寒痢 / 522
deficiency cold in the bladder 膀胱虚寒 / 114
deficiency cold in the lower energizer 下焦虚寒 / 215
deficiency cold in the middle energizer 中焦虚寒 / 215
deficiency cold in the triple energizer 三焦虚寒 / 214
deficiency cold in the upper energizer 上焦虚寒 / 214
deficiency-cold in yang brightness (*fu*-organs) 阳明虚寒 / 115
deficiency-cold of lung *qi* 肺气虚寒 / 109
deficiency cold syndrome/pattern 虚寒证 / 172
deficiency complicated by excess 虚中夹实 / 84
deficiency-excess in complexity 虚实夹杂 / 84
deficiency-excess pattern identification 虚实辨证 / 169
deficiency-excess syndrome differentiation 虚实辨证 / 169
deficiency-exploiting pathogen 虚邪 / 63
deficiency fire 虚火 / 91
deficiency fire flaming upward 虚火上炎 / 90
deficiency-fire pharyngitis 虚火喉痹 / 629
deficiency fire syndrome/pattern 虚火证 / 172
deficiency-fire tonsillitis 虚火乳蛾 / 629
deficiency-fire toothache 虚火牙痛 / 632
deficiency heat 虚热 / 90
deficiency-heat-clearing formula 清虚热剂 / 369
deficiency-heat-clearing medicinal/drug 清虚热药 / 288
deficiency heat syndrome/pattern 虚热证 / 172
deficiency in both the exterior and interior 表里俱虚 / 85
deficiency in both the heart and

spleen 心脾两虚 / 101
deficiency in both the lung and kidney 肺肾两虚 / 102
deficiency in both the spleen and lung 脾肺两虚 / 106
deficiency of both *qi* and blood 气血两虚 / 96
deficiency or excess of the exterior and interior 表里虚实 / 82
deficiency syndrome/pattern of both the heart and spleen 心脾两虚证 / 202
deficiency syndrome/pattern of both the spleen and lung 脾肺两虚证 / 207
deficiency syndrome/pattern 虚证 / 170
Degelatinated Deer-horn 鹿角霜 / 346
delirious speech 谵语 / 140
delirium 谵妄 / 124
delivery 分娩 / 568
dementia 痴呆 / 536
Dendrobium 石斛 / 343
Dendrobium Eyesight-improving Pills 石斛夜光丸 / 396
Dens Draconis 龙齿 / 337
dental caries 齿龋 / 632
dental decay 齿蠹 / 632
dental transition 齿更 / 632
depletion of the lower origin 下元亏损 / 112
depressant formula 降剂 / 360
depressed *qi* transforming into fire 气郁化火 / 93
depression 癫，郁病 / 534，549
depression and stagnation of *qi* movement 气机郁滞 / 93
depressive disease 郁病 / 549
depressive-manic psychosis 癫狂 / 534
depressive psychosis 癫病 / 534
derangement of meridian/channel *qi* 经气逆乱 / 114
dermal needle therapy 皮肤针疗法 / 450
dermal needle 皮肤针 / 449
dermatitis medicamentosa 药毒 / 603
Deserted House Medical Talks 冷庐医话 / 702
Desert-living Cistanche 肉苁蓉 / 346
desiccating formula 燥剂 / 360
desire only to sleep 但欲寐 / 155
detention of afterbirth 胞衣不下，息胞 / 570
deteriorated otopyorrhea 脓耳变证 / 623
deteriorated syndrome/pattern 变证 / 116
Detoxicant Coptis Decoction 黄连解毒汤 / 368
Detoxicant Pills of Lonicera and Forsythia 银翘解毒丸 / 381
detoxication 解毒 / 270
deviated eye and mouth 口眼㖞斜 / 127
deviated tongue 舌歪，歪斜舌 / 133
deviation 出偏 / 505
deviation of *qigong* 气功偏差 / 505
deviation of the mouth 口僻 / 537
devitalized middle yang 中阳不振 / 108
diabetes 消渴（病）/ 551
diabetes in children 小儿消渴 / 589
diagnosis 诊断 / 122
diagnostic method 诊法 / 123
diagnostic significance of the five colors 五色主病 / 126
diagnostics 诊断学 / 122
diaphoretic exterior-releasing medicinal/drug 发汗解表药 / 287
diaphoretic method 汗法 / 225
diaphragm 膈 / 42
diarrhea 泄泻，下利 / 149，50，545
diarrhea (disease) 泄泻（病）/ 545
diarrhea during menstruation 经行泄泻 / 563
diarrhea with undigested food 下利清谷 / 150，545
Dicang (ST 4) 地仓 / 411
Dictionary of Chinese Medicine 中国医学大辞典 / 705
Dictionary of Chinese Pharmaceutics 中国药学大辞典 / 705
diet therapy 食疗 / 274
dietary irregularities 饮食不节 / 70
dietary partiality 饮食偏嗜 / 153
dietary prohibitions 食忌 / 284
dietary prohibitions during medication 服药食忌 / 284
different treatments for the same disease 同病异治 / 218
difficult labor 产难，难产 / 569
difficult painful urination 小便涩痛 / 151
diffuse palatitis 飞扬喉 / 631
digestant (medicinal/drug) 消食药 / 291
digestant and evacuant medicinal/drug 消导药 / 291
digestant formula 消食剂 / 379
digging 抠法 / 481
digital circular rubbing manipulation 指摩法 / 650

digital gangrene 脱疽 / 595
digital point pressure therapy 点穴疗法 / 490
Dihuang Pills 地黄丸 / 389
Diji (SP 8) 地机 / 415
dimness of vision 瞑眩 / 146
Ding Ganren 丁甘仁 / 681
Ding Zezhou 丁泽周 / 681
Dingchuan (EX-B 1) 定喘 / 441
Dingchuan Decoction 定喘汤 / 375
Dingchuan Pills 定喘丸 / 383
Dingxiang Shidi Decoction 丁香柿蒂汤 / 376
diphtheria 白喉，白缠喉 / 585
direct attack 直中 / 116
direct contact moxibustion 着肤灸 / 465
Direct Explanation of the Treatise on Cold Damage Diseases 伤寒论直解 / 685
direct moxibustion 明灸，直接灸 / 465
direct needling 直针刺 / 461
directing *qi* downward 降气，下气 / 254
directing *qi* downward and eliminating phlegm 下气消痰 / 253
directing *qi* downward and resolving phlegm 降气化痰 / 253
directing *qi* downward to relieve dyspnea 降气平喘 / 254
directing *qi* downward to stop hiccupping 降气止呃 / 254
directing to the affected meridian/channel or site 引经报使 / 358
directional reinforcement and reduction 迎随补泻 / 457
directional reinforcing-reducing method 迎随补泻法 / 457
discharge-arresting medicinal/drug 收涩药 / 294
discharging fire with bitter-cold 苦寒泻火 / 231
disease 疾病 / 122
disease cause pattern identification 病因辨证 / 191
disease cause syndrome differentiation 病因辨证 / 191
disease differentiation 辨病 / 122
disease identification 诊病 / 122
disease involving both the exterior and interior 表里同病 / 83
disease of both defense and nutrient (aspects) 卫营同病 / 86
disease of both defense and *qi* (aspects) 卫气同病 / 86
disease patterns of the six meridians/channels 六经病证 / 175
diseases of pregnancy 妊娠病 / 566
diseases of the six meridians/channels 六经病 / 175
disequilibrium between physique and *qi* 形气相失 / 3，126
disharmony between nutrient and defense *qi* 营卫不和 / 86
disharmony of liver *qi* 肝气不和 / 97
disharmony of *qi* and blood 气血失调 / 95
disharmony of the thoroughfare and conception vessels 冲任失［不］调 / 114
disinhibiting *qi* 利气 / 252
dislocation 脱位，脱骱，脱臼，脱髎 / 637
disorder of *qi* movement 气机失调 / 93
dispelling cold and resolving phlegm 祛寒化痰 / 258
dispelling dampness 祛湿 / 259
dispelling dampness with bland diuretics 淡渗祛湿 / 260
dispelling phlegm 祛痰 / 258
dispelling stasis to activate blood 祛瘀活血 / 256
dispelling stasis to promote regeneration 祛瘀生新 / 257
dispelling stasis to reduce swelling 祛瘀消肿 / 256
dispelling stasis to stop bleeding 祛瘀止血 / 258
dispelling stasis to unblock collaterals 祛瘀通络 / 257
dispelling summerheat and resolving dampness 祛暑化湿 / 232
dispelling wind 祛风 / 227
dispelling wind and clearing heat 祛风清热 / 227
dispelling wind and dissipating cold 祛风散寒 / 227
dispelling wind and promoting diuresis 祛风行水 / 228
dispelling wind and releasing the exterior 祛风解表 / 227
dispelling wind and relieving spasm 祛风解痉 / 228
dispelling wind and removing dampness 祛风除湿 / 227
dispelling wind and removing dampness to relieve pain 祛风除湿止痛 / 227
dispelling wind and resolving phlegm 祛风化痰 / 227
dispelling wind and unblocking collaterals 祛风通络 / 228
dispelling wind to relieve itching

祛风止痒 / 228
dispelling wind to relieve pain 祛风止痛 / 227
dispensing a prescription 配方 / 357
dispersing abscesses and boils 消痈散疖 / 270
dispersing abscesses and nodules 消痈散结 / 270
dispersing formula 宣剂 / 360
dispersing swelling to relieve pain 消肿止痛 / 271
dispersing wind 疏风 / 226
dispersing wind and clearing heat 疏风清热 / 226
dispersing wind and clearing the lung 疏风清肺 / 226
dispersing wind and discharging heat 疏风泄热 / 226
dispersing wind and dissipating cold 疏风散寒 / 226
dispersing wind and harmonizing the nutrient (aspect) 疏风和营 / 227
dispersing wind and releasing the exterior 疏风解表 / 226
dispersing wind and releasing the flesh 疏风解肌 / 226
dispersing wind and ventilating the lung 疏风宣肺 / 227
dispersing wind-heat 疏散风热 / 225
dispersing wind to alleviate edema 疏风消肿 / 227
dispersing wind to promote eruption 疏风透疹 / 226
dispersing wind to relieve itching 疏风止痒 / 227
dispersion and purgation 开泄 / 229
dispersion with the pungent and purgation with the bitter 辛开苦泄 / 229
displacement of fractured ends 断端移位 / 635
disposable needle 一次性针 / 452
dissipating cold and resolving retained fluid 散寒化饮 / 259
dissipating cold 散寒 / 226
dissolution 溶化 / 282
dissolving calculi 化石 / 272
dissolving fish bone 消骨鲠 / 271
distal bleeding 远血 / 550
distal gingival abscess 牙龄［咬］痈 / 633
distant-local point combination 远近配穴法 / 448
distant needling 远道刺 / 460
distending pain 胀痛 / 147
distending pain in the breasts during menstruation 经行乳房胀痛 / 563
distension of the eyeball 睛胀 / 622
Distension-relieving Pills 越鞠丸 / 387
distillate 露，露剂 / 281
distress below the heart 心下急 / 156
distress in the heart 心中懊侬 / 124
distributing *qi* 布气 / 504
disturbance in ascending and descending 升降失常 / 94
disturbance of *qi* movement 气机不利 / 93
disturbance of *qi* transformation 气化不利 / 93
Dittany Root-bark 白鲜皮 / 308
diuretic hydragogue (medicinal/drug) 利尿逐水药 / 290
Divaricate Saposhnikovia Root 防风 / 295
divergent collateral vessel 别络 / 407
Diverse-color Cinquefoil 翻白草 / 310
Divine Axis 灵枢 / 684
Diwuhui (GB 42) 地五会 / 431
dizziness 眩晕 / 146，532
dizziness during menstruation 经行眩晕 / 562
dizziness with dimmed vision 眩冒 / 146
dizziness with dimmed vision and shaking 徇蒙招尤 / 146
dizziness with shaking 掉眩 / 146
Dodder Seed 菟丝子 / 347
Dogbane Leaf 罗布麻叶 / 305
dominant *qi* 主气 / 18
dominant circuit 主运 / 18
dorsal carbuncle 发背 / 594
dorsoventral boundary (of the hand or foot) 赤白肉际 / 52
dorsum nasi 鼻梁 / 39
dorsum of the nose 鼻柱 / 39
dosage 剂量 / 280
dosage form 剂型 / 280
dotted nebula 星翳 / 612
double cross-legged sitting 双盘坐 / 495
double-handed needle insertion 双手进针法 / 453
double-nine yang exercise 九九阳功 / 503
double tongue 重舌 / 133，633
Doubleteeth Pubescent Angelica Root 独活 / 314
down 毫毛 / 41
down-hanging elbows 垂肘 / 494
downpour of dampness-heat 湿热下注 / 89

downward-pressing posture 下按式 / 496
dragged shoulder 牵拉肩 / 646
dragging 揪法 / 483
dragging for congestion 揪痧 / 486
dragging pain 掣痛 / 148
Dragon's Blood 血竭 / 355
Dragon's Bone 龙骨 / 337
Dragon's Teeth 龙齿 / 337
dragon-mouth gesture 龙衔式 / 505
drainage needling 大泻刺 / 460
draining dampness with bland diuretics 淡渗利湿 / 260
draining dampness 利湿，渗湿 / 260
drastic hydragogue 峻下逐水药 / 289
drastic pungent-cool formula 辛凉重剂 / 362
drastic purgation 峻下 / 236
Drastic Purgative Decoction 大承气汤 / 364
drawing out pus and removing putridity 提脓去腐 / 269
drawing out pus and toxins 提脓拔毒 / 269
drawing out toxins 拔毒 / 269
dream emission 梦遗 / 155
dreamfulness 多梦 / 155
dredging the pleurodiaphragmatic space 开达膜［募］原 / 238
dribbling after voiding 余沥不尽 / 151
dribbling urination 小便淋漓 / 151
dribbling with wet cheeks 滞颐 / 579
Dried Ginger 干姜 / 317
Dried Tangerine Peel 陈皮 / 325
dripping pill 滴丸 / 280
drool 涎 / 58
drooling 流涎 / 578
drooling from the corner of the mouth 口角流涎 / 136
drooping nebula 垂帘翳 / 619
drooping pannus 赤膜下垂 / 619
drooping the shoulders 沉肩 / 493
dropping the elbows 坠肘 / 493
drowsy filthy attack 闷痧 / 583
drug eruption 药毒 / 603
drumskin pulse 革脉 / 162
dry blood consumption 干血痨 / 530
dry choleraic turmoil 干霍乱 / 522
dry cough 干咳 / 142，525
dry cracked lips 口唇干裂 / 136
dry deafness 干聋 / 625
dry mouth 口干 / 149
dry nose 鼻燥 / 626
dry orifice syndrome/pattern 燥干清窍证 / 198
dry ringworm 干癣 / 605
dry teeth 齿燥 / 137
dry (tongue) coating/fur 燥苔 / 135
drying dampness 燥湿 / 260
drying dampness and relieving itching 燥湿止痒 / 267
drying dampness and resolving phlegm 燥湿化痰 / 258
drying dampness to invigorate the spleen 燥湿健脾 / 260
drying dampness with bitter-cold 苦寒燥湿 / 260
drying dampness with bitter-warm 苦温燥湿 / 244
drying dampness with bitter-warmth 苦温燥湿 / 260
dryness 燥 / 66
dryness accumulation syndrome/pattern 燥结证 / 198
dryness accumulation 燥结 / 92
dryness affecting the clear orifices 燥干清窍 / 90
dryness and discomfort of the eyes 眼珠干涩 / 128
Dryness-clearing Lung-saving Decoction 清燥救肺汤 / 378
dryness damaging body fluid 燥伤津液 / 90
dryness damaging lung *qi* 燥伤肺气 / 89
dryness-fire 燥火 / 66，68
dryness-heat in yang brightness (*fu*-organs) 阳明燥热 / 115
dryness-heat 燥热 / 66，68
dryness in the mouth with no desire to drink 口干不欲饮 / 149
dryness (infantile) malnutrition 干疳 / 580
dryness (infantile) malnutrition syndrome 干疳证 / 580
dryness-phlegm syndrome/pattern 燥痰证 / 189
dryness *qi* transforming into cold 燥气寒化 / 90
dryness *qi* transforming into heat 燥气化热 / 90
dryness *qi* 燥气 / 66
dryness transformation 燥化 / 92
dryness-treating formula 治燥剂 / 378
dual deficiency of yin-yang 阴阳两虚 / 80
Dubi (ST 35) 犊鼻 / 414
Duhuo Jisheng Decoction 独活寄生汤 / 377
Duiduan (GV 27) 兑端 / 435
dull pain 隐痛 / 148
Dushu (BL 16) 督俞 / 420

dusty complexion 面尘 / 125
Dutchmanspipe Fruit 马兜铃 / 303
Dutchmanspipe Root 青木香 / 321
Duyin (EX-LE 11) 独阴 / 444
Dwarf Lilyturf Root 麦冬 / 343
dwarfism 侏儒 / 590
Dyers Woad Leaf 大青叶 / 311
dynamic *qigong* 动功 / 492
dysentery 痢疾 / 521
dysentery with purulent and bloody stools 下利［痢］脓血 / 150
dysfunction in essence storage 封藏失职 / 112
dysfunction of lung *qi* 肺气不利 / 109
dysfunction of meridian/channel passages 经隧失职 / 114
dysfunction of the large intestine in conveyance 大肠传导失职 / 110
dysfunction of the spleen in transportation 脾失健运 / 105
dysmenorrhea 痛经 / 560
Dysmenorrhea Pills 痛经丸 / 394
dyspepsia 伤食，食积 / 543，582
dyspepsia syndrome 伤食证 / 543
dysphagia 噎嗝，膈噎 / 543
dyspnea 喘，上气 / 140，526，527
dyspnea (disease) 喘病 / 527
dyspnea of deficiency type 虚喘 / 527
dyspnea of excess type 实喘 / 527
dyspnea (syndrome) 喘证 / 527
dyspnea with reversed flow of *qi* 喘逆 / 141
dystocia 产难，难产 / 569

E

ear 耳 / 45
ear acupoints 耳穴 / 473
ear acupuncture 耳针 / 472
ear acupuncture therapy 耳针疗法 / 472
ear block 耳闭 / 623
ear boil 耳疔 / 623
ear distension 耳胀 / 623
ear exercise 耳功 / 501，505
ear fistula 耳瘘 / 625
ear furuncle 耳疖 / 623
ear-hole 耳孔 / 45
ear pile 耳痔 / 625
ear-point massotherapy 耳穴推拿疗法 / 490
ear polyp 耳菌，耳蕈 / 625
ear protuberance 耳挺 / 625
ear sore 耳疮 / 623
eardrum 耳膜 / 45
earlobe 耳垂 / 45，473
early leakage of amniotic fluid 试水 / 569
early periods due to blood heat 血热经行先期 / 557
early periods due to *qi* deficiency 气虚经行先期 / 557
early periods 月经提前，月经先期，经行先期，经水先期，经早 / 157，557
ear-point massotherapy 耳穴推拿疗法 / 490
earth failing to control water 土不制水 / 14
earth-featured person 土形之人 / 73
earth generating metal 土生金 / 11
earth restricting water 土克水 / 12
earthly branches 地支 / 18
Earthworm 地龙 / 339
earwax 耵聍 / 625
easing joint movement 通利关节 / 269
easing the joint 通利关节 / 654
eclampsia 子痫，子冒 / 566，567
eclampsia (in pregnancy) 妊娠痫证 / 566
eclipsed lunar sore 月蚀疮 / 623
Eclipta 墨旱莲 / 330
eczema 湿疮，湿疹 / 603
eczema of the external ear 旋耳疮，月蚀疮 / 623
eczematous dermatitis of the eyelid 风赤疮痍，风赤疮疾 / 614
edema 水肿 / 138，548
edema-alleviating diuretic (medicinal/drug) 利水消肿药 / 290
edema due to yang deficiency 阳虚水泛 / 86
edema during menstruation 经期水肿 / 562
edema in children 小儿浮肿，小儿水肿 / 590
edema of deficiency type 虚肿 / 548
edema of pregnancy 妊娠肿胀 / 568
edema of the eye sockets 目窠肿 / 128
edema of the eyelids 目胞浮肿 / 128
edema syndrome/pattern 水气证 / 189
edema under the eyes 目下肿 / 128
edematous disease 水肿病 / 548
edge of the tongue 舌边 / 39
effective formula 良方 / 357
Effective Prescriptions 本事方 / 691

Effective Prescriptions for Universal Relief 普济本事方 / 691
Effective Prescriptions for Women 妇人良方 / 695
Effective Prescriptions Handed Down for Generations 世医得效方 / 692
effervescent tablet 泡腾片 / 280
efflux diarrhea 滑泄 / 545
effulgent life gate fire 命门火旺 / 111
egret's cough 鹭鸶咳 / 586
eight bone-setting manipulations 正骨八法 / 638
eight confluence points 八脉交会穴 / 439
eight-diagram walking 八卦步 / 496
eight extra meridians/channels 奇经八脉 / 405
eight influential points 八会穴 / 439
Eight-ingredient Rectification Powder 八正散 / 380
Eight-precious Motherwort Pills 八珍益母丸 / 395
eight principles 八纲 / 168
eight-principle pattern identification 八纲辨证 / 168
eight-principle syndrome differentiation 八纲辨证 / 168
eight regions of the eye 八廓 / 44，607
eight-section brocade 八段锦 / 502
eight signs of infantile convulsions 惊风八候 / 574
eight therapeutic methods 八法 / 225
eight transverse markings 八溪 / 52
Eight-treasure Decoction 八珍汤 / 372
Eight-treasure Pills 八珍丸 / 388
eighteen antagonisms 十八反 / 359
elbow-kneading manipulation 肘揉法 / 648
elbow-pressing manipulation 肘按法 / 651
elbow pushing manipulation 肘推法 / 648
electric moxibustion 电灸，电热灸 / 467
electric moxibustion device 电灸器 / 467
electric ophthalmia 电光伤目 / 621
electric stimulator 电针仪 / 470
electro-acupuncture 电针 / 470
electro-acupuncture anesthesia 电针麻醉 / 470
electro-acupuncture therapy 电针疗法 / 470
elevating formula 升剂 / 360
elevating the middle *qi* 升提中气 / 246
elevating yang 升阳 / 247
elevating yang to cure drooping 升阳举陷 / 247
eliminating jaundice 退黄 / 269
eliminating mass 消痞 / 252
eliminating phlegm 豁痰 / 259
eliminating phlegm to arouse the brain 豁痰醒脑 / 267
eliminating phlegm to induce resuscitation 豁痰开窍 / 267
eliminating stagnant blood by catharsis 攻下逐瘀 / 238
eliminating the pathogenic (factors) 祛邪 / 219
eliminating the pathogenic with reinforcement of the healthy 祛邪兼扶正 / 220
eliminating the stale and the stagnant 去菀陈莝 / 237
elimination followed by reinforcement 先攻后补 / 220
elimination for reinforcement 寓补于攻 / 220
elimination from within 内消 / 269
elixir field 丹田 / 42，497
Elsholtzia Herb 香薷 / 296
Elshotzia Powder 香薷散 / 361
Elucidation of Massotherapy for Children 小儿推拿广意 / 696
Elucidation of Massotherapy 推拿广意 / 696
Elucidation of the Fourteen Meridians/ Channels 十四经发挥 / 699
elutriation 水飞 / 276
emaciation with sagging flesh 大肉陷下 / 126
emergency purgation 急下 / 236
emergency purgation to preserve fluid 急下存津 / 237
emergency purgation to preserve yin 急下存阴 / 236
emesis 吐法 / 267
emetic (medicinal/drug) 催吐药，涌吐药 / 294
emetic method 吐法 / 267
eminence-rubbing manipulation 鱼际擦法 / 650
emission of outgoing *qi* 发放外气 / 504
emission of *qi* 发气 / 504
emission of trained *qi* 发功 / 504
emmeniopathy 月经病 / 557
emolliating the liver 柔肝 / 265
empty pain 空痛 / 148
encrusted skin 肌肤甲错 / 139
endemic goiter in children 小儿

瘿气 / 589
endogenous cause 内因 / 62
endogenous damage 内伤 / 69
endogenous toxin 内毒 / 69
endogenous-wind-extinguishing formula 平熄内风剂 / 377
Endothelium Corneum Gigeriae Galli 鸡内金 / 352
engendering fluid 生津 / 264
engendering fluid with sweet-cold 甘寒生津 / 264
English Walnut Seed 核桃仁 / 346
enlarged tongue 胖大舌 / 132
enlivening the spleen 醒脾 / 245
entering quiescence 入静 / 493
entering the interior and exiting to the exterior 表里出入 / 82
entering the interior from the exterior 由表入里 / 82
entrance doors 户门 / 40
entwining throat infection 缠喉风 / 630
entwining throat wind 缠喉风 / 630
enuresis 失溲，遗尿（病）/ 151，553，590
enuresis in children 小儿遗尿 / 590
Ephedra 麻黄 / 295
Ephedra Decoction 麻黄汤 / 361
Ephedra Root 麻黄根 / 348
epidemic 时行 / 514
epidemic conjunctivitis 天行赤目，天行赤眼 / 616
epidemic cough 疫咳 / 586
epidemic dysentery 时疫痢，疫痢 / 522
epidemic erythema 疫痧 / 585
epidemic fulminant red eye 天行暴赤 / 616
epidemic kerato-conjunctivitis 天行赤目暴翳 / 616
epidemic parotitis 痄腮 / 585
epidemic pathogen 疠气，戾气，时行戾气 / 63，514
epidemic red eye 天行赤目，天行赤眼 / 616
epidemic red eye with fulminant nebula 天行赤目暴翳 / 616
epidemic summer fever in children 小儿暑温 / 582
epidemic swollen-head infection 大头瘟 / 520
epidemic throat diseases 疫喉 / 585
epidemic toad-like infection 虾蟆瘟 / 520
epidemic toxic dysentery 疫毒痢 / 522
epidemic toxin 疫毒 / 63
epigastric fullness 心下满 / 156
epigastric fullness with counterflow 心下逆满 / 156
epigastric pain 脘痛，胃脘痛 / 147，152
epigastric pain (disease) 胃脘痛（病）/ 542
epigastric rigidity 心下硬 / 156
epigastric stuffiness 心下痞 / 156，542
epigastric stuffiness and rigidity 心下痞硬 / 156
epiglottis 会厌，吸门 / 40，41
epilepsy 癫痫 / 535，589
epilepsy (disease) 痫病 / 534
epilepsy (in older children) 颠疾 / 589
epilepsy (in younger children) 痫证 / 589
epilepsy (syndrome) 痫证 / 534
Epimedium Herb 淫羊藿 / 346
epiphora 不时泪溢 / 611
episcleritis 火疳，火疡 / 617
epistaxis 鼻衄 / 130，550，627
epistaxis during menstruation 经行衄血 / 562
equilibrium between physique and *qi* 形气相得 / 3，126
Erbai (EX-UE 2) 二白 / 442
Erchen Decoction 二陈汤 / 380
Erheliao (TE 22) 耳和髎 / 428
Erjian (EX-HN 6) 耳尖 / 440
Erjian (LI 2) 二间 / 409
Erlong Zuoci Pills 耳聋左慈丸 / 397
Ermen (TE 21) 耳门 / 428
Ermu Ningsou Pills［Tablets］二母宁嗽丸 / 382
erosion of the canthal eyelid 眦帷赤烂 / 614
erosion of the lips 口唇糜烂 / 136
erosion of the palpebral margin 风弦赤烂，睑弦赤烂，眼缘赤烂 / 613
erosion of the throat with erythema 烂喉丹痧 / 585
erroneous administration of purgatives 误下 / 238
eructation 嗳气 / 153
Erxian Decoction 二仙汤 / 373
erysipelas 丹毒，火丹 / 593
erysipelas facialis 大头瘟 / 520
erythema multiforme 猫眼疮 / 601
erythema nodosum 瓜藤缠 / 601
erythroderma neonatorum 胎赤 / 576
essence 精 / 2，56
essence chamber 精室 / 49
Essence of External Medicine 外科精要 / 697
Essence of the Silvery Sea 银海精微 / 698
essence, *qi*, and mind 精、气、神 / 498

essence-blood 精血 / 56
essence-marrow depletion 精髓空虚 / 111
Essential Prescriptions Worth a Thousand Pieces of Gold for Emergencies 备急千金要方 / 690
Essential Prescriptions Worth a Thousand Pieces of Gold 千金要方 / 690
essential *qi* 精气 / 2，54
Essential Readings for Medical Professionals 医宗必读 / 704
Essentials for Diagnosticians 诊家枢要 / 686
Essentials of External Medicine 外科精义 / 697
Essentials of Materia Medica 本草备要 / 689
Essentials of Obstetrics from the Treasury of Household Hygiene 卫生家宝产科备要 / 695
essentials of posture management 调身要领 / 493
Essentials of the Canon of Medicine 内经知要 / 684
Essentials of the Internal Classic 内经知要 / 684
ethereal soul 魂 / 57
Eucommia Bark 杜仲 / 347
Eupolyphaga seu Steleophaga 䗪虫 / 333
European Verbena Herb 马鞭草 / 334
evacuating pus 排脓 / 269
evacuating pus and eliminating swelling 排脓消肿 / 269
evacuating pus and expelling toxins 排脓托毒 / 269
evacuating pus from within 托里排脓 / 269
evaluation via kneading-pressing 搏捺皮相 / 648
even-numbered formula/prescription 偶方 / 356
Ever-effective Decoction 一贯煎 / 373
eversion 外翻 / 656
evil reactions 走火入魔 / 505
Evodia Decoction 吴茱萸汤 / 370
Evodia Fruit 吴茱萸 / 318
examination of the eye 察目 / 128
exanthem 痧 / 583
exathema subitum 奶麻 / 584
excess amniotic fluid 胎水肿满 / 567
excess cold 实寒 / 90
excess cold syndrome/pattern 实寒证 / 172，194
excess complicated by deficiency 实中夹虚 / 84
excess fire 实火 / 90
excess fire in the liver meridian/channel 肝经实火 / 98
excess fire syndrome/pattern 实火证 / 173，198
excess heat 实热 / 90
excess heat in the large intestine (meridian/channel) 大肠实热 / 111
excess heat in the lower energizer 下焦实热 / 215
excess heat in the middle energizer 中焦实热 / 215
excess heat in the triple energizer 三焦实热 / 215
excess heat in the upper energizer 上焦实热 / 215
excess heat syndrome/pattern 实热证 / 173
excess in both the exterior and interior 表里俱实 / 85
excess of sexual activity 房事过度 / 71
excess syndrome/pattern 实证 / 170
excessive *qi* 淫气 / 63
excessive sweating 多汗 / 144
excessiveness in the stomach and intestines 胃家实 / 523
excessiveness in yang brightness *fu*-organ 阳明腑实 / 115
exfoliative cheilitis 唇风 / 633
exhaustion of meridian/channel *qi* 经气衰竭 / 114
exhaustion of *tiangui* 天癸竭 / 556
exiting to the exterior from the interior 由里出表 / 83
Exocarpium Benincasae 冬瓜皮 / 321
Exocarpium Citri Grandis 化橘红 / 327
Exocarpium Citri Rubrum 橘红 / 325
exogenous cause 外因 / 62
exogenous-dryness-dispersing formula 轻宣外燥剂 / 378
exogenous-wind-dispersing formula 疏散外风剂 / 377
exophthalmos 眼球突出 / 128
expectorant，antitussive and antiasthmatic 化痰止咳平喘药 / 292
expediting child delivery 催生 / 268
expelling calculi 排石 / 272
expelling intestinal worms and dissipating accumulation 驱虫消积 / 271
expelling pathogens 达邪，透邪 / 229
expelling pathogens through the

exterior and clearing heat 透表清热 / 229
expelling pathogens through the exterior 透表 / 228
expelling pus from sores 托疮 / 269
expelling retained fluid by catharsis 泻下逐饮 / 237
expelling retained water 攻逐水饮，泻水逐饮 / 237
expelling through the exterior and removing from the interior 透泄 / 229
expelling toxins 托毒 / 269
expelling water 逐水 / 237
expelling water by catharsis 泻下逐水 / 237
expelling worms 驱虫 / 271
expiry sweating 绝汗 / 145
exposure of dental root 齿挺 / 633
exposure of dental root 牙宣 / 633
expulsion from within 内托 / 269
expulsion method 托法 / 269
Exsiccated Sodium Sulfate 玄明粉 / 353
extension through the passes toward the nail 透关射甲 / 138
exterior and interior 表里 / 169
exterior cold 表寒 / 82
exterior cold and interior heat 表寒里热 / 83
exterior cold syndrome/pattern 表寒证 / 170
exterior dampness syndrome/pattern 表湿证 / 196
exterior deficiency 表虚 / 82
exterior deficiency and interior excess 表虚里实 / 83
exterior deficiency syndrome/pattern 表虚证 / 170
exterior-effusing medicinal/drug 发表药 / 287
exterior excess 表实 / 82
exterior excess and interior deficiency 表实里虚 / 84
exterior excess syndrome/pattern 表实证 / 170
exterior heat 表热 / 82
exterior heat and interior cold 表热里寒 / 83
exterior heat syndrome/pattern 表热证 / 170
exterior-interior meridian/channel point combination 表里经配穴法 / 447
exterior-interior pattern identification 表里辨证 / 169
exterior-interior point combination 表里配穴法 / 447
exterior-interior releasing formula 表里双解剂 / 366
exterior-interior syndrome differentiation 表里辨证 / 169
exterior-interior transmission 表里传 / 116
exterior-releasing formula 解表剂 / 361
exterior-releasing medicinal/drug 解表药 / 287
exterior syndrome/pattern 表证 / 169
exterior wind-cold syndrome/pattern 风寒表证 / 192
external abscess 外痈 / 593
external acoustic meatus 耳道，耳窍 / 45
external application 外敷 / 272
external blowing 外吹 / 596
"external blowing" mastitis 外吹乳痈 / 596
external cause 外因 / 62
external channel 外经 / 400
external cold 外寒 / 64
external contraction 外感 / 62, 519
external dampness 外湿 / 65
external disease 外证 / 591
external dryness 外燥 / 66
external dryness syndrome/pattern 外燥证 / 197
external exercise 外功 / 492
external fixation 外固定 / 640
external genitals 阴器 / 49
external hemorrhoid 外痔 / 599
external malleolus 核骨，外踝 / 50
external meridian 外踝 / 50
external opening of the ear / 473
external ophthalmopathy 外障 / 612
external pathogen 外邪 / 62
external therapy 外治法 / 272
external treatment 外治 / 272
external urethral orifice (of the female) 廷孔 / 49
external wind 外风 / 64
external wind syndrome/pattern 外风证 / 191
externally contracted cough 外感咳嗽 / 525
externally contracted headache 外感头痛 / 533
externally contracted lumbago 外感腰痛 / 553
extinguishing wind 熄［息］风 / 265
extinguishing wind and resolving phlegm 熄［息］风化痰 / 259
extinguishing wind to arrest

convulsions 熄［息］风定痉 / 266
extinguishing wind to arrest epilepsy 熄［息］风定痫 / 266
extinguishing wind to relieve convulsions 熄［息］风解痉 / 266
extra conductant ingredient 药引子 / 358
extra-ocular muscles 眼带 / 610
extra points 经外穴 / 439
extracorporeal cosmic cycle 离体周天 / 500
extracorporeal heavenly circuit 离体周天 / 500
Extractum Malti 饴糖 / 342
extraordinary organs 奇恒之腑 / 24
extreme heat engendering wind 热极生风 / 88，103
extreme heat producing wind 热极生风 / 103
extreme yang resembling yin 阳极似阴 / 7
extreme yin resembling yang 阴极似阳 / 7
extremely abnormal pulse 脉悬绝 / 165
extremely poisonous, moderately poisonous, slightly poisonous and non-poisonous (medicinals) 大毒、常毒、小毒、无毒 / 279
exuberance and debilitation between pathogenic and healthy *qi* 邪正盛衰 / 78
exuberance of heart fire 心火亢盛 / 101
exuberant fire-heat syndrome/pattern 火热炽盛证 / 173
exuberant heat damaging fluid 热盛伤津 / 88
exuberant heat stirring up wind 热盛风动 / 88
exuberant wood overrestricting earth 木旺乘土 / 13
exuberant yang repelling yin 阳盛格阴 / 79
exuberant yin repelling yang 阴盛格阳 / 80
exudative eczema 浸淫疮 / 603
eye 目 / 43
eye connector 目系 / 45
eye dropping 点眼 / 273
eye exercise 眼功，目功 / 501，506
eye gum 目眵 / 610
eye gum and tears 眵泪 / 611
eye (infantile) malnutrition 眼疳 / 581
eye itching 目痒 / 622
eye pain 目痛 / 610
eye socket 目眶 / 43，608
eyeball 目珠，眼珠 / 610
eyelid 眼睑，胞睑，目胞，目裹 / 607

F

facial acupuncture 面针 / 477
facial acupuncture therapy 面针疗法 / 478
facial erysipelas 抱头火丹 / 594
facing a wall 面壁 / 499
Faeces Trogopterorum 五灵脂 / 332
failure of bladder retention 膀胱失约 / 113
failure of blood to nourish sinews/tendons 血不养筋 / 95
failure of *qi* to control the blood 气不摄血 / 95
failure of *qi* transformation 气化无权 / 93
failure of the mind to keep to its abode 神不守舍 / 100
failure of water to transform into *qi* 水不化气 / 93
failure to cry in the newborn 初生不啼 / 574
failure to suck in the newborn 初生不乳 / 574
faint low voice 语声低微 / 140
faint pulse 微脉 / 161
fainting 昏厥 / 538
fainting during acupuncture 晕针 / 463
fainting during moxibustion 晕灸 / 467
falling into static state 入静 / 493
false cold 假寒 / 91
false heat 假热 / 91
false labor 弄胎 / 569
false vitality 假神 / 123
Fangfeng Tongsheng Pills 防风通圣丸 / 382
Fangfeng Tongsheng Powder 防风通圣散 / 366
farsightedness 能远怯近症 / 621
fascicular keratitis 风轮赤豆 / 619
fasting exercise 辟谷功 / 503
fat infertility 脂塞不孕 / 566
fat person 膏人 / 75
fat sore肥疮 / 604
fat tumor 肉瘤 / 598
fat-congealed nebula 凝脂翳 / 618
faucial abscess 喉关痈 / 629
faucial isthmus 喉关 / 40，628
favorable complexion 善色 / 124
favorable syndrome/pattern of

measles 麻疹顺证 / 584
favus 肥疮 / 604
fear 恐 / 70
fearful throbbing 怔忡 / 151, 530
Feather Cockscomb Seed 青葙子 / 304
febrile convulsions 热甚发痉 / 538
febrile disease 热病 / 515
feeble breathing 呼吸气微 / 140
feeble pulse 虚脉 / 161
feeding (infantile) malnutrition 食疳 / 581
feeding on *qi* instead of food 却谷食气 / 503
Feishu (BL 13) 肺俞 / 419
Feiyang (BL 58) 飞阳 / 423
Fel Ursi 熊胆 / 339
felon 瘭疽 / 594
female *zang* organs 牝脏 / 20
femur 髀骨 / 51
Fengchi (GB 20) 风池 / 430
Fengfu (GV 16) 风府 / 434
Fenglong (ST 40) 丰隆 / 414
Fengmen (BL 12) 风门 / 419
Fengshi (GB 31) 风市 / 431
Fennel Fruit 小茴香 / 318
fermentation 发酵 / 278
Fermented Soybean 淡豆豉 / 298
fetal breathing 胎息 / 497
fetal cold 胎寒 / 576
fetal endowment 胎禀 / 576
fetal feebleness 胎怯 / 576
fetal feeding 胎食 / 494
fetal heat 胎热 / 576
fetal origin 胎元 / 566
fetal redness 胎赤 / 576
fetal toxicosis 胎毒 / 576
fetal toxin 胎毒 / 69
fetal weakness 胎弱 / 576
fetid vaginal discharge 带下臭秽 / 158
fever 发热 / 143
fever at blood aspect 血热 / 95
fever at night 夜热 / 582
fever due to fright 惊热 / 583
fever during menstruation 经行发热 / 562
fever of deficiency type 虚热 / 530
fever with chills 发热恶寒 / 143
fever with hypochondriac mass 癖热 / 583
fever without chills 但热不寒 / 143
feverish sensation in the palms and soles 手足心热 / 144
fevers in children 小儿诸热 / 582
fibula 外辅骨 / 51
Field Thistle 小蓟 / 328
fifteen collateral vessels 十五络脉 / 407
fifth-watch cough 五更咳 / 526
fifth-watch diarrhea 五更泄 / 545
Figwort Root 玄参 / 306
Figwortflower Picrorhiza Rhizome 胡黄连 / 308
filiform needle 毫针 / 449
filiform wart 线瘊 / 600
filling for the stuffed 塞因塞用 / 221
filthy attack in children 小儿发痧 / 583
filthy turbidity 秽浊 / 72
fine pulse 细脉 / 161
Fineleaf Schizonepeta Herb 荆芥 / 295
Fineleaf Schizonepeta Spike 荆芥穗 / 296
finger-breadth body-*cun* 横指同身寸 / 445
finger-breadth body-inch 横指同身寸 / 445
Finger Citron 佛手 / 326
finger-combining pinching manipulation 合指捏法 / 652
finger-kneading manipulation 指揉法 / 647
finger-pressing manipulation 指按法 / 651
finger-pressing massage 指压推拿 / 490
finger-pressing *tuina* 指压推拿 / 490
finger-pressure anesthesia 指压麻醉 / 479
finger-pressure conduction of qi 指压行气法 / 459
finger-pressure therapy 指压疗法 / 479
finger puncture 指针法 / 481
finger-pushing manipulation 指推法 / 648
fingernail pressing 掐法 / 480
fingernail-pressing needle insertion 指切进针法 / 453
fire 火 / 66
fire amenorrhea 火邪经闭 / 559
fire cupping 火罐法 / 468
fire damaging blood vessels 火伤血络 / 90
fire failing to generate earth 火不生土 / 13
fire-featured person 火形之人 / 73
fire generating earth 火生土 / 11
fire-insertion cupping 投火法 / 468
fire needle 火针 / 450
fire needling therapy 火针疗法 / 450
fire phlegm 火痰 / 528
fire processing 火制 / 276

fire-rack cupping 架火法 / 468
fire restricting metal 火克金 / 12
fire toxin 火毒 / 68
fire toxin syndrome/pattern 火毒证 / 198
fire ulcer (of the eye) 火疳，火疡 / 617
firm pulse 牢脉 / 162
first yang 一阳 / 400
first yin 一阴 / 399
fish-swimming pulse 鱼翔脉 / 163
fissure of the tongue 舌裂 / 133
fissured fracture 骨错缝 / 646
fissured tongue 裂纹舌 / 133
fist-kneading manipulation 拳揉法 / 647
fist-striking manipulation 拳击法 / 649
fistula 漏 / 591
five (infantile) malnutrition syndromes 五疳 / 580
five circuits and six *qi* 五运六气 / 17
five circuits 五运 / 17
five colors 五色 / 125
five directions 五方 / 14
five elements/phases 五行 / 11
five-element/phase theory 五行学说 / 11
five emotions 五志 / 26，69
five emotions/minds in excess 五志过极 / 70
five evolutive phases 五化 / 14
five fauna-mimic frolics 五禽戏 / 502
Five-ingredient Decoction with Milkvetch and Cassia Twig 黄芪桂枝五物汤 / 370
five kinds of edema 五水 / 549
five kinds of liquid 五液 / 58
five kinds of overstrain 五劳 / 529
five kinds of retardation 五迟 / 577
five kinds of stranguria 五淋 / 552
five minds 五志 / 26，69
five needling methods 五刺 / 459
five orbiculi 五轮 / 43，607
five *qi* 五气 / 14
five seasons 五时 / 14
Five-seed Pill 五仁丸 / 364
five (sense) organs 五官 / 14，38
five tastes (flavors) 五味 / 279
five transport points 五输穴 / 437
five-transport-points combination 五输配穴法 / 448
five types of flaccidity 五软 / 578
five types of stiffness 五硬 / 578
five viscera 五脏 / 20
five voices 五声 / 14
five yin-yang dispositions 阴阳五态人 / 74
five *zang* organs 五脏 / 20
fixation of pubic cartilage 交骨不开 / 570
fixation pad 固定垫 / 641
fixation with cotton pads 棉枕固定 / 640
fixation with one pad 一垫固定法 / 641
fixation with three pads 三垫固定法 / 641
fixation with two pads 二垫固定法 / 641
fixed arthralgia 着痹 / 540
fixed impediment 着痹 / 540
fixed pain 固定痛 / 148
flaccid tongue 舌痿，痿软舌 / 133
flaring of the nares 鼻翼煽动 / 130
flash-fire cupping 闪火法 / 468
flash ophthalmia 电光伤目 / 621
flat pad 平垫 / 641
flat-palm gesture 平掌式 / 504
flat wart 扁瘊 / 600
Flatstem Milkvetch Seed 沙苑子 / 344
flavor predilection 五味偏嗜 / 70
Fleeceflower Root 何首乌 / 344
Fleeceflower Stem 首乌藤 / 336
flesh 肉 / 41
flesh atrophy-flaccidity 肉痿 / 539
flesh orbiculus 肉轮 / 44，607
fleshy goiter 肉瘿 / 597
flexing 屈法 / 485
flexing-stretching manipulation 屈伸法 / 653
flicking 弹击法 / 484
flicking-in insertion 弹入法 / 453
flicking manipulation 弹法 / 651
flicking stone pulse 弹石脉 / 163
floaters 蛛丝飘浮 / 612
floating pulse at both yin and yang 脉阴阳俱浮 / 164
floating pulse 浮脉 / 160
floccillation 捻衣摸床，循衣摸床 / 124
flooding 血崩 / 561
flooding and spotting 崩漏 / 561
flooding syndrome 崩证 / 561
Flos Albiziae 合欢花 / 336
Flos Buddlejae 密蒙花 / 305
Flos Campsis 凌霄花 / 332
Flos Carthami 红花 / 330
Flos Caryophylli 丁香 / 318
Flos Chrysanthemi Indici 野菊花 / 311
Flos Chrysanthemi 菊花 / 297

Flos Daturae 洋金花 / 303
Flos Eriocauli 谷精草 / 304
Flos Farfarae 款冬花 / 301
Flos Genkwa 芫花 / 324
Flos Inulae 旋覆花 / 299
Flos Lonicerae 金银花 / 310
Flos Magnoliae Officinalis 厚朴花 / 327
Flos Magnoliae 辛夷 / 296
Flos Mume 梅花 / 327
Flos Rosae Chinensis 月季花 / 332
Flos Sophorae Immaturus 槐米 / 329
Flos Sophorae 槐花 / 329
"flowing fire" 流火 / 594
"flowing phlegm" 流痰 / 596
fluid 津 / 58
fluid collapse 津脱 / 81，550
fluid collapse syndrome/pattern 液脱证 / 187
fluid consumption syndrome/pattern 津伤证 / 187
fluid deficiency syndrome/pattern 津液亏损证，津液亏虚证 / 187
fluid depletion with blood dryness 津亏血燥 / 81
fluid depletion with exuberant fire 津亏火炽 / 81
fluid depletion with retained heat 津亏热结 / 81
fluid exhaustion 亡津液 / 81
fluid exhaustion with intestinal dryness 津枯肠燥 / 90
fluid inadequacy syndrome/pattern 津亏证 / 187
fluid insufficiency of visceral organs 脏腑津亏 / 81
fluid *qi* 津气 / 54
fluid-*qi* deficiency syndrome/pattern 津气亏虚证 / 187
fluid retention 饮，水饮 / 527
fluid retention syndrome/pattern 饮证 / 188，528
flushing phlegm away 涤痰 / 259
flusteredness 心慌 / 151
fly-wing-like shadow 蝇翅黑花 / 620
"flying door" 飞门 / 39
flying fly shadow 蝇影飞越 / 620
fog floating before the eye 云雾移睛 / 620
Folium Apocyni Veneti 罗布麻叶 / 305
Folium Artemisiae Argyi 艾叶 / 318
Folium Eriobotryae 枇杷叶 / 301
Folium et Flos Wikstroemiae Chamaedaphnis 黄芫花 / 324
Folium et Ramulus Cotini 黄栌 / 309
Folium Isatidis 大青叶 / 311
Folium Liriodendra Tracheotomy 臭梧桐叶 / 316
Folium Mori 桑叶 / 297
Folium Nelumbinis 荷叶 / 320
Folium Perillae 紫苏叶 / 296
Folium Polygoni Tinctorii 蓼大青叶 / 311
Folium Pyrrosiae 石韦 / 323
Folium Rhododendri Daurici 满山红 / 302
Folium Sennae 番泻叶 / 352
folk recipe/formula 土方 / 357
folk treatment 土法 / 357
follicular conjunctivitis 粟疮 / 613
following one's own breathing 随息 / 498
fontanel 囟，囟门 / 42
food and drink 水谷 / 53
food damage 伤食 / 543
food damage syndrome 伤食证 / 543
food damage vomiting 伤食吐 / 587
food-denial dysentery 噤口痢 / 522
food essence 水谷精微，水谷之精 / 57
food-induced epilepsy 食痫 / 589
food partiality 嗜偏食 / 544
food *qi* 谷气 / 53
food-restricting exercise 辟谷功 / 503
food retention 停食，宿食，食积 / 543，544，582
food-retention abdominal pain 食积腹痛 / 546，588
food-retention night sweating 食积盗汗 / 586
food retention syndrome/pattern 食积证 / 199
food retention with chills and fever 食积寒热 / 583
food-retention vomiting 积吐 / 587
food stagnation 食滞 / 543
food taboo 忌口 / 284
foot acupuncture 足针 / 478
foot acupuncture therapy 足针疗法 / 478
forceful lifting and light thrusting 重提轻插 / 457
forceful thrusting and light lifting 重插轻提 / 456
forehead 额 / 43
forehead corner 额角 / 43
foreign body entering the eye 异物入目 / 621
forgetfulness 健忘，善忘 / 146，535
form of the tongue 舌形 / 132

formula 方剂 / 356
formulae in rhyme 汤头歌 / 358
Formulary of the Bureau of People's Welfare Pharmacy 太平惠民和剂局方 / 691
Formulary of the Bureau of Pharmacy 和剂局方 / 691
Fortune Eupatorium Herb 佩兰 / 319
Fortune's Drynaria Rhizome 骨碎补 / 347
foulage 搓法 / 647
four examinations 四诊 / 123
Four-Medicinal Decoction 四物汤 / 371
Four-miracle Pill 四神丸 / 374
four natures 四气 / 279
four properties 四性 / 279
four reservoirs 四海 / 25
four seas 四海 / 25
Fourleaf Ladybell Root 南沙参 / 300
Fourstamen Stephania Root 防己 / 317
fourteen categories of formulae 十四剂 / 360
fourteen meridians/channels 十四经 / 400
foxy odor 狐臭 / 605
fracture 骨折 / 635
fracture from a fall 踠跌 / 635
fracture of the nose bridge 鼻梁骨折 / 628
fracture with broken tendon 折骨绝筋 / 635
fracture with split skin 折骨列肤 / 635
Fragrant Solomonseal Rhizome 玉竹 / 343
Franchet Groundcherry Fruit 锦灯笼 / 313
Frankincense 乳香 / 334
freckle 雀斑 / 601
freeing milk flow 通乳 / 268
freeing *qi* 通气 / 252
frenetic stirring of the ministerial fire 相火妄动 / 112
frequent nictitation 目连劄 / 614
frequent sighing 善太息 / 141
frequent urination 尿频，小便频数 / 150
Fresh Ginger 生姜 / 295
fresh nebula 新翳 / 612
fright 惊 / 70
fright epilepsy 惊痫 / 535，589
fright (infantile) malnutrition 惊疳 / 581
fright palpitations 惊悸 / 530
fright seizure 客忤 / 577
fright vomiting 惊吐 / 587
Fritillary-Loquat Syrup 川贝枇杷糖浆 / 382
frons 额颅 / 43
frostbite 冻疮，冻风 / 605，606
frosting 制霜 / 278
frothy sputum 痰如泡沫 / 137
Fructus Amomi Rotundus 豆蔻 / 319
Fructus Amomi 砂仁 / 319
Fructus Arctii 牛蒡子 / 297
Fructus Aristolochiae 马兜铃 / 303
Fructus Aurantii Immaturus 枳实 / 325
Fructus Aurantii 枳壳 / 325
Fructus Bruceae 鸦胆子 / 308
Fructus Canarii 青果 / 313
Fructus Cannabis 火麻仁 / 352
Fructus Carotae 南鹤虱 / 354
Fructus Carpesii 鹤虱 / 353
Fructus Chaenomelis 木瓜 / 314
Fructus Chebulae 诃子 / 349
Fructus Citri Sarcodactylis 佛手 / 326
Fructus Citri 香橼 / 326
Fructus Cnidii 蛇床子 / 355
Fructus Corni 山茱萸 / 343
Fructus Crataegi 山楂 / 351
Fructus Crataegi Preparatus 焦山楂 / 351
Fructus Evodiae 吴茱萸 / 318
Fructus Foeniculi 小茴香 / 318
Fructus Forsythiae 连翘 / 310
Fructus Gardeniae 栀子 / 310
Fructus Hippophae 沙棘 / 301
Fructus Hordei Germinatus 麦芽 / 351
Fructus Hordei Germinatus Preparatus 焦麦芽 / 351
Fructus Jujubae 大枣 / 341
Fructus Kochiae 地肤子 / 322
Fructus Leonuri 茺蔚子 / 334
Fructus Ligustri Lucidi 女贞子 / 344
Fructus Liquidambaris 路路通 / 323
Fructus Litseae 荜澄茄 / 318
Fructus Lycii 枸杞子 / 343
Fructus Malvae 冬葵果 / 322
Fructus Momordicae 罗汉果 / 301
Fructus Mori 桑椹 / 345
Fructus Mume 乌梅 / 349
Fructus Oryzae Germinatus 稻芽 / 351
Fructus Perillae 紫苏子 / 303
Fructus Piperis Longi 荜拨 / 319
Fructus Piperis 胡椒 / 318
Fructus Polygoni Orientalis 水红花子 / 332
Fructus Psoraleae 补骨脂 / 347
Fructus Quisqualis 使君子 / 353
Fructus Rosae Laevigatae 金樱子 / 351

Fructus Rubi 覆盆子 / 351
Fructus Schisandrae 五味子 / 350
Fructus Setariae Germinatus 谷芽 / 351
Fructus Sophorae 槐角 / 329
Fructus Toosendan 川楝子 / 328
Fructus Tribuli 蒺藜 / 339
Fructus Trichosanthis 瓜蒌 / 299
Fructus Tritici Levis 浮小麦 / 348
Fructus Tsaoko 草果 / 320
Fructus Viticis 蔓荆子 / 297
Fructus Xanthii 苍耳子 / 296
fu organ 腑 / 20
fu organ for water communication 中渎之腑 / 27
fu organ of conveyance 传导之腑 / 27
fu-organ *qi* 腑气 / 54
fu (-organ) stroke 中腑 / 537
fu-organ syndrome/pattern 腑证 / 178
fu organ with clear juice 中清之腑 / 27
fu organ with refined juice 中精之腑 / 27
fu organs of conveyance and transformation 传化之腑 / 26
Fu Qing Zhu Nü Ke 傅青主女科 / 695
Fu Qingzhu 傅青主 / 674
Fu Qingzhu's Obstetrics and Gynecology 傅青主女科 / 695
Fu Ren Da Quan Liang Fang 妇人大全良方 / 695
Fu Ren Liang Fang 妇人良方 / 695
Fu Renyu 傅仁宇 / 673
Fu Shan 傅山 / 674
Fu Yunke 傅允科 / 673
Fu'ai (SP 16) 腹哀 / 416
Fubai (GB 10) 浮白 / 429
Fufang Chuanbeijing Tablets 复方川贝精片 / 382
Fufang Danshen Tablets 复方丹参片 / 393
Fufen (BL 41) 附分 / 421
Fujie (SP 14) 腹结 / 415
Fuke Shiwei Tablets 妇科十味片 / 395
Fuliu (KI 7) 复溜 / 424
fullness below the heart 心下满 / 156
fulminant conjunctivitis 暴发火眼 / 616
fulminant diarrhea (disease) 暴泻（病） / 545
fulminant epilepsy 暴痫 / 589
fulminant jaundice 急黄 / 523
fulminant red eye with nebula formation 暴赤生翳 / 616
fuming and steaming 熏蒸 / 272
fuming-washing therapy 熏洗疗法 / 274
functional training 练功 / 653
Funneled Physochlaina Root 华山参 / 304
furuncle 疖 / 591
furunculosis 疖病 / 592
Fushe (SP 13) 府舍 / 415
Futonggu (KI 20) 腹通谷 / 425
Futu (LI 18) 扶突 / 411
Futu (ST 32) 伏兔 / 413
Fuxi (BL 38) 浮郄 / 421
Fuyang (BL 59) 跗阳 / 423
Fuzi Lizhong Pills 附子理中丸 / 387

G

Gadfly 虻虫 / 333
galactorrhea 乳汁自出，乳溢 / 573
Galla Chinensis 五倍子 / 348
gallbladder cough 胆咳 / 525
gallbladder distension 胆胀（病） / 547
gallbladder fire syndrome/pattern 胆火证 / 212
gallbladder heat 胆热 / 104
gallbladder heat syndrome/pattern 胆热证 / 211
gallbladder insufficiency with timidity 胆虚气怯 / 104
gallbladder meridian/channel (GB) 足少阳胆经 / 404
gallbladder meridian/channel of foot lesser yang 足少阳胆经 / 404
gallbladder *qi* 胆气 / 55
gallbladder *qi* deficiency 胆气虚 / 104
gallbladder *qi* deficiency syndrome/pattern 胆气虚证 / 211
gallbladder 胆 / 23
galvano-acupuncture 电针 / 470
Gambir Plant 钩藤 / 338
Gan Mai Dazao Decoction 甘麦大枣汤 / 381
gangrene of the extremities 脱骨疽 / 595
Ganmao Qingre Granules 感冒清热冲剂 / 381
Ganmao Tuire Granules 感冒退热冲剂 / 381
Ganoderma Lucidum 灵芝 / 337
Ganshu (BL 18) 肝俞 / 420
Gao Meigu 高梅孤 / 671
Gao Wu 高武 / 671
Gaohuang (BL 43) 膏肓 / 422
Garden Burnet Root 地榆 / 329
gargling 含漱 / 273
gargling with saliva 漱津 / 506
garlic-interposed moxibustion 隔

蒜灸 / 466
gas gangrene 烂疔 / 592
gastric upset 嘈杂 / 153，543
Gastrodia Pills 天麻丸 / 393
Gastrodia Tuber 天麻 / 338
Gastrodia-Uncaria Decoction 天麻钩藤饮 / 378
Ge Hong 葛洪 / 659
Ge Kejiu 葛可久 / 667
Ge Qiansun 葛乾孙 / 667
Ge Zhi Yu Lun 格致余论 / 701
Ge Zhichuan 葛稚川 / 660
Gecko 蛤蚧 / 348
Gegen Huangqin Huanglian Decoction 葛根黄芩黄连汤 / 367
Geguan (BL 46) 膈关 / 422
Gemma Agrimoniae 鹤草芽 / 354
general aching during menstruation 经行身痛 / 562
General Discussion of Cold Damage Diseases 伤寒总病论 / 685
generalized fever 身热 / 143
generalized itching 身痒 / 147
generalized pain 身痛 / 147
generation among the five elements/phases 五行相生 / 11
Generation and Resolution Decoction 生化汤 / 376
generation and transformation 生化 / 2
generation of cold from the interior 寒从中生 / 91
Gengnian'an Tablets 更年安 / 395
genital pain 阴器痛 / 147
genital sweating 阴汗 / 145
Gentian Liver-purging Decoction 龙胆泻肝汤 / 368
gentle moxibustion 温和灸 / 464
genuine fire 真火 / 23
genuine origin insufficiency syndrome/pattern 真元亏虚证 / 212
genuine *qi* 真气 / 53，500
genuine water 真水 / 22
genuine yang 真阳 / 23
genuine yin 真阴 / 22
genuine yin insufficiency 真阴不足 / 112
geo-authentic materia medica 道地药材 / 275
geographic tongue 地图舌 / 579
Germinated Barley 麦芽 / 351
Geshu (BL 17) 膈俞 / 420
getting rid of mental distractions 排除杂念 / 499
ghost gate 鬼门 / 42
Giant Knotweed Rhizome 虎杖 / 309
Giant Typhonium Tuber 白附子 / 299
ginger-interposed moxibustion 隔姜灸 / 465
gingival abscess 牙痈 / 633
gingival eruption 马牙 / 579
gingival recession 齿龈宣露，食床，牙宣 / 633
Ginkgo Seed 白果 / 301
Ginseng 人参 / 340
Ginseng-Aconite Injection 参附注射液 / 391
Ginseng-Antler Life-preserving Pills 参茸卫生丸 / 391
Ginseng-Antler Restorative Tablets 参茸固本片 / 391
Ginseng Nutritive Pills 人参养荣丸 / 391
Ginseng-Perilla Decoction 参苏饮 / 363
Ginseng-Poria-Atractylodes Pills 参苓白术丸 / 388
Ginseng-Poria-Atractylodes Powder 参苓白术散 / 371
Ginseng Restorative Pills 人参再造丸 / 391
Ginseng Spleen-strengthening Pills 人参健脾丸 / 388
glabella 眉心 / 43
Glabrous Greenbrier Rhizome 土茯苓 / 309
glass cup 玻璃罐 / 467
Glauber's Salt 芒硝 / 352
glide cupping 推罐 / 469
globus hystericus 梅核气 / 631
Glory Bower Leaf 臭梧桐叶 / 316
Glossy Privet Fruit 女贞子 / 344
glue 胶 / 282
gluteal abscess 臀痈 / 594
goiter 瘿 / 597
goiter with varicose veins 筋瘿 / 597
Golden Larch Bark 土荆皮 / 355
Golden Mirror of Medicine 医宗金鉴 / 705
Golden Powder for Alleviation 如意金黄散 / 396
Golden Thread 黄连 / 307
Golden-chamber Kidney *Qi* pill 金匮肾气丸 / 373
Golden-lock Semen-securing Pill 金锁固精丸 / 374
Gong Qingxuan 龚庆宣 / 660
Gong Tingxian 龚廷贤 / 672
Gong Yunlin 龚云林 / 672
Gongsun (SP 4) 公孙 / 415
gonorrhea 淋病 / 551
Gordon Euryale Seed 芡实 / 349
governor vessel (GV) 督脉 / 405
gradual reduction 慢性复位 / 642
Grand Torreya Seed 榧子 / 353

granular intradermal needle 颗粒型皮内针 / 450
granular pharyngitis 帘珠喉痹 / 629
granules 颗粒剂 / 282
grasping 拿法 / 483
grasping and pinching 拿捏法 / 483
grasping *Hegu* (LI 4) 拿合谷 / 489
grasping manipulation 拿法 / 651
grasping the feet with both hands 双手攀足式 / 653
grasping the neck 拿颈项 / 488
grasping with the whole hand 抓法 / 483
Grass-leaved Sweetflag Rhizome 石菖蒲 / 335
gravid aphonia 子喑 / 568
gravid edema 子肿 / 568
gravid oppression 子悬 / 567
gravidic cough 子嗽 / 568
gravidic stranguria 子淋 / 567
gravidic vertigo 子晕 / 566
gravidic vexation 子烦 / 567
gravidity 重身 / 564
gray (tongue) coating/fur 灰苔 / 135
greasy (tongue) coating/fur 腻苔 / 135
great collateral vessel of the spleen 脾之大络 / 407
Great Compendium of Acupuncture and Moxibustion 针灸大成 / 699
great dripping sweating 大汗淋漓 / 144
greater yang blood accumulation syndrome/pattern 太阳蓄血证 / 176
greater yang cold damage syndrome/pattern 太阳伤寒证 / 175
greater yang cold damage 太阳伤寒 / 176
greater yang disease 太阳病 / 175
greater yang disease pattern 太阳病证 / 175
greater yang *fu*-organ disease 太阳腑病 / 176
greater yang *fu*-organ syndrome/pattern 太阳腑证 / 176
greater yang meridian/channel disease 太阳经病 / 175
greater yang meridian/channel syndrome/pattern 太阳经证 / 175
greater yang syndrome 太阳病证 / 175
greater yang water accumulation syndrome/pattern 太阳蓄水证 / 176
greater yang wind attack 太阳中风 / 175
greater yang wind attack syndrome/pattern 太阳中风证 / 175
greater yin disease 太阴病 / 177
greater yin disease pattern/syndrome 太阴病证 / 177
Green Tangerine Peel 青皮 / 325
greenish glaucoma 绿风内障，绿风 / 619，620
grinding of teeth 龂齿 / 632
Grosvenor Momordica Fruit 罗汉果 / 301
Ground Beetle 䗪虫 / 333
ground garlic moxibustion 蒜泥灸 / 466
growth fever 变蒸 / 583
Gryllotalpa 蝼蛄 / 323
Gu Jin Tu Shu Ji Cheng Yi Bu Quan Lu 古今图书集成医部全录 / 704
Gu Jin Yi An An 古今医案按 / 702
Gu Jin Yi Tong 古今医统 / 703
Gu Jin Yi Tong Da Quan 古今医统大全 / 703
Gualou Xiebai Banxia Decoction 瓜蒌薤白半夏汤 / 375
Guanchong (TE 1) 关冲 / 426
Guangming (GB 37) 光明 / 431
Guanmen (ST 22) 关门 / 413
Guanxin Suhe Pills 冠心苏合丸 / 393
Guanyuan (CV 4) 关元 / 435
Guanyuanshu (BL 26) 关元俞 / 420
guest circuit 客运 / 18
guest *qi* 客气 / 18
Gui Lu Erxian Glue 龟鹿二仙胶 / 373
guide ingredient 使药 / 358
Guifu Dihuang Pills 桂附地黄丸 / 390
Guilai (ST 29) 归来 / 413
Guilingji Capsules 龟龄集 / 390
Guipi Decoction 归脾汤 / 372
Guizhi Decoction 桂枝汤 / 361
Gujing Pill 固精丸 / 374
gum bleeding 齿衄 / 550
gum 龈 / 39
gum (in the eyes) 眵 / 610
Guogong Wine 国公酒 / 393
gynecomastia 乳疬 / 597
Gypsum Fibrosum 石膏 / 304
Gypsum 石膏 / 304

H

habitual abortion 滑胎 / 569
Haematitum 赭石 / 339
Haiquan (EX-HN 11) 海泉 / 440
hairline 发际 / 42

hairline boil 发际疮 / 592
Hairvein Agrimonia Herb 仙鹤草 / 328
Hairy Deer-horn 鹿茸 / 345
half needling 半刺 / 459
half-exterior half-interior 半表半里 / 83
half-exterior half-interior syndrome/pattern 半表半里证 / 171
half-squatting walking 矮步 / 496
halitosis 口臭 / 142
Halloysitum Rubrum 赤石脂 / 349
hammering 捶法 / 485
hammering the lower back 捶腰背 / 489
Han Mao 韩懋 / 668
Han Shi Yi Tong 韩氏医通 / 701
Han's General Medicine 韩氏医通 / 701
hand acupuncture 手针 / 478
hand acupuncture therapy 手针疗法 / 478
hand bones 手骨 / 47
hand-holding needle insertion 夹持进针法 / 453
handle-flicking method 弹柄法 / 455
handle of the needle 针柄 / 449
handle-scrapng method 刮柄法 / 455
handle-twisting method 搓柄法 / 455
handle-waggling method 摇柄法 / 455
hand-pressing postural stake-standing exercise 下按式站桩功 / 502
Hanyan (GB 4) 颔厌 / 428
Hao Qin Qingdan Decoction 蒿芩清胆汤 / 365
hard mass in the abdomen 腹中硬块 / 154
hard *qigong* 硬气功 / 492
hardness of hearing 重听 / 624
harelip 兔唇 / 590
harmonizing blood to extinguish wind 和血熄风 / 239
harmonizing blood to prevent abortion 和血安胎 / 239
harmonizing blood to regulate menstruation 和血调经 / 239
harmonizing blood to relieve pain 和血止痛 / 239
harmonizing formula 和解剂 / 365
harmonizing lesser yang meridian/channel 和解少阳 / 238
harmonizing method 和法，和解法 / 238
harmonizing *qi* and blood 调和气血 / 239
harmonizing *shaoyang* meridian/channel 和解少阳 / 238
harmonizing the exterior and interior 和解表里 / 238
harmonizing the liver and spleen 调和肝脾 / 239
harmonizing the liver and stomach 调和肝胃 / 239
harmonizing the middle 和中 / 238
harmonizing the nutrient 和营 / 239
harmonizing the nutrient and activating blood 和营活血 / 240
harmonizing the nutrient and defense 调和营卫 / 229
harmonizing the nutrient to promote regeneration 和营生新 / 240
harmonizing the nutrient to relieve pain 和营止痛 / 240
harmonizing the spleen and stomach 调和脾胃 / 238
harmonizing the stomach 和胃 / 238
harmony between physique and spirit 形与神俱 / 3
harmony in the mouth 口中和 / 154
Hawksbill Shell 玳瑁 / 339
Hawthorn Fruit 山楂 / 351
He Bingyuan 何炳元 / 680
He Ji Ju Fang 和剂局方 / 691
He Lianchen 何廉臣 / 681
He Mengyao 何梦瑶 / 676
He Xichi 何西池 / 677
head erysipelas 抱头火丹 / 594
head upright 头正 / 493
head wind 头风 / 146，533
headache 头痛 / 146，533
headache and painful stiff neck 头项强痛 / 146
headache during menstruation 经行头痛 / 562
Head-clearing Pills 脑立清 / 385
headed phlegmon 有头疽 / 594
head-face exercise 头面功 / 500
healing stone 砭石 / 451
health-ball massage 保健球按摩 / 490
health-preserving exercise 保健功 / 505
Health-restoring Agastache Powder 藿香正气散 / 379
healthy *qi* 正气 / 54
healthy-*qi*-reinforcing exterior-releasing formula 扶正解表剂 / 363
heart 心 / 20

heart atrophy-flaccidity 心痿 / 539
heart blood 心血 / 21
heart blood deficiency 心血虚 / 99
heart blood deficiency insomnia 心血虚不得卧 / 535
heart blood deficiency syndrome/pattern 心血（亏）虚证 / 200
heart blood stasis (and obstruction) 心血瘀阻 / 99
heart blood stasis syndrome/pattern 心血瘀阻证 / 200
heart consumption 心劳 / 529
heart cough 心咳 / 524
heart deficiency 心虚 / 99
heart edema / 549
heart fire flaming upward 心火上炎 / 101
heart fire 心火 / 21
heart impediment 心痹 / 541
heart (infantile) malnutrition 心疳 / 581
heart insufficiency amenorrhea 心虚经闭 / 559
heart-kidney interaction 心肾相交 / 27
heart-kidney non-interaction syndrome/pattern 心肾不交证 / 202
heart-kidney non-interaction 心肾不交 / 101
heart meridian/channel (HT) 手少阴心经 / 402
heart meridian/channel cough 心经咳嗽 / 524
heart meridian/channel of hand lesser yin 手少阴心经 / 402
heart-nourishing tranquilizer 养心安神药 / 293
heart-nourishing tranquilizing medicinal/drug 养心安神药 / 293
heart pain 心痛 / 530
heart pain with cold limbs 厥心痛 / 530
heart *qi* 心气 / 21，54
heart *qi* deficiency insomnia 心气虚不得卧 / 535
heart *qi* deficiency syndrome/pattern 心气（亏）虚证 / 200
heart *qi* deficiency 心气虚 / 99
heart *qi* insufficiency 心气不足 / 99
heart-regulation exercise 理心功 / 501
heart shifting heat to the small intestine 心移热于小肠 / 101
Heart-tonifying Tranquilizing Pills 安神补心丸 / 385
heart vessel obstruction syndrome/pattern 心脉痹阻证 / 201
heart yang 心阳 / 21
heart yang deficiency 心阳虚 / 100
heart yang deficiency syndrome/pattern 心阳（亏）虚证 / 200
heart yang collapse syndrome/pattern 心阳虚脱证 / 200
heart yin 心阴 / 21
heart yin deficiency 心阴虚 / 99
heart yin deficiency syndrome/pattern 心阴（亏）虚证 / 201
heartburn 烧心 / 153
Heartleaf Houttuynia Herb 鱼腥草 / 311
heat 热 / 66
heat accumulation 热结 / 87
heat accumulation in the interior 热邪内结 / 87
heat accumulation in the lower energizer 热结下焦 / 87
heat accumulation (retention) in the bladder 热积［结］膀胱 / 113
heat accumulation with intestinal dryness 热结肠燥 / 110
heat arthralgia 热痹 / 540
heat-clearing and blood-cooling medicinal/drug 清热凉血药 / 288
heat-clearing and dampness-drying medicinal/drug 清热燥湿药 / 288
heat-clearing and fire-purging medicinal/drug 清热泻火药 / 288
heat-clearing and toxicity-relieving medicinal/drug 清热解毒药 / 288
heat-clearing dampness-dispelling formula 清热祛湿剂 / 379
heat-clearing formula 清热剂 / 367
heat-clearing medicinal/drug 清热药 / 288
heat-clearing method 清法 / 230
heat-clearing therapy 清热法 / 230
heat-clearing toxin-counteracting formula 清热解毒剂 / 368
heat choleraic turmoil 热霍乱 / 523
heat constipation 热秘 / 544
heat dacryorrhea 热泪 / 615
heat damaging lung vessels 热伤肺络 / 110
heat damaging muscles and sinews/tendons 热伤筋脉 / 88
heat damaging the mind 热伤神明 / 100

heat diarrhea 热泻 / 545
heat distressing the large intestine 热迫大肠 / 86
heat enabling frenetic movement of blood 血热妄行 / 95
heat entering nutrient-blood 热入营血 / 87
heat entering the blood aspect 热入血分 / 87
heat entering the blood chamber 热入血室 / 87
heat entering the pericardium 热入心包 / 86
heat epilepsy 热痫 / 590
heat filthy attack 热痧 / 583
heat hiding in the thoroughfare and conception vessels 热伏冲任 / 87
heat impediment 热痹 / 540
heat in both the exterior and interior 表里俱热 / 83
heat in the stomach 胃中热 / 108
heat miasmic malaria 热瘴 / 521
heat pathogen 热邪 / 67
heat pathogen obstructing the lung 热邪阻肺 / 86
heat phlegm 热痰 / 528
heat-phlegm syndrome/pattern 热痰证 / 189
heat scorching kidney yin 热灼肾阴 / 88
heat sore 热疮 / 600
heat stranguria 热淋 / 552
heat syncope 热厥 / 538
heat syndrome of the gravida 胎热 / 568
heat syndrome/pattern 热证 / 169
heat toxin 热毒 / 68
heat toxin in the blood aspect 血分热毒 / 87
heat toxin syndrome/pattern 热毒证 / 198
heat transformation 热化 / 92
heat transformation of lesser yin 少阴热化 / 116
heat transformation syndrome/pattern of lesser yin 少阴热化证 / 177
heat vomiting 热呕，热吐 / 542，586
heat wheezing 热哮 / 527
heating for the hot 热因热用 / 221
heatstroke 中暑 / 517
heatstroke dizziness 中暑眩晕 / 533
heatstroke vertigo 中暑眩晕 / 533
heavenly circuit exercise 周天功 / 501
heavenly circuit 周天 / 500
heavenly stems 天干 / 18
heavy body 身重 / 147
heavy breathing 呼吸气粗 / 140
heavy formula 大方，重剂 / 357，360
heavy head and light feet 头重脚轻 / 146
heavy-headedness 头重 / 146
heavy pain 重痛 / 148
heavy reinforcing-reducing method 大补大泻法 / 458
Heche Dazao Pills 河车大造丸 / 389
Heding (EX-LE 2) 鹤顶 / 443
heel 踵 / 50
heel pain 足跟痛 / 147
Hegu (LI 4) 合谷 / 410
Heliao (LI 19) 禾髎 / 411
Heliao (TE 22) 和髎 / 428
helix 耳轮 / 45，472
helix cauda 耳轮尾 / 472
helix crus 耳轮脚 / 472
helix notch 轮屏切迹 / 473
helix tubercle 耳轮结节 / 472
helminthic amenorrhea 虫积经闭 / 559
hemangioma 血瘤 / 598
hematemesis 呕血，吐血 / 152，550
hematemesis and epistaxis during menstruation 经行吐衄 / 562
hematemesis during menstruation 经行吐血 / 562
Hematite 赭石 / 339
hematochezia 便血 / 550
hematuria 尿血，溲血 / 151，550
hemihidrosis 半身汗出 / 145
hemilateral anhidrosis 半身无汗 / 145
hemilateral head wind 偏头风 / 146，533
hemilateral headache 偏头痛 / 146，533
hemilateral sagging 偏坠 / 600
hemiplegia 半身不遂，偏枯 / 537
hemiplegia with wry mouth 㖞僻不遂 / 537
hemoptysis with coughing 咳血 / 550
hemoptysis without coughing 咯血 / 550
hemoptysis 咯血 / 137
hemorrhage 失血 / 549
hemorrhagic syndrome 血证 / 549
hemorrhoid 痔 / 598
hemospermia 血精 / 552
hemostasis 止血 / 257
hemostatic (medicinal/drug) 止血药 / 291
Hemp Seed 火麻仁 / 352

Hemp-seed Pill 麻子仁丸 / 365
Henbane Seed 天仙子 / 303
Henggu (KI 11) 横骨 / 424
Herba Abri 鸡骨草 / 308
Herba Agastachis 藿香 / 319
Herba Agrimoniae 仙鹤草 / 328
Herba Andrographitis 穿心莲 / 312
Herba Artemisiae Annuae 青蒿 / 307
Herba Artemisiae Scopariae 茵陈 / 309
Herba Asari 细辛 / 296
Herba Capsellae 荠菜 / 329
Herba Centipedae 鹅不食草 / 296
Herba Cirsii 小蓟 / 328
Herba Cistanchis 肉苁蓉 / 346
Herba Commelinae 鸭跖草 / 312
Herba Cymbopogonis 芸香草 / 304
Herba Cynomorii 锁阳 / 346
Herba Dendrobii 石斛 / 343
Herba Dianthi 瞿麦 / 322
Herba Ecliptae 墨旱莲 / 330
Herba Elshotziae 香薷 / 296
Herba Ephedrae 麻黄 / 295
Herba Epimedii 淫羊藿 / 346
Herba Equiseti Hiemalis 木贼 / 305
Herba Erodii seu Geranii 老鹳草 / 316
Herba Eupatorii 佩兰 / 319
Herba Euphorbiae Humifusae 地锦草 / 309
Herba Houttuyniae 鱼腥草 / 311
Herba Humuli Scandentis 葎草 / 313
Herba Inulae 金沸草 / 299
Herba Leonuri 益母草 / 334
Herba Lobeliae Chinensis 半边莲 / 312
Herba Lophatheri 淡竹叶 / 305
Herba Lycopi 泽兰 / 334
Herba Lycopodii 伸筋草 / 316
Herba Lysimachiae 金钱草 / 322
Herba Menthae 薄荷 / 297
Herba Oldenlandiae 白花蛇舌草 / 312
Herba Orostachyos 瓦松 / 330
Herba Patriniae 败酱草 / 312
Herba Plantaginis 车前草 / 320
Herba Pogostemonis 广藿香 / 319
Herba Polygoni Avicularis 萹蓄 / 322
Herba Portulacae 马齿苋 / 309
Herba Potentillae Discoloris 翻白草 / 310
Herba Pyrolae 鹿衔草 / 345
Herba Schizonepetae Carbonisata 荆芥炭 / 296
Herba Schizonepetae 荆芥 / 295
Herba Scutellariae Barbatae 半枝莲 / 312
Herba Sedi 垂盆草 / 309
Herba Selaginellae 卷柏 / 332
Herba seu Radix Cirsii Japonici 大蓟 / 328
Herba Siegesbeckiae 豨莶草 / 314
Herba Solani Nigri 龙葵 / 312
Herba Spirodelae 浮萍 / 298
Herba Taraxaci 蒲公英 / 311
Herba Verbenae 马鞭草 / 334
Herba Violae 紫花地丁 / 311
herbal drugs 草药 / 275
herbal medicinals 草药 / 275
hernia 疝，疝气，小肠气 / 554
Heron's Bill or Wilford Ganesbill Herb 老鹳草 / 316
herpes febrilis 热疮 / 600
herpes zoster 蛇串疮 / 600
Heterophylly Falsestarwort Root 太子参 / 340
Heyang (BL 55) 合阳 / 422
hiccough 呃逆 / 153，543
hiccup 哕 /153，543
hidden pulse 伏脉 / 160
high fever 壮热 / 143
high-low pad 高低垫 / 641
Himalayan Teasel Root 续断 / 347
hipbone 髁骨，胯骨，髋骨 / 51
Hippocampus 海马 / 348
hircismus 腋臭 / 605
Hirudo 水蛭 / 333
hitting with the knuckle 笃击法 / 481
hives 隐（瘾）疹 / 603
hives during menstruation 经行风疹块 / 563
hives during menstruation 经行瘖 / 563
hoarseness 声嗄，嘶嗄 / 140
Hogfennel Root 前胡 / 300
hold-carrying 端法 / 639
holding a rope and standing on a pile of bricks 攀索叠砖 / 642
holding tight 扼法 / 484
holding，lifting，and restoring to the right location 端提捺正 / 639
hollow pulse 芤脉 / 162
Holy Benevolent Prescriptions 圣惠方 / 691
Honey 蜂蜜 / 352
honeyed pill 蜜丸 / 280
Honeysuckle Flower 金银花 / 310
Honeysuckle Stem 忍冬藤 / 310
hordeolum 针眼，偷针，土疳，土疡 / 612，613
horizontal insertion 平刺 / 454

horseman's stance 骑马式 / 495
horse-spleen wind 马脾风 / 586
hot-compress medicinal 熨药 / 642
hot compression 热罨 / 272
hot compression with rubbing 熨法 / 272
hot sweats 热汗 / 144
Houding (GV 19) 后顶 / 434
hour-prescription of points 纳支法，纳子法 / 459，459
house of blood 血之府 / 25
house of intelligence 精明之府 / 42
house of marrow 髓之府 / 25
house of sinews/tendons 筋之府 / 50
house of the kidney 肾之府 / 27
house of the original spirit 元神之府 / 25
Houxi (SI 3) 后溪 / 417
Hu Sihui 忽思慧 / 667
Hua Boren 滑伯仁 / 667
Hua Fu 华旉 / 659
Hua Shou 滑寿 / 667
Hua Tuo 华佗 / 659
Huagai (CV 20) 华盖 / 436
Huang Di Nei Jing Ling Shu Jing 黄帝内经灵枢经 / 683
Huang Di Nei Jing Ling Shu Zhu Zheng Fa Wei 黄帝内经灵枢注证发微 / 684
Huang Di Nei Jing 黄帝内经 / 683
Huang Di Nei Jing Su Wen 黄帝内经素问 / 683
Huang Di Nei Jing Su Wen Zhu Zheng Fa Wei 黄帝内经素问注证发微 / 684
Huang Ting Jing 黄庭经 / 700
Huangdi's Internal Classic 黄帝内经 / 683
Huangfu Mi 皇甫谧 / 659
Huangfu Shi'an 皇甫士安 / 659
Huanglian Jiedu Decoction 黄连解毒汤 / 368
Huangmen (BL 51) 肓门 / 422
Huangqi Guizhi Wuwu Decoction 黄芪桂枝五物汤 / 370
Huangshu (KI 16) 肓俞 / 425
Huangtu Decoction 黄土汤 / 377
Huantiao (GB 30) 环跳 / 430
Huaroumen (ST 24) 滑肉门 / 413
Huatuo Zaizao Pills 华佗再造丸 / 394
Huiyang (BL 35) 会阳 / 421
Huiyin (CV 1) 会阴 / 435
Huizong (TE 7) 会宗 / 427
Human Placenta 紫河车 / 342
humeral region 臑 / 47
humerus 臑骨 / 47
humpback 龟背 / 578
Hunmen (BL 47) 魂门 / 422
Huo Luan Lun 霍乱论 / 694
Huoxiang Zhengqi Powder 藿香正气散 / 379
hydatidiform mole 葡萄胎 / 567
hydragogue formula 逐水剂 / 365
hydramnios 子满 / 567
hydro-acupuncture 水针 / 470
hydrocephalus 解颅 / 577
hydrocephalus (disease) 解颅病 / 577
hydrocele 水疝 / 599
hydrogogue therapy 逐水 / 237
hyperactive kidney fire 肾火偏亢 / 111
hyperactivity of liver yang 肝阳亢盛 / 98
hyperemesis gravidarum 妊娠呕吐 / 566
hyperemia of subconjunctival capillaries 赤丝虬脉，白睛虬脉 / 617，618
hyperemia of the bulbar conjunctiva 白睛红赤 / 611
hyperhidrosis 多汗 / 144
hypermenorrhea 月经过多，经水过多，月水过多 / 157，560，561
hyperopia 远视 / 621
hypertrophy of the tonsil 石蛾 / 629
hypochondriac pain 胁痛(病) / 546
hypochondriac pain 胁痛，季胁痛，胁下痛 / 146，547
hypochondriac region 季肋 / 48
hypochondrium 季胁，季肋 / 48
hypogalactia 缺乳 / 572
Hypoglaucous Yam Rhizome 粉萆薢 / 322
hypomenorrhea 月经过少 / 157，558
hypopyon 黄脓上冲，黄膜上冲，黄液上冲 / 618
hysteria 脏躁 / 535

I

icterus neonatorum 胎黄，胎黄病 / 576
ileocecal conjunction 阑门 / 41
illness 疾病 / 122
Illustrated Internal Qigong Exercise 内功图说 / 700
Illustrated Manual of Acupoints on the Bronze Figure 铜人俞穴针灸图经 / 699
Illustrated Supplement to the Classified Classic 类经图翼 / 684

imaginary breathing 意呼吸 / 498
imaginary concentration 存想 / 499
imbalance between cold and heat 寒热失调 / 90
Immature Orange Fruit 枳实 / 325
immature yin-yang 稚阴稚阳 / 574
impacted cerumen 耵耳 / 625
impaired preservation of the mind 心神失养 / 100
impairment of gastric harmony and down-sending 胃失和降 / 108
impediment disease 痹(病) / 540
impetigo 黄水疮 / 604
Important Formula for Painful Diarrhea 痛泻要方 / 366
impotence 阳萎 / 156，552
improper diet and overstrain 饮食劳倦 / 70
improving auditory acuity 聪耳 / 271
improving *qi* reception to relieve asthma 纳气平喘 / 242
improving the appetite 开胃 / 246
improving the eyesight 明目 / 271
improving the hearing 聪耳 / 271
impure *qi* 杂气 / 63
inability to lie flat 不得偃卧 / 141
inability to lift the shoulder and arm 肩不举 / 147
inability to sleep 不得眠，不得卧 / 155，535
inborn fire 先天之火 / 27
incessant discharge of lochia 恶露不止 / 570
"inch opening" 寸口 / 159
inch，bar and cubit 寸、关、尺 / 158
incised wound 金创，金疮，金疡 / 605，635
incision therapy 割治疗法 / 478
incompatibility 相反 / 359
incongruity of pulses with the seasons 脉逆四时 / 164
increasing fluid to induce laxation 增液通下 / 237
Indian Bread 茯苓 / 320
Indian Bread with Pine 茯神 / 337
Indian Madder Root 茜草 / 328
Indian Trumpetflower Seed 木蝴蝶 / 303
indications of the color of the nose 鼻色主病 / 130
indigestion diarrhea 伤食泄泻，伤食泻，食泻 / 545，588
indigestion 食积 / 582
Indigo Naturalis 青黛 / 311
Indigoplant Leaf 蓼大青叶 / 311
indirect moxibustion 间接灸 / 465
individual palpation 单按 / 159
individual's normal complexion 主色 / 124
inducing defecation 导便 / 273
inducing diuresis 利尿，利水 / 260
inducing diuresis to alleviate edema 利水消肿 / 261
inducing diuresis to drain dampness 利水渗湿 / 260
inducing diuresis to expel dampness 利水除湿 / 260
inducing *qi* 导气 / 455
inducing resuscitation 开窍 / 266
inducing resuscitation with aromatics 芳香开窍 / 266
inducing sedation and calming the mind 镇静安神 / 265
inducing sweating to release the exterior 发汗解表 / 225
induction of acupuncture anesthesia 针麻诱导 / 470
infantile asthma 小儿哮喘 / 577
infantile clonic convulsions 婴儿瘛疭 / 575
infantile cold-dampness diarrhea 小儿寒湿泻 / 587
infantile convulsions 惊风 / 574
infantile convulsions with abdominal pain 惊风腹痛 / 576
infantile convulsions with vexing thirst 惊风烦渴 / 576
infantile convulsive disease 惊风病 / 574
infantile convulsive seizure 惊风抽搐 / 575
infantile dampness-heat diarrhea 小儿湿热泻 / 587
infantile diarrhea 小儿泄泻 / 587
infantile dyspepsia 伤乳，乳积 / 577，582
infantile eczema 婴儿湿疮 / 604
infantile fire diarrhea 小儿火泻 / 587
infantile heat diarrhea 小儿热泻 / 587
infantile massotherapy 小儿推拿疗法 / 486
infantile paralysis 小儿麻痹 / 590
infantile slobbering 小儿多涎 / 578
infantile *tuina*-therapy 小儿推拿疗法 / 486
infantile vomiting 小儿呕吐 / 586

inferior auricular root 下耳根 / 473
inferior crus of the antihelix 对耳轮下脚 / 472
inferior-grade medicinal 下品 / 280
infertility 不孕 / 565
infertility due to jealousy 嫉妒不孕 / 565
inflammatory swelling of the eyelid 胞肿如桃 / 614
inflammed eye 火眼 / 616
influenza 时行感冒 / 515
infracardio-supradiaphragmatic space 膏肓 / 42
infrared moxibustion 红外线灸 / 467
infusion granules 冲服剂，冲剂 / 282
ingredient combination in formula/prescription 方剂配伍 / 358
inguinal abscess 胯腹痈 / 593
inhalation 吸入 / 272
inhibited bladder 膀胱不利 / 113
inhibited *qi* transformation 气化不利 / 93
inhibited urination 小便不利 / 151
inhibiting relationship 相恶 / 359
inhibition and generation among the five elements/phases 五行制化 / 12
injury-induced labor 伤产 / 569
innate essence 先天之精 / 57
innate *qi* 先天之气 / 53
inner aspect of the arm 臂内廉 / 47
inner canthus 内眦，目内眦 / 44，608
inner-canthus dacryopyorrhea 大眦脓漏 / 615
inner elixir 内丹 / 498
inner elixir art 内丹术 / 499
inner elixir exercise 内丹功 / 498
inner nourishing exercise 内养功 / 500
inner *qi* 内气 / 500
inner scene 内景 / 493
innominate toxic swelling 无名肿毒 / 594
inquiry 问诊 / 142
inquiry about cold and heat 问寒热 / 142
inquiry about menstruation and leukorrhea 问妇女经带 / 156
inquiry about sleep 问睡眠 / 155
inquiry about stools 问大便 / 149
inquiry about stools and urine 问二便 / 149
inquiry about sweating 问汗 / 144
inquiry about taste in the mouth 问口味 / 154
inquiry about the chest and abdomen 问胸腹 / 151
inquiry about the head and body 问头身 / 146
inquiry about the onset of illness 问起病 / 142
inquiry about the present illness 问现证 / 142
inquiry about thirst and drink 问渴饮 / 148
inquiry about urine 问小便 / 150
insect bite 毒虫咬伤 / 606
insect dermatitis 虫咬皮炎 / 603
insect or animal bite 虫兽伤 / 71
insecurity of bladder *qi* 脬气不固 / 113
insecurity of defense *qi* 卫气不固 / 85
insecurity of exterior *qi* 表气不固 / 85
insecurity of fetus 胎元不固 / 569
insecurity of heart *qi* 心气不固 / 99
insecurity of kidney *qi* 肾气不固 / 112
insecurity of the lower origin 下元不固 / 112
insecurity of the thoroughfare and conception vessels 冲任不固 / 114
insensitivity of the skin 肌肤不仁 / 147
insensitivity 不仁 / 148
insertion method 塞法 / 273
insomnia 失眠 / 155，535
inspection 望诊 / 123
inspection of finger venules 望指纹 / 138
inspection of sputum 望痰 / 137
inspection of the complexion 望色 / 124
inspection of the ear 望耳 / 129
inspection of the eye 望目 / 128
inspection of the nose 望鼻 / 129
inspection of the physique 望形体 / 126
inspection of the posture 望姿态 / 127
inspection of the signal orifices 审苗窍 / 128
inspection of the skin 望皮肤 / 138
inspection of the teeth 望齿 / 137
inspection of the tongue 望舌 / 130
inspection of the white of the eye 白睛色诊 / 129

inspection of vitality 望神 / 123
instep 跗，足跗 / 51
instep edema 跗肿 / 139
Instructions to Coroner 洗冤集录 / 700
insufficiency of both *qi* and blood 气血两亏 / 96
insufficiency of healthy *qi* and excessiveness of pathogenic *qi* 正虚邪实 / 78
insufficiency of heart blood 心血不足 / 99
insufficiency of heart yang 心阳不足 / 100
insufficiency of heart yin 心阴不足 / 100
insufficiency of middle *qi* 中气不足 / 108
insufficiency of vital *qi* 神气不足 / 123
insufflating into the nose 搐鼻 / 273
insufflation into the throat 吹药 / 273
intemperance in sexual life 房事不节 / 71
intense heart-fire syndrome/pattern 心火炽［亢］盛证 / 201
intense lung heat 肺热炽盛 / 102
intense lung heat syndrome/pattern 肺热炽盛证 / 204
intense stomach fire 胃火炽盛 / 108
intense stomach fire syndrome/pattern 胃火炽盛证 / 208
intense stomach heat 胃热壅盛 / 108
intense stomach heat syndrome/pattern 胃热壅盛证 / 208
interior cold 里寒 / 82
interior cold syndrome/pattern 里寒证 / 170
interior deficiency 里虚 / 82
interior deficiency cold syndrome/pattern 里虚寒证 / 170
interior deficiency heat syndrome/pattern 里虚热证 / 171
interior edema 里水 / 549
interior excess 里实 / 82
interior excess syndrome/pattern 里实证 / 171
interior heat 里热 / 82
interior heat syndrome/pattern 里热证 / 170
interior syndrome/pattern 里证 / 169
interior-warming formula 温里剂 / 369
interior-warming medicinal/drug 温里药 / 290
intermediate *qi* 间气 / 18
intermenstrual bleeding 经间期出血 / 560
intermittent dysentery 休息痢 / 522
intermuscular needling 分刺 / 460
internal abscess 内痈 / 593
internal blazing of heart fire 心火内炽 / 101
"internal blowing" 内吹 / 596
"internal blowing" mastitis 内吹乳痈 / 596
internal cause 内因 / 62
Internal Classic 内经 / 683
internal cold 内寒 / 64
internal damage cough 内伤咳嗽 / 526
internal damage fever 内伤发热 / 530
internal damage headache 内伤头痛 / 533
internal damage lumbago 内伤腰痛 / 553
internal dampness 内湿 / 65
internal deflagration of heart fire 心火内焚 / 101
internal dryness 内燥 / 66
internal dryness syndrome/pattern 内燥证 / 197
internal exercise 内功 / 491
internal exercise massage 内功推拿 / 490
internal exercise *tuina* 内功推拿 / 490
internal fixation 内固定 / 642
internal hemorrhoid 内痔 / 599
internal malleolus 合骨，内踝 / 50
internal ophthalmopathy 内障 / 612
internal retention of dampness-heat 湿热内蕴 / 89
internal stirring of liver wind 肝风内动 / 103
internal wind 内风 / 64
interposed moxibustion 隔物灸，间隔灸 / 465
interrupting malaria 截疟 / 271
interstitial keratitis 混睛障 / 618
interstitial striae 腠［凑］理 / 41
intertragic notch 屏间切迹 / 473
interweaving of cold and heat 厥热胜复 / 116
intestinal abscess 肠痈 / 546
intestinal fluid depletion syndrome/pattern 肠燥津亏证 / 187
intestinal impediment 肠痹 / 542
intestinal parasitosis 虫积 / 582
intestinal *qi* colic 盘肠气痛 / 588
intestine-astringing antidiarrheal formula 涩肠固脱剂 / 374

intolerance of cold 畏寒 / 143
intradermal needle 皮内针 / 450
intradermal needle therapy 皮内针疗法 / 450
intramammary abscess 乳疽 / 597
Introduction to Medicine 医学入门 / 703
intruding pathogen 客邪 / 62
Inula Flower 旋覆花 / 299
Inula Herb 金沸草 / 299
Inula-Haematite Decoction 旋复代赭汤 / 376
invalid eyelid 睑废 / 614
inversion 内翻 / 656
inverted menstruation 逆经 / 560
Investigations of Medical Prescriptions 医方考 / 692
invigorating the pulse 通脉 / 241
invigorating the spleen 健脾 / 245
invigorating the spleen and draining dampness 健脾利湿 / 245
invigorating the spleen and harmonizing the stomach 健脾和胃 / 245
invigorating the spleen and inducing diuresis 健脾利水 / 245
invigorating the spleen and nourishing the blood 健脾养血 / 246
invigorating the spleen and replenishing *qi* 健脾益气 / 246
invigorating the spleen and tonifying the lung 健脾补肺 / 246
invigorating the spleen to arrest diarrhea 健脾止泻 / 246
invigorating the spleen to arrest leukorrhea 健脾止带 / 246
invigorating the spleen to dispel dampness 健脾祛湿 / 245
invigorating the spleen to promote digestion 健脾消食 / 245
invigorating the spleen to resolve dampness 健脾化湿 / 245
invigorating the spleen to resolve phlegm 健脾化痰 / 245
invigorating the stomach 健胃 / 246
invigorating the stomach to stop vomiting 健胃止呕 / 246
invigorating yang 壮阳 / 251
invisible phlegm 无形之痰 / 71
inward invasion 内陷 / 94，595
inward invasion of fire 火陷 / 596
inward invasion of measles 麻毒内攻 / 584
inward invasion of sore toxin 疮毒内陷 / 596
inward transmission of exterior heat 表热传里 / 83
inward vision 内视 / 493
iris 虹彩，睛帘 / 609
Iron Mirror of Pediatrics 幼科铁镜 / 696
iron-crotch exercise 铁裆功 / 502
irregular menstrual cycle 月经先后无定期，经行先后无定期 / 157，558
irregular periods 经乱，月经先后无定期，经行先后无定期 / 157，558
irregular rapid pulse 促脉 / 162
irregular recurrent fever 客热 / 583
irregularly intermittent pulse 结脉 / 162
irritation and pain of the bulbar conjunctiva 白睛涩痛 / 611
Isatis Root 板蓝根 / 310
Isatis-root Granules 板蓝根冲剂 / 381
ischuria 癃闭 / 552

J

Jack Bean 刀豆 / 328
Jack-in-the-Pulpit Tuber 天南星 / 298
Jade-screen Liquid 玉屏风口服液 / 383
Jade-screen Powder 玉屏风散 / 371
Japanese Ampelopsis Root 白蔹 / 312
Japanese Climbing-fern Spores 海金沙 / 323
Japanese Pagodatree Pod 槐角 / 329
Japanese Thistle 大蓟 / 328
Japanese Yam 穿山龙 / 316
jaundice 黄疸 / 523
Java Brucea Fruit 鸦胆子 / 308
jaw 颌 / 46
Ji Sheng Fang 济生方 / 691
Ji Yin Gang Mu 济阴纲目 / 695
Jiache (ST 6) 颊车 / 411
Jiaji (EX-B 2) 夹脊 / 441
Jiajian Weirui Decoction 加减葳蕤汤 / 363
Jian Zhen 鉴真 / 661
Jianjing (GB 21) 肩井 / 430
Jianli (CV 11) 建里 / 436
Jianliao (TE 14) 肩髎 / 427
Jianshi (PC 5) 间使 / 426
Jianwaishu (SI 14) 肩外俞 / 418
Jianyu (LI 15) 肩髃 / 410
Jianzhen (SI 9) 肩贞 / 418

Jianzhongshu (SI 15) 肩中俞 / 418
Jiaosun (TE 20) 角孙 / 428
Jiaoxin (KI 8) 交信 / 424
Jiawei Wuyao Decoction 加味乌药汤 / 375
Jiawei Xiaoyao Pills 加味逍遥丸 / 386
Jie Wei Yuan Sou 解围元薮 / 697
Jiexi (ST 41) 解溪 / 414
Jimai (LR 12) 急脉 / 433
Jimen (SP 11) 箕门 / 415
Jin Gui Yao Lue Fang Lun 金匮要略方论 / 686
Jin Gui Yao Lue Xin Dian 金匮要略心典 / 686
Jin Gui Yao Lue 金匮要略 / 686
Jin Gui Yi 金匮翼 / 686
Jinbuhuan Plaster 金不换膏 / 395
Jing Shi Zheng Lei Bei Ji Ben Cao 经史证类备急本草 / 688
Jing Xiao Chan Bao 经效产宝 / 694
Jing Yue Quan Shu 景岳全书 / 704
Jingbailao (EX-HN 15) 颈白劳 / 440
Jingfang Baidu Powder 荆防败毒散 / 363
Jinggu (BL 64) 京骨 / 423
Jingmen (GB 25) 京门 / 430
Jingming (BL 1) 睛明 / 418
Jingqu (LU 8) 经渠 / 409
Jingui Shenqi Pill 金匮肾气丸 / 373
Jinjin (EX-HN 12) 金津 / 440
Jinlingzi Powder 金铃子散 / 375
Jinmen (BL 63) 金门 / 423
Jinsuo (GV 8) 筋缩 / 433
Jinsuo Gujing Pill 金锁固精丸 / 374
Jiquan (HT 1) 极泉 / 416
Jiu Huang Ben Cao 救荒本草 / 688
Jiuwei (CV 15) 鸠尾 / 436
Jiuwei Qianghuo Decoction 九味羌活汤 / 361
Jizhong (GV 6) 脊中 / 433
Job's-tears Seed 薏苡仁 / 321
joined valley needling 合谷刺 / 460
joint 骨解 / 52
joint needling 关刺 / 460
joint reduction 入臼 / 642
joint-running wind 历节风 / 540
joy 喜 / 69
Ju Fang Fa Hui 局方发挥 / 692
Jueyinshu (BL 14) 厥阴俞 / 419
Jugu (LI 16) 巨骨 / 410
Juhong Pills 橘红丸［片］/ 383
Jujube 大枣 / 341
Juliao (GB 29) 居髎 / 430
Juliao (ST 3) 巨髎 / 411
Jupi Zhuru Decoction 橘皮竹茹汤 / 376
Juquan (EX-HN 10) 聚泉 / 440
Juque (CV 14) 巨阙 / 436

K

Kadsura Pepper Stem 海风藤 / 315
Kansui Root 甘遂 / 324
Katsumada Galangal Seed 草豆蔻 / 320
Ke Qin 柯琴 / 675
Ke Yunbo 柯韵伯 / 675
keeping *qi* 守气 / 456
keeping the head upright as if carrying something on the top 头如顶物 / 493
keeping the waist and abdomen relaxed 舒腰松腹 / 494
Kelp or Tangle 昆布 / 300
keratic pannus 血翳包睛 / 619
keratomalacia 疳眼，疳积上目 / 621
Key Link of Medicine 医贯 / 702
Key to the Therapeutics of Children's Diseases 小儿药证直诀 / 696
kidney 肾 / 22
kidney atrophy-flaccidity 肾痿 / 540
kidney consumption 肾劳 / 529
kidney cough 肾咳 / 525
kidney deficiency 肾虚 / 111
kidney deficiency diarrhea 肾虚泄泻 / 545
kidney deficiency syndrome/pattern 肾虚证 / 212
kidney deficiency with water flooding 肾虚水泛 / 113
kidney edema 肾水 / 549
kidney essence 肾精 / 57
kidney essence insufficiency syndrome/pattern 肾精亏虚证 / 212
kidney essence insufficiency 肾精不足 / 112
kidney failing to receive *qi* 肾不纳气 / 113
kidney (infantile) malnutrition 肾疳 / 540
kidney insufficiency 肾亏 / 111
kidney insuffciency dysmenorrhea 肾虚痛经 / 560
kidney insufficiency amenorrhea 肾虚经闭 / 559
kidney insufficiency diarrhea 肾虚泻 / 588
kidney insufficiency dizziness 肾虚眩晕 / 532

kidney insufficiency habitual abortion 肾虚滑胎 / 570
kidney insufficiency hypomenorrhea 肾虚月经过少 / 558
kidney insufficiency infertility 肾虚不孕 / 565
kidney insufficiency leukorrhagia 肾虚带下 / 564
kidney-insufficiency lumbago 肾虚腰痛 / 554
kidney insufficiency metrorrhagia and metrostaxis 肾虚崩漏 / 561
kidney-insufficiency tinnitus 肾虚耳鸣 / 624
kidney insufficiency vertigo 肾虚眩晕 / 532
kidney impediment 肾痹 / 541
kidney meridian/channel (KI) 足少阴肾经 / 403
kidney meridian/channel cold-dampness syndrome/pattern 肾经寒湿证 / 213
kidney meridian/channel cough 肾经咳嗽 / 525
kidney meridian/channel of foot lesser yin 足少阴肾经 / 403
kidney *qi* 肾气 / 55
kidney *qi* deficiency syndrome/pattern 肾气（亏）虚证 / 212
kidney *qi* deficiency 肾气虚 / 111
kidney *qi* insecurity syndrome/pattern 肾气不固证 / 212
kidney *qi* insufficiency 肾气不足 / 111
Kidney *qi* Pill 肾气丸 / 373
kidney wasting-thirst 肾消 / 551
kidney water 肾水 / 22
kidney water insufficiency 肾水不足 / 112
kidney-water insufficiency syndrome/pattern 肾水亏虚证 / 212
kidney yang 肾阳 / 23
kidney yang deficiency syndrome/pattern 肾阳虚证 / 213
kidney yang deficiency 肾阳虚 / 112
kidney yang insufficiency 肾阳不足 / 113
kidney-yang tonic 补肾阳药 / 293
kidney yin 肾阴 / 22
kidney yin deficiency 肾阴虚 / 112
kidney yin deficiency syndrome/pattern 肾阴虚证 / 212
kidney yin insufficiency 肾阴不足 / 112
killing worms 杀虫 / 272
kneading 揉法 / 480
kneading *Cuanzhu* (BL 2) 揉攒竹 / 487
kneading *Jiache* (ST 6) 揉颊车 / 488
kneading manipulation 揉法 / 647
kneading-pressing (the fractured ends) close 搏捺相近 / 648
kneading restoration 搏令平正 / 648
kneading *Sibai* (ST 2) 揉四白 / 487
kneading the knees 揉膝 / 506
kneading the shoulders 揉肩 / 506
kneading the sides of the small of the back 揉腰眼 / 489
knee 膝 / 49
knee-pushing (reduction) 膝顶 / 639
knee-pushing thoracic pulling manipulation 膝顶扳胸椎法 / 653
kneecap 膝髌 / 50
knocks and falls 跌打损伤 / 71
knuckle-patting manipulation 指节拍法 / 649
Kongzui (LU 6) 孔最 / 409
Kou Ping 寇平 / 668
Kou Zongshi 寇宗奭 / 663
Kouheliao (LI 19) 口禾髎 / 411
Kuangu (EX-LE 1) 髋骨 / 443
Kudzuvine Root 葛根 / 297
Kufang (ST 14) 库房 / 412
Kunlun (BL 60) 昆仑 / 423
Kusnezoff Monkshood Root 草乌 / 314
kyphosi 龟背 / 578

L

labor 临产 / 568
lacerated wound 撕裂伤 / 646
laceration 撕裂伤 / 646
lack of proper postnatal care 后天失调 / 73
lack of vitality 少神 / 123
lacquer dermatitis 漆疮 / 603
lacrimal gland 泪泉 / 609
lacrimal point 泪点 / 609
lacrimal punctum 泪窍，泪堂 / 43，609
lacrimation induced by wind 迎风流泪 / 611
lactational malnutrition 哺乳疳 / 582
Lalang Grass Rhizome 白茅根 / 307
Lameness Granules 尪痹颗粒 / 393
lameness impediment 尪痹 / 541
Lan Shi Mi Cang 兰室秘藏 / 701

lance needle 锋针 / 452
Lanwei (EX-LE 7) 阑尾 / 443
Laogong (PC 8) 劳宫 / 426
Laphatherum-Gypsum Decoction 竹叶石膏汤 / 367
Lapis Micae Aureus 金礞石 / 301
large cone moxibustion 大炷灸 / 465
Large Haw Pills 大山楂丸 / 387
large heavenly circuit 大周天 / 500
large heavenly circuit exercise 大周天功 / 502
large intestine 大肠 / 24
large intestinal cold accumulation 大肠寒结 / 110
large intestinal cold accumulation syndrome/pattern 大肠寒结证 / 208
large intestinal cough 大肠咳 / 525
large intestinal dampness-heat 大肠湿热 / 111
large intestinal dampness-heat syndrome/pattern 大肠湿热证 / 208
large intestinal deficiency cold 大肠虚寒 / 111
large intestinal deficiency cold syndrome/pattern 大肠虚寒证 / 208
large intestinal fluid depletion 大肠津［液］亏 / 81，111
large intestinal fluid insufficiency syndrome/pattern 大肠津［液］亏证 / 208
large intestinal heat accumulation 大肠热结 / 110
large intestinal heat accumulation syndrome/pattern 大肠热结证 / 208
large intestine meridian/channel of hand yang brightness (LI) 手阳明大肠经 / 400
large joints 大节 / 52
large needle 大针 / 452
large pulse 大脉 / 162
Large Yin-nourishing Pills 大补阴丸 / 389
Largehead Atractylodes Rhizome 白术 / 341
Large-leaf Gentian Root 秦艽 / 314
Largetrifoliolious Bugbane Rhizome 升麻 / 298
laryngeal prominence 结喉 / 46
laryngopharynx 咽喉 / 40
laser acupuncture 激光针 / 470
Lasiosphaera seu Calvatia 马勃 / 313
"last radiance of the setting sun" 回光返照 / 123
late afternoon fever 日晡发热 / 519
late afternoon tidal fever 日晡潮热 / 144，519
late periods 经迟，经行后期，月经后期，经水后期，月经错后 / 157，557
late periods due to blood cold 血寒经行后期 / 558
late periods due to blood deficiency 血虚经行后期 / 558
late periods due to *qi* stagnation 气滞经行后期 / 558
latent breathing 潜呼吸 / 497
latent fluid retention 伏饮 / 528
latent heat 伏热 / 88
latent heat in the interior 伏热在里 / 88
latent menstruation 暗经 / 556
latent pathogen 伏邪 / 64
latent *qi* 伏气 / 63，515
latent-*qi* warm disease 伏气温病 / 515
latent summerheat 伏暑 / 518
latent summerheat disease 伏暑病 / 518
lateral canthus 目锐眦，锐眦 / 607，608
lateral canthus (of the eye) 目锐眦 / 44
lateral line 1 of the forehead (MS 2) 额旁1线 / 471
lateral line 1 of the vertex (MS 8) 顶旁1线 / 471
lateral line 2 of the forehead (MS 3) 额旁2线 / 471
lateral line 2 of the vertex (MS 9) 顶旁2线 / 471
lateral line 3 of the forehead (MS 4) 额旁3线 / 471
lateral lower abdomen 少腹 / 48
lateral malleolus 外踝 / 50
lateral pectoral region 胁 / 47
lateral recumbent posture 侧卧式 / 495
laterally-rotating reduction of cervical vertebra 颈椎侧旋复位法 / 652
lateropectoral pain 胁痛(病) / 546
laxation 缓下 / 236
laxative (medicinal/drug) 润下药 / 289
leaking sweating 漏汗 / 145
leaning sitting 靠坐 / 495
leaven 曲 / 282
Leech 水蛭 / 333
leg pulling 扳腿推拿手法 / 485
leg-pulling manipulation 拉腿手法 / 486
leg *qi* 脚气 / 539
leg training 腿功 / 653
leg weakness 脚弱 / 539

leg-straightening traction 挺腿拔伸 / 640
Lei Feng 雷丰 / 681
Lei Gong Pao Zhi Lun 雷公炮炙论 / 689
Lei Gong Yao Xing Fu 雷公药性赋 / 689
Lei Gong 雷公 / 658
Lei Jing Tu Yi 类经图翼 / 684
Lei Jing 类经 / 684
Lei Shaoyi 雷少逸 / 681
Lei Xiao 雷敩 / 660
Lei Zheng Zhi Cai 类证治裁 / 694
Lei's Nature of Drugs in Songs 雷公药性赋 / 689
Lei's Treatise on Medicinal Processing 雷公炮炙论 / 689
Lemongrass 芸香草 / 304
Leng Lu Yi Hua 冷庐医话 / 702
lengthened menstrual cycles 经期错后 / 557
Lenitive Pill 保和丸 / 379
lens 精珠 / 610
leopard-spot needling 豹文刺 / 459
leprosy 麻风，大风，疠风，癞病 / 605
Lesser Galangal Rhizome 高良姜 / 318
lesser yang disease 少阳病 / 177
lesser yang disease pattern 少阳病证 / 177
lesser-yang-harmonizing formula 和解少阳剂 / 365
lesser yang syndrome 少阳病证 / 177
lesser yin disease 少阴病 / 177
lesser yin disease pattern 少阴病证 / 177
lesser yin syndrome 少阴病证 / 177
lethargic sleeping with the eyes open 昏睡露睛 / 129
leukorrhea 白带，带下 / 158，563，564
leukorrheal diseases 带下病 / 564
Li Binhu 李濒湖 / 670
Li Dongbi 李东壁 / 670
Li Dongyuan 李东垣 / 665
Li Gao 李杲 / 665
Li Lian 李濂 / 669
Li Mingzhi 李明之 / 665
Li Shang Xu Duan Mi Fang 理伤续断秘方 / 697
Li Shicai 李士材 / 673
Li Shizhen 李时珍 / 670
Li Xing'an 李惺庵 / 675
Li Xiuzhi 李修之 / 675
Li Yan 李梴 / 669
Li Yongcui 李用粹 / 675
Li Yue Pian Wen 理瀹骈文 / 693
Li Zhengyu 李正宇 / 671
Li Zhongli 李中立 / 671
Li Zhongzi 李中梓 / 673
liability to change from excess to deficiency and vice versa 易虚易实 / 574
liability to change from heat to cold and vice versa 易寒易热 / 574
Liang Fu Pill 良附丸 / 375
Liangmen (ST 21) 梁门 / 413
Liangqiu (ST 34) 梁丘 / 414
Lianquan (CV 23) 廉泉 / 437
Licorice Root 甘草 / 340
Lidui (ST 45) 厉兑 / 414
lienteric diarrhea 飧泄［泻］/ 545
Lieque (LU 7) 列缺 / 409
life fire 命火 / 27
life gate 命门之火 / 27
life gate fire 命门之火 / 27
life pass 命关 / 138
Life-saving Manual of Diagnosis and Treatment of External Diseases 外科证治全生集 / 698
lifting 提法 / 639
lifting and stretching 提伸法 / 485
lifting, pressing, holding, and squeezing 提按端挤 / 638
lifting-thrusting method 提插法 / 455
lifting-thrusting reinforcement and reduction 提插补泻 / 456
lifting-thrusting reinforcement-reduction method 提插补泻法 / 456
ligation therapy 结扎疗法 / 273
light (diaphoretic) formula 轻剂 / 360
light red tongue 淡红舌 / 131
Light Wheat 浮小麦 / 348
Light-yellow Sophora Root 苦参 / 308
Lignum Aquilariae Resinatum 沉香 / 327
Lignum Dalbergiae Odoriferae 降香 / 327
Lignum Santali Albi 檀香 / 326
Lignum Sappan 苏木 / 333
Ligou (LR 5) 蠡沟 / 432
Ligustrazine Injection 川芎嗪注射液 / 394
Lilac Daphne Flower Bud 芫花 / 324
Liliac Pink Herb 瞿麦 / 322
Lily Bulb 百合 / 302
"lily disease" 百合病 / 534
Lilyturf-Magnoliavine Rehmannia Pills 麦味地黄丸 / 390
"limb-pressing" 按跷 / 433
Limonite 禹余粮 / 349

Limonitum 禹余粮 / 349
Lin Peiqin 林佩琴 / 679
Lin Xitong 林羲桐 / 679
Lin Yunhe 林云和 / 679
Lin Zheng Zhi Nan Yi An 临证指南医案 / 702
Ling Shu 灵枢 / 684
Lingdao (HT 4) 灵道 / 416
Lingtai (GV 10) 灵台 / 434
lingual hyperplasia 雀舌 / 634
Lingxu (KI 24) 灵墟 / 425
lip 唇 / 39
lip abscess 唇疽 / 634
lip cancer 茧唇，唇菌 / 598，634
lip pustule 唇疔 / 634
lip sore 唇疮 / 634
lipoma 肉瘤 / 598
liquid 液 / 58
liquid collapse 液脱 / 550
listening and smelling examination 闻诊 / 139
listening to the sounds 闻声音 / 139
little tongue 小舌 / 628
Liu Fang 刘昉 / 663
Liu Juanzi Gui Yi Fang 刘涓子鬼遗方 / 697
Liu Juanzi's Ghost-Bequeathed Prescriptions 刘涓子鬼遗方 / 697
Liu Ke Zheng Zhi Zhun Sheng 六科证治准绳 / 704
Liu Shouzhen 刘守真 / 664
Liu Wansu 刘完素 / 664
Liu Yi Powder 六一散 / 369
Liushen Pills 六神丸 / 395
Liuwei Dihuang Decoction 六味地黄汤 / 372
Liuwei Dihuang Pills 六味地黄丸 / 389
liver 肝 / 21
liver atrophy-flaccidity 肝痿 / 539
liver blood 肝血 / 21
liver blood deficiency 肝血虚 / 97
liver blood deficiency syndrome/pattern 肝血（亏）虚证 / 209
liver blood insufficiency 肝血不足 / 97
liver cold 肝寒 / 103
liver cold syndrome/pattern 肝寒证 / 209
liver consumption 肝劳 / 529
liver cough 肝咳 / 524
liver deficiency cold 肝虚寒 / 97
liver deficiency cold syndrome/pattern 肝虚寒证 / 209
liver depression 肝郁 / 103
liver depression and spleen insufficiency 肝郁脾虚 / 104
liver depression infertility 肝郁不孕 / 565
liver depression syndrome/pattern 肝郁证 / 210
liver-depressive hypochondriac pain 肝郁胁痛 / 531
liver edema 肝水 / 549
liver-emolliating medicinal/drug 柔肝药 / 294
liver fire 肝火 / 103
liver fire dizziness 肝火眩晕 / 532
liver fire insomnia 肝火不得卧 / 535
liver fire syndrome 肝火证 / 209
liver-fire tinnitus 肝火耳鸣 / 624
liver fire vertigo 肝火眩晕 / 532
liver-gallbladder dampness-heat syndrome/pattern 肝胆湿热证 / 211
liver-gallbladder dampness-heat 肝胆湿热 / 104
liver heat 肝热 / 103
liver impediment 肝痹 / 541
liver (infantile) malnutrition 肝疳 / 581
liver-kidney yin deficiency syndrome/pattern 肝肾阴虚证 / 211
liver-kidney yin deficiency 肝肾阴虚 / 104
liver meridian/channel (LR) 足厥阴肝经 / 405
liver meridian/channel cough 肝经咳嗽 / 524
liver meridian/channel of foot reverting yin 足厥阴肝经 / 405
liver-pacifying and wind-extinguishing medicinal/drug 平肝熄［息］风药 / 293
liver-pacifying and yang-suppressing medicinal/drug 平肝抑阳药 / 293
liver *qi* 肝气 / 21，54
liver *qi* deficiency 肝气虚 / 96
liver *qi* deficiency syndrome/pattern 肝气（亏）虚证 / 209
liver *qi* depression 肝气郁结 / 97
liver *qi* depression syndrome/pattern 肝气郁结证 / 210
liver *qi* hypochondriac pain 肝气胁痛 / 531
liver *qi* insufficiency 肝气不足 / 96
liver *qi* invading the spleen 肝气犯脾 / 98，104
liver *qi* invading the stomach 肝气犯胃 / 97，103
liver *qi* stagnation 肝气郁结 / 97

liver *qi* stagnation syndrome/pattern 肝气郁结证 / 210
liver-*qi* stomachache 肝胃气痛 / 542
liver-soothing and vision-improving exercise 疏肝明目功 / 502
Liver-soothing Pills 舒肝丸 / 386
liver-spleen disharmony 肝脾不和 / 104
liver-spleen disharmony syndrome/pattern 肝脾不和证 / 211
liver-spleen harmonizing formula 调和肝脾剂 / 365
liver stagnation 肝郁 / 103
liver stagnation and spleen insufficiency 肝郁脾虚 / 104
liver stagnation syndrome/pattern 肝郁证 / 210
liver-stomach disharmony 肝胃不和 / 103
liver-stomach disharmony syndrome/pattern 肝胃不和证 / 210
Liver-warming Decoction 暖肝煎 / 375
liver wind 肝风 / 103
liver yang 肝阳 / 21
liver yang deficiency syndrome/pattern 肝阳（亏）虚证 / 209
liver yang deficiency 肝阳虚 / 97
liver yang dizziness 肝阳眩晕 / 532
liver-yang headache 肝阳头痛 / 534
liver-yang hyperactivity syndrome 肝阳亢盛证 / 210
liver yang transforming into fire 肝阳化火 / 98
liver yang transforming into wind 肝阳化风 / 103
liver yang vertigo 肝阳眩晕 / 532
liver yin 肝阴 / 21
liver yin deficiency 肝阴虚 / 97
liver yin deficiency syndrome/pattern 肝阴（亏）虚证 / 209
liver yin insufficiency 肝阴不足 / 97
Lizhong Decoction 理中汤 / 369
location of point by bone measurement 骨度分寸定穴法 / 445
lochia 恶露 / 570
lochiorrhea 产后恶露不绝 / 570
locked abdomen 锁肚 / 575
lockjaw 口噤，噤风 / 136，575
long illness 宿疾 / 524
Long Mu's Recondite Treatise on Ophthalmology 秘传眼科龙木论 / 698
long needle 长针 / 452
Long-noded Pit Viper 蕲蛇 / 315
Long Pepper 荜拨 / 319
long pulse 长脉 / 162
long voiding of clear urine 小便清长 / 150
Longan Aril 龙眼肉 / 342
Longdan Xiegan Decoction 龙胆泻肝汤 / 368
Longevity and Health Preservation 寿世保元 / 703
Longevity Capsules 龟龄集 / 390
Longstamen Onion 薤白 / 326
Lonicera-Forsythia Powder 银翘散 / 362
Lonicera-Scutellaria-Forsythia Oral Liquid 双黄连口服液 / 383
Lonicera-Scutellariae Oral Liquid 银黄口服液 / 383
looking at a wall 壁观 / 499
loose bowels 便溏 / 149
loose stool 溏便 / 149
loose teeth 齿摇 / 137
loosening clothes 宽解衣带 / 493
Lophatherum Herb 淡竹叶 / 305
Loquat Leaf 枇杷叶 / 301
loss of blood 夺血，失血 / 549
loss of bulk and shedding of flesh 破䐃脱肉 / 127
loss of consciousness 不省人事 / 124
loss of smell 鼻不闻香臭 / 130
loss of vitality 失神 / 123
loss of voice 失音 / 140
Lotus Leaf 荷叶 / 320
Lotus Plumule 莲子心 / 305
Lotus Rhizome Node 藕节 / 330
Lotus Seed 莲子 / 349
Lotus Stamen 莲须 / 349
lotus tongue 莲花舌 / 634
Lou Gongshuang 楼公爽 / 667
Lou Ying 楼英 / 667
Lougu (SP 7) 漏谷 / 415
lower abdomen 小腹 / 48
lower abdominal cramp 少腹拘急 / 154
lower abdominal fullness 小腹满 / 154
lower abdominal numbness 小腹不仁 / 154
lower abdominal rigidity and fullness 少腹硬满 / 154
lower back 腰 / 49
lower cheek 颐 / 46
lower confluent points 下合穴 / 439
lower *dantian* 下丹田 / 497
lower elixir field 下丹田 / 497

lower energizer 下焦 / 24
lower-energizer dampness-heat syndrome/pattern 下焦湿热证 / 182
lower energizer deficiency cold 下焦虚寒 / 215
lower energizer excess heat 下焦实热 / 215
lower-energizer syndrome/pattern 下焦病证 / 181
lower eyelid 下睑，目下胞 / 45，609
lower eyelid margin 目下弦 / 609
lower-lateral line of the occiput (MS 14) 枕下旁线 / 472
lower limb exercise 下肢功 / 501
lower obstruction 下膈 / 543
lower orifices 下窍 / 38
lower palpebral musculature 目下纲，目下网 / 608
lower sea points 下合穴 / 439
lower stomach cavity 下脘 / 24
lower wasting-thirst 下消 / 551
lozenge 锭，锭剂 / 281
Lu He 卢和 / 669
Lu Jiuzhi 陆九芝 / 680
Lu Maoxiu 陆懋修 / 680
Lu Yitian 陆以湉 / 681
Lu Yuanlei 陆渊雷 / 682
lubricant laxation 润下 / 236
lubricant laxative formula 润下剂 / 364
lubricating formula 滑剂 / 360
Lucid Ganoderma 灵芝 / 337
Luffa Vegetable Sponge 丝瓜络 / 316
lumbago 腰痛 / 147，553
lumbar aching 腰酸，腰痠 / 147
lumbar bone 腰骨 / 50
lumbar extending-counterpulling manipulation 后伸扳腰法 / 653
lumbar pain 腰痛 / 147
lumbar pulling manipulation 扳腰椎法 / 653
lumbar rotating reduction manipulation 腰椎旋转复位法 / 653
lumbar weakness 腰软 / 554
lumbodorsal carbuncle 搭手 / 594
Lumbricus 地龙 / 339
lumbus 腰 / 49
lung 肺 / 22
lung abscess 肺痈 / 528
lung-astringing antitussive formula 敛肺止咳剂 / 374
lung atrophy 肺萎［痿］/ 528
lung consumption 肺劳 / 529
lung cough 肺咳 / 525
lung deficiency 肺虚 / 102
lung-defense *qi* deficiency syndrome 肺卫气虚（不固）证 / 202
lung deficiency cold syndrome/pattern 肺虚寒证 / 203
lung-deficiency cough 肺虚咳嗽 / 526
lung deficiency heat syndrome/pattern 肺虚热证 / 203
lung distension 肺胀 / 528
lung dryness 肺燥 / 102
lung edema 肺水 / 549
lung excess 肺实 / 102
lung failing in purification 肺失清肃 / 109
lung failing to distribute fluid 肺津不布 / 109
lung fire 肺火 / 102
lung fire syndrome/pattern 肺火证 / 204
lung fluid 肺津 / 22
lung fluid depletion syndrome/pattern 肺燥津伤证 / 187
lung fluid depletion 肺津亏损 / 81
lung heat 肺热 / 102
lung-kidney *qi* deficiency syndrome/pattern 肺肾气虚证 / 205
lung-kidney *qi* deficiency 肺肾气虚 / 102
lung-kidney yang deficiency syndrome/pattern 肺肾阳虚证 / 205
lung-kidney yang deficiency 肺肾阳虚 / 102
lung-kidney yin deficiency 肺肾阴虚 / 102
lung-kidney yin deficiency syndrome/pattern 肺肾阴虚证 / 204
lung impediment 肺痹 / 541
lung (infantile) malnutrition 肺疳 / 581
lung inflammation with dyspnea and cough 肺炎喘嗽 / 586
lung-intestine astringent (medicinal/drug) 敛肺涩肠药 / 294
lung meridian/channel (LU) 手太阴肺经 / 400
lung meridian/channel cough 肺经咳嗽 / 525
lung meridian/channel of hand greater yin 手太阴肺经 / 400
lung phthisis 肺痨 / 529
Lung-purging Powder 泻白散 / 368
lung *qi* 肺气 / 22，55
lung *qi* deficiency syndrome/pattern 肺气虚证 / 202
lung *qi* deficiency 肺气虚 / 109
lung *qi* failing in dispersion 肺气不宣 / 109
lung *qi* insufficiency 肺气不足 / 109

lung-regulation exercise 理肺功 / 501
lung system 肺系 / 40
Lung-ventilating Pills [Tablets] 通宣理肺丸［片］/ 382
lung wasting-thirst 肺消 / 551
lung wind with phlegmatic dyspnea 肺风痰喘 / 585
lung yang 肺阳 / 22
lung yang deficiency 肺阳虚 / 109
lung yang deficiency syndrome/pattern 肺阳虚证 / 203
lung yin 肺阴 / 22
lung yin deficiency 肺阴虚 / 109
lung yin deficiency syndrome/pattern 肺阴虚证 / 203
lung yin insufficiency 肺阴不足 / 109
Luo Qianfu 罗谦甫 / 666
Luo Tianyi 罗天益 / 666
Luoque (BL 8) 络却 / 419
lupus erythematosus 红蝴蝶疮 / 601
lusterless eyes 两眼无光 / 128
luxation 脱位 / 637
Luxi (TE 19) 颅息 / 428
luxuriant, withered, tough and tender-soft 荣枯老嫩 / 131
Lychee Seed 荔枝核 / 327
lying on one's side with the knees drawn up 踡［蜷］卧缩足 / 127
lying posture 卧式 / 495
lying supine with the legs outstretched 仰卧伸足 / 127

M

Ma Shi 马莳 / 670
Ma Xing Shi Gan Decoction 麻杏石甘汤 / 362
maceration 泡 / 276
macrocosmic cycle 大周天 / 500
macula 斑 / 139，591
macule and papule 斑疹 / 139
maculo-papule 斑疹 / 139
magnetic bead therapy 磁珠疗法 / 478
Magnetite 磁石 / 336
Magnetitum 磁石 / 336
magpie bridge 鹊桥 / 494
Mahuang Decoction 麻黄汤 / 361
Mai Jing 脉经 / 686
Maimendong Decoction 麦门冬汤 / 378
Maiwei Dihuang Pills 麦味地黄丸 / 390
Major Bupleurum Decoction 大柴胡汤 / 366
major chest bind 大结胸 / 519
major formula 大方 / 357
major syncope 大厥 / 538
major thoracic accumulation 大结胸 / 519
malar eminence 颧 / 45
malaria 疟，疟病，疟疾 / 520
malarial accumulation 疟积 / 521
malarial lump 疟痞 / 521
malarial mass 疟母 / 521
Malaytea Scurfpea Fruit 补骨脂 / 347
male urinary meatus 精窍 / 49
male viscera 牡脏 / 20
male *zang* organs 牡脏 / 20
malign *qi* 恶气 / 63
malnutrition 疳 / 580
malnutrition-accumulation syndrome 疳积证 / 580
malnutrition disease 疳病 / 580
(infantile) malnutrition involving the eyes 眼疳 / 581
(infantile) malnutrition involving the heart 心疳 / 581
(infantile) malnutrition involving the kidney 肾疳 / 581
(infantile) malnutrition involving the liver 肝疳 / 581
(infantile) malnutrition involving the lung 肺疳 / 581
(infantile) malnutrition involving the spleen 脾疳 / 580
malnutrition *qi* syndrome 疳气证 / 580
malnutrition *qi* 疳气 / 580
malnutrition syndrome 疳证 / 580
malnutrition with accumulation 疳积 / 580
Malt Extract 饴糖 / 342
mammary cancer 乳岩 / 598
mammary fistula 乳漏 / 597
mammary hyperplasia 乳癖 / 597
mammary phlegm 乳痰 / 597
mammary phthisis 乳痨 / 597
management of breath 调息 / 497
management of *qi* 调气 / 497
management of the mind 调心 / 498
Manchurian Dutchmanspipe Stem 关木通 / 321
Manchurian Lilac Bark 暴马子皮 / 303
Manchurian Wild Ginger 细辛 / 296
mandibular angle 颊车，曲牙 / 46
mandibular arch 曲颊 / 46
mania 躁狂，狂 / 124，534
manic psychosis 狂病 / 534
manic raving 狂言 / 140
manipulating the needle to await *qi* 行针候气 / 456
Mantid Egg Capsule 桑螵蛸 / 350

manual correction 捺正 / 640
manual restoration 纳入原位 / 640
manual restoration 徒手整复 / 491
manual traction 手法牵引 / 642
manubrium of the sternum 上横骨 / 47
Maren Pills 麻仁丸 / 386
Maren Runchang Pills 麻仁润肠丸 / 386
Margarita 珍珠 / 337
margin of the eyelid 目弦 / 44, 608
margin of the lower eyelid 目下弦 / 45
margin of the tongue 舌边 / 130
margin of the upper eyelid 目上弦 / 45
marginal blepharitis 风弦赤烂，睑弦赤烂，眼缘赤烂 / 613
marrow 髓 / 25
martial-art *qigong* 武术气功 / 492
Massa Fermentata Medicinalis 神曲 / 351
massage 按摩 / 480
massage along the meridian/channel 循按法，循法 / 455
massage manipulation 按摩手法 / 480
massage practitioner 按摩师 / 480
massage therapy with ointment 膏摩疗法 / 274
massaging *Zusanli* (ST36) 按摩足三里 / 489
masseur 按摩师 / 480
masseuse 按摩师 / 480
massotherapy 按摩疗法 / 480
mastauxy in children 乳疬 / 597
mastoid bone 完骨 / 623
mastoid process 完骨 / 46
Materia Medica for Decoctions 汤液本草 / 688
Materia Medica for Relief of Famine 救荒本草 / 688
Materia Medica of Diet Therapy 食疗本草 / 687
materia medica 本草，药材 / 275
maxillary osteomyelitis 骨槽风 / 633
Maziren Pill 麻子仁丸 / 365
measles toxin 麻毒 / 69
measles toxin attacking the eyes 麻毒攻目 / 584
measles toxin blocking the lung 麻毒闭肺 / 584
measles toxin entering the nutrient aspect 麻毒入营 / 584
measles toxin penetrating into the lung 麻毒陷肺 / 584
measles 麻疹，痧子 / 584
mechanical induction of vomiting 探吐 / 267
mechanism of disease 病机 / 78
medial canthus 内眦，目内眦 / 44，608
medial-lateral point combination 内外配穴法 / 448
medial malleolus 内踝 / 50
medial suppurative osteomyelitis 咬骨疽 / 595
medical *qigong* 医用气功 / 492
Medical Records as a Guide to Clinical Practice 临证指南医案 / 702
medicated cupping 药罐 / 469
medicated diet 药膳 / 507
Medicated Leaven 神曲 / 351
medicated immersion 溻浴 / 273
medicated porridge 药粥 / 507
medicated spill therapy 药捻疗法 / 274
medicated tea 茶剂，药茶 / 282，507
medicated thread therapy 药线疗法 / 274
medicated wine 药酒，酒剂 / 281，507
Medicinal Cyathula Root 川牛膝 / 331
"medicinal guide" 药引子 / 358
medicinal ingredients (in a prescription) 药味 / 278
Medicinal Magnolia Bark 厚朴 / 325
medicinal massage 药摩 / 490
medicinal moxibustion 药物灸 / 466
medicinal powder 药面 / 282
medicinal properties 药性 / 279
medicinal slices 饮片 / 282
medicinal substance 药材 / 275
medicinal wine 药酒，酒剂 / 281
medicinals contraindicated during pregnancy 妊娠禁忌药 / 284
meditating fixation 禅定 / 500
medium-grade medicinal 中品 / 279
Medulla Junci 灯心草 / 323
Medulla Tetrapanacis 通草 / 321
megacaput pad 大头垫 / 641
Meichong (BL 3) 眉冲 / 419
Mel 蜂蜜 / 352
melting 烊化 / 283
Meng Shen 孟诜 / 661
menopause 经断，经绝，经水断绝 / 157，158
menopausal diseases 绝经前后诸病 / 563
menopausal syndromes 断经前

后诸证 / 563
menorrhagia 月经过多，经崩 / 157，563
menostaxis 经期延长 / 559
menstrual blood 经血 / 556
menstrual body pain 经行身痛 / 562
menstrual diarrhea 经行泄泻，经来泄泻 / 563
menstrual discharge 经水 / 556
menstrual disease 月经病 / 557
menstrual disorders, leukorrheal diseases, gravid troubles, and parturition problems 经带胎产 / 556
menstrual dizziness 经行眩晕 / 562
menstrual dripping 经漏 / 561
menstrual edema 经行浮肿，经期水肿 / 562
menstrual epistaxis 经行衄血 / 562
menstrual fever 经行发热，经来发热 / 562
menstrual flooding 经崩 / 561
menstrual headache 经行头痛 / 562
menstrual hematemesis 经行吐血 / 562
menstrual hematemesis and epistaxis 经行吐衄 / 562
menstrual irregularities 月经不调，月水不调，经水不调 / 557
menstrual mental disorder 经行情志异常 / 563
menstrual oral ulcer 经行口糜 / 563
menstrual urticaria 经行隐疹 / 563
menstruation during pregnancy 垢胎，激经，盛胎 / 566
menstruation 月经，月事，月水，月信 / 157，556
mental confusion 昏蒙，神志昏愦［溃］/ 123，124
mental disorder 神乱 / 124
meridian/channel and collateral 经络 / 398
meridian/channel divergence 经别 / 407
meridian/channel induced disease 是动病 / 408
meridian/channel needling 经刺 / 460
meridian/channel pattern identification 经络辨证 / 215，408
meridian/channel point 经穴 / 437，408
meridian/channel *qi* 经络之气，经气 / 55
meridian/channel-*qi*-connecting point combination 通经接气配穴法 / 449
meridian/channel sinew 经筋 / 406
meridian/channel syndrome differentiation 经络辨证 / 215，408
meridian/channel syndrome 经络证候 / 408
meridian/channel transmission 传经 / 116
meridian/channel tropism 归经 / 279
meridian/channel-warming cold-dispersing formula 温经散寒剂 / 370
meridian passage 经隧 / 398
meridian stroke 中经 / 537
meridian syndrome/pattern 经证 / 178
meridian-warming hemostatic (medicinal/drug) 温经止血药 / 291
meridians 经脉 / 398
metal-featured person 金形之人 / 74
metal generating water 金生水 / 11
metal needle 金针 / 452
metal restricting wood 金克木 / 12
metal ulcer (of the eye) 金疳，金疡 / 617
metamorphopsia 视直为曲 / 621
metastatic abscess 流注 / 595
metastatic abscess of the iliac fossa 髂窝流注 / 595
metatarsal bones 跗骨 / 52
metatarsus 跖 / 50
method of making a decoction 煎药法 / 283
method of reinforcement and reduction 补泻法 / 456
metrorrhagia 血崩 / 561
metrorrhagia and metrostaxis 崩漏 / 561
metrostaxis 漏下 / 561
metrorrhagic syndrome 崩证 / 561
Mi Chuan Yan Ke Long Mu Lun 秘传眼科龙木论 / 698
Miao Xiyong 缪希雍 / 672
Miao Zhongchun 缪仲淳 / 672
miasma 瘴气 / 72，520
miasmic malaria 瘴疟 / 520，521
miasmic toxin 瘴毒 / 72，521
Mica-schist 金礞石 / 301
microcosmic cycle 小周天 / 500
microwave acumoxibustion 微波针灸 / 470

microwave acupuncture therapy 微波针灸疗法 / 470
middle *dantian* 中丹田 / 496
middle elixir field 中丹田 / 496
middle energizer 中焦 / 24
middle energizer dampness-heat 中焦湿热 / 106
middle-energizer dampness-heat syndrome/pattern 中焦湿热证 / 181，207
middle energizer deficiency cold 中焦虚寒 / 215
middle energizer excess heat 中焦实热 / 215
middle-energizer syndrome/pattern 中焦病证 / 181
middle finger body-*cun* 中指同身寸 / 444
middle finger body-inch 中指同身寸 / 444
middle-finger-propping gesture 中指独立式 / 505
middle fullness 中满 / 154
middle line of the forehead (MS 1) 额中线 / 471
middle line of the vertex (MS 5) 顶中线 / 471
middle of the mentolabial groove 承浆 / 46
middle of the tongue 舌中 / 130
middle *qi* 中气 / 56
middle *qi* sinking syndrome/pattern 中气下陷证 / 206
Middle-reinforcing *Qi*-replenishing Pills 补中益气丸 / 388
middle stomach cavity 中脘 / 23
middle wasting-thirst 中消 / 551
mid-frons 天庭 / 43
midnight-midday ebb flow 子午流注 / 459
midnight-midday ebb flow acupuncture 子午流注针法 / 459
migraine 偏头痛，偏头风 / 146，533
migratory arthralgia 行痹 / 540
migratory impediment 行痹 / 540
mild fever 微热 / 144
mild fire 文火 / 283
mild formula 小方 / 357
mild (infantile) malnutrition 疳气 / 580
mild moxibustion 温和灸 / 464
mild pungent-cool formula 辛凉轻剂 / 362
mild purgation 轻下 / 237
Mild Purgative Decoction 小承气汤 / 364
miliaria 痱（子）/ 601
miliaria alba 白痦 / 139
miliaria crystalline 晶痦 / 139
milk damage vomiting 伤乳吐 / 587
milk damage 伤乳 / 577
milk lichen 奶癣 / 604
milk regurgitation 溢乳 / 577，587
milk retention 乳积 / 582
milk vomiting 呕乳 / 587
Milkvetch Root 黄芪 / 340
millet sore 粟疮 / 613
Millet Sprout 谷芽 / 351
mind 神 / 2，57
Mind-tonic Pills 补心丹 / 385
Mind-tonic Pills of Arborvitae Seed 柏子养心丸 / 385
Ming Yi Bie Lu 名医别录 / 687
Ming Yi Lei An 名医类案 / 702
Ming Yi Za Zhu 明医杂著 / 701
Mingmen 命门 / 23
Mingmen (GV 4) 命门 / 433
minister ingredient 臣药 / 358
ministerial fire 相火 / 27
Minor Center-constructing Decoction 小建中汤 / 370
minor chest bind 小结胸 / 519
Minor Decoction of Blue Dragon 小青龙汤 / 361
minor formula 小方 / 357
Minor Panacea 小金丸［丹］/ 395
minor thoracic accumulation 小结胸 / 519
Minor/Mild Bupleurum Decoction 小柴胡汤 / 365
minute pellet 微丸 / 280
miosis 瞳神缩小，瞳神紧小，瞳神细小 / 619
Miraculous Pills of Six Ingredients 六神丸 / 395
Miraculous Powder of Saposhnikovia 防风通圣散 / 366
Miraculous Saposhnikovia Pills 防风通圣丸 / 382
mirror tongue 镜面舌 / 136
miscarriage 小产 / 569
miscellaneous diseases 杂病 / 524
miscellaneous internal diseases 内科杂病 / 524
Miscellaneous Records of Famous Physicians 名医别录 / 687
missed labor 死胎不下，胎死不下 / 567
mixed hemorrhoid 内外痔 / 599
moderate pulse 缓脉 / 161
moderate pungent-cool formula 辛凉平剂 / 362
Modified Carefree Pills 加味逍遥丸 / 386
Modified Solomon's Seal Decoction 加减葳蕤汤 / 363
moist (tongue) coating/fur 润苔 / 135

moistening 润 / 276
moistening and resolving dryness-phlegm 润化燥痰 / 258
moistening (dryness) 润燥 / 263
moistening dryness and resolving phlegm 润燥化痰 / 258
moistening dryness to relax the bowels 润燥通便 / 237
moistening dryness to relieve itching 润燥止痒 / 267
moistening (dryness) with sweet-cold 甘寒润燥 / 263
moistening formula 湿剂 / 360
moistening the intestines 润肠 / 236
moistening the intestines to relax the bowels 润肠通便 / 237
moistening the intestines to relieve constipation 润肠通便 / 263
moistening the lung 润肺 / 263
moistening the lung and engendering fluid 润肺生津 / 264
moistening the lung and resolving phlegm 润肺化痰 / 258
moistening the lung to relieve cough 润肺止咳 / 264
Mole Cricket 蝼蛄 / 323
mole cricket boil 蝼蛄疖 / 592
molluscum contagiosum 鼠乳 / 600
monocular blindness 眇目 / 622
monthly discharge 月水 / 556
"monthly matter" 月事 / 556
"monthly message" 月信 / 556
moodiness during menstruation 经行情志异常 / 563
morbid complexion 病色 / 124
morbid fire 邪火 / 70
Morinda Root 巴戟天 / 347
morning sickness 恶阻，妊娠恶阻 / 566
Morus-Chrysanthemum Decoction 桑菊饮 / 362
Moschus 麝香 / 335
mother (element/phase) 母 / 13
mother (element/phase) *qi* 母气 / 13
"mother-child relationship" in the five elements/phases 五行母子相及 / 13
mother-son point combination 子母配穴法 / 448
mother-son reinforcing and reducing method 子母补泻法 / 458
Mother Root of Common Monkshood 川乌 / 314
Motherwort Fruit 茺蔚子 / 334
Motherwort Herb 益母草 / 334
motility of the tongue 舌态 / 133
motion within quiescence 静中有动 / 492
motive *qi* between the kidneys 肾间动气 / 54
mountain miasma 山岚瘴气 / 72
Mountain Spicy Fruit 荜澄茄 / 318
"mouse nipple" 鼠乳 / 600
mouth 口 / 39
mouth odor 口气 / 142
moving mouth 口动 / 136
moving *qi* and activating blood 行气活血 / 253
moving *qi* and resolving phlegm 行气化痰 / 253
moving *qi* to activate blood 行气活血 / 253
moving *qi* to relieve pain 行气止痛 / 253
moving *qi* to relieve stuffiness 行气消痞 / 253
moving *qi* to soothe the chest 行气宽胸 / 253
moving *qi* to soothe the middle 行气宽中 / 253
moving *qi* to unblock collaterals 行气通络 / 254
moving *qi* 行气，运气 / 252, 503
moxa (Artemisia vulgaris) 艾 / 463
moxa burner 温灸器 / 464
moxa-burner moxibustion 温灸器灸 / 466
moxa cone 艾炷 / 463
moxa-cone moxibustion 艾炷灸 / 464
moxa floss 艾绒 / 463
moxa roll 艾卷 / 464
moxa-roll moxibustion 艾卷灸 / 464
moxa stick 艾条 / 464
moxa-stick moxibustion 艾条灸 / 464
moxibustion 灸，灸法，灸疗法 / 463
moxibustion contraindication 灸禁，灸忌 / 467
moxibustion-prohibited point 禁灸穴 / 467
moxibustion with an ignited moxa roll 艾卷灸 / 464
moxibustion with moxa stick 艾条灸 / 464
Muchuang (GB 16) 目窗 / 429
mud ball 泥丸 / 496
muffled cough 咳声不扬 / 141
Mugua Pills 木瓜丸 / 392
Mulberry Fruit 桑椹 / 345
Mulberry Leaf 桑叶 / 297
Mulberry Mistletoe 桑寄生 / 344
Mulberry Twig 桑枝 / 315
Muli Powder 牡蛎散 / 374
multi-featured pulse 相兼脉象 / 163

multiple abscesses of summerheat-dampness 暑湿流注 / 516
multiple arthralgia 历节风 / 540
mumps 痄腮 / 585
murky eye nebula 混睛外障，混睛障 / 619
murky nebula 混障症 / 619
muscae volitantes 蛛丝飘浮 / 612
muscle 肌 / 41
muscle boundary 分肉 / 41
muscle contracture 筋缩 / 643
muscle flaccidity 筋痿 / 643
muscle impediment 肌痹 / 541
muscular striae 肌腠 / 41
muscular twitching 筋惕肉瞤/ 127
muscle-wasting diabetes 消肌 / 589
musculotendinous nodulation 筋结 / 643
musculotendinous rupture 筋断 / 643
musculotendinous softening 筋柔 / 643
musculotendinous thickening 筋粗 / 643
Musk 麝香 / 335
mutual contention of wind and dampness 风湿相搏 / 89
mutual impairment between yin and yang 阴阳互损 / 7
mutual incitement of wind and fire 风火相煽 / 89
mutual reinforcement 相须 / 358
mutual rooting of yin and yang 阴阳互根 / 5
mutual transformation of essence and *qi* 精气互化 / 2
Muxiang Shunqi Pills 木香顺气丸 / 387
mydriasis 瞳神散大 / 619
Mylabris 斑蝥 / 355
myopia 近视 / 621
Myrrh 没药 / 334
Myrrha 没药 / 334

N

Nacre 珍珠母 / 337
Nan Jing Ben Yi 难经本义 / 684
Nan Jing 难经 / 684
Nan Ya Tang Yi Shu Quan Ji 南雅堂医书全集 / 705
Nao Li Qing 脑立清 / 385
Naohu (GV 17) 脑户 / 434
Naohui (TE 13) 臑会 / 427
Naokong (GB 19) 脑空 / 430
Naoshu (SI 10) 臑俞 / 418
nape 项 / 46
nape exercise 项功 / 506
Nardus Root 甘松 / 326
nasal boil 鼻疔 / 626
nasal breathing 鼻吸鼻呼 / 497
nasal congestion 鼻塞，鼻窍不利 / 626
nasal disease 鼻病 / 626
nasal discharge 鼻涕 / 626
nasal obstruction in common cold 伤风鼻塞 / 626
nasal orifice 鼻窍 / 38
nasal passage 鼻隧 / 39
nasal polyp 鼻息肉，鼻菌，鼻痔，鼻赘 / 627
nasal polyposis 鼻息肉病 / 627
nasal sore 鼻疮，鼻疳，鼻疳疮 / 626
nasal vestibule 鼻前庭 / 626
nasal vestibulitis 鼻疮，鼻疳，鼻疳疮 / 626
nasopharynx 颃颡 / 40，628
Native Achyranthes Root 土牛膝 / 313
Natrii Sulfas 芒硝 / 352
Natrii Sulfas Exsiccatus 玄明粉 / 353
natural breathing 自然呼吸 / 497
Natural Indigo 青黛 / 311
natural life span 天年 / 18
natural moxibustion 天灸 / 466
natural stake-standing exercise 自然站桩功 / 502
natural standing posture 自然站式 / 495
Nature of the Drugs of the Pearl Bag in Songs 珍珠囊药性赋 / 689
nausea 恶心 / 152
navel breathing 脐呼吸 / 497
nearsightedness 能近怯远症 / 621
nebula 翳 / 612
neck 颈 / 46
neck bone 颈骨 / 50
neck exercise 颈项功 / 501
neck relaxed 颈松 / 493
necrotizing therapy for hemorrhoids 枯痔法 / 273
needle cataractopiesis 金针拨障法 / 479
needle couching 金针拨障法 / 479
needle-direction conduction of *qi* 针向行气法 / 459
needle-embedding therapy 埋针疗法 / 450
needle-flying insertion 飞入法 / 453
needle insertion 进针 / 452
needle insertion during coughing 随咳进针法 / 454
needle insertion method 进针法 / 452
needle insertion with tube 管针

进针法 / 454
needle manipulation 行针，运针 / 454
needle retention 留针 / 462
needle-retreating method 退法 / 463
needle roller 滚刺［针］筒 / 452
needle root 针根 / 449
needle withdrawal 出针，起针 / 462
needle withdrawal method 出针法，起针法 / 462
needling hand 刺手 / 453
needling-prohibited point 禁针穴 / 463
needling sensation 针感 / 456
Nei Gong Tu Shuo 内功图说 / 700
Nei Jing 内经 / 683
Nei Jing Zhi Yao 内经知要 / 684
Neiguan (PC 6) 内关 / 426
Neihuajian (EX-LE 8) 内踝尖 / 443
Neiting (ST 44) 内庭 / 414
Neixiyan (EX-LE 4) 内膝眼 / 443
Neiyingxiang (EX-HN 9) 内迎香 / 440
neonatal cough 百晬内嗽 / 577
neonatal epilepsy 胎痫 / 590
neonatal jaundice (disease) 胎黄病 / 576
neonatal jaundice 胎疸，胎黄 / 576
neonatal tetanus 脐风 / 575
neurodermatitis 牛皮癣 / 602
neutral reinforcement and reduction 平补平泻 / 458
neutral reinforcing-reducing method 平补平泻法 / 458
neutralizing 相杀 / 359
Newly Revised Materia Medica (of Tang) 新修本草 / 687
Ni Weide 倪维德 / 667
Ni Zhongxian 倪仲贤 / 667
nictitation 目劄 / 614
Nidus Vespae 蜂房 / 356
night blindness 雀盲 / 621
night crying 夜啼 / 577
night crying due to cold 寒夜啼 / 577
night crying due to fright 客忤夜啼 / 577
night crying due to heat 热夜啼 / 577
night sweats 盗汗 / 144，531
night sweating after childbirth 产后盗汗 / 571
night sweating in yin deficiency 阴虚盗汗 / 532
nine classical needles 九针 / 451
Nine-ingredient Decoction with Notopterygium 九味羌活汤 / 361
nine needling methods 九刺 / 460
nine orifices 九窍 / 38
nineteen guiding rules of pathomechanism 病机十九条 / 78
nineteen incompatibilities 十九畏 / 359
nipple wind 乳头风 / 596
Niuhuang Jiangya Pills 牛黄降压丸 / 384
Niuhuang Jiedu Pills [Tablets] 牛黄解毒丸［片］/ 384
Niuhuang Qingxin Pills [Tablets] 牛黄清心丸［片］/ 384
Niuhuang Shangqing Pills 牛黄上清丸 / 384
“no clothes-changing” 不更衣 / 149
no desire to eat despite hunger 饥不欲食 / 153
nocturnal emission 梦遗 / 155，552
nodular vegetation of the ear 耳痔 / 625
nodule in the breast 乳中结核 / 597
Nodus Nelumbinis Rhizomatis 藕节 / 330
noma 走马疳，走马牙疳 / 633
non-acclimatization 水土不服 / 72
non-contraction of heart *qi* 心气不收 / 99
non-exo-endogenous cause 不内外因 / 62
non-festering inward invasion 干陷 / 595
non-inflammatory edema of the eyelid 胞虚如球，脾虚如球 / 614
non-pustulating moxibustion 非化脓灸 / 465
non-scarring moxibustion 无瘢痕灸 / 465
non-transmission 不传 / 116
normal breathing 平息 / 159
normal circuit *qi* 平气 / 18
normal complexion 常色 / 124
normal pulse 常脉，平脉 / 160
normal transmission 顺传 / 179
nose acupuncture 鼻针 / 477
nose acupuncture therapy 鼻针疗法 / 477
nose 鼻 / 38
nose stem 鼻柱 / 626
nose-teeth exercise 鼻齿功 / 501
nose tip 鼻尖 / 626
nosebleed 鼻衄，鼻出血，鼻沥血 / 130，627，628
nostril 鼻孔，鼻前孔 / 38，626
Notopterygium Rhizome or Root 羌活 / 313

nourishing blood 养血 / 247
nourishing blood and dispelling wind 养血祛风 / 228
nourishing blood and emolliating the liver 养血柔肝 / 265
nourishing blood and releasing the exterior 养血解表 / 230
nourishing blood to extinguish wind 养血熄［息］风 / 239，266
nourishing blood to moisten dryness 养血润燥 / 263
nourishing blood to moisten the intestines 养血润肠 / 263
nourishing heart blood 补养心血 / 247
nourishing heart yin 养心阴 / 248
nourishing liver yin 养肝阴 / 248
nourishing lung yin 养肺阴 / 249
nourishing stomach yin 养胃阴 / 249
nourishing the heart 养心 / 248
nourishing the heart to calm the mind 养心安神 / 264
nourishing the liver 养肝 / 265
nourishing the liver and kidney 滋养肝肾 / 248
nourishing the lung and kidney 滋补肺肾 / 249
nourishing the stomach 养胃 / 249
nourishing the stomach to produce fluid 养胃生津 / 249
nourishing yin 养阴，育阴 / 248
nourishing yin and releasing the exterior 养阴解表 / 230
nourishing yin and subduing yang 滋阴潜阳 / 265
nourishing yin to extinguish wind 滋阴熄［息］风 / 266
nourishing yin to moisten dryness 养阴润燥 / 263
nourishing yin to moisten the lung 养阴润肺 / 263
Nü Ke Bai Wen 女科百问 / 695
Nü Ke Jing Lun 女科经纶 / 695
Nuangan Decoction 暖肝煎 / 375
nulliparous vaginal orifice 龙门 / 555
numbness 麻木 / 148，537
numbness of the mouth 口不仁 / 155
numbness of the skin 肌肤麻木 / 147
Nutgrass Galingale Rhizome 香附 / 326
Nutmeg 肉豆蔻 / 349
nutrient 营 / 56
nutrient aspect 营分 / 56
nutrient aspect syndrome/pattern 营分证 / 179
nutrient-blood 营血 / 56
nutrient-blood-aspect heat-clearing formula 清营凉血剂 / 367
Nutrient-clearing Decoction 清营汤 / 367
nutrient *qi* 营气 / 54
nutrient yin 营阴 / 54
Nux Vomica 马钱子 / 316
nyctalopia 雀盲 / 621

O

obesity infertility 肥胖不孕 / 565
oblique insertion 斜刺 / 454
oblique lumbar pulling manipulation 斜扳腰椎法 / 653
oblique-running pulse 斜飞脉 / 163
Obscured Homalomena Rhizome 千年健 / 315
obstinate disease 固［痼］疾 / 524
obstinate phlegm 顽痰 / 72，528
obstruction-removing formula 通剂 / 359
obstructive sensation below the heart 心下支结 / 156
obstructive throat wind
obtaining *qi* 得气 / 456
occipital bone 玉枕骨，枕骨 / 46
occult disease 隐疾 / 524
ocular connector 目本，目系，眼系 / 610
ocular contusion 撞击伤目 / 621
odd-numbered formula/prescription 奇方 / 356
offensive breath smell 口气臭秽 / 142
offensive purgative (medicinal/drug) 攻下药 / 289
Officinal Magnolia Flower 厚朴花 / 327
oily sweat 油汗，汗出如油 / 145，146
ointment massage 膏摩 / 490
ointment 软膏 / 281
old disease 宿疾 / 524
Oldenlandia 白花蛇舌草 / 312
Olibanum 乳香 / 334
oligogalactia 缺乳 / 572
oligomenorrhea 月经后期 / 557
oliguria 少尿 / 150
ominous throat abscess 猛疽 / 629
omphalelcosis 脐疮 / 578
Omphalia 雷丸 / 353
omphalitis 脐痈 / 593
omphalorrhagia 脐血 / 578

omphalorrhea 脐湿 / 578
One Hundred Questions on Women's Diseases 女科百问 / 695
Oötheca Mantidis 桑螵蛸 / 350
open-closed reinforcement and reduction 开阖补泻 / 457
open-closed reinforcement-reduction method 开阖补泻法 / 457
open fracture 折骨列肤 / 635
"opening of smelling" 畜门 / 625
opening of the nasal cavity 鼻洞 / 38
opening of the pharynx 咽门 / 40
opening sweat pores 开鬼门 / 229
opening the "ghost gates" 开鬼门 / 229
opening the orifices 开窍 / 266
Ophicalcite 花蕊石 / 329
Ophicalcitum 花蕊石 / 329
Ophiopogon Decoction 麦门冬汤 / 378
ophryon 印堂，阙中，阙 / 43
ophthalmology 眼科（学） / 607
ophthalmopathy 障 / 612
opisthotonus 角弓反张 / 127
oral erosion 口糜 / 633
oral sore 口疳 / 580
oral ulcer during menstruation 经行口糜 / 563
Orange Fruit 枳壳 / 325
orbit bone 目眶骨 / 608
orbit 目眶 / 43，608
ordinary malaria 正疟 / 520
organ of conveyance 传导之官 / 27
organs containing visible substances 形脏 / 24
Oriental Wormwood Decoction 茵陈蒿汤 / 379
Orientvine Stem 青风藤 / 317
orifice 孔窍 / 38
orifice-opening medicinal/drug 开窍药 / 293
orifice pyorrhea 窍漏 / 615
original *qi* 元气，原气 / 53
original yang 元阳 / 23
original yang insufficiency 元阳亏虚 / 113
original yin 元阴 / 22
Orthodox Commentary of Medicine 医学正傳 / 703
Orthodox Manual of External Medicine 外科正宗 / 698
orthodromic abdominal breathing 顺腹式呼吸 / 497
orthopedics 正骨（科） / 635
Os Draconis Ustum 煅龙骨 / 350
Os Draconis 龙骨 / 337
Os Sepiae 海螵蛸 / 350
osteoma 骨瘤 / 598
osteopathy 骨病 / 654
Ostrea Powder 牡蛎散 / 374
otogenic intracranial infection 黄耳伤寒 / 624
otology 耳科（学） / 623
otopyorrhea 脓耳，聤耳 / 623
otopyorrhea with facial paralysis 脓耳口眼㖞斜 / 624
otopyorrheal vertigo 脓耳眩晕 / 625
outer aspect of the arm 臂外廉 / 47
outer canthus 外眦，目外眦 / 44，608
out-going *qi* 外气 / 500
Oven-earth Decoction 黄土汤 / 377
over-consumption of heart nutrient 心营过耗 / 100
overindulgence in raw and cold food 贪食生冷 / 70
overlapping of diseases 并病 / 178
overlapping of two yang diseases 二阳并病 / 178
over-restriction among the five elements/phases 五行相乘 / 12
overstrain 劳倦，劳伤 / 71
overstrain stranguria 劳淋 / 552
Oyster Shell 牡蛎 / 338

P

pacifying the liver 平肝 / 265
pacifying the liver and subduing yang 平肝潜阳 / 265
pacifying the liver to extinguish wind 平肝熄［息］风 / 266
Pagodatree Flower 槐花 / 329
Pagodatree Flower-bud 槐米 / 329
pain below the heart 心下痛 / 152
pain in the stomach 脘痛 / 152
pain of unfixed location 痛无定处 / 148
painful and swollen testis 睾丸肿痛 / 600
painful gum swelling 齿龈肿痛 / 137
painful menstruation 经行腹痛，痛经 / 158，560
painful swollen gum 齿龈肿痛 / 634
paired needling 偶刺 / 461
pairing of visceral organs 脏腑相合 / 26
pairing of *zang* and *fu* organs 脏腑相合 / 26

palatine uvula 悬雍垂 / 40
Pale Butterfly-bush Flower 密蒙花 / 305
pale complexion 面色苍白 / 125
pale helices 耳轮淡白 / 129
pale tongue 舌淡，淡白舌 / 131
pale white complexion 面色淡白 / 125
palm-kneading manipulation 掌揉法 / 647
palm measurement 一夫法 / 445
palm-pressing manipulation 掌按法 / 651
palm-pushing manipulation 掌推法 / 648
palm-pushing thoracic pulling manipulation 掌推扳胸椎法 / 652
palm-rubbing manipulation 掌擦法 / 650
palm-striking manipulation 掌击法 / 649
palm-to-palm pushing-pulling conduction of *qi* 对掌推拉导气 / 503
palmar circular rubbing manipulation 掌摩法 / 650
palmar infection 手心毒，掌心毒 / 592
palmar pustule 手心毒，掌心毒，托盘疔 / 592
Palmleaf Raspberry Fruit 覆盆子 / 351
palms and soles 五心烦热 / 144
palpating 摸法 / 482
palpation 按诊，切诊 / 158，165
palpation of the chest and abdomen 按胸腹 / 165
palpation of the epigastrium and abdomen 按脘腹 / 165
palpation of the forearm 按尺肤 / 165
palpation of the hands and feet 按手足 / 165
palpation of the skin 按肌肤 / 165
palpebra 胞睑，眼睑，胞脸，目胞，目裹 / 44，607
palpebral conjunctiva 睑内 / 45，609
palpebral margin 睑弦 / 44，608
palpitations 心悸 / 151，530
palpitations below the heart 心下悸 / 151
Pang Anshi 庞安时 / 662
Pangguangshu (BL 28) 膀胱俞 / 420
Pangolin Scale 穿山甲 / 333
Paniculate Swallowwort Root 徐长卿 / 317
pannus 赤膜，红膜，白膜蔽睛 / 612，617
panting 喘，喘促，喘急 / 140，141
Pao Zhi Da Quan 炮炙大全 / 689
papule 丘疹 / 591
paradoxical treatment 反治 / 220
paralytic strabismus 风牵偏视 / 622
paraphrasia 错语 / 140
parasitic abdominal pain 虫积腹痛 / 546，588
parasitic epilepsy 虫痫 / 590
parasitic toxin 蛊毒 / 69
parasitic worms 诸虫 / 72
parched teeth 齿焦 / 137
Paris Rhizome 重楼 / 311
parous vaginal orifice 胞门 / 555
partition of the tongue 舌的分部 / 130
parturition 分娩 / 568
parturient diseases 临产病 / 569
parturient vaginal orifice 产门 / 555
paste 膏，膏剂 / 281
pasted pill 糊丸 / 280
pastil 锭，锭剂 / 281
patella 膝髌 / 50
pathogen 邪，邪气 / 62
pathogeneses of six meridians/channels 六经病机 / 115
pathogenesis of *jueyin* (reverting yin) disease 厥阴病机 / 116
pathogenesis of *shaoyang* (lesser yang) disease 少阳病机 / 115
pathogenesis of *shaoyin* (lesser yin) disease 少阴病机 / 115
pathogenesis of *taiyang* (greater yang) disease 太阳病机 / 115
pathogenesis of *taiyin* (greater yin) disease 太阴病机 / 115
pathogenesis of the exterior and interior 表里病机 / 81
pathogenesis of *yangming* (yang brightness) disease 阳明病机 / 115
pathogenesis of *zang-fu* organs 脏腑病机 / 96
pathogenic cold 寒邪 / 64
pathogenic dampness 湿邪 / 65
pathogenic dryness 燥邪 / 66
pathogenic fire 火邪 / 66
pathogenic heat 热邪 / 67
pathogenic *qi* 邪气 / 62
pathogenic summerheat 暑邪 / 65
pathogenic warmth 温邪 / 67
pathogenic water 水气 / 66
pathogenic wind 风邪 / 64
pathogenic wind-cold 风寒邪气 / 67
pathogenic wind-cold-dampness

风寒湿邪 / 68
pathogenic wind-dampness 风湿邪气 / 68
pathogenic wind-heat 风热邪气 / 67
pathogenic wind-warmth 风温邪气 / 67
pathological diathesis 病理体质 / 74
pathological state of a disease 病能［态］/ 78
pathomechanism 病机 / 78
Patient Dock Root 牛西西 / 330
Patrinia 败酱草 / 312
pattern identification 辨证 / 122，168
pattern identification and treatment 辨证施治 / 218
pattern identification of gastro-intestinal diseases 胃肠病辨证 / 207
pattern identification of heart diseases 心病辨证 / 200
pattern identification of kidney and bladder diseases 肾膀胱病辨证 / 212
pattern identification of liver and gallbladder diseases 肝胆病辨证 / 208
pattern identification of lung diseases 肺病辨证 / 202
pattern identification of spleen diseases 脾病辨证 / 205
pattern manifestation 证候 / 168
pattern type 证型 / 168
patting 拍法 / 483
patting stick 振挺 / 654
patting-striking manipulation 拍击法 / 649
peach-like eyelid swelling 胞肿如桃 / 614
Peach Seed 桃仁 / 330
Pearl 珍珠 / 337
pecking 啄击法 / 484
pecking manipulation 啄法 / 650
pecking moxibustion 雀啄灸 / 464
pectoral muscle 臆 / 47
pectoral *qi* 宗气 / 54
peeled tongue 光剥舌 / 136
peeling coating/fur 剥苔 / 135
peeling of the tongue coating/fur 舌苔脱落 / 135
Peking Euphorbia Root 京大戟 / 324
pellet 丹，丹剂 / 281
penetration needling 透刺 / 454
penial cancer 肾岩 / 598
penis 阴茎，茎 / 49
penis and testes 茎垂 / 49
pensiveness 思 / 69
Pepper Fruit 胡椒 / 318
Peppermint 薄荷 / 297
Pepperweed Seed 葶苈子 / 303
perianal abscess 肠痔 / 599
peri-ankle manipulation 抱踝手法 / 648
peri-auricular sore 旋耳疮 / 623
pericardial fluid retention syndrome/pattern 饮停心包证 / 188
pericardium meridian/channel (PC) 手厥阴心包经 / 404
pericardium meridian/channel of hand reverting yin 手厥阴心包经 / 404
pericardium 心包 / 23
Pericarpium Arecae 大腹皮 / 321
Pericarpium Citri Reticulatae Viride 青皮 / 325
Pericarpium Citri Reticulatae 陈皮 / 325
Pericarpium Granati 石榴皮 / 349
Pericarpium Lagenariae 葫芦 / 323
Pericarpium Papaveris 罂粟壳 / 302，350
Pericarpium Zanthoxy 花椒 / 318
Perilla Fruit 紫苏子 / 303
Perilla Leaf 紫苏叶 / 296
Perilla Stem 紫苏梗 / 326
perineum 会阴 / 48
Periostracum Cicadae 蝉蜕 / 298
Periostracum Serpentis 蛇蜕 / 315
peripatellapexor 抱膝器 / 641
peri-umbilical abdomen 脐腹 / 48
perlèche 燕口疮 / 579
perpendicular insertion 直刺 / 454
perpendicular penetration 直透 / 454
Persimmon Calyx 柿蒂 / 328
person of greater yang 太阳之人 / 74
person of greater yin 太阴之人 / 74
person of lesser yang 少阳之人 / 74
person of lesser yin 少阴之人 / 74
pertussis 百日咳 / 586
pestilence 温［瘟］疫 / 515
pestilent boil 疫疔 / 592
pestilential *qi* 疠气，戾气 / 63
pestilential toxin 疫毒 / 63
pestilential toxin syndrome/pattern 疫毒证 / 200
petaloid gum 齿龈结瓣 / 634
petaloid nebula with sunken center 花翳白陷 / 618
Petiolus Trachycarpi Carbonisatus 棕榈炭 / 329
Pharbitis Seed 牵牛子 / 323

pharyngitis 咽痹，喉痹 / 629，630

pharyngolaryngology 咽喉科学 / 628

pharynx 咽，嗌，喉嗌 / 40，628

pharynx impediment 咽痹 / 629

philtrum 人中 / 46

phlegm 痰 / 71

phlegm clouding the mind 痰蒙心神 / 100

phlegm clouding the pericardium 痰蒙心包 / 100

phlegm constipation 痰秘 / 544

phlegm cough 痰咳 / 526

phlegm cyst 痰包 / 634

phlegm-dampness 痰湿 / 72

phlegm-dampness cough 痰湿咳嗽 / 526

phlegm-dampness diathesis 痰湿质 / 75

phlegm-dampness infertility 痰湿不孕 / 565

phlegm-dampness obstructing the lung 痰湿阻肺 / 110

phlegm-dispelling formula 祛痰剂 / 380

phlegm dyspnea 痰喘 / 527

phlegm epilepsy 痰痫 / 590

phlegm-fire harassing the heart 痰火扰心 / 101

phlegm-fire tinnitus 痰火耳鸣 / 624

phlegm-fluid retention 痰饮 / 528

phlegm-heat blocking the lung 痰热闭肺 / 110

phlegm misting the heart orifices 痰迷心窍 / 100

phlegm node on the eyelid 胞生痰核 / 613

phlegm rale 痰鸣 / 141

phlegm stuffiness 痰痞 / 542

phlegm syncope 痰厥 / 538

phlegm syndrome/pattern 痰证 / 189

phlegm turbidity 痰浊 / 72

phlegmon 发，疽 / 594

phlegmon of the dorsum of the foot 足发背 / 594

phlegmon of the dorsum of the hand 手发背 / 594

phlegmonous mastitis 乳发 / 596

phlegm-resolving medicinal/drug 化痰药 / 292

phlegm-resolving, cough-stopping and asthma-relieving medicinal/drug 化痰止咳平喘药 / 292

phlegm-turbidity headache 痰浊头痛 / 533

phlegm-turbidity obstructing the lung 痰浊阻肺 / 110

phlegm-turbidity syndrome 痰浊证 / 189

phlyctenular conjunctivitis 金疳，金疡 / 617

phlyctenular kerato-conjunctivitis 白膜侵睛 / 617

photophobia 羞明，畏明，羞明畏日 / 610

phthisis 劳［痨］瘵 / 529

phthisis (disease) 痨病 / 529

phthisis sore 疮痨 / 596

physique and *qi* 形气 / 3

physique predominating *qi* 形胜气 / 126

physique 形，形体 / 2，57

Pi Wei Lun 脾胃论 / 694

Pianli (LI 6) 偏历 / 410

Pigen (EX-B 4) 痞根 / 441

pigeon chest 鸡胸 / 578

pigmentary retinopathy 高风内障，高风雀目 / 620，621

pile 痔 / 598

pile-driving standing posture 震桩式 / 503

pill 丸，丸剂 / 280

Pills of Five Kinds of Seeds for Offsprings 五子衍宗丸 / 389

pinching 捏法，捏积 / 482，486

pinching along the spine 捏脊 / 486

pinching and lifting 拧法 / 481

pinching manipulation 捏法 / 652

pinching needle insertion 提捏进针法 / 453

pinching the glabella 拧眉心 / 487

pinching therapy 撮痧疗法，抓痧疗法 / 469，470

pine-bark lichen 松皮癣 / 602

Pinellia Heart-purging Decoction 半夏泻心汤 / 366

Pinellia Tuber 半夏 / 298

Pinellia-Magnolia Decoction 半夏厚朴汤 / 375

pinguecula 黄油障，黄油证 / 618

Pingwei Powder 平胃散 / 379

Pipewort Flower 谷精草 / 304

Pishu (BL 20) 脾俞 / 420

pityriasis rosea 风热疮 / 602

Placenta Hominis 紫河车 / 342

placenta 人胞 / 555

Plain Questions 素问 / 683

Plain Questions of Huangdi's Internal Classic 黄帝内经素问 / 683

Plain Questions of Yellow Emperor's Canon of Medicine 黄帝内经素问 / 683

plain sitting 平坐 / 495

Plantain Herb 车前草 / 320

Plantain Seed 车前子 / 320

plantar pustule 足底疔 / 592
plantar wart 跖疣 / 600
plaster dermatitis 膏药风 / 603
Plastrum Testudinis 龟板 / 345
Platycodon Root 桔梗 / 299
pleural fluid retention 悬饮 / 528
pleurodiaphragmatic interspace 膜原 / 42
plum-blossom needle 梅花针 / 450
plump, fat and stout persons 肥膏肉人 / 75
Plum Flower 梅花 / 327
plump person 肥人，脂人 / 75
"plum-stone *qi*" 梅核气 / 535
plump tongue 舌胖 / 132
plump tongue body 舌体胖大 / 132
Plumula Nelumbinis 莲子心 / 305
Pohu (BL 42) 魄户 / 421
point combination 配穴法 / 447
point combination of the same meridian/channel 本经配穴法 / 447
point-hitting 点击法 / 481
point pressing 点法 / 481
point selection according to pattern identification 辨证选穴法 / 446
point selection according to symptoms 对症选穴法 / 446
point selection according to syndrome differentiation 辨证选穴法 / 446
points of the bladder meridian/channel 足太阳膀胱经穴 / 418
points of the conception vessel 任脉穴 / 435
points of the gallbladder meridian/channel 足少阳胆经穴 / 428
points of the governor vessel 督脉穴 / 433
points of the head and neck 头颈部穴 / 439
points of the heart meridian/channel 手少阴心经穴，足少阴肾经穴 / 416，423
points of the large intestine meridian/channel 手阳明大肠经穴 / 409
points of the liver meridian/channel 足厥阴肝经穴 / 432
points of the lower extremities 下肢穴 / 443
points of the lung meridian/channel 手太阴肺经穴 / 408
points of the pericardium meridian/channel 手厥阴心包经穴 / 425
points of the small intestine meridian/channel 手太阳小肠经穴 / 417
points of the spleen meridian/channel 足太阴脾经穴 / 414
points of the stomach meridian/channel 足阳明胃经穴 / 411
points of the triple energizer meridian/channel 手少阳三焦经穴 / 426
points of the upper extremities 上肢穴 / 442
points on the back 背部穴 / 441
points on the chest and abdomen 胸腹部穴 / 441
poisoning 中毒 / 72
Pokeberry Root 商陆 / 324
poking 拨法 / 485
poliomyelitis 小儿麻痹 / 590
Pollen Typhae 蒲黄 / 332
Pollen Typhae Carbonisatum 蒲黄炭 / 333
polymenorrhea 月经先期 / 557
polyphagia with frequent hunger 多食善饥 / 153
Polyporus 猪苓 / 320
polyuria 多尿 / 150
Pomegranate Rind 石榴皮 / 349
popliteal fossa 腘 / 50
popliteal sore 委中毒 / 593
Poppy Capsule 罂粟壳 / 302，350
Popular Prescriptions in Verse 时方歌括 / 693
Poria cum Radice Pino 茯神 / 337
Poria 茯苓 / 320
post-patellar fossa 膝腘 / 50
postauricular abscess 耳根痈 / 624
postauricular infection 耳根毒 / 624
postauricular phlegmon 耳后发 / 625
postauricular subperiosteal abscess 耳后附骨痈 / 624
posterior hairline 后发际 / 42
posterior oblique line of the vertex-temporal (MS 7) 顶颞后斜线 / 471
posterior splint 后侧夹板 / 640
posterior temporal line (MS 11) 颞后线 / 471
posterior yin 后阴 / 48
postmenopausal hemorrhage 经断复来 / 563
postnatal *qi* 后天之气 / 53
postpartum abdominal distension 产后腹胀 / 572
postpartum abdominal pain 产后腹痛 / 572
postpartum arthralgia 产后痹证 / 572
postpartum convulsions 产后病痉，产后痉证 / 572

postpartum convulsive disease 产后痉病 / 572
postpartum depression and dizziness 产后郁冒 / 571
postpartum diseases 产后病 / 570
postpartum dyschezia 产后大便难 / 571
postpartum edema 产后水肿 / 572
postpartum fainting 产后血晕 / 571
postpartum fever 产后发热 / 571
postpartum galactorrhea 产后乳汁自出 / 573
postpartum general aching 产后身痛 / 571
postpartum headache 产后头痛 / 571
postpartum hematuria 产后尿血 / 571
postpartum hypochondriac pain 产后胁痛 / 572
postpartum hypogalactia 产后缺乳 / 572
postpartum incontinence of urine 产后小便失禁 / 571
postpartum lumbago 产后腰痛 / 572
postpartum metrorrhagia 产后血崩 / 571
postpartum oligogalactia 产后缺乳 / 572
postpartum palpitations 产后怔忡 / 571
postpartum retention of urine 产后小便不通 / 571
postpartum warm disease 产后病温 / 571
posture management 身法，调身 / 493
posturization 姿式 / 493
pottery cup 陶罐 / 467
pounding 捣法，捣击法 / 481
pouring diarrhea 注泄，泄注 / 150
powder 散，散剂 / 280，281
Powder of Five Medicinals with Poria 五苓散 / 379
pox 痘 / 584
practicing *qigong* 练功 / 499
prancing to conduct *qi* in a burst 腾跃爆发导气 / 504
precedence of pulse over symptoms 舍症从脉 / 165
precedence of symptoms over pulse 舍脉从症 / 165
Precious Writings of Bianque 扁鹊心书 / 700
precordial pain radiating to the back 心痛彻背 / 151
precordial sweating 心汗 / 145
preference for pressing 喜按 / 166
pregnancy 妊娠 / 564
pregnancy mastitis 内吹乳痈 / 596
pregnancy pulse 喜脉 / 163
premature amniotic rupture 沥胞生，沥浆生，沥浆产 / 569
premature ejaculation 早泄 / 156，552
premature rupture of fetal membrane 胞衣先破 / 569
premature whitening of the hair 须发早白 / 139
premenstrual syndrome 经行情志异常 / 563
prenatal *qi* 先天之气 / 53
preparation form 剂型 / 280
Prepared Daughter Root of Common Monkshood 附子 / 317
Prepared Dried Ginger 炮姜 / 318
Prepared Fleeceflower Root 制何首乌 / 344
Prepared Licorice Root 炙甘草 / 341
Prepared Mother Root of Common Monkshood 制川乌 / 314
Prepared Rehmannia Root 熟地黄 / 342
prescription 药方，方剂 / 356
Prescriptions for Succoring the Sick 济生方 / 691
Prescriptions for Universal Relief 普济方 / 692
Prescriptions in Rhymes 汤头歌诀 / 692
presence of vitality 得神 / 123
preservation of the breath 存息 / 498
preservation of the mind 存神 / 498
preservation of thought 存想 / 499
pressing 按法 / 159，480
pressing and kneading *Fengchi* (GB 20) 按揉风池 / 489
pressing and kneading the neck 按揉颈项 / 488
pressing and pinching the nose bridge 按捏鼻梁 / 488
pressing down with the foot 足蹬 / 639
pressing-grasping 捺法 / 483
pressing hand 押手 / 453
pressing manipulation 按法 / 651
pressing moxibustion 实按灸 / 466
pressing the auricular points 按压耳穴 / 488

pressing the ear orifice 按捺耳窍 / 488
pressing the four canthi 按目四眦 / 487
pressing the spine 夹脊 / 506
pressing the temples 按太阳 / 487
pressing *Yingxiang* (LI 20) 按迎香 / 488
pressure pad 压垫，压力垫 / 641
prevalent seasonal epidemic 天行时疫 / 514
preventing miscarriage 安胎 / 268
preventive treatment 治未病 / 219
Priceless Plaster 金不换膏 / 395
pricking method 挑刺法 / 449
prickles on the tongue 舌起芒刺 / 132
prickly heat 痱(子) / 601
prickly tongue 芒刺舌 / 133
Prickly-ash Peel 花椒 / 318
primary infertility 全不产 / 565
primary-secondary point combination 主应配穴法 / 448
Prince's-feather Fruit 水红花子 / 332
principal, adjuvant, auxiliary and conductant 主辅佐引 / 358
Principles and Prohibitions of the Medical Profession 医门法律 / 701
Principles of Buddhist Cultivation 修习止观坐禅法要 / 700
Principles of Correct Diet 饮膳正要 / 689
Principles of Gynecology and Obstetrics 女科经纶 / 695
processing (of materia medica) 炮制，炮炙，修治 / 275
processing of medicinal substances 药材炮制 / 275
profuse clear urine 尿清长 / 150
profuse dreaming 多梦 / 155
profuse menstruation 月水过多，月经过多 / 157，560
profuse nasal bleeding 鼻洪 / 628
profuse sputum 痰多 / 137
profuse sweating 大汗 / 144
progressive deafness 渐聋 / 625
prolapse of the rectum 脱肛 / 599
prolapse of the uterus 阴挺 / 564
prolonged menstruation 经期延长 / 559
prominent muscle 胂 / 47
promoting digestion 消食 / 251
promoting digestion and relieving distension 消食下气 / 252
promoting digestion and removing (food) stagnation 消食导滞 / 251
promoting digestion and resolving (food) stagnation 消食化滞 / 251
promoting digestion to harmonize the middle (energizer) 消食和中 / 252
promoting digestion to harmonize the stomach 消食和胃 / 252
promoting eruption 透疹 / 229
promoting eruption of macules 透斑 / 229
promoting lactation 下乳 / 268
promoting rupture 溃坚 / 270
promoting suppuration 攻溃 / 270
promoting suppuration to regenerate flesh 煨脓长肉 / 270
promoting tissue regeneration 生肌 / 270
promoting tissue regeneration and closing the wound 生肌收口 / 270
promoting tissue regeneration and wound healing 生肌敛疮 / 270
property and flavor 气味，性味 / 278
propping with a lever 杠杆支撑 / 639
prostatic hypertrophy 精癃 / 600
protracted dysentery 迁延痢 / 522
protruding and waggling of tongue 吐弄舌 / 134
protruding bone 高骨 / 51
protruding tongue 吐舌 / 134
protrusion of the eyeball 眼球突出 / 128
proven formula 验方 / 357
proximal bleeding 近血 / 550
proximate needling 傍针刺 / 462
pruritus vulvae 阴痒 / 147
Pseudobulbus Cremastrae seu Pleiones 山慈菇 / 300
pseudo-cold 假寒 / 91
pseudo-heat 假热 / 91
pseudopregnancy 鬼胎 / 567
pseudopterygium 流金凌木 / 615
psoriasis 白疕 / 602
pterygium 胬肉扳睛，胬肉攀睛，胬肉侵睛 / 615
Pu Ji Ben Shi Fang 普济本事方 / 691
Pu Ji Fang 普济方 / 692
Pubescent Angelica and Loranthus Decoction 独活寄生汤 / 377
Pubescent Holly Root 毛冬青 / 334

pubic bone 横骨 / 48
pubic symphysis 曲骨 / 48
Pucan (BL 61) 仆参 / 423
Pueraria-Scutellaria-Coptis Decoction 葛根黄芩黄连汤 / 367
puerperal epidemic febrile disease 产后病温 / 571
puerperal mastitis 外吹乳痈 / 596
puerperal phthisis 蓐劳 / 572
puerperal tetanus 蓐风 / 572
Puff-ball 马勃 / 313
puffiness of the eyelids 目窠上微肿 / 128
puffy face 面浮 / 125
Puji Xiaodu Decoction 普济消毒饮 / 368
pulling 扯法，扳法 / 483，485
pulling and stretching 引伸法 / 485
Pulling-aright Powder 牵正散 / 377
pulling for congestion 扯痧 / 486
pulling-kneading reduction 拔伸捏正 / 640
pulling manipulation 扳法 / 652
pulling pain 掣痛 / 148
pulling-pushing manipulation 牵推法 / 642
pulling, stretching and traction 拔伸牵引 / 638
pulling-stretching manipulation 拔伸法 / 653
pulling-stretching reduction 拔伸复位 / 640
Pulsatilla Decoction 白头翁汤 / 369
Pulse-activating Drink 生脉饮 / 389
Pulse Classic 脉经 / 686
pulse condition 脉象 / 158
pulse diagnosis 脉诊 / 158
pulse manifestation 脉象 / 158
pulse on the back of the wrist 反关脉 / 163
pulse taking 切脉 / 158
pulse-taking with one finger 单按 / 159
pulse-taking with three fingers 总按 / 159
pulse-to-disease correspondence 脉象主病 / 158
pulse with root 脉有根 / 164
pulse with stomach *qi* 脉有胃气 / 164
pulse with vitality 脉有神 / 164
pulse without stomach *qi* 脉无胃气 / 164
Pummelo Peel 化橘红 / 327
Pumpkin Seed 南瓜子 / 353
Puncture-vine Caltrop Fruit 蒺藜 / 339
puncturing and moxibustion 刺灸法 / 444
puncturing (technique) 刺法 / 444
pungent-cool exterior-releasing formula 辛凉解表剂 / 362
pungent-cool exterior-releasing medicinal/drug 辛凉解表药 / 288
pungent-warm exterior-releasing formula 辛温解表剂 / 361
pungent-warm exterior-releasing medicinal/drug 辛温解表药 / 288
pupil 金井，瞳人，瞳仁，瞳子，瞳神 / 609
pupil and intra-ocular tissues 瞳神 / 609
pupillary metamorphosis 瞳人干缺，瞳神干缺，瞳神缺陷 / 619
pure yang constitution 纯阳之体 / 574
purgation 泻下，攻下，通下 / 236
purgative (medicinal/drug) 泻下药 / 289
purgative formula 泄剂，泻下剂 / 360，363
purgative method 下法 / 235
purging for the diarrhetic 通因通用 / 221
purging heart fire 泻心火 / 234
purging heat to preserve fluids 泄热存津 / 231
purging heat with bitter-cold 苦寒泄热 / 231
purging the heart 泻心 / 234
purging the liver 泻肝 / 233
purging the lung 泻肺 / 235
purging the lung to relieve dyspnea 泻肺平喘 / 235
Purple Cowry Shell 紫贝齿 / 337
purple lips 唇紫 / 136
Purple Rock Salt 紫硇砂 / 355
Purple Snowy Powder 紫雪 / 392
purple tongue 紫舌 / 131
purpura 紫斑 / 550
pursed mouth 撮口，口撮 / 136，575
Purslane Herb 马齿苋 / 309
purulent and bloody stool 脓血便 / 150
purulent keratitis 凝脂翳 / 618
purulent toxin syndrome/pattern 脓毒证 / 199
pushing 推法 / 159，482
pushing manipulation 推法 / 648
pushing-pulling 推扳手法 / 486
pushing upwards with both hands 双手托天式 / 654

pushing with the knee 膝顶 / 639
pustulating moxibustion 化脓灸 / 465
pustule 脓疱 / 591
putrid belching 嗳腐 / 153
putrid-blood-induced heart crisis 败血冲心 / 570
putrid-blood-induced lung crisis 败血冲肺 / 570
putrid-blood-induced stomach crisis 败血冲胃 / 571
pylorus 幽门 / 41
pyosepticemia 走黄 / 595
Pyrite 自然铜 / 335
Pyritum 自然铜 / 335
Pyrola Herb 鹿衔草 / 345

Q

qi 气 / 2，53
qi-accumulation abdominal pain 气积腹痛 / 588
qi activity 气机 / 2，56
qi-aspect heat-clearing formula 清气分热剂 / 367
qi aspect 气分 / 56
qi aspect syndrome/pattern 气分证 / 179
qi block syndrome/pattern 气闭证 / 182
qi blockage 气闭 / 94
qi-blood deficiency diathesis 气血两虚质 / 75
qi-blood deficiency dysmenorrhea 气血虚弱痛经 / 560
qi-blood pattern identification 气血辨证 / 182
qi-blood stagnation syndrome/pattern 气血瘀滞证 / 186
qi-blood syndrome differentiation 气血辨证 / 182
qi-blood tonifying formula 气血双补剂 / 372
Qi Bo 岐伯 / 658
qi collapse 气脱 / 93
qi collapse syndrome/pattern 气脱证 / 182
qi-concentrated single-finger pushing manipulation 一指禅推法 / 648
qi-concentrated single-finger pushing therapy 一指禅推拿疗法 / 648
qi-conducting method 行气法 / 459
qi constipation 气秘 / 544
qi counterflow 气逆 / 94
qi counterflow syndrome/pattern 气逆证 / 182
qi deficiency 气虚 / 92
qi deficiency and blood stasis 气虚血瘀 / 96
qi-deficiency common cold 气虚感冒 / 516
qi-deficiency cough 气虚咳嗽 / 526
qi deficiency dizziness 气虚眩晕 / 532
qi deficiency failing to control the blood 气虚不摄 / 94
qi deficiency habitual abortion 气虚滑胎 / 569
qi-deficiency headache 气虚头痛 / 534
qi deficiency metrorrhagia and metrostaxis 气虚崩漏 / 561
qi deficiency syndrome/pattern 气虚证 / 182
qi deficiency vertigo 气虚眩晕 / 532
qi deficiency with abdominal fullness 气虚中满 / 95
qi-deficient early periods 气虚经行先期 / 557
qi depression 气郁 / 93
qi depression syndrome/pattern 气郁证 / 182
qi-descending formula 降气剂 / 375
Qi Dezhi 齐德之 / 666
qi dysphagia 气鬲 / 586
qi-emitting hand gesture 发气手势 / 504
qi goiter 气瘿 / 597
qi-hastening method 催气法 / 454
qi (infantile) malnutrition 气疳 / 581
qi movement 气机 / 2，56
qi-moving formula 行气剂 / 374
qi-moving medicinal/drug 行气药 / 291
qi nebula 气翳 / 619
qi of water and grain; *qi* of food and drink 水谷之气 / 53
qi of *zang* organs 脏气 / 26
"*qi* opening" 气口 / 160
qi orbiculus 气轮 / 44，607
qi pass 气关 / 138
qi pathway 气街 / 48
"*qi* portal" 气门 / 41
qi predominating physique 气胜形 / 126
qi-regulating formula 理气剂 / 374
qi-regulating medicinal/drug 理气药 / 290
qi sinking 气陷 / 94
qi sinking metrorrhagia 气陷血崩 / 561
qi sinking syndrome/pattern 气陷证 / 182
qi-stagnant abdominal pain 气滞腹痛 / 546
Qi-stagnant Gastralgia Relieving Granules 气滞胃痛颗粒 / 387

qi-stagnant late periods 气滞经行后期 / 558
qi stagnation 气滞 / 93
qi stagnation and blood stasis 气滞血瘀 / 96
qi stagnation due to congealing cold 寒凝气滞 / 94
qi stagnation dysmenorrhea 气滞痛经 / 560
qi-stagnation lumbago 气滞腰痛 / 554
qi stagnation metrorrhagia 气郁血崩 / 562
qi stagnation syndrome/pattern 气滞证 / 182
qi stranguria 气淋 / 552
qi stuffiness 气痞 / 542
qi syncope 气厥 / 538
qi tonic 补气药 / 293
qi-tonifying formula 补气剂 / 371
qi-tonifying medicinal/drug 补气药 / 293
qi transformation 气化 / 2，56
qi tumor 气瘤 / 598
Qi Xiao Liang Fang 奇效良方 / 692
qi-yin insufficiency syndrome/pattern 气阴亏虚证 / 184
Qi Zhongfu 齐仲甫 / 664
Qian Jin Yao Fang 千金要方 / 690
Qian Jin Yi Fang 千金翼方 / 690
Qian Yi 钱乙 / 662
Qian Zhongyang 钱仲阳 / 662
Qianding (GV 21) 前顶 / 435
Qiangjian (GV 18) 强间 / 434
Qiangu (SI 2) 前谷 / 417
Qianzheng Powder 牵正散 / 377
Qichong (ST 30) 气冲 / 413
Qiduan (EX-LE 12) 气端 / 444
qigong therapy 气功疗法 / 492
qigong 气功 / 491
Qihai (CV 6) 气海 / 435
Qihaishu (BL 24) 气海俞 / 420
Qihu (ST 13) 气户 / 412
Qiju Dihuang Pills 杞菊地黄丸 / 389
Qili Powder 七厘散 / 396
Qimen (LR 14) 期门 / 433
Qin Yueren 秦越人 / 658
Qinggu Powder 清骨散 / 369
Qinghao Biejia Decoction 青蒿鳖甲汤 / 369
Qingkailing Injection 清开灵注射液 / 384
Qinglengyuan (TE 11) 清冷渊 / 427
Qingling (HT 2) 青灵 / 416
Qingwei Powder 清胃散 / 368
Qingying Decoction 清营汤 / 367
Qingzao Jiufei Decoction 清燥救肺汤 / 378
Qipi Pills 启脾丸 / 387
Qishe (ST 11) 气舍 / 412
Qiuhou (EX-HN 7) 球后 / 440
Qiuxu (GB 40) 丘墟 / 431
Qixue (KI 13) 气穴 / 424
Qizhi Weitong Granules 气滞胃痛颗粒 / 387
Quan Guo Zhong Cao Yao Hui Bian 全国中草药汇编 / 690
Quanliao (SI 18) 颧髎 / 418
Quanlu Pills 全鹿丸 / 390
Qubin (GB 7) 曲鬓 / 429
Qucha (*Quchai*) (BL 4) 曲差 / 419
Quchi (LI 11) 曲池 / 410
quenching 淬 / 278
quenching thirst 止渴 / 267
Quepen (ST 12) 缺盆 / 412
Qugu (CV 2) 曲骨 / 435
quick-acting formula 急方 / 357
Quick-acting Heart-saving Pills 速效救心丸 / 394
quick pricking 点刺 / 449
quick-slow reinforcement and reduction 疾徐补泻 / 457
quick-slow reinforcing-reducing method 疾徐补泻法 / 458
quick withdrawal of the needle 迅速出针法，快速起针法 / 462，463
quiescence within motion 动中有静 / 492
quieting ascaris 安蛔 / 271
quieting ascaris to relieve pain 安蛔定痛 / 271
Ququan (LR 8) 曲泉 / 432
Quyuan (SI 13) 曲垣 / 418
Quze (PC 3) 曲泽 / 426

R

rabid dog bite 癫狗咬伤 / 71
racing pulse 疾脉 / 162
Radish Seed 莱菔子 / 352
Radix Acanthopanacis Senticosi 刺五加 / 341
Radix Achyranthis Asperae 土牛膝 / 313
Radix Achyranthis Bidentatae 牛膝 / 344
Radix Aconiti 川乌 / 314
Radix Aconiti Kusnezoffii 草乌 / 314
Radix Aconiti Lateralis Preparata 附子 / 317
Radix Aconiti Preparata 制川乌 / 314
Radix Adenophorae 南沙参 / 300
Radix Ampelopsis 白蔹 / 312
Radix Angelicae Dahuricae 白芷 / 295

Radix Angelicae Pubescentis 独活 / 314
Radix Angelicae Sinensis 当归 / 342
Radix Aristolochiae 青木香 / 321
Radix Arnebiae seu Lithospermi 紫草 / 306
Radix Asparagi 天冬 / 343
Radix Asteris 紫菀 / 299
Radix Astragali 黄芪 / 340
Radix Aucklandiae 木香 / 326
Radix Berberidis 三颗针 / 307
Radix Boehmeriae 苎麻根 / 329
Radix Bupleuri 柴胡 / 297
Radix Clematidis 威灵仙 / 314
Radix Codonopsis 党参 / 340
Radix Curcumae 郁金 / 331
Radix Cyathulae 川牛膝 / 331
Radix Cynanchi Atrati 白薇 / 307
Radix Cynanchi Paniculati 徐长卿 / 317
Radix Dichroae 常山 / 298
Radix Dipsaci 续断 / 347
Radix Ephedrae 麻黄根 / 348
Radix et Rhizoma Nardostachyos 甘松 / 326
Radix et Rhizoma Rhei 大黄 / 352
Radix Euphorbiae Ebractealatae 狼毒 / 324
Radix Euphorbiae Kansui 甘遂 / 324
Radix Euphorbiae Pekinensis 京大戟 / 324
Radix Gentianae 龙胆 / 308
Radix Gentianae Macrophyllae 秦艽 / 314
Radix Ginseng 人参 / 340
Radix Glehniae 北沙参 / 343
Radix Glycyrrhizae 甘草 / 340
Radix Glycyrrhizae Preparata 炙甘草 / 341
Radix Hedysari 红芪 / 340
Radix Isatidis 板蓝根 / 310
Radix Linderae 乌药 / 326
Radix llicis Pubescentis 毛冬青 / 334
Radix Morindae Officinalis 巴戟天 / 347
radix nasi 鼻根，頞，山根 / 39，626
Radix Notoginseng 三七 / 328
Radix Ophiopogonis 麦冬 / 343
Radix Paeoniae Alba 白芍 / 342
Radix Paeoniae Rubra 赤芍 / 306
Radix Panacis Quinquefolii 西洋参 / 343
Radix Peucedani 前胡 / 300
Radix Physochlainae 华山参 / 304
Radix Phytolaccae 商陆 / 324
Radix Platycodi 桔梗 / 299
Radix Polygalae 远志 / 336
Radix Polygoni Multiflori 何首乌 / 344
Radix Polygoni Multiflori Preparata 制何首乌 / 344
Radix Pseudostellariae 太子参 / 340
Radix Puerariae 葛根 / 297
Radix Pulsatillae 白头翁 / 308
Radix Rehmanniae Praeparata 熟地黄 / 342
Radix Rehmanniae 地黄 / 306
Radix Rhapontici 漏芦 / 312
Radix Rubiae 茜草 / 328
Radix Rumecis Patientiae 牛西西 / 330
Radix Salviae Miltiorrhizae 丹参 / 331
Radix Sanguisorbae 地榆 / 329
Radix Saposhnikoviae 防风 / 295
Radix Scrophulariae 玄参 / 306
Radix Scutellariae 黄芩 / 307
Radix Sophorae Flavescentis 苦参 / 308
Radix Sophorae Tonkinensis 山豆根 / 313
Radix Stellariae 银柴胡 / 306
Radix Stemonae 百部 / 302
Radix Stephaniae Tetrandrae 防己 / 317
Radix Trichosanthis 天花粉 / 300
Radix Zanthoxyli 两面针 / 333
raising the middle *qi* 升举中气 / 246
Ramie Root 苎麻根 / 329
Ramulus Cinnamomi 桂枝 / 295
Ramulus Mori 桑枝 / 315
Ramulus Taxilli 桑寄生 / 344
Ramulus Uncariae cum Uncis 钩藤 / 338
Rangoon-creeper Fruit 使君子 / 353
Rangu (KI 2) 然谷 / 424
rapid pulse 数脉 / 160
rapping 拳击法 / 483
rash 疹，痧 / 139，583，591
real headache 真头痛 / 533
real heart pain 真心痛 / 530
real stroke 真中 / 536
real wind stroke 真中风 / 536
Realgar 雄黄 / 354
Realgar 雄黄 / 354
recent contraction 新感 / 515
recent illness 新病 / 515
recipe 方剂 / 356
Recordings of the Art of Health and Life Preservation 养性延命录 / 700
Records of Traditional Chinese and Western Medicine in Combination 医学衷中参西

录 / 702
Recovery from All Ailments 万病回春 / 703
rectal polyp 息肉痔 / 599
rectovesical fistula 交肠 / 599
recurrent headache 头风 / 533
red discoloration 赤色 / 126
red discoloration of the white of the eye 白睛红赤 / 129
"red dragon stirring the sea" 赤龙搅海 / 506
red dysentery 赤痢 / 522
red eye 赤眼 / 616
Red Halloysite 赤石脂 / 349
red-hot needling 焠刺 / 460
red membrane 赤膜，红膜 / 612
red nose 赤鼻 / 601
Red Peony Root 赤芍 / 306
red-streaked boil 红丝疔 / 592
red swollen helices 耳轮红肿 / 129
Red Tangerine Peel 橘红 / 325
Red Tangerine Pills 橘红丸 / 383
red tongue 红舌，舌红 / 131
red vessels crossing the eye 赤脉贯睛/ 612
red vessels invading the eye 赤脉侵睛 / 612
red vessels passing the eye 赤脉传睛 / 611
red-white dysentery 赤白痢 / 522
reddened complexion 面红 / 125
reddish leukorrhea 赤白带 / 564
reddish vaginal discharge 赤白带下 / 158
redness and swelling of the bulbar conjunctiva 白睛赤肿 / 611
redness of the white of the eye 白睛红赤 / 611
Redness-removing Powder 导赤散 / 368
reduction 整复，复位 / 638，642
reduction of fracture 断骨接整 / 638
Reed Rhizome 芦根 / 305
referred testicular pain 控睾 / 154
refined essence 精微 / 57
refined juice 精汁 / 57
refusal of pressure 拒按 / 166
regular edema 正水 / 549
regular meridians/channels 正经 / 398
regularly intermittent pulse 代脉 / 162
regulating blood 理血 / 256
regulating menstruation 调经 / 268
regulating *qi* and activating blood 理气活血 / 253
regulating *qi* and blood 调理气血 / 239
regulating *qi* and harmonizing blood 理气和血 / 239
regulating *qi* and harmonizing the stomach 理气和胃 / 238
regulating *qi* and invigorating the spleen 理气健脾 / 253
regulating *qi* and relieving depression 理气解郁 / 255
regulating *qi* and removing stagnation 理气导滞 / 255
regulating *qi* and resolving blood stasis 理气化瘀 / 256
regulating *qi* and resolving dampness 理气化湿 / 255
regulating *qi* and resolving phlegm 理气化痰 / 253
regulating *qi* to activate blood 理气活血 / 253
regulating *qi* to promote menstrual discharge 理气通经 / 256
regulating *qi* to quiet the fetus 理气安胎 / 256
regulating *qi* to relieve distension 理气消胀 / 255
regulating *qi* to relieve pain 理气止痛 / 252，256
regulating *qi* to relieve stuffiness 理气消痞 / 253
regulating *qi* 理气 / 252
regulating the middle 理中 / 238
regurgitation 反胃，胃反 / 152，543
Rehmannia Pills 地黄丸 / 389
Rehmannia Root 地黄 / 306
reinforcement and reduction manipulations in massotherapy 推拿的补泻手法 / 490
reinforcement and reduction manipulations in *tuina* therapy 推拿的补泻手法 / 490
reinforcement followed by elimination 先补后攻 / 220
reinforcement-reduction by choosing direction 择向补泻法 / 491
reinforcement-reduction by massaging along or against the meridian/channel 迎随顺逆补泻法 / 491
reinforcement-reduction by varying the force and speed 轻重徐疾补泻法 / 491
reinforcemnt for elimination 寓攻于补 / 220
reinforcing fire to generate earth 补火生土 / 251
reinforcing healthy *qi* and

releasing the exterior 扶正解表 / 230
reinforcing relationship 相须 / 358
reinforcing the healthy (*qi*) 扶正 / 219
reinforcing the healthy and eliminating the pathogenic 扶正祛邪 / 219
reinforcing the healthy and strengthening the base 扶正固本 / 220
reinforcing the healthy with elimination of the pathogenic 扶正兼祛邪 / 219
reinforcing yang 扶阳 / 250
rejoining 接法 / 639
relapse due to diet 食复 / 71
relapse due to overexertion 劳复 / 71
relapse due to sex 女劳复 / 71
relaxation 松 / 493
relaxation exercise 放松功 / 500
relaxed stomach 胃缓 / 546
relaxing and purging 通泄 / 237
relaxing needling 恢刺 / 461
relaxing tendons and activating collaterals 舒筋活络 / 257
relaxing tendons and harmonizing collaterals 舒筋和络 / 257
relaxing tendons and unblocking collaterals 舒筋通络 / 257
relaxing tendons to relieve pain 舒筋止痛 / 257
relaxing the bowels 通便 / 236
relaxing the bowels and purging heat 通腑泄热 / 237
releasing both the exterior and interior 表里双解 / 230
releasing the exterior 解表 / 225
releasing the exterior and clearing heat 解表清热 / 225
releasing the exterior and clearing the lung 解表清肺 / 225
releasing the exterior and moistening dryness 疏表润燥 / 227
releasing the exterior to promote eruption 解表透疹 / 226
releasing the exterior with pungent-cool (medicinals) 辛凉解表 / 225
releasing the exterior with pungent-warm (medicinals) 辛温解表 / 225
releasing the flesh 解肌 / 225
releasing the flesh and clearing heat 解肌清热 / 226
releasing the flesh to promote eruption 解肌透疹 / 226
releasing the flesh to relieve the exterior 解肌发表 / 226
relieving cough and resolving phlegm 止咳化痰 / 264
relieving distension 消胀 / 252
relieving dryness with bitter-warm 苦温平燥 / 244
relieving fainting 止晕 / 267
relieving fever with sweet-warm 甘温除热 / 244
relieving itching 止痒 / 267
relieving pain 止痛 / 267
relieving sore throat 利咽 / 271
relieving spasm 止痉 / 268
relieving stranguria 通淋 / 268
relieving stuffy nose 通鼻，通鼻窍 / 271
relieving swelling 消肿 / 252
relieving swelling and redness 消肿退红 / 252
relieving vexation and thirst 除烦止渴 / 231
removal of fire toxin 去火毒 / 278
removing accumulation 消积 / 252
removing accumulation and relieving distension 消积除胀 / 252
removing alcoholic toxins 解酒毒 / 270
"removing firewood from under the cauldron" 釜底抽薪 / 237
removing impediment and unblocking yang 宣痹通阳 / 241
removing nebula 退目翳 / 271
removing nebula to improve vision 退翳明目 / 271
removing necrotic tissue 去腐肉 / 269
removing toxins 解毒 / 270
removing toxins and promoting subsidence of swelling 解毒消肿 / 270
removing toxins to promote eruption 解毒透疹 / 226
Renewal of the Treatise on Cold Damage Diseases 伤寒来苏集 / 685
Renshen Jianpi Pills 人参健脾丸 / 388
Renshen Yangrong Pills 人参养荣丸 / 391
Renshen Zaizao Pills 人参再造丸 / 391
Renying (ST 9) 人迎 / 412
repeated lifting-thrust method 捣法 / 455
repeated shallow needling 赞刺 / 462
replenishing kidney *qi* 补益肾气 / 249
replenishing kidney yin 滋补肾

阴，滋肾阴 / 249，250
replenishing lung *qi* 补益肺气 / 247
replenishing lung yin 补养肺阴 / 249
replenishing *qi* 益气 / 244
replenishing *qi* and engendering fluid 益气生津 / 264
replenishing *qi* and releasing the exterior 益气解表 / 230
replenishing *qi* to arrest bleeding 补气摄血 / 258
replenishing *qi* to calm the mind 益气安神 / 264
replenishing *qi* to stop bleeding 补气止血 / 258
replenishing the kidney to calm the mind 益肾宁神 / 264
replenishing the kidney 滋肾 / 250
replenishing the middle *qi* 补益中气 / 246
replenishing water to moisten wood 滋水涵木 / 248
replenishing yin 益阴，滋阴 / 248
replenishing yin and clearing heat 滋阴清热 / 250
replenishing yin and cooling the blood 滋阴凉血 / 250
replenishing yin and inducing diuresis 滋阴利水 / 250
replenishing yin and reducing fire 滋阴降火 / 250
replenishing yin and releasing the exterior 滋阴解表 / 230
replenishing yin and tonifying blood 滋阴补血 / 250
replenishing yin to moisten dryness 滋阴润燥 / 250
replenishing yin to moisten the lung 滋阴润肺 / 249
replenishing yin to suppress yang 滋阴抑阳 / 250
replete pulse 实脉 / 161
reproductive essence 生殖之精 / 57
repulsion of yang 格阳 / 80
repulsion of yin 格阴 / 79
rescuing yang 救阳 / 240
reservoir of blood 血海 / 25
reservoir of food and drink 水谷之海 / 26
reservoir of *qi* 气海 / 25
residual heat syndrome/pattern 余热未清证 / 180
resolution 消法 / 251
resolving dampness 化湿 / 259
resolving dampness with aromatics 芳香化湿 / 259
resolving method 消法 / 251
resolving phlegm 化痰 / 258
resolving phlegm to induce resuscitation 化痰开窍 / 267
resolving phlegm to ventilate the lung 化痰宣肺 / 228
resolving putridity 化腐 / 269
resolving retained fluid 化饮 / 259
resolving retained fluid and releasing the exterior 化饮解表 / 230
resolving retained fluid to calm the heart 化饮宁心 / 259
resolving retained fluid to soothe the chest 化饮宽胸 / 259
resolving turbidity with aromatics 芳香化浊 / 259
respiration 呼吸 / 140
respiratory reinforcement and reduction 呼吸补泻 / 457
respiratory reinforcing-reducing method 呼吸补泻法 / 457
restlessness of heart *qi* 心气不宁 / 99
Restorative Pills 再造丸，华佗再造丸 / 391，394
Restorative Placenta Pills 河车大造丸 / 389
restoring yang 回阳 / 240
restoring yang from collapse 回阳救逆 / 240
restraining relationship 相畏 / 359
restriction among the five elements/phases 五行相克 / 12
retained cupping 留罐，坐罐 / 469
retained fluid attacking the heart 水气凌心 / 101
retained fluid 饮，水饮 / 72，527
retaining the needle to await *qi* 留针候气 / 456
retardation of hair-growth 发迟 / 578
retardation of speaking 语迟 / 578
retardation of standing 立迟 / 577
retardation of tooth-eruption 齿迟 / 578
retardation of walking 行迟 / 578
retching 干呕 / 152
retention of lochia 恶露不下 / 570
Retinervus Luffae Fructus 丝瓜络 / 316
retropharyngeal abscess 里喉痈，咽后痈 / 629
retropharynx 咽底，喉底 / 40，628

reunion after separation 离而复合 / 640
reunion of fractured bone and tendon 续筋接骨 / 640
reunion of the bone, muscle and ligament 接骨续筋 / 639
Revealing the Mystery of External Medicine 外科启玄 / 697
Revealing the Mystery of the Origin (of Eye Diseases) 原［元］机启微 / 698
reverse rotation 回旋 / 639
reversed cold of hands and feet 手足厥冷，手足逆冷，四逆 / 538
reversed restriction of water on asthenic earth 土虚水侮 / 14
reverting yin disease 厥阴病 / 178
reverting yin disease pattern 厥阴病证 / 177
reverting yin syndrome 厥阴病证 / 177
Revised Zhenghe Classical Classified Materia Medica for Emergencies 重修政和经史证类备急本草 / 688
revolving moxibustion 回旋灸 / 464
revolving the ears 旋耳 / 488
rhagades 皲裂疮 / 601
rhagas 皲裂 / 601
Rheumatic-pain-relieving Plaster 伤湿止痛膏 / 396
Rhinoceros Horn 犀角 / 305
rhinology 鼻科（学）/ 625
rhinorrhea with turbid discharge 鼻渊，脑漏，脑渗，脑崩，控脑砂 / 627
Rhizoma Acori Tatarinowii 石菖蒲 / 335
Rhizoma Alismatis 泽泻 / 320
Rhizoma Alpiniae Officinarum 高良姜 / 318
Rhizoma Anemarrhenae 知母 / 304
Rhizoma Arisaematis 天南星 / 298
Rhizoma Atractylodis Macrocephalae 白术 / 341
Rhizoma Atractylodis 苍术 / 319
Rhizoma Belamcandae 射干 / 313
Rhizoma Bistortae 拳参 / 309
Rhizoma Bletillae 白及 / 328
Rhizoma Cibotii 狗脊 / 347
Rhizoma Cimicifugae 升麻 / 298
Rhizoma Coptidis 黄连 / 307
Rhizoma Corydalis 延胡索 / 332
Rhizoma Curculiginis 仙茅 / 346
Rhizoma Curcumae 莪术 / 331
Rhizoma Curcumae Longae 姜黄 / 331
Rhizoma Cynanchi Stauntonii 白前 / 301
Rhizoma Cyperi 香附 / 326
Rhizoma Dioscoreae 山药 / 341
Rhizoma Dioscoreae Bulbiferae 黄药子 / 301
Rhizoma Dioscoreae Hypoglaucae 粉萆薢 / 322
Rhizoma Dioscoreae Nipponicae 穿山龙 / 316
Rhizoma Dioscoreae Septemlobae 萆薢 / 322
Rhizoma Drynariae 骨碎补 / 347
Rhizoma Gastrodiae 天麻 / 338
Rhizoma Homalomenae 千年健 / 315
Rhizoma Imperatae 白茅根 / 307
Rhizoma Ligustici 藁本 / 296
Rhizoma Menispermi 北豆根 / 313
Rhizoma Paridis 重楼 / 311
Rhizoma Phragmitis 芦根 / 305
Rhizoma Picrorhizae 胡黄连 / 308
Rhizoma Pinelliae 半夏 / 298
Rhizoma Polygonati 黄精 / 341
Rhizoma Polygonati Odorati 玉竹 / 343
Rhizoma Polygoni Cuspidati 虎杖 / 309
Rhizoma seu Radix Notopterygii 羌活 / 313
Rhizoma Smilacis Glabrae 土茯苓 / 309
Rhizoma Sparganii 三棱 / 334
Rhizoma Typhonii 白附子 / 299
Rhizoma Valerianae 缬草 / 337
Rhizoma Wenyujin Concisa 片姜黄 / 331
Rhizoma Zingiberis 干姜 / 317
Rhizoma Zingiberis Preparata 炮姜 / 318
Rhizoma Zingiberis Recens 生姜 / 295
Rhizome Chuanxiong 川芎 / 330
Rhubarb 大黄 / 352
Rhubarb-Aconite Decoction 大黄附子汤 / 364
Rhubarb-Peony Decoction 大黄牡丹汤 / 364
Rhubarb-Scutellaria-Coptis Tablets 三黄片 / 384
rhythmic stepping 踏跳法 / 486
Rice Bean 赤小豆 / 323
Rice-grain Sprout 稻芽 / 351
Ricepaper-plant Pith 通草 / 321
rich and flavored food 膏粱厚味 / 70
right-left point combination 左右配穴法 / 447
rigidity below the heart 心下坚，心下硬 / 156

rigidity of the neck 项强 / 127
rigor 寒战 / 143
ringworm 癣 / 604
rinsing 漂 / 276
rise and decline between pathogenic and healthy *qi* 邪正消长 / 78
Riyue (GB 24) 日月 / 430
roasting (in hot ashes) 煨 / 276
roborant exercise 强壮功 / 500
rocking and tapping 摇摆触碰 / 638
rod-striking manipulation 棒击法 / 650
rodstroking 棒击法 / 485
roller needle therapy 滚刺疗法 / 452
rotating 摇法 / 485
rolling 滚法 / 481
rolling manipulation 滚法 / 649
rolling massage 滚法推拿 / 490
rolling *tuina* 滚法推拿 / 490
roof-leaking pulse 屋漏脉 / 163
Roof Stonecrop 瓦松 / 330
root 本 / 219
root of the nose 山根 / 626
root of the tongue 舌根 / 131
rooted (tongue) coating/fur 有根苔 / 136
rootless (tongue) coating/fur 无根苔 / 136
rosacea 酒皶鼻 / 601
roseola infantum 奶麻 / 584
Rosewood 降香 / 327
rosy clouds shining on the cornea 红霞映日 / 619
rotating 摇法 / 652
rotating, bending and stretching 旋转屈伸 / 638
rotating manipulation 摇法 / 652
rough coating/fur 糙苔 / 135
Round Cardamom Fruit 豆蔻 / 319
Round Cardamom Seed 蔻仁 / 319
round-pointed needle 圆针 / 451
round ringworm 圆癣 / 604
round-sharp needle 圆利针 / 452
routine treatment 正治 / 220
"rowing upstream" 逆流挽舟 / 230
Ru Men Shi Qin 儒门事亲 / 701
rubbing 擦法 / 482
rubbing and stroking the arm 摩击上肢 / 489
rubbing *dantian* 擦丹田 / 506
rubbing manipulation 擦法 / 650
rubbing the abdomen 摩腹 / 489
rubbing the face 摩面，擦面 / 487
rubbing the forehead to the top 存泥丸 / 487
rubbing the inner kidney 搓内肾 / 506
rubbing the navel 摩脐 / 489
rubbing the neck 摩颈项 / 488
rubbing the nose 擦鼻 / 506
rubbing the waist 搓腰 / 506
rubbing with ointment 膏摩 / 273
rubbing *Yongquan* (KI 1) 擦涌泉 / 490，506
rubella 风疹 / 583
Rugen (ST 18) 乳根 / 412
Rules for the Use of Drugs 用药法象 / 689
running nose with sneezing 鼽嚏 / 627
running nose 鼻臭证 / 627
"running piglet" 奔豚 / 535
"running piglet *qi*" 奔豚气 / 535
rupture 断裂伤 / 646
ruptured wound 断裂伤 / 646
ruptured wound of the eyeball 真睛破损 / 621
"rushing gate" 贲门 / 41
Ruyi Jinhuang Powder 如意金黄散 / 396
Ruzhong (ST 17) 乳中 / 412

S

sacral region 尻 / 51
sacrococcygeal region 尾骶 / 51
sacrococcyx 尾骶骨 / 51
sacromiobrachial functional training 肩臂功 / 653
sacrum 尻骨 / 51
Safflower 红花 / 330
Saffron 西红花 / 330
Sal Ammoniac 白硇砂，硇砂 / 355
Sal Ammoniacum 白硇砂 / 355
Sal Ammoniacum 硇砂 / 355
Sal Purpureum 紫硇砂 / 355
saliva 涎 / 58
saliva-swallowing 胎食 / 494
sallow complexion 面色萎黄 / 125
sallow complexion with emaciation 面黄肌瘦 / 125
sallow disease 萎黄病 / 547
sallowness 萎黄 / 125，547
salt-interposed moxibustion 隔盐灸 / 466
salty taste in the mouth 口咸 / 155
same treatment for different diseases 异病同治 / 218
San Yin Ji Yi Bing Zheng Fang Lun 三因极一病证方论 / 687
Sanchi 三七 / 328
Sandalwood 檀香 / 326
Sang Ju Yin 桑菊饮 / 362
Sanguis Draconis 血竭 / 355
Sanhuang Tablets 三黄片 / 384

Sanjian (LI 3) 三间 / 409
Sanjiaoshu (BL 22) 三焦俞 / 420
Sanyangluo (TE 8) 三阳络 / 427
Sanyinjiao (SP 6) 三阴交 / 415
Sappan Wood 苏木 / 333
Sargassum 海藻 / 300
saving from collapse 救脱 / 240
scabies 疥疮，疥癞 / 603
scald and burn 烫火伤 / 71
scalp acupuncture lines 头穴线 / 471
scalp acupuncture therapy 头针疗法，头皮针疗法 / 471
scalp acupuncture 头针，头皮针 / 470
scaly dry helices 耳轮甲错 / 129
scaly nebula with sunken center 白陷鱼鳞 / 618
scant inhibited menorrhea 月经涩少，经水涩少 / 558
scant menorrhea 月经过少 / 558
scant semen 精少 / 553
scanty dark urine 尿短赤 / 150
scanty menstruation 月经过少 / 157
scapha 耳舟 / 473
scapula 肩胛 / 47
scapular cellulitis 肩胛疽 / 594
scarlatina angionosa 烂喉丹痧 / 520
scarlatina 丹痧，喉痧，烂喉痧 / 520
scarlet fever 疫痧，疫喉痧，丹痧 / 520，585
scarring moxibustion 瘢痕灸 / 465
scattered needling 散刺 / 449
scattered pulse 散脉 / 162
Schizonepeta-Saposhnikovia Antiphlogistic Powder 荆防败毒散 / 363
sclerederma neonatorum 硬肿症 / 576
Scolopendra 蜈蚣 / 338
Scorpio 全蝎 / 338
Scorpion 全蝎 / 338
scraping 刮法 / 481
scraping bar 刮痧板 / 469
scraping the orbital rims 刮眼眶 / 487
scraping therapy 刮痧疗法 / 469
scraping to congestion 刮痧 / 481
scratching 挠法 / 482
"screen gate" 阑门 / 41
scrofula 瘰疬 / 596
scrotal abscess 囊痈 / 599
scrotal eczema 肾囊风 / 603
scrotum 阴囊，肾囊 / 49
scurrying pain 窜痛 / 148
scurrying pain 走窜痛 / 148
Sea-ear Shell 石决明 / 339
Sea-Horse 海马 / 348
sea of blood 血海 / 25
sea of marrow 髓海 / 25
sea of *qi* 气海 / 25
sea points 合穴 / 438
Seabuckthorn Fruit 沙棘 / 301
searching 寻法 / 159
seasonal diseases 时病，时令病 / 514
seasonal epidemic 时疫 / 514
seasonal epidemic pathogen 时行戾气 / 63
seasonal menstruation 季经 / 556
seasonal pathogen 时邪 / 62
seasonal pestilential *qi*;
seasonal toxin 时毒 / 514
seat sore 坐板疮 / 592
Seaweed 海藻 / 300
sebaceous cyst 粉瘤，脂瘤 / 598
seborrhea 面游风 / 602
seborrhea sicca 白屑风 / 602
seborrheic dermatitis 面游风 / 602
second yang 二阳 / 400
second yin 二阴 / 399
secondary infertility 断绪 / 565
secret formula 秘方，禁方 / 357
secret formula handed down in a family 祖传秘方 / 357
Secret Principles of Massotherapy for Children 小儿推拿秘旨 / 696
secretion from the five *zang* organs 五脏化液 / 58
Secrets of Treating Wounds and Rejoining Fractures Handed Down by an Immortal 仙授理伤续断秘方 / 697
Secrets of Treating Wounds and Rejoining Fractures 理伤续断秘方 / 697
sedative or tranquilizing formula 安神剂 / 380
selection of adjacent points 邻近选穴法 / 446
selection of distant points 远道选穴法 / 446
selection of local points 局部选穴法 / 446
selection of points 选穴法，取穴法 / 445，446
selection of points along the affected meridian/channel 循经选穴法 / 446
selection of points on other meridian(s)/channel(s) 异经选穴法，他经选穴法 / 446
selection of points on the exterior-interiorly related meridians/channels 表里选穴

法 / 446
selection of points opposite to the affected area 对应选穴法 / 446
Semen Abutili 苘麻子 / 322
Semen Aesculi 娑罗子 / 327
Semen Allii Tuberosi 韭菜子 / 348
Semen Alpiniae Katsumadai 草豆蔻 / 320
Semen Alpiniae Oxyphyllae 益智仁 / 346
Semen Amomi Rotundus 蔻仁 / 319
Semen Arecae 槟榔 / 353
Semen Armeniacae Amarum 苦杏仁 / 301
Semen Astragali Complanati 沙苑子 / 344
Semen Canavaliae 刀豆 / 328
Semen Cassiae 决明子 / 304
Semen Celosiae 青葙子 / 304
Semen Citri Reticulatae 橘核 / 325
Semen Coicis 薏苡仁 / 321
Semen Crotonis Pulveratum 巴豆霜 / 324
Semen Crotonis 巴豆 / 355
Semen Cucurbitae 南瓜子 / 353
Semen Cuscutae 菟丝子 / 347
Semen Euphorbiae 千金子 / 355
Semen Euryales 芡实 / 349
Semen Ginkgo 白果 / 301
Semen Hyoscyami 天仙子 / 303
Semen Juglandis 核桃仁 / 346
Semen Lablab Album 白扁豆 / 341
Semen Lepidii seu Descurainiae 葶苈子 / 303
Semen Litchi 荔枝核 / 327
Semen Myristicae 肉豆蔻 / 349
Semen Nelumbinis 莲子 / 349
Semen Oroxyli 木蝴蝶 / 303
Semen Persicae 桃仁 / 330
Semen Pharbitidis 牵牛子 / 323
Semen Phaseoli 赤小豆 / 323
Semen Plantaginis 车前子 / 320
Semen Platycladi 柏子仁 / 337
Semen Pruni 郁李仁 / 352
Semen Raphani 莱菔子 / 352
Semen Sesami Nigrum 黑芝麻 / 345
Semen Sinapis Albae 白芥子 / 299
Semen Sojae Preparatum 淡豆豉 / 298
Semen Sterculiae Lychnophorae 胖大海 / 303
Semen Strychni 马钱子 / 316
Semen Torreyae 榧子 / 353
Semen Trigonellae 葫芦巴 / 347
Semen Vaccariae 王不留行 / 333
Semen Ziziphi Spinosae 酸枣仁 / 336
semen-astringing enuresis-arresting formula 涩精止遗剂 / 374
Semen-securing Pill 固精丸 / 374
seminal emission 遗精 / 552
seminal turbidity 精浊 / 599
semi-recumbent posture 半卧式 / 495
Senna Leaf 番泻叶 / 352
sensation of filthy *qi* 秽气气感 / 505
sensation of genuine *qi* 真气气感 / 505
sensation of *qi* 气感 / 505
separate bones by squeezing 夹挤分骨 / 638
separation before reunion 欲合先离 / 640
separation of yin and yang 阴阳离决 / 6
sequelae of wind stroke 中风后遗症 / 537
sequential meridian/channel transmission 循经传 / 116
sequential transmission 顺传 / 179，515
“serene gate” 幽门 / 41
set formula 成方 / 356
settling and subduing 镇潜 / 265
settling fright 镇惊 / 264
settling fright and calming the mind 镇惊安神 / 264
settling the heart and calming the mind 镇心安神 / 264
settling the liver and subduing yang 镇肝潜阳 / 265
settling the liver to extinguish wind 镇肝熄［息］风 / 266
settling tranquilizer 重镇安神药 / 293
settling tranquilizing formula 重镇安神剂 / 380
settling tranquilizing medicinal/drug 重镇安神药 / 293
seven emotions 七情 / 69
seven gates 七冲门 / 40
Seven-lobed Yam Rhizome 绵萆薢 / 322
seven moribund pulses 七绝脉，七死脉 / 163
seven- or eight-year-old child 龆龀 / 574
seven orifices 七窍 / 38
seven paradoxical pulses 七怪脉 / 163
seven portals 七冲门 / 40
seven-star exercise 七星功 / 503
seven-star needle 七星针 / 450
severe epistaxis 脑衄 / 628
severe palpitations 怔忡 / 151

sex-stimulating substance 天癸 / 556
sexual consumption 房劳 / 71
shaft-flicking method 努法，弩法 / 455
shaking manipulation 抖法 / 651
shallow insertion 浅刺 / 454
shallow surround needling 扬刺 / 461
Shang Han Guan Zhu Ji 伤寒贯珠集 / 686
Shang Han Lai Su Ji 伤寒来苏集 / 685
Shang Han Lei Fang 伤寒类方 / 685
Shang Han Lun 伤寒论 / 685
Shang Han Lun Zhi Jie 伤寒论直解 / 685
Shang Han Ming Li Lun 伤寒明理论 / 685
Shang Han Za Bing Lun 伤寒杂病论 / 685
Shang Han Zhi Zhang 伤寒指掌 / 685
Shang Han Zong Bing Lun 伤寒总病论 / 685
Shang Ke Bu Yao 伤科补要 / 698
Shang Ke Hui Zuan 伤科汇纂 / 698
Shangguan (GB 3) 上关 / 428
Shangjuxu (ST 37) 上巨虚 / 414
Shanglian (LI 9) 上廉 / 410
Shangliao (BL 31) 上髎 / 421
Shangqiu (SP 5) 商丘 / 415
Shangqu (KI 17) 商曲 / 425
Shangshi Zhitong Plaster 伤湿止痛膏 / 396
Shangwan (CV 13) 上脘 / 436
Shangxing (GV 23) 上星 / 435
Shangyang (LI 1) 商阳 / 409
Shangyingxiang (EX-HN 8) 上迎香 / 440
shank bone 骺骨 / 51
shank erysipelas 流火 / 594
shank sore 臁疮 / 595
Shaochong (HT 9) 少冲 / 417
Shaofu (HT 8) 少府 / 417
Shaohai (HT 3) 少海 / 416
Shaoshang (LU 11) 少商 / 409
shaoyang person 少阳之人 / 74
shaoyang-harmonizing formula 和解少阳剂 / 365
shaoyin person 少阴之人 / 74
Shaoze (SI 1) 少泽 / 417
Sharpleaf Galangal Seed 益智仁 / 346
shear needle 镵针 / 451
Shearer's Pyrrosia Leaf石韦 / 323
Shedan Chenpi Powder 蛇胆陈皮散 / 382
Shedan Chuanbei Powder 蛇胆川贝散 / 382
Shen Cunzhong 沈存中 / 662
Shen Jin'ao 沈金鳌 / 677
Shen Kuo 沈括 / 662
Shen Nong Ben Cao Jing 神农本草经 / 687
Shen Nong's Herbal 神农本草经 / 687
Shen Nong's Materia Medica 神农本草经 / 687
Shen Qianlü 沈芊绿 / 677
Shen Shi Yao Han 审视瑶函 / 698
Shen Su Yin 参苏饮 / 363
Shen Zhiwen 沈之问 / 669
Shencang (KI 25) 神藏 / 425
Shendao (GV 11) 神道 / 434
Shenfeng (KI 23) 神封 / 425
Shenfu Injection 参附注射液 / 391
Sheng Hui Fang 圣惠方 / 691
Sheng Ji Zong Lu 圣济总录 / 703
Shenghua Decoction 生化汤 / 376
Shengma Gegen Decoction 升麻葛根汤 / 363
Shengmai Drink 生脉饮 / 389
Shenling Baizhu Pills 参苓白术丸 / 388
Shenling Baizhu Powder 参苓白术散 / 371
Shenmai (BL 62) 申脉 / 423
Shenmen (HT 7) 神门 / 417
Shenqi Pill 肾气丸 / 373
Shenque (CV 8) 神阙 / 436
Shenrong Guben Tablets 参茸固本片 / 391
Shenrong Weisheng Pills 参茸卫生丸 / 391
Shenshu (BL 23) 肾俞 / 420
Shentang (BL 44) 神堂 / 422
Shenting (GV 24) 神庭 / 435
Shenzhu (GV 12) 身柱 / 434
Shepherd's Purse 荠菜 / 329
Shi Bing Lun 时病论 / 694
Shi Fang Ge Kuo 时方歌括 / 693
Shi Liao Ben Cao 食疗本草 / 687
Shi Si Jing Fa Hui 十四经发挥 / 699
Shi Yao Shen Shu 十药神书 / 694
Shi Yi De Xiao Fang 世医得效方 / 692
Shidou (SP 17) 食窦 / 416
shifting 挪法 / 482
Shiguan (KI 18) 石关 / 425
Shihu Yeguang Pills 石斛夜光丸 / 396

Shimen (CV 5) 石门 / 435
shin 胫 / 50
shinbone 胫骨，骭骨 / 50，51
shingles 火带疮 / 600
Shinyleaf Pricklyash Root 两面针 / 333
Shiqizhui (EX-B 8) 十七椎 / 441
Shiquan Dabu Decoction 十全大补汤 / 372
Shiquan Dabu Pills 十全大补丸 / 388
shiver sweating 战汗 / 531
shiver 战栗 / 143
shivery sweating 战汗 / 145
Shixuan (EX-UE 11) 十宣 / 443
Shizao Decoction 十枣汤 / 365
shooting through the passes to the nail 通关射甲 / 138
short pulse 短脉 / 162
short thrust needling 短刺 / 461
short voiding of dark urine 小便短赤 / 151
shortage of *qi* 少气 / 141，526
shortened menstrual cycles 经行先期 / 557
shortened tongue 舌短 / 134
shortness of breath 短气 / 141，526
Shou Shi Bao Yuan 寿世保元 / 703
shoulder 肩 / 46
shoulder-arm exercise 肩臂功 / 501，653
shoulder blade 肩胛 / 47
shoulder pain 肩痛 / 147
Shousanli (LI 10) 手三里 / 410
Shouwuli (LI 13) 手五里 / 410
shrimp-darting pulse 虾游脉 / 163
shrinking the chest and straightening the back 含胸拔背 / 494
Shrub Chaste-tree Fruit 蔓荆子 / 297
Shuaigu (GB 8) 率谷 / 429
Shuanghuanlian Oral Liquid 双黄连口服液 / 383
Shufu (KI 27) 俞府 / 425
Shugan Pills 舒肝丸 / 386
Shugu (BL 65) 束骨 / 423
Shuidao (ST 28) 水道 / 413
Shuifen (CV 9) 水分 / 436
Shuigou (GV 26) 水沟 / 435
Shuiquan (KI 5) 水泉 / 424
Shuitu (ST 10) 水突 / 412
Si Zhen Jue Wei 四诊抉微 / 686
Sibai (ST 2) 四白 / 411
Siberian Cocklebur Fruit 苍耳子 / 296
sickness 疾病 / 122
side of the tongue 舌旁 / 39
sideburns 锐发 / 43
side-rubbing manipulation 侧擦法 / 651
Sidu (TE 9) 四渎 / 427
Siegesbeckia Herb 豨莶草 / 314
Siegesbeckia Pills 豨莶丸 / 393
Sifeng (EX-UE 10) 四缝 / 443
sighing 太息 / 141
sign 征候 / 122
signal orifices 苗窍 / 38
Sijunzi Decoction 四君子汤 / 371
silent sitting 静坐 / 505
Silktree Albizia Bark 合欢皮 / 336
silver needle 银针 / 452
Siman (KI 14) 四满 / 424
simmering 熬 / 278
simmering in a bath 炖 / 278
simple abdominal distension 单腹胀 / 547
simple formula/prescription 单方 / 356
simultaneous elimination and reinforcement 攻补兼施 / 220
simultaneous palpation 总按 / 159
simultaneous vomiting and diarrhea 上吐下泻 / 150
simultaneous yin-yang tonifying formula 阴阳并补剂 / 373
sinew 筋 / 42
sinew atrophy-flaccidity 筋痿 / 539
sinew impediment 筋痹 / 541
sinew-transforming exercise 易筋功 / 503
sinew tumor 筋瘤 / 598
single cross-legged sitting 单盘坐 / 495
single-featured pulse 单一脉象 / 163
single-finger meditation gesture 一指禅式 / 504
single-finger meditation manipulation 一指禅功 / 482
single-finger meditation massage 一指禅推拿 / 490
single-finger meditation pushing 一指禅推法 / 482
single-finger meditation *tuina* 一指禅推拿 / 490
single-handed needle insertion 单手进针法 / 453
single-handed rotating reduction of cervical vertebra 颈椎单人旋转复位法 / 652
Sini Decoction 四逆汤 / 370
Sini Powder 四逆散 / 366
Sinkiang Fritillary Bulb 伊贝母 / 302
sinking 下陷 / 94
sinking of spleen *qi* 脾气下陷 / 94
sinking of the middle *qi* 中气下陷 / 94
sinusitis 鼻渊，脑漏，脑渗，脑崩，控脑砂 / 627

Sishen Pill 四神丸 / 374
Sishencong (EX-HN 1) 四神聪 / 439
sitting in forgetfulness 坐忘 / 498
sitting posture 坐式 / 494
sitting reduction 坐式复位 / 642
Siwu Decoction 四物汤 / 371
six bowels 六腑 / 20
six excesses 六淫 / 62
six *fu* organs 六腑 / 20
Six-ingredient Rehmannia Decoction 六味地黄汤 / 372
Six-ingredient Rehmannia Pills 六味地黄丸 / 389
six meridians/channels 六经 / 399
six-meridian/channel pattern identification 六经辨证 / 175
six-meridian/channel syndrome differentiation 六经辨证 / 175
six *qi* 六气 / 17，62
six stagnations 六郁 / 70
Six-to-one Powder 六一散 / 369
six yang meridians/channels 六阳脉 / 400
six yin meridians/channels 六阴脉 / 400
Sixteen Medical Works by Chen Xiuyuan 陈修圆医书十六种 / 705
Sizhukong (TE 23) 丝竹空 / 428
skeleton 百骸 / 50
skin and body hair 皮毛 / 41
skin edema 皮水 / 549
skin impediment 皮痹 / 541
skin numbness 皮痹 / 602
skin-spreading needle insertion 舒张进针法 / 453
skip-over meridian/channel transmission 越经传 / 116
skipping pulse 促脉 / 162
"sleeping silkworm beneath the eye" 目下有卧蚕 / 128
sleeplessness 不寐 / 155
Slenderstyle Acanthopanax Bark 五加皮 / 316
slicing 切片 / 276
slide cupping 走罐 / 469
slimming exercise 减肥功 / 503
slimy (tongue) coating/fur 腻苔，滑苔 / 135
slippery pulse 滑脉 / 161
slobbery nausea 泛恶 / 152
sloppy stool 溏便/ 149
slow-acting formula 缓方 / 357
slow fire 慢火 / 283
slow pulse 迟脉 / 160
sluggish speech 语言謇涩 / 140
sluggish tongue 舌謇［蹇］/ 133
small canthus 小眦 / 608
Small Centipeda Herb 鹅不食草 / 296
small cone moxibustion 小炷灸 / 465
small heavenly circuit 小周天 / 500
small heavenly circuit exercise 小周天功 / 501
small intestine 小肠 / 24
small intestinal cough 小肠咳 / 525
small intestinal deficiency cold 小肠虚寒 / 101
small intestinal excess heat 小肠实热 / 101
small intestinal excess heat syndrome/pattern 小肠实热证 / 202
small intestine meridian/channel (SI) 手太阳小肠经 / 402
small intestine meridian/channel of hand greater yang 手太阳小肠经 / 402
"small tongue" 小舌 / 40
smallpox 天花 / 585
smell of breath 口气 / 142
smelling odors 嗅气味 / 142
Smoked Plum 乌梅 / 349
Smoketree Twig 黄栌 / 309
Snake-bile and Tangerine-peel Powder 蛇胆陈皮散 / 382
Snake-bile and Tendrilled-Fritillary Powder 蛇胆川贝散 / 382
snake-body felon 蛇肚疔 / 592
snake-body whitlow 蛇肚疔 / 592
snake-eye felon 蛇眼疔 / 592
snake-eye whitlow 蛇眼疔 / 592
Snake-gourd Root 天花粉 / 300
snake-head felon 蛇头疔 / 592
snake-head whitlow 蛇头疔 / 592
Snake Slough 蛇蜕 / 315
Snakegourd Fruit 瓜蒌 / 299
snapping finger 弹响指 / 647
snivel 涕 / 58
snow-white mouth 雪口 / 579
soaking 泡 / 276
Sodium Sulfate 芒硝 / 352
soft extract 煎膏，膏滋 / 281
soft pulse 软脉 / 161
soft *qigong* 软气功 / 492
soft tissue injury 筋伤 / 643
soggy pulse 濡脉 / 161
soliloquy 独语 / 140
solitary yang floating upward 孤阳上越 / 80
Solomonseal Rhizome 黄精 / 341
somniloquy 呓语 / 140
somnolence 嗜卧，嗜睡 / 155，535
Son Huifu 宋惠父 / 665

Song Ci 宋慈 / 665
Songaria Cynomorium Herb 锁阳 / 346
soothing the chest 宽胸 / 254
soothing the chest and dissipating stagnation 宽胸散结 / 254
soothing the liver 疏肝 / 255
soothing the liver and harmonizing the spleen 疏肝和脾 / 255
soothing the liver and harmonizing the stomach 疏肝和胃 / 255
soothing the liver and invigorating the spleen 疏肝健脾 / 255
soothing the liver and nourishing blood 疏肝养血 / 255
soothing the liver and regulating *qi* 疏肝理气 / 255
soothing the liver and regulating the spleen 疏肝理脾 / 255
soothing the liver and relieving depression 疏肝解郁 / 255
soothing the middle and dissipating stagnation 宽中散结 / 254
sore 疮 / 591
sore and ulcer 疮疡 / 591
sore throat 咽喉肿痛 / 629
sorrow 悲 / 69
"sounding the celestial drum" 鸣天鼓 / 488
sour breath 口气酸臭 / 142
sour taste in the mouth 口酸 / 155
Source of Relief 解围元薮 / 697
source-connecting point combination 原络配穴法 / 447
source points 原穴 / 438
sovereign fire 君火 / 21
sovereign ingredient 君药 / 358
sovereign, minister, adjuvant and courier 君臣佐使 / 358
sparrow's blindness 雀盲 / 621
sparrow's cataract 雀目内障 / 622
sparrow's vision 雀目 / 622
special but irregular recipe 偏方 / 357
specific points 特定穴 / 437
spermatorrhea 滑精（病）/ 155，552
sphygmology 脉学 / 158
Spica Prunellae 夏枯草 / 305
Spica Schizonepetae 荆芥穗 / 296
spider nevus 血缕 / 601
Spikemoss 卷柏 / 332
Spikenard Root甘松 / 326
spilling of dampness-toxin 湿毒流注 / 89
Spina Gleditsiae 皂角刺 / 333
spine 脊 / 50
Spine Date Seed 酸枣仁 / 336
Spiny Amomum Fruit 砂仁 / 319
Spiny Jujube Seed Decoction 酸枣仁汤 / 381
spirit 神，精神 / 2，57
spiritless eyes 神光耗散 / 128
Spiritual Pivot 灵枢 / 684
Spiritual Pivot of Huangdi's Internal Classsic 黄帝内经灵枢经 / 683
*Spiritual Pivot of Yellow Emperor's Canon of Medicine*黄帝内经灵枢经 / 683
spitting of blood 吐血 / 152
spittle 唾 / 58
spleen 脾 / 21
Spleen-activating Pills 启脾丸 / 387
spleen atrophy-flaccidity 脾痿 / 539
spleen consumption 脾劳 / 529
spleen cough 脾咳 / 525
spleen deficiency 脾虚 / 104
spleen deficiency cold syndrome/pattern 脾虚寒证 / 205
spleen deficiency diarrhea 脾虚泄泻 / 545
spleen deficiency generating phlegm 脾虚生痰 / 106
spleen deficiency generating wind 脾虚生风 / 106
spleen deficiency syndrome/pattern with sinking of *qi* 脾虚气陷证 / 206
spleen deficiency syndrome/pattern 脾虚证 / 205
spleen deficiency with dampness encumbrance 脾虚湿困 / 105
spleen edema 脾水 / 549
spleen failing to control blood 脾不统血 / 105
spleen impediment 脾痹 / 541
spleen (infantile) malnutrition 脾疳 / 580
spleen insufficiency amenorrhea 脾虚经闭 / 559
spleen-insufficiency diarrhea 脾虚泻 / 588
spleen insufficiency leukorrhagia 脾虚带下 / 564
spleen insufficiency with sinking of *qi* 脾虚气陷 / 94
spleen-kidney deficiency cold 脾肾虚寒 / 107
spleen-kidney deficiency cold syndrome/pattern 脾肾虚寒证 / 207
spleen-kidney yang deficiency 脾肾阳虚 / 107
spleen-kidney yang deficiency syndrome/pattern 脾肾阳虚证 / 207

spleen-lung *qi* deficiency 脾肺气虚 / 106
spleen-lung *qi* deficiency syndrome/pattern 脾肺气虚证 / 207
spleen meridian/channel (SP) 足太阴脾经 / 401
spleen meridian/channel cough 脾经咳嗽 / 524
spleen meridian/channel of foot greater yin 足太阴脾经 / 401
spleen *qi* 脾气 / 21，54
spleen *qi* deficiency 脾气虚 / 104
spleen *qi* deficiency syndrome/pattern 脾气虚证 / 205
spleen *qi* failing to ascend 脾气不升 / 106
spleen *qi* insufficiency 脾气不足 / 105
spleen *qi* sinking syndrome/pattern 脾气下陷证 / 206
spleen-regulation exercise 理脾功 / 501
Spleen-restoring Decoction 归脾汤 / 372
spleen-stomach dampness-heat syndrome/pattern 脾胃湿热证 / 206
spleen-stomach dampness-heat 脾胃湿热 / 106
spleen-stomach deficiency cold syndrome/pattern 脾胃虚寒证 / 205
spleen-stomach deficiency cold 脾胃虚寒 / 106
spleen-stomach yang deficiency syndrome/pattern 脾胃阳虚证 / 205
spleen-stomach yang deficiency 脾胃阳虚 / 106
Spleen-warming Decoction 温脾汤 / 364
spleen wasting-thirst 脾消 / 551
spleen yang 脾阳 / 22
spleen yang deficiency 脾阳虚 / 105
spleen yang deficiency syndrome/pattern 脾阳虚证 / 205
spleen yang insufficiency 脾阳不振 / 105
spleen yin 脾阴 / 22
spleen yin deficiency 脾阴虚 / 105
spleen yin deficiency syndrome/pattern 脾阴虚证 / 205
splenic constipation 脾约 / 544
splintage 夹板固定 / 640
splintage therapy 夹板固定疗法 / 640
spontaneous harmonization of yin and yang 阴阳自和 / 6
spontaneous seminal emission 滑精 / 155
spontaneous sweating 自汗 / 144，531
spontaneous sweating after childbirth 产后自汗 / 571
spontaneous sweating in *qi* deficiency 气虚自汗 / 531
spontaneous sweating in yang deficiency 阳虚自汗 / 531
spoon-like needle 锃针 / 451
Spora Lygodii 海金沙 / 323
spotted tongue 点刺舌 / 132
spotting 漏下 / 561
sprain 扭伤 / 646
spreading-claw gesture 探爪式 / 504
spring points 荥穴 / 437
spring warmth 春温 / 516
spring warmth disease 春温病 / 516
sprouting 发芽 / 278
Squama Manitis 穿山甲 / 333
squeezing 挤法 / 484
squint 眼珠牵斜，目偏视 / 128，622
stagnant fire 郁火 / 70
stabbing pain 刺痛 / 148
stagnant dampness transforming into fire 湿郁化火 / 89
stagnant dampness transforming into heat 湿郁化热 / 89
stagnant heat 瘀热 / 88
stagnant heat in the blood aspect 血分瘀热 / 88
stagnant heat in the liver meridian/channel 肝经郁热 / 98
stagnation of meridian/channel *qi* 经气郁滞 / 114
stained (tongue) coating/fur 染苔 / 135
stainless steel needle 不锈钢针 / 452
stake-standing exercise 站桩功 / 502
Stamen Nelumbinis 莲须 / 349
stamping 跷法 / 486
Standards of Syndrome/Pattern Identification and Treatment 证治准绳 / 703
Standards of Syndrome/Pattern Identification and Treatment in Six Branches of Medicine 六科证治准绳 / 704
standing posture 站式 / 495
star-cluster nebula 聚星障 / 618
staring sideways 横目斜视 / 129
staring straight ahead 瞪目直视 / 129
Starwort Root 银柴胡 / 306
stasis-resolving hemostatic (medicinal/drug) 化瘀止血药 / 291
stasis-resolving medicinal/drug

化瘀药 / 292
static blood 瘀血 / 71
static blood obstruction syndrome/pattern 瘀血阻滞证 / 185
static-dynamic *qigong* 动静相兼功 / 492
static *qigong* 静功 / 491
steady withdrawal of the needle 平稳出针法 / 462
stealthy wind 贼风 / 63
steaming 蒸 / 278
Stemona Root 百部 / 302
sterility 不育 / 553
sticking of the needle 滞针 / 463
sticking the tongue against the palate 舌抵上腭 / 494
sticky eye gum and tears 眵泪胶粘 / 611
sticky slimy sensation in the mouth 口黏腻 / 155
Stiff Silkworm 僵蚕 / 338
stiff tongue 强硬舌，舌强 / 133
Stigma Croci 西红花 / 330
Stigma Maydis 玉米须 / 323
stiletto needle 铍针 / 452
stimulant 开窍药 / 293
stimulated menses 激经 / 566
stimulating lactation 催乳 / 268
stimulating menstrual discharge 通经 / 268
stink 腥臭气 / 142
Stink-bug 九香虫 / 327
stir-baking 炒 / 277
stir-baking at a high temperature 炮 / 277
stir-baking to brown 炒焦 / 277
stir-baking to charcoal 炒炭 / 277
stir-baking to cracking 炒爆 / 277
stir-baking to dryness 微炒 / 277
stir-baking to yellowish 炒黄 / 277
stir-baking with adjuvant 加辅料炒 / 277
stir-baking with fluid adjuvant 炙 / 277
stir-baking with ginger 姜炙 / 277
stir-baking with honey 蜜炙 / 277
stir-baking with vinegar 醋炙 / 277
stir-baking with wine 酒炙 / 277
stir-baking without adjuvant 清炒 / 277
stirred pulse 动脉 / 162
stirring the tongue 搅舌 / 488
stomach 胃 / 23
stomach cavity 胃脘，脘 / 23
Stomach-clearing Powder 清胃散 / 368
stomach cold 胃寒 / 107
stomach cough 胃咳 / 525
stomach deficiency 胃虚 / 107
stomach deficiency cold 胃虚寒 / 107
stomach deficiency cold syndrome/pattern 胃虚寒证 / 207
stomach disharmony 胃不和 / 108
stomach excess cold 胃实寒 / 107
stomach excess cold syndrome/pattern 胃实寒证 / 207
stomach fire 胃火 / 108
stomach-fire toothache 胃火牙痛 / 632
stomach fire syndrome 胃火证 / 208
stomach fluid 胃津 / 24
stomach fluid depletion 胃津亏损 / 81
stomach fluid depletion syndrome/pattern 胃燥津亏证 / 187
stomach heat 胃热 / 107
stomach heat vomiting 胃热呕吐 / 586
stomach heat with accelerated digestion 胃热消［杀］谷 / 92，108
stomach-insufficiency sweating 胃虚汗 / 586
stomach meridian/channel (ST) 足阳明胃经 / 401
stomach meridian/channel of foot yang brightness 足阳明胃经 / 401
Stomach-pacifying Powder 平胃散 / 379
stomach *qi* 胃气 / 24，55
stomach *qi* deficiency 胃气虚 / 107
stomach *qi* deficiency syndrome/pattern 胃气虚证 / 207
stomach *qi* disharmony 胃气不和 / 108
stomach *qi* failing to descend 胃气不降 / 108
stomach *qi*，vitality，and root 胃、神、根 / 164
stomach reflux 胃反，反胃 / 543
stomach stuffiness 胃痞 / 542
stomach wasting-thirst 胃消 / 551
stomach yang 胃阳 / 24
stomach yang deficiency 胃阳虚 / 107
stomach yang deficiency syndrome/pattern 胃阳虚证 / 207
stomach yin deficiency syndrome/pattern 胃阴虚证 / 207
stomach yin 胃阴 / 24
stomach yin deficiency 胃阴虚 / 107
stomach yin insufficiency 胃阴

不足 / 107
stomachache 胃痛 / 152
stomatology and dentistry 口齿科（学） / 632
stone needle 砭石 / 451
stony edema 石水 / 549
stony goiter 石瘿 / 597
"stony moth" 石蛾 / 629
stools sometimes loose and sometimes bound 溏结不调 / 149
stopping bleeding 止血 / 257
stopping hiccups 止呃 / 267
storage of the five *zang* organs 五脏所藏 / 26
Storax 苏合香 / 335
Storax Pills 苏合香丸 / 392
stout person 肉人 / 75
strabismus 眼珠牵斜，目偏视，偏斜瞻视 / 128，622
straining at stool 下坠 / 156
stranguria 淋（证） / 551
stranguria in pregnancy 妊娠小便淋痛 / 567
stranguria-relieving diuretic (medicinal/drug) 利尿通淋药 / 290
stranguria-relieving medicinal/drug 通淋药 / 290
stranguria with turbid discharge 淋浊 / 551
strawberry tongue 杨莓舌 / 585
Stream-reducing Pill 缩泉丸 / 374
strengthening the kidney 固肾 / 262
strengthening the kidney to arrest emission 固肾涩精 / 262
strengthening the kidney to check leukorrhagia 固肾止带 / 262
strengthening the kidney to reduce urination 固肾缩尿 / 262
strengthening the muscles and bones 强筋健骨 / 251
strengthening the thoroughfare vessel and stopping leukorrhagia 固冲止带 / 263
stretching 伸法 / 485
stretching the waist and keeping the hips sunk 伸腰沉胯 / 494
string-like pulse 弦脉 / 162
striking 击法 / 484
striking manipulation 击法 / 649
striking the lower limb 击下肢 / 489
Stringy Stonecrop Herb 垂盆草 / 309
stroke 卒中 / 536
strong defense *qi* with weak nutrient 卫强营弱 / 86
strong fire 急火，武火 / 283
struggle between healthy and pathogenic *qi* 正邪分争，正邪相争 / 78
stubborn lichen 顽癣 / 602
study of the pulse 脉学 / 158
stuffiness 痞 / 542
stuffiness and fullness 痞满 / 156
stuffiness and rigidity below the heart 心下痞硬 / 156
stuffiness below the heart 心下痞 / 156
stuffiness of deficiency type 虚痞 / 542
stuffiness of excess type 实痞 / 542
stuffy lump 痞块 / 547
stuffy nose 鼻塞，鼻窍不利，鼻窒 / 626，627
stuffy pain 闷痛 / 147
stye 针眼，偷针，土疳，土疡 / 612，613
styptic formula 止血剂 / 377
Styrax 苏合香 / 335
Su Gong 苏恭 / 661
Su Jing 苏敬 / 661
Su Shen Liang Fang 苏沈良方 / 691
Su Shi 苏轼 / 662
Su Song 苏颂 / 662
Su Wen 素问 / 683
Suanzaoren Decoction 酸枣仁汤 / 381
subconjunctival ecchymosis 白睛溢血 / 617
subcutaneous fluid retention 溢饮 / 528
subcutaneous node 结核 / 591
subduing yang and extinguishing wind 潜阳熄风 / 265
subduing yang 潜阳 / 265
Suberect Spatholobus Stem 鸡血藤 / 332
sublingual blood stasis syndrome/pattern 血瘀舌下证 / 185
sublingual collateral vessel 舌下脉络 / 131
sublingual cyst 舌下痰包 / 634
sublingual swelling 重舌 / 633
submandibular abscess 颌下痈 / 629
submerged fever 身热不扬 / 144
Subtle Meaning of the Jade Swivel 玉机微义 / 701
successive trigger needling 报刺 / 461
Succinum 琥珀 / 336
suction cup 抽气罐 / 468
suction cupping 抽气罐法 / 468
sudamina 晶 / 139
sudden attack of bulbar conjunctivitis 暴风客热 / 616
sudden attack of wind-heat on

the eye 暴风客热 / 616
sudden blindness 暴盲 / 620
sudden collapse of heart yang 心阳暴脱 / 100
sudden deafness 暴聋，卒聋 / 624
sudden dyspnea 暴喘 / 586
sudden flooding 暴崩 / 561
sudden heart pain 卒心痛 / 531
sudden hoarseness or aphonia 暴喑，卒喑 / 630
sudden illness 暴病 / 515
sudden infantile diarrhea 小儿暴泻，小儿卒利 / 587
sudden onset of throat impediment 卒喉痹 / 630
sudden protrusion of the eyeball 突起睛高，睛高突起 / 622
sudden redness of the bulbar conjunctiva 白睛暴赤 / 611
sudden syncope 薄厥 / 538
sudden throbbing of a pulse 脉暴出 / 164
Suhexiang Pills 苏合香丸 / 392
Sulfur 硫黄 / 354
Suliao (GV 25) 素髎 / 435
summer affliction 苦夏 / 582
summer fever 夏季热 / 582
summer fever disease 夏季热病 / 582
summer non-acclimation 疰夏 / 582
summer non-acclimation disease 疰夏病 / 582
summerheat 暑，暑热 / 65
summerheat affection 冒暑，感暑 / 516，517
summerheat boil 暑疖 / 592
summerheat-clearing formula 清热祛暑剂 / 369
summerheat convulsion 暑痉 / 517
summerheat damage 伤暑 / 517
summerheat-dampness 暑湿 / 65
summerheat-dampness syndrome/pattern 暑湿证 / 195
summerheat disease 暑病 / 517
summerheat dizziness 感暑眩晕 / 532
summerheat entering *yangming* (yang brightness) 暑入阳明 / 517
summerheat epilepsy 暑痫 / 517
summerheat filth 暑秽 / 516
summerheat filth disease 暑秽病 / 516
summerheat malaria 暑疟 / 521
summerheat phthisis 暑瘵 / 517
summerheat *qi* 暑气 / 65
summerheat stroke 中暑 / 517
summerheat syncope 暑厥 / 517
summerheat syncope syndrome/pattern 暑厥证 / 517
summerheat syndrome/pattern 暑证，暑热证 / 195
summerheat vertigo 感暑眩晕 / 532
summerheat-warmth 暑温 / 517
summerheat-warmth disease 暑温病 / 517
summerheat-wind 暑风 / 517
summerheat-wind syndrome/pattern 暑风证 / 517
Sun Dongsu 孙东宿 / 669
Sun Simiao 孙思邈 / 661
Sun Wenyuan 孙文垣 / 669
Sun Yikui 孙一奎 / 669
sunken eyes 眼珠塌陷 / 128
sunken eye sockets 眼窝凹陷 / 128
sunken fontanel 囟陷 / 577
sunken pulse 沉脉 / 160
Suoquan Pill 缩泉丸 / 374
superficial collateral vessel 浮络 / 407
superficial needling 毛刺，浮刺 / 460，461
superficial punctate keratitis 聚星障 / 618
superficial thrombophlebitis 青蛇毒 / 606
superficies-consolidating anhidrotic 固表止汗药 / 294
superficies-consolidating sweating-arresting formula 固表止汗剂 / 374
superficies-releasing medicinal/drug 解表药 / 287
superior auricular root 上耳根 / 473
superior crus of the antihelix 对耳轮上脚 / 472
supine posture 仰卧式 / 495
Supplement to Diagnosis and Treatment 证治汇补 / 694
Supplement to the Classified Medical Records of Distinguished Physicians 续名医类案 / 702
Supplement to the Essential Prescriptions Worth a Thousand Pieces of Gold 千金翼方 / 690
Supplement to Traumatology 伤科补要 / 698
Supplementary Treatise on Knowledge from Practice 格致余论 / 701
Supplemented Lindera Decoction 加味乌药汤 / 375
supplementing fire and invigorating yang 补火壮阳 / 251
supplementing water to inhibit yang 壮水制阳 / 250
Supplements to Commentaries on the Synopsis of the Golden Chamber 金匮翼 / 686

supporting and lifting 托提法 / 484
supporting board 托板 / 640
supporting yang 助阳 / 250
supporting yang and releasing the exterior 助阳解表 / 230
suppository 栓剂 / 282
suppressing relationship 相杀 / 359
suppressing upward perversion of *qi* (and directing *qi* downward) 降逆下气 / 254
suppressing upward perversion of *qi* to relieve cough and dyspnea 降逆止咳平喘 / 254
suppressing upward perversion of *qi* to relieve dyspnea 降逆平喘 / 254
suppressing upward perversion of *qi* to stop hiccupping 降逆止呃 / 254
suppressing upward perversion of *qi* to stop vomiting 降逆止呕 / 254
suppurative coxitis 环跳疽 / 595
suppurative osteomyelitis 附骨疽 / 595
suppurative otitis media 脓耳，聤耳 / 623
suppurative parotitis 发颐 / 594
supraclavicular fossa 缺盆 / 47
supraduction 两眼翻上 / 129
supra-ophryon area 阙上 / 43
supra-orbital ridge 眉棱骨 / 43
suprapubic margin 毛际 / 48
supratragic notch 屏上切迹 / 473
surging pulse 洪脉 / 161
suspended moxibustion 悬灸，悬起灸 / 464
sustained pressing 按压法 / 480
Suxiao Jiuxin Pills 速效救心丸 / 394
sweat 汗 / 58
sweat pore 元府，玄府 / 41
sweating-arresting and superficies-strengthening medicinal/drug 敛汗固表药 / 294
sweating disease 汗病 / 531
sweating forehead 额汗 / 145
sweating hands and feet 手足汗 / 145
sweating head 头汗 / 145
sweating in shock 脱汗 / 531
sweating palms and soles 手足心汗 / 145
sweating syndrome 汗证 / 531
sweet taste in the mouth 口甘，口甜 / 155
Sweet Wormwood Herb 青蒿 / 307
Sweetvetch Root 红芪 / 340
swelling 肿胀 / 138
swelling (sore) 肿疡 / 591
swelling of the tongue 舌肿 / 133
swift digestion with rapid hunger 消谷善饥 / 153
swift lifting and slow thrusting 紧提慢按 / 457
swift pulse 疾脉 / 162
swift thrusting and slow lifting 紧按慢提 / 456
swollen cheek 腮肿 / 585
swollen eyelid 胞肿 / 614
swollen feet 脚肿 / 138
swollen tongue 肿胀舌 / 132
swollen uvula 悬雍肿 / 630
sword needle 剑针 / 452
sword-thrusting gesture 剑决式 / 504
symblepharon 睑粘睛珠，睥肉粘轮 / 613
symptom 症状 / 122
syncope 厥，厥证 / 537
syncope from terror 惊厥 / 575
syndrome 证 / 168
syndrome differentiation 辨证 / 122，168
syndrome differentiation and treatment 辨证施治 / 218
syndrome differentiation of gastro-intestinal diseases 胃肠病辨证 / 207
syndrome differentiation of heart diseases 心病辨证 / 200
syndrome differentiation of kidney and bladder diseases 肾膀胱病辨证 / 212
syndrome differentiation of liver and gallbladder diseases 肝胆病辨证 / 208
syndrome differentiation of lung diseases 肺病辨证 / 202
syndrome differentiation of spleen diseases 脾病辨证 / 205
syndrome manifestation 证候 / 168
syndrome of gallbladder insufficiency with timidity 胆虚气怯证 / 211
syndrome type 证型 / 168
syndrome/pattern of accumulated heat in the uterus 胞宫积热证 / 213
syndrome/pattern of accumulated pathogenic heat in the lung 邪热壅肺证 / 204
syndrome/pattern of ascendant hyperactivity of liver yang 肝阳上亢证 / 209
syndrome/pattern of blood deficiency and cold congealing

血虚寒凝证 / 184
syndrome/pattern of blood deficiency and external contraction 血虚外感证 / 184
syndrome/pattern of blood deficiency and wind-dryness 血虚风燥证 / 184
syndrome/pattern of blood deficiency complicated by stasis 血虚挟瘀证 / 184
syndrome/pattern of blood deficiency generating wind 血虚生［动］风证 / 184
syndrome/pattern of blood deficiency with dryness of skin and generation of wind 血虚肤燥生风证 / 185
syndrome/pattern of blood deficiency with internal heat 血虚内热证 / 184
syndrome/pattern of blood heat stirring blood 血热动血证 / 180
syndrome/pattern of blood heat with dryness transformation 血热化燥证 / 180
syndrome/pattern of blood heat with raging wind 血热风盛证 / 180
syndrome/pattern of blood stasis with water retention 血瘀水停证 / 186
syndrome/pattern of blood stasis with wind-dryness 血瘀风燥证 / 185
syndrome/pattern of both defense and nutrient aspects 卫营同病证 / 179
syndrome/pattern of both defense and *qi* aspects 卫气同病证 / 179
syndrome/pattern of cold congealing in the uterus 寒凝胞宫证 / 194，213
syndrome/pattern of cold pathogen invading the stomach 寒邪犯胃证 / 208
syndrome/pattern of cold stagnating in the heart vessels 寒滞心脉证 / 194
syndrome/pattern of cold stagnating in the liver meridian/channel 寒滞肝脉证 / 211
syndrome/pattern of cold stagnating in the meridians/channels 寒滞经脉证 / 195
syndrome/pattern of cold stagnating in the stomach and intestines 寒滞胃肠证 / 194
syndrome/pattern of cold-dampness encumbering the spleen 寒湿困脾证 / 206
syndrome/pattern of cold-dominant agonizing arthralgia 寒胜痛痹证 / 195
syndrome/pattern of cold-fluid retention in the lung 寒饮停肺证 / 188
syndrome/pattern of cold-fluid retention in the stomach 寒饮停胃证 / 188
syndrome/pattern of cold-phlegm obstructing the lung 寒痰阻肺证 / 203
syndrome/pattern of combined phlegm and *qi* 痰气互［郁］结证 / 190
syndrome/pattern of congealing cold with blood stasis 寒凝血瘀证 / 194
syndrome/pattern of dampness encumbering spleen yang 湿困脾阳证 / 206
syndrome/pattern of dampness-heat accumulating in the spleen 湿热蕴脾证 / 197
syndrome/pattern of dampness-heat in the liver meridian/channel 肝经湿热证 / 211
syndrome/pattern of dampness-heat invading the ear 湿热犯耳证 / 197
syndrome/pattern of dampness-heat obstructing arthralgia 湿热阻痹证 / 197
syndrome/pattern of dampness-heat obstructing the semen chamber 湿热阻滞精室证 / 214
syndrome/pattern of dampness-heat steaming the lip 湿热蒸唇证 / 196
syndrome/pattern of dampness-heat steaming the mouth 湿热蒸口证 / 196
syndrome/pattern of dampness-heat steaming the teeth 湿热蒸齿证 / 197
syndrome/pattern of dampness-heat steaming the tongue 湿热蒸舌证 / 197
syndrome/pattern of dampness obstructing the middle energizer 湿阻中焦证 / 206
syndrome/pattern of dampness-prevailing agonizing arthralgia 湿胜着痹证 / 196
syndrome/pattern of deficiency of both heart *qi* and heart blood 心气血两虚证 / 200
syndrome/pattern of deficiency of both *qi* and yin 气阴两虚证 / 183

syndrome/pattern of downpouring dampness-heat 湿热下注证 / 197
syndrome/pattern of dryness pathogen invading [damaging] the lung 燥邪犯［伤］肺证 / 198
syndrome/pattern of dual blaze of *qi*-blood aspects 气血两燔证 / 180
syndrome/pattern of dual blaze of *qi*-nutrient aspects 气营两燔证 / 180
syndrome/pattern of exterior cold and interior heat 表寒里热证 / 171
syndrome/pattern of exterior deficiency and interior excess 表虚里实证 / 171
syndrome/pattern of exterior excess and interior deficiency 表实里虚证 / 171
syndrome/pattern of exterior heat and interior cold 表热里寒证 / 171
syndrome/pattern of external invasion of wind-dampness 风湿外袭证 / 194
syndrome/pattern of external invasion of wind-heat 风热外袭证 / 192
syndrome/pattern of external invasion of wind pathogen 风邪外袭证 / 191
syndrome/pattern of extreme heat engendering wind 热极生风证 / 210
syndrome/pattern of exuberant heat with bleeding 热盛动血证 / 180
syndrome/pattern of fire harassing the mind 火扰心神证 / 201
syndrome/pattern of fire toxin attacking the throat 火毒攻喉证 / 199
syndrome/pattern of fire toxin attacking the tongue 火毒攻舌证 / 199
syndrome/pattern of fluid depletion with retained heat 津亏热结证 / 187
syndrome/pattern of heat accumulatiom with intestinal dryness 热结肠燥证 / 208
syndrome/pattern of heat entering nutrient-blood 热入营血证 / 180
syndrome/pattern of heat entering the blood chamber 热入血室证 / 214
syndrome/pattern of heat entering the pericardium 热入［闭］心包证 / 180
syndrome/pattern of heat harassing the mind 热扰心神证 / 201
syndrome/pattern of heat obstructing arthralgia 热邪阻痹证 / 198
syndrome/pattern of heat toxin attacking the throat 热毒攻喉证 / 199
syndrome/pattern of heat toxin attacking the tongue 热毒攻舌证 / 199
syndrome/pattern of heat toxin blocking the lung 热毒闭肺证 / 204
syndrome/pattern of insecurity of thoroughfare and conception vessels 冲任不固证 / 215
syndrome/pattern of interior retention of cold-fluid 寒饮内停证 / 188
syndrome/pattern of interior retention of milk 乳食内积证 / 199
syndrome/pattern of interior retention of water-fluid 水饮内停证 / 187
syndrome/pattern of internal accumulation of summerheat and dampness 暑湿内蕴证 / 195
syndrome/pattern of internal block of phlegm-heat 痰热内闭证 / 190
syndrome/pattern of internal harassment of phlegm-heat 痰热内扰证 / 190
syndrome/pattern of internal obstruction of cold-dampness 寒湿内阻证 / 196
syndrome/pattern of internal stagnation of summerheat 暑热内郁证 / 195
syndrome/pattern of internal stirring of liver wind 肝风内动证 / 210
syndrome/pattern of inward invasion of fire toxin 火毒内陷证 / 198
syndrome/pattern of inward invasion of heat toxin 热毒内陷证 / 198
syndrome/pattern of kidney deficiency with water flooding 肾虚水泛证 / 213
syndrome/pattern of kidney yin deficiency with effulgent fire 肾阴虚火旺证 / 212
syndrome/pattern of lingering

phlegm nodules 痰核留结证 / 190
syndrome/pattern of liver depression and spleen insufficiency 肝郁脾虚证 / 211
syndrome/pattern of liver fire blazing in the ear 肝火燔耳证 / 209
syndrome/pattern of liver fire invading the head 肝火犯头证 / 209
syndrome/pattern of liver *qi* invading the spleen 肝气犯脾证 / 210
syndrome/pattern of liver *qi* invading the stomach 肝气犯胃证 / 210
syndrome/pattern of liver stagnation and spleen insufficiency 肝郁脾虚证 / 211
syndrome/pattern of liver yang transforming into wind 肝阳化风证 / 210
syndrome/pattern of lung dryness with constipation 肺燥肠闭证 / 204
syndrome/pattern of obstruction by wind-cold-dampness 风寒湿阻证 / 192
syndrome/pattern of phlegm and static blood 瘀痰证 / 190
syndrome/pattern of phlegm clouding the mind 痰蒙心神证 / 201
syndrome/pattern of phlegm obstructing the semen chamber 痰阻精室证 / 214
syndrome/pattern of phlegm-dampness invading the ear 痰湿犯耳证 / 190
syndrome/pattern of phlegm-dampness obstructing the lung 痰湿阻肺证 / 203
syndrome/pattern of phlegm-dampness obstructing the semen chamber 痰湿阻滞精室证 / 214
syndrome/pattern of phlegm-fire harassing the heart 痰火扰心证 / 201
syndrome/pattern of phlegm-fire harassing the mind 痰火扰神证 / 201
syndrome/pattern of phlegm-heat accumulating in the lung 痰热壅［蕴］肺证 / 204
syndrome/pattern of phlegm-heat blocking the lung 痰热闭肺证 / 204
syndrome/pattern of phlegm-heat stirring wind 痰热动风证 / 190
syndrome/pattern of phlegm-turbidity invading the head 痰浊犯头证 / 190
syndrome/pattern of phlegm-turbidity obstructing the lung 痰浊阻肺证 / 203
syndrome/pattern of *qi* block with syncope 气闭神厥证 / 202
syndrome/pattern of *qi* collapse following bleeding 气随血脱证 / 186
syndrome/pattern of *qi* deficiency and blood stasis 气虚血瘀证 / 186
syndrome/pattern of *qi* deficiency and stagnation 气虚气滞证 / 183
syndrome/pattern of *qi* deficiency with dampness obstruction 气虚湿阻［困］证 / 183
syndrome/pattern of *qi* deficiency with external contraction 气虚外感证 / 183
syndrome/pattern of *qi* deficiency with fever 气虚发热证 / 183
syndrome/pattern of *qi* deficiency with hearing loss 气虚耳窍失充证 / 183
syndrome/pattern of *qi* deficiency with smell loss 气虚鼻窍失充证 / 183
syndrome/pattern of *qi* deficiency with water retention 气虚水停证 / 183
syndrome/pattern of *qi* failing to control blood 气不摄［统］血证 / 186
syndrome/pattern of *qi* stagnation and blood stasis 气滞血瘀证 / 186
syndrome/pattern of *qi* stagnation and phlegm coagulation in the throat 气滞痰凝咽喉证 / 186
syndrome/pattern of *qi* stagnation with water retention 气滞水停证 / 188
syndrome/pattern of *qi*-blood dual deficiency 气血两虚证 / 186
syndrome/pattern of retained fluid attacking the heart 水气凌心证 / 202
syndrome/pattern of spleen deficiency with dampness encumbrance 脾虚湿困证 / 206
syndrome/pattern of spleen deficiency with phlegm-dampness 脾虚痰湿证 / 206

syndrome/pattern of spleen deficiency with stirred wind 脾虚动风证 / 206
syndrome/pattern of static blood invading the head 瘀血犯头证 / 185
syndrome/pattern of static blood obstructing the brain collateral 瘀阻脑络证 / 201
syndrome/pattern of static blood obstructing the uterus 瘀阻胞宫证 / 214
syndrome/pattern of stomach cold with fluid retention 胃寒饮停证 / 188
syndrome/pattern of sudden collapse of heart yang 心阳暴脱证 / 200
syndrome/pattern of summerheat blocking the mental activity 暑热闭神证 / 196
syndrome/pattern of summerheat blocking the *qi* activity 暑闭气机证 / 196
syndrome/pattern of summerheat damaging the lung vessel 暑伤肺络证 / 204
syndrome/pattern of summerheat-dampness attacking the exterior 暑湿袭表证 / 195
syndrome/pattern of summerheat entering *yangming* (yang brightness) 暑入阳明证 / 518
syndrome/pattern of summerheat impairing the fluid and *qi* 暑伤津气证 / 195
syndrome/pattern of summerheat stirring wind 暑热动风证 / 195
syndrome/pattern of the kidney failing to receive *qi* 肾不纳气证 / 213
syndrome/pattern of thoroughfare-conception-vessel disorder 冲任失［不］调证 / 215
syndrome/pattern of toxic fire attacking the lip 毒火攻唇证 / 198
syndrome/pattern of toxic fire attacking the mouth 毒火攻口证 / 199
syndrome/pattern of transmission of heart heat to the bladder 心移热膀胱证 / 202
syndrome/pattern of transmission of heart heat to the small intestine 心移热小肠证 / 202
syndrome/pattern of true cold with false heat 真寒假热证 / 174
syndrome/pattern of true deficiency with false excess 真虚假实证 / 174
syndrome/pattern of true excess with false deficiency 真实假虚证 / 174
syndrome/pattern of true heat with false cold 真热假寒证 / 174
syndrome/pattern of up-flaming liver fire 肝火上炎证 / 210
syndrome/pattern of wind attacking the loose exterior 风袭表疏证 / 191
syndrome/pattern of wind-cold attacking the collaterals 风寒袭络证 / 192
syndrome/pattern of wind-cold attacking the exterior 风寒袭表证 / 192
syndrome/pattern of wind-cold attacking the lung 水寒射肺证，风寒袭肺证 / 192，203，205
syndrome/pattern of wind-cold attacking the nose 风寒袭鼻证 / 192
syndrome/pattern of wind-cold attacking the throat 风寒袭喉［咽］证 / 192
syndrome/pattern of wind-cold fettering the lung 风寒束肺证 / 203
syndrome/pattern of wind-cold invading the head 风寒犯头证 / 192
syndrome/pattern of wind-dampness attacking the exterior 风湿袭表证 / 194
syndrome/pattern of wind-dampness invading the eye 风湿凌目证 / 194
syndrome/pattern of wind-dampness invading the head 风湿犯头证 / 194
syndrome/pattern of wind-dryness attacking the exterior 风燥袭表证 / 194
syndrome/pattern of wind-fire attacking the eye 风火攻目证 / 193
syndrome/pattern of wind-heat attacking the eye 风热攻目证 / 193
syndrome/pattern of wind-heat blocking the lung 风热闭肺证 / 193
syndrome/pattern of wind-heat in the liver meridian/channel 肝经风热证 / 211
syndrome/pattern of wind-heat invading the ear 风热犯耳证 / 193
syndrome/pattern of wind-heat invading the eye 风热犯目证 / 193

syndrome/pattern of wind-heat invading the head 风热犯头证 / 193
syndrome/pattern of wind-heat invading the lung 风热犯肺证 / 193，203
syndrome/pattern of wind-heat invading the nose 风热犯鼻证 / 193
syndrome/pattern of wind-heat invading the throat 风热侵喉［咽］证 / 193
syndrome/pattern of wind pathogen attacking the collaterals 风邪袭络证 / 191
syndrome/pattern of wind pathogen invading the exterior 风邪犯表证 / 191
syndrome/pattern of wind-prevailing migratory arthralgia 风胜行痹证 / 191
syndrome/pattern of wind striking the meridians/channels 风中经络证 / 191
syndrome/pattern of wind-water combat 风水相搏证 / 188
syndrome/pattern of yin deficiency with effulgent fire 阴虚火旺证 / 172
syndrome/pattern of yin deficiency with internal heat 阴虚内热证 / 172
syndrome/pattern of yin deficiency with lung dryness 阴虚肺燥证 / 204
syndrome/pattern of yin deficiency with stirring wind 阴虚动风证 / 210
syndrome/pattern of yin deficiency with unmoistenable throat 阴虚咽喉失濡证 / 203
syndrome/pattern manifestation 证候 / 122
syndrome/pattern type 证型 / 122
syndromes of the six meridians/channels 六经病证 / 175
Synopsis of Prescriptions of the Golden Chamber 金匮要略方论 / 686
Synopsis of the Golden Chamber 金匮要略 / 686
syrup 糖浆 / 281
Systematic Compilation of the Internal Classic 类经 / 684
systremma 抽筋 / 127
Szechwan Chinaberry 川楝子 / 328
Szechwan Chinaberry Bark 苦楝皮 / 353
Szechwan Lovage Rhizome 川芎 / 330

T

T-shaped (infantile) malnutrition 丁奚疳 / 580
Tabanus 虻虫 / 333
Tabashir 天竺黄 / 300
tablet 片，片剂 / 282
Tai Ping Sheng Hui Fang 太平圣惠方 / 691
Taibai (SP 3) 太白 / 415
Taichong (LR 3) 太冲 / 432
taiji walking 太极步 / 496
Taiping Holy Benevolent Prescriptions 太平圣惠方 / 691
Tai Ping Hui Min He Ji Ju Fang 太平惠民和剂局方 / 691
Taixi (KI 3) 太溪 / 424
Taiyang (EX-HN 5) 太阳 / 440
taiyang person 太阳之人 / 74
Taiyi (ST 23) 太乙 / 413
taiyin person 太阴之人 / 74
Taiyuan (LU 9) 太渊 / 409
taking measures that are suited to the place 因地制宜 / 17
taking measures that are suited to the time 因时制宜 / 17
taking up with fingers 撮法 / 484
Talc 滑石 / 321
Talcum 滑石 / 321
Tang Ben Cao 唐本草 / 687
Tang Rongchuan 唐容川 / 680
Tang Shenwei 唐慎微 / 663
Tang Shenyuan 唐审元 / 663
Tang Tou Ge Jue 汤头歌诀 / 692
Tang Ye Ben Cao 汤液本草 / 688
Tang Zonghai 唐宗海 / 680
Tangerine Seed 橘核 / 325
Tangshen 党参 / 340
Tansy Mustard Seed 葶苈子 / 303
Tao Hongjing 陶弘景 / 660
Tao Tongming 陶通明 / 660
Taodao (GV 13) 陶道 / 434
Taoist *qigong* 道家气功 / 492
tapping 叩［扣］法 / 484
tapping the head 击头 / 487
tapping the teeth 叩［扣］齿 / 488
tarsal plate 目纲 / 44
tarsi of the eyelid 目纲 / 608
Tartarian Aster Root 紫菀 / 299
tastelessness in the mouth 口中无味 / 154
tea 茶 / 282
tears 泪 / 58
teeth grinding 龂齿，齿龂 / 579，632
temperance in eating and drinking 饮食有节 / 507

temporal region 太阳 / 43
ten categories of formulae 十剂 / 359
Ten-Dates Decoction 十枣汤 / 365
ten health-preserving routines 养生十常 / 507
Ten-ingredient Gynecological Tables 妇科十味片 / 395
ten items of avoidance for sleep 睡眠十忌 / 507
ten questions 十问 / 142
tendon 筋 / 42
tendon-plucking 弹筋 / 485
tendon-plucking manipulation 弹筋法 / 651
tendon-regulating manipulation 理筋手法 / 647
tendon regulation 理筋 / 647
tendon restoration 筋正 / 647
tendon reunion 筋合 / 647
tendon separation 分筋 / 647
tendon-stroking along the bone 顺骨捋筋 / 640
ten-year-old child 稚子 / 574
Tendrilleaf Fritillary Bulb 川贝母 / 302
tenesmus 里急后重，下坠 / 150，156
tense pulse at both yin and yang 脉阴阳俱紧 / 164
tense pulse 紧脉 / 162
Terminalia Fruit 诃子 / 349
terminating lactation 断乳，回乳 / 268
Terra Flava Usta 伏龙肝 / 349
terrestrial effect 在泉 / 18
tertiary collateral vessel 孙络 / 407
Tested Treasures of Obstetrics 经效产宝 / 694
testicle 睾 / 49
testicular abscess 子痈 / 599
testicular atrophy 睾丸萎缩 / 600
testing labor 试胎，试月 / 568
testis 睾 / 49
tetanus 金疮痉，破伤风 / 605
Thallus Laminariae seu Eckloniae 昆布 / 300
The ABC Classic of Acupuncture and Moxibustion 针灸甲乙经 / 699
The Complete Book of Effective Prescriptions for Women 妇人大全良方 / 695
The Essentials of Four Diagnostic Examinations 四诊抉微 / 686
The Genuine Meaning of the Classic of Difficulties 难经本义 / 684
the incidental 标 / 219
the radical 本 / 219
The Tang Materia Medica 唐本草 / 687
thelorrhagia 乳衄 / 597
thenar collateral vessel 鱼络 / 407
theory of essential *qi* 精气学说 / 2
theory of meridians/channels and collaterals 经络学说 / 398
theory of physical constitution 体质学说 / 73
theory of the circuits and *qi* 运气学说 / 17
thick (tongue) coating/fur 厚苔 / 135
thigh 股，髀 / 49，51
thigh cellulitis 股疽 / 594
thigh swelling 股肿 / 606
thigh yang cellulitis 股阳疽 / 595
thigh yin cellulitis 股阴疽 / 595
thighbone 楗，髀骨 / 51
Thin-leaf Milkwort Root 远志 / 336
thin nasal discharge 鼻流清涕 / 130
thin pulse 细脉 / 161
thin tongue 瘦薄舌 / 132
thin (tongue) coating/fur 薄苔 / 135
thin white sputum 痰稀白 / 137
thin white (tongue) coating/fur 薄白苔 / 134
thin yellow (tongue) coating 薄黄苔 / 134
third molar tooth 真牙 / 632
thirst 口渴 / 148
thirst with frequent drinking 口渴引饮 / 149
thirst with preference for cold drinks 口渴喜冷 / 149
thoracic accumulation 结胸 / 519
thoracic accumulation of blood 血结胸 / 520
thoracic accumulation of cold 寒结胸 / 520
thoracic center 膻中 / 47
thoracic fluid retention 支饮 / 528
thoracic fluid retention syndrome/pattern 饮停胸胁证 / 188
thoracic oppression 胸闷 / 156
thoracic pulling manipulation 扳胸椎法 / 652
Thoracic Stasis-expelling Decoction 血府逐瘀汤 / 376
thoracic stuffiness 胸痞 / 156
Thorny Acathopanax Root 刺五加 / 341
Thorough Understanding of

Cold Damage 伤寒指掌 / 685
thoroughfare vessel (TV) 冲脉 / 406
thought 意，思 / 57，69
threaded ligation therapy 挂线疗法 / 273
thready pulse 细脉 / 161
threatened miscarriage 胎动不安 / 568
three categories of disease cause 三因 / 62
three-circle posture 三圆式 / 496
three-contact posture 三接式 / 495
three-edged needle 三棱针 / 449
three-edged needle therapy 三棱针疗法 / 449
three grades of medicinals 三品 / 279
three kinds of arthralgia 三痹 / 540
three kinds of impediment 三痹 / 540
three kinds of postpartum collapses 产后三脱 / 570
three passes 三关 / 138
three-point aligning conduction of *qi* 三点拉线导气 / 504
three-point circle-drawing conduction of *qi* 三点求圆导气 / 504
three positions and nine pulse-takings 三部九候 / 159
three postpartum crises 产后三冲 / 570
three postpartum diseases 产后三病 / 570
three postpartum emergencies 产后三急 / 570
three signs of neonatal tetanus 脐风三证 / 575
three therapeutic methods 三法 / 225
three treasures 三宝 / 2
three types of wasting-thirst; three types of diabetes 三消 / 551
three yang 三阳 / 399
three yang meridians/channels of the foot 足三阳经 / 399
three yang meridians/channels of the hand 手三阳经 / 399
three yin 三阴 / 399
three yin meridians/channels of the foot 足三阴经 / 399
three yin meridians/channels of the hand 手三阴经 / 399
throat 咽喉 / 40
throat abscess 喉痈 / 629
throat-anus-genital syndrome 狐惑 / 547
throat-blocking abscess 锁喉痈 / 593
throat-blocking infection 锁喉毒 / 593
throat cancer 喉岩，喉菌 / 631
throat impediment 喉痹 / 629，630
throat infection with erythema 喉痧 / 585
throat moth 喉蛾 / 628
throat necrosis 喉疳 / 631
throat tinea with moth-eaten holes 天白蚁 / 629
throat wind 喉风 / 630
throbbing below the umbilicus 脐下悸，脐下悸动 / 154
throbbing palpitations 心动悸 / 151
thrush 鹅口疮 / 579，634
thrusting insertion 插入法 / 453
thumb body-*cun* 拇指同身寸 / 445
thumb body-inch 拇指同身寸 / 445
thumb web 虎口 / 52
thumbtack intradermal needle 图钉型皮内针 / 450
thumbtack needle 揿针 / 450
Thunbery Fritillary Bulb 浙贝母 / 302
Thunder Ball 雷丸 / 353
thunder head wind 雷头风 / 533
thunder-fire miraculous moxibustion 雷火神针 / 466
thunderous borborygmus 腹中雷鸣 / 154
thyroiditis 瘿痈 / 597
Tianchi (PC 1) 天池 / 425
Tianchong (GB 9) 天冲 / 429
Tianchuang (SI 16) 天窗 / 418
Tianding (LI 17) 天鼎 / 411
Tianfu (LU 3) 天府 / 408
tiangui 天癸 / 556
Tianjing (TE 10) 天井 / 427
Tianliao (TE 15) 天髎 / 427
Tianma Gouteng Decoction 天麻钩藤饮 / 378
Tianma Pills 天麻丸 / 393
Tianquan (PC 2) 天泉 / 426
Tianrong (SI 17) 天容 / 418
Tianshu (ST 25) 天枢 / 413
Tiantu (CV 22) 天突 / 437
Tianxi (SP 18) 天溪 / 416
Tianyou (TE 16) 天牖 / 427
Tianzhu (BL 10) 天柱 / 419
Tianzong (SI 11) 天宗 / 418
Tiaokou (ST 38) 条口 / 414
tibia 胫骨 / 50，51
tic of the eyelid 胞轮振跳，睥轮振跳 / 614
tidal fever 潮热 / 144，519
"tiger's mouth" 虎口 / 52

tiger-striding exercise 虎步功 / 502
tight pulse 紧脉 / 162
tinea 癣 / 604
tinea alba 白秃疮 / 604
tinea circinata 圆癣 / 604
tinea corporis 风癣 / 604
tinea cruris 股癣 / 604
tinea favosa 肥疮 / 604
tinea-like erosion of the throat 喉癣 / 629
tinea manuum 鹅掌风 / 604
tinea pedis 脚气疮，脚湿气 / 604
tinea unguium 鹅爪风 / 605
tinea versicolor 紫白癜风 / 605
Tinggong (SI 19) 听宫 / 418
Tinghui (GB 2) 听会 / 428
tinnitus 耳鸣 / 624
tip 标 / 219
tip of the needle 针尖 / 449
tip of the nose 鼻尖 / 38
tip of the tongue 舌尖，舌端 / 39，130
to be decocted alone 单煎 / 283
to be decocted first 先煎 / 283
to be decocted later 后下 / 283
to be decocted separately 另煎，别煮 / 283
to be decocted with wrapping 包煎 / 283
to be dissolved in the mouth 噙化 / 284
to be swallowed 吞服 / 284
to be taken after mixing 调服 / 283
to be taken at a draught 顿服 / 284
to be taken before bed-time 临睡前服 / 284
to be taken cold 冷服 / 284
to be taken frequently 频服 / 284
to be taken hot 热服 / 284
to be taken in the early morning 平旦服 / 284
to be taken infused 冲服 / 283
to be taken midway between meals 食远服 / 284
to be taken on an empty stomach 空腹服 / 284
to be taken warm 温服 / 284
to be taken with fluid 送服 / 284
Toad Venom 蟾酥 / 356
Tokay Gecko 蛤蚧 / 348
Tokyo Violet Herb 紫花地丁 / 311
Tong Ren Shu Xue Zhen Jiu Tu Jing 铜人俞穴针灸图经 / 699
Tongjing Pills 痛经丸 / 394
Tongli (HT 5) 通里 / 416
Tongtian (BL 7) 通天 / 419
tongue 舌 / 39
tongue abscess 舌痈 / 634
tongue body 舌体 / 131
tongue cancer 舌菌 / 598，634
tongue coating 舌苔 / 134
tongue coating/fur color 苔色 / 134
tongue color 舌色 / 131
tongue diagnosis 舌诊 / 130
tongue exercise 舌功 / 505
tongue fur 舌苔 / 134
tongue manifestations 舌象 / 130
tongue proper 舌体 / 131
tongue propping 柱舌 / 494
tongue propping the palate 舌柱上腭 / 494
tongue pustule 舌疔 / 634
tongue sore 舌疮 / 634
tongue spirit 舌神 / 131
tongue texture 舌质 / 131
tongue-tie 结舌 / 579
tongue with ecchymosis 舌有瘀斑 / 132
tongue with purple spots 舌有瘀点 / 132
tongue with teeth-marks 舌有齿痕 / 132
Tongxie Yaofang 痛泻要方 / 366
Tongxuan Lifei Pills [Tablets] 通宣理肺丸［片］ / 382
Tongziliao (GB 1) 瞳子髎 / 428
tonic 补养药，补益药 / 293
tonic convulsions 刚痉 / 127
tonification 补法 / 244
tonifying and nourishing medicinal/drug 补养药 / 293
tonifying and replenishing heart *qi* 补益心气 / 244
tonifying and replenishing medicinal/drug 补益药 / 293
tonifying blood 补血 / 247
tonifying formula 补剂，补益剂 / 360，371
tonifying heart yin 补心阴 / 248
tonifying kidney yin 补肾阴 / 250
tonifying liver yin 补肝阴 / 248
tonifying lung yin 补肺阴 / 249
tonifying method 补法 / 244
tonifying *qi* 补气 / 244
tonifying *qi* and blood 补益气血 / 247
tonifying *qi* and generating blood 补气生血 / 247
tonifying *qi* and nourishing blood 补气养血 / 247
tonifying *qi* to strengthen the superficies 补气固表 / 244
tonifying stomach yin 补胃阴 / 249
tonifying the heart and replenishing *qi* 补心益气 / 244
tonifying the heart and spleen 补益心脾 / 247
tonifying the kidney 补肾 / 249

tonifying the kidney and reinforcing the lung 补肾益肺 / 251

tonifying the kidney and replenishing *qi* 补肾益气 / 249

tonifying the kidney and supporting yang 补肾助阳 / 251

tonifying the kidney to arrest emission 补肾固精 / 250

tonifying the kidney to calm the mind 补肾安神 / 264

tonifying the kidney to improve inspiration 补肾纳气 / 251

tonifying the kidney to strengthen the bones 补肾健骨 / 251

tonifying the liver and kidney 补益肝肾 / 248

tonifying the lung 补肺 / 247

tonifying the lung and replenishing *qi* 补肺益气 / 247

tonifying the middle and replenishing *qi* 补中益气 / 246

tonifying the spleen 补脾 / 245

tonifying the spleen and replenishing *qi* 补脾益气 / 246

tonifying the spleen to replenish the lung 补脾益肺 / 247

tonifying tranquilizing formula 补养安神剂 / 380

tonifying yang 补阳 / 250

tonifying yin 补阴 / 248

tonsil 喉核 / 628

tonsillitis 乳蛾 / 628

tonsils 喉核 / 40

Toosendan Powder 金铃子散 / 375

tooth 齿 / 39

tooth-marked tongue 齿痕舌 / 132

toothache 牙痛 / 632

top-grade medicinal 上品 / 279

tortoise chest 龟胸 / 578

Tortoise Plastron 龟板 / 345

Tortoise Shell 龟甲 / 345

touching 举法 / 159

touching, pressing and searching 举、按、寻 / 158

Toulinqi (GB 15) 头临泣 / 429

Touqiaoyin (GB 11) 头窍阴 / 429

Touwei (ST 8) 头维 / 412

toxic dampness leukorrhagia 湿毒带下 / 564

toxic swelling 肿毒 / 591

toxin 毒 / 68

trachoma 椒疮 / 613

trachomatous pannus 赤膜下垂 / 619

tracing 循法 / 159

traction 拉法，牵拉法 / 639

traction therapy 牵引疗法 / 642

tragus 耳门，耳屏 / 45，473

training of the mind 练神 / 498

training *qi* 练气 / 503

tranquilizer 安神药 / 293

tranquilizing medicinal/drug 安神药 / 293

transformation into dryness 化燥 / 92

transformation into fire 化火 / 92

transformation into heat 化热 / 92

transformation into wind 化风 / 92

transformation of stomach heat into fire 胃热化火 / 92

transformation of the five emotions/minds into fire 五志化火 / 70

transformation of the sour-sweet into yin 酸甘化阴 / 248

transmission and change 传变 / 116

transmission of pathogenic heat into the interior 热邪传里 / 83

transmission of sensation along the meridian/channel 循经感传 / 458

transport-alarm point combination 俞募配穴法 / 448

transport needling 输刺 / 460

transport-source point combination 俞原配穴法 / 448

transverse counterflow of liver *qi* 肝气横逆 / 97

transverse insertion 横刺 / 454

transverse pad 横垫 / 641

transverse penetration 横透 / 454

trauma 疡 / 635

trauma and fracture 折疡 / 635

traumatic cataract 惊震内障 / 620

traumatic injury to the eyeball 物损真睛 / 621

traumato-orthopedics 骨伤科（学） / 635

traumato-orthopedist 疡医 / 635

traumatology 伤科 / 635

tray-like palmar infection 托盘疔 / 592

treading 踩法 / 485

treading manipulation 踩跷法 / 652

treading-stamping 踩跷法 / 486

Treasure of Obstetrics 产宝 / 695

Treasured Classic 中藏经 / 700

treating diarrhea with diuretics 利小便，实大便 / 261

treating disease from the root 治病求本 / 219

treating diseases of the left with

points on the right, and vice versa 左病右取，右病左取 / 221
treating the incidental 治标 / 219
treating the incidental and radical simultaneously 标本同治 / 219
treating the incidental and radical together 标本兼治 / 219
treating the lower for the upper, and treating the upper for the lower 上病下取，下病上取 / 221
treating the radical 治本 / 219
treating wind and resolving phlegm 治风化痰 / 259
treating yang for yin diseases 阴病治阳 / 221
treating yin for yang diseases 阳病治阴 / 221
Treatise on Blood Syndromes 血证论 / 694
Treatise on Causes and Manifestations of Diseases 诸病源侯总论 / 687
Treatise on Choleric Turmoil 霍乱论 / 694
Treatise on Cold Damage and Miscellaneous Diseases 伤寒杂病论 / 685
Treatise on Cold Damage Diseases 伤寒论 / 685
Treatise on Medical Prescriptions 医方论 / 693
Treatise on Pestilence 温疫论 / 693
Treatise on Seasonal Diseases 时病论 / 694
Treatise on Smallpox and Measles in Children 小儿痘疹方论 / 696
Treatise on the Spleen and Stomach 脾胃论 / 694
Treatise on the Three Categories of Pathogenic Factors and Prescriptions 三因极一病证方论 / 687
Treatise on Warm-heat Diseases 温热论 / 693
treatment according to individual 因人制宜 / 218
treatment according to place 因地制宜 / 218
treatment according to time 因时制宜 / 218
treatment according to time, place and individual 因时、因地、因人制宜 / 218
Tree Peony Bark 牡丹皮 / 306
Tree-of-heaven Bark 椿皮 / 308
trembling 振掉 / 540
trembling method 震颤法 / 455
trembling mouth 口振 / 136
trembling of the extremities 手足颤动 / 127
trembling tongue 颤动舌，舌战 / 133
tremor 颤震［振］/ 540
tri-monthly menstruation 居经 / 556
tri-tabular massotherapy 三板推拿疗法 / 486
tri-tabular *tuina*-therapy 三板推拿疗法 / 486
triangular fossa 三角窝 / 472
trichiasis 倒睫，睫毛倒入 / 613
trichiasis and entropion 倒睫拳毛 / 613
Trichosanthes-Allium-Pinellia Decoction 瓜蒌薤白半夏汤 / 375
triple combination of yang meridian/channel diseases 三阳合病 / 178
triple energizer 三焦 / 24
triple energizer cough 三焦咳 / 525
triple-energizer dampness-heat syndrome/pattern 三焦湿热证 / 181
triple energizer deficiency cold 三焦虚寒 / 214
triple energizer excess heat 三焦实热 / 215
triple energizer meridian/channel (TE) 手三焦经 / 404
triple energizer meridian/channel of hand lesser yang 手少阳三焦经 / 404
triple-energizer syndrome differentiation 三焦辨证 / 181
triple-energizer pattern identification 三焦辨证 / 181
triple needling 齐刺 / 461
triple-round stake-standing exercise 三圆站桩功 / 502
tripod-shaped splint fixation 鼎式夹板固定 / 640
trismus 口噤 / 537
trochanter 髀枢 / 51
Trogopterus Dung 五灵脂 / 332
true cold with false heat 真寒假热 / 92
true deficiency with false excess 真虚假实 / 85
true excess with false deficiency 真实假虚 / 85
true headache 真头痛 / 533
true heat with false cold 真热假寒 / 92
true or false cold and heat 寒热真假 / 91
true or false deficiency and excess 虚实真假 / 84
true stroke 真中 / 536
true visceral color 真脏色 / 126

true visceral pulse 真脏脉 / 165
true wind stroke 真中风 / 536
Trumpetcreeper Flower 凌霄花 / 332
trunk of the antihelix 对耳轮体 / 472
Tsaoko 草果 / 320
Tuber Onion Seed 韭菜子 / 348
tuberculosis of epididymis 子痰 / 599
Tui Na Guang Yi 推拿广意 / 696
tuina therapy 推拿疗法 / 480
tuina 推拿 / 480
tumor 瘤 / 598
tumor of the throat 喉瘤 / 631
turbid diabetes 消浊 / 589
turbid nasal discharge 鼻流浊涕 / 130
turbid pathogen 浊邪 / 72
turbid *qi* 浊气 / 55
turbid redness of the white of the eye 白睛混赤 / 611
turbid urine (disease) 尿浊 / 551
turbid yin 浊阴 / 57
Turmeric 姜黄 / 331
Turmeric Root Tuber 郁金 / 331
turning to the opposite 折顶 / 639
Turtle Shell 鳖甲 / 345
twelve categories of formulae 十二剂 / 360
twelve channels 十二经 / 398
twelve cutaneous regions 十二皮部 / 407
twelve joints 十二节 / 52
twelve meridian/channel divergences 十二经别 / 407
twelve meridian/channel sinews 十二经筋 / 406
twelve meridians十二经 / 398
twelve meridians/channels 十二经脉 / 398
twelve needling methods 十二刺 / 461
twenty-eight pulses 二十八脉 / 160
twirling method 捻转法 / 454
twirling reinforcement and reduction 捻转补泻 / 457
twirling reinforcing-reducing method 捻转补泻法 / 457
twisting 捻法 / 481
twisting for congestion 扭痧 / 486
twisting manipulation 搓法 / 647
twisting rubbing 搓法 / 484
twitching of the body 身瞤动 / 127
Two-elixir Decoction 二仙汤 / 373
Two-elixir Glue of Tortoise Plastron and Deer Horn 龟鹿二仙胶 / 373
two private parts 二阴 / 48
two yin 二阴 / 48
Twoteethed Achyranthes Root 牛膝 / 344
tympanic pulse 革脉 / 162
tympanites 气臌（病） / 547
typical edema 正水 / 549

U

ulcer 溃疡，疡 / 591
ulcerated ear 耳疳 / 625
ulcerated gangrene 烂疔 / 592
ulceration of the palpebral margin 睑弦糜烂 / 614
ulcerative gingivitis 牙疳 / 633
ulcerative keratitis 白陷鱼鳞，花翳白陷 / 618
ulcerative marginal blepharitis 睑弦糜烂 / 614
ulcerative stomatitis 口糜 / 579
Umbellate Polypore 猪苓 / 320
umbilical abscess 脐痈 / 593
umbilical bleeding 脐血 / 578
umbilical cold diarrhea 脐寒泻 / 588
umbilical cord 脐带 / 566
umbilical dampness 脐湿 / 578
umbilical eczema 脐疮 / 603
umbilical fistula 脐漏 / 593
umbilical hernia 脐疝 / 578
umbilical protrusion 脐突 / 578
umbilical sore 脐疮 / 578，593
umbilicus 神阙 / 48
unblocking and promoting blood flow 通利血脉 / 268
unblocking collaterals to relieve pain 通络止痛 / 268
unblocking meridians/channels and activating collaterals 通经活络 / 268
unblocking meridians/channels to relieve pain 通经止痛 / 268
unblocking the interior 通里 / 236
unblocking yang 通阳 / 240
Unbracteolated Euphorbia Root 狼毒 / 324
unconscious murmuring 郑声 / 140
unconsciousness 神志不清 / 123
undigested food (in stool) 完谷不化 / 149
unfavorable complexion 恶色 / 125
unfavorable syndrome/pattern of measles 麻疹逆证 / 584
ungratifying diarrhea 泻下不爽 / 149
Uniflower Swisscentaury Root 漏芦 / 312
unilateral swollen testicle 差颓［癞］/ 578
unilateral tonsillitis 单蛾 / 628

union bone 交骨 / 49
Universal Antitoxic Decoction 普济消毒饮 / 368
unsmooth pulse 涩脉 / 161
untwining rope pulse 解索脉 / 163
ununited skull 解颅 / 577
ununited skull (disease) 解颅病 / 577
up-flaming heart-fire syndrome/pattern 心火上炎证 / 201
up-flaming of liver fire 肝火上炎 / 98
up-flaming of stomach fire 胃火上炎 / 108
up-rising of fire 上火 / 519
updated formula 时方 / 357
upper arm 肱 / 47
upper cold and lower heat 上寒下热 / 91
upper-cold and lower-heat syndrome/pattern 上寒下热证 / 171
upper *dantian* 上丹田 / 496
upper deficiency and lower excess 上虚下实 / 84
upper-deficiency and lower-excess syndrome/pattern 上虚下实证 / 172
upper diabetes 消上 / 589
upper elixir field 上丹田 / 496
upper energizer 上焦 / 24
upper-energizer dampness-heat syndrome/pattern 上焦湿热证 / 181
upper energizer deficiency cold 上焦虚寒 / 214
upper energizer excess heat 上焦实热 / 215
upper-energizer syndrome/pattern 上焦病证 / 181
upper excess and lower deficiency 上实下虚 / 84
upper-excess and lower-deficiency syndrome/pattern 上实下虚证 / 172
upper eyelid 目上胞，上睑 / 44，608
upper eyelid margin 目上弦 / 609
upper heat and lower cold 上热下寒 / 91
upper-heat and lower-cold syndrome/pattern 上热下寒证 / 172
upper-lateral line of the occiput (MS 13) 枕上旁线 / 472
upper-lower point combination 上下配穴法 / 447
upper-middle line of the occiput (MS 12) 枕上正中线 / 471
upper obstruction 上膈 / 543
upper orifices 上窍 / 38
upper palpebral musculature 目上纲，目上网 / 608
upper preponderance and lower deficiency 上盛下虚 / 84
upper stomach cavity 上脘 / 23
upper wasting-thirst 上消 / 551
upsurging of the yellow fluid 黄液上冲 / 618
upsurging of the yellow membrane 黄膜上冲 / 618
upsurging of the yellow pus 黄脓上冲 / 618
upward counterflow of liver *qi* 肝气上逆 / 98
upward counterflow of lung *qi* 肺气上逆 / 109
upward counterflow of stomach *qi* 胃气上逆 / 108
upward reversal of fetal *qi* 胎气上逆 / 567
upward-staring convulsions 天钓 / 575
urinary incontinence 小便失禁 / 151
urolithic stranguria 砂（石）淋，石淋 / 552
urticaria 风瘾疹 / 603
urticaria during menstruation 经行隐疹 / 563
use of corrigents 反佐 / 221
using a corrigent 反佐 / 358
Ussuri Fritillary Bulb 平贝母 / 302
uterine collateral vessel 胞络 / 407
uterine dampness-heat syndrome/pattern 胞宫湿热证 / 214
uterine deficiency-cold syndrome/pattern 胞宫虚寒证 / 213
uterine flooding 崩中 / 561
uterine obstruction 胞阻 / 566
uterine vessel 胞脉 / 407
uterus 胞，胞宫，胞脏，女子胞，血脏，子宫，女子胞 / 25，555，556
uterus coldness infertility 宫冷不孕，胞寒不孕 / 565
uvula 蒂丁，蒂中，悬雍垂 / 40，628
uvular abscess 悬痈 / 630
uvular hematoma 悬旗小舌 / 630
uvular wind 悬旗风 / 630
uvulitis 悬雍肿 / 630

V

vacuous pulse 虚脉 / 161
vagina 阴道，子肠 / 555
vaginal bleeding during pregnancy 胎漏 / 569
vaginal discharge 带下 / 563
vaginal orifice 阴门，阴户 / 49

vaginal orifice (of a paturient) 产门 / 48
Valerian Rhizome 缬草 / 337
varicella 水痘 / 584
varied normal complexion 客色 / 124
variola 痘疮 / 585
Variorum of the Classic of Materia Medica 本草经集注 / 687
varix 筋瘤 / 598
vascular spider 血缕 / 601
Venenum Bufonis 蟾酥 / 356
venomous snake bite 毒蛇咬伤 / 606
ventilating the lung and directing *qi* downward 宣肺降气 / 228
ventilating the lung and resolving phlegm 宣肺化痰 / 228
ventilating the lung and resolving retained fluid 宣肺化饮 / 228
ventilating the lung to relieve cough and dyspnea 宣肺止咳平喘 / 228
ventilating the lung to relieve cough 宣肺止咳 / 228
ventilating the lung to relieve dyspnea 宣肺平喘 / 228
ventilating the lung 宣肺 / 228
ventro-dorsal point combination 腹背配穴法 / 447
verruca 疣 / 600
verruca filiformis 丝状疣 / 600
verruca plana 扁瘊 / 600
verruca plantaris 跖疣 / 600
verruca vulgaris 疣目 / 600
vertex 巅 / 42
vertex cranii 巅顶 / 42
vertical palm-striking manipulation 劈法 / 649
vertigo in pregnancy 妊娠眩晕 / 566
vesicle 水疱，疱疹 / 139，591
vesiculating moxibustion 发泡灸 / 466
vesiculation 发泡 / 273
vessel 脉 / 25
vessel atrophy-flaccidity 脉痿 / 539
vessel impediment 脉痹 / 541
"vessel opening" 脉口 / 160
vexation 心烦 / 124
vexation and agitation 烦躁 / 124
vexation during pregnancy 妊娠心烦 / 567
vexation of deficiency type 虚烦 / 529
vexing fever 烦热 / 144
vexing heat in the chest 五心烦热 / 144
vexing thirst 烦渴 / 149
vibrating 颤法，振法 / 484
vibrissa 鼻毛 / 39
vicarious menstruation 倒经 / 560
Vietnamese Sophora Root 山豆根 / 313
Virgate Wormwood Herb 茵陈 / 309
virginal orifice 玉门 / 555
viscera and bowels 脏腑 / 20
visceral cold diarrhea 脏寒泻 / 588
visceral convulsions 内钓 / 575
visceral exhaustion color 真脏色 / 126
visceral exhaustion pulse 真脏脉 / 165
visceral manifestation 脏象 / 20，26
visceral manifestation theory 脏象学说 / 20
visceral pattern identification 脏腑辨证 / 200
visceral *qi* 脏气 / 26
visceral stroke 中脏 / 536
visceral syncope 脏厥 / 538
visceral syndrome differentiation 脏腑辨证 / 200
viscus 脏 / 20
viscus for fetus 胞脏 / 25
viscus for offspring 子脏 / 25
viscus-induced disease 所生病 / 408
visible phlegm 有形之痰 / 71
vision obstruction 障 / 612
vitality 神 / 2
vitiligo 白癜风，白驳风 / 602
vitreous 神膏 / 610
vitreous opacity 云雾移睛 / 620
voice 语声 / 139
vomiting 呕吐 / 542
vomiting fecal matter 吐矢 / 544
vomiting in the evening of food eaten in the morning 朝食暮吐 / 152
vomiting in the morning of food eaten the previous evening 暮食朝吐 / 152
vomiting of clear mucus 呕吐清涎 / 152
vomiting of milk 呕乳 / 577
vomiting of pregnancy 妊娠呕吐 / 566
vomiting of retained food 呕吐宿食 / 152
vomiting of sour fetid matter 呕吐酸腐 / 152
vomiting right after eating 食已即吐 / 153
vomiting with fright 夹惊吐 / 587

vulva 阴户 / 555

W

waggling tongue 弄舌 / 134
Wai Ke Da Cheng 外科大成 / 698
Wai Ke Jing Yao 外科精要 / 697
Wai Ke Jing Yi 外科精义 / 697
Wai Ke qi Xuan 外科启玄 / 697
Wai Ke Zheng Zhi Quan Sheng Ji 外科证治全生集 / 698
Wai Ke Zheng Zong 外科正宗 / 698
Wai Tai Mi Yao 外台秘要 / 690
Waiguan (TE 5) 外关 / 427
Waihuaijian (EX-LE 9) 外踝尖 / 443
Wailaogong (EX-UE 8) 外劳宫 / 442
Wailing (ST 26) 外陵 / 413
Waiqiu (GB 36) 外丘 / 431
waist exercise 腰部功 / 501
walking posture 走式 / 496
Wan Bing Hui Chun 万病回春 / 703
Wan Mi Zhai Yi Xue Quan Shu 万密斋医学全书 / 703
Wan Mizhai 万密斋 / 670
Wan Quan 万全 / 670
Wan Shi Nü Ke 万氏女科 / 695
Wan's Gynecology and Obstetrics 万氏女科 / 695
wandering erysipelas 赤游丹 / 594
wandering pain 游走痛 / 148
Wang Ang 汪昂 / 674
Wang Bing 王冰 / 661
Wang Haizang 王海藏 / 666
Wang Haogu 王好古 / 666
Wang Ji 汪机 / 668
Wang Jinzhi 王进之 / 666
Wang Kentang 王肯堂 / 671
Wang Lun 王纶 / 668
Wang Mengying 王孟英 / 680
Wang Qingren 王清任 / 678
Wang Ren'an 汪讱安 / 674
Wang Shixiong 王士雄 / 680
Wang Shuhe 王叔和 / 659
Wang Sun'an 王损庵 / 671
Wang Tailin 王泰林 / 679
Wang Tao 王焘 / 661
Wang Weide 王惟德 / 662
Wang Weiyi 王维一 / 662
Wang Xi 王熙 / 659
Wang Xingzhi 汪省之 / 668
Wang Xugao 王旭高 / 679
Wang Xunchen 王勋臣 / 678
Wang Yutai 王宇泰 / 671
Wang Zhizhong 王执中 / 664
Wangbi Granules 尪痹颗粒 / 393
Wangu (GB 12) 完骨 / 429
Wangu (SI 4) 腕骨 / 417
warm disease 温病 / 515
warm dryness 温燥，温燥 / 66
warm dryness disease 温燥病 / 519
warm-dryness syndrome/pattern 温燥证 / 197
warm malaria 温疟 / 520
warm pathogen 温邪 / 514
warm pathogen invading the lung 温邪犯肺 / 85
warm purgation 温下 / 236
warm purgation of cold accumulation 温下寒积 / 236
warm purgative formula 温下剂 / 364
warm tear shedding induced by wind 迎风热泪 / 611
warm toxin 温毒 / 514
warming and resolving cold-phlegm 温化寒痰 / 258
warming and tonifying kidney yang 温补肾阳 / 242
warming and tonifying stomach yang 温补胃阳 / 241
warming and tonifying the life gate 温补命门 / 251
warming and tonifying the spleen and kidney 温补脾肾 / 243
warming and tonifying the spleen and stomach 温补脾胃 / 246
warming and unblocking the meridians/channels and collaterals 温经通络 / 243
warming formula 热剂 / 360
warming heart yang 温心阳 / 240
warming kidney yang 温肾阳 / 242
warming method 温法 / 240
warming needle moxibustion 温针灸 / 466
warming over fire 热烘 / 272
warming phlegm-resolving medicinal/drug 温化寒痰药 / 292
warming purgative (medicinal/drug) 温下药 / 289
warming the interior 温里 / 240
warming the interior and dispelling cold 温里祛寒 / 244
warming the interior and dissipating cold 温里散寒 / 244
warming the kidney 温肾 / 242
warming the kidney to improve *qi* reception 温肾纳气 / 242

warming the kidney to induce diuresis 温肾利水 / 261
warming the kidney to invigorate yang 温肾壮阳 / 242
warming the kidney to reduce urination 温肾缩尿 / 242
warming the kidney to resolve phlegm 温肾化痰 / 242
warming the kidney to resolve retained fluid 温肾化饮 / 243
warming the kidney to stop diarrhea 温肾止泻 / 242
warming the liver 温肝 / 240
warming the lung 温肺 / 242
warming the lung and dissipating cold 温肺散寒 / 242
warming the lung and resolving phlegm 温肺化痰 / 242
warming the lung and resolving retained fluid 温肺化饮 / 242
warming the meridians/channels 温经 / 243
warming the meridians/channels and activating blood 温经活血 / 243
warming the meridians/channels and dispelling cold 温经祛寒 / 243
warming the meridians/channels and dissipating cold 温经散寒 / 243
warming the meridians/channels and nourishing blood 温经养血 / 244
warming the meridians/channels and restoring yang 温经回阳 / 243
warming the meridians/channels and supporting yang 温经扶阳 / 243
warming the meridians/channels and the uterus 温经暖宫 / 243
warming the meridians/channels and unblocking yang 温经通阳 / 243
warming the meridians/channels to move stagnation 温经行滞 / 243
warming the meridians/channels to relieve pain 温经止痛 / 244
warming the middle 温中 / 241
warming the middle and dispelling cold 温中祛寒，温中散寒 / 241
warming the middle and harmonizing the stomach 温中和胃 / 241
warming the middle and moving *qi* 温中行气 / 241
warming the middle to relieve pain 温中止痛 / 242
warming the middle to stop diarrhea 温中止泻 / 242
warming the middle to stop vomiting 温中止呕，温中止吐 / 241
warming the spleen 温脾 / 241
warming the stomach 温胃 / 241
warming the stomach to stop vomiting 温胃止呕 / 241
warming the stomach to suppress upward counterflow of *qi* 温胃降逆 / 241
warming the uterus 暖宫 / 243
warming yang 温阳 / 240
warming yang to drain dampness 温阳利湿 / 261
warming yang to induce diuresis 温阳利水 / 261
warming yang to promote urination 温阳行水 / 261
warmth-heat 温热 / 67
warmth pathogen 温邪 / 67
wart 疣，瘊子 / 600
wart eye 疣目 / 600
washing 洗 / 276
washing by gargling 漱涤 / 273
Wasp's Nest 蜂房 / 356
wasting thirst 消渴（病）/ 551
water and grain 水谷 / 53
water-cold attacking the lung 水寒射肺 / 103
water distension 水胀 / 548
water failing to nourish wood 水不涵木 / 14
water-featured person 水形之人 / 74
water-fire coordination 水火相济 / 27
water-fire processing 水火共制 / 276
water generating wood 水生木 / 12
water orbiculus 水轮 / 44，607
Water-plantain Rhizome 泽泻 / 320
water processing 水制 / 276
water *qi* 水气 / 548
water-*qi* syndrome/pattern 水气证 / 189
water restricting fire 水克火 / 12
water retention syndrome/pattern 水停证 / 189
watered pill 水丸 / 280
watering of the eyes from time to time 不时泪溢 / 611
watery diarrhea 水泻 / 150
watery diarrhea with blood and mucus 泄注赤白 / 150
watery lienteric diarrhea 飧水泻 / 588
waxed pill 蜡丸 / 280

waxing and waning of yin and yang 阴阳消长 / 6
weak defense *qi* with strong nutrient 卫弱营强 / 86
weak pulse 弱脉 / 161
Weeping Forsythia Fruit 连翘 / 310
Wei Dazhai 危达斋 / 666
Wei Liuzhou 魏柳洲 / 675
Wei Sheng Jia Bao Chan Ke Bei Yao 卫生家宝产科备要 / 695
Wei Yilin 危亦林 / 665
Wei Zhixiu 魏之琇 / 675
Weicang (BL 50) 胃仓 / 422
Weidao (GB 28) 维道 / 430
Weishu (BL 21) 胃俞 / 420
Weiwanxiashu (EX-B 3) 胃脘下俞 / 441
Weiyang (BL 39) 委阳 / 421
Weizhong (BL 40) 委中 / 421
well points 井穴 / 437
Wen Bing Tiao Bian 温病条辨 / 693
Wen Re Jing Wei 温热经纬 / 693
Wen Re Lun 温热论 / 693
Wen Yi Lun 温疫论 / 693
Wenliu (LI 7) 温溜 / 410
Wenpi Decoction 温脾汤 / 364
Wenyujin Concise Rhizome 片姜黄 / 331
what the different tastes act on 五味所入 / 280
wheal 风团 / 603
wheat-grain-sized cone moxibustion 麦粒灸 / 465
wheatgrain intradermal needle 麦粒型皮内针 / 450
wheezing 哮 / 141，527
wheezing disease 哮病 / 527
wheezing dyspnea 喘鸣 / 141
whisking 拂法 / 483
white bald 白秃 / 604
white bald scalp sore 白秃疮 / 604
white discoloration 白色 / 126
white dysentery 白痢 / 522
white greasy (tongue) coating/fur 白腻苔 / 134
White Hyacinth Bean 白扁豆 / 341
white kernel 白仁 / 45，609
white membrane covering the eye 白膜蔽睛 / 617
white membrane invading the eye 白膜侵睛 / 617
White Mulberry Root-bark 桑白皮 / 303
white mustard moxibustion 白芥子灸 / 467
White Mustard Seed 白芥子 / 299
white of the eye 白睛，白珠 / 45，609
white ooze 白淫 / 552
White Peony Root 白芍 / 342
White Pharbitis Seed 白丑 / 324
White Phoenix Pills 乌鸡白凤丸 / 394
white ringworm 白秃疮 / 604
white sandy (tongue) coating/fur 白砂苔 / 135
white slimy (tongue) coating/fur 白腻苔 / 134
White Tiger Decoction 白虎汤 / 367
"white tiger shaking its head" 白虎摇头法 / 458
white (tongue) coating/fur 白苔 / 134
white vaginal discharge 白带 / 564
white xerotic disease 白涩病 / 617
white xerotic syndrome 白涩症 / 617
whitlow 瘭疽 / 594
whole abdomen 大腹 / 48
whooping cough 百日咳，顿咳 / 586
Wild Aconite Root 草乌 / 314
Wild Chrysanthemum Flower 野菊花 / 311
will 志 / 58
Willowleaf Swallowwort Rhizome 白前 / 301
wind 风 / 64
wind arthralgia 风痹 / 540
wind attacking blood vessel 风中血脉 / 89
wind-cold attacking the lung 风寒袭肺 / 109
wind-cold common cold 风寒感冒 / 516
wind-cold cough 风寒咳嗽 / 525
wind-cold dispersing medicinal/drug 发散风寒药 / 287
wind-cold dizziness 风寒眩晕 / 532
wind-cold fettering the exterior 风寒束表 / 88
wind-cold fettering the lung 风寒束肺 / 110
wind-cold headache 风寒头痛 / 533
wind-cold lumbago 风寒腰痛 / 553
wind-cold pathogen 风寒邪气 / 67
wind-cold pharyngitis 风寒喉痹 / 629
wind-cold syndrome/pattern 风寒证 / 191
wind-cold toothache 风寒牙痛 / 632
wind-cold vertigo 风寒眩晕 / 532
wind-cold 风寒 / 67

wind-cold-dampness 风寒湿 / 68
wind-dampness 风湿 / 68
wind-dampness-dispelling and cold-dispersing medicinal/drug 祛风湿散寒药 / 289
wind-dampness-dispelling and heat-clearing medicinal/drug 祛风湿清热药 / 289
wind-dampness-dispelling and tendon-bone-strengthening medicinal/drug 祛风湿强筋骨药 / 289
wind-dampness-dispelling medicinal/drug 祛风湿药 / 289
wind-dampness headache 风湿头痛 / 533
wind-dampness lumbago 风湿腰痛 / 553
wind-dampness pathogen 风湿邪气 / 68
wind-dampness syndrome/pattern 风湿证 / 193
wind-dryness 风燥 / 64，68
wind-dryness cough 风燥咳嗽 / 526
wind edema 风水 / 549
wind epilepsy 风痫 / 589
wind-extinguishing and spasm-controlling medicinal/drug 熄［息］风止痉药 / 293
wind-extinguishing formula 熄风剂 / 378
wind-fire 风火 / 67
wind-fire eye 风火眼 / 615
wind-fire painful eye 风火眼痛 / 616
wind-fire toothache 风火牙痛 / 632
wind-fire whirling internally 风火内旋 / 89
wind-heat 风热 / 67
wind-heat common cold 风热感冒 / 516
wind-heat cough 风热咳嗽 / 525
wind-heat dispersing medicinal/drug 发散风热药 / 287
wind-heat dizziness 风热眩晕 / 532
wind-heat exterior syndrome/pattern 风热表证 / 192
wind-heat eye 风热眼 / 616
wind-heat headache 风热头痛 / 533
wind-heat in the liver meridian/channel 肝经风热 / 98
wind-heat invading the lung 风热犯肺 / 110
wind-heat lumbago 风热腰痛 / 553
wind-heat pathogen 风热邪气 / 67
wind-heat pharyngitis 风热喉痹 / 629
wind-heat sore 风热疮 / 602
wind-heat syndrome/pattern 风热证 / 192
wind-heat tinnitus 风热耳鸣 / 624
wind-heat tonsillitis 风热乳蛾 / 628
wind-heat toothache 风热牙痛 / 632
wind-heat ulcerative gingivitis 风热牙疳 / 633
wind-heat vertigo 风热眩晕 / 532
wind impediment 风痹 / 540
wind-induced squint 风牵偏视 / 622
wind itch 风痒 / 602
wind orbiculus 风轮 / 44，607
wind-orbiculus red bean 风轮赤豆 / 619
wind pass 风关 / 138
wind-phlegm 风痰 / 64
wind-phlegm dizziness 风痰眩晕 / 532
wind-phlegm headache 风痰头痛 / 534
wind-phlegm syndrome/pattern 风痰证 / 189
wind-phlegm vertigo 风痰眩晕 / 532
wind pruritus 风瘙痒 / 603
wind rash 风痧 / 584
wind red sore of the eyelid 风赤疮痍，风赤疮疾 / 614
wind-warmth 风温 / 67
wind-toxin syndrome/pattern 风毒证 / 199
wind-treating formula 治风剂 / 377
wind-warmth (disease) 风温 / 516
wind-warmth disease 风温病 / 516
wind-warmth pathogen 风温邪气 / 67
wind stroke 中风 / 536
wind stroke disease 中风病 / 536
winter warmth 冬温 / 519
wiping (with the palm or thumb) 抹法 / 482
wiping the forehead (with fingers) 抹前额 / 487
wiry pulse 弦脉 / 162
wisdom tooth 真牙，智齿 / 39
withdrawal of the needle 引针 / 462
withdrawal of the needle with gentle twirling 轻捻出针法 / 462
withered teeth 齿槁 / 137
withering of the helices 耳轮干枯 / 129
Wolfberry-Chrysanthemum

Rehmannia Pills 杞菊地黄丸 / 389
womb 胞宫，女子胞 / 25
Wonderful Well-tried Prescriptions 奇效良方 / 692
wood-featured person 木形之人 / 73
wood fire tormenting metal 木火刑金 / 13
wood generating fire 木生火 / 11
wood overrestricting asthenic earth 土虚木乘 / 13
wood overrestricting earth 木乘土 / 13
wood restricting earth 木克土 / 12
wooden tongue 木舌 / 134，579
word-articulating breathing 吐字呼吸 / 497
worm accumulation (syndrome/pattern) 虫积（证）/ 199，547
worm accumulation 虫积 / 582
worm-expelling medicinal/drug 驱虫药 / 294
wrap-decoct 包煎 / 283
wriggling of the extremities 手足蠕动 / 127
wringing the hands 洗手 / 489
wrist artery 寸口脉 / 160
wry mouth 口㖞，口僻/ 127，136，537
Wu Anye 吴安业 / 680
Wu Jutong 吴鞠通 / 678
Wu Qijun 吴其浚 / 679
Wu Shangxian 吴尚先 / 679
Wu Shiji 吴师机 / 680
Wu Shuqing 武叔卿 / 673
Wu Tang 吴瑭 / 678
Wu Youke 吴又可 / 672
Wu Youxing 吴有性 / 672
Wu Yuezhai 吴瀹斋 / 679
Wu Zhiwang 武之望 / 673
Wuchu (BL 5) 五处 / 419
Wuji Baifeng Pills 乌鸡白凤丸 / 394
Wuling Powder 五苓散 / 379
Wuren Pill 五仁丸 / 364
Wushu (GB 27) 五枢 / 430
Wuyi (ST 15) 屋翳 / 412
Wuzhuyu Decoction 吴茱萸汤 / 370
Wuzi Yanzong Pills 五子衍宗丸 / 389

X

Xi Yuan Ji Lu 洗冤集录 / 700
Xiabai (LU 4) 侠白 / 409
Xiaguan (ST 7) 下关 / 411
Xiajishu (EX-B 5) 下极俞 / 441
Xiajuxu (ST 39) 下巨虚 / 414
Xialian (LI 8) 下廉 / 410
Xialiao (BL 34) 下髎 / 421
Xian Shou Li Shang Xu Duan Mi Fang 仙授理伤续断秘方 / 697
Xianglian Pills 香连丸 / 386
Xiangru Powder 香薷散 / 361
Xiangsha Liujun Pills 香砂六君丸 / 388
Xiangsha Yangwei Pills 香砂养胃丸 / 387
Xiangu (ST 43) 陷谷 / 414
Xiao Chaihu Decoction 小柴胡汤 / 365
Xiao Chengqi Decoction 小承气汤 / 364
Xiao Er Dou Zhen Fang Lun 小儿痘疹方论 / 696
Xiao Er Tui Na Guang Yi 小儿推拿广意 / 696
Xiao Er Tui Na Mi Zhi 小儿推拿秘旨 / 696
Xiao Er Yao Zheng Zhi Jue 小儿药证直诀 / 696
Xiao Gengliu 萧赓六 / 675
Xiao Jianzhong Decoction 小建中汤 / 370
Xiao Qinglong Decoction 小青龙汤 / 361
Xiao'er Ganmao Granules 小儿感冒冲剂 / 381
Xiaochangshu (BL 27) 小肠俞 / 420
Xiaogukong (EX-UE 6) 小骨空 / 442
Xiaohai (SI 8) 小海 / 417
Xiaohuoluo Pills 小活络丸［丹］/ 392
Xiaoji Decoction 小蓟饮子 / 37
Xiaojin Pills 小金丸［丹］/ 395
Xiaoluo (TE 12) 消泺 / 427
Xiaoyao Pills 逍遥丸 / 386
Xiaoyao Powder 逍遥散 / 366
Xiawan (CV 10) 下脘 / 436
Xiaxi (GB 43) 侠溪 / 432
Xie Guan 谢观 / 682
Xiebai Powder 泻白散 / 368
Xiguan (LR 7) 膝关 / 432
Xihuang Pill 西黄丸 / 384
Xijiao Dihuang Decoction 犀角地黄汤 / 367
Ximen (PC 4) 郄门 / 426
Xin Xiu Ben Cao 新修本草 / 687
Xing Su Powder 杏苏散 / 378
Xingjian (LR 2) 行间 / 432
Xinhui (GV 22) 囟会 / 435
Xinshu (BL 15) 心俞 / 419
Xiong Daoxuan 熊道轩 / 668
Xiong Zongli 熊宗立 / 668
Xiongxiang (SP 19) 胸乡 / 416
xiphoid process 鸠尾 / 47

Xiu Xi Zhi Guan Zuo Chan Fa Yao 修习止观坐禅法要 / 700
Xixian Pills 豨莶丸 / 393
Xiyan (EX-LE 5) 膝眼 / 443
Xiyangguan (GB 33) 膝阳关 / 431
Xu Chunfu 徐春甫 / 669
Xu Dachun 徐大椿 / 676
Xu Daye 徐大业 / 676
Xu Lingtai 徐灵胎 / 676
Xu Ming Yi Lei An 续名医类案 / 702
Xu Ruyuan 徐汝元 / 669
Xu Shimao 徐士茂 / 660
Xu Shuwei 许叔微 / 663
Xu Zhicai 徐之才 / 660
Xuanfu Daizhe Decoction 旋复代赭汤 / 376
Xuanji (CV 21) 璇玑 / 436
Xuanli (GB 6) 悬厘 / 429
Xuanlu (GB 5) 悬颅 / 429
Xuanshu (GV 5) 悬枢 / 433
Xuanzhong (GB 39) 悬钟 / 431
Xue Ji 薛己 / 668
Xue Kai 薛铠 / 668
Xue Liangwu 薛良武 / 668
Xue Shengbai 薛生白 / 676
Xue Xinfu 薛新甫 / 669
Xue Xue 薛雪 / 676
Xue Zheng Lun 血证论 / 694
Xuefu Zhuyu Decoction 血府逐瘀汤 / 376
Xuehai (SP 10) 血海 / 415
Xuezhining Pills 血脂宁丸 / 385
Xuli 虚里 / 47

Y

Yamen (GV 15) 哑门 / 434
Yan Ke Da Quan 眼科大全 / 699
Yan Shi Ji Sheng Fang 严氏济生方 / 692
Yan Yonghe 严用和 / 665
Yan's Prescriptions for Succoring the Sick 严氏济生方 / 692
yang 阳 / 5
yang blockage of wind stroke 中风阳闭 / 536
yang brightness disease 阳明病 / 176
yang brightness disease pattern 阳明病证 / 176
yang brightness syndrome 阳明病证 / 176
yang brightness *fu*-organ disease 阳明腑病 / 177
yang brightness *fu*-organ syndrome/pattern 阳明腑证 / 177
yang brightness meridian/channel disease 阳明经病 / 176
yang brightness meridian/channel syndrome/pattern 阳明经证 / 176
yang collapse 阳脱，脱阳 / 80
yang collapse syndrome/pattern 阳脱证 / 173
yang collateral 阳络 / 407
yang deficiency 阳虚 / 79
yang-deficiency common cold 阳虚感冒 / 516
yang deficiency diathesis 阳虚质 / 75
yang-deficiency fever 阳虚发热 / 530
yang deficiency syndrome/pattern 阳虚证 / 173
yang deficiency with water flood 阳虚水泛 / 86
yang deficiency with yin exuberance 阳虚阴盛 / 78
yang disease 阳病 / 515
yang edema 阳水 / 548
yang epilepsy 阳痫 / 535，589
yang exhaustion 亡阳 / 80
yang exhaustion syndrome/pattern 亡阳证 / 173
yang exuberance 阳盛 / 78
Yang-harmonizing Decoction 阳和汤 / 370
yang-heat diathesis 阳热质 / 74
yang heel vessel (YangHV) 阳跷脉 / 406
yang heel vessel syndrome/pattern 阳跷脉病证 / 216
yang impairment affecting yin 阳损及阴 / 7
yang jaundice 阳黄 / 523
Yang Jishi 杨济时 / 671
Yang Jizhou 杨继洲 / 671
yang link vessel (YangLV) 阳维脉 / 406
yang link vessel syndrome/pattern 阳维脉病证 / 216
yang macule 阳斑 / 139
yang meridians/channels 阳经 / 399
yang pathogen 阳邪 / 63
yang-preponderant constitution 偏阳质 / 73
yang *qi* 阳气 / 55
yang-restoring emergency formula 回阳救逆剂 / 370
Yang-restoring Pill 右归丸 / 373
Yang Shangshan 杨上善 / 660
yang summerheat 阳暑 / 517
yang sweats 阳汗 / 145
yang syndrome/pattern 阳证 / 168
yang syndrome/pattern resembling yin 阳证似阴 / 174
yang tonic 补阳药 / 293
Yang-tonifying Five-tenths-restoring Decoction 补阳还

五汤 / 376
yang-tonifying formula 补阳剂 / 373
yang-tonifying medicinal/drug 补阳药 / 293
yang viscera 阳脏 / 20
yang within yang 阳中之阳 / 5
yang within yin 阴中之阳 / 5
Yang Xing Yan Ming Lu 养性延命录 / 700
yang *zang* organs 阳脏 / 20
Yangbai (GB 14) 阳白 / 429
Yangchi (TE 4) 阳池 / 426
Yangfu (GB 38) 阳辅 / 431
Yanggang (BL 48) 阳纲 / 422
Yanggu (SI 5) 阳谷 / 417
Yanghe Decoction 阳和汤 / 370
Yangjiao (GB 35) 阳交 / 431
Yanglao (SI 6) 养老 / 417
Yanglingquan (GB 34) 阳陵泉 / 431
Yangxi (LI 5) 阳溪 / 410
Yangxue Shengfa Capsules 养血生发胶囊 / 396
Yangyin Qingfei Decoction 养阴清肺汤 / 378
Yangyin Qingfei Extract 养阴清肺膏 / 383
Yanhusuo 延胡索 / 332
Yaoqi (EX-B 9) 腰奇 / 442
Yaoshu (GV 2) 腰俞 / 433
Yaotongdian (EX-UE 7) 腰痛点 / 442
Yaoyan (EX-B 7) 腰眼 / 441
Yaoyangguan (GV 3) 腰阳关 / 433
Yaoyi (EX-B 6) 腰宜 / 441
Ye Gui 叶桂 / 675
Ye Tianshi 叶天士 / 675
Ye Xiangyan 叶香岩 / 675
yellow discoloration of the white of the eye 白睛发黄 / 129
yellow discoloration 发黄，黄色 /125，139，523
Yellow Emperor's Canon of Medicine 黄帝内经 / 683
Yellow Genkwa Leaf and Flower 黄芫花 / 324
yellow greasy (tongue) coating/fur 黄腻苔 / 134
yellow kernel 黄仁 / 610
yellow puffiness 黄胖 / 139
yellow slimy (tongue) coating/fur 黄腻苔 / 134
yellow sputum 痰黄 / 137
yellow sweat 黄汗 / 531
yellow (tongue) coating/fur 黄苔 / 134
yellow-water sore 黄水疮 / 604
yellowish glaucoma 黄风，黄风内障 / 620
yellowish lens 黄精 / 610
yellowish leukorrhea 黄带 / 564
yellowish puffiness 黄胖 / 547
yellowish puffy disease 黄胖病 / 547
yellowish vaginal discharge 黄带 / 158
Yemen (TE 2) 液门 / 426
Yerbadetajo Herb 墨旱莲 / 330
"Yes-no" point 阿是穴 / 444
Yi Fang Ji Jie 医方集解 / 692
Yi Fang Kao 医方考 / 692
Yi Fang Lun 医方论 / 693
Yi Guan 医贯 / 702
Yi He 医和 / 658
Yi Lin Gai Cuo 医林改错 / 702
Yi Men Fa Lü 医门法律 / 701
Yi Xue Ru Men 医学入门 / 703
Yi Xue Xin Wu 医学心悟 / 704
Yi Xue Zheng Zhuan 医学正傳 / 703
Yi Xue Zhong Zhong Can Xi Lu 医学衷中参西录 / 702
Yi Zong Bi Du 医宗必读 / 704
Yi Zong Jin Jian 医宗金鉴 / 705
Yifeng (TE 17) 翳风 / 428
Yiguan Decoction 一贯煎 / 373
Yiming (EX-HN 14) 翳明 / 440
yin 阴 / 5
yin and yang 阴阳 / 5
yin bind 阴结 / 545
yin blockage of wind stroke 中风阴闭 / 536
yin-cold diathesis 阴寒质 / 75
yin collapse 脱阴，阴脱 / 80，81
yin collapse syndrome/pattern 阴脱证 / 173
yin collateral 阴络 / 407
yin convulsions 阴痫 / 589
yin deficiency 阴虚 / 79
yin-deficiency common cold 阴虚感冒 / 516
yin deficiency diathesis 阴虚质 / 75
yin-deficiency fever 阴虚发热 / 530
yin deficiency syndrome/pattern 阴虚证 / 173
yin-deficiency tidal fever 阴虚潮热 / 519
yin deficiency with effulgent fire 阴虚火旺 / 79
yin deficiency with lung dryness 阴虚肺燥 / 102
yin deficiency with stirring wind 阴虚风动 / 103
yin deficiency with yang hyperactivity 阴虚阳亢 / 79
yin disease 阴病 / 514
yin edema 阴水 / 549
yin epilepsy 阴痫 / 535，589
yin exhaustion 亡阴 / 80
yin exhaustion and yang collapse 阴竭阳脱 / 80

yin exhaustion syndrome/pattern 亡阴证 / 173
yin exuberance 阴盛 / 79
yin exuberance with yang debilitation 阴盛阳衰 / 78
yin fluid insufficiency syndrome/pattern 阴液亏虚证 / 173
Yin Hai Jing Wei 银海精微 / 698
yin heel vessel (YinHV) 阴跷脉 / 406
yin heel vessel syndrome/pattern 阴跷脉病证 / 216
yin impairment affecting yang 阴损及阳 / 7
yin jaundice 阴黄 / 523
yin link vessel (YinLV) 阴维脉 / 406
yin link vessel syndrome/pattern 阴维脉病证 / 216
yin liquid 阴液 / 58
yin macule 阴斑 / 139
yin malaria 牝疟 / 521
yin meridians/channels 阴经 / 399
yin needling 阴刺 / 462
Yin-nourishing and Lung-clearing Decoction 养阴清肺汤 / 378
Yin-nourishing Lung-clearing Extract 养阴清肺膏 / 383
yin-nourishing medicinal/drug 养阴药 / 294
yin pathogen 阴邪 / 63
yin-preponderant constitution 偏阴质 / 73
yin *qi* 阴气 / 55
Yin Qiao Powder 银翘散 / 362
yin-replenishing formula 补阴剂 / 372
yin-replenishing medicinal/drug 滋阴药 / 294
yin-replenishing moistening formula 滋阴润燥剂 / 378
Yin-restoring Pill 左归丸 / 372
Yin Shan Zheng Yao 饮膳正要 / 689
yin summerheat 阴暑 / 517
yin syndrome/pattern 阴证 / 168
yin syndrome/pattern resembling yang 阴证似阳 / 173
yin tonic 补阴药 / 294
yin-tonifying medicinal/drug 补阴药 / 294
yin viscera 牝脏，阴脏 / 20
yin within yang 阳中之阴 / 5
yin within yin 阴中之阴 / 5
yin-yang balance 阴阳平衡 / 6
yin-yang conversion 阴阳转化 / 6
yin-yang disharmony 阴阳不和，阴阳失调 / 6
yin-yang harmony 阴阳调和 / 6
yin-yang imbalance 阴阳乖戾 / 6
yin-yang interaction 阴阳交感 / 5
yin-yang interdependence 阴阳互根 / 5
yin-yang opposition 阴阳对立 / 6
yin-yang pattern identification 阴阳辨证 / 168
yin-yang point combination 阴阳配穴法 / 447
yin-yang repulsion 阴阳格拒 / 79
yin-yang syndrome differentiation 阴阳辨证 / 168
yin-yang theory 阴阳学说 / 5
yin-yang transmission 阴阳易 / 553
yin *zang* organs 阴脏 / 20
Yinbai (SP 1) 隐白 / 415
Yinbao (LR 9) 阴包 / 432
Yinchenhao Decoction 茵陈蒿汤 / 379
Yindu (KI 19) 阴都 / 425
Yingchuang (ST 16) 膺窗 / 412
Yingu (KI 10) 阴谷 / 424
Yingxiang (LI 20) 迎香 / 411
Yinhuang Oral Liquid 银黄口服液 / 383
Yinjiao (CV 7) 阴交 / 436
Yinjiao (GV 28) 龈交 / 435
Yinlian (LR 11) 阴廉 / 433
Yinlingquan (SP 9) 阴陵泉 / 415
Yinmen (BL 37) 殷门 / 421
Yinqiao Jiedu Pills 银翘解毒丸 / 381
Yinshi (ST 33) 阴市 / 414
Yintang (EX-HN 3) 印堂 / 440
Yishe (BL 49) 意舍 / 422
Yixi (BL 45) 谚譆 / 422
Yinxi (HT 6) 阴郄 / 416
Yong Yao Fa Xiang 用药法象 / 416
Yongquan (KI 1) 涌泉 / 423
You Gui Pill 右归丸 / 373
You Ke Tie Jing 幼科铁镜 / 696
You Yi 尤怡 / 675
You You Ji Cheng 幼幼集成 / 696
You You Xin Shu 幼幼新书 / 696
You Zaijing 尤在泾 / 676
Youmen (KI 21) 幽门 / 425
Yu Chang 喻昌 / 673
Yu Ji Wei Yi 玉机微义 / 701
Yu Jiayan 喻嘉言 / 673
Yu Lin 余霖 / 678
Yu Tianmin 虞天民 / 668
Yu Tuan 虞抟 / 668
Yuan Ji Qi Wei 原［元］机启微 / 698
Yuanhu Zhitong Tablets 元胡止痛片 / 393
Yuanye (GB 22) 渊液 / 430
Yueju Pills 越鞠丸 / 387
Yuji (LU 10) 鱼际 / 409
Yun Shujue 恽树珏 / 682
Yun Tieqiao 恽铁樵 / 682
Yunmen (LU 2) 云门 / 408

Yupingfeng Oral Liquid 玉屏风口服液 / 383
Yupingfeng Powder 玉屏风散 / 371
Yutang (CV 18) 玉堂 / 436
Yuyao (EX-HN 4) 鱼腰 / 440
Yuye (EX-HN 13) 玉液 / 440
Yuzhen (BL 9) 玉枕 / 419
Yuzhong (KI 26) 彧中 / 425

Z

Zaizao Pills 再造丸 / 391
Zan Yin 昝殷 / 662
zang-fu heat-clearing formula 清脏腑热剂 / 368
zang-fu insufficiency tinnitus 脏腑虚损耳鸣 / 624
zang-fu organs 脏腑 / 20
zang organ 脏 / 20
zang-organ qi 脏气 / 54
zang (-organ) stroke 中脏/ 536
Zaocys 乌梢蛇 / 315
Zedoary Rhizome 莪术 / 331
Zeng Shirong 曾世荣 / 666
Zhang Congzheng 张从正 / 664
Zhang Ji 张机 / 658
Zhang Jiebin 张介宾 / 672
Zhang Jiegu 张洁古 / 664
Zhang Jingyue 张景岳 / 672
Zhang Lu 张璐 / 674
Zhang Luyu 张路玉 / 674
Zhang Nan 章楠 / 678
Zhang Sanxi 张三锡 / 670
Zhang Shanlei 张山雷 / 682
Zhang Shi Yi Tong 张氏医通 / 704
Zhang Shiwan 张石顽 / 674
Zhang Shoufu 张寿甫 / 681
Zhang Shouyi 张寿颐 / 681
Zhang Xiaoshan 张筱衫 / 680
Zhang Xichun 张锡纯 / 681
Zhang Yin'an 张隐庵 / 674
Zhang Yuansu 张元素 / 664
Zhang Zhenjun 张振鋆 / 680
Zhang Zhicong 张志聪 / 674
Zhang Zhongjing 张仲景 / 659
Zhang Zihe 张子和 / 664
Zhang's Treatise on General Medicine 张氏医通 / 704
Zhangmen (LR 13) 章门 / 433
Zhao Shuxuan 赵恕轩 / 677
Zhao Xianke 赵献可 / 671
Zhao Xuemin 赵学敏 / 677
Zhao Yangkui 赵养葵 / 671
Zhaohai (KI 6) 照海 / 424
Zhejin (GB 23) 辄筋 / 430
Zhen Ben Yi Shu Ji Cheng 珍本医书集成 / 705
Zhen Ci Ma Zui 针刺麻醉 / 699
Zhen Jia Shu Yao 诊家枢要 / 686
Zhen Jiu Da Cheng 针灸大成 / 699
Zhen Jiu Jia Yi Jing 针灸甲乙经 / 699
Zhen Jiu Ju Ying 针灸聚英 / 699
Zhen Jiu Wen Da 针灸问答 / 699
Zhen Jiu Wen Dui 针灸问对 / 699
Zhen Jiu Zi Sheng Jing 针灸资生经 / 699
Zhen Quan 甄权 / 660
Zhen Zhu Nang Yao Xing Fu 珍珠囊药性赋 / 689
Zheng Han 郑瀚 / 677
Zheng He Ben Cao 政和本草 / 688
Zheng Honggang 郑宏纲 / 677
Zheng Lei Ben Cao 证类本草 / 688
Zheng Meijian 郑梅涧 / 677
Zheng Ruoxi 郑若溪 / 678
Zheng Zhi Hui Bu 证治汇补 / 694
Zheng Zhi Zhun Sheng 证治准绳 / 703
Zhenghe Materia Medica 政和本草 / 688
Zhengying (GB 17) 正营 / 429
Zhenwu Decoction 真武汤 / 380
Zhi Wu Ming Shi Tu Kao Chang Bian 植物名实图考长编 / 690
Zhi Wu Ming Shi Tu Kao 植物名实图考 / 689
Zhibai Dihuang Pills 知柏地黄丸 / 390
Zhibian (BL 54) 秩边 / 422
Zhigou (TE 6) 支沟 / 427
Zhishi (BL 52) 志室 / 422
Zhisou Powder 止嗽散 / 361
Zhiyang (GV 9) 至阳 / 434
Zhiyin (BL 67) 至阴 / 423
Zhizheng (SI 7) 支正 / 417
Zhong Guo Yao Xue Da Ci Dian 中国药学大辞典 / 705
Zhong Guo Yi Xue Da Cheng 中国医学大成 / 705
Zhong Guo Yi Xue Da Ci Dian 中国医学大辞典 / 705
Zhong Zang Jing 中藏经 / 700
Zhongchong (PC 9) 中冲 / 426
Zhongdu (GB 32) 中渎 / 431
Zhongdu (LR 6) 中都 / 432
Zhongfeng (LR 4) 中封 / 432
Zhongfu (LU 1) 中府 / 408
Zhongji (CV 3) 中极 / 435
Zhongkui (EX-UE 4) 中魁 / 442
Zhongliao (BL 33) 中髎 / 421
Zhonglushu (BL 29) 中膂俞 / 421

Zhongquan (EX-UE 3) 中泉 / 442
Zhongshu (GV 7) 中枢 / 433
Zhongting (CV 16) 中庭 / 436
Zhongwan (CV 12) 中脘 / 436
Zhongzhu (KI 15) 中注 / 424
Zhongzhu (TE 3) 中渚 / 426
Zhou Hou Bei Ji Fang 肘后备急方 / 690
Zhou Yi Can Tong Qi 周易参同契 / 700
Zhoujian (EX-UE 1) 肘尖 / 442
Zhouliao (LI 12) 肘髎 / 410
Zhourong (SP 20) 周荣 / 416
Zhu Bing Yuan Hou Zong Lun 诸病源候总论 / 687
Zhu Danxi 朱丹溪 / 666
Zhu Peiwen 朱沛文 / 679
Zhu Zhenheng 朱震亨 / 666
Zhubin (KI 9) 筑宾 / 424
Zhusha Anshen Pill 朱砂安神丸 / 385
Zhuye Shigao Decoction 竹叶石膏汤 / 367
Zigong (CV 19) 紫宫 / 436
Zigong (EX-CA 1) 子宫 / 441
Zixue Powder 紫雪 / 392
zoster 蛇丹，缠腰蛇丹，缠腰火丹 / 600
Zulinqi (GB 41) 足临泣 / 431
Zuo Gui Pill 左归丸 / 372
Zuoci's Deafness Pills 耳聋左慈丸 / 397
Zuqiaoyin (GB 44) 足窍阴 / 432
Zusanli (ST 36) 足三里 / 414
Zutonggu (BL 66) 足通谷 / 423
Zuwuli (LR 10) 足五里 / 433

后　记

术语是概念的符号，每一个学科或行业都有自己的术语。术语享有至高的地位：建立一门学科或行业的关键在于术语，而了解、学习这门学科或行业的关键也在于掌握其术语。

虽然术语如此重要，但 20 世纪 70 年代以前，中医术语的翻译只停留在小范围内，而且非常零散。其实，针灸早于 17 世纪就流行于欧洲了，这让我们很容易想象到那时一定做了大量的翻译工作。“acupuncture”一词的确是在那个时候被“造”出来的，“acus”来源于拉丁语，是“针”的意思，而“puncture”则是“用尖锐的器具刺”的意思。可以说，“acupuncture”是中医术语英译最早、最典型的案例之一。可除此之外，基本上没什么中医概念被译成西文。

相比之下，自 19 世纪初叶西医传入中国后的短短数十年时间内，西医名词术语就被翻译成了中文，而且其标准很快就取得了里程碑式的成就。1908 年，标志着医学名词翻译初步统一的《高氏医学词汇》（*Cousland's English-Chinese Medical Lexicon*）问世，依据标准名词而编译的医学教材在这个时期相继问世，中国的西医学随后进入了高速发展时期。

与发展于近代的西医不同的是，中医早在两千多年前就已经在“阴阳五行”、“气血经络”等理论的基础上建立起来。由于它发源于独特的中国文化，其思想体系与西方科学、哲学区别很大。准确地翻译一个中医术语是一项难度极高的任务，它需要译者从中医思想、汉字演变以及西方思维、西方医学、英文表达等诸多方面进行推敲，方可找到恰当的解释。在东西方文化相互生疏的年代，中医术语的翻译是一项不可能完成的任务。因此，尽管中医的针灸技术早在几百年前就走出国门传到欧洲，但中医的思想却依然留守在国内直到 20 世纪 70 年代。

完成中医术语的翻译需要两个先决条件：第一，东西方在思想、医学、文字等领域达到相当程度的相互了解，积累相当多的文献资料；第二，有人能够从这些文献资料中分析、提炼、总结和提出最合理的释义。

我父亲就诞生于东西方文化初步交融的时代！他从小接受了中西文化的双重洗礼——先是中英双语教育，成为西医专家后又转而研究中医。他勤奋好学，几乎在他接触到的每个领域都是佼佼者，在东西方文字、医学、哲学等方面的把握能力让他成为完成这项艰巨

任务的合适人选 。在 20 世纪 70 年代末，他响应国家对外开放政策，踏上了中医名词术语翻译的漫长历程。从 1978 年起，他与英文教授黄孝楷一起着手钻研，他们主编的《汉英常用中医药词汇》(*Common Terms of Traditional Chinese Medicine in English*) 于 1980 年出版并由《中西医结合杂志》连载。1984 年该书由香港商务印书馆改名为 *Dictionary of Traditional Chinese Medicine* 向国外发行。1987 年卫生部指派我父亲参与《汉英医学大词典》中医部分的修订工作，使该词典得以顺利出版。为此，他不仅在 1987 年受到卫生部的嘉奖，而且在 1994 年又由于读者的好评而再次受到卫生部的表彰。1999 年他受命于国家中医药管理局，进行“中医药名词术语英译标准化”课题的研究。他除了将研究结果编制成《中医药常用名词术语英译》外，还编写了《新编汉英中医药分类词典》(2002)，本书即为后者的第二版。

伴随中医名词术语翻译的出现，多种中医教材被译成西文，中医学术终于走出了国门！随着世界范围内越来越多的研究者关注中医，中医将会发展得更快，不断更新中医名词术语也将是下一步的任务。我们希望这部作品不仅给普通读者提供一个工具，还能够给更新术语翻译的后来者提供可靠的参考。

谢方

2019 年 8 月 2 日，于成都

Afterword

A term is the label of a concept. Any discipline or industry has been assigned terminology of its own. In fact, terminology occupies the supreme position since it is the key to both building and learning a discipline or an industry.

Despite the importance of terminology, only a very small number of sporadic TCM terms were translated into English before the 70s of the 20th century. In fact, a needle manipulation therapy from China was once popular in Europe as early as the 17th century, which prompts us to imagine that a lot of translational work must have been done during that period. The word *acupuncture* was indeed coined to describe the technique, in which the prefix "acu" comes from the Latin word *acus* meaning "needle", and "puncture" means "the act of piercing with a pointed instrument or object". And the word *acupuncture* became one of the earliest and most typical examples of the translation of TCM terms. But other than that, not much had been done in terms of interpreting TCM concepts in a western language.

In contrast, within several decades after the introduction of western medicine into China, which took place in the early 19th century, western medical terms were translated from English to Chinese and the standardization of terminology soon reached a milestone accomplishment. In 1908, *Cousland's Egnlish-Chinese Medical Lexicon* was published, indicating the preliminary unification of western medical terms in Chinese. Guided under the principles of the standard translation of terminology, Chinese versions of western medical textbooks came into being. Consequently, China entered a rapid growth period in the fields of western medicine.

Unlike western medicine which was developed in modern times, TCM was well established over 2,000 years ago, with its theoretic backgrounds being yin and yang, *qi* and blood, and meridian channels and collaterals. The unique Chinese culture that nurtured TCM has almost ensured a huge gap between its logic and that of the western culture dominated by modern science and philosophy. So, accurately translating a TCM term into English is a tremendous task. It requires a translator to evaluate the factors from the aspects of TCM thoughts, etymology of Chinese characters, western thoughts, western medicine, and English language, before he or she can locate the most suitable translation. It was thus a mission impossible to complete in the years when the East and West were unfamiliar with each other. So, although the technique of acupuncture was delivered out of China to Europe several hundred years ago, the TCM thoughts behind it had still been locked within until the 1970s.

Two prerequisites are needed for the completion of TCM terminology translation: first, the East and West should reach mutual understanding on thoughts, medical concepts, and languages to such a degree that sufficient amount of literature is available; second, there should be scholars who are able to analyze the literature, extract and summarize the useful information, and propose and rationalize the most suitable translations and explanations.

My father was born in the time when the Eastern and Western cultures began to have full contact with each other. He was brain-washed by both Eastern and Western cultures. For example, he was educated in both Chinese and English languages, became an expert in western medicine and then focused on TCM research. With a curious mind and eagerness to learn, he has always been the leader in every area he is engaged in. His diverse talents in such areas as Chinese and western languages, philosophies, and disciplines of medicine have made him the perfect candidate for the challenging task.

In the 1970s, he started the long journey of TCM terminology translation, following the national policy of "opening to the outside world". In 1978, he began to work with professor Huang Xiaokai on *Common Terms of Traditional Chinese Medicine in English*, which was published as a book in 1980 and also as serial articles in *Chinese Journal of Integrated Traditional and Western Medicine* since 1981. In 1984, the book was assigned a new title, *Dictionary of Traditional Chinese Medicine*, and was republished and distributed abroad by Hong Kong Commercial Press. In 1987, my father was appointed by the Ministry of Health to revise the TCM section of *The Chinese-English Medical Dictionary.* To thank him for his contribution that enabled the publication of the dictionary in a timely manner, he was awarded by the Ministry of Health in 1987. In 1994, the Ministry of Health issued him another award due to immensely positive responses to the dictionary from readers. In 1999, appointed by the State Administration of Traditional Chinese Medicine of the P. R. C., he started research programs on the standardization of English translation of TCM terminology. Besides *English Translation of Common Terms in Traditional Chinese Medicine*, he compiled *Classified Dictionary of Traditional Chinese Medicine (New Edition)* in 2002. This book is the second version of the latter.

With the advent of English translation of TCM terminology, numerous TCM teaching materials have been translated into western languages. Finally, TCM went abroad academically. The pace of TCM development is expected to be boosted since researchers from all over the world have been paying attention to it. With TCM development, unremittingly updating its terminology will become the future task. We hope that this book will provide not only a tool for general readers but also a reliable reference in the updating endeavors of the followers.

Fang Xie

In Chengdu

Aug. 2, 2019

图书在版编目（CIP）数据

新编汉英中医药分类词典 / 谢竹藩，谢方编著. --
2版. —北京：外文出版社，2018.11
ISBN 978-7-119-11782-9

Ⅰ. ①新… Ⅱ. ①谢… ②谢… Ⅲ. ①中国医药学—
词典—汉、英 Ⅳ. ①R2-61

中国版本图书馆 CIP 数据核字（2018）第 278847 号

策划指导：胡开敏
责任编辑：熊冰頔
英文审定：Paul White
英文编辑：严　晶
封面设计：蔡　荣
装帧设计：邱　彬
印刷监制：章云天

新编汉英中医药分类词典（第二版）

谢竹藩　谢方　编著

出 版 人：徐　步
出版发行：外文出版社有限责任公司
地　　址：北京市西城区百万庄大街24号　　**邮政编码：**100037
网　　址：http://www.flp.com.cn　　**电子邮箱：**flp@cipg.org.cn
电　　话：008610-68320579（总编室）　　008610-68996064（编辑部）
008610-68995852（发行部）　　008610-68996183（投稿电话）
制　　版：北京易拍宝文化发展有限公司
印　　刷：北京通州皇家印刷厂
经　　销：新华书店/ 外文书店
开　　本：787mm × 1092mm　1/16　　**印　　张：**68
版　　次：2019 年 8 月第 1 版第 1 次印刷
书　　号：ISBN 978-7-119-11782-9
定　　价：198.00 元（精装）
